PAIN MEDICINE

PAIN MEDICINE

AN INTERDISCIPLINARY CASE-BASED APPROACH

EDITED BY

Salim M. Hayek, MD
PROFESSOR OF ANESTHESIOLOGY
CASE WESTERN RESERVE UNIVERSITY
CHIEF, DIVISION OF PAIN MEDICINE
UNIVERSITY HOSPITALS OF CLEVELAND
CLEVELAND, OHIO

Binit J. Shah, MD, FAPA
DIRECTOR, INTENSIVE CARE UNIT
OHIO HOSPITAL FOR PSYCHIATRY
COLUMBUS, OHIO

Mehul J. Desai, MD, MPH
DIRECTOR, SPINE, PAIN MEDICINE & RESEARCH
METRO ORTHOPEDICS AND SPORTS THERAPY
SILVER SPRING, MARYLAND

Thomas C. Chelimsky, MD
PROFESSOR OF NEUROLOGY
MEDICAL COLLEGE OF WISCONSIN
MILWAUKEE, WISCONSIN

OXFORD
UNIVERSITY PRESS

.FORD
/ERSITY PRESS

ord University Press is a department of the University of
ford. It furthers the University's objective of excellence in research,
ıolarship, and education by publishing worldwide.

)xford New York
Auckland Cape Town Dar es Salaam Hong Kong Karachi
Kuala Lumpur Madrid Melbourne Mexico City Nairobi
New Delhi Shanghai Taipei Toronto

With offices in
Argentina Austria Brazil Chile Czech Republic France Greece
Guatemala Hungary Italy Japan Poland Portugal Singapore
South Korea Switzerland Thailand Turkey Ukraine Vietnam

Oxford is a registered trademark of Oxford University Press
in the UK and certain other countries.

Published in the United States of America by
Oxford University Press
198 Madison Avenue, New York, NY 10016

Library of Congress Cataloging-in-Publication Data
Pain medicine (Hayek)
Pain medicine : an interdisciplinary case-based approach / edited by Salim M. Hayek, Binit J. Shah, Mehul J. Desai, Thomas C. Chelimsky.
p ; cm.
Includes bibliographical references and index.
ISBN 978–0–19–993148–4 (alk. paper)
I. Hayek, Salim M., editor. II. Shah, Binit J., editor. III. Desai, Mehul J., editor. IV. Chelimsky, Thomas C., editor. V. Title.
[DNLM: 1. Pain Management. 2. Chronic Pain—therapy. WL 704.6]
RB127
616′.0472—dc23
2014040913

9 8 7 6 5 4 3 2
Printed in the United States of America
on acid-free paper

To our families
To our patients
To the healthcare workers, students, residents, and fellows in-training in Pain Medicine
In Memory of Howard Smith

Salim Hayek
Binit Shah
Mehul Desai
Thomas Chelimsky

To my mentor, Salim Hayek, who has guided, encouraged, and supported me in every step of my career. I owe my successes to you.To my wife, Rupa, who has sacrificed so that I might succeed, challenged me that I might be a better man, and loved me that I might live.

—BJS

To my fellow co-editors, who provided me this opportunity and inspired me with their Herculean efforts. To Sophia and Milan, you motivate me every day to make you both as proud of me as I am of you.

—MJD

To my colleagues who wrote this book, and all who have inspired and taught me every day in each conversation about a suffering person we treat together, to my wife Gisela and two children Miriam and Hannah who are so patient with me, and to God, the greatest teacher and pain fighter of all.

—TCC

IN MEMORIAM

It would have been very unusual for Howard S. Smith not to complete a project. Howard was the consummate academician, having completed three different residencies, authored more than 100 articles and book chapters, and edited more than 10 books, including this one. He could not have accomplished these things without having perseverance and being meticulous. Yet, it would be easy for someone to not know these things about Howard. He was sincere, humble, and down-to-earth, qualities that unfortunately are somewhat unusual among super-achievers, which is a term that personifies Howard Smith.

It is somewhat ironic that what we may remember most about Howard is not his plethora of accomplishments, but rather his empathy, compassion, and infectious laugh that made everyone around him smile. His presence at conferences meant not only that there would be astute observations on the latest trends in pain medicine, but that there would also be someone who would listen intently to all sides of a debate, show compassion to minority viewpoints, and mediate seemingly irreconcilable differences of opinion.

Howard's departure came as a shock to his many friends, his family, and the medical community, all of whom had come to love and admire him. He was chosen as an editor for this book because of his incomparable work ethic, intellect, reliability, and dedication. Although we are saddened that he will not see this textbook come to fruition, we take some consolation in the fact that this book represents the ideals that Howard emulated in his life: an evidence-based compendium of the principles and practice of pain medicine.

We hereby dedicate this book to the memory of Howard Smith, whose keen insight and gentle demeanor touched everyone he met.

Salim M. Hayek
Binit J. Shah
Mehul J. Desai
Thomas C. Chelimsky
Steven Cohen

CONTENTS

Foreword by James P. Rathmell xi

Preface xiii

Contributors xv

SECTION I
NEUROPATHIC PAIN

1. Small Fiber Neuropathy 3
   Kamal Chemali, Salim M. Hayek, and Thomas C. Chelimsky
2. Postherpetic Neuralgia 16
   Srinivasa N. Raja, Ronen Shechter, and Raimy Amasha
3. Trigeminal Neuralgia and Other Facial Pain Conditions 38
   Kevin E. Vorenkamp, Afton L. Hassett, Gregory M. Figg, Jennifer Sweet, and Jonathan Miller
4. Carpal Tunnel Syndrome 60
   Bashar Katirji and Binit J. Shah

SECTION II
MUSCLE, JOINT, AND TENDON PAIN

5. Myofascial Pain Syndrome 69
   Robert Gerwin
6. Pain of Rheumatological Disease 89
   David G. Borenstein, Philip Appel, and Joseph Signorino
7. Tendinopathies 110
   Troy Henning and Jeanne M. Lackamp

SECTION III
SPINE AND RELATED DISORDERS

8. Discogenic Pain 127
   Irina L. Melnik, Richard Derby, Binit J. Shah, and Jason Eubanks
9. Lumbar Facet Pain 146
   Michael Gofeld, James P. Robinson, John G. Hanlon, and Binit J. Shah
10. Sacroiliac Joint Pain 160
    Samuel L. Holmes, Steven P. Cohen, Michael-Flynn L. Cullen, Christopher D. Kenny, Harold J. Wain, and S. Avery Davis
11. Lumbar Spinal Stenosis 183
    John D. Markman and Kiran Nandigam
12. Lumbar Disc Displacement 196
    Mehul J. Desai, Jeffrey D. Petersohn, Joseph O'Brien, Mathew Cyriac, and Chili Lati
13. Postlaminectomy Syndrome 213
    Krishna Kumar, Syed Rizvi, and Binit J. Shah
14. Piriformis Syndrome 238
    W. Evan Rivers, Honorio T. Benzon, and Binit J. Shah
15. Whiplash Associated Disorder and Cervical Facet Pain 247
    Jeffrey D. Petersohn, Girish Padmanabhan, and Mehul J. Desai
16. Cervical Radicular Pain 258
    Jan Van Zundert, Dieter M. J. Peuskens, Peter Hallet, Koen Van Boxem, and Binit J. Shah
17. Thoracic Back Pain 264
    Shrif Costandi, Yashar Eshraghi, and Nagy Mekhail

SECTION IV
VISCERAL PAIN

18. Pain from Chronic Pancreatitis 289
    Leonardo Kapural, Martine Puylaert, R. Matthew Walsh, and Giries W. Sweis
19. Chronic Pelvic Pain 297
    Thomas C. Chelimsky, Jeffrey Janata, Sawsan As-Sanie, Frank F. Tu, and Denniz Zolnoun
20. Chronic Refractory Angina 303
    Philippe Mavrocordatos, Dag Söderström, and Mike J. L. DeJongste

SECTION V
PERSISTENT POSTSURGICAL PAIN

21. Postsurgical Thoracic Pain 321
    Dalia H. Elmofty, Asokumar Buvanendran, and Jennifer Moore Brandstetter
22. Post-Herniorrhaphy Pain 337
    David A. Edwards, James P. Rathmell, and Binit J. Shah

SECTION VI
CANCER-RELATED PAIN

23. Palliative Cancer Pain 355
    Mellar P. Davis, Harold Goforth, and Pam Gamier

SECTION VII
OTHER DISORDERS

24. Headache 381
Hossein Ansari and Samer Narouze

25. Complex Regional Pain Syndrome (CRPS) 390
Salim M. Hayek, Binit J. Shah, Mehul J. Desai, Howard S. Smith, and Thomas C. Chelimsky

26. Fibromyalgia 407
Howard S. Smith, Kim D. Jones, Daniel J. Clauw, and Binit J. Shah

Index 421

FOREWORD

John Bonica (February 16, 1917–August 15, 1994) was an anesthesiologist and is recognized as the founding father of pain management, a field that has now evolved into the well-recognized medical specialty called Pain Medicine. After completing residency in 1944, Bonica joined the Unites States Army and was appointed Chief of Anesthesiology at Madigan Army Medical Center in Fort Lewis, Washington. For the next three years, he gained firsthand experience while treating painful injuries in World War II veterans. As an anesthesiologist, Bonica found that the tools at his disposal, opioid analgesics and peripheral nerve blocks using local anesthetics, were just a small part of what was needed to adequately diagnose and treat patients with complex, chronic painful disorders. He went on to pioneer the concept of bringing multiple medical specialists together to evaluate patients and construct a comprehensive treatment plan for each patient. Thus, the multidisciplinary approach to pain management was born. The original approach was to have each patient evaluated by a number of different specialists, usually an anesthesiologist or other physician would act as the team leader, often a surgical specialist would be involved, and the team always had a psychiatrist or psychologist and a physical therapist. Programs emerged around the world, many of which were based at rehabilitation facilities and they admitted patients for treatment during lengthy inpatient hospitalizations. Research about the effectiveness of this comprehensive approach emerged, demonstrating sustainable improvements in pain and function: Yes, the multidisciplinary rehabilitation approach really works. But there was a problem. Getting so many specialists together and coordinating care in this comprehensive fashion takes a lot of time and requires many different specialists, so it is expensive. Insurance providers began to deny coverage for comprehensive pain care and the approach fell out of favor in the 1980s.

Even as the cumbersome multidisciplinary programs like the one that John Bonica built during his long academic career at the University of Washington were in decline, modern training in the area of pain management began to emerge. The interest of anesthesiologists in pain management emerged largely from the use of analgesics and regional anesthesia to control pain in the immediate postoperative period. It was clear that many patients did gain some relief from chronic pain conditions when specific neural structures were blocked. Specific treatments emerged from this paradigm, most notably epidural injection of corticosteroids for lumbar radicular pain. Formal accredited training programs for physicians seeking to subspecialize in pain management began in the United States in 1993. This fellowship training added a single year to anesthesiology training and was often technically focused on interventional. While there was some lip service given to the overall multidisciplinary treatment of pain, many early pain specialists entered practice offering largely technical services (they were known as "block docs"). The true benefit of multidisciplinary pain care was lost.

By the late 1990s, it was clear that physicians from disciplines other than anesthesiology also wanted access to subspecialty training in pain management, which by that time had adopted the broader name of Pain Medicine. It was not until 2007 that the requirements for training programs were finally changed to ensure that all pain specialists would gain exposure to disciplines beyond anesthesiology during their subspecialty training. They would be required to have some minimal exposure to psychiatry, physical medicine and rehabilitation, and neurology. The excessive focus on interventions has gradually subsided and a new and refreshing recognition has taken hold: that each patient with chronic pain may well benefit from a broad range of treatment options that include rehabilitation, psychology, and involvement of other disciplines in coordinated plans of care. The term "multidisciplinary" has been gradually overtaken by the term "interdisciplinary" in recent years, and this is fitting. Instead of calling on experts from multiple disciplines to work together to formulate a treatment plan, modern pain training and pain care are more often organized so that a pain specialist actually delivers care across traditional boundaries. The anesthesiologist must gain sufficient skills in neurology to care for patients with headaches and the neurologist must gain sufficient skills in performing neural blockade to provide the treatments pain patients will need.

So, it is inspiring to see a book appear that embraces the interdisciplinary approach and presents in-depth discussions of common and unusual chronic pain conditions in a case-based fashion that emphasizes interdisciplinary pain care. Drs. Hayek, Shah, Desai, and Chelimsky have created just such a text in *Pain Medicine: An Interdisciplinary Case-based Approach*. Each chapter is built around a well-described patient with the disorder that is being discussed in that chapter. The cases are detailed and realistic. Each case is followed by a number of questions that the authors then address in detail. The questions posed are the very ones a pain specialist will have to master in order to effectively care for patients with that specific painful disorder. Every chapter crosses more than one discipline and discusses the broad array of treatment techniques that can be brought to bear on that specific painful condition. This novel approach is a powerful way for practitioners to acquire state-of-the-art information about the causes, evaluation, and treatment of pain. This interdisciplinary, case-based approach will allow pain practitioners, new and experienced alike, to bring the very best care to their patients suffering with pain.

James P. Rathmell, MD
Massachusetts General Hospital
Harvard Medical School
Boston, Massachusetts
December 2014

PREFACE

Although it is no secret that chronic pain is a major healthcare problem of epidemic proportions, its management is far from perfect. In the United States, chronic pain has an estimated prevalence of greater that 30% and is one of the main reasons for seeking medical care. The direct and indirect economic costs of chronic pain are astronomical. Chronic pain is challenging not only because of complex pathophysiological processes but also because it affects all facets of life: physical, emotional, psychological, economic, and social. Hence, many experts consider chronic pain not a mere symptom but a disease entity in itself. This constellation poses particular challenges in the management of chronic pain and requires integration of multiple, and often simultaneous, approaches to optimize patient outcomes.

Interdisciplinary clinical medicine involves bringing together the input of multiple healthcare specialists of different backgrounds in the care of complex patients. Patients benefit from the contribution of experts from different clinical backgrounds who address their problems in an integrated and concurrent fashion. The resultant comprehensive patient care may be more successful at managing and solving patient problems that are beyond the proficiency and training of a single provider. The benefits, however, are not limited to the patients. Clinicians learn from the cross-pollination of knowledge and exchange of clinical experiences and skills.

This concept has been embraced in medical education, and particularly in pain medicine. Indeed, the Accreditation Council for Graduate Medical Education (ACGME) has mandated multidisciplinary training of fellows in accredited programs in pain medicine since 2007. Greater exposure of trainees to the disciplines of neurology, physical medicine and rehabilitation, and psychiatry/psychology, in addition to anesthesiology is now routine. Innovation in educational experience is highly encouraged, including training in cancer pain, palliative care, and pediatric pain. Specific training requirements are also delineated for the interventional track trainees.

Interdisciplinary medicine, although ideal, may be difficult to practice. Team members must learn to appreciate the differing perspectives and accede to work with each other. In addition, interdisciplinary practice has been criticized as inefficient. Nonetheless, it carries a very high and perhaps underestimated value, both from the perspective of physician education and job satisfaction and the perspective of patient outcomes and quality of care.

This textbook embraces the spirit and implementation of interdisciplinary pain medicine practice. Common chronic pain conditions are tackled in-depth using a vignette-based approach and contributions from multiple authors from different disciplines in each chapter. Although neither interdisciplinary practice nor interdisciplinary book writing are easy feats, the editors believe they are worth the effort. We believe the readers and students of pain medicine will agree.

CONTRIBUTORS

Raimy Amasha, MD
Department of Anesthesiology
Johns Hopkins University, School of Medicine
Baltimore, Maryland

Hossein Ansari, MD
Medical Director, Headache Center
Neurology and Neuroscience Associates
Akron, Ohio

Philip R. Appel, PhD, FASCH
Director, Psychological Services
MedStar National Rehabilitation Network
Washington, DC

Sawsan As-Sanie, MD
Assistant Professor of Obstetrics & Gynecology
University of Michigan Health System
Ann Arbor, Michigan

Honorio T. Benzon, MD
Professor of Anesthesiology
Northwestern University Feinberg School of Medicine
Chicago, Illinois

David G. Borenstein, MD, MACP, MACR
Clinical Professor of Medicine
The George Washington University Medical Center
Partner, Arthritis and Rheumatism Associates
Washington, DC

Asokumar Buvanendran, MD
Director of Orthopedic Anesthesia
Professor of Anesthesiology
Rush University Medical Center
Chicago, Illinois

Kamal Chemali, MD
Associate Professor of Neurology
Eastern Virginia Medical School
Director Neuromuscular and Autonomic Center
Director Music and Medicine Center
Sentara Healthcare
Norfolk, Virginia

Daniel J. Clauw, MD
Professor of Anesthesiology, Medicine, and Psychiatry
Director of the Chronic Pain and Fatigue Research Center
University of Michigan
Ann Arbor, Michigan

Steven P. Cohen, MD
Professor of Anesthesiology, Pain Medicine Division
Department of Anesthesiology & Critical Care Medicine
Johns Hopkins School of Medicine
Baltimore, Maryland
Professor of Anesthesiology
Walter Reed National Military Medical Center
Uniformed Services University of the Health Sciences
Bethesda, Maryland

Shrif Costandi, MD
Department of Pain Management
Cleveland Clinic
Cleveland, Ohio

Michael-Flynn L. Cullen, MD
Resident Physician of Physical Medicine & Rehabilitation
Walter Reed National Military Medical Center
Bethesda, Maryland

Mathew Cyriac, MD
Department of Orthopaedic Surgery
School of Medicine and Health Sciences
The George Washington University
Washington, DC

Mellar P. Davis, MD, FCCP, FAAHPM
Harry R. Horvitz Center for Palliative Medicine
Division of Solid Tumor
Taussig Cancer Institute
Cleveland Clinic
Cleveland, Ohio

S. Avery Davis, MD
Chief of Physical Medicine and Rehabilitation Service
Walter Reed National Military Medical Center
Bethesda, Maryland

Mike J. L. DeJongste, MD, PhD, FESC
Department of Cardiology
University of Groningen
University Hospital of Groningen
Groningen, The Netherlands

Richard Derby, MD
Medical Director
Spinal Diagnostics and Treatment Center
Daly City, California

David A. Edwards, MD, PhD
Division of Pain Medicine
Department of Anesthesia, Critical Care and Pain Medicine
Harvard Medical School
Massachusetts General Hospital
Boston, Massachusetts

Dalia H. Elmofty, MD
Assistant Professor of Anesthesia & Critical Care
University of Chicago
Chicago, Illinois

Yashar Eshraghi, MD
Department of Pain Management
Cleveland Clinic
Cleveland, Ohio

Jason Eubanks, MD
Assistant Professor of Orthopedics
Case Western Reserve University
University Hospitals Case Medical Center
Cleveland, Ohio

Gregory M. Figg, MD
Associate, Columbus Neurology and Neurosurgery
Columbus, Ohio

Pam Gamier, RN, BSN, CHPN
Harry R. Horvitz Center for Palliative Medicine
Division of Solid Tumor
Taussig Cancer Institute
Cleveland Clinic
Cleveland, Ohio

Robert Gerwin, MD, FAAN
Medical Director and President
Pain and Rehabilitation Medicine
Bethesda, Maryland

Michael Gofeld, MD
Department of Anesthesia
St. Michael's Hospital
Toronto, Ontario

Harold Goforth, MD
Harry R. Horvitz Center for Palliative Medicine
Division of Solid Tumor
Taussig Cancer Institute
Cleveland Clinic
Cleveland, Ohio

Peter Hallet, MD
Department of Anesthesiology
Multidisciplinary Pain Center
Ziekenhuis Oost-Limburg
Genk, Belgium

John G. Hanlon, MD, FRCPC
Assistant Professor of Anesthesia
University of Toronto
St. Michael's Hospital
Toronto, Ontario, Canada

Afton L. Hassett, PsyD
Associate Research Scientist
Department of Anesthesiology
University of Michigan Medical School
Ann Arbor, Michigan

Troy Henning, DO
Assistant Professor of Physical Medicine & Rehabilitation
University of Michigan Health System
Ann Arbor, Michigan

Samuel L. Holmes, MD
Fellow, Pain Medicine
Walter Reed National Military Medical Center
Bethesda, Maryland

Jeffrey Janata, PhD
Associate Professor of Psychiatry
Case Western Reserve University School of Medicine
Division Chief of Psychology
University Hospitals Case Medical Center
Cleveland, Ohio

Kim D. Jones, RNC, PhD, FNP
Associate Professor of Nursing
Oregon Health & Science University
Portland, Oregon

Leonardo Kapural, MD, PhD
Carolinas Pain Institute at Brookstown
Wake Forest Baptist Health
Winston-Salem, North Carolina

Bashar Katirji, MD, FACP
Neuromuscular Center
Neurological Institute
University Hospitals Case Medical Center
Case Western Reserve University
School of Medicine
Cleveland, Ohio

Christopher D. Kenny, DO
Resident Physician of Physical Medicine & Rehabilitation
Walter Reed National Military Medical Center
Bethesda, Maryland

Krishna Kumar, MBBS, MS, FRCSC
Department of Neurosurgery
University of Saskatchewan
Regina General Hospital
Regina, Saskatchewan, Canada

Jeanne M. Lackamp, MD
Assistant Professor of Psychiatry
Division of Psychiatry and Medicine
University Hospitals Case Medical Center
Cleveland, Ohio

Chili Lati, MSPT, CSCS
Physical Therapist
Vital Physical Therapy, LLC
Washington, DC

John D. Markman, MD
Director, Neuromedicine Pain Management Center and Translational Pain Research
Departments of Neurosurgery and Neurology
University of Rochester School of Medicine and Dentistry
Rochester, New York

Philippe Mavrocordatos, MD
Department of Anesthesiology and Pain Medicine
Multidisciplinary Pain Center—Clinique Cecil
Lausanne, Switzerland

Nagy Mekhail, MD, PhD
Carl E. Wasmuth Endowed Chair and Director, Evidence Based Pain Medicine Research
Department of Pain Management
Cleveland Clinic
Cleveland, Ohio

Irina L. Melnik, MD
Spinal Diagnostics and Treatment Center
Daly City, California
Comprehensive Spine and Sports
Mill Valley, California

Jonathan Miller, MD
Director, Functional and Restorative Neurosurgery
Department of Neurosurgery
University Hospitals Case Medical Center
Cleveland, Ohio

Jennifer Moore Brandstetter, MD
Senior Instructor
Department of Psychiatry
Division of Psychiatry and Medicine
University Hospitals Case Medical Center
Cleveland, Ohio

Kiran Nandigam, BS, MBA
University of Rochester School of Medicine and Dentistry
Rochester, New York

Samer Narouze, MD, PhD
Clinical Professor of Anesthesiology
Ohio University College of Medicine
Clinical Professor of Neurological Surgery
Ohio State University
Chairman, Center for Pain Medicine
Summa Western Reserve Hospital
Cuyahoga Falls, Ohio

Joseph O'Brien, MD, MPH
Department of Orthopaedic Surgery
The George Washington University
Washington, DC

Girish Padmanabhan, DPT, OCS, Cert MDT
Director, Outpatient Rehabilitation Center
The George Washington University Hospital
Washington, DC

Jeffrey D. Petersohn, MD
Advanced Spine and Orthopedic Institute
Shore Medical Center
Somers Point, New Jersey

Dieter M. J. Peuskens, MD
Department of Neurosurgery
Multidisciplinary Pain Center
Ziekenhuis Oost-Limburg
Genk, Belgium

Martine Puylaert, MD, FIPP
Department of Anesthesiology
Multidisciplinary Pain Center
Ziekenhuis Oost-Limburg
Genk, Belgium

Srinivasa N. Raja, MD
Director, Pain Medicine Division
Professor of Anesthesiology/Critical Care Medicine
and Professor of Neurology
Johns Hopkins University
Baltimore, Maryland

James P. Rathmell, MD
Division of Pain Medicine
Department of Anesthesia, Critical Care and Pain Medicine
Harvard Medical School
Massachusetts General Hospital
Boston, Massachusetts

W. Evan Rivers, DO
University of New Mexico
Albuquerque, New Mexico

Syed Rizvi, MD
Department of Neurology
University of Saskatchewan
Regina General Hospital
Regina, Saskatchewan, Canada

James P. Robinson, MD
Clinical Professor of Physical Medicine and Rehabilitation
University of Washington
UW Medicine Center for Pain Relief
Seattle, Washington

Ronen Shechter, MD
Assistant Professor of Anesthesiology
Johns Hopkins University, School of Medicine
Baltimore, Maryland

Joseph Signorino, PT, DPT
Physical Therapist
Outpatient Rehabilitation Center
The George Washington University Hospital
Washington, DC

Howard S. Smith, MD
Professor of Anesthesiology, Internal Medicine, and Physical Medicine and Rehabilitation
Albany Medical College
Albany, New York

Dag Söderström, MD
Consultant Psychiatrist
Cecil Clinic and Riviera Hospital
Lausanne University
Multidisciplinary Pain Center—Clinique Cecil
Lausanne, Switzerland

Jennifer Sweet, MD
Associate, Functional and Restorative Neurosurgery
Department of Neurosurgery
University Hospitals Case Medical Center
Cleveland, Ohio

Giries W. Sweis, PsyD, MHS
Neurological Center for Pain
Cleveland Clinic
Cleveland, Ohio

Frank F. Tu, MD, MPH
Associate Professor of Obstetrics & Gynecology
Northwestern University Feinberg School of Medicine
North Shore University Health System
Chicago, Illinois

Koen Van Boxem, MD
Department of Anesthesiology & Pain Management
Maastricht University Medical Center
The Netherlands
Department of Anesthesiology
Critical Care and Multidisciplinary Pain Center
Sint-Jozefkliniek Bornem en Willebroek, Belgium

Nicole Van den Hecke, MD
Department of Anesthesiology
Multidisciplinary Pain Center
Ziekenhuis Oost-Limburg
Genk, Belgium

Jan Van Zundert, MD, PhD, FIPP
Head of Multidisciplinary Pain Center
Department of Anesthesiology
Ziekenhuis Oost-Limburg
Genk, Belgium

Kevin E. Vorenkamp, MD
Associate, Department of Anesthesiology and Pain Medicine
Virginia Mason Medical Center
Seattle, Washington

Harold J. Wain, PhD
Chief of Psychiatry Consultation Liaison Service
Walter Reed National Military Medical Center
Bethesda, Maryland

R. Matthew Walsh, MD, FACS
Department of General Surgery
Cleveland Clinic
Cleveland, Ohio

Denniz Zolnoun, MD, MPH
Associate Professor of Obstetrics and Gynecology
University of North Carolina
Chapel Hill, North Carolina

SECTION I

NEUROPATHIC PAIN

1.

SMALL FIBER NEUROPATHY

Kamal Chemali, Salim Hayek, and Thomas C. Chelimsky

CASE PRESENTATION

A 48-year-old man presents to the clinic because of a burning sensation in both toes that started 3 months ago and has progressed to involve the entire foot up to the ankle. He denies any past medical history but has gained 25 lbs in the past year due to overeating and inactivity.

On examination, motor strength is normal. He has a mild sensory gradient to pinprick and temperature in stocking distribution to the ankles, bilaterally and symmetrically. Vibration and joint position sense are intact. Reflexes are graded at 2+ NINDS (classification of the National Institute of Neurological Disorders and Stroke) at the knees and 1+ NINDS at the ankles. His gait is normal, and the Romberg test is negative.

QUESTIONS

1. What is the definition and pathophysiology of small fiber neuropathy (SFN)?
2. How does one evaluate the patient with autonomic SFN?
3. What are the differential diagnosis and the testing recommendations for SFN?
4. How does one manage SFN?
   a. Pain management
   b. Practical checklist for management of orthostasis

WHAT IS THE DEFINITION AND PATHOPHYSIOLOGY OF SFN?

It is not uncommon in chronic pain or neurologic practices to encounter cases of peripheral polyneuropathy (PN) that affect small fibers mediating autonomic and pain functions. Actually, it is thought that most patients with a PN have some degree of small fiber impairment[1] that often goes underrecognized. Autonomic dysfunction most often accompanies a PN involving the unmyelinated small C and Aδ fibers. We refer to this component as *small fiber neuropathy* (SFN). SFN presents with two basic types of complaints: those involving primarily autonomic nerves, with complaints of loss of function (also referred to as *negative* symptoms) such as numbness, orthostatic hypotension (OH), or bowel and bladder dysfunction, and those involving primarily pain nerves, with gain of function (also referred to as *positive* symptoms) complaints such as burning pain, tightness, paresthesiaes, and the like. Many SFNs present with both types of complaints. This case-based review will revisit the most common forms of SFN, emphasizing their manifestations, evaluation, and management.

This presentation is a classic example of a peripheral neuropathy affecting nerve fibers mediating perception of pain and temperature more than other sensory modalities. Small, unmyelinated C fibers and thinly myelinated Aδ fibers subserve two major categories of signals: (1) *afferent* signals, including somatic and visceral pain, visceral state (e.g., baroreceptor, chemoreceptor, etc.), and temperature; and (2) *efferent autonomic* signals, including sympathetic and parasympathetic nerves to all organs and their vascular beds and enteric nerves in the gut. In particular, these fibers innervate the skin epidermis, the subcutaneous vascular bed, and the sweat glands in the dermis. Exaggerated and ectopic discharges of epidermal C fibers (somatic C fibers) result from an insult to the axon, resulting in a painful burning or tingling sensation. These are termed "positive" neuropathic symptoms because they result from pathologic *hyperactivity* of the nerve cell. As the disease underlying the C fiber attack progresses, the C fibers degenerate and "negative" symptoms, such as loss of pin or temperature sensation, will appear, resulting from pathologic *hypoactivity*. Clinically, positive and negative symptoms differ in that positive symptoms draw attention to themselves, whereas negative symptoms only manifest once a person realizes he or she cannot perform a specific function. Involvement of the C fibers to the subcutaneous vascular bed will produce vasomotor changes, warmth, redness or paleness, and possibly edema. Involvement of sweat gland C fibers (sudomotor fibers) may result in abnormal sweat output, such as hyper- or hypohidrosis. In approaching SFN clinically, a first step is to determine if both afferent (sensory) and efferent (autonomic) C fibers are involved or if the disorder affects only one fiber type. For example, the presence of vasomotor changes and sudomotor symptoms concomitant with somatic symptoms suggests a generalized disorder involving all C fibers. Autonomic C-fiber involvement can be ascertained by testing autonomic functions such as the cardiovascular, pupillary, sudomotor, or other functions. Involvement may extend to the gastrointestinal tract, including endocrine pancreas, perhaps contributing to weight gain. This patient's assessment should always include a thorough evaluation for diabetes or glucose intolerance with a 2- or 3-hour glucose tolerance test (discussed in detail later in the chapter).

Upon further questioning, the patient recognizes that his feet turn red at times, with blotchy skin. He reports that they are hypersensitive to touch and hurt when in contact with the bed sheet. He denies any change in the sweating pattern of his feet, although he thinks that they feel very hot and dry at times. He acknowledges that, more often than not, he feels lightheaded when he stands up quickly from a chair or from bed in the morning, but he does not pass out. He denies any gastrointestinal changes, but has been unable to maintain an erection for the past 6 months.

This additional information was not volunteered by the patient and would have been missed had the examiner not asked these specific questions. Patients often do not put these symptoms together with the sensory complaints or even with one another. The picture now suggests that a generalized dysautonomia constitutes a part of this SFN. The orthostatic lightheadedness may suggest hypotension and a sympathetic deficit at the level of the peripheral vasculature. Peripheral blood vessels constrict under the influence of the sympathetic nervous system. In normal conditions, a sympathetic surge causes vasoconstriction as a reflex reaction to standing and venous pooling that results from a transient drop in blood pressure (BP). This baroreflex allows the BP to return to baseline within seconds. In the case of a peripheral sympathetic deficit at the level of the peripheral vasculature, reflex vasoconstriction does not occur effectively, leading to a drop in BP and orthostatic symptoms, such as lightheadedness and, in severe cases, syncope. Erectile dysfunction results from a peripheral parasympathetic denervation of penile arteries and of the corpus cavernosum.[2] Clinically, this patient is now suspected to have both autonomic and sensory SFN.

Additional examination reveals a heart rate of 100 beats per minute (bpm), the presence of hypersensitivity to pinprick, tactile allodynia, and vasomotor changes at both feet symmetrically. Pupils are at 6 mm in darkness and constrict to 5 mm sluggishly. No other abnormalities are noted.

The effect of a dysfunction of the autonomic nervous system (ANS) on end organs is the result of a loss of balance between its two limbs, the sympathetic and parasympathetic nervous systems. The former causes the heart to race, whereas the latter slows heart rate. Similarly, the pupil is under the balanced influence of these two systems. The parasympathetic system causes pupillary constriction, and the sympathetic system causes pupillary dilation. A decrease in parasympathetic tone at the pupil leads to a relative increase in sympathetic tone, resulting in mydriasis with sluggish pupillary constriction. It therefore now becomes clear that this patient presents with a possible cardiovagal abnormality at the heart leading to baseline tachycardia and parasympathetic dysfunction at the pupil leading to a relative mydriasis and poor constriction. These changes are at the heart of ANS testing discussed later in the chapter.

In addition, sympathetic dysfunction at the peripheral nerves, dorsal root ganglia (DRG) and the dorsal horns of the spinal cord leads to sensitization and allodynia. Injury to the peripheral C fibers engenders a cascade of events, with changes in the types of channels expressed on the membrane. Sick C fibers have sodium channels with a lower threshold and a shorter refractory period, thus allowing more easily triggered and higher frequency discharge, and some inactivation of some potassium channels destabilizes the membrane, resulting in disturbed nerve axon potential traffic along the fiber. In cases where injury to the nerve is severe enough to encourage significant expression of nerve growth factor in the DRG, sympathetic fibers may form nonphysiologic synapses with DRG cells and permit sympathetic stimulation of nociceptive sensory afferent cells. This mechanism opens a window in the role of the ANS in the generation and perpetuation of pain.[3] Further changes in processing occur at the dorsal horn in the spinal cord, resulting in further up-regulation of nociceptive signals at the level of the dorsal horns.[4]

In summary, the diagnosis of SFN with sensory and autonomic features, both sympathetic and parasympathetic at different end organs, results from the careful review of this patient's history along with a detailed neurologic examination focusing on the sensory and autonomic aspects of small fiber functions.

HOW TO EVALUATE THE PATIENT WITH AUTONOMIC SFN

The evaluation of a patient suspected of having a SFN consists of (1) establishing the diagnosis of peripheral polyneuropathy, (2) assessing for the presence of a measurable dysautonomia, and (3) searching for an etiology.

CONFIRMING THE SUSPICION OF SFN

Four tests are available: the electrodiagnostic test (EDX), the autonomic screen including a quantitative sudomotor axon reflex test (QSART), the intra epidermal nerve fiber density (IENFD), and quantitative sensory testing.

Electrodiagnostic Test (EDX)

Formerly known as the electromyogram (EMG), the EDX consists of two parts: nerve conduction studies and a needle electrode examination. Technical details can be found elsewhere.[5] It is aimed essentially at diagnosing lesions affecting the large myelinated nerve fibers. The EDX is therefore expected to be normal or only minimally abnormal in a peripheral polyneuropathy of the pure small fiber type.

Quantitative Sudomotor Axon Reflex Test (QSART)

This method tests the sympathetic cholinergic postganglionic sudomotor nerve.[15] As its name implies, it consists of stimulating the sudomotor (sweat) nerve in one location and recording the sweat response at a distance. The underlying principle relies on stimulation of the nerve terminal (innervating a sweat gland), thus producing a retrograde action potential along the axon until it reaches a collateral (branching) axon that innervates a different sweat gland. The action potential will then spread along this collateral and induce a release of acetylcholine at its terminal, which in turn will produce a sweat response that is recorded and quantitated. An abnormal QSART can therefore be produced by an abnormality at any of the following five anatomical locations:

Point 1: the stimulated presynaptic sudomotor nerve terminal

Point 2: the postganglionic sudomotor nerve axon

Point 3: the collateral axon

Point 4: the collateral axon terminal or the synaptic cleft

Point 5: the sweat gland from which the sweat response is recorded

This test is widely employed as a sensitive marker of distal autonomic neuropathy because the response depends on the integrity of the postganglionic segment of the sudomotor nerve. Because it is quantitative, distal-to-proximal gradients can also be detected, giving it good resolution for early disease. In SFN, it is abnormal in 50–80% of patients.[6,7] Recent publications have called into question the true "normality" of the test in healthy control subjects. Although it is still too early to draw firm conclusions, modifications of the procedure or of the healthy control values may be needed.[7a]

This test is abnormal in the following conditions:

- Diabetic small fiber sensory neuropathy,[6] where it is quite sensitive
- Complex regional pain syndrome (CRPS; reflex sympathetic dystrophy), where it may be exaggerated or reduced[8]
- Aging (only mildly decreased responses)[9]
- Generalized conditions affecting the ANS, such as generalized autonomic failure,[10] postural orthostatic tachycardia syndrome (POTS),[11] parkinsonism-plus and cerebellar disorders with dysautonomia,[12] multiple system atrophy (MSA), and progressive autonomic failure (PAF).[13] Note should be made of the latter conditions, in which theory suggesting a normal QSART response is contradicted by the findings. Postganglionic degeneration has been suggested as an explanation.
- Concomitant use of certain medications, particularly anticholinergic medications and tricyclic antidepressants,[14] although in our hands these drug effects are mild to moderate at most

The test is gender-sensitive. Generally, females have lower sweat responses than do males.[15] The QSART is considered a highly sensitive test for the detection of a postganglionic autonomic neuropathy.

Intra-epidermal Nerve Fiber Density (IENFD)

In the past decade, reports of the use of punch skin biopsy and the quantification of IENFD as a diagnostic tool in peripheral neuropathy has flourished. First developed at the Karolinska Institute in Sweden,[16] this technique received further refinement by the major centers that pioneered its use in clinical practice, mainly the University of Minnesota [17] and Johns Hopkins University.[18] This technique allows the visualization of epidermal, dermal, and autonomic sudomotor nerve fibers surrounding sweat glands. Recently, guidelines on the use of skin biopsy in peripheral neuropathy were developed by a Task Force under the auspices of the European Federations of Neurological Societies (EFNS). These include[19]:

A. 3 mm punch biopsy. This biopsy is safe, causes minimal bleeding, and does not need stitches if proper care is taken. The recommended biopsy sites are the distal leg and the proximal thigh. These sites allow the assessment of a distal peripheral neuropathy and give information about a length-dependent process.

B. Staining with protein gene product (PGP) 9.5, a ubiquitin carboxyl-terminal hydrolase, which stains all types of axons. The biopsy specimen is immediately fixed in a cold fixative (2% PLP) for up to 24 h at 4°C, then kept in a cryoprotective solution for one night and serially cut with a freezing microtome or a cryostat. Each biopsy yields about 55 vertical 50 μm sections.

The immunostaining methods commonly used are bright-field immunohistochemistry and indirect immunofluorescence with or without confocal microscopy. Quantification of IENFD is performed on images formed by stacking 16 sections of consecutive 2 μm sections for a standard linear length of epidermis from 1 to 3 mm.

IENF should be counted at high magnification (40×) in at least three sections per biopsy. Only fibers that cross the dermis-epidermis barrier should be counted, excluding secondary branching. This is controversial because some centers include free nerve fragments within the epidermis in the count, even if they do not cross the barrier. To calculate the IENFD, the number of counted fibers in a section is divided by the length of the section and expressed as #IENF/mm.[20]

C. Diagnostic efficiency and predictive values of skin biopsy with linear quantification of IENF in the diagnosis of SFN is very high. Bright-field microscopy was used to determine cutoff values or epidermal densities, but immunofluorescence is an acceptable method for counting fibers. Normative age, gender, ethnic, and anatomical site-matched data are available and should be used. Normal IENF density in the lower leg ranged in different studies between 17.4 ± 7.4 and 33.0 ± 7.9/mm.

D. Assessment of morphological changes such as axonal swellings, branching, and fragmentation may have a predictive value in the progression of the neuropathy. Whether one can diagnose a SFN based on swellings alone is not clear.

E. There is a correlation between skin biopsy and other neurophysiological tests (mainly sural nerve conduction studies in large fiber neuropathies), whereas IENF density is more sensitive than EMG in diagnosing SFN. A linear correlation between the medial plantar sensory nerve potential amplitude and IENF density has been reported.[21] IENF density inversely correlated more closely with warm and heat-pain threshold than with cooling threshold on quantitative sensory testing (QST).[22,23] A significant correlation occurs between decreased IENF density and abnormal QSART,[24] which matches our own experience.

The overall conclusion is that skin biopsy is more sensitive that either sural nerve conduction studies or sural nerve biopsy for the diagnosis of SFN and correlates well with QSART, heat-pain threshold on QST, and possibly with medial plantar nerve conduction studies. It should only be performed in certified cutaneous nerve laboratories by trained personnel.

Most recently, researchers at the University of Minnesota suggested the use of the suction skin blister method, a minimally invasive technique, as a potential diagnostic tool to investigate SFNs. It was found to be comparable to skin biopsy for determining epidermal nerve fiber density.[25]

Recommendation:

- Skin biopsy as first-line diagnostic test for SFN if the electrodiagnostic examination (EDX or EMG) is normal. If the EDX examination is consistent with the diagnosis of peripheral neuropathy, this is an indication of large fiber involvement and therefore the skin biopsy may provide more second-line than first-line diagnostic information.

The next tests may provide additional diagnostic information in difficult cases.

Quantitative Sensory Testing (QST)

Described in detail by Fruhstorfer et al.,[26] this technique consists of measuring cold, warm, and heat pain detection thresholds by applying alternating heat and cold stimuli to the skin and asking the patient to activate a switch as soon as cold, warm, or pain are perceived. The results are compared to sex- and age-matched published normative values, and results above the 95th percentile are considered abnormal. There has been an increased interest recently in this technique, comparing its sensitivity to IENFD in the detection of SFN. Results vary, but, in a recent study on 67 patients with pure SFN, QST detected fewer than 50% of cases, which is consistent with our experience.[27] In addition, QST cannot localize the lesion, since disruption of small thermosensitive fibers at any point in their course, including near the thalamus, may alter detection thresholds.

Thermoregulatory Sweat Test (TST)

The TST tests the integrity of the entire central and peripheral sudomotor pathway. Under the term "central" are included the preganglionic sympathetic fibers, the intermediolateral cell columns, the bulbospinal pathways, and the hypothalamus. The term "peripheral" encompasses the postganglionic sudomotor fibers and the sympathetic chain.[28] The test is based on the assumption that the maximal sweat response is directly proportional to the local skin temperature and the core temperature.[28] Therefore, the test consists of passively raising the body core and skin temperature in a sweat chamber, under constant conditions of ambient air temperature and humidity using infrared lamps, and visually evaluating the distribution of sweat production over the different regions of the body ("sweat pattern"). Thermoregulatory sweat production is age- and sex-dependant,[29] and the TST is no exception. Several sweat patterns have been described in normal individuals and in different dysautonomias, and knowledge of these patterns is important for a correct diagnosis. The most typical patterns are the "peripheral" pattern, indicating loss in a stocking-glove distribution, and its mirror-image, the "central" pattern, with preservation of sweating over the distal extremities. Other patterns include "radicular," with stripes of absent sweating marking particular dermatomes, particularly over the thorax, as seen in a ganglionitis or radiculitis, and "patchy," with loss of sweating in patches, as would occur in leprosy. A myelopathic pattern indicates loss of sweating clearly demarcated below a particular level. Excellent detailed reviews are available.[28]

CONFIRMING THE PRESENCE OF A MEASURABLE DYSAUTONOMIA

Confirmation is achieved in the autonomic laboratory by performing tests of autonomic function. Sudomotor autonomic function is performed with the QSART and TST, but the presence of dysautonomia is also assessed at different levels and organs, mainly the heart and vasculature.

The heart and its different structures are innervated by both the sympathetic and parasympathetic nervous systems. Similarly, the peripheral vasculature receives fibers from both arms of the ANS. However, sympathetic fibers have a predominant action at the level of the peripheral vasculature, whereas the parasympathetic has little influence.

The responses of the heart and peripheral blood vessels to the different tests described here are reflex compensatory responses. In other terms, a decrease in BP leads to a reflex increase in heart rate (HR) and a reflex vasoconstriction, whereas the opposite is true with an increase in BP. Afferent fibers of this reflex pathway originate at the level of the baroreceptors of the carotid sinus, arterial walls, aortic arch, cardiac mechanoreceptors, and pulmonary stretch receptors. An increase in afferent activity leads to a decrease in sympathetic efferent activity, an increase of parasympathetic efferent activity, or both, and vice versa.[30]

Photoplethysmographic Blood Pressure Recordings

Photoplethysmographic recordings use an infrared sensor applied to the finger within a finger cuff to record its blood volume. Through a computerized servosystem, the BP is recorded beat-to-beat and accurately reflects intra-arterial pressures.[31] This technique has proved useful in detecting sudden changes in hemodynamics as a result of autonomic compensatory reflex. It is commonly used in the deep breathing test, the Valsalva maneuver (VM), and the tilt test.

Heart Rate Response to Deep Breathing (HR_{DB})

Heart rate variability to deep breathing, one of the most commonly performed tests of cardiac autonomic innervation, is simple to perform and provides a sensitive, specific, and reproducible indirect measure of cardiac vagal nerve function.[32,33]

Heart rate variability measurements are derived from a regular strip of an electrocardiogram (ECG) performed while the patient is breathing deeply in the supine position.[32]

The VM

Another commonly used test of cardiovascular autonomic function is the heart rate response to the VM. It consists of a precisely timed forced expiration against resistance followed by release of pressure, which leads to a series of hemodynamic changes that are recorded and analyzed. These changes are classically divided into four phases, of which only phase II (forced expiration phase) and IV (release phase) are of clinical significance.[34] The Valsalva ratio, a sensitive, specific, and reproducible measure of autonomic function,[33] is defined as a ratio of the highest heart rate during phase II (sympathetic) to the lowest heart rate during phase IV (parasympathetic). The VM is a good indicator of both parasympathetic and sympathetic failure.

Head-up Tilt Table Test (HUT)

HUT differs from standing because (a) it is passive and hence requires no cortical motor command, and (b) it is usually performed at 70 not 90 degrees, thus reducing the action of the calf and thigh muscle pumps. It is therefore more sensitive than standing as a test of orthostatic tolerance. The patient lies supine horizontally on a pivoting table while BP and HR are measured for as long as it takes to obtain a solid, consistent baseline (minimum of 5–10 min). The patient is then tilted head-up to 70 degrees, and changes in HR and BP are measured continuously for 10–40 minutes depending on the test indication. The patient is returned to the supine position, and the same vital signs are recorded until they match the initial baseline. Generally, there is an initial drop in systolic BP by 5–10 mm Hg and a rise in diastolic BP by the same amount. Similarly, HR increases gradually, usually by less than 20 bpm. HR variation with tilting reflects the integrity of parasympathetic cardiovagal function and sympathetic cardioadrenergic function, whereas BP variation reflects the state of sympathetic cardiovascular function. This test constitutes the gold standard in assessing reflex (neurocardiogenic) syncope, neurally mediated (or vasovagal) syncope, postural tachycardia syndrome (POTS), and OH.[35]

Autonomic testing in this patient reveals the following: QSART shows a reduction of sweat output at the foot and distal leg. Skin biopsy reveals a reduction in IENFD at the distal leg and proximal leg. Cardiovascular autonomic tests show an abnormally low I:E ratio during the HR_{DB} test and a reduced Valsalva ratio reflecting the presence of a cardiovagal deficit. HUT is normal. The conclusion is that this evaluation is consistent with a SFN involving (1) sensory fibers (skin biopsy), (2) sudomotor efferent autonomic fibers (reduced axon reflex sweat output), and (3) cardiac parasympathetic vagal fibers (low deep breathing response).

SEARCHING FOR AN ETIOLOGY

The ultimate goal of the evaluation of an SFN is to reverse or stabilize the disorder by providing an effective treatment based on an accurate diagnosis. Treating the neuropathy includes treating the underlying cause when known. If a potential etiology is uncovered, the neuropathy will be considered as caused by that etiology despite the fact that the causative link can never really be proved, and it will be termed as such (e.g., diabetic autonomic SFN, amyloidotic SFN, autoimmune autonomic SFN, etc.). If no etiology can be found, the autonomic SFN will be termed "idiopathic." In our experience, the latter constitutes about 30% of all autonomic SFN.

WHAT ARE THE DIFFERENTIAL DIAGNOSIS AND THE TESTING RECOMMENDATIONS OF SFN?

METABOLIC, TOXIC, AND GENETIC CAUSES

Diabetes Mellitus

Small fibers are often the first peripheral nerves to be affected in diabetes mellitus and are affected in 50–70% of patients,[31] and diabetes mellitus/glucose intolerance is the most common disorder associated with a SFN, accounting for about 50% of cases of SFN.[38] They manifest clinically as "positive symptoms," such as subjective sensation of burning, coldness, shooting pains, or tightness in the distal extremities. Impaired glucose tolerance (IGT) by itself or impaired fasting glucose (IFG) in the absence of true diabetes is frequently associated with SFN. This has been shown in the past few years in several studies.[36–39] Recently, a study by Hoffman-Snyder et al. showed that a 2-hour oral glucose tolerance test (OGTT) is superior to fasting glucose in diagnosing SFN due to glucose dysmetabolism.[38] Furthermore, a progression study showed that small fibers were most affected in patients with IGT without diabetes, whereas patients with diabetes had more involvement of large fibers.[40] Since IGT is frequently a precursor to diabetes, these findings not only point to a dose-response relationship between the severity of glucose dysmetabolism and the degree of peripheral neuropathy, but they also suggest that there may be a progression from small fiber involvement early in the disease to large fiber involvement later on as the disease progresses. Although the association between IGT and SFN is almost certain, it remains unclear whether IGT is an independent causative factor as opposed to being covariant with other factors belonging to the so-called *metabolic syndrome*.[41] IGT is associated both with sensory SFN and an autonomic SFN, with sudomotor fibers possibly being the first to be affected.[42,43] According to the American Diabetes Association (ADA) criteria, an OGTT is considered as normal if fasting blood glucose levels are less than 110 mg/dL and 2-hour postglucose challenge levels are less than 140 mg/dL. IGT was defined as 2-hour post-glucose (75 g oral load) challenge level between 140 mg/dL and 200 mg/dL,[44] following ingestion of 75 g of glucose, normally after fasting for 6–12 consecutive hours. Impaired fasting glucose was redefined by the revised ADA criteria from 2003 as fasting serum glucose between 100 mg/dL and 126 mg/dL.[45]

Recommendations:

- Obtain a 2-hour OGTT (75 g of glucose) in every patient with SFN symptomatology.
- Do not rely on the HbA1c as a diagnostic test for diabetic SFN because this index may be normal and the patient still have IGT.
- Favor the OGTT over simply fasting glucose in the workup of SFN

The patient underwent the entire etiological workup consisting of extensive fasting blood work. All tests returned negative or normal, except for an abnormal glucose tolerance test, suggesting the diagnosis of previously undiagnosed diabetes mellitus. An HbA1c was obtained and was 7.1%, confirming this diagnosis.

Hyperlipidemia

A study of six patients by McManis et al.[46] suggested a real association between hyperlipidemia (particularly hypertriglyceridemia [HTG]) and SFN, with little written since. Our experience links the two conditions because we sometimes see isolated HTG in patients who otherwise would be diagnosed as idiopathic SFN. HTG is known to be associated with IGT, and both are now part of the so-called metabolic syndrome.[47] However, we think that isolated HTG in patients with SFN is a real finding and should be studied more carefully because HTG is a treatable condition and the neuropathy may reverse. Another uncertainty is about the triglyceride levels needed to cause SFN. In McManis' study, patients had elevated levels of more than 800 mg/dL. Mild to moderately elevated levels (200–400 mg/dL) should be studied for their effect on peripheral C and Aδ fibers.

Recommendation:

- Obtain a triglyceride level in every patient with SFN and treat if elevated (>200 mg/dL).

Alcohol and Toxins

Alcohol abuse has been well established as a cause of peripheral neuropathy, and about 60% of alcoholics are affected. A recent study by Zambelis et al. has tried to differentiate between small fiber and large fiber neuropathy in alcoholism. In their study of 98 patients, they found about 12% of their patients to be affected by SFN alone, 20% to have a large fiber neuropathy, and 25% to have a mixed polyneuropathy.[48] It is generally agreed that the longer the duration of alcohol abuse, the more likely it is to have large fibers affected. A recent study suggested that mediators of the hypothalamic-pituitary and sympathoadrenal stress axes act on sensory neurons in the induction and maintenance of alcohol-induced painful peripheral neuropathy, and this painful neuropathy is successfully blocked in experimental rats by adrenal medullectomy and the administration of a glucocorticoid receptor antagonist, mifepristone.[49]

According to the excellent review by Lacomis on SFN, among the most common toxins only metronidazole has been associated to SFN. We also have experience with taclipaxel producing an autonomic neuropathy, with most other chemotherapeutic and environmental toxins causing large fiber neuropathy.[50]

Recommendations:

- Obtain urine and blood toxicology screens if you suspect alcoholism in a patient with SFN.
- Inquire about all medications the patient is taking currently and has taken in the past, including toxic and occupational exposure.

Thyroid Abnormalities

The medical literature does not establish a clear cause-effect relationship between SFN and thyroid disorders. However, a recent study from Norway reported the presence of SFN symptoms in patients with hypothyroidism.[51]

Recommendation:

- Obtaining thyroid function tests in patients with SFN is not an absolute recommendation.

Vitamin B_{12} Deficiency

Although deficiency in cobalamin most often produces a large fiber neuropathy, and there is no documented clear cause-effect relationship between B_{12} deficiency and somatic

SFN, it is nonetheless known that autonomic neuropathy can occur in the context of vitamin B_{12} deficiency. Beitzke et al., in a study of 21 nondiabetic patients with this deficiency, found that these patients had abnormal autonomic cardiovascular reflexes similar to those in patients with diabetic autonomic neuropathy.[52] In addition, B_{12} deficiency may be directly associated with OH through a non-neuropathic mechanism. This may occur suddenly after general anesthesia and requires rapid B_{12} replacement. However, whether a deficiency in vitamin B_{12} can cause an autonomic peripheral painful SFN is not known.

Recommendation:

- There is no solid evidence of an association between SFN and vitamin B_{12} deficiency, but if autonomic symptoms and signs are present, getting a B_{12} level is reasonable, with aggressive replacement if the level is below 350 ng/dL.

Hereditary Causes

The existence of a strong family history of SFN in patients with SFN has been reported by several authors.[6,24,53] The most common hereditary conditions associated with SFN are the hereditary sensory autonomic neuropathies (HSAN) I–V. HSAN III is also known as *familial dysautonomia*, a disorder in which the visceral afferent sensors such as baro- and chemoreceptors are particularly affected, resulting in very characteristic autonomic features with large fluctuations in BP and abdominal pain. These have been extensively reviewed.[53a]

Fabry's disease is a rare X-linked recessive condition caused by a reduction of lysosomal α-galactosidase A and consecutive storage of glycolipids (e.g., in the brain, kidney, skin, and nerve fibers). Cardinal neurologic findings are hypohidrosis, painful episodes, and peripheral neuropathy. It is associated with severe somatic and visceral burning pain and has a characteristic skin lesion called *angiokeratoma corporis* (scaly red to red-blue macules over the chest). The small fibers in this condition have been extensively studied and show a preferential loss of C and Aδ fibers, as manifested by severe impairment of thermal and preserved vibratory and mechanical discrimination.[54–56] This seems to be true even in heterozygous states (carrier females).[57]

Porphyria includes several inborn errors of metabolism, all affecting the formation of heme. They may present with cutaneous, hepatic, or neurologic manifestations. Three disorders have neurologic manifestations that include an autonomic neuropathy: acute intermittent porphyria, hereditary coproporphyria, and variegate porphyria. Measuring δ-amino levulinic acid and porphyrobilinogen in both urine and serum at the time of a porphyric crisis provides a diagnostic screen. Specific genetic testing can be ordered for the specific suspected porphyria.

Recent evidence has begun to link autonomic neuropathy to mitochondrial disorders. Although unequivocal evidence of this link has yet to emerge, a mitochondrial polymorphism has been linked to pediatric cyclic vomiting syndrome (but not adult) and to forms of migraine.[57a]

We also mention here the "familial burning feet syndrome," a condition of unknown genetics.

Recommendations:

- Inquire about family history of SFN and cardiac, liver, and kidney disease in every patient with this disorder, as well as evidence of mitochondrial manifestations such as seizures, proximal muscle weakness, and loss of hearing and vision.
- Inspect the skin of all patients with SFN.

Erythromelalgia

This is a clinical syndrome characterized by intermittent or constant heat, redness, and pain affecting the lower extremities in a bilateral and symmetrical fashion. Typically, there is a specific temperature sensitivity, such that above a certain temperature (e.g., 58°F), the limbs become intolerable. Patients are known to bathe their feet in ice water to relieve the burning, which often leads to ice burns and sometimes difficult to manage ulcerations. A mutation of the SCN9A gene coding for the α subunit of the NaV1.7 sodium channel causes the disorder in about 15% of cases. Mutations produce a temperature-sensitive increase in channel function, allowing more sodium to cross the neuron membrane and resulting in a lower opening threshold.[57b] This form of SFN is associated with abnormal adrenergic and sudomotor functions on autonomic testing.[58] The disorder may sometimes responds to mexiletine or sympathetic blockade.

Recommendation:

- Consider this diagnosis in the presence of a temperature-sensitive autonomic SFN associated with marked erythema of the limbs.
- Gene testing is not commercially available, but a family history is strongly suggestive of the diagnosis.
- Consider mexiletine for symptom management.

INFECTIOUS AND IMMUNOLOGIC CAUSES

Sjögren Syndrome

Among the connective tissue diseases, SS has probably the strongest association with SFN and overall represents the second most common cause after diabetes. This condition presents with sicca symptoms consistent mainly of dryness of the eyes and mouth. Known complications are sensory polyneuropathy, axonal sensorimotor polyneuropathy, and sensory neuronopathy. In a study by Lopate et al. that compared patients with SS with controls, small fibers (including autonomic) were much more affected in the patient group than were large fibers.[59] In another study by Chai et al., 80% of a cohort of patients with SS were shown to have an SFN; however, a large percentage of these patients showed a "non-dying back" SFN process on skin biopsy suggesting a small fiber ganglionopathy.[60,61] These and other studies have emphasized the predominance of SFN or ganglionopathy in SS over any other type of neuropathy. As importantly, autonomic manifestations were described to be widely present in SS-related polyneuropathies.[61]

Recommendations:

- Include SSA and SSB antibodies (usually part of the ANA panel) in the workup of SFN.
- Pursue the diagnosis of SS with salivary gland biopsy if sicca symptoms are present, even if there is another obvious cause of SFN, if there are autonomic manifestations associated or if there is evidence of nondistal SFN clinically on skin biopsy or QSART.

Monoclonal Gammopathy

As in most other disorders mentioned in this section, a cause-effect relationship has not been proved between monoclonal gammopathy and SFN. However the association appears to be too frequent to occur by chance alone (1 in 44 patients in one study[53]). The association is more frequent when the monoclonal gammopathy is a manifestation of amyloidosis (AL), addressed in the next section.

AL

Primary AL makes up approximately 90% of all amyloid cases. Its incidence is estimated at about 0.9 per 100,000. It affects usually elderly patients, with a median age of 65. It is caused by proliferation or deposition of light chains in tissues.[62]

SFN is the earliest form of neuropathy in this disease.[63] Autonomic dysfunction is very common.[64] In a recent study, various clinical patterns of peripheral neuropathy in amyloidosis were found, the most common form being a generalized autonomic failure and polyneuropathy with pain in 62% of patients. All patients were found to have a moderately severe generalized autonomic failure even if symptoms of dysautonomia were not present.[65] Most patients complain of weakness and fatigue, and the neuropathy is relentlessly progressive and later affects motor and sensory large fibers. AL is associated with carpal tunnel syndrome in up to 20%. Liver, renal, and cardiac disease are often present. A large tongue may be a clinical clue.

In 50% of cases, a serum monoclonal protein of the IgA or IgG type is found, and, when a urine M-protein analysis is also obtained, this percentage rises to 90%. Multiple myeloma can be present. However, the definitive diagnosis requires tissue: a bone marrow biopsy generally gives a diagnosis in 50% of cases (amyloid stains positive with Congo red). An abdominal fat pad aspirate yields a diagnosis in 70–80% of cases. The combination of bone marrow biopsy and fat aspirate raises this number to 90%. A sural nerve biopsy can be positive in up to 85% of cases.

The familial form (transthyretin gene mutation) forms about 5% of all cases. It is similar to AL in its clinical presentation, but severe weight loss and M-protein spike are absent and the age of onset is younger. Orthotopic liver transplant may cure the disorder and is recommended as early as possible in the course of the disease,[66] thus the importance of early diagnosis.

Recommendations:

- Consider amyloidosis in patients who present first with SFN symptoms then progress rapidly to motor and sensory large fiber neuropathy. Carpal tunnel syndrome and a large tongue may be clinical clues.
- Consider amyloidosis in every patient with autonomic dysfunction and peripheral neuropathy, especially of the small fiber type.

Celiac Disease

The association of this disease with peripheral neuropathy is known. However, a recent report by Brannagan et al. described the presence of an asymmetrical, non-length dependent SFN in eight patients with celiac disease, sometimes involving the face. Four of these patients improved with a gluten-free diet.[67] In our experience, we have similarly encountered several patients with SFN who did not have any other abnormalities except elevated antigliadin antibodies (IgA and IgG). Interestingly, one of these patients presented with an asymmetrical SFN that resembled CRPS I, associated with unilateral allodynia of one foot, and this patient turned out to have markedly reduced intraepidermal nerve fibers on skin biopsy of the affected foot compared to the contralateral foot despite the presence of SFN-symptoms in the latter.

Recommendation:

- Even though the evidence is not solid, we think the association between these two conditions is real, and we recommend including trans-glutaminase or antiendomysial IgA antibodies in the second-tier workup of a SFN.

OTHER AUTOIMMUNE, INFLAMMATORY, INFECTIOUS CAUSES

SFN may occur in the context of inflammatory or autoimmune disease.[68,69] Although SFN is occasionally associated with a true vasculitis,[70] this disease usually presents as a large fiber mononeuropathy multiplex, not SFN. Infectious illnesses, mainly human immunodeficiency virus (HIV),[71–73] have also been described as a cause of SFN. Antinerve antibodies have not been useful in diagnosing an autoimmune cause of SFN.[53] Gorson and Ropper described improvement of the symptoms in some of their idiopathic patients with intravenous immunoglobulins (IVIg), suggesting the possibility of an autoimmune pathophysiology.[74] We have had a similar experience with certain patients with SFN associated with certain autoimmune diseases, but a large-scale double-blinded, placebo-controlled study of the effect of IVIg in the treatment of SFN is lacking.

Recommendations:

- Obtain an ANA blood panel as well as an erythrocyte sedimentation rate (ESR), a C reactive protein (CRP), and an HIV test (in the appropriate context) in the first-tier workup of a SFN.

- We do not recommend obtaining antinerve antibodies or viral titers in the blood or cerebrospinal fluid in the routine workup of SFN because supportive evidence is poor.
- Consider IVIg therapy if an autoimmune association is strongly suspected based on acute or subacute onset 2–6 weeks after a viral or other infectious process or an immunization.

HIV

The relationship between SFN and HIV infection has been extensively studied. It is well-known that HIV-1 causes different types of peripheral neuropathy, including an SFN but also an acute polyradiculoneuropathy mimicking the Guillain-Barré syndrome, which is a large fiber neuropathy.[23]

Lyme Disease

Lyme disease may be associated with SFN, but more often is associated with small fiber polyradiculopathy, a logical extension of the disorder's predilection for producing disease at the root entry zone. Although no formal reports specifically address this pathophysiology, one found that 50% of their patients with Lyme (12/24) had an asymmetric painful radicular syndrome.[74a] Another report reviews five patients with POTS after a Lyme infection.[74b]

Idiopathic

Earlier literature that did not specifically include OGTT and other rarer causes in the workup of these patients considered the idiopathic category as most common. In 1999, Periquet et al.[53] found an "idiopathic" diagnosis in 93% of patients with SFN. However, this study did not specifically look for IGT, and the definition of SFN was not as strict as today. Nevertheless, in our experience, idiopathic SFN can safely be considered to represent at least 30% of all SFN. In our experience and others',[74] it generally tends to evolve very slowly and to not develop into a large fiber neuropathy.

Recommendations:

- Do not call a SFN "idiopathic" unless you have proved that the patient does not have any of the more and less common causes of SFN. Do not forget the OGTT!
- Refer the patient to a tertiary care center if the etiology was not found for more elaborate evaluation of the diagnosis.

HOW TO MANAGE AUTONOMIC SFN

The management of autonomic SFN is divided into etiological management and symptomatic management. As mentioned earlier, etiological management consists in treating the underlying causes, if found. However, a major part of the treatment of this condition remains symptomatic management. This consists mainly of pain management and management of orthostatic symptoms, when present.

PAIN MANAGEMENT

Burning pain may be one of the primary complaints of a patient with SFN. It is critical to recall that successful management of chronic pain aims at treating the dysfunction associated with the pain, not just the pain, and that this dysfunction may be a much greater source of disability to the patient than the pain itself. This includes associated depression, anxiety, loss of self-esteem, sleeplessness, and more. Thus, the primary goal of the approach is a more meaningful and satisfying life for the patient. The management tools that can help the patient toward this goal fall into three categories. First, the patient must learn the purpose, limitations, and proper use of medications and be empowered to participate in educated self-management decisions. In parallel, when anesthetic blocks or neuromodulation approaches are suggested, the patient must understand their realistic limitations, purpose, and the patient's own active role in deriving maximal benefit. Second, the patient's lifestyle must be altered to incorporate pain and stress management strategies. Examples include self-pacing of activity levels, avoidance of pain-reinforcing behavior, reduction in covert pain signals (sometimes called "pain behaviors"), improved open communication about pain, and finally, when appropriate, relaxation and biofeedback. Third, overall functional level and physical fitness must be gently and gradually increased if the patient is to return to a productive life. Not only can a deconditioned patient not perform in the more strenuous daily activities, but his or her muscles are more susceptible to spasm and even injury, both of which further increase pain.

The choice of medications is large. The particular agents selected depend in large part on the specific quality of pain (Table 1.1) and desired side effects. For example, a patient with sleep disturbance would benefit from a tricyclic agent through an improved sleep pattern and pain reduction. The mainstay of treatment involves some combination of an anticonvulsant[75] and a tricyclic agent,[76] with additional medications added to address remaining symptoms (e.g., mexiletine[75,77,78] and flecainide for the treatment of chronic neuropathic pain[79]).

A word about the tricyclics. Although slightly more complex to manage initially, once a well-tolerated regimen is established, they are probably more effective and less expensive than any other agent used in the management of pain. For all agents except trazodone, a typical adult dose may be 75–150 mg, whereas a geriatric dose might range from 10 to 50 mg. These are only guidelines. Some "tricks of the trade" include:

1. Push the drug to the maximal tolerated dose, not stopping at a predetermined dose level and using gradual increases every second or third day until either an unacceptable side effect (causing discontinuance) or the desired benefit ensue.

Table 1.1 **SELECTED AGENTS FOR PAIN MANAGEMENT IN AUTONOMIC SMALL FIBER NEUROPATHY**

SYMPTOM	LIKELY MECHANISM	DRUG TYPE
Burning pain	Peripheral sensitization; Dorsal horn reorganization	Tricyclic antidepressant
Aching pain	Peripheral activation of C-nociceptors; inflammation	Nonsteroidal anti-inflammatory agent
Shooting pain	Ephaptic transmission	Anticonvulsant; oral local anesthetic
Allodynia	To heat: peripheral sensitization; To mechanical stimuli: central sensitization	Anesthetic creams Capsaicin cream Ketamine-clonidine cream
Vasomotor Sudomotor	Sympathetically maintained component	α-Adrenergic blockers; steroids[91]
Tinel's sign	Neuroma; Fascicular disruption with ephaptic transmission; nerve sprout	Clonidine patch over Tinel's site
Parathesiae	Same as Tinel's sign; also dorsal horn and higher central neural reorganization	Anticonvulsant; oral local anesthetic

2. A guide for this titration: if a person does not have a dry mouth from the anticholinergic effect of these agents, they probably do not have significant levels in their central nervous system.
3. Most agents should be prescribed in the evening with intent to provide sound sleep; the onset of action may be delayed, and patients should fine-tune dose timing for the onset to coincide with the time they wish to go to sleep. This may be 2 or even 3 hours before bedtime. Earlier timing also allows for a higher dosage since it will have worn off by the time the patient awakens.
4. Always check an EKG before prescribing to exclude a prolonged QT syndrome that contraindicates these agents, as well as another EKG once the goal dose is reached.
5. Check blood levels if doses greater than 2 mg/Kg are required due to poor absorption or rapid metabolism; this should be suspected if the patient does not develop a dry mouth.
6. Dose titration and timing should aim for a sound night of sleep with drug effect gone after less than 1 hour after awakening.
7. Choice of agent: amitriptyline—most effective, but most side effects, try first in the young adult; imipramine—may be tolerated during the day and given three times per day, particularly helpful in complex regional pain; the milder counterparts of these first two agents (nortriptyline and desipramine, respectively) may be better tolerated in the older patient; doxepin has the most anticholinergic properties for sleep effect, and less α-adrenergic blockade makes it easier to tolerate if someone has orthostatic intolerance. Protriptyline has some stimulant properties and may be given in the morning in some patients.

It is crucial that all pain-relieving medications be prescribed in a time-contingent, not pain-contingent, fashion (i.e., "scheduled" not "as needed"). Scheduled dosing provides constant levels of analgesic throughout the day; provides analgesia as the pain is beginning, not after hopelessly high levels have been reached; and takes much of the decision making out of the patient's hands, thus reducing focus on pain levels and reducing the risk of improper use and addiction. Compared to "as needed" dosing, scheduled dosing has been shown to reduce total drug used and enhance pain relief. If patients have difficulty with this concept, the analogy with treatment of high BP, which also fluctuates from day to day, can be quite helpful.

Neuromodulation interventions benefit some patients with continued significant nonresponsive neuropathic pain. These interventions include neurostimulation, which is commonly employed in painful peripheral neuropathy. Transcutaneous electrical nerve stimulation (TENS) reduces pain scores more than sham in patients with mild to moderate pain from diabetic neuropathy.[80–82] For patients with more severe pain, treatment with spinal cord stimulation (SCS) is effective for those with diabetic neuropathy. Kumar and colleagues reported clinical effectiveness of SCS in a case series published in 1996.[83] Around the same time, Tesfaye and colleagues reported a prospective study on SCS in 10 patients with refractory painful diabetic neuropathy in the absence of peripheral vascular disease. The average duration of diabetes was 12 years, and mean duration of pain was 5 years. The mean visual analog pain scale score (VAS) prior to SCS trial was 62.5 mm despite anticonvulsants and antidepressants for all patients. Nurses tracked pain levels every 4 hours for 2 days immediately prior to the SCS trial. All patients were implanted with a single midline epidural percutaneous quadripolar trial lead. Half the patients were subjected to a 2-day trial with a placebo controller attached to the SCS lead, followed by 2 days of active stimulation; and the other five patients were subjected to the reverse paradigm, with active stimulation preceding placebo stimulation. Patients experiencing greater than 50% pain relief with active stimulation were considered to have a successful outcome of the trial and were implanted with a generator and followed for 14 months. As such, 8 of 10 patients undergoing SCS trial went on to have the generator implanted. One patient died 2 months following the implant due to unrelated causes, and another patient ceased to maintain pain relief 4 months after the implant and was explanted (although pain scores continued to be reported). The other six patients experienced significant pain relief while using the stimulator as their sole analgesic modality. There were also improvements in exercise tolerance at

3 months and 6 months after implant but not at the 1-month mark. There were no improvements in electrophysiological tests, vibration perception-threshold, or glycemic control.[84] Patients were followed up for up to 8.5 years, and pain scores were assessed with the stimulator off and with the stimulator on. Among surviving patients, pain scores with the stimulator off were similar to original pain scores prior to implantation of the SCS, whereas pain scores continued to be low with the SCS on, with reduced analgesic medication use compared to preimplantation. The authors of this study suggested that SCS can provide long-term relief of painful diabetic neuropathy with little associated morbidity.[85]

A prospective open-label study examined SCS effects on pain and microcirculation in 11 patients with refractory painful diabetic neuropathy. Greater than 50% pain relief was achieved in nine patients who received the permanent implant. VAS pain scores decreased from an average 77 mm to 34 mm; for six of the patients, SCS was the sole treatment for pain. However, no changes in blood flow as measured by Doppler flowmetry were noted in this 30-month study.[86] Limitations of these studies include small sample size and lack of comparative effectiveness to other interventions. Nonetheless, SCS appears to be an attractive reversible option in patients with refractory painful neuropathies. Other forms of neuromodulation, such as peripheral nerve stimulation and intrathecal drug delivery, have been used only anecdotally in painful peripheral neuropathies.

PRACTICAL CHECKLIST FOR MANAGEMENT OF ORTHOSTASIS

For a detailed and in-depth review of the management of OH, the reader is referred to a recent chapter on autonomic disorders.[86a]

The management of orthostatic disorders (OH or POTS) is primarily nonpharmacologic. The first and simplest step consists of increasing central fluid volume with salt and fluids. In the absence of comorbid hypertension, one usually provides 2 g of salt supplementation (pill form) in the morning and again in the early afternoon, aiming for 24 h sodium levels of 170 meq or more. Daily fluid intake should approximate 1 gallon. Elevation of the head of the bed at night using two bricks under the legs (not using pillows; which does not place the legs below the heart level) reduces nocturnal microgravity and increases available central volume upon awakening. A 16 oz glass of water will increase BP by about 30–40 mm Hg for about 1 hour and can be very helpful upon arising in the morning, before medications can take effect.[86b] High-pressure (40 mm Hg) fitted thigh-high stockings will increase BP and considerably improve venous return. Finally, a set of exercises will critically improve overall well-being and central venous volumes, including water jogging or water aerobics in shoulder-high water (BP is maintained by the hydrostatic pressure of the water upon the lower body (caution must be used when exiting the pool); self-tilt exercises[86c] consisting of standing in a carpeted environment without sharp objects (in case of a fall), back against the wall, feet 1–2 feet from the wall (mimicking a 70-degree tilt) twice per day for 10 minutes each time; and specific physical countermaneuvers[86d] such as squatting, contracting the leg muscles, crossing the legs, or lifting one leg onto a chair.

Several medications are available for management as well, but these will not provide much benefit without first implementing the nonpharmacologic measures. Midodrine,[87] a pure $\alpha 1$ adrenergic agonist can be given three times per day because of its short duration of action. It raises BP by 10–20 mm Hg and does not cross into the brain. Caution is critical with concomitant supine hypertension, and the patient should be instructed never to lie flat within 4 hours of administration. Its use is mainly in OH, rarely in POTS. Fludrocortisone, a mineral corticoid with an aldosterone-like action at high dose, increases volume. At low dose (<0.2 mg/d) it sensitizes α receptors.[88] We often prescribe a half-tablet every other day for this effect. Pyridostigmine[89,90] increases ganglionic sympathetic traffic, which happens mainly in the upright position, and therefore rarely produces supine hypertension. β-blockade can reduce the epinephrine dilator effect on veins and improve venous return. Nadolol, propranolol, and other nonspecific β-blockers are best.

REFERENCES

1. Freeman R. Autonomic peripheral neuropathy. *Neurol Clin.* 2007;25:277–301.
2. Melman A, Rehman J. Pathophysiology of erectile dysfunction. *Mol Urol.* 1999;3:87–102.
3. Jänig W. Relationship between pain and autonomic phenomena in headache and other pain conditions. *Cephalalgia.* 2003;23(Suppl 1):43–48.
4. Mendell JR, Sahenk Z. Clinical practice. Painful sensory neuropathy. *N Engl J Med.* 2003;348:1243–1255.
5. Chémali KR, Tsao B. Electrodiagnostic testing of nerves and muscles: when, why, and how to order. *Cleve Clin J Med.* 2005;72:37–48.
6. Stewart JD, Low PA, Fealey RD. Distal small fiber neuropathy: results of tests of sweating and autonomic cardiovascular reflexes. *Muscle Nerve.* 1992;15:661–665.
7. Tobin K, Giuliani MJ, Lacomis D. Comparison of different modalities for detection of small fiber neuropathy. *Clin Neurophysiol.* 1999;110:1909–1912.

7a. Chelimsky G, McCabe NP, Janata J, et al. Autonomic testing of women with interstitial cystitis/bladder pain syndrome. *Clinical Autonomic Research.* 2014;24:161–166. PMID 24781351.

8. Chelimsky TC, Low PA, Naessens JM, Wilson PR, Amadio PC, O'Brien PC. Value of autonomic testing in reflex sympathetic dystrophy. *Mayo Clin Proc.* 1995;70:1029–1040.
9. Low PA, Opfer-Gehrking TL, Proper CJ, Zimmerman I. The effect of aging on cardiac autonomic and postganglionic sudomotor function. *Muscle Nerve.* 1990;13:152–157.
10. Low PA. Composite autonomic scoring scale for laboratory quantification of generalized autonomic failure. *Mayo Clin Proc.* 1993;68:748–752.
11. Schondorf R, Low PA. Idiopathic postural orthostatic tachycardia syndrome: an attenuated form of acute pandysautonomia? *Neurology.* 1993;43:132–137.
12. Sandroni P, Ahlskog JE, Fealey RD, Low PA. Autonomic involvement in extrapyramidal and cerebellar disorders. *Clin Auton Res.* 1991;1:147–155.
13. Cohen J, Low P, Fealey R, Sheps S, Jiang NS. Somatic and autonomic function in progressive autonomic failure and multiple system atrophy. *Ann Neurol.* 1987;22:692–699.

14. Low PA, Opfer-Gehrking TL. Differential effects of amitriptyline on sudomotor, cardiovagal, and adrenergic function in human subjects. *Muscle Nerve.* 1992;15:1340–1344.
15. Low PA, Caskey PE, Tuck RR, Fealey RD, Dyck PJ. Quantitative sudomotor axon reflex test in normal and neuropathic subjects. *Ann Neurol.* 1983;14:573–580.
16. Wang L, Hilliges M, Jernberg T, Wiegleb-Edstrom D, Johansson O. Protein gene product 9.5-immunoreactive nerve fibres and cells in human skin. *Cell Tissue Res.* 1990;261:25–33.
17. Kennedy WR, Wendelschafer-Crabb G. The innervation of human epidermis. *J Neurol Sci.* 1993;115:184–190.
18. McCarthy BG, Hsieh ST, Stocks A, et al. Cutaneous innervation in sensory neuropathies: evaluation by skin biopsy. *Neurology.* 1995;45:1848–1855.
19. Lauria G, Cornblath DR, Johansson O, et al. EFNS guidelines on the use of skin biopsy in the diagnosis of peripheral neuropathy. *Eur J Neurol.* 2005;12:747–758.
20. Kennedy WR, Wendelschafer-Crabb G, Polydefkis M, McArthur J. Pathology and quantitation of cutaneous nerves. In: Dyck PJ, Thomas PK, eds. *Peripheral Neuropathy.* 4th ed. Philadelphia: Saunders; 2005: 869–896.
21. Herrmann DN, Ferguson ML, Pannoni V, Barbano RL, Stanton M, Logigian EL. Plantar nerve AP and skin biopsy in sensory neuropathies with normal routine conduction studies. *Neurology.* 2004;63:879–885.
22. Pan CL, Lin YH, Lin WM, Tai TY, Hsieh ST. Degeneration of nociceptive nerve terminals in human peripheral neuropathy. *Neuroreport.* 2001;12:787–792.
23. Pan CL, Tseng TJ, Lin YH, Chiang MC, Lin WM, Hsieh ST. Cutaneous innervation in Guillain-Barre syndrome: pathology and clinical correlations. *Brain.* 2003;126:386–397.
24. Novak V, Freimer ML, Kissel JT, et al. Autonomic impairment in painful neuropathy. *Neurology.* 2001;56:861–868.
25. Panoutsopoulou IG, Wendelschafer-Crabb G, Hodges JS, Kennedy WR. Skin blister and skin biopsy to quantify epidermal nerves. A comparative study. *Neurology.* 2008. 72:1205-10.
26. Fruhstorfer H, Lindblom U, Schmidt WC. Method for quantitative estimation of thermal thresholds in patients. *J Neurol Neurosurg Psychiatry.* 1976;39:1071–1075.
27. Devigili G, Tugnoli V, Penza P, et al. The diagnostic criteria for small fibre neuropathy: from symptoms to neuropathology. *Brain.* 2008;131:1912–1925.
28. Fealey R. Thermoregulatory Sweat Test. In: Low P, ed., *Clinical Autonomic Disorders.* 2nd ed. Philadelphia: Lippincott-Raven; 1997:245–257.
29. Foster KG, Ellis FP, Dore C, Exton-Smith AN, Weiner JS. Sweat responses in the aged. *Age Ageing.* 1976;5:91–101.
30. Ravits J. AAEM Minimonograph #48. *Muscle Nerve.* 1997;20:919–937.
31. Low PA. Laboratory evaluation of autonomic function. *Suppl Clin Neurophysiol.* 2004;57:358–368.
32. Bennett T, Fentem PH, Fitton D, Hampton JR, Hosking DJ, Riggott PA. Assessment of vagal control of the heart in diabetes. Measures of R-R interval variation under different conditions. *Br Heart J.* 1977;39:25–28.
33. Freeman R. Noninvasive Evaluation of Heart Rate Variability. In: Low P, ed., *Clinical Autonomic Disorders.* Philadelphia: Lippincott-Raven; 1997:297–308.
34. Sandroni P, Benarroch EE, Low PA. Pharmacological dissection of components of the Valsalva maneuver in adrenergic failure. *J Appl Physiol.* 1991;71:1563–1567.
35. Gibbons C, Freeman R. The evaluation of small fiber function-autonomic and quantitative sensory testing. *Neurol Clin.* 2004;22:683–702, vii.
36. Singleton JR, Smith AG, Bromberg MB. Increased prevalence of impaired glucose tolerance in patients with painful sensory neuropathy. *Diabetes Care.* 2001;24:1448–1453.
37. Singleton JR, Smith AG, Bromberg MB. Painful sensory polyneuropathy associated with impaired glucose tolerance. *Muscle Nerve.* 2001;24:1225–1228.
38. Hoffman-Snyder C, Smith BE, Ross MA, Hernandez J, Bosch EP. Value of the oral glucose tolerance test in the evaluation of chronic idiopathic axonal polyneuropathy. *Arch Neurol.* 2006;63:1075–1079.
39. Smith AG, Ramachandran P, Tripp S, Singleton JR. Epidermal nerve innervation in impaired glucose tolerance and diabetes-associated neuropathy. *Neurology.* 2001;57:1701–1704.
40. Sumner CJ, Sheth S, Griffin JW, Cornblath DR, Polydefkis M. The spectrum of neuropathy in diabetes and impaired glucose tolerance. *Neurology.* 2003;60:108–111.
41. Smith AG, Singleton JR. Impaired glucose tolerance and neuropathy. *Neurologist.* 2008;14:23–29.
42. Isak B, Oflazoglu B, Tanridag T, Yitmen I, Us O. Evaluation of peripheral and autonomic neuropathy among patients with newly diagnosed impaired glucose tolerance. *Diabetes Metab Res Rev.* 2008;24:563–569.
43. Grandinetti A, Chow DC, Sletten DM, et al. Impaired glucose tolerance is associated with postganglionic sudomotor impairment. *Clin Auton Res.* 2007;17:231–233.
44. Report of the Expert Committee on the Diagnosis and Classification of Diabetes Mellitus. *Diabetes Care.* 1997;20:1183–1197.
45. Genuth S, Alberti KG, Bennett P, et al. Follow-up report on the diagnosis of diabetes mellitus. *Diabetes Care.* 2003;26:3160–3167.
46. McManis PGMF, Windebank AJMD, Kiziltan MMD. Neuropathy associated with hyperlipidemia. *Neurology.* November 1994;44:2185–2186.
47. Pittenger GL, Mehrabyan A, Simmons K, et al. Small fiber neuropathy is associated with the metabolic syndrome. *Metab Syndr Relat Disord.* 2005;3:113–121.
48. Zambelis T, Karandreas N, Tzavellas E, Kokotis P, Liappas J. Large and small fiber neuropathy in chronic alcohol-dependent subjects. *J Peripher Nerv Syst.* 2005;10:375–381.
49. Dina OA, Khasar SG, Alessandri-Haber N, Green PG, Messing RO, Levine JD. Alcohol-induced stress in painful alcoholic neuropathy. *Eur J Neurosci.* 2008;27:83–92.
50. Lacomis D. Small-fiber neuropathy. *Muscle Nerve.* 2002;26:173–188.
51. Orstavik K, Norheim I, Jorum E. Pain and small-fiber neuropathy in patients with hypothyroidism. *Neurology.* 2006;67:786–791.
52. Beitzke M, Pfister P, Fortin J, Skrabal F. Autonomic dysfunction and hemodynamics in vitamin B12 deficiency. *Auton Neurosci.* 2002;97:45–54.
53. Periquet MI, Novak V, Collins MP, et al. Painful sensory neuropathy: prospective evaluation using skin biopsy. *Neurology.* 1999;53:1641–1647.
53a. Axelrod FB. Genetic autonomic disorders. Semin Pediatr Neurol. 2013 20:3–11.
54. Scott LJ, Griffin JW, Luciano C, et al. Quantitative analysis of epidermal innervation in Fabry disease. *Neurology.* 1999;52:1249–1254.
55. Dutsch M, Marthol H, Stemper B, Brys M, Haendl T, Hilz MJ. Small fiber dysfunction predominates in Fabry neuropathy. *J Clin Neurophysiol.* 2002;19:575–586.
56. Maag R, Binder A, Baron R. Assessment of pain and somatosensory function in Fabry disease: early diagnosis. *Clin Ther.* 2008;30(Suppl B):S52–53.
57. Laaksonen SM, Roytta M, Jaaskelainen SK, Kantola I, Penttinen M, Falck B. Neuropathic symptoms and findings in women with Fabry disease. *Clin Neurophysiol.* 2008;119:1365–1372.
57a. Zaki EA, Freilinger T, Klopstock T, et al.Two common mitochondrial DNA polymorphisms are highly associated with migraine headache and cyclic vomiting syndrome. Cephalalgia. 2009;29:719–728.
57b. Dib-Hajj SD, Cummins TR, Black JA, Waxman SG. Sodium channels in normal and pathological pain. Annu Rev Neurosci. 2010;33:325–347.
58. Davis MD, Sandroni P, Rooke TW, Low PA. Erythromelalgia: vasculopathy, neuropathy, or both? A prospective study of vascular and neurophysiologic studies in erythromelalgia. *Arch Dermatol.* 2003;139:1337–1343.

59. Lopate G, Pestronk A, Al-Lozi M, et al. Peripheral neuropathy in an outpatient cohort of patients with Sjogren's syndrome. *Muscle Nerve*. 2006;33:672–676.
60. Chai J, Herrmann DN, Stanton M, Barbano RL, Logigian EL. Painful small-fiber neuropathy in Sjogren syndrome. *Neurology*. 2005;65:925–927.
61. Mori K, Iijima M, Koike H, et al. The wide spectrum of clinical manifestations in Sjogren's syndrome-associated neuropathy. *Brain*. 2005;128:2518–2534.
62. Gertz MA, Kyle RA. Primary systemic amyloidosis--a diagnostic primer. *Mayo Clin Proc*. 1989;64:1505–1519.
63. Kyle R, Dyck P. Amyloidosis and neuropathy. In: Dyck P, Thomas P, eds., *Peripheral Neuropathy*. 3rd ed. Philadelphia: Saunders; 1993:1294–1307.
64. Ito T, Sakakibara R, Yamamoto T, et al. Urinary dysfunction and autonomic control in amyloid neuropathy. *Clin Auton Res*. 2006;16:66–71.
65. Wang AK, Fealey RD, Gehrking TL, Low PA. Patterns of neuropathy and autonomic failure in patients with amyloidosis. *Mayo Clin Proc*. 2008;83:1226–1230.
66. Plante-Bordeneuve V. [The diagnosis and management of familial amyloid polyneuropathy]. *Rev Neurol (Paris)*. 2006;162:1138–1146.
67. Brannagan TH, 3rd, Hays AP, Chin SS, et al. Small-fiber neuropathy/neuronopathy associated with celiac disease: skin biopsy findings. *Arch Neurol*. 2005;62:1574–1578.
68. McDermott W, Kelkar P, Parry G. "Cryptogenic" painful neuropathy: is there an inflammatory basis? *Neurology*. 2000;54 (Suppl 3):A71.
69. Suarez GA, Fealey RD, Camilleri M, Low PA. Idiopathic autonomic neuropathy: clinical, neurophysiologic, and follow-up studies on 27 patients. *Neurology*. 1994;44:1675–1682.
70. Lacomis D, Giuliani MJ, Steen V, Powell HC. Small fiber neuropathy and vasculitis. *Arthritis Rheum*. 1997;40:1173–1177.
71. Holland NR, Crawford TO, Hauer P, Cornblath DR, Griffin JW, McArthur JC. Small-fiber sensory neuropathies: clinical course and neuropathology of idiopathic cases. *Ann Neurol*. 1998;44:47–59.
72. Polydefkis M, Yiannoutsos CT, Cohen BA, et al. Reduced intraepidermal nerve fiber density in HIV-associated sensory neuropathy. *Neurology*. 2002;58:115–119.
73. Herrmann DN, McDermott MP, Sowden JE, et al. Is skin biopsy a predictor of transition to symptomatic HIV neuropathy? A longitudinal study. *Neurology*. 2006;66:857–861.
74. Gorson KC, Ropper AH. Idiopathic distal small fiber neuropathy. *Acta Neurologica Scandinavica*. 1995;92:376–382.
74a. Logigian EL, Steere AC. Clinical and electrophysiologic findings in chronic neuropathy of Lyme disease. Neurology. 1992;42:303–311.
74b. Kanjwal K, Karabin B, Kanjwal Y, Grubb BP. Postural orthostatic tachycardia syndrome following Lyme disease. *Cardiol J*. 2011;18:63–66.
75. Dworkin RH, O'Connor AB, Backonja M, et al. Pharmacologic management of neuropathic pain: evidence-based recommendations. *Pain*. 2007;132:237–251.
76. Max MB, Lynch SA, Muir J, Shoaf SE, Smoller B, Dubner R. Effects of desipramine, amitriptyline, and fluoxetine on pain in diabetic neuropathy. *N Engl J Med*. 1992;326:1250–1256.
77. Carroll IR, Kaplan KM, Mackey SC. Mexiletine therapy for chronic pain: survival analysis identifies factors predicting clinical success. *J Pain Symptom Manage*. 2008;35:321–326.
78. Tremont-Lukats IW, Challapalli V, McNicol ED, Lau J, Carr DB. Systemic administration of local anesthetics to relieve neuropathic pain: a systematic review and meta-analysis. *Anesth Analg*. 2005;101:1738–1749.
79. von Gunten CF, Eappen S, Cleary JF, et al. Flecainide for the treatment of chronic neuropathic pain: a Phase II trial. *Palliat Med*. 2007;21:667–672.
80. Kumar D, Alvaro MS, Julka IS, Marshall HJ. Diabetic peripheral neuropathy. Effectiveness of electrotherapy and amitriptyline for symptomatic relief. *Diabetes Care*. 1998;21:1322–1325.
81. Kumar D, Marshall HJ. Diabetic peripheral neuropathy: amelioration of pain with transcutaneous electrostimulation. *Diabetes Care*. 1997;20:1702–1705.
82. Forst T, Nguyen M, Forst S, Disselhoff B, Pohlmann T, Pfutzner A. Impact of low frequency transcutaneous electrical nerve stimulation on symptomatic diabetic neuropathy using the new Salutaris device. *Diabetes Nutr Metab*. 2004;17:163–168.
83. Kumar K, Toth C, Nath RK. Spinal cord stimulation for chronic pain in peripheral neuropathy. *Surg Neurol*. 1996;46:363–369.
84. Tesfaye S, Watt J, Benbow SJ, Pang KA, Miles J, MacFarlane IA. Electrical spinal-cord stimulation for painful diabetic peripheral neuropathy. *Lancet*. 1996;348:1698–1701.
85. Daousi C, Benbow SJ, MacFarlane IA. Electrical spinal cord stimulation in the long-term treatment of chronic painful diabetic neuropathy. *Diabet Med*. 2005;22:393–398.
86. de Vos CC, Rajan V, Steenbergen W, van der Aa HE, Buschman HP. Effect and safety of spinal cord stimulation for treatment of chronic pain caused by diabetic neuropathy. *J Diabetes Complications*. 2009;23:40–45.
86a. Chelimsky T, Robertson D, Chelimsky G, Disorders of the autonomic nervous system. In: Daroff RB, Fenichel GM, Jankovic J, Mazziotta JC, *Neurology in Clinical Practice*. 6th ed. Philadelphia: Elsevier; 2012:2040–2044.
86b. Shannon JR, Diedrich A, Biaggioni I, et al. Water drinking as a treatment for orthostatic syndromes. *Am J Med*. 2002;112:355–360.
86c. Ector H, Reybrouck T, Heidbuchel H, Gewillig M, Van de Werf F. Tilt training: a new treatment for recurrent neurocardiogenic syncope and severe orthostatic intolerance. *Pacing Clin Electrophysiol*. 1998;21:193–196.
86d. Bouvette CM, McPhee BR, Opfer-Gehrking TL, Low PA. Role of physical countermaneuvers in the management of orthostatic hypotension: efficacy and biofeedback augmentation. *Mayo Clin Proc*. 1996;71:847–853.
87. Jankovic J, Gilden JL, Hiner BC, et al. Neurogenic orthostatic hypotension: a double-blind, placebo-controlled study with midodrine. *Am J Med*. 1993;95:38–48.
88. Davies IB, Bannister RG, Sever PS, Wilcox CS. Fludrocortisone in the treatment of postural hypotension: altered sensitivity to pressor agents [proceedings]. *Br J Clin Pharmacol*. 1978;6:444P–445P.
89. Singer W, Opfer-Gehrking TL, McPhee BR, Hilz MJ, Bharucha AE, Low PA. Acetylcholinesterase inhibition: a novel approach in the treatment of neurogenic orthostatic hypotension. *J Neurol Neurosurg Psychiatry*. 2003;74:1294–1298.
90. Singer W, Sandroni P, Opfer-Gehrking TL, et al. Pyridostigmine treatment trial in neurogenic orthostatic hypotension. *Arch Neurol*. 2006;63:513–518.
91. Kingery WS, A critical review of controlled clinical trials for peripheral neuropathic pain and complex regional pain syndromes. *Pain*. 1997;73(2):123–139.

2.

POSTHERPETIC NEURALGIA

Srinivasa N. Raja, Ronen Shechter, and Raimy Amsaha

CASE PRESENTATION

A 78-year-old man with intense left-sided chest pain is admitted to the hospital for cardiac monitoring. Twenty-four hours after admission, a vesicular rash is noted over the T5–6 dermatome on the left. The pain is reported as burning, constant, and severe. The pain prevents the patient from lying on his left side and is not relieved by acetaminophen or nonsteroidal anti-inflammatory drugs (NSAIDs). The patient underwent testing that confirmed herpes zoster (HZ) infection. He was ultimately discharged on oral oxycodone 5 mg TID with modest analgesia reported. He is referred to the Interdisciplinary Pain Medicine Clinic.

Past medical history is significant for hypertension.

Review of systems is significant only as noted above.

On examination, the patient weighs 90 kg and is 185 cm tall. His examination is significant for allodynia over the left side of the chest wall, as well as for decreased sensation to light touch in the T5 and T6 dermatomes.

A review of the initial case presentation reveals that the patient fits the classic description of an acute HZ attack. The patient is elderly (70s), with a well-demarcated rash (T5–6 dermatome) on the left thorax (a common location for HZ). As this chapter will explain, it is not uncommon for intense, localized pain to precede the vesicular rash. Moreover, an understanding of the pathophysiology of HZ will help explain how allodynia and decreased touch sensation may coexist. The prodrome of chest pain prior to appearance of a rash in this elderly population may sometimes be mistaken initially for an acute myocardial infarction.

QUESTIONS

1. What is the etiological agent of HZ?
2. What are the clinical manifestations?
3. What is the natural history of this condition and what phases exist?
4. What is the incidence and prevalence of HZ and postherpetic neuralgia (PHN)?
5. How has vaccination affected incidence and prevalence of HZ and PHN?
6. What predisposes a patient to have an HZ rash?
7. Why is the HZ rash painful?
8. What increases the risk of a patient having prolonged or chronic pain?
9. Why is PHN painful?
10. How are the various phases of this painful condition managed?
11. What are the guidelines for PHN prevention?

WHAT IS THE ETIOLOGICAL AGENT OF HZ?

The varicella-zoster virus (VZV), a member of the herpes virus family, is a double-stranded DNA virus (Figure 2.1). Infection with VZV causes two distinct disease states: chickenpox and zoster. Chickenpox occurs after a primary infection with the VZV. The virus subsequently resides in a latent form in dorsal root and cranial nerve ganglia. HZ (also known as shingles) results from reactivation of the virus from a dormant sensory ganglion years later.[1,2] Although the two disease states share the same viral progenitor, the clinical presentations of chickenpox and shingles are different. A typical case of chickenpox may be a young child with a widespread papular rash, vesicles, and crusted lesions. In contrast, an older adult with a painful, well-demarcated vesicular rash that is limited to the trunk or face in a unilateral dermatomal pattern depicts a typical case of shingles.[3]

The notion that shingles is a distinct disease state apart from chickenpox dates as far back as the Middle Ages.[4] However, our understanding of how VZV could manifest as two vastly different clinical presentations is more recent. In the 19th century, Head and Campbell used cadaveric studies to correlate skin affected by the zoster rash with scarring and degeneration in the trigeminal and dorsal root ganglia (DRG). This research led to a landmark paper in the journal *Brain,* which also introduced the concept of the dermatome.[3]

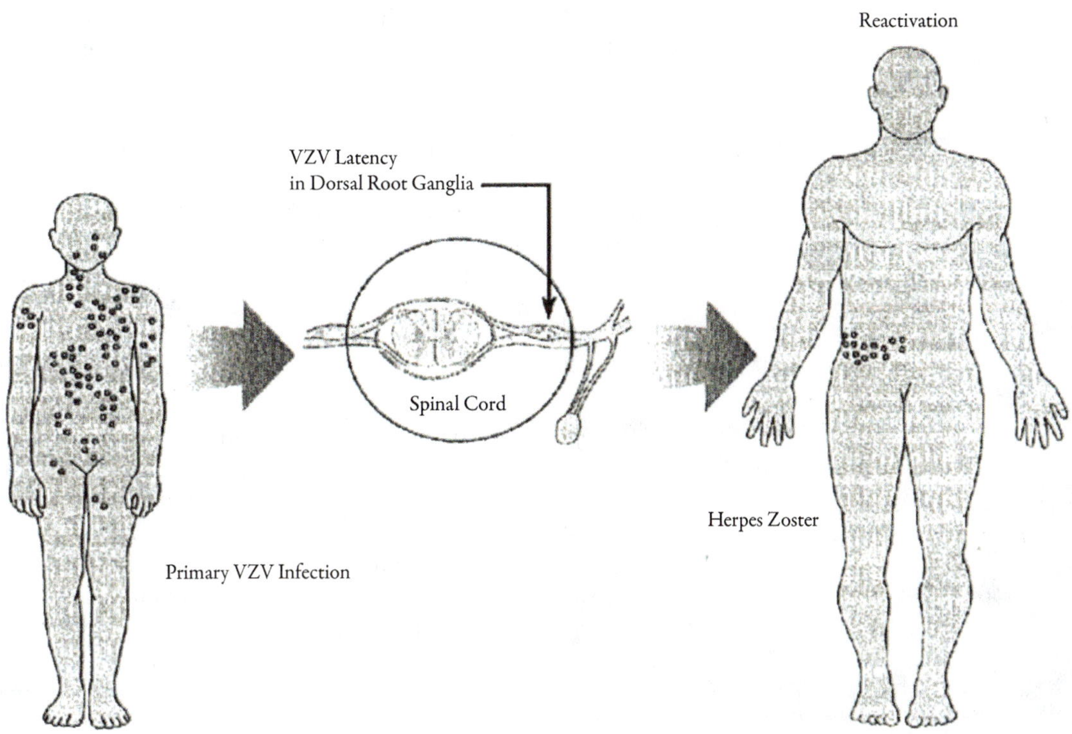

Figure 2.1 Primary varicella-zoster virus (VZV) infection typically occurs in childhood. Viral latency occurs in the dorsal root ganglia. Later in life, virus often reactivates in a thoracic or V1 trigeminal nerve distribution causing secondary infection known as herpes zoster. From Arvin, AM. Varicella-zoster virus. In: Knipe DM, Howley PM, eds. *Fields Virology*. Vol. 2. 4th ed. Philadelphia: Lippincott Williams and Wilkins; 2001: 2731–2767.

Hope-Simpson, a general practitioner in the United Kingdom, introduced the latency hypothesis in the mid-1900s, suggesting that HZ is due to the reactivation of a latent varicella infection in a sensory ganglion.[3,5] Hope-Simpson further hypothesized that viral latency is maintained by immunocompetence and that this immunocompetence could be boosted by periodic subclinical reactivations and exposures to exogenous virus. However, at times when immunocompetence falls below a critical threshold, the virus can be reactivated.[5]

WHAT ARE THE CLINICAL MANIFESTATIONS?

Abnormal localized skin sensations may precede the HZ skin eruption by 1–5 days and are known as a prodrome (Figure 2.2). These abnormal skin sensations may range from itching and tingling to severe burning and pain.[6] During the prodromal period, patients may also report headache, photophobia, low-grade fever, malaise, and regional lymph node enlargement.[7]

After the prodrome, the HZ rash typically manifests as macules and papules on an erythematous base. The clustered vesicles invade in a unilateral dermatomal distribution that does not cross the midline.[7] The two most common sites for the rash to occur include the mid to low thoracic region and the ophthalmic branch of the trigeminal nerve[8] (Figure 2.3). The HZ vesicles continue to form for 3–5 days and evolve through stages of pustulation, ulceration, and crusting. Healing occurs over a period of 2–4 weeks.[7,9] In approximately 20% of immunocompetent individuals, lesions may overlap adjacent dermatomes; however, simultaneous involvement of noncontiguous dermatomes is exceedingly rare and more common in immunocompromised patients. As the HZ rash heals, it may produce scarring and pigment changes in the skin.[8] Occasionally, the vesicles may become superinfected and lead to cellulitis that may require antibiotic therapy. Rarely, acute HZ may present as searing pain without a rash, a condition known as zoster sine herpete.[10,11]

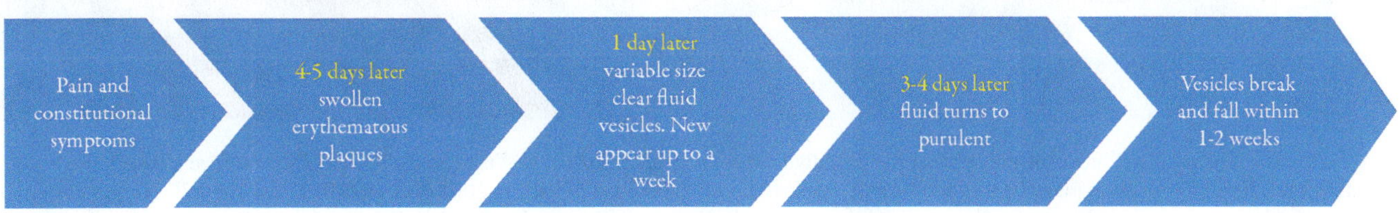

Figure 2.2 Progression of acute herpes zoster symptoms and rash.

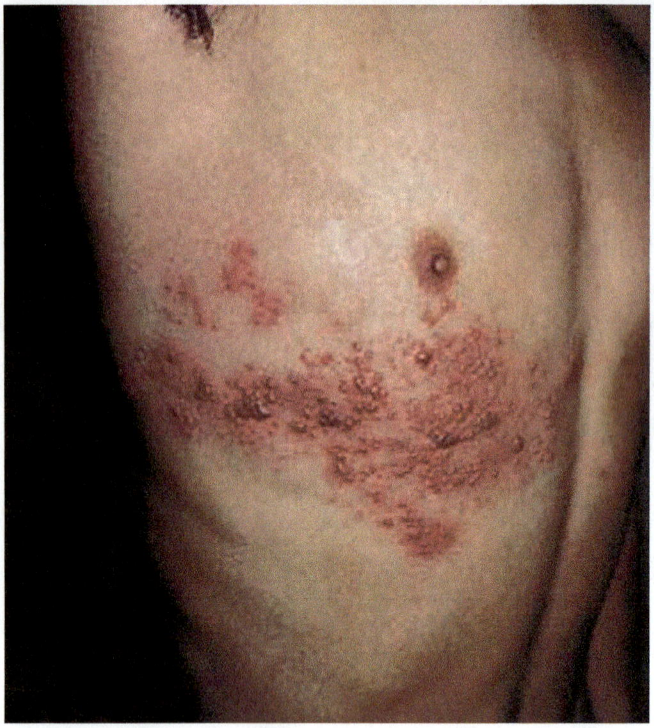

Figure 2.3 Herpes zoster, classic dermatomal distribution. Reprinted with permission from James WD, Berger T, Elston D. *Andrew's Disease of the Skin: Clinical Dermatology*. New York: Elsevier Health Sciences, 2011; 372.

HZ ophthalmicus occurs in about 10–20%[12] of cases and involves the ophthalmic branch (V1) of the trigeminal nerve (cranial nerve [CN] V) (Figure 2.4). Involvement of the maxillary (V2) and mandibular (V3) branches of the trigeminal nerve is five times less common than involvement of the ophthalmic branch. The prodromal symptoms include headache and preauricular lymphadenopathy. Ocular involvement most commonly affects the cornea and uvea.[13] Because the ophthalmic branch sends branches to the tentorium, meningeal signs may develop. In addition, because the ophthalmic branch is connected to the occulomotor (CN III) and abducens (CN VI), patients may present with ocular palsies. The ophthalmic division has three main branches—nasociliary, lacrimal, and frontal. Of these, the frontal nerve is the most commonly involved. Hutchinson's sign, the presence of vesicles on the tip, side, or root of the nose, indicates involvement of the nasociliary branch and is a predictor of ocular involvement.[14]

Ramsay-Hunt syndrome is a reactivation of latent VZV at the geniculate ganglion and results in facial nerve (CN VII) involvement (Figure 2.5). Clinically, it presents as herpetic eruption on the external auditory meatus and is called zoster oticus. Patients with this presentation may experience unilateral loss of taste on the anterior two-thirds of the tongue. The adjacent motor branches of the facial nerve (CN VII) and the vestibulocochlear nerve (CN VIII) may be inflamed and result in facial palsy, tinnitus, hearing loss, nausea, vomiting, vertigo and nystagmus.

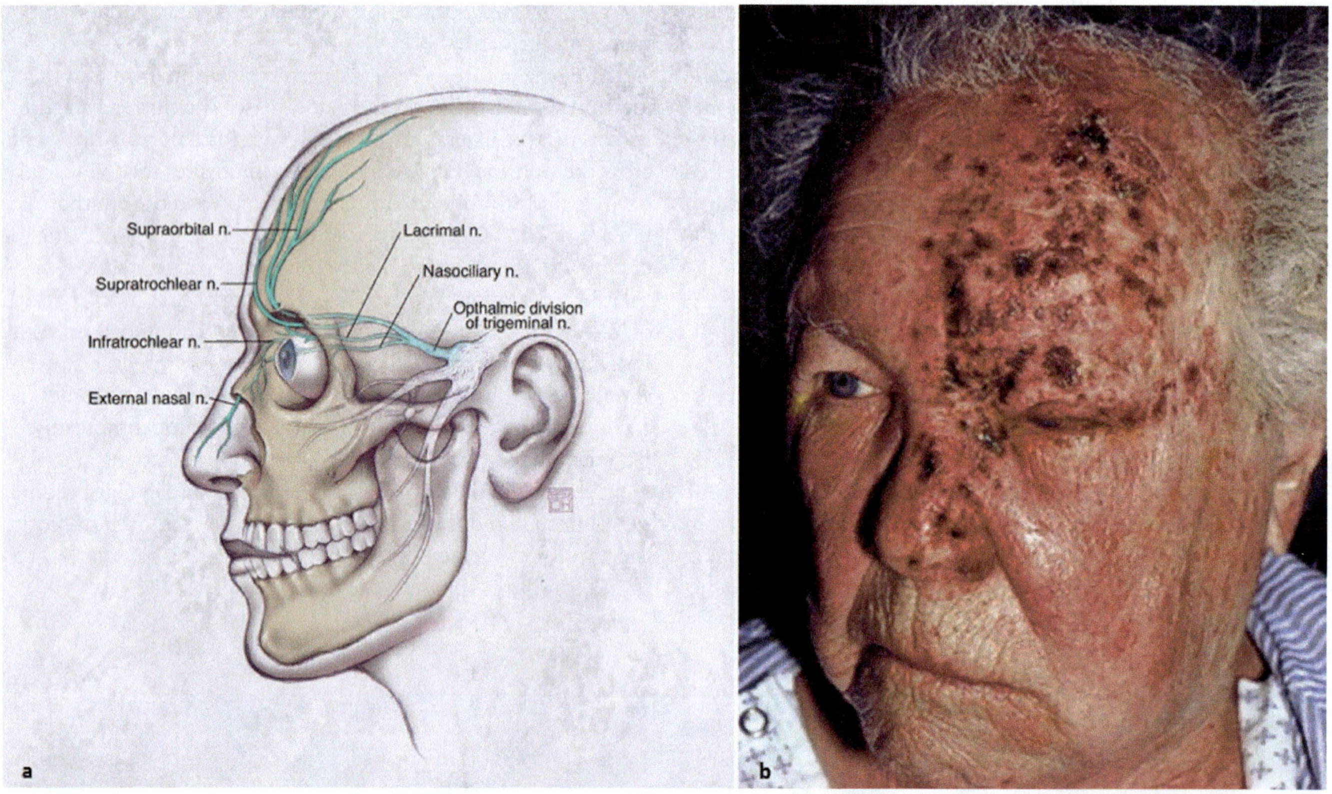

Figure 2.4 A. The sensory distribution of the ophthalmic (V_1) division of the trigeminal nerve. From Shaikh S, Ta CN, Stanford University Medical Center. Evaluation and management of herpes zoster ophthalmicus. *Am Fam Physician*. 2002 Nov 1;66(9):1723–1730. B. Herpes zoster, involvement of V1 dermatome. Reprinted with permission from James WD, Berger T, Elson D. *Andrew's Disease of the Skin: Clinical Dermatology*. New York: Elsevier Health Sciences, 2011; 373.

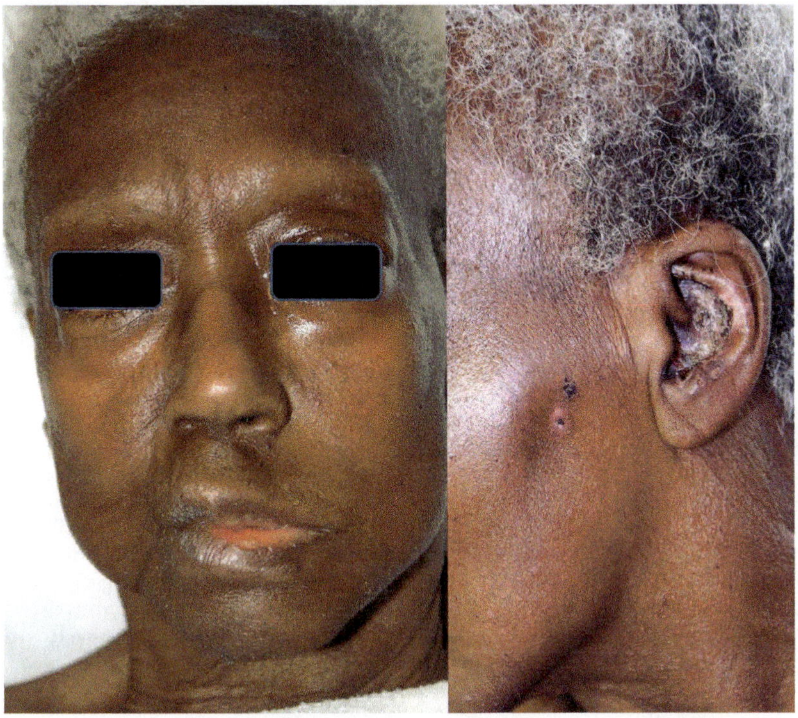

Figure 2.5 Ramsay-Hunt syndrome. Note the healing vesicular eruptions in the ear and the face and the ipsilateral facial nerve palsy. Courtesy Srinivasa N. Raja, MD.

Other clinical consequences of VZV reactivation may be divided into neurologic, ophthalmic, cutaneous, and disseminated disease.

NEUROLOGIC

PHN is the most common neurologic complication that causes major morbidity. Although historic definitions of PHN differ, the currently accepted definition is pain that persists beyond 3 months after the acute rash. The pain is usually in the rash distribution and can be constant or intermittent, with burning, aching, throbbing, stabbing, and shooting qualities. It is often difficult to treat and may last for years, with occasional remissions. PHN may result in physical inactivity, decreased social involvement, insomnia, chronic fatigue, and depression.

Patients with varicella zoster vasculopathy, also referred to as granulomatous angitis, present with fever, headaches, change in mental status, focal neurologic deficits, and occasionally no rash. Its prevalence is unknown, although patients with this condition have been reported to have a 31% increased risk for stroke within 1 year; the risk may be even higher in patients with zoster ophthalmicus.[15] Patients with varicella zoster meningitis, meningoencephalitis, and cerebellitis have been described and present occasionally without a rash.[16–18] The etiology in these cases of aseptic meningitis is confirmed by the detection of VZV DNA and anti-VZV antibody in cerebrospinal fluid.

Myelopathy in immunocompetent patients usually presents weeks after the acute illness as spastic paresis with occasional sensory or sphincter function changes; it is usually treated with steroids.[19] In immunocompromised patients, it may present as slow, progressive sensory and motor deficits. Some of these patients will respond to intravenous acyclovir.[20]

Occasionally, in addition to involvement of sensory nerve fibers, HZ may cause inflammation of the motor and autonomic fibers that are in close proximity or spread to the ventral root horn. Patients will present with motor paresis or autonomic changes in the infected dermatome. The weakness usually develops 2–3 weeks after the rash starts and may last for several weeks. Rarely, when the S2, S3, or S4 dermatomes are involved, the reactivated virus may affect the adjacent autonomic nerves, leading to neurogenic bladder.

OCULAR

In addition to causing scarring of the eyelids, HZ can affect various parts of the eye globe and cause sight-threatening processes such as corneal keratitis, corneal perforation, glaucoma, uveitis, retinal necrosis, and optic nerve neuritis.

CUTANEOUS

In the elderly and in immunocompromised and malnourished patients, the skin involvement tends to be more extensive and aggressive, with diffuse vesiculation and possibly skin necrosis, which scars upon healing. In addition, there is the risk of cellulitis secondary to bacterial superinfection.

DISSEMINATED

Viremia may develop and lead to involvement of other organs beyond the dermatomal skin rash. In some cases, organ failure may lead to death. However, viremia is confined mostly to immunocompromised patients.

WHAT IS THE NATURAL HISTORY OF THIS CONDITION AND WHAT PHASES EXIST?

The pain associated with an HZ attack has generally been classified into three phases: acute, subacute, and chronic or PHN. However the exact point at which one phase ends and the next phase begins is a topic of debate. Generally, the first phase, acute HZ pain, is closely associated with an HZ attack and occurs within the first 30 days after rash onset. The pain that occurs with acute HZ has been commonly described as a continuous, burning or throbbing pain, and sharp.[11,21,22] The second phase, subacute herpetic neuralgia, signifies pain that persists beyond the acute phase but resolves before a diagnosis of PHN can be made. The third phase, chronic or PHN, may signify pain that persists for 90–120 days or more after rash onset.[23–25] However, at present, the timeline from HZ rash resolution until diagnosis of PHN is not unanimously accepted in the scientific community. Some scientists and clinicians denote PHN as pain that exists beyond resolution of the HZ rash.[26] Persistent pain is the most common complication of HZ. The pain associated with PHN can continue for months or years.[10]

Applying what we know of the natural history of HZ to our clinical scenario from the patient's hospital admission to the Interdisciplinary Pain Medicine Clinic, we can see the disease progression from prodrome to acute HZ to PHN. The patient presented to the hospital with pain 24 hours before rash eruption (prodrome). The rash erupted (acute HZ attack) in the mid-thoracic region and was described as burning, constant, and severe. By the time the patient presented to the Interdisciplinary Pain Clinic, the patient no longer exhibited the vesicular rash (presumably crusted over and resolved). Persistent pain beyond acute HZ attack is regarded by many to classify as PHN. The patient is now presenting to the clinic with sensory descriptors consistent with PHN, including but not limited to allodynia and decreased touch sensation.

WHAT IS THE INCIDENCE AND PREVALENCE OF HZ AND PHN?

HZ has the highest incidence of all neurologic diseases, occurring in approximately 1 million Americans each year.[27,28] A fundamental epidemiologic feature of HZ is a marked increase in incidence with aging. In population-based studies, the incidence of HZ in persons of all ages is 1.2–4.8 cases

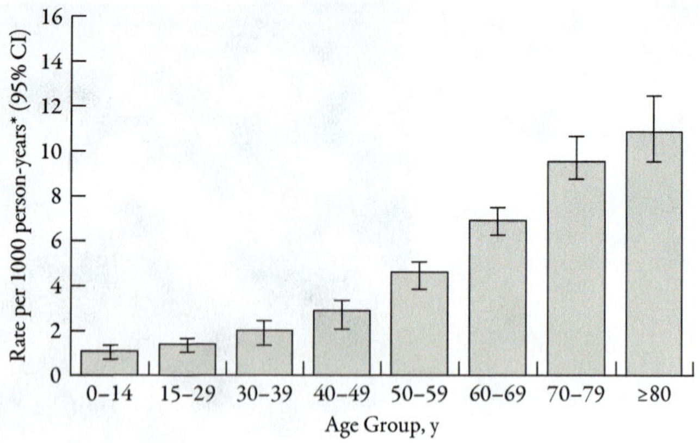

Figure 2.6 Age-specific incidence rates (across both sexes) of herpes zoster from a healthcare claims database of more than 2.8 million individuals for 2000–2001, sex-adjusted to the 2000 U.S. population. Approximately 40–50% of the 1 million new cases of herpes zoster that occur each year develop in individuals who are 60 years of age or older. Reprinted from Insinga, RP et al. The incidence of herpes zoster in a United States administrative database. *J Gen Intern Med.* 2005;20:748–753, with permission from Springer.

per 1,000 persons per year. The incidence of HZ is low among individuals younger than 40 years, ranging from 0.9–1.9 cases per 1,000 patient-years, but it begins to climb thereafter (Figure 2.6). The incidence of HZ in individuals older than 60 years is 7.2–11.8 cases per 1,000 per year.[29] The age at which the sharpest increase in HZ occurs is 50–60 years, although the slope continues its upward course in decades above 60 years.[29]

There is an estimated 20% lifetime risk of developing HZ,[30] and the disease may afflict nearly 50% of all people who live to 85 years of age.[6] Recurrence of an HZ episode is rare in immunocompetent patients and is estimated to be 1–6%.[27] The likely reason for this low recurrence rate is that patients with competent immune systems have a boost in cell-mediated immunity after an HZ insult.[27]

PHN is the most common complication of HZ. Behind neuropathic low back pain and diabetic neuropathy, PHN is the third most common cause of neuropathic pain in the United States.[31] PHN is of varying duration and develops in approximately 9–34% of individuals with HZ, depending on the definition used and population studied.[10]

As the worldwide population ages, the proportion of the over-65 population in industrialized nations is projected to double from 15% today to nearly 30% by 2050.[32] Consequently PHN may grow in prevalence. Epidemiologic studies of PHN indicate that the risk of having continued pain at 12 months is five times higher in patients who are 80 years of age than in younger patients. In fact, almost half of patients older than 70 years describe pain lasting over a year after the onset of the HZ rash (Figure 2.7).

In Figure 2.6, we can see that the age of our patient (78 years) predisposes him to development of HZ. Moreover, as Figure 2.7 illustrates, this individual is also at increased risk for neurologic sequelae after acute HZ resolution, specifically, PHN.

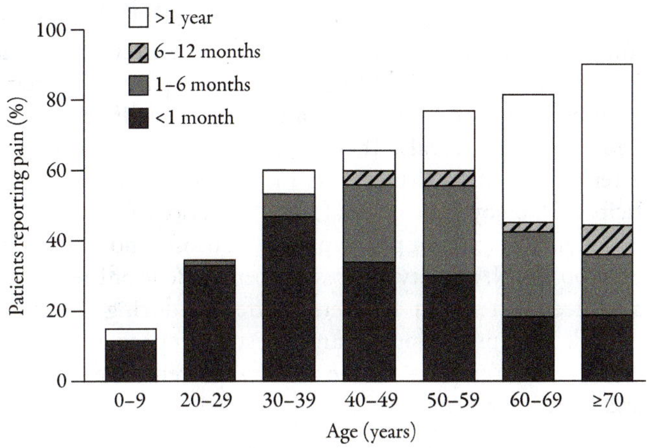

Figure 2.7 Prevalence of postherpetic neuralgia symptoms in patients who had acute herpes zoster, according to age.
Reproduced from Kost RG, Straus, SE. Postherpetic neuralgia-pathogenesis, treatment, and prevention. *N Engl J Med.* 1996, Jul 4;335(1):32–42, with permission from the Massachusetts Medical Society.

HOW HAS VACCINATION AFFECTED INCIDENCE AND PREVALENCE OF HZ AND PHN?

Similar to the live varicella vaccine, a live zoster vaccine was introduced within the last decade that was purported to be safe and effective clinically (Figure 2.8).

In a prospective, double-blind, placebo-controlled trial of attenuated VZV vaccine designed to prevent zoster and PHN in men and women over the age of 60,[28] healthy adults 60 years and older (median 69 years) were vaccinated with placebo or an attenuated Oka/Merck-VZV vaccine containing 18,700 to 60,000 plaque-forming units of virus (considerably greater than the approximately 1,350 plaque-forming units in the Oka/Merck-VZV vaccine administered to American children since 1995). More than 38,000 recipients of the zoster vaccine were followed closely for 3 years.

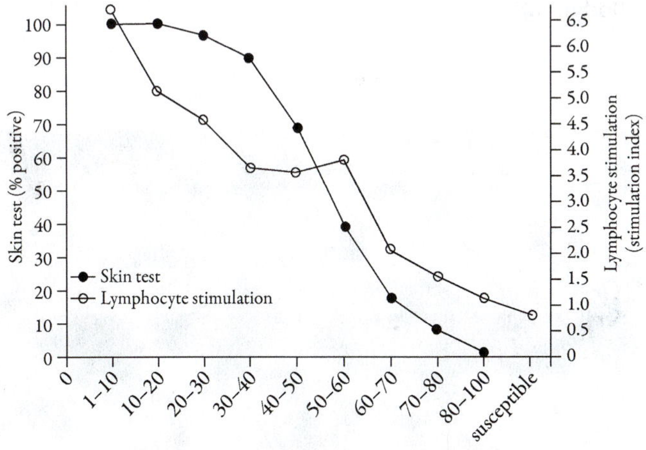

Figure 2.8 Varicella-zoster virus-specific cell-mediated immunity declines with age. Reprinted from Gruber, MF. Maternal immunization: US FDA regulatory considerations. *Vaccine* 2003;21:3487–3491, with permission from Elsevier.

The incidence of HZ in the placebo group was 11.1 per 1,000-person years, approximating the results of previously published US population data.[33] Compared with the placebo group, the zoster vaccine had a significant effect on HZ incidence. According to the study, the vaccination reduced the incidence of HZ by 51% and the incidence of PHN by 66%.[28]

Overall, serious adverse effects and deaths occurred in 1.4% of both vaccine and placebo recipients. In more than 6,000 subjects who kept daily diaries of minor adverse effects for 42 days, 48% of vaccine recipients reported injection site erythema, pain or tenderness, swelling, and pruritus, compared with 16% of placebo recipients. The relative impact of these side effects on the elderly (age >70) compared with younger patients was not examined.[28]

Even if every healthy adult in the US over the age 60 years received the zoster vaccine, it is estimated that approximately 500,000 patients would develop HZ annually and that about 200,000 of those would experience PHN and associated complications.[34] Furthermore, because the zoster vaccine has not been approved for immunocompromised individuals, reactivation in this population continues unabated.[34]

WHAT PREDISPOSES A PATIENT TO HAVE AN HZ RASH?

After the initial VZV infection, an individual with intact cell-mediated immunity restricts the virus to specific ganglia. However, owing to a variety of circumstances, an individual's cell-mediated immunity may no longer be sufficient to stave off reactivation. Predisposing factors for an HZ rash include advanced age, medications (e.g., immunosuppressants), infection (e.g., HIV, AIDS), hematologic malignancies, previous organ transplantation (e.g., bone marrow transplant), and autoimmune diseases.[2] Stress, both psychological and physical, may also play a role in reactivation of the VZV virus.[3] Other possible risk factors include physical trauma at the involved dermatome, diabetes, female gender, and Caucasian race.[35–38]

WHY IS THE HZ RASH PAINFUL?

In HZ, VZV, originating in the DRG or trigeminal neuron, travels antidromically to sensory terminals in the skin. The subsequent rash is accompanied by a robust inflammatory response and release of mediators that sensitize pain-specific sensory fibers (nociceptors), thus lowering their activation threshold. These sensitized nociceptors respond to innocuous stimuli (allodynia) or have an increased response to painful stimuli (hyperalgesia). Moreover, these irritable nociceptors may also develop spontaneous activity that is manifested as ongoing pain in the absence of an exogenous stimulus.[39]

WHAT INCREASES THE RISK OF A PATIENT HAVING PROLONGED OR CHRONIC PAIN?

Several risk factors and predisposing conditions for the transition from acute HZ to PHN have been identified. Many of these overlap with the risk factors for an acute zoster episode. In addition to increased age, other risk factors for progression to PHN include intensity and duration of pain during the acute zoster episode, greater HZ rash severity, greater neurosensory disturbances during acute zoster, a more pronounced zoster immune response, psychosocial distress, and immunocompromised state (including HIV and history of transplantation).[27,40–43] Other risk factors were determined by comparing patients with HZ who developed PHN with HZ patients who did not develop PHN (controlling for rash duration). Such studies also identified female gender as a risk factor to be included.[40] It is important to note that the location and number of affected dermatomes of the rash and involvement of the trigeminal nerve were not found to be risk factors.[40] However, other studies have found an increased risk of PHN among individuals with ophthalmic zoster, which affects the first division of the trigeminal nerve.[44]

Knowledge of potential risk factors has limited benefit in predicting PHN in individual patients; however, if a patient has multiple risk factors, clinicians and scientists are better able to predict if progression to PHN is more likely. For example, as reported by Jung et al.,[40] PHN developed in almost half of all female patients older than 60 years who had a prodrome, severe rash, and acute HZ pain. In addition, PHN was unlikely to develop in patients who did not have any of these risk factors; PHN developed in only 5–10% of patients who had none of these risk factors.

Review of the risk factor categories that predispose patients to develop PHN is worthwhile. For example, as Jung et al. reported in combined data from 855 participants, adjoining the risk factors of age (>60 years), severe acute pain, severe rash, prodrome, and female gender provided 0.97 specificity, 0.15 sensitivity, 0.88 negative predictive value, and 0.47 positive predictive value. In contrast, the same study showed that adjoining age (>50 years), severe acute pain, severe rash, and prodrome yielded a decrease in specificity (0.92), increase in sensitivity (0.32), increase in negative predictive value (0.9), and decrease in positive predictive value (0.38). Identifying those variables that increase the risk of PHN or chronic pain may enable patients to be identified who may benefit from preventive strategies and early, aggressive intervention. The importance of this point cannot be overstated because PHN causes not only physical debilitation, but psychological as well. Hess et al.[45] reported that PHN is the number one cause of intractable pain in the elderly and the leading cause of suicide in chronic pain patients over the age of 70.

Drolet et al.[46] assessed the impact of HZ and PHN on health-related quality of life. From October 2005 to July 2006, they recruited 261 outpatients aged 50 years or older from clinical practice, all within 2 weeks of HZ rash onset. They used assessment tools such as the Zoster Brief Pain Inventory and EuroQol EQ-5D to measure pain interference with activities of daily living and quality of life at weekly and monthly intervals. Their group reported that acute HZ interfered in all health aspects including sleep (64% of participants), enjoyment of life (58% of participants), and general activities (53% of participants). In those who went on to develop PHN, anxiety, depression, enjoyment of life, mood, and sleep were most frequently affected during the PHN period. This psychological and lifestyle impact of HZ and PHN further emphasizes the need for preventative strategies and early intervention.[46]

Identifiable risk factors for the patient in our clinical vignette for progression to PHN after acute HZ include advanced age (70s), presence of a prodrome, and severe pain. Being of male gender and having the rash cover the T5 and T6 dermatomes have not been identified as risk factors for progression to PHN.

WHY IS PHN PAINFUL?

After the initial stage of HZ eruption, inflammation is present in the DRG that progresses to loss of neurons and scarring of the dorsal horn centrally, as well as in the peripheral nerve (Figures 2.9 and 2.10).

Thus, PHN pain may result from aberrant activity of the remaining peripheral sensitized nociceptors, deafferentation, central reorganization, or possibly a combination of these processes,[47,48] Based on its neural mechanisms for pain, PHN has been classified into subtypes: (1) the irritable nociceptor group, which include patients who display hyperalgesia; (2) the deafferentation group, which includes patients who suffer from persistent pain in a region of sensory loss (anesthesia dolorosa); and (3) the central reorganization group, in which patients have mechanical allodynia.[49]

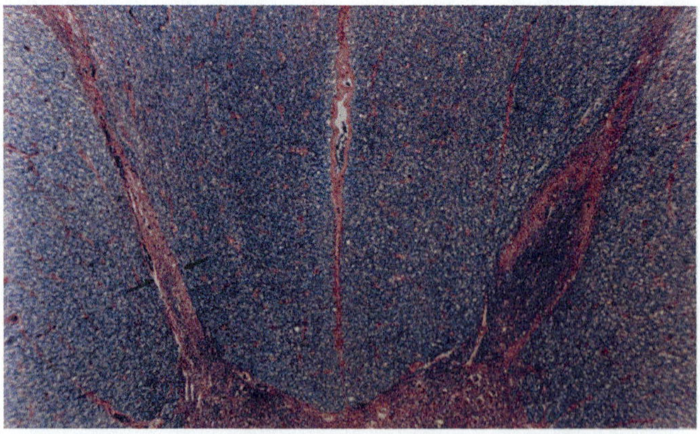

Figure 2.9 Atrophy of dorsal horn of the spinal cord in postherpetic neuralgia. Courtesy C. Peter N. Watson, MD, FRCPC.

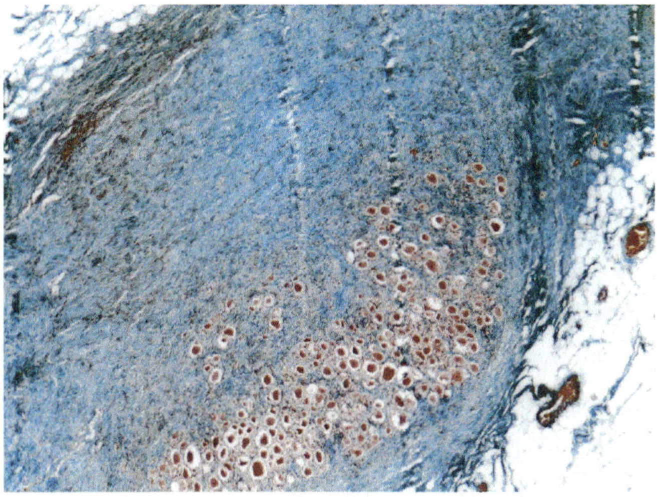

Figure 2.10 Scarring in the dorsal root ganglia with postherpetic neuralgia. Courtesy C. Peter N. Watson, MD, FRCPC.

HOW ARE THE VARIOUS PHASES OF THIS PAINFUL CONDITION MANAGED?

A number of randomized studies and case series have examined the potential treatment strategies for the management of pain associated with acute HZ and PHN. The goals of the treatment strategies for the acute phase of HZ and PHN differ and therefore will be discussed separately. Table 2.1 summarizes the current available guidelines for the treatment of neuropathic pain and PHN.

Medications include therapies that involve delivery of drugs by mouth or intravenously, whereas interventional/surgical procedures include any other methods of treatment. In general, the literature is less extensive with regard to procedures than to medications, and most of the evidence is from case reports, with few randomized controlled studies. Procedures can be divided based on medication used, delivery method utilized, energy applied, tissue targeted, and reversibility.

Nonablative injections with local anesthetics block peripheral and central nervous system (CNS) targets; the use of steroid injections has been mentioned as well. With the exception of sympathetic ganglion blocks (stellate, thoracic, and lumbar), all blocks affect both the somatic and autonomic nervous systems. Rarely, a block is used to treat a nonpainful post-shingles complication, such as a sphenopalatine ganglion block to treat bradycardia and sinus arrest.[50] Much less of the literature is devoted to other injected medications. Electrical stimulation-induced neuromodulation, such as spinal cord stimulation (SCS) has been used clinically. The mechanisms of action of SCS is not completely clear, but probably involves at-level stimulation changes, as well as antegrade and retrograde effects on peripheral, spinal, and supraspinal nervous systems.[51] Data to support surgical/ablative procedures in the treatment of PHN pain are weak. Last, external treatment such as radiation and cryoanalgesia have been suggested as potentially beneficial.

Therapies that do not target the nervous system will not be described in detail but may include myofascial trigger point injections,[52] as well as procedures to treat other post-shingles complications, most commonly those that involve the eye.

The objectives of treating acute HZ are to control pain, hasten rash healing, and prevent complications such as PHN.

MEDICATIONS

Pain Control and Potential Hastening of Rash Healing

Antivirals

Nucleoside analogues are a group of medications that inhibit viral replication by blocking its chain synthesis. Antiviral medications used most commonly against VZV are the guanosine analogues and include acyclovir, famciclovir, and valacyclovir, which differ in their pharmacokinetics. The first drug in this group to be studied was acyclovir, which was first administered intravenously and later found to be as effective when taken orally.[53] It reduces the acute phase rash, duration of new lesion formation, and pain.[54–56] Famciclovir and valacyclovir have better pharmacokinetics than does acyclovir and therefore require only three doses per day compared to five with acyclovir. Both drugs relieve acute phase pain and hasten rash healing;[57–59] they are also better than acyclovir with regard to acute pain relief,[60] A fourth drug that is still awaiting full approval by the FDA is valomacyclovir. Also a guanosine analogue, it requires only once-daily dosing.[61] All of the guanosine analogues are well tolerated, and their common adverse effects are nausea, constipation, and headache.

Although the current recommendation is to start therapy within 72 hours of rash onset, no randomized controlled trial has verified this time frame. Some recommend using antiviral medications even if the rash has been present for more than 72 hours.[62,63] This empirical rule of treatment initiation does not apply to HZ ophthalmicus, for which it is always recommended.[63]

Opioids

Opioids were found to be effective for treating acute shingles pain in a randomized, placebo-controlled trial.[64] The most significant pain relief was achieved within the first 8 days ($p = 0.01$); significant pain relief was not shown over longer time periods, probably because pain resolved in most of the patients. The common adverse effects of opioids are constipation, nausea, vomiting, sedation, dizziness, and change in mental status. All of these adverse effects improve over time except for constipation, which requires bowel prophylaxis.

N-methyl D-aspartate (NMDA) Antagonists

NMDA receptors are critical in the induction and maintenance of pain. In a double-blind, placebo-controlled trial of amantadine in patients with acute HZ, a smaller proportion of patients in the treatment group had pain than in the placebo group at 28 days; skin healing did not differ between the

Table 2.1 SUMMARY OF NEUROPATHIC AND POSTHERPETIC NEURALGIA PAIN THERAPY GUIDELINES

SOCIETY	GROUP	FIRST AUTHOR, YEAR OF PUBLICATION, SEARCH YEARS	CONDITIONS	BASIS OF RECOMMENDATIONS	SPECIFIC LINES FOR NEUROPATHIC PAIN THERAPY	SPECIFIC LINES/ EVIDENCE FOR PHN THERAPY
EFNS	EFNS Task Force	Attal et al., 2010, 1966–2009[235]	Neuropathic pain separated per conditions	Classification of evidence and recommendation grading adhere to EFNS standard (Brainin et al., 2004)		First: 1. TCA 2. Gabapentin/pregabalin 3. Topical lidocaine Second or Third: 1. Capsaicin 2. Opioids
IASP	NeuPSIG	Dworkin et al., 2007 and 2010, 1960–2007[236,237]	Neuropathic pain as a group	1. Quality of evidence 2. Clinical efficacy 3. Adverse effects 4. Impact on health-related quality of life 5. Convenience 6. Cost	First: 1. TCA/SNRI 2. Gabapentin/pregablin 3. Topical lidocaine Second: 1. Opioids 2. Tramadol Third: 1. Antiepileptic 2. SSRI 3. Mexiletine 4. NMDA receptor antagonist 5. Topical capsaicin	TCA—positive Duloxetine—not available Venlafexine—negative Gabapentin—positive Pregabalin—both positive and negative Topical lidocaine—positive Opioids—positive Tramadol—positive
Canadian Pain Society	NeuPSIG	Moulin DE et al., 2007, not specified[238]	Neuropathic pain as a group	1. Quality of evidence 2. Analgesic efficacy (NNT) 3. Side-effect profile 4. Ease of use 5. Cost	First: 1. TCA 2. Gabapentin/pregabalin 3. Carbamazepine (trigeminal neuralgia) Second: 1. SNRI 2. Topical lidocaine Third: 1. Opioids 2. Tramadol Fourth 1. Cannabinoids (not in USA) 2. Methadone 3. SSRIs 4. Antiepileptic (lamotrigine, topiramate, valproic acid) 5. Miscellaneous agents (mexiletine, clonidine)	
American Academy of Neurology		Dubinsky et al., 2004, 1960–2003[239]	PHN	1. Quality of evidence 2. Therapeutic level (ARR, NNT) 3. Adverse effect (NNH)		First: 1. TCA 2. Gabapentin/pregabalin 3. Topical lidocaine 4. Oxycodone/morphine/CR Second: 1. Capsaicin 2. Aspirin cream or ointment 3. Intrathecal methylprednisolone No efficacy: 1. Acupuncture 2. Benzydamine cream 3. Dextromethorphan 4. Indomethacin 5. Lorazepam 6. Epidural methylprednisolone 7. Vincristine iontophoresis 8. Vitamin E 9. Zimelidine (SSRI)

ARR, absolute risk reduction; CR, controlled release; EFNS, European Federation of Neurological Societies; IASP, International Association for the Study of Pain; NeuPSIG, Neuropathic pain special interest group; NNT, number needed to treat; NNH, number needed to harm; PHN, postherpetic neuralgia; SNRI, serotonin-norepinephrine reuptake inhibitor; SSRI, selective serotonin reuptake inhibitor; TCA, tricyclic antidepressant two groups.[65] Unfortunately, this group of drugs can cause significant adverse effects, particularly sedation, ataxia, and nausea.

Cimetidine

Some evidence suggests that H_2 receptor activation may inhibit different functions within the immune system.[66] In a double-blinded, controlled study of patients with acute HZ, the cimetidine-treated group had faster resolution of pain and cutaneous lesions than did the placebo-treated group.[67]

Levodopa

Levodopa is used for conditions in which dopamine is deficient, such as Parkinson disease and restless legs syndrome. It also has been found to relieve central pain that is common in these conditions. In a rat model of neuropathic pain, systemic or intrathecal administration of levodopa decreased tactile allodynia and thermal hyperalgesia.[68] Kernbaus and Hauchecorne[69] found in a double-blind, placebo-controlled study of patients with HZ that levodopa with benserazide (L-amino acid decarboxylase inhibitor) decreased pain and healing time significantly compared to placebo, particularly in high-risk groups (those >65 years old or with ophthalmic zoster).

Adenosine Derivatives

As purinergic receptors are involved in pain transduction peripherally and pain transmission centrally,[70] adenosine derivatives have been studied in HZ-induced pain. Sklar et al.[71] showed that shingles patients treated with gel-sustained intramuscular adenosine monophosphate had less incidence of pain at 4 weeks than did patients treated with placebo.

Gabapentin

Gabapentin, despite its name, binds to the $\alpha_2\delta$ subunit of voltage-gated calcium channels in the CNS. It causes a decrease in excitatory neurotransmitter release. In addition, it possibly inhibits binding of thrombospondin, an astrocyte-secreted protein that promotes CNS synaptogenesis, to the same $\alpha_2\delta$ subunit, decreasing new excitatory synapse formation.[72] A single dose of gabapentin in patients with acute HZ decreased pain severity and the area of allodynia compared to placebo at every time point from 1.5 to 6 hours after it was taken.[73] In contrast, in another randomized, placebo-controlled trial, gabapentin did not improve pain relief compared to placebo in patients with shingles who were treated with famciclovir.[64] Neither study examined the effect of gabapentin on PHN development.

In a pooled analysis of adverse effects of gabapentin, the most common were transient dizziness and somnolence that was not dose-dependent. Peripheral edema incidence was increased with doses higher than 1,800 mg/d.[74]

Topical Lidocaine

Lidocaine, an amide local anesthetic, blocks sodium channels, which in turn blocks impulse propagation. Use of lidocaine during acute HZ was found to effectively decrease both resting spontaneous pain and activity-induced pain.[75]

Topical Aspirin

Skin rash and pain resolved more quickly in patients who received a topical aspirin/diethyl ether (ADE) preparation than in those who received placebo and compared to resolution rates reported in the literature.[76,77] Other topical aspirin preparations, such as those including chloroform and moisturizer, were also effective.[78,79]

Other Topical Medications

Dextranomer, a high-molecular-weight dextran derivative used mostly for decubitus ulcers, may be useful also in HZ lesions.[80]

Vitamin C

Vitamin C, or L-ascorbic acid, is an antioxidant that is consumed quickly by immune cells during infections. In a multicenter prospective cohort study, adding intravenous vitamin C to standard therapy possibly improved healing and pain in shingles patients.[81]

Interferon

Interferons are a group of glycoproteins that are released from infected host cells. After binding to receptors, interferon promotes the death of the infected host cell by inhibiting protein synthesis, increasing p53-induced apoptosis, and increasing exposure to cytotoxic T cells and NK cells.[82] Because different viruses, including VZV,[83] have developed resistance to interferon, and because its common side effects include fever, nausea, and leucopenia, interferon is not a first-line treatment for acute HZ. However, in a randomized study, interferon-α was equally effective to acyclovir at rash healing and reducing pain severity and duration. Additionally, it decreased dissemination in immunosuppressed patients.[84,85] In addition to systemic administration, there have been case reports of it being used topically[86] and intralesionally.[87]

Other Topical Medications

Topical acyclovir 5% cream was not found to be better than placebo at either healing the rash or reducing acute pain.[88]

Systemic NSAIDs

Systemic aspirin was found inferior to topical aspirin at providing pain relief.[79]

PHN Prevention

Tricyclic Antidepressants (TCAs)

TCAs were first discovered in the early 1950s and named for their chemical structure. They have been used to treat depression but have been found to be effective for pain. TCAs are divided into two general classes, the tertiary and the secondary amines. The tertiary amines (amitriptyline, imipramine, and doxepin) have a greater inhibitory effect on serotonin than on norepinephrine, causing more sedation and anticholinergic effects. In contrast, the secondary amines (nortriptyline, desipramine) cause greater increases in norepinephrine levels and are associated with less sedating and anticholinergic adverse effects. Amoxapine (tricyclic dibenzoxazepine) and maprotiline (tetracyclic) are different structurally but have many similarities to TCAs. Bowsher[89] showed in a randomized, double-blind, placebo-controlled trial decreased odds ratio of pain at 6 months after acute zoster when amitriptyline was added to the antiviral therapy. Due to their anticholinergic properties, the common adverse effects of TCAs are dry mouth, dizziness, sedation, constipation, urinary retention, blurred vision, weight gain, and orthostatic hypotension. In addition, they may cause prolonged QT interval and should be used cautiously in patients with cardiac arrhythmias.

Antivirals

Some randomized controlled studies support the view that acyclovir decreases the incidence of PHN,[54,,90–92] but others question its role in preventing PHN.[55] Consequently, a definitive conclusion cannot be derived from the existing meta-analyses. Earlier meta-analyses supported the utility of acyclovir in preventing PHN,[56,93] but a more recent Cochrane review[94] fails to show acyclovir effectiveness. Nonetheless, one study demonstrated that famciclovir significantly reduced the prevalence of PHN, defined as pain beyond 3 months after the acute rash.[95] Valacyclovir was found to be as effective.[59]

Topical Aspirin

The use of topical aspirin/ADE preparation decreased the incidence of patients developing PHN compared to that reported in the literature.[76]

Systemic Steroids

Although earlier studies showed that systemic steroids might lower the rate of PHN if used in the acute phase of HZ,[96,97] later studies and meta-analyses showed that oral corticosteroid therapy does not prevent PHN.[92,98–100]

PHN Therapy

TCAs

Strong evidence supports the use of TCAs in treating PHN.[101,102] When different TCAs were compared, desipramine produced more pain relief than did amitriptyline,[103] whereas amitriptyline and nortriptyline were comparable with regard to pain relief, mood, disability, satisfaction, and preference.[48]

Gabapentin

In pooled meta-analyses, gabapentin was found to be effective in treating PHN pain,[101,104] and, interestingly, it was most effective for sharp, dull, and itchy pain qualities and less effective for hot, cold, deep, or surface pain qualities.[105] Similar efficacy was found with the gastric-retentive gabapentin.[106] Gabapentin enacarbil solves problems related to unpredictable and saturable gabapentin absorption by utilizing high-capacity transporters expressed throughout the intestine and was found to be effective.[107] Gabapentin was equally efficacious to nortriptyline in treating PHN pain and improving sleep[108]; a combination of the two drugs was better than each one alone.[109]

Pregabalin

The mechanism of action of pregabalin is similar to that of gabapentin, but it differs in its pharmacokinetics. Compared to gabapentin's less predictable zero-order absorption, pregabalin has first-order absorption with stable 90% bioavailability at different doses.[110] In addition, the pain relief is usually noticed within 48 hours,[111] which is earlier than with gabapentin. A Cochrane review of pregabalin's role in acute and chronic pain in adults[112] calculated relative benefit and numbers needed to treat (NNT) at different doses (150–600 mg/d) in the treatment of PHN. The analysis showed greater pain relief and lower NNT as the daily dose increased, which unfortunately was associated with more adverse events. Interestingly, pregabalin at 150 mg/d was effective for PHN but not for other pain syndromes. Pregabalin was also found to be effective in treating PHN in two pooled meta-analyses.[101,104]

Opioids

Although an early study did not find opioids to be effective in treating PHN pain,[113] later evidence indicates that opioids may be beneficial,[114] particularly for steady pain, paroxysmal spontaneous pain, and allodynia.[48] When opioids (morphine or methadone), TCAs (nortriptyline or desipramine), and placebo were compared, pain was decreased significantly more in both treatment groups than in the placebo group ($p < 0.001$), and patients preferred opioids over the other groups.[47] Meta-analysis of the available studies reconfirmed opioid efficacy in treating patients with PHN.[101,104] Gilron et al.[115] found that patients who received an opioid and gabapentin in combination had lower mean daily pain and McGill Pain Questionnaire scores than did patients who received either therapy alone. Although opioids have a positive effect on PHN pain, their chronic use poses difficulties such as adverse effects (endocrine, immunologic), dependency, and tolerance. As a result, some guidelines recommend the use of opioids only as a second- or even third-line therapy.

Tramadol

Tramadol, which is a weak μ-opioid receptor agonist and an inhibitor of monoamine (serotonin and norepinephrine) reuptake, was found to be effective in a randomized controlled trial. It provided significantly more pain relief compared to placebo ($p = 0.012$) and was associated with less need for rescue pain medication ($p = 0.022$).[116] In addition to the common adverse effects of opioids, concomitant use of tramadol with selective serotonin reuptake inhibitors (SSRIs), serotonin-norepinephrine reuptake inhibitors (SNRIs), and monoamine oxidase inhibitors may increase the risk of serotonin syndrome.

Intravenous Lidocaine and Oral Mexiletine

Intravenous lidocaine 0.5 mg/kg/h and 2.5 mg/kg/h decreased the dynamic pressure-provoked pain and area of allodynia but not the visual analog scale (VAS) score for ongoing pain compared to placebo.[117] Unfortunately, this study did not assess lidocaine's effect beyond the time of therapy. In another study, intravenous lidocaine decreased both spontaneous pain and mechanical allodynia (static and dynamic) compared to placebo, but did not appear to affect thermal hyperalgesia. Interestingly, patients who suffered from mechanical allodynia experienced more spontaneous pain relief with intravenous lidocaine or oral mexiletine.[118]

Topical Lidocaine

Lidocaine 5% gel or patch alone was found to be effective in treating PHN pain.[119–121] When it was combined with pregabalin, additive pain relief was achieved.[122,123] In a randomized, open-label, multicenter study that compared the effectiveness of pregabalin and topical lidocaine, a larger percentage of patients receiving topical lidocaine 5% reported a 2-point or greater decrease in pain on a 0–10-point scale at 4 weeks of therapy. In addition, the patients who received lidocaine had a lower incidence of adverse effects.[122] In a separate study, a novel 8% lidocaine spray with possible shorter latency was described as safe and effective for use as a rescue therapy for PHN pain.[124]

Topical lidocaine is safe to use because blood concentrations remain low.[75,120] Cardiovascular, respiratory, or neurologic adverse reactions have not been reported. The most common adverse reaction reported (in up to 13.6% of patients) is skin irritation, which may be caused by the patch itself.[121]

Capsaicin

Capsaicin was first extracted in 1816 from the genus *Capsicum*, a member of which is the chili pepper. Capsaicin is a highly selective agonist for the $TRPV_1$ receptor. Topical application of capsaicin 0.075% induces pain relief and improves function in PHN patients[125] even with prolonged use.[126] One 60-minute application of capsaicin 8% was shown to provide a prolonged decrease in pain from baseline on a numerical pain rating scale for up to 12 weeks of follow-up.[127] Pain relief was achieved regardless of concomitant systemic antineuropathic pain medication use.[128] Topical capsaicin causes short-term mild to moderate erythema and pain on the day of treatment, which can be minimized by pretreatment with a topical local anesthetic.

NMDA Antagonists

Meta-analysis has shown that NMDA antagonists are effective in treating PHN.[101] Intravenous ketamine decreased mechanical allodynia and wind-up pain.[129] It has been found to be effective with prolonged use through different routes of delivery, including intravenous, subcutaneous, intramuscular, and oral.[130,131] Unfortunately, as described earlier, NMDA antagonists can cause significant adverse effects, thus making the relative risk possibly higher than the relative benefit.

Magnesium

Because magnesium blocks NMDA receptors that are involved in the development of hyperalgesia, Brill et al.[132] conducted a double-blind, placebo-controlled, crossover study in seven PHN patients. Intravenous magnesium decreased VAS pain scores significantly more than did saline at 20 and 30 minutes postinfusion and was well tolerated.

Clonidine

Clonidine is an $\alpha 2$ agonist that may modulate pain transmission in the dorsal horn. In a randomized, double-blind, crossover study, Max et al.[113] compared pain relief and side effects in PHN patients given a single oral dose of clonidine 0.2 mg, codeine 120 mg, ibuprofen 800 mg, or placebo. Clonidine was the only treatment that provided a statistically significant decrease in pain compared to placebo. Its benefit peaked at 3–4 hours after use. However, the clonidine group had the highest rate of side effects, the most common of which were sleepiness, dizziness, dry mouth, and headache.

Vitamin C

Chen et al.[133] found that plasma vitamin C levels were significantly lower in PHN patients than in healthy volunteers. In a double-blind study, they compared the effects of intravenous vitamin C treatment with placebo (saline) treatment for patients with PHN. Spontaneous pain decreased significantly more in the vitamin C-treated group than in the saline-treated group, but no difference was observed in brush-evoked pain.

Adenosine Derivatives

Moriyama et al.[134] showed in a randomized, controlled, single-blind trial that intravenous adenosine triphosphate (ATP) decreased spontaneous pain and allodynia compared to baseline, whereas the placebo did not. The intravenous ATP induced pain relief that developed slowly, lasted for a median time of 9 hours, and correlated with ketamine therapy responsiveness.[135] Adverse effects were uncommon (nausea and nonischemic chest discomfort) and resolved within a few minutes after slowing the rate of transfusion.

There is limited evidence to show that divalproex sodium,[136] levetiracetam,[137] carbamazepine,[138] or oxcarbazepine[139] can be effective in relieving PHN pain.

Topical Aspirin

The use of a topical aspirin/ADE preparation resulted in decreased PHN pain compared to placebo[77] and was comparable to topical lidocaine for PHN.[140]

Prostaglandin E1 (PGE1)

PGE1 has vasodilatory properties and has been studied in PHN with the hope that improving blood circulation may relieve pain. Intravenous PGE1 followed by oral PGE1 therapy decreased VAS scores of PHN patients for rest pain and tactile allodynia.[141] In a randomized, double-blind, placebo-controlled, crossover study, both treatment and placebo groups experienced improved ongoing pain, but greater reduction was reported in the PGE1-treated group.[142] The most common adverse reactions reported in these studies were nausea and diarrhea.

Interferon

No strong evidence is available for the use of interferon to treat PHN except a case series of two patients who were treated successfully with interferon-γ.[143]

SSRI/SNRI

Neither SSRIs nor SNRIs were found to be effective for treating PHN pain.[103,144]

Other Topical Medications

Topical benzydamine 3%,[145] amitriptyline 2%, and ketamine 1%[146] were no more effective than placebo for treating patients with PHN.

Systemic NSAIDs

One dose of ibuprofen 800 mg was found to be less effective than placebo for decreasing PHN pain in a randomized, double-blind, crossover study.[113]

Other Medications

In a single-blind controlled study, epidural morphine was ineffective compared to placebo at reducing PHN pain and produced more side effects.[147]

INTERVENTIONAL/SURGICAL TREATMENTS

Pain Control and Potential Hastening of Rash Healing

Sympathetic Ganglion Block

Sympathectomy alone can be achieved by blocking the stellate ganglion or the paravertebral sympathetic chain. Theoretically, it can also be achieved by using low concentrations of local anesthetics at other targets. Local anesthetics have been administered as a single[148] or series[149] of injections to treat acute shingles. According to Colding,[149] the pain relief started 10–15 minutes after the block and usually lasted for 8–12 hours. Additionally, the pain was less intense when it returned. Interestingly, he found that if the block was given within the first 2 weeks of the acute rash, 90% of patients responded to it compared to only 40% response beyond that time frame. Winnie and Hartwell[150] reported similar findings, although the cutoff period after the acute rash was 2 months.

Combined Somatic and Sympathetic Block

Local infiltration with local anesthetics during the acute phase was shown to effectively relieve HZ pain.[151] Targeting specific nerves or plexuses, such as the trigeminal nerve and its branches,[152] occipital nerve, cervical plexus,[153] paravertebral space block,[154] intercostal nerves, and "three-in-one block,"[155] also was reported to be effective at relieving pain in the acute phase. With neuroaxial injections, high thoracic epidural local anesthetic therapy was found to be as effective as stellate ganglion blocks for achieving pain relief in shingles.[156] Data indicate that continuous epidural infusion is better than intermittent injections.[157] A prospective study showed that acute pain was shorter when local anesthetic epidural injections were used in combination with acyclovir[158] or famciclovir[159] than when antiviral therapy was used alone.

Neuromodulation

Transcutaneous electrical nerve stimulation (TENS),[160] percutaneous electrical nerve stimulation,[161] and spinal cord stimulation[162,163] have been used successfully in shingles to alleviate pain.

External Therapy

Ultraviolet B (UVB) spectrum combined with antiviral therapy[164] and UVA light on shingles lesions pretreated with chlorinated neutral red solution[165] accelerated acute shingles pain relief.

PHN Prevention

Sympathetic Ganglion Block with Steroids

Makharita et al.[166] found in a randomized controlled study that two stellate ganglion blocks with steroids given within 2 weeks of acute rash onset lowered the incidence of PHN and increased patient satisfaction at 3 and 6 months.

Combined Somatic and Sympathetic Block with Steroids

In a randomized controlled study, Ji et al.[167] reported a significantly lower incidence of pain at up to 1 year of follow-up in patients who were treated with repeat paravertebral local anesthetics and steroid injections. Although adding a single epidural local anesthetic and steroid injection did not change the PHN incidence,[168] repeat epidural local anesthetic and steroid injections were found to significantly decrease the incidence of pain at 1 year.[169]

Combined Somatic and Sympathetic Block Without Steroids

Local anesthetics alone infiltrated into the painful area during the acute phase of HZ did not prevent PHN from developing.[151]

PHN Therapy

PHN patients who received intrathecal steroid injections experienced long-lasting pain relief, whereas those who received intrathecal lidocaine or no treatment had little to no decrease in pain.[170] Although no adhesive arachnoiditis was reported in any of the study patients, this therapy is not commonly utilized. Interestingly, the pain relief correlated with a decrease in cerebrospinal fluid interleukin-8 levels, supporting chronic inflammation etiology.

Combined Somatic and Sympathetic Block

In contrast to the low efficacy of pure sympathectomy in treating PHN, field block with local anesthetics and steroids was reported to eliminate PHN pain for a prolonged period.

Although the long effect may be explained by the natural history of the process, it may also be attributed to the steroids.[171] Paravertebral space block also has been used to treat PHN successfully,[172] as has epidural space block with local anesthetics alone.[173]

Steroid Injection

In a case series of 37 patients with PHN who were treated with a series of three epidural steroid injections, Forrest[174] reported that the mean VAS pain score was reduced significantly from pretreatment value and was maintained for at least 1 year of follow-up. This finding is contrary to the short-term pain relief from epidural steroid injection reported by Kikuchi et al. [175] Adding intrathecal midazolam to epidural steroid injections may prolong the pain relief achieved by each one alone.[176]

Botulinum Toxin Injection

Botulinum toxin A inhibits release of acetylcholine at the neuromuscular junction, as well as from peripheral parasympathetic and sudomotor sympathetic nerve terminals. After a few case reports of successful PHN pain relief with subcutaneously injected botulinum toxin A[177–179] compared VAS scores and sleeping time among patients who were administered subcutaneous botulinum toxin, lidocaine 0.5%, and saline. All groups showed improvement from pretreatment, but the group that received botulinum toxin A group showed the most significant improvement.

Magnesium Injection

A case report described successful PHN pain relief with epidural transforaminal injection of magnesium.[180]

Neuromodulation

Scrambler therapy, which electrically stimulates multiple points over a large area, was found in a small randomized trial to be effective for treatment of neuropathic pain, including PHN.[181] TENS[182] and STS (implanted field stimulation) applied to lateral thoracic,[183] subscapular, and paraspinal areas[184] also were reported to be effective at reducing PHN pain. When a specific nerve can be targeted, the stimulation electrode can be surgically implanted near the involved nerve. Supraorbital, infraorbital,[185] occipital, [186] and even DRG[187] electrical nerve stimulation have been reported to provide pain relief and reduce analgesic use in this population.

Several case reports described favorable results with dorsal column stimulation in PHN patients,[188–190] but, based on a survey by Shimoji et al.,[191] the percentage of patients who achieved more than 50% pain relief was significantly lower among patients with PHN than among those with complex regional pain syndrome (CRPS), especially with long-term use.[192] Other more central and invasive targets for electrical neuromodulation that have been reported as possible treatment for PHN pain include epidural motor cortex,[193–195] ventral posterior lateral thalamic nucleus, periventricular gray area, and periaqueductal gray area.[196,197]

Surgical/Ablation

Because the purpose of the surgical and ablative procedures is to eliminate the source of the pain, prevent its transmission, or change the pain perception, these procedures are usually irreversible and riskier than nonablative injections, neuromodulation, or external therapies. Therefore, these procedures do not have a role in acute shingles pain management. Nonetheless, before nonablative procedures became prevalent, multiple case reports and series that described excision of the painful area, neurectomy, ganglionectomy (DRG and gasserian nucleus), dorsal root/postgasserian nerve ablation, dorsal root entry zone (DREZ) lesion, cordotomy, and intracranial lesioning reported variable success and complications. Skin resection down to the muscle fascia is not a good option because pain may worsen over the time.[198,199] Ablating a peripheral nerve after a favorable block trial is limited only to sensory nerves or intercostal nerves. The results of cryoablation were not promising[200]; success was as high as 42% at 6 weeks but decreased to 3% at 6 months, a rate lower than that for nonherpetic indications.[201] Pulsed radiofrequency, which is not always defined as an ablative procedure, is used successfully in our clinic to treat facial PHN pain and has been reported by Kim et al.[202]

A case series by Lauretti et al.[203] and a case report by Benzon et al.[204] described the use of dorsal root chemical neurolysis for PHN involving thoracic dermatomes. γ-Knife ablation of the retrogasserian nucleus nerve, which may be considered as the equivalent of the dorsal roots, was found successful in fewer than 50% of patients.[205]

DREZ ablation at the spinal or trigeminal nucleus caudalis levels by different modalities, such as thermal coagulation or CO_2 laser, has been reported with variable outcomes and complication rates.[206,207] Prolonged favorable outcomes ranged from as high as 50–60%[208,209] to 20%.[210] The most common major complication from this procedure was upper motor neuron dysfunction, which may lead to long-term disability. Other minor complications included hypoesthesia, gait ataxia, and paresthesia.

Disrupting the spinothalamic tract surgically can be achieved by anterolateral cordotomy and myelotomy. Cordotomy was performed originally by Spiller and Martin (1912), and since then it has evolved into a percutaneous procedure. Its use in PHN patients has been reported in several case series.[211,212] Trigeminal tractotomy (targeting the trigeminal descending tract in the medulla) and trigeminal nucleotomy (targeting the nucleus caudalis) have been described in small case series[212,213] of patients with PHN of the face. Myelotomy, which originally was believed to interrupt the decussating fibers, is believed today to ablate the ascending nonspecific polysynaptic pathway around the central region that is related mostly to visceral pain. Although the procedure is not believed to be effective for PHN, Schvarcz[214] reported treating PHN patients (2 out of 3) successfully. Complications from these ablation procedures may be caused by incorrect localization of the needle or unintended enlargement of the ablated lesion.

Central nervous system lesions may involve thalamotomy, cingulotomy, prefrontal leucotomy, and other central locations. Young et al.[215] described 10 patients (two of whom suffered from PHN) who were treated with γ-knife thalamotomy (intralaminar nuclei, lateral portion of the medial dorsal nucleus, and parafascicular nuclei). Good to excellent pain relief was achieved in 70% of the patients. Cingulate cortex is involved in pain processing,[216] and because it lacks somatotopic presentation, cingulotomy has been tried in cases of intractable pain in any part of the body. Unfortunately, this procedure has been unsuccessful for PHN.[217] Prefrontal leukotomy was first defined as "psychosurgery" because it had a calming effect and involved disrupting fiber projection from cingulate gyrus and dorsomedial thalamus to frontal cortex. After it was reported that the procedure relieved pain, Elithorn et al.[218] performed bilateral prefrontal leucotomy in 25 patients (five with PHN), a third of whom experienced pain improvement. Because it has a devastating effect on intellectual performance and social activities, prefrontal leucotomy is not considered today for treatment of pain.

Radiation and External Therapies

Low-power He:Ne laser was reported safe and effective in decreasing PHN pain.[219] Cryoanalgesia with topically applied local liquid nitrogen spray over the painful dermatomes was also effective.[220]

Sympathetic Ganglion Block

Nurmikko et al.[221] showed that sympathetic blocks most likely had no significant role in treating PHN pain compared to favorable results produced with somatic blocks.

Radiation

UVB irradiation over the painful dermatomes failed to provide significant pain relief in five patients with PHN.[222]

COMPLEMENTARY AND ALTERNATIVE TREATMENTS

Acupuncture and Moxibustion

Inserting solid needles into acupuncture points is believed by Traditional Chinese Medicine to correct imbalance in the flow of energy (*qi*). Acupuncture has been used for acute HZ pain as well as for PHN. Moxibustion is also a TCM technique in which the same acupuncture points are warmed (directly or indirectly) to have the same effect on the flow of *qi*. In shingles patients who were treated with antiviral medication, acupuncture was compared to standard pharmacologic therapy (pregabalin, opioids, and epidural/perineural local anesthetics) and was found to be as effective in reducing pain and the incidence of PHN at 3 months.[223] Acupuncture as a treatment for PHN pain was not found to be effective in a small randomized, single-blind, controlled trial.[224]

Wet Cupping

There are eight types of cupping therapies in which horn, bamboo, or glass cups are applied to the skin to create negative pressure. Among the different techniques, wet cupping is the most common and involves a small bleeding incision. TCM believes that cupping regulates the flow of blood and *qi*, and helps to draw out pathogenic factors. In a systematic review, wet cupping was found to be very effective in acute HZ, although the study's results might be questionable.[225]

Herbal

Case reports have described patients with HZ who have obtained significant pain relief after ingestion of an herbal formula containing *Ganoderma lucidum*[226] and accelerated rash healing with Tasmanian *Undaria pinnatifida*, which is a commonly eaten seaweed in Japan.[227] Another topical medication is *Clinacanthus nutans*, a small tropical shrub in Asia that is believed to have antiviral, analgesic, and anti-inflammatory properties. In a small study, its use led to faster pain relief and lesion healing compared to placebo.[228]

Combinations of TCM

Hui et al.[229] studied the efficacy of complementary and alternative medicine in treating PHN with a duration of greater than 30 days. They compared TCM techniques (acupuncture, cupping and bleeding) combined with neural therapy (1% procaine injection) to a wait-list group who started the same therapy 3 weeks later. The pain in both groups on an 11-point pain scale was comparable at baseline. After 3 weeks of treatment, the pain level was significantly lower in the first-treated group.

PSYCHOSOCIAL TREATMENT AND REHABILITATION

Jensen et al. [230] reviewed the impact of neuropathic pain on quality of life and found that the presence and severity of neuropathic pain correlates strongly with impairment in physical, emotional, and social functioning, as well as with a decrease in global quality of life. The data indicate that patients with neuropathic pain should be assessed periodically for health-related quality of life to determine whether therapies that reduce pain also indirectly improve the quality of life and to tailor specific psychosocial treatments that can directly improve these modalities. Specifically, cognitive restructuring and self-hypnosis showed promising results for neuropathic pain patients by potentially improving the patients' sense of control and decreasing their sense of helplessness.

Chronic neuropathic pain syndromes require a comprehensive treatment strategy and should include nonpharmacologic modalities that may facilitate functional restoration and decrease disability. Sleep should be normalized, and psychological referral is recommended. Patients should be assessed with physical therapy to determine whether treatment can provide neuromuscular rehabilitation. Desensitization and possible TENS trials also may be beneficial.[231] In a case report by Tashiro et al.,[231] a patient with HZ-induced T12–L1 segmental paresis that led to pseudohernia, scoliosis, and gait disturbances exhibited dramatic improvement in function after 4 months of rehabilitation that included thoracolumbosacral soft orthosis, muscle reeducation, strengthening of trunk and extremity muscles, and gait exercise. In addition, at a later stage of recovery, occupational and vocational rehabilitation may facilitate return to the independent premorbid function level.

WHAT ARE THE GUIDELINES FOR PHN PREVENTION?

Prevention of VZV reactivation with vaccination may be the best way to avoid acute zoster and the zoster-associated pain. However, once acute zoster is diagnosed, it is reasonable to treat patients aggressively to relieve the acute pain and possibly decrease the risk of PHN. Nucleoside analogues should be given within the first 72 hours of rash. In addition, treatment with amitriptyline, gabapentin, opioids, and nerve blocks may also help to prevent ongoing pain. Systemic steroids are likely ineffective.

For established PHN, published guidelines are summarized in Table 2.1. The guidelines rank TCA, gabapentinoids, and topical lidocaine alone or combined as the first-line therapies. Opioids are effective treatment for PHN, but their side effects, tolerance development, and risk of addiction place them as a second-line therapy by some of the guidelines. The use of topical agents, such as capsaicin and aspirin, is attractive because of their limited adverse effects. In refractory cases, therapeutic trials with other agents, such as divalproex sodium, levetiracetam, carbamazepine, or oxcarbazepine have been recommended. Intrathecal steroid injection was also reported to be effective, but due to the potential risks of adhesive arachnoiditis, it is not commonly utilized. Last, neuromodulation is an attractive modality but its effectiveness in PHN treatment has been less well studied compared to CRPS.

CONCLUSION: PUTATIVE PAIN MECHANISMS BASED ON PATHOLOGY, CLINICAL FEATURES, AND PHARMACODYNAMICS AND THE IMPLICATIONS

Considerable information is available about the pathology of PHN. It has been known for more than 100 years that acute hemorrhagic inflammation is present in one DRG at the stage of HZ eruption.[232] Inflammation then extends distally as well as proximally into the spinal cord.[233] After months, the DRG exhibits significant scarring and loss of neurons, and the spinal cord dorsal horn exhibits atrophy and scarring (Figures 2.9 and 2.10).[233,234] Some patients have persistent inflammatory cells.[234] An assessment of the nerve fiber population in the peripheral nerve after the eruption of HZ shows a predominance of small (some probably pain-conducting) fibers and a deficiency in large myelinated (pain-inhibitory) fibers.[233,234] However, this predominance of small fibers may be due in part to regenerating sprouts from a variety of sensory neurons that transmit pressure and vibration as well as pain and temperature. Furthermore, although shingles and PHN are associated with unilateral clinical findings, with the rash, distribution, and residual scarring associated with only one ganglion, contralateral pathologic findings in the same skin segment have been shown.

PHN pain has three main features. Patients describe a constant, steady, burning pain; electric shock-like pains reminiscent of trigeminal neuralgia (TN); and skin that is often very sensitive or painful. The physical examination often reveals pain to summating touch stimuli such as skin stroking (dynamic mechanical allodynia) and excessive pain from pinprick (hyperalgesia) or cold stimuli over areas wider than the single ganglion usually thought to be the site of the eruption and pathology.

We know little about dysfunction associated with these clinical and pathologic findings. We can only hypothesize that excessive ectopic activity in injured peripheral nerve fibers and ganglion cells drives central activity that results in pain from nonpainful stimuli and expansion of the receptive fields of second-order neurons in the spinal cord due to activation of latent connections with adjacent dermatomes. Unfortunately, this knowledge has not led to useful changes in medical or surgical therapy.

For most patients, surgery does not rectify the disordered pain signaling. Surgery may relieve the sensitivity of the skin, but it usually does not alleviate the steady and shock-like pain. Surgical procedures are likely ineffective because the damage is to the spinal cord, nerve root, and ganglion, areas that cannot be accessed easily. Surgical treatment can worsen the situation by producing anesthesia dolorosa (pain in a numb area) or provide temporary relief at best.

Differing pharmacodynamics of the various drugs used to treat PHN and the limitations of monotherapy provide a rationale for using combinations of drugs, which may also limit adverse effects by enabling the use of lower doses. TCAs and SNRIs potentiate the inhibitory neurotransmitters norepinephrine and serotonin in pain-inhibitory pathways that descend from the brainstem to the spinal cord, gabapentinoids are presynaptic $\alpha_2\delta$ calcium channel modulators, and opioids act on spinal and brainstem opioid receptors. Despite this specific knowledge regarding pharmacodynamics, a good mechanism-based treatment continues to elude us. Although the shock-like pain component resembles that of TN, the sodium channel blocker carbamazepine (the closest we have to a mechanism-based treatment that is successful in TN) is usually a failure in PHN. Drugs such as TCAs, gabapentinoids, and opioids affect indiscriminately all features of the pain—that is, the steady burning, shock-like pain, and sensitivity of the skin (allodynia). Monotherapy or combination therapy can provide moderate improvement in only half to two-thirds of patient with established PHN, and very few have complete relief. Perhaps one reason for the intractability is the severe damage to the dorsal horn of the spinal cord (Figures 2.9 and 2.10) Hence, the receptors for pain-inhibitory drugs such as opioids, TCAs, and gabapentinoids might be damaged or destroyed. This scenario argues very strongly for prevention of HZ by vaccination and by the early, aggressive treatment of HZ with antivirals and analgesics in an attempt to prevent this disease.

REFERENCES

1. Dworkin RH, Gnann JW, Oaklander AL, Raja SN, Schmader KE, Whitley RJ. Diagnosis and assessment of pain associated with herpes zoster and postherpetic neuralgia. *J Pain*. 2008;9:S37–S44.
2. Gnann JW, Whitley RJ. Clinical practice. Herpes zoster. *N Engl J Med*. 2002;347:340–346.
3. Bennett GT, Watson CP. Herpes zoster and postherpetic neuralgia: past, present and future. *Pain Res Manage*. 2009;14:275–282.
4. Abraham N, Murray J. The belt of roses from hell: historical aspects of herpes zoster and postherpetic neuralgia. In: Watson CPN, Gershon AA, eds. *Herpes Zoster and Postherpetic Neuralgia*. Amsterdam: Elsevier; 2001:20–23.
5. Hope-Simpson R. The nature of herpes zoster: a long-term study and a new hypothesis. *Proc R Soc Med*. 1965;58:9–20.
6. Johnson RW, Dworkin RH. Treatment of herpes zoster and postherpetic neuralgia. *Br Med J*. 2003;326.
7. Gnann JW. Varicella-zoster virus: atypical presentations and unusual complications. *Journal of Infectious Diseases*. 2002;186:S91–S98.
8. Weinberg JM, Scheinfeld NS. Cutaneous infections in the elderly: diagnosis and management. *Dermato Ther*. 2003;16:195–205.
9. Weaver B. Herpes zoster overview: natural history and incidence. *J Am Osteopath Assoc*. 2009;109:S2–S6.
10. Dworkin RH, Portenoy RK. Pain and its persistence in herpes zoster. *Pain*. 1996;67:241–251.
11. Gilden DH, Kleinschmidt-DeMasters BK, LaGuardia JJ, Mahalingam R, Cohrs RJ. Neurologic complications of the reactivation of varicella-zoster virus. *N Engl J Med*. 2000;342:635–645.
12. Ragozzino MW, Melton LJ, Kurland LT, Chu CP, Perry HO. Population-based study of herpes zoster and its sequelae. *Medicine* (Baltimore). 1982;61:310–316.
13. Womack LW, Liesegang TJ. Complications of herpes zoster ophthalmicus. *Arch Opthamol*. 1983;101:42–45.
14. Zaal M, Völker-Dieben H, D'Amaro J. Prognostic value of Hutchinson's sign in acute herpes zoster ophthalmicus. *Graefe's Arch Clin Exp Ophthalmol*. 2003;241:187–191.
15. Kang JH, Ho JD, Chen YH, Lin HC. Increased risk of stroke after a herpes zoster attack: a population-based follow-up study. *Stroke*. 2009;40:3443–3448.
16. Cunha BA, Warren-Favorito H, Mickail N. Unusually severe varicella zoster (VZV) virus viral (aseptic) meningitis in an unimmunized, immunocompetent host with chickenpox. *Heart Lung*. 2011;40:349–351.
17. Klein NC, McDermott B, Cunha BA. Varicella-zoster virus meningoencephalitis in an immunocompetent patient without a rash. *Scand J Infect Dis*. 2010;42631–633.
18. Suzuki Y, Kanno A, Minami M, Ogawa K, Oishi M, Kamei S. Case of acute cerebellitis as a result of varicella zoster virus infection without skin manifestations. *Geriatr Gerontol Int*. 2012;12:756–757.
19. Celik Y, Tabak F, Mert A, Çelik AD, Aktuğlu Y. Transverse myelitis caused by varicella. *Clin Neurol Neurosurg*. 2001;103:260–261.
20. Hung CH, Chang KH, Kuo HC, et al. Features of varicella zoster virus myelitis and dependence on immune status. *J Neurol Sci*. 2012;318:19–24.
21. Haanpaa M, Hükkinen V, Nurmikko T. Motor involvement in acute herpes zoster. *Muscle Nerv*. 1997;20:1433–1438.
22. Liesegang TJ. Varicella-zoster virus eye disease. *Cornea*. 1999;18:511–531.
23. Arani RB, Soong SJ, Weiss HL, et al. Phase specific analysis of herpes zoster associated pain data: a new statistical approach. *Stat Med*. 2001;20:2429–2439.
24. Desmond RA, Weiss HL, Arani RB, et al. Clinical applications for change-point analysis of herpes zoster pain. *J Pain Symptom Manage*. 2002;23:510–516.
25. Dworkin RH, Portenoy RK. Proposed classification of herpes zoster pain. *Lancet*. 1994;343:1648.
26. Christo PJ, Hobelmann G, Maine DN. Post-herpetic neuralgia in older adults: evidence-based approaches to clinical management. *Drugs Aging*. 2007;24.
27. Weaver B. The burden of herpes zoster and postherpetic neuralgia in the United States. *JAOA*. 2007;107(3 Suppl 1):S2–7.
28. Oxman MN, Levin MJ, Johnson GR, et al. A vaccine to prevent herpes zoster and postherpetic neuralgia in older adults. *N Engl J Med*. 2005;352:2271–2284.
29. Schmader K, Gnann JW Jr, Watson CP. The epidemiological, clinical, and pathological rationale for the herpes zoster vaccine. J Infect Dis. 2008;197 (Suppl 2):S207–15.
30. Douglas MW, Johnson RW, Cunningham AL. Tolerability of treatments for postherpetic neuralgia. *Drug Saf*. 2004;27:1217–1233.
31. Bennett GT. Neuropathic pain: new insights, new interventions. *Hosp Pract*. 1998;33:95–98.
32. Kinsella K, Velkoff VA. *An aging world*. Washington, DC: US Census Bureau: US Government Printing Office. 2001.
33. Donahue JG, Choo PW, Manson JE, Platt R. The incidence of herpes zoster. *Arch Intern Med*. 1995;155:1605–1609.
34. Mueller NH, Gilden DH, Cohrs RJ, Mahalingam R, Nagel MA. Varicella zoster virus infection: clinical features, molecular pathogenesis of disease, and latency. *Neurol Clin*. 2008;26:675–697.
35. Thomas SL, Wheeler JH, Hall AJ. Case-control study of the effect of mechanical trauma on the risk of herpes zoster. *Br Med J*. 2004;328:439.
36. Schmader K, George LK, Burchett BM, Pieper CF. Race and stress in the incidence of herpes zoster in older adults. *J Am Geriatr Soc*. 1998;46:973–977.
37. Heymann AD, Chodick G, Karpati T, et al. Diabetes as a risk factor for herpes zoster infection: results of a population-based study in Israel. *Infection*. 2008;36:226–230.
38. Thomas SL, Hall AJ. What does epidemiology tell us about risk factors for herpes zoster? *Lancet Infect Dis*. 2004;4:26–33.
39. Bennett GT. Hypotheses on the pathogenesis of herpes zoster-associated pain. *Ann Neurol*. 1994;35:S38–S41.
40. Jung BF, Johnson RW, Griffin DRJ, Dworkin RH. Risk factors for postherpetic neuralgia in patients with herpes zoster. *Neurology*. 2004;62:1545–1551.
41. Dworkin RH, Schmader KE. The epidemiology and natural history of herpes zoster and postherpetic neuralgia. In: Watson CP, Gershon AA, eds. *Herpes Zoster and Postherpetic Neuralgia*. 2nd ed. New York: Elsevier; 2001: 39–64.
42. Katz J, Cooper EM, Walther RR, Sweeney EW, Dworkin RH. Acute pain in herpes zoster and its impact on health-related quality of life. *Clin Infect Dis*. 2004;39:342–348.
43. Wood MJ, Easterbrook P. Shingles, scourge of the elderly: the acute illness. In: Sacks SL, Straus SE, Whitley, RJ, Griffiths PD, eds. *Clinical Management of Herpes Zoster*. Washington, DC: IOS Press; 1995:193–209.
44. Opstelten W, Mauritz JW, de Wit NJ, van Wijck AJ, Stalman WA, van Essen GA. Herpes zoster and postherpetic neuralgia: incidence and risk indicators using a general practice research database. *Fam Pract*. 2002;19:471–475.
45. Hess TM, Lutz LJ, Nauss LA, Lamer TJ. Treatment of acute herpetic neuralgia. A case report and review of the literature. *Minn Med*. 1990;73:37–40.

46. Drolet BC, Lorenzi NM. Translational research: understanding the continuum from bench to bedside. *Transl Res*. 2011;157:1–5.
47. Raja SN, Haythornthwaite JA, Pappagallo M, et al. Opioids versus antidepressants in postherpetic neuralgia: a randomized, placebo-controlled trial. *Neurology*. 2002;59:1015–1021.
48. Watson CP, Babul N. Efficacy of oxycodone in neuropathic pain: a randomized trial in postherpetic neuralgia. *Neurology*. 1998;50:1837–1841.
49. Rowbotham MC, Petersen KL, Fields HL. Is postherpetic neuralgia more than one disorder? *Pain Forum*. 1998;7:231–237.
50. Saberski L, Ahmad M, Wiske P. Sphenopalatine ganglion block for treatment of sinus arrest in postherpetic neuralgia. *Headache: J Head Face Pain*. 1999;39:42–44.
51. Guan Y. Spinal cord stimulation: neurophysiological and neurochemical mechanisms of action. *Curr Pain Headache Rep*. 2012;16:217–225.
52. Chen SM, Chen JT, Kuan TS, Hong CZ. Myofascial trigger points in intercostal muscles secondary to herpes zoster infection of the intercostal nerve. *Arch Phys Med Rehab*. 1998;79:336–338.
53. Peterslund NA, Esmann V, Ipsen J, Christensen KD, Petersen CM. Oral and intravenous acyclovir are equally effective in herpes zoster. *J Antimicrob Chemother*. 1984;14:185–189.
54. Morton P, Thomson AN. Oral acyclovir in the treatment of herpes zoster in general practice. *N Z Med J*. 1989;102:93–95.
55. Wood MJ, Ogan PH, McKendrick MW, Care CD, McGill JI, Webb EM. Efficacy of oral acyclovir treatment of acute herpes zoster. *Am J Med*. 1988;85:79–83.
56. Wood MJ, Kay R, Dworkin RH, Soong SJ, Whitley RJ. Oral acyclovir therapy accelerates pain resolution in patients with herpes zoster: a meta-analysis of placebo-controlled trials. *Clin Infect Dis*. 1996;22:341–347.
57. Tyring S, Barbarash RA, Nahlik JE. Famciclovir for the treatment of acute herpes zoster: effects on acute disease and postherpetic neuralgia: a randomized, double-blind, placebo-controlled trial. *Ann Intern Med*. 1995;123:89–96.
58. Degreef H. Famciclovir, a new oral antiherpes drug: results of the first controlled clinical study demonstrating its efficacy and safety in the treatment of uncomplicated herpes zoster in immunocompetent patients. *Int J Antimicrob Agents*. 1994;4:241–246.
59. Tyring SK, Beutner KR, Tucker BA, Anderson WC, Crooks RJ. Antiviral therapy for herpes zoster: randomized, controlled clinical trial of valacyclovir and famciclovir therapy in immunocompetent patients 50 years and older. *Arch Fam Med*. 2000;9:863–869.
60. McDonald EM, deKock J, Ram FS. Antivirals for management of herpes zoster including ophthalmicus: a systematic review of high-quality randomized controlled trials. *Antivir Ther*. 2012;17:255–264.
61. Tyring SK, Plunkett S, Scribner AR, et al. Valomaciclovir versus valacyclovir for the treatment of acute herpes zoster in immunocompetent adults: a randomized, double-blind, active-controlled trial. *J Med Virol*. 2012;84:1224–1232.
62. Dworkin RH, Johnson RW, Breuer J, et al. Recommendations for the management of herpes zoster. *Clin Infect Dis*. 2007;44:S1–S26.
63. Opstelten W, Eekhof J, Neven AK, Verheij T. Treatment of herpes zoster. *Can Fam Physician*. 2008;54:373–377.
64. Dworkin RH, Barbano RL, Tyring SK, et al. A randomized, placebo-controlled trial of oxycodone and of gabapentin for acute pain in herpes zoster. *Pain*. 2009;142:209–217.
65. Galbraith AW. Treatment of acute herpes zoster with amantadine hydrochloride (Symmetrel). *Br Med J*. 1973;4:693–695.
66. Jutel M, Akdis M, Akdis CA. Histamine, histamine receptors and their role in immune pathology. *Clin Exp Allergy*. 2009;39:1786–1800.
67. Miller A, Harel D, Laor A, Lahat N. Cimetidine as an immunomodulator in the treatment of herpes zoster. *J Neuroimmunol*. 1989; 22:69–76.
68. Cobacho N, De la Calle JL, González-Escalada JR, Paíno CL. Levodopa analgesia in experimental neuropathic pain. *Brain Res Bull*. 2010;83:304–309.
69. Kernbaum S, Hauchecorne J. Administration of levodopa for relief of herpes zoster pain. *JAMA*. 1981;246:132–134.
70. Burnstock G. Purinergic receptors and pain. *Curr Pharm Des*. 2009;15:1717–1735.
71. Sklar SH, Blue WT, Alexander EJ, Bodian CA. Herpes zoster: the treatment and prevention of neuralgia with adenosine monophosphate. *JAMA*. 1985;253:1427–1430.
72. Eroglu Ç, Allen NJ, Susman MW, et al. Gabapentin receptor +¦2+¦-1 is a neuronal thrombospondin receptor responsible for excitatory CNS synaptogenesis. *Cell*. 2009;139:380–392.
73. Berry JD, Petersen KL. A single dose of gabapentin reduces acute pain and allodynia in patients with herpes zoster. *Neurology*. 2005;65:444–447.
74. Parsons B, Tive L, Huang S. Gabapentin: a pooled analysis of adverse events from three clinical trials in patients with postherpetic neuralgia. *Am J Geriatr Pharmacotherapy*. 2004;2:157–162.
75. Campbell BJ, Rowbotham M, Davies PS, Jacob P, Benowitz NL. Systemic absorption of topical lidocaine in normal volunteers, patients with post-herpetic neuralgia, and patients with acute herpes zoster. *J Pharm Sci*. 2002;91:1343–1350.
76. De Benedittis G., Besana F, Lorenzetti A, A new topical treatment for acute herpetic neuralgia and post-herpetic neuralgia: the aspirin/diethyl ether mixture. An open-label study plus a double-blind controlled clinical trial. *Pain*. 1992;48:383–390.
77. De Benedittis G, Lorenzetti A. Topical aspirin/diethyl ether mixture versus indomethacin and diclofenac/diethyl ether mixtures for acute herpetic neuralgia and postherpetic neuralgia: a double-blind crossover placebo-controlled study. *Pain*. 1996;65:45–51.
78. Kochar DK, Agarwal RP, Joshi A, Kumawat BL. Herpes zoster and post-herpetic neuralgia—a clinical trial of aspirin in chloroform for anodyne. *J Assoc Physicians India*. 1998;46:337–340.
79. Balakrishnan S, Bhushan K, Bhargava VK, Pandhi P. A randomized parallel trial of topical aspirin-moisturizer solution vs. oral aspirin for acute herpetic neuralgia. *Int J Dermatol*. 2001;40:535–538.
80. Parish LC, Witkowski JA. Dextranomer in dermatologic conditions. Int J Dermatol 1979; 18: 480–484.
81. Schencking M, Vollbracht C, Weiss G, et al. Intravenous vitamin C in the treatment of shingles: results of a multicenter prospective cohort study. *Med Sci Monit*. 2012;18:CR 215–CR 224.
82. Fensterl V, Sen GC. Interferons and viral infections. *BioFactors*. 2009;35:14–20.
83. Ambagala APN, Cohen JI. Varicella-zoster virus IE63, a major viral latency protein, is required to inhibit the alpha interferon-induced antiviral response. *Journal of Virology*. 2007;81:7844–7851.
84. Duschet P, Schwarz T, Soyer P, Henk A, Hausmaninger H, Gschnait F. Treatment of herpes zoster. Recombinant alpha interferon versus acyclovir. *Int J Dermatol*. 1988;27:193–197.
85. Winston DJ, Eron LJ, Ho M, et al. Recombinant interferon alpha-2a for treatment of herpes zoster in immunosuppressed patients with cancer. *Am J Med*. 1988;85:147–151.
86. Miyoshi H, Hirotsuji N, Kino T, Katsu K. Interferon alpha gel for herpes zoster. *Dermatol*. 1997;194:306.
87. Rossi S W. The treatment of acyclovir-resistant herpes zoster with trifluorothymidine and interferon alfa. *Arch Dermatol*. 1995;131:24–26.
88. Mandal BK, Dunbar EM, Ellis ME, Ellis J, Dowd P. A double-masked, placebo-controlled trial of acyclovir cream in immunocompetent patients with herpes zoster. *J Infect*. 1988;17:57–63.
89. Bowsher D. The effects of pre-emptive treatment of postherpetic neuralgia with amitriptyline: a randomized, double-blind, placebo-controlled trial. *J Pain Symptom Manage*. 1997;13:327–331.
90. Huff C, Bean B, Balfour HH Jr, et al. Therapy of herpes zoster with oral acyclovir. *Am J Med*. 1988;85:84–89.
91. Harding SP, Porter SM. Oral acyclovir in herpes zoster ophthalmicus. *Curr Eye Res*. 1991;10:177–182.
92. Whitley RJ, Weiss H, Gnann J, et al. Acyclovir with and without Prednisone for the treatment of herpes zoster: a randomized, placebo-controlled trial. *Ann Intern Med*. 1996;125:376–383.

93. Riopelle JM, Naraghi M, Grush KP. The effect of treating herpes zoster with oral acyclovir in preventing postherpetic neuralgia: a meta-analysis. *Arch Intern Med.* 1997;157:909–912.
94. Li Q, Chen N, Yang J, et al. Antiviral treatment for preventing postherpetic neuralgia. *Cochrane Database Syst Rev.* 2009;15:CD006866.
95. Dworkin RH, Boon RJ, Griffin DRG, Phung D. Postherpetic Neuralgia: impact of famciclovir, age, rash severity, and acute pain in herpes zoster patients. *J Infect Dis.* 1998;178:S76–S80.
96. Eaglstein WH, Katz R, Brown JA.. The effects of early corticosteroid therapy on the skin eruption and pain of herpes zoster. *JAMA.* 1970;211:1681–1683.
97. Keczkes K, Basheer AM. Do corticosteroids prevent post-herpetic neuralgia? *Br J Dermatol.* 1980;102:551–555.
98. Esmann V, Kroon S, Peterslund NA, et al. Prednisolone does not prevent post-herpetic neuralgia. *Lancet.* 1987;330:126–129.
99. Wood MJ, Johnson RW, McKendrick MW, Taylor J, Mandal BK, Crooks J. A randomized trial of Acyclovir for 7 days or 21 days with and without Prednisolone for treatment of acute herpes zoster. *N Engl J Med.* 1994;330:896–900.
100. Chen N, Yang M, He L, Zhang D, Zhou M, Zhu C. Corticosteroids for preventing postherpetic neuralgia. *Cochrane Database Syst Rev.* 2010;8:CD005582
101. Hempenstall K, Nurmikko TJ, Johnson RW, A'Hern RP, Rice ASC. Analgesic therapy in postherpetic neuralgia: a quantitative systematic review. *PLoS Med.* 2005;2:628–644.
102. Saarto T, Wiffen PJ. Antidepressants for neuropathic pain: a Cochrane review. *J Neurol Neurosurg Psychiatry.* 2010;81:1372–1373.
103. Rowbotham MC, Reisner LA, Davies PS, Fields HL. Treatment response in antidepressant-naive postherpetic neuralgia patients: double-blind, randomized trial. *J Pain.* 2005;6:741–746.
104. Edelsberg JS, Lord C, Oster G. Systematic review and meta-analysis of efficacy, safety, and tolerability data from randomized controlled trials of drugs used to treat postherpetic neuralgia. *Ann Pharmacother.* 2011;45:1483–1490.
105. Jensen MP, Chiang YK, Wu J. Assessment of pain quality in a clinical trial of gabapentin extended release for postherpetic neuralgia. *Clin J Pain.* 2009;25:286–292.
106. Irving G, Jensen M, Cramer M, et al. Efficacy and tolerability of gastric-retentive gabapentin for the treatment of postherpetic neuralgia: results of a double-blind, randomized, placebo-controlled clinical trial. *Clin J Pain.* 2009;25:185–192.
107. Backonja MM, Canafax DM, Cundy KC. Efficacy of gabapentin enacarbil vs placebo in patients with postherpetic neuralgia and a pharmacokinetic comparison with oral gabapentin. *Pain Med.* 2011;12:1098–1108.
108. Chandra K, Shafiq N, Paindhi P, Gupta S, Malhotra S. Gabapentin versus nortriptyline in post-herpetic neuralgia patients: a randomized, double-blind clinical trial—the GONIP trial. *Int J Clin Pharmacol Ther.* 2006;44:358–363.
109. Gilron I, Bailey JM, Tu D, Holden RR, Jackson AC, Houlden RL. Nortriptyline and gabapentin, alone and in combination for neuropathic pain: a double-blind, randomised controlled crossover trial. *Lancet.* 2010;374:1252–1261.
110. Bockbrader HN, Wesche D, Miller R, Chapel S, Janiczek N, Burger P. A comparison of the pharmacokinetics and pharmacodynamics of Pregabalin and Gabapentin. *Clin Pharmacokinet.* 2010; 49(10):661–669.
111. Sharma U, Griesing T, Emir B, Young JP Jr. Time to onset of neuropathic pain reduction: a retrospective analysis of data from nine controlled trials of pregabalin for painful diabetic peripheral neuropathy and postherpetic neuralgia. *Am J Ther.* 2010;17:577–585.
112. Moore RA, Straube S, Wiffen PJ, Derry S, McQuay HJ. Pregabalin for acute and chronic pain in adults. *Cochrane Database Syst Rev.* 2009;8:CD007076.
113. Max MB, Schafer SC, Culnane M, Dubner R, Gracely RH. Association of pain relief with drug side effects in postherpetic neuralgia: a single-dose study of clonidine, codeine, ibuprofen, and placebo. *Clin Pharm Ther.* 1988;43:363–371.
114. Rowbotham MC, Reisner-Keller LA, Fields HL. Both intravenous lidocaine and morphine reduce the pain of postherpetic neuralgia. *Neurology.* 1991;41:1024–1028.
115. Gilron I, Bailey JM, Tu D, Holden RR, Weaver DF, Houlden RL. Morphine, Gabapentin, or their combination for neuropathic pain. *N Engl J Med.* 2005;352:1324–1334.
116. Boureau F, Legallicier P, Kabir-Ahmadi M. Tramadol in post-herpetic neuralgia: a randomized, double-blind, placebo-controlled trial. *Pain.* 2003;104:323–331.
117. Baranowski AP, De Courcey J, Bonello E. A trial of intravenous lidocaine on the pain and allodynia of postherpetic neuralgia. *J Pain Symptom Manage.* 1999;17:429–433.
118. Attal N, Rouaud J, Brasseur L, Chauvin M, Bouhassira D. Systemic lidocaine in pain due to peripheral nerve injury and predictors of response. *Neurology.* 2004;62:218–225.
119. Rowbotham MC, Davies PS, Fields HL. Topical lidocaine gel relieves postherpetic neuralgia. *Ann Neurol.* 1995;37:246–253.
120. Rowbotham MC, Davies PS, Verkempinck C, Galer BS. Lidocaine patch: double-blind controlled study of a new treatment method for post-herpetic neuralgia. *Pain.* 1996;65:39–44.
121. Binder A, Bruxelle J, Rogers P, Hans G, Boesl I, Baron R. Topical 5% Lidocaine (Lignocaine) medicated plaster treatment for post-herpetic neuralgia: results of a double-blind, placebo-controlled, multinational efficacy and safety trial. *Clin Drug Investig.* 2009;29:393–408.
122. Baron R, Mayoral V, Leijon G, Binder A, Steigerwald I, Serpell M. 5% lidocaine medicated plaster versus pregabalin in post-herpetic neuralgia and diabetic polyneuropathy: an open-label, non-inferiority two-stage RCT study. *Curr Med Res Opin.* 2009;25:1663–1676.
123. Rehm S, Binder A, Baron R. Post-herpetic neuralgia: 5% lidocaine medicated plaster, pregabalin, or a combination of both? A randomized, open, clinical effectiveness study. *Curr Med Res Opin.* 2010;26:1607–1619.
124. Kanai A, Kumaki C, Niki Y, Suzuki A, Tazawa T, Okamoto H. Efficacy of a metered-dose 8% Lidocaine pump spray for patients with post-herpetic neuralgia. *Pain Med.* 2009;10:902–909.
125. Bernstein JE, Korman NJ, Bickers DR, Dahl MV, Millikan LE. Topical capsaicin treatment of chronic postherpetic neuralgia. *J Am Acad Dermatol.* 1989; 21:265–270.
126. Watson CP, Tyler KL, Bickers DR, Millikan LE, Smith S, Coleman E. A randomized vehicle-controlled trial of topical capsaicin in the treatment of postherpetic neuralgia. *Clin Ther.* 1993;15:510–526.
127. Backonja MM, Malan TP, Vanhove GF, Tobias JK. NGX-4010, a high-concentration capsaicin patch, for the treatment of postherpetic neuralgia: a randomized, double-blind, controlled study with an open-label extension. *Pain Med.* 2010;11:600–608.
128. Irving G, Backonja M, Rauck R, Webster LR, Tobias JK, Vanhove GF. NGX-4010, a capsaicin 8% dermal patch, administered alone or in combination with systemic neuropathic pain medications, reduces pain in patients with postherpetic neuralgia. *Clin J Pain.* 2012;28:101–107.
129. Eide PK, Jorum E, Stubhaug A. Relief of post-herpetic neuralgia with the N-methyl-D-aspartic acid receptor antagonist ketamine: a double-blind, cross-over comparison with morphine and placebo. *Pain.* 1994;58:347–354.
130. Eide PK, Stubhaug A, Øye I, Breivik H. Continuous subcutaneous administration of the N-methyl-d-aspartic acid (NMDA) receptor antagonist ketamine in the treatment of post-herpetic neuralgia. *Pain.* 1995;61:221–228.
131. Klepstad P, Borchgrevink PC. Four years' treatment with ketamine and a trial of dextromethorphan in a patient with severe post-herpetic neuralgia. *Acta Anaesthesiol Scand.* 1997;41:422–426.

132. Brill S, Sedgwick PM, Hamann W, di Vadi PP. Efficacy of intravenous magnesium in neuropathic pain. *Br J Anaesth.* 2002;89:711–714.
133. Chen JY, Chang CY, Feng PH, Chu CC, So EC, Hu ML. Plasma vitamin C is lower in postherpetic neuralgia patients and administration of vitamin C reduces spontaneous pain but not brush-evoked pain. *Clin J Pain.* 2009;25.
134. Moriyama M, Kitamura A, Ikezaki H, et al. Systemic ATP infusion improves spontaneous pain and tactile allodynia, but not tactile hypesthesia, in patients with postherpetic neuralgia. *J Anesth.* 2004; 18:177–180.
135. Hayashida M, Fukuda Ki, Fukunaga A, et al. Analgesic effect of intravenous ATP on postherpetic neuralgia in comparison with responses to intravenous ketamine and lidocaine. *J Anesth.* 2005;19:31–35.
136. Kochar DK, Garg P, Bumb RA, et al. Divalproex sodium in the management of post-herpetic neuralgia: a randomized double-blind placebo-controlled study. *QJ Med.* 2005;98:29–34.
137. Rowbotham MC, Manville NS, Ren J. Pilot tolerability and effectiveness study of levetiracetam for postherpetic neuralgia. *Neurology.* 2003;61:866–867.
138. Gerson GR, Jones RB, Luscombe DK. Studies on the concomitant use of carbamazepine and clomipramine for the relief of post-herpetic neuralgia. *Postgrad Med J.* 1977;53:104–109.
139. Criscuolo S, Auletta C, Lippi S, Brogi F, Brogi A. Oxcarbazepine monotherapy in postherpetic neuralgia unresponsive to carbamazepine and gabapentin. *Acta Neurol Scand.* 2005;111:229–232.
140. Tajti J, Szok D, Vecsei L. Topical acetylsalicylic acid versus lidocaine for postherpetic neuralgia: results of a double-blind comparative clinical trial. *Neurobiology* (Bp). 1999;7:103–108.
141. Kanai A, Osawa S, Suzuki A, Ishimaru R, Hoka S. Effectiveness of prostaglandin E1 for the treatment of patients with neuropathic pain following herpes zoster. *Pain Med.* 2007;8:36–40.
142. Kanai A, Wang G, Hoshi K, Okamoto H. Effects of intravenous prostaglandin E1 on pain and body temperature in patients with post-herpetic neuralgia. *Pain Med.* 2010;11:609–616.
143. Usuki K, Kitamura K, Urabe A, Takaku F. Herpes zoster, postherpetic neuralgia, and interferon-gamma. *Ann Intern Med.* 1988;108:643–644.
144. Grothe DR, Scheckner B, Albano D. Treatment of pain syndromes with venlafaxine. *Pharmacother: J Hum Pharmacol Drug Ther.* 2004;24:621–629.
145. McQuay HJ, Carroll D, Moxon A, Glynn CJ, Moore RA. Benzydamine cream for the treatment of post-herpetic neuralgia: minimum duration of treatment periods in a cross-over trial. *Pain.* 1990;40:131–135.
146. Lynch ME, Clark AJ, Sawynok J, Sullivan MJ. Topical 2% amitriptyline and 1% ketamine in neuropathic pain syndromes: a randomized, double-blind, placebo-controlled trial. *Anesthesiol.* 2005;103:140–146.
147. Watt JW, Wiles JR, Bowsher DR. Epidural morphine for postherpetic neuralgia. *Anaesthesiology.* 1996;51:647–651.
148. Harding SP, Lipton JR, Wells JC, Campbell JA. Relief of acute pain in herpes zoster ophthalmicus by stellate ganglion block. *Br Med J.* 1986;292.
149. Colding A. Treatment of pain: organization of a pain clinic: treatment of acute herpes zoster. *Proc R Soc Med.* 1973;66:541–543.
150. Winnie AP, Hartwell PW. Relationship between time of treatment of acute herpes zoster with sympathetic blockade and prevention of post-herpetic neuralgia: clinical support for a new theory of the mechanism by which sympathetic blockade provides therapeutic benefit. *Reg Anesth.* 1993;18:277–282.
151. Riopelle JM, Naraghi M, Grush KP. Chronic neuralgia incidence following local anesthetic therapy for herpes zoster. *Arch Dermatol.* 1984;120: 747–750.
152. Gain P, Thuret G, Chiquet C, Navez ML, Pascal J. Frontal and nasal nerve blocks in the treatment of severe pain in acute ophthalmic zoster. *Anesth Analg.* 2002;95:503.
153. Hardy D. Relief of pain in acute herpes zoster by nerve blocks and possible prevention of post-herpetic neuralgia. *Can J Anaesth.* 2005;52:186–190.
154. Rosenak SS. Paravertebral procaine block for the treatment of herpes zoster. *NY State J Med.* 1956;56:2684–2687.
155. Hadzic A, Vloka JD, Saff GN, Hertz R, Thys DM. The "three-in-one block" for treatment of pain in a patient with acute herpes zoster infection. *Reg Anesth.* 1997;22:575–578.
156. Higa K, Hori K, Harasawa I, Hirata K, Dan K. High thoracic epidural block relieves acute herpetic pain involving the trigeminal and cervical regions: comparison with effects of stellate ganglion block. *Reg Anesth Pain Med.* 1998;23:25–29.
157. Manabe H, Dan K, Hirata K, et al. Optimum pain relief with continuous epidural infusion of local anesthetics shortens the duration of zoster-associated pain. *Clin J Pain.* 2004;20:302–308.
158. Hwang SK. The effects of epidural blockade on the acute pain in herpes zoster. *Arch Dermatol.* 1999;135:1359–1364.
159. Ahn HJ, Lim HK, Lee YB, et al. The effects of famciclovir and epidural block in the treatment of herpes zoster. *J Dermatol.* 2001;28:208–216.
160. Kolsek M. TENS—an alternative to antiviral drugs for acute herpes zoster treatment and postherpetic neuralgia prevention. *Swiss Med Wkly.* 2012;17:w13229.
161. Ahmed HE, Craig WF, White PF, et al. Percutaneous electrical nerve stimulation: an alternative to antiviral drugs for acute herpes zoster. *Anesth Analg.* 1998;87:911–914.
162. Moriyama K. Effect of temporary spinal cord stimulation on postherpetic neuralgia in the thoracic nerve area. *Neuromodulation.* 2009;12:39–43.
163. Yanamoto F, Murakawa K. The effects of temporary spinal cord stimulation (or spinal nerve root stimulation) on the management of early postherpetic neuralgia from one to six months of its onset. *Neuromodulation.* 2012;15:151–154.
164. Hadi Aziz Jalali M, Ansarin H, Soltani-Arabshahi R. Broad-band ultraviolet B phototherapy in zoster patients may reduce the incidence and severity of postherpetic neuralgia. *Photodermatol Photoimmunol Photomed.* 2006;22:232–237.
165. Martin WJ, Stoneburner J. Symptomatic relief of herpetic skin lesions utilizing an energy-based approach to healing. *Exp Mol Pathol.* 2005;78:131–134.
166. Makharita MY, Amr YM, El-Bayoumy Y. Effect of early stellate ganglion blockade for facial pain from acute herpes zoster and incidence of postherpetic neuralgia. *Pain Physician.* 2012;15:467–474.
167. Ji G, Niu J, Shi Y, Hou L, Lu Y, Xiong L. The effectiveness of repetitive paravertebral injections with local anesthetics and steroids for the prevention of postherpetic neuralgia in patients with acute herpes zoster. *Anesth Analg.* 2009;109:1651–1655.
168. van Wijck AJ, Opstelten W, Moons KG, et al. The PINE study of epidural steroids and local anaesthetics to prevent postherpetic neuralgia: a randomised controlled trial. *Lancet.* 2006;367:219–224.
169. Pasqualucci A, Pasqualucci V, Galla F, et al. Prevention of post-herpetic neuralgia: acyclovir and prednisolone versus epidural local anesthetic and methylprednisolone. *Acta Anaesthesiol Scand.* 2000;44:910–918.
170. Kotani N, Kushikata T, Hashimoto H, et al. Intrathecal methylprednisolone for intractable postherpetic neuralgia. *N Engl J Med.* 2000;343:1514–1519.
171. Bhargava R, Bhargava S, Haldia KN, Bhargava P. Jaipur block in postherpetic neuralgia. *Int J Dermatol.* 1998;37:465–468.
172. Naja ZM, Maaliki H, Al-Tannir MA, El-Rajab M, Ziade F, Zeidan A. Repetitive paravertebral nerve block using a catheter technique for pain relief in post-herpetic neuralgia. *Br J Anaesth.* 2006;96:381–383.
173. Kang FC, Chang PJ, Chen HP, Tsai YC. Patient-controlled epidural analgesia for postherpetic neuralgia in an HIV-infected patient as a therapeutic ambulatory modality. *Acta Anaesthesiol Sin.* 1998;36:235–239.

174. Forrest J. The response to epidural steroid injections in chronic dorsal root pain. *Can Anaesth Soc J* 1980;27:40–46.
175. Kikuchi A, Kotani N, Sato T, Takamura K, Sakai I, Matsuki A. Comparative therapeutic evaluation of intrathecal versus epidural methylprednisolone for long-term analgesia in patients with intractable postherpetic neuralgia. *Reg Anesth Pain Med.* 1999;24:287–293.
176. Dureja GP, Usmani H, Khan M, Tahseen M, Jamal A. Efficacy of intrathecal midazolam with or without epidural methylprednisolone for management of post-herpetic neuralgia involving lumbosacral dermatomes. *Pain Physician.* 2010;13:213–221.
177. Hsu-Tang L, Shen-Kou T, Ming-Chang K, Hu JS. Botulinum toxin A relieved neuropathic pain in a case of post-herpetic neuralgia. *Pain Med.* 2006;7:89–91.
178. Sotiriou E, Apalla Z, Panagiotidou D, Ioannidis D. Severe post-herpetic neuralgia successfully treated with botulinum toxin A: three case reports. *Acta Derm Venereol.* 2009;89:214–215.
179. Xiao L, Mackey S, Hui H, Xong D, Zhang Q, Zhang D. Subcutaneous injection of botulinum toxin A is beneficial in postherpetic neuralgia. *Pain Med.* 2010;11:1827–1833.
180. Yu HK, Le JH, Cho SH, Kim YI. Relief of postherpetic neuralgia with transforaminal epidural injection of magnesium—a case report. *Korean J Pain.* 2011;24:53–56.
181. Marineo G, Iorno V, Gandini C, Moschini V, Smith TJ. Scrambler therapy may relieve chronic neuropathic pain more effectively than guideline-based drug management: results of a pilot, randomized, controlled trial. *J Pain Symptom Manage.* 2012;43:87–95.
182. Barbarisi M, Aurilio C, Pace MC, et al. Pregabalin and transcutaneous electrical nerve stimulation for postherpetic neuralgia treatment. Clin J Pain. 2010;26:567–572.
183. Kouroukli I, Neofytos D, Panaretou V, et al. Peripheral subcutaneous stimulation for the treatment of intractable postherpetic neuralgia: two case reports and literature review. *Pain Pract.* 2009;9:225–229.
184. Yakovlev AE, Peterson AT. Peripheral nerve stimulation in treatment of intractable postherpetic neuralgia. *Neuromodulation.* 2007;10:373–375.
185. Johnson MD, Burchiel KJ. Peripheral stimulation for treatment of trigeminal postherpetic neuralgia and trigeminal posttraumatic neuropathic pain: a pilot study. *Neurosurgery.* 2004;55:135–141.
186. Rodrigo-Royo MD, Azcona JM, Quero J, Lorente MC, Acin P, Azcona J. Peripheral neurostimulation in the management of cervicogenic headache: four case reports. *Neuromodulation.* 2005;8:241–248.
187. Lynch PJ, McJunkin T, Eross E, Gooch S, Maloney J. Case report: successful epiradicular peripheral nerve stimulation of the C2 dorsal root ganglion for postherpetic neuralgia. *Neuromodulation.* 2011;14:58–61.
188. Sanchez-Ledesman MJ, Garcia-March G, Diaz-Cascajo P, Gomez-Moreta J, Broseta J. Spinal cord stimulation in deafferentation pain. *Stereotact Funct Neurosurg.* 1989;53:40–45.
189. Meglio M, Cioni B, Prezioso A, Talamonti G. Spinal cord stimulation (SCS) in the treatment of postherpetic pain. *Acta Neurochir Suppl* (Wein). 1989;46:65–66.
190. Harke H, Gretenkort P, Ladleif HU, Koester P, Rahman S. Spinal cord stimulation in postherpetic neuralgia and in acute herpes zoster pain. *Anesth Analg.* 2002;94:694–700.
191. Shimoji K, Hokari T, Kano T, et al. Management of intractable pain with percutaneous epidural spinal cord stimulation: differences in pain-relieving effects among diseases and sites of pain. *Anesth Analg.* 1993;77:110–116.
192. Kumar K, Toth C, Nath RK. Spinal cord stimulation for chronic pain in peripheral neuropathy. *Surg Neurol.* 1996;46:363–369.
193. Ebel H, Rust D, Tronnier V, Boker D, Kunze S. Chronic precentral stimulation in trigeminal neuropathic pain. *Acta Neurochir.* 1996;138:1300–1306.
194. Brown JA, Pilitsis JG. Motor cortex stimulation for central and neuropathic facial pain: a prospective study of 10 patients and observations of enhanced sensory and motor function during stimulation. *Neurosurgery.* 2005;56.
195. Lefaucheur JP, Drouot X, Cunin P, et al. Motor cortex stimulation for the treatment of refractory peripheral neuropathic pain. *Brain,* 2009;132:1463–1471.
196. Green AL, Nandi D, Armstrong G, Carter H, Aziz T. Post-herpetic trigeminal neuralgia treated with deep brain stimulation. *J Clin Neurosci.* 2003;10:512–514.
197. Owen SL, Green AL, Nandi DD, Bittar RG, Wang S, Aziz TZ. Deep brain stimulation for neuropathic pain. *Acta Neurochir.* 2007;97:111–116.
198. Petersen KL, Rice FL, Suess F, Berro M, Rowbotham MC. Relief of post-herpetic neuralgia by surgical removal of painful skin. *Pain.* 2002;98:119–126.
199. Petersen KL, Rowbotham MC. Relief of post-herpetic neuralgia by surgical removal of painful skin. *Pain.* 2007;131:214–218.
200. Jones MJ, Murrin KR. Intercostal block with cryotherapy. *Ann R Coll Surg Engl.* 1987;69:261–262.
201. Barnard D, Lloyd J, Evans J. Cryoanalgesia in the management of chronic facial pain. *J Maxillofac Surg.* 1981;9:101–102.
202. Kim SH, Shin JW, Leem JG, Suh JH. Pulsed radiofrequency treatment of the anterior ethmoidal nerve under nasal endoscopic guidance for the treatment of postherpetic neuralgia. *Anaesthesia.* 2011;66:1057–1058.
203. Lauretti GR, Trevelin WR, Frade LC, Lima IC. Spinal alcohol neurolysis for intractable thoracic postherpetic neuralgia after test bupivacaine spinal analgesia. *Anesthesiology.* 2004;101: 244–247.
204. Benzon HT, Chekka K, Darnule A, Chung B, Wille O, Malik K. Evidence-based case report: the prevention and management of postherpetic neuralgia with emphasis on interventional procedures. *Reg Anesth Pain Med.* 2009;34.
205. Urgosik D, Vymazal J, Vladyka V, Liscak R. Treatment of postherpetic trigeminal neuralgia with the Leksell gamma knife. *J Neurosurg.* 2000;93:165–168.
206. Kanpolat Y., Tuna H, Bozkurt M, Elhan AH. Spinal and nucleus caudalis dorsal root entry zone operations for chronic pain. *Neurosurgery.* 2008;62:235–42; discussion 242–244.
207. Samreen N, Friedman WA. Nucleus caudalis dorsal root entry zone lesions: a clinical-radiographic case report. *Stereotact Funct Neurosurg.* 2009;87:314–321.
208. Friedman AH, Nashold BS, Ovelmen-Levitt J. Dorsal root entry zone lesions for the treatment of post-herpetic neuralgia. *J Neurosurg.* 1984;60:1258–1262.
209. Young RF. Clinical experience with radiofrequency and laser DREZ lesions. *J Neurosurg.* 1990;72:715–720.
210. Rath SA, Braun V, Soliman N, Antoniadis G, Richter HP. Results of DREZ coagulations for pain related to plexus lesions, spinal cord injuries and postherpetic neuralgia. *Acta Neurochir Suppl* (Wien). 1996;138:364–369.
211. Kim SH, Lee KH, Kim SC, Chung SS, Lee KC, Lee HJ. Percutaneous cervical radiofrequency cordotomy for intractable pain. *Yonsei Med J.* 1975;16:72–82.
212. Kanpolat Y. The surgical treatment of chronic pain: destructive therapies in the spinal cord. *Neurosurg Clin N Am.* 2004;15:307–317.
213. Hitchcock ER, Schvarcz JR. Stereotaxic trigeminal tractotomy for post-herpetic facial pain. *J Neurosurg.* 1972;37:412–417.
214. Schvarcz JR. Stereotactic extralemniscal myelotomy. *J Neurol Neurosurg Psychiatry.* 1976;39:53–57.
215. Young RF, Jacques DS, Rand RW, Copcutt BR. Medial thalamotomy with the Leksell Gamma Knife for treatment of chronic pain. *Acta Neurochir.* 1994; 62(suppl):105–110.
216. Vogt BA, Derbyshire S, Jones AK. Pain processing in four regions of human cingulate cortex localized with co-registered PET and MR imaging. *Eur J Neurosci.* 1996;8:1461–1473.

217. Ballantine HT Jr, Giriunas IE. Treatment of intractable psychiatric illness and chronic pain by stereotactic cingulotomy. In Schmidek HH, Sweet WH, eds. *Operative neurosurgical techniques. indications, methods, and results.* Philadelphia: WB Saunders; 1988:1069–1075.
218. Elithorn A, Glithero E, Slater E. Leucotomy for pain. *J Neurol Neurosurg Psychiatry.* 1958;21:249–261.
219. Lijima K, Shimoyama N., Shimoyama M, Mizuguchi T. Evaluation of analgesic effect of low-power He:Ne laser on postherpetic neuralgia using VAS and modified McGill pain questionnaire. *J Clin Laser Med Surg.* 1991;9:121–126.
220. Calandria L. Cryoanalgesia for post-herpetic neuralgia: a new treatment. *Int J Dermatol.* 2011;50:746–750.
221. Nurmikko T, Wells C, Bowsher D. Pain and allodynia in postherpetic neuralgia: role of somatic and sympathetic nervous systems. *Acta Neurol Scand.* 1991;84:146–152.
222. Jalili MH, Ansarin H, Soltani-Arabshahi R. Broad-band ultraviolet B phototherapy in zoster patients may reduce the incidence and severity of postherpetic neuralgia. *Photodermatol Photoimmunol Photomed.* 2006;22:232–237.
223. Ursini T, Tontodonati M, Manzoli L, et al. Acupuncture for the treatment of severe acute pain in herpes zoster: results of a nested, open-label, randomized trial in the VZV pain study. *BMC Comp Alt Med.* 2011;11:46.
224. Lewith GT, Field J, Machin D. Acupuncture compared with placebo in post-herpetic pain. *Pain.* 1983;17:361–368.
225. Cao H, Zhu C, Liu J. Wet cupping therapy for treatment of herpes zoster: a systematic review of randomized controlled trials. *Altern Ther Health Med.* 2010;16:48–54.
226. Hijikata Y, Yasuhara A, Sahashi Y. Effect of an herbal formula containing Ganoderma lucidum on reduction of herpes zoster pain: a pilot clinical trial. *Am J Chin Med.* 2005;33:517–523.
227. Cooper R, Dragar C, Elliot K, Fitton JH, Godwin J, Thompson K. GFS, a preparation of Tasmanian Undaria pinnatifida is associated with healing and inhibition of reactivation of herpes. *BMC Comp Alt Med.* 2002;2:11.
228. Sangkitporn S, Chaiwat S, Balachandra K, Na-Ayudhaya TD, Bunjob M, Jayavasu C. Treatment of herpes zoster with Clinacanthus nutans (bi phaya yaw) extract. *J Md Assoc Thai.* 1995;78:624–627.
229. Hui F, Boyle E, Vayda E, Glazier R. A randomized controlled trial of a multifaceted integrated complementary—alternative therapy for chronic herpes zoster-related pain. *Altern Med Rev.* 2012;17:57–68.
230. Jensen MP, Chodroff MJ, Dworkin RH. The impact of neuropathic pain on health-related quality of life: review and implications. *Neurology.* 2007;68:1178–1182.
231. Tashiro S, Akaboshi K, Kobayashi Y, Mori T, Nagata M, Liu M. Herpes zoster-induced trunk muscle paresis presenting with abdominal wall pseudohernia, scoliosis, and gait disturbance and its rehabilitation: a case report. *Arch Phys Med Rehab.* 2010;91:321–325.
232. Head H, Campbell HW. The pathology of herpes zoster and its bearing on sensory localization. *Brain.* 1900;23:353–523.
233. Watson CPN, Morshead C, Van der Kooy D, Deck J, Evans RJ. Post-herpetic neuralgia: post-mortem analysis of a case. *Pain.* 1988;34:129–138.
234. Watson CP, Watt VR, Chipman M, et al. The prognosis with postherpetic neuralgia. *Pain.* 1991;46:195–199.
235. Attal N, Cruccu G, Baron R, et al. EFNS guidelines on the pharmacological treatment of neuropathic pain: 2010 revision. *Eur J Neurol.* 2010;17:1113–e88.
236. Dworkin RH, O'Connor AB, Backonja M, et al. Pharmacologic management of neuropathic pain: evidence-based recommendations. *Pain.* 2007;132:237–251.
237. Dworkin RH, O'Connor AB, Audette J, et al. Recommendations for the pharmacological management of neuropathic pain: an overview and literature update. *Mayo Clin Proc.* 2010;85:S3–S14.
238. Moulin DE, Clark AJ, Gilron I, et al. Pharmacological management of chronic neuropathic pain—consensus statement and guidelines from the Canadian Pain Society. *Pain Res Manage.* 2007;12:13–21.
239. Dubinsky RM, Kabbani H, El-Chami Z, Boutwell C, Ali H. Practice parameter: treatment of postherpetic neuralgia: an evidence-based report of the quality standards subcommittee of the American Academy of Neurology. *Neurology.* 2004;63:959–965.

3.

TRIGEMINAL NEURALGIA AND OTHER FACIAL PAIN CONDITIONS

Kevin E. Vorenkamp, Afton L. Hassett, Gregory M. Figg, Jennifer Sweet, and Jonathan Miller

CASE PRESENTATION

A 45-year-old female executive presents with right-sided headache of 6-month duration. The pain started spontaneously in the right cheek area and, following dental work, became more frequent and intense. The pain is described as constant burning with occasional spasms. It is made worse by chewing. It is occasionally associated with eyelid twitching but not lacrimation or sensitivity to light. It is not relieved by acetaminophen or nonsteroidal anti-inflammatory drugs (NSAIDs). The patient is currently on cyclobenzaprine and oxycodone. The pain and the analgesics have been interfering with her focus and work and have affected her mood negatively. She blames previous physicians for "mishandling her pain." She is referred to the Interdisciplinary Pain Medicine Clinic.

Past medical history is significant for obsessive-compulsive behavior.

Social history is significant for being divorced within the last year. She drinks alcohol socially and denies illicit drugs or smoking.

Review of systems is significant for the medications listed above.

On examination, the patient weighs 92 kg and is 186 cm tall. Her neurologic examination is significant for occasional twitching in the right cheek and eyelid. She has an audible click when opening the jaw and mild decreased sensation over the right cheek and mandible.

QUESTIONS

1. What is the differential diagnosis of facial pain in this case?
   a. What are the most common neuropathic facial pain conditions?
   b. What further history may be useful in making the diagnosis?
   c. What diagnostic studies may be helpful?
2. What anatomical structures are involved with facial pain?
3. What is the pathophysiology of the facial pain diagnoses?
4. What are the common comorbidities of the facial pain diagnoses?
5. How are the patient's medications managed in facial pain diagnoses?
6. What other approaches may be considered for managing this patient?
   a. Behavioral approaches
   b. Microvascular decompression (MVD)
   c. Ablative procedures
   d. Rehabilitation

WHAT IS THE DIFFERENTIAL DIAGNOSIS OF FACIAL PAIN IN THIS CASE?

The differential diagnosis for facial pain in this patient is extensive. Chronic facial pain may result from a diverse assortment of causes including trauma, structural abnormalities (temporomandibular joint, neurovascular compression, etc.), infections, tumors, central nervous system (CNS) disease, and primary headache disorders, or it may reflect referred pain from the neck.

Facial pain can be due to neuropathic pain syndromes that result from unintentional trauma, deafferentation, and cephalic neuralgias. Some of the more common cephalic neuralgias include trigeminal neuralgia (TN), tic convulsif (combined trigeminal neuralgia and hemifacial spasm), geniculate neuralgia, glossopharyngeal neuralgia, and occipital neuralgia. Persistent idiopathic facial pain (PIFP), incorporating the previous diagnosis of atypical facial pain, represents an idiopathic facial pain condition that does not have the clinical characteristics of particular cranial neuralgias.

In classic trigeminal neuralgia (CTN), there are no accompanying laboratory or radiographic abnormalities. Although gross motor or sensory abnormalities are not typically found on physical examination, more sensitive tests such as quantitative sensory testing and blink reflex studies reveal abnormal responses in most patients. Although TN and PIFP are two of the most common etiologies of paroxysmal facial pain, other "red flag" conditions (tumor, infection, vascular abnormality/dissection, fracture, and intracranial hemorrhage) must first be excluded. Additionally, other comorbidities, such as demyelinating, autoimmune or neuromuscular conditions, should be identified. When patients exhibit abnormalities such as sensory loss in the fifth cranial nerve (CN) distribution, weakness in the muscles of mastication, or abnormality of any other CN, consideration of a lesion involving the trigeminal ganglion, main sensory root, or root entry zone in the pons must be given. Herpetic infections of the trigeminal nerve can produce symptoms of neuralgia that affect the geniculate ganglion of the facial nerve, as in Ramsay-Hunt syndrome. Isolated involvement of the ophthalmic division (V1) warrants further questioning regarding a prior rash in that area. Similarly, multiple sclerosis (MS), a demyelinating disease, can elicit symptoms of unilateral or occasionally bilateral trigeminal neuralgia. Bilateral symptoms of paroxysmal facial pain typical of TN increase suspicion of MS. In addition to TN, there is a set of primary headache disorders that may warrant consideration.

Inflammation is a well-established pain generator, and inflammatory disorders play a major role in many facial pain syndromes. One example is Tolosa-Hunt, which affects the contents of the superior orbital fissure including the first and second divisions of the trigeminal nerve. Other examples include pseudotumor of the orbit, Raeder's paratrigeminal neuralgia, and optic neuritis.[1] Vascular syndromes such as migraine, cluster headache and other trigeminal autonomic cephalalgias (TACs), and giant cell arteritis account for many cases of facial pain. Extracranial and intracranial neoplasms such as schwannomas, meningiomas, and epidermoids must also be considered in the differential diagnosis.[2] Finally, musculoskeletal conditions such as temporomandibular joint disorders may cause dull, aching pain or tenderness, often worsened with jaw movement. Pathology affecting the teeth or gums may result in deep, sharp pain triggered by eating. This can also be seen with infectious processes such as Gradenigo's syndrome or apical petrositis, or more common infections involving the ears, sinuses, and mastoids.

WHAT ARE THE MOST COMMON NEUROPATHIC FACIAL PAIN CONDITIONS?

Neuropathic Pain

Neuropathic pain is a condition that results from disease or injury to nociceptive neurons (A-δ and C fibers) within the central or peripheral nervous system.[3] This is distinct from nociceptive pain, which is caused by activation of pain receptors. Neural fibers affected in neuropathic pain may show evidence of demyelination and dysfunction of ion channels, leading to alterations in neurotransmitters and second-messenger systems. This results in spontaneous action potentials, ephaptic transmission, and nuclear hyperexcitability of pain fibers.[4] Patients experience symptoms ranging from constant burning and aching pain to severe, paroxysmal shock-like pain in the distribution of the affected nerve. Neuropathic pain may be distinguished from other pain syndromes by the following criteria: (1) pain and sensory symptoms persist beyond the expected period of healing; (2) neurological sensory signs may present as negative sensory phenomena or positive sensory phenomena such as pain, dysesthesia, and hyperalgesia; and (3) negative and positive motor and autonomic signs may also be present.[5]

Neuropathic pain syndromes account for many cases of facial pain, and it is essential to differentiate between the various disorders in order to accurately diagnose and treat patients. The importance of obtaining a thorough patient history and physical examination cannot be overemphasized. The aim of this chapter is to provide a model for workup of patients with neuropathic facial pain, particularly trigeminal and glossopharyngeal neuralgia, using the clinical vignette as a guide.

Neuropathic Facial Pain

TN

Facial pain syndromes such as trigeminal and glossopharyngeal neuralgia are classified as peripheral neuropathic pain disorders because they most commonly arise from injury related to neurovascular compression at their respective root entry zone.[6] Of the facial pain disorders, TN is the most common, with an estimated 15,000 new cases per year in the United States.[7] Worldwide incidence of new patients is commonly reported in the range of 4–27/100,000 (0.004%)[8]; however, a recent population based study of 3,336 people in Essen, Germany, found a lifetime prevalence nearly 100 times greater (10/3336, 0.3%)[9] than the prior estimates. This incidence increases with older age—90% of cases begin after age 40—and with the female gender (1.5:1).[7,10] Classically, TN has been defined as paroxysmal episodes of sharp, lancinating pain with exacerbations and remissions following the distribution of the trigeminal nerve, pain precipitated by tactile stimuli, and pain that is idiopathic without neurological deficit or mass lesion on magnetic resonance imaging (MRI).[11] Typically, the attacks of pain last only seconds, but the pain may be repetitive at short intervals so that the individual attacks blur into one another. After many attacks, the patient may describe a residual lingering facial pain.

The etiology of TN is often due to vascular compression of the nerve at the brainstem or distally. There are two types of TN with identical clinical features: (1) CTN [1] and (2) symptomatic TN (if a structural lesion other than vascular compression is identified as etiology).[12] Figure 3.1 compares the characteristics and treatment responsiveness

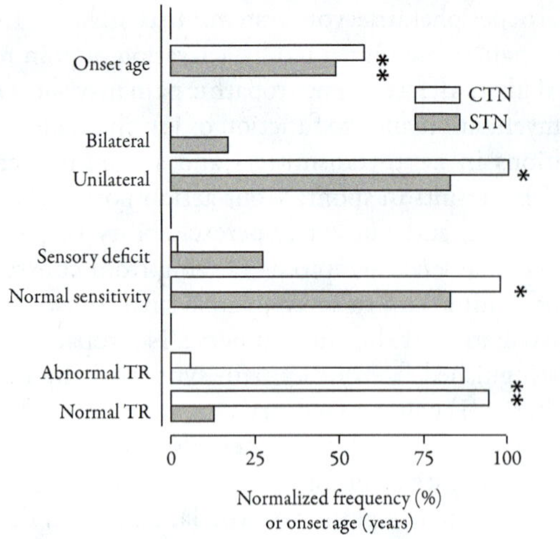

Figure 3.1 Mean age and relative frequency of clinical characteristics and abnormal trigeminal reflexes in classic trigeminal neuralgia (CTN) and symptomatic trigeminal neuralgia (STN). Reprinted with permission from Gronseth G, Cruccu G, Alksne J, Argoff C, Brainin M, Burchiel K, et al. Practice parameter: the diagnostic evaluation and treatment of trigeminal neuralgia (an evidence-based review): report of the Quality Standards subcommittee of the American Academy of Neurology and the European Federation of Neurological Societies. *Neurology*. 2008; 71:1183–1190.

of patients with CTN and symptomatic TN (STN). More recently, the third edition of the international classification of headache disorders (ICHD-3) has been released and divides trigeminal neuralgia into classical trigeminal neuralgia and trigeminal neuropathy (Boxes 3.1 and 3.2)[13]. For the purposes of this chapter, we will continue to discuss characterics under the prior ICHD-II diagnoses which coincide

Box 3.1 ICHD-III DIAGNOSTIC CRITERIA FOR CLASSICAL TRIGEMINAL NEURALGIA

A. At least three attacks of unilateral facial pain fulfilling criteria B and C
B. Occurring in one or more divisions of the trigeminal nerve, with no radiation beyond the trigeminal distribution
C. Pain has at least three of the following characteristics:
   1. recurring in paroxysmal attacks lasting from a fraction of a second to 2 minutes
   2. severe intensity
   3. electric shock-like, shooting, stabbing, or sharp in quality
   4. precipitated by innocuous stimuli to the affected side of the face
D. No clinically evident neurological deficit
E. Not better accounted for by another ICHD-3 diagnosis

ICHD, The International Classification of Headache Disorder

Adapted from Headache Classification Subcommittee of the International Headache Society. The International Classification of Headache Disorders, 3rd edition. *Cephalalgia*. 2013;33(9):629-808.

Box 3.2 ICHD-III DIAGNOSTIC CRITERIA FOR PAINFUL TRIGEMINAL NEUROPATHY ATTRIBUTED TO OTHER DISORDER

1. Head and/or facial pain with the characteristics of *Classical trigeminal neuralgia* with or without concomitant persistent facial pain, but not necessarily unilateral
2. A disorder, other than those described above but known to be capable of causing painful trigeminal neuropathy, has been diagnosed
3. Pain has developed after onset of the disorder, or led to its discovery
4. Not better accounted for by another ICHD-3 diagnosis

Adapted from Headache Classification Subcommittee of the International Headache Society. The International Classification of Headache Disorders, 3d ed. *Cephalalgia*. 2013;33(9):629–808.

with the relevant literature. Whereas average age of onset does little to differentiate CTN from STN, presence of bilateral symptoms, sensory deficit, and especially an abnormal trigeminal reflex all suggest STN, as demonstrated in Figure 3.1.[14]

The symptoms of both types of TN consist of pain in one or more branches of the trigeminal nerve, most commonly involving the maxillary (V2) and/or mandibular (V3) divisions (Table 3.1[7]). The pain rarely occurs bilaterally and more commonly affects the right side (59–66%). If the pain is bilateral, a central cause such as MS should be considered. Between paroxysms, the patient is usually pain-free, but a dull, continuous pain may persist in some long-standing cases, suggesting a role for central sensitization.[15] A painful paroxysm is often triggered by non-noxious stimuli (touch, movement, wind exposure, brushing teeth, shaving, chewing, and swallowing) and is usually followed by a refractory period during which pain cannot be triggered. Such triggers are often on the anterior aspect of the face, especially the nasolabial fold and the side of the chin (Figure 3.2[16]).

Table 3.1 PAIN DISTRIBUTION IN TRIGEMINAL NEURALGIA

TRIGEMINAL NERVE BRANCH AFFECTED (PAIN)	PERCENTAGE (%) OF PATIENTS
V1 only	4
V2 only	17
V3 only	15
V1 + V2	14
V2 + V3	32
V1 + V2 + V3	17

Modified and used with permission from Rozen TD. Trigeminal neuralgia and glossopharyngeal neuralgia. *Neurol Clin*. 2004;22:185–206.[7]

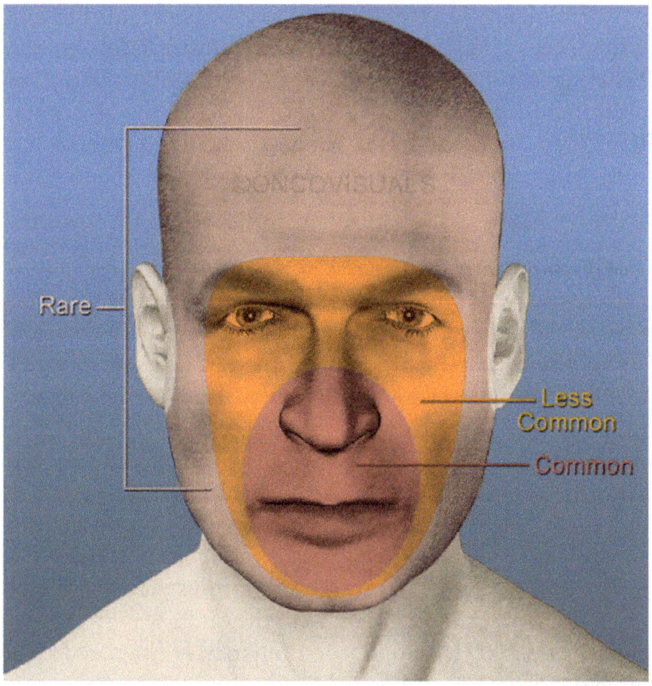

Figure 3.2 Trigger areas for trigeminal neuralgia pain. Reprinted with permission from American Society of Anesthesiology and American Society of Regional Anesthesia and Pain Medicine self-assessment module for pain medicine, 2012.

The pain frequently evokes spasm of the muscle of the face on the affected side. Nicolaus André, a French surgeon, coined the term "*tic douloureux*" to describe the violent reactions that his patients displayed in response to their characteristically intense bouts of pain.[17]

However, although the symptoms of typical TN are distinctive, in many individuals, the syndrome can present in an atypical manner. In these instances, patients can experience aching and throbbing pain that is long in duration or even constant. Alternatively, patients may complain of both a continuous underlying discomfort, which may or may not be triggered in onset, and a severe, paroxysmal pain with any number of additional sensory findings. Thus, over time, the term "atypical TN" has become an umbrella phrase under which all facial pain disorders differing from typical TN fell. PIFP is now the more appropriate diagnosis for this condition.

Various classification schematics have been devised to aid physicians in the diagnosis and management of facial pain disorders. One such system frequently employed by neurosurgeons describes two types of TN and distinguishes between TN and neuropathic facial pain.[18] Type 1 TN is characterized by an idiopathic, spontaneous onset of sharp, electric pain in one or more distributions of the trigeminal nerve, with clear triggers and distinct episodes separated by pain-free periods. This relapsing and remitting sequence, along with the intense quality of the pain must be the predominant symptom for more than 50% of the time. In contrast, in type 2 TN an idiopathic, constant, aching and throbbing pain is the primary symptom more than 50% of the time.[18] Type 2 TN may now be regarded as PIFP and will be referred to as such for the remainder of the chapter. The type of TN with which a patient presents can serve as a predictive measure of outcome following surgical intervention.[19]

This classification system also differentiates between TN and other nonidiopathic facial pain syndromes: trigeminal deafferentation pain, post-herpetic TN, and atypical facial pain. As mentioned earlier, symptomatic TN is caused by demyelination of the trigeminal nerve due to MS or another identified structural lesion other than vascular compression. Trigeminal deafferentation pain is a by-product of an intentional lesioning procedure such as a neurectomy, rhizotomy, tractotomy, or other form of denervation. These patients frequently complain of a feeling of burning or crawling. The most severe form of this is *anesthesia dolorosa*, in which patients have an unrelenting pain in the area of the face that lacks sensation.[20] Postherpetic TN can occur following a herpes infection and tends to present in the ophthalmic division of the trigeminal nerve. Finally, atypical facial pain refers to somatoform pain disorder in which patients have psychogenic facial pain. Formal psychological testing is necessary to establish the diagnosis of atypical facial pain.[20] As noted earlier, the term "atypical facial pain" is no longer a proper diagnosis, and PIFP may be used when diagnostic criteria are met.

Tic Convulsif

Tic convulsif is a condition in which patients have clinical findings consistent with TN along with involuntary contractions of the face as seen in hemifacial spasm. This can be explained by vascular compression at the root entry zone of both the fifth and seventh CNs or, less likely, by compression at only one site in the setting of aberrant innervation between the trigeminal and facial nerves.[21]

PIFP

Another consideration in cases where diagnostic criteria of TN are not met is PIFP. PIFP, previously termed "atypical facial pain," is described as a persistent facial pain that does not have the classical characteristics of cranial neuralgias and for which there is no obvious cause (Box 3.3[13]). As noted earlier, ICHD-III now incorporates the diagnosis of trigeminal neuropathy, which would now capture many patients with the prior diagnosis of PIFP; however, we will

Box 3.3 ICHD-III DIAGNOSTIC CRITERIA FOR PERSISTENT IDIOPATHIC FACIAL PAIN

Pain in the face, present on a daily basis, satisfying criteria B and C
Pain is confined at onset to a limited area on one side of the face, is deep and poorly localized
Pain is not associated with sensory loss or other physical signs
Clinical and imaging investigations do not demonstrate any relevant abnormalities of the face

ICHD, The International Classification of Headache Disorder

Adapted from Headache Classification Subcommittee of the International Headache Society. The International Classification of Headache Disorders, 3rd edition. *Cephalalgia*. 2013;33(9):629-808.

continue to use the ICHD-II criteria for PIFP in this chapter. Although the estimated incidence has been (under-) reported as 1/100,000,[22] Mueller showed 1/3,336 in their study.[9] The same study found that TN had a ten times greater lifetime prevalence than PIFP in the same population. The diagnosis is made following exclusion of other possible causes and if pain is present daily (for all or most of the day) and is fairly localized. Pain is usually in the maxilla, but may extend to the eyes, nose, cheeks, and temple. By definition, neurological and physical examination findings should be normal; however, abnormalities are often appreciated on more sensitive tests, including blink reflex (BR) and quantitative sensory testing (QST) assessments,[23] as demonstrated in Table 3.2.

Table 3.2 **CLINICAL FEATURES OF TRIGEMINAL NEURALGIA AND PERSISTENT IDIOPATHIC FACIAL PAIN**

FEATURE	TRIGEMINAL NEURALGIA (TN)	PERSISTENT IDIOPATHIC FACIAL PAIN (PIFP)/ ATYPICAL FACIAL PAIN
Age of Onset (years)	>50	Variable
Gender (Female: Male)	1.5–2:1	2–4:1
Frequency	Intermittent	Constant, fluctuates
Pain-Free Intervals	Always	Rarely, Never
Description	Electric, stabbing, shooting	Burning, aching
Precipitation Factors	Triggered, non-noxious	Rarely triggered
Causative Factors	Vascular, Multiple Sclerosis, Tumor	Idiopathic,[b] Tumor, Infection, Trauma, Mechanical
Normal BR and QST[a]	0%	25%
Abnormal QST[a]		
Thermal hypoesthesia	100%	45%
Warm allodynia	–	10%
BR changes[a]		
Abnormal BR	58%	15%
Deficient habituation (excitability)	33%	35%

[a]BR, blink reflex; QST, quantitative sensory testing.

[b]By definition, PIFP cannot be attributed to identifiable structural abnormalities such as tumor or infection.

Data from Forsell H, Tenovuo O, Silvoniemi P, Jaaskelainen SK. Differences and similarities between atypical facial pain and trigeminal neuropathic pain. *Neurology.* 2007;69:1451–1459, modified and used with permission from Vorenkamp KE. Interventional procedures for facial pain. *Curr Pain Headache Rep.* 2012;17:308. Epub ahead of print.

Additionally, particular attention to ruling out metastatic lung cancer is noted, as well as other differential diagnoses, including cervicogenic headache. Table 3.2[23,24] illustrates some of the differences between the characteristics of TN and PIFP. Compared with TN, patients with PIFP benefit less from medications, interventional procedures, and open surgical techniques.

Glossopharyngeal Neuralgia

Patients with glossopharyngeal neuralgia often describe pain in the throat, tonsillar region, posterior third of the tongue, larynx, nasopharynx, and pinna of the ear. Glossopharyngeal neuralgia produces symptoms of severe, lancinating, paroxysmal pain deep in the throat that is triggered by tactile stimuli such as swallowing or coughing. The symptoms can vary and frequently involve different dermatomal territories supplied by the ninth CN. For instance, patients may experience pain primarily in the ear that later spreads to the throat, referred to as the *tympanic form*. Conversely, symptoms may initially be felt in the throat and then extend to the ear, as seen in the *oropharyngeal form*.[21] It is not uncommon to have associated vagal nerve symptoms as well, which can result in syncopal events and bradycardia. The diagnosis of glossopharyngeal neuralgia can be confirmed by temporary resolution of symptoms with the application of 10% topical cocaine to the trigger zone.[21]

TACs

Consideration of the diagnosis of the TACs should be given in any circumstance under which unilateral facial pain is accompanied by autonomic features such as lacrimation, conjunctival injection, or nasal symptoms. Included within this category are cluster headache, paroxysmal hemicrania, and short-lasting unilateral neuralgiform headache attacks with conjunctival injection and tearing (SUNCT)/short-lasting unilateral neuralgiform headache attacks with cranial autonomic features (SUNA). In addition to these entities, hemicrania continua may exhibit many similar characteristics. The TACs are distinguished predominantly by the frequency of attacks and duration of symptoms, and diagnosis of one versus another may lead to a change in treatment plan because they respond to specific treatments in each case (Table 3.3[25]). Proper diagnosis will assist in the choice of appropriate treatment and allow the clinician and patient to understand the prognosis for successful treatment. As a rule, cluster headache has the longest attack duration with lowest attack frequency. Paroxysmal hemicrania is of intermediate duration and frequency, and the SUNCT/SUNA attacks are the shortest in duration, but have the greatest attack frequency. Hemicrania continua is by definition continuous, but may have frequent exacerbations accompanied by autonomic symptoms.

WHAT FURTHER HISTORY MAY BE USEFUL IN MAKING THE DIAGNOSIS?

The description of the distribution of the pain is paramount in the proper diagnosis. Patients with glossopharyngeal neuralgia often describe pain in the throat, tonsillar region,

Table 3.3 CLINICAL CHARACTERISTICS USED TO DIFFERENTIATE CLUSTER HEADACHE FROM PAROXYSMAL HEMICRANIA AND SUNCT/SUNA

	CLUSTER HEADACHE	PAROXYSMAL HEMICRANIA	SUNCT/SUNA
Sex ratio	3 Males to 1 Female	Males = Females	1.5 Males to 1 Female
Pain			
Quality	Sharp/stab/throb	Sharp/stab/throb	Sharp/stab/throb
Severity	Very severe	Very severe	Severe
Distribution	V1 > C2 > V2 > V3	V1 > C2 > V2 > V3	V1 > C2 > V2 > V3
Attacks			
frequency (per day)	1–8	11	100
length (minutes)	30–180	2–30	1–10
Triggers			
alcohol	+++	+	–
nitroglycerin	+++	+	–
cutaneous	–	–	+++
Agitation/restlessness	90%	80%	65%
Episodic versus chronic	90:10	35:65	10:90
Circadian/circannual periodicity	Present	Absent	Absent
Treatment effects			
oxygen	70%	No effect	No effect
sumatriptan (6 mg)	90%	20%	<10%
indomethacin	No effect	100%	No effect
Migraine features with attacks			
nausea	50%	40%	25%
photophobia/phonophobia	65%	65%	25%

SUNCT/SUNA, Short-lasting unilateral neuralgiform headache attacks with conjunctival injection and tearing/short-lasting unilateral neuralgiform headache attacks with cranial autonomic features; C, cervical; V, trigeminal.

Reprinted with permission from Goadsby P. Trigeminal autonomic cephalalgias. *Continuum.* 2012;18(4):883–895.

posterior third of the tongue, larynx, nasopharynx, and pinna of the ear. More commonly, the trigeminal nerve, CN V, is involved, and, most commonly, the pain affects the maxillary (V2) and/or mandibular (V3) branches. Patients will describe the pain as electric shock-like, shooting, or lancinating. Typically, the attacks of pain last only seconds, but the pain may be repetitive at short intervals so that the individual attacks blur into one another. After many attacks, the patient may describe a residual lingering facial pain.

Although there is often overlap between the signs and symptoms of the conditions, a series of six questions has been proposed to differentiate between the types of orofacial pain:[26]

1. Does the pain occur in attacks?
2. Are most of the attacks of a short duration (seconds to minutes)?
3. Do you sometimes have extremely short attacks?
4. Are the attacks unilateral?
5. Do the attacks occur in the distribution of the trigeminal nerve?
6. Are there unilateral autonomous symptoms?

Many aspects of the history of the patient in the sample vignette are consistent with TN. First, her pain was spontaneous in onset, without a clear inciting event. She also has specific triggers that elicit her symptoms, namely, chewing food. However, the patient's pain has qualities of both TN and PIFP, since she has constant burning pain in addition to episodic spasms. It would thus be helpful to ask the patient which symptoms predominate.

The patient also presents with motor findings consisting of involuntary twitching. This is compatible with symptoms of hemifacial spasm, seen with neurovascular compression of the seventh CN. The combination of TN symptoms with hemifacial spasms is referred to as tic convulsif, and this is high on the differential diagnosis in the clinical vignette. PIFP, on the other hand, may account for more of the constant aching pain that she describes, but does not typically present with the twitching the patient describes, although a secondary myofascial component cannot be excluded.

WHAT DIAGNOSTIC STUDIES MAY BE HELPFUL?

Although the diagnosis of TN remains a clinical one, various imaging modalities are available to aid in both the diagnosis and determination of treatment for TN. Findings on neurologic examination are essentially normal in patients with classic TN, although abnormalities are noted with BR, and QST commonly reveals thermal hypoesthesia.[23] Gross abnormalities on neurologic examination are more indicative of symptomatic TN. Investigation for a symptomatic cause is suggested in the event of any focal neurological examination finding and particularly in the case of facial sensory loss. Differential diagnosis includes MS, basilar artery aneurysm, neoplasm, arterial or venous compression, syringobulbia, and brainstem infarction. MRI with and without contrast and vascular imaging are reasonable studies in this setting. Although the presence of vascular compression on MRI may determine subsequent treatment approaches, it is worthwhile to note that compressing blood vessels are seen in one-third of asymptomatic patients.[14]

Since the arrival of MRI, clinicians have been able to identify compression of the trigeminal nerve by tumors or large blood vessels preoperatively. However, the ability to visualize subtleties, such as mild indentation of the nerve by finer arteries or veins, has only recently emerged. Balanced fast-field echo (BFFE) images allow for very high-resolution T2-weighted images with substantial contrast between the bright cerebrospinal fluid (CSF) and the darker structures of the brain, nerves, vessels, and bones (Figure 3.3). Three-dimensional high-resolution time-of-flight MR angiography and postgadolinium spoiled gradient (SPGR) MRI can be used to distinguish between the neurovascular structures. Technological advancements such as these allow clinicians to formulate accurate diagnoses and devise better treatment strategies.

Clinical Correlate

In the case of the patient in the vignette, the use of sophisticated imaging modalities may help support a suspected diagnosis of TN or tic convulsif. By obtaining MR imaging and performing postprocessing image fusion and reconstruction, one might see vascular compression of both the fifth and seventh CNs, which might have significant implications on treatment options, particularly if MVD is thought likely to relieve her symptoms. Determining the type of TN from which a patient suffers and radiographic confirmation of the underlying etiology may help establish potential candidacy for surgery. Conversely, if vascular compression or other structural abnormality were not apparent, the patient would have PIFP, although further workup may be indicated.

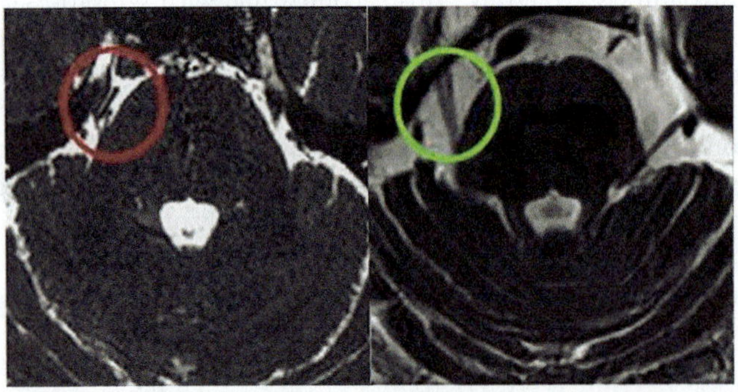

Figure 3.3 (Left) Balanced fast-field echo magnetic resonance image (MRI) demonstrating vascular compression of the trigeminal nerve as it exits the pons. (Right) Balanced fast-field echo MRI of noncompressed trigeminal nerve exiting pons.

WHAT ANATOMICAL STRUCTURES ARE INVOLVED WITH FACIAL PAIN?

ANATOMY OF HEAD PAIN

A multitude of anatomical structures are potentially responsible for head pain. The brain parenchyma is insensate, but the dura mater, dural vessels, proximal cerebral arteries, venous sinuses, tendons, face, eyes, ears, scalp, oropharynx, and sinuses are potentially painful. Transmission of this pain can occur through the upper cervical nerve roots or the CNs, specifically CN III, IV, V, VII, IX, and X. Of particular interest is CN V, the trigeminal nerve. The interconnections of this CN are complex and include somatic and autonomic components. The trigeminal nerve or fifth cranial nerve (CN V) is the largest among the facial nerves, and its branches provide the cutaneous innervation of the head and face. It also innervates muscles that move the lower jaw.

The trigeminal (Gasserian) ganglion, located in the middle cranial fossa, was named after Johann Lorentz Gasser (1723–1765), a Viennese anatomist.[27] The ganglion occupies a CSF-containing cavity (Meckel's cave) in the dura mater, with the dura covering the posterior two-thirds of the ganglion. The ganglion, formed by the fusion of a series of midpontine rootlets, is located near the apex of the petrous part of the temporal bone. The ganglion is bound medially by the cavernous sinus and optic and trochlear nerves, superiorly by the temporal lobe, and posteriorly by the brainstem. The ganglion interfaces with the autonomic nervous system through several ganglia and also through communicating nerves. These include the ciliary, sphenopalatine, otic, and submaxillary ganglia and the oculomotor, facial, and glossopharyngeal nerves (Figure 3.4).

Unmyelinated C fibers pass through the trigeminal (Gasserian) ganglion, enter the pons, and proceed to the trigeminal nucleus caudalis. This structure runs from the medulla down into the region of the third cervical segment, where it blends into the dorsal horn to form the trigeminocervical complex. This arrangement explains the phenomenon of head pain referred from cervical pathology. Fibers from the upper cervical roots enter the trigeminal nucleus caudalis, which sends fibers rostrally to the thalamus and collaterals to the autonomic nuclei in the brainstem and hypothalamus. Thalamic neurons then project to the somatosensory cortex and to the limbic system. Additionally, there is a polysynaptic connection to the parasympathetic superior salivatory nucleus in the pons. This nucleus innervates meningeal vessels and the contents of the nasal sinuses and eyes. Because of

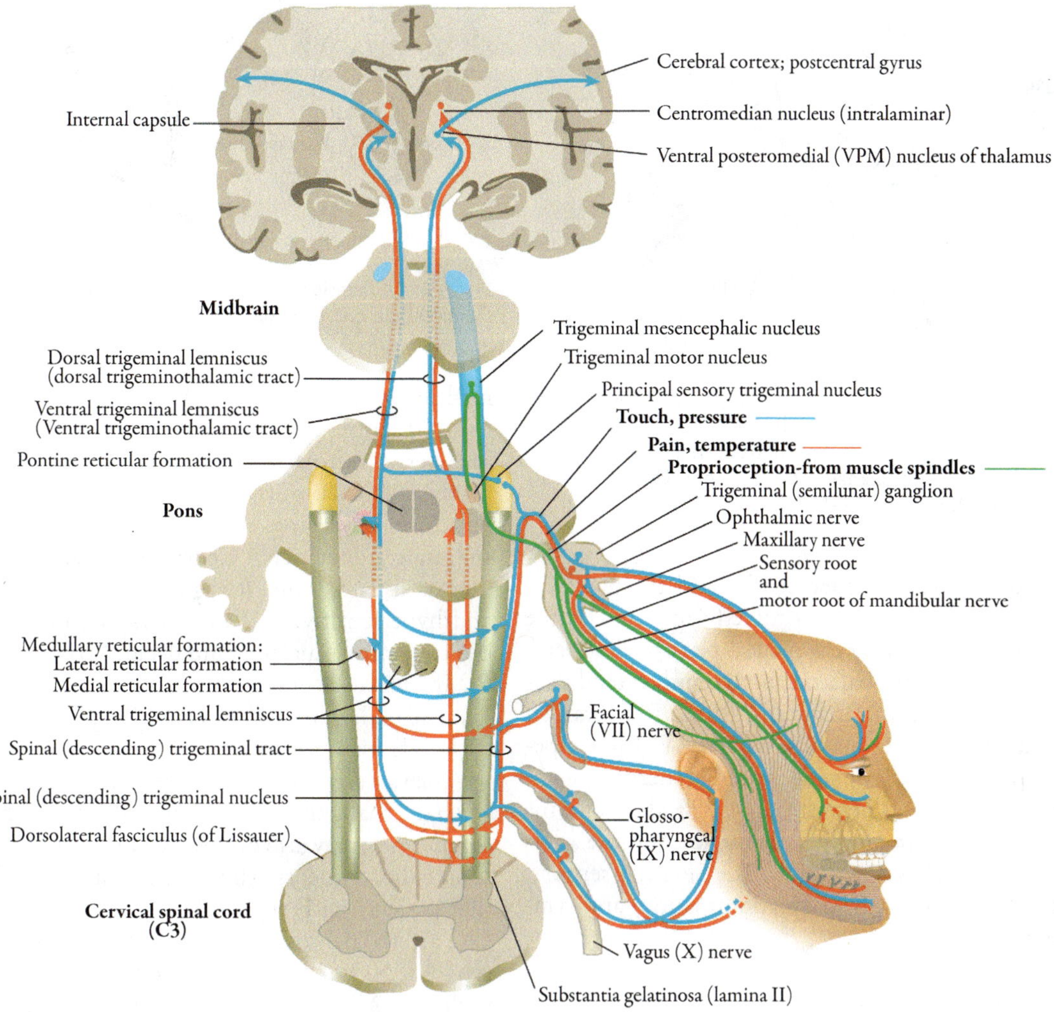

Figure 3.4 Anatomy of head pain and pain transmission. Adapted with permissions from Schmidt-Wilcke T, Hierlmeier S, Leinisch E. Altered regional brain morphology in patients with chronic facial pain. *Headache* 2010;50(8):1278–1285.

this complex arrangement, head and facial pain may be difficult to localize.

ANATOMY OF THE TRIGEMINAL (GASSERIAN) GANGLION AND TRIGEMINAL NERVES

The trigeminal ganglion has three major divisions: ophthalmic (V1), maxillary (V2), and mandibular (V3). These are located dorsally, intermediate, and ventrally, respectively, within the middle cranial fossa.

The ophthalmic division (V1), upon exiting the ganglion, passes into the orbit via the superior orbital fissure, thus making the V1 division a poor target for blockade once it leaves the ganglion. The ophthalmic division (V1) branches into the supraorbital, supratrochlear, and nasociliary nerves that provide sensory innervation from the forehead and nose. The maxillary division (V2) exits the middle cranial fossa via the foramen rotundum, and it then crosses the pterygopalatine fossa (PPF), thus making it amenable to percutaneous approaches, before entering the orbit through the inferior orbital fissure. The infraorbital, superior alveolar, palatine, and zygomatic nerves, all arising from V2, carry sensory information from the maxilla and overlying skin, nasal cavity, palate, nasopharynx, and meninges of the anterior and middle cranial fossa. The mandibular division (V3) exits the middle cranial fossa via the foramen ovale and then divides into the buccal, lingual, inferior alveolar, and auriculotemporal nerves. In addition to the sensory input from these nerves, the motor component of V3 innervates the muscles of mastication, tensor tympani, tensor veli palatine, mylohyoid, and anterior belly of the digastric. Sensory input of the lower face (including chin, teeth, gums, and anterior two-thirds of tongue) is primarily communicated via the mandibular division, with the exception of a small area covering the angle and lower body of the ramus of the mandible and parts of the ear, all of which are innervated by cervical nerves.

SPHENOPALATINE GANGLION (SPG) NEUROANATOMY

The SPG is the largest extracranial nervous structure and is located within the PPF (Figure 3.5). The PPF is an

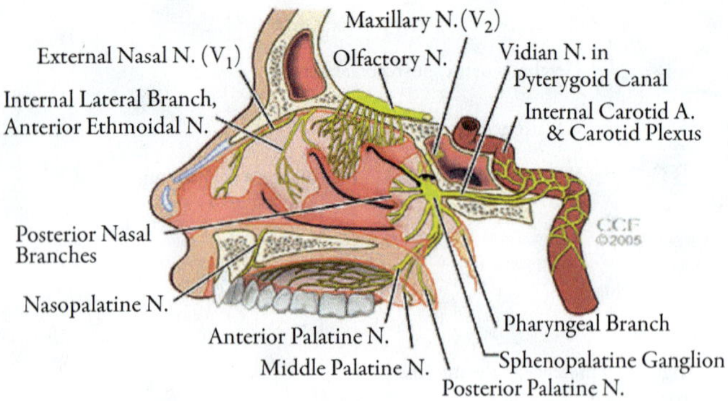

Figure 3.5 Anatomy of the sphenopalatine ganglion within the pterygopalatine fossa. Reprinted with permission from Narouze S, Kapural L, Casanova J, Mekhail N. Sphenopalatine ganglion radiofrequency ablation for the management of chronic cluster headache. *Headache*. 2009;49(4):571–577.

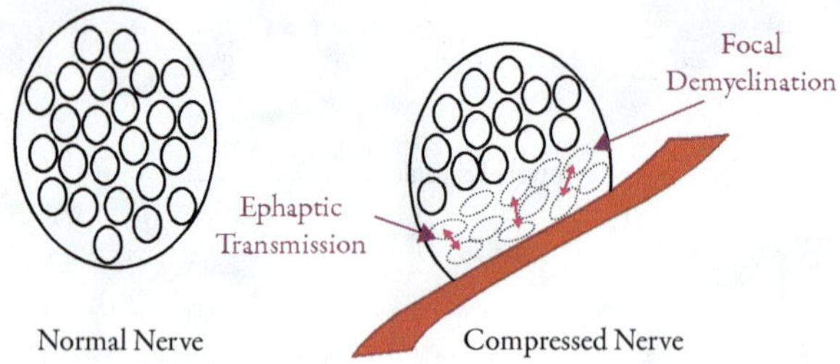

Figure 3.6 Ephaptic transmission due to focal demyelination of nerve from vascular compression.

upside-down pyramidal space located behind the posterior wall of the maxillary sinus. It is bordered superiorly by the sphenoid sinus, posteriorly by the medial plate of the pterygoid process, medially by palatine bone, and, laterally, it communicates with the infratemporal fossa. The foramen rotundum with the exiting maxillary nerve (V2) lies superior laterally; inferior medially runs the vidian nerve (greater petrosal and deep petrosal nerves).[28] The PPF also contains the internal maxillary artery and its branches, and the afferent and efferent branches of the SPG. The SPG has sensory, motor, and rich parasympathetic (predominantly) and sympathetic components.

WHAT IS THE PATHOPHYSIOLOGY OF THE FACIAL PAIN DIAGNOSES?

The pathogenesis of TN remains incompletely understood. Both peripheral and central dysfunction likely play a role. The etiology of TN is likely related to demyelination of sensory axons in the dorsal root entry zone of the trigeminal nerve caused by continuous or pulsatile vascular compression.[29] It is thought that long-standing impingement of the trigeminal nerve from aberrant blood vessels results in faulty myelination and, ultimately, in demyelination of the nerve thus leading to an increased firing rate in the trigeminal primary afferents. This in turn facilitates the development of ectopic action potential sites causing spontaneous bursts of activity in the dorsal root entry zone.[30] This may also negatively affect the function of inhibitory mechanisms in the trigeminal brainstem complex. The net resulting increased excitability of the trigeminal brainstem complex can then lead to a response usually reserved for noxious stimuli happening even with non-noxious tactile stimuli. This would explain the phenomenon of pain triggered by a sensory stimulus to the skin, mucosa, or teeth innervated by the ipsilateral trigeminal nerve. The demyelination of nociceptive pain fibers augments the function of ion channels, neurotransmitters, and second-messenger systems, producing spontaneous action potentials, ephaptic transmission, and nuclear hyperexcitability[4] (Figure 3.6). The idea of repetitive and spontaneous firing of action potentials in demyelinated nerves is further supported by the responsiveness of TN to the administration of antiepileptic medications, many of which lower the excitability of neurons by decreasing sodium conductance.[30] Centrally, it is suggested that there is increased paroxysmal firing of wide dynamic range neurons and hypersensitivity of low-threshold mechanoreceptors in the trigeminal nucleus caudalis and trigeminal nucleus oralis. The presence of refractory, continued volleys of pain after nerve stimulation suggests central hypersensitivity, and many of the effective treatments are predominantly centrally active.

The vascular structure compressing the nerve is frequently arterial, usually the superior cerebellar artery; however, venous compression may also occur[31] (Figure 3.7). In one study of 144 consecutive patients who underwent MVD,[32] it was found that patients with type 1 TN were nearly twice as likely to have arterial neurovascular compression as those patients with type 2 TN. Furthermore, although the majority of patients with type 2 TN were found to have arterial compression, the incidence of venous compression in these patients was almost equal to that of the impingement from an artery. Patients with type 2 TN were also five times more likely to have no neurovascular compression as patients with type 1 TN.[33]

Although it is clear that vascular compression of the trigeminal nerve is present in the majority of patients with TN, the extent to which neurovascular compression exists in patients without TN is less obvious. In a radiographic study of patients with and without TN, the incidence of vascular

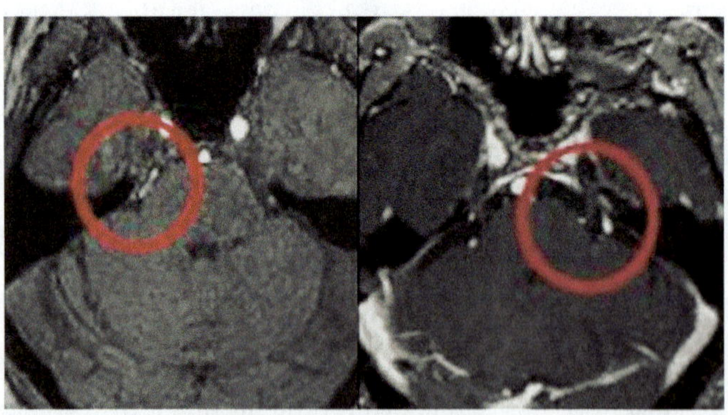

Figure 3.7 Magnetic resonance angiography (left) and postgadolinium magnetic resonance imaging (right) revealing compression of the trigeminal nerve from the superior cerebellar artery (SCA).

compression of the trigeminal nerve was found to be highest on the ipsilateral side of symptomatic patients, and the severity of indentation and proximal compression of the nerve was found to be predictive of TN.[31] TN may also be attributed to pathologies that create crowding of the posterior fossa, such as Chiari malformation.[34] Mechanisms by which Chiari malformations may produce symptoms of TN include vascular compression due to a small posterior fossa, stretching of the trigeminal nerve resulting in demyelination, microischemic changes on the trigeminal nerve, direct compression on the brainstem, and hyperexcitability of sensory fibers arising from the trigeminal nucleus as they descend to C2 in the setting of a cervical syrinx associated with Chiari malformations.[34]

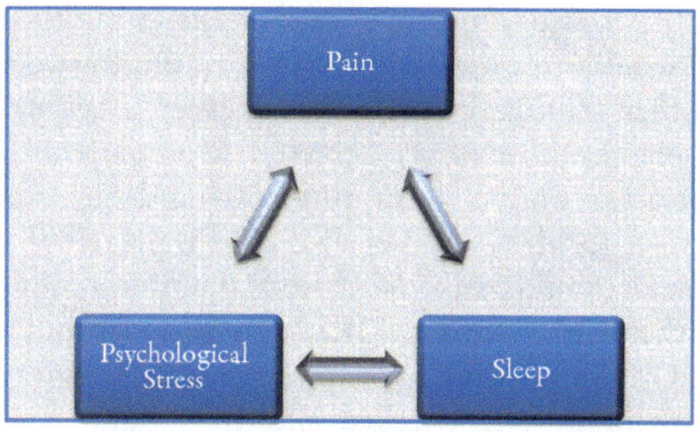

Figure 3.8 Pain, sleep, and psychological stress such as depression and anxiety have interactive and additive effects. Negative effects in any of the three domains will negatively impact the other two domains.

WHAT ARE THE COMMON COMORBIDITIES OF THE FACIAL PAIN DIAGNOSES?

Psychological comorbidities are common in patients with orofacial pain. Up to 30% of these patients may have anxiety disorder, and PIFP is associated with multiple psychiatric comorbidities.[35] Remich and Blasberg reported 68% of patients with PIFP having various psychiatric disorders, including affective, somatoform, and psychosis.[36] A recent study of patients with PIFP reported regional differences in gray matter density/volume in several areas, including the ipsilateral anterior cingulate gyrus and insular cortex.[37] These areas are known to play a critical role in antinociception and anticipation for a variety of pain experiences.[38] This study also found thinning in somatosensory and motor cortex, believed to be areas specific to face pain. Similar models have been described for TN.[39] It is still not entirely clear whether these changes are a result of the underlying pain condition versus a predisposing factor for its development, but these studies demonstrate reproducible altered brain morphology in patients with chronic facial pain.

As with any chronic pain condition, psychological and behavioral factors likely play a pivotal role in the severity and maintenance of pain, concomitant symptoms, and level of functioning. Having persistent facial pain can be frustrating for patients, and they may experience feelings of isolation, hopelessness, and being misunderstood. Not surprisingly, depression is common in these patients, affecting as many as half, whereas anxiety has been observed in up to 30% of chronic orofacial pain patients.[35] The direction of this relationship is not fully understood, but the impact of psychiatric comorbidity on pain severity is clear. Psychological distress is associated with worse pain in several types of orofacial pain[40,41] likely having both direct (e.g., neuroendocrine changes) and indirect effects on pain (i.e., behaviors that promote pain like inactivity or poor treatment adherence).

The prevalence of psychiatric disorders may vary across different chronic facial pain populations.[40,41] A study comparing patients with TN to those with atypical facial pain found that the TN patients had higher levels of depressive and anxiety symptoms.[41] Moreover, 46.7% of the TN patients were categorized as having severe depressive symptoms. These findings are consistent with the broader literature showing rates of depression to be as high as 50% in other chronic pain populations.[42–44] Regardless of diagnostic category, the assessment of psychiatric comorbidity should be a standard aspect of the evaluation; however, even when such comorbidities are observed, patients frequently do not follow physician recommendations to seek care from a mental health professional.[41] Thus, addressing psychiatric comorbidity is often left to the treating physician. Failing to address depression, anxiety, and other psychiatric disorders can derail treatment of pain, and functioning and sleep can all be affected in a manner that is reciprocal and multiplicative (Figure 3.8).

In addition to substantial overlap between orofacial pain and psychiatric comorbidity, there is significant overlap between orofacial pain and other chronic pain conditions such as fibromyalgia.[45] Recognizing when pain is no longer regional but is more widespread in nature can inform a mechanistic approach to treatment. Orofacial pain has been considered one of a number of chronic pain conditions in which prominent CNS mechanisms (as opposed to, or in addition to, peripheral damage) play an important role in pain perception.[46,47] CNS mechanisms include diffuse hyperalgesia or allodynia, and/or a lack of endogenous descending analgesic activity, as has been observed in fibromyalgia.[48–50] Furthermore, CNS sensitivity is thought to mediate other common symptoms including fatigue, problems with thinking, poor sleep, and psychiatric comorbidities. This same constellation of symptoms has been observed in patients with chronic orofacial pain.[45,51] Addressing these painful and persistent conditions requires more comprehensive evaluation and management that take into consideration potential mechanisms underlying the pain and other symptoms.

HOW ARE THE PATIENT'S MEDICATIONS MANAGED IN FACIAL PAIN DIAGNOSES?

In the case of the patient in the vignette, the first therapeutic intervention should be to optimize her medications. The patient has not yet had a trial of anticonvulsive therapy, and I would recommend a trial of carbamazepine. Often these medications are started at a low dose and then slowly tapered up over the course of one to several weeks to minimize side effects. I would start the patient at 100 mg one to two times a day and then increase by 100–200 mg every 3 days until significant pain improvement is achieved. Most patients achieve satisfactory relief when taking 400–800 mg/d, but some need higher doses for desired relief. If dosage is greater than 800 mg/d, then it should be divided three or four times daily (TID/QID) rather than twice daily (BID). The patient should have a baseline CBC, LFTs, and basic metabolic profile (with creatinine and sodium level) checked, and this should be repeated after 1 month and again every 6–12 months. If the patient has continued facial spasms, then I may consider the addition of baclofen at 5–10 mg up to three times daily (TID).

Pharmacologic therapy with antiepileptic drugs (AEDs) can reduce TN pain in nearly 90% of these patients, at least initially, and is thus the primary treatment modality for all newly diagnosed cases.[10] Carbamazepine (alternatively, oxcarbazepine) is considered first-line therapy, although the addition of baclofen and/or lamotrigine may be of increased benefit.[52] The American Academy of Neurology has established a practice guideline with regards to medication therapy for CTN.[13]

Carbamazepine is effective for controlling pain in patients with CTN (multiple class I and II studies). Carbamazepine decreases sodium and potassium conductance, thus reducing the spontaneous activity of A-δ and C fibers. Oxcarbazepine is probably effective for treating pain in CTN (three class II studies). Baclofen, lamotrigine, and pimozide, particularly in combination with carbamazepine or oxcarbazepine, are possibly effective for controlling pain in patients with CTN (single class II study for each drug). Topical ophthalmic anesthesia is probably ineffective for controlling pain in patients with CTN (single class I study). There is insufficient evidence to support or refute the efficacy of clonazepam, gabapentin, phenytoin, tizanidine, topical capsaicin, and valproate for controlling pain in patients with CTN. Similarly, phenytoin inhibits sodium channels, preventing glutamate release from presynaptic cells and lessening the spontaneous discharge of injured nociceptive neurons. Other antiepileptic medications, such as benzodiazepines and gabapentin, act either directly or indirectly to increase the effects of γ-aminobutyric acid (GABA) in the brain and spinal cord, while also influencing ion channels.[4]

Drowsiness is a common initial side effect of carbamazepine, but often will abate with time. Other side effects include dizziness, nausea, vomiting, nystagmus, ataxia, and diplopia. In the elderly, carbamazepine may activate latent psychosis and cause agitation. Hematologic side effects can occur in 2–6% of patients and may include leukopenia and aplastic anemia. As such, CBC and liver and renal function should be monitored early in therapy.

Rozen[7] set forth a list of suggestions with regards to medication management in the case of TN:

1. Do not overtreat. Look for remission, and taper the drug if the patient has been pain-free for 4–6 weeks. Recurrence is not uncommon.
2. Chronic anticonvulsant therapy, especially in an older population, can cause cognitive impairment. Use the smallest pain-relieving dose available.
3. Many TN patients become less responsive to medication with time. Try the drug to its fullest potential, recognize changes in pharmacokinetics, and adjust doses accordingly.
4. Minimize medication side effects by carefully titrating doses throughout the day, avoiding peaks and troughs.
5. Aim for monotherapy, but polypharmacy is an acceptable and successful treatment scheme in TN.

These medications appear less effective in patients with PIFP; however, often a trial of amitriptyline, venlafaxine, fluoxetine, or AEDs is indicated.[24,53]

WHAT OTHER APPROACHES MAY BE CONSIDERED FOR MANAGING THIS PATIENT?

BEHAVIORAL APPROACHES

Psychological treatment is essential for patients with orofacial pain. A report from the Institute of Medicine addressing the monumental problem that is chronic noncancer pain noted that "interdisciplinary, biopsychosocial approaches are the most promising for treating patients with persistent pain."[54] However, the authors also warned that "costly procedures often are performed when other actions should be considered, such as prevention, counseling, and facilitation of self-care, which are common features of successful treatment."[54] These recommendations are based on studies that have shown that physical activity/exercise, cognitive-behavioral therapy (CBT), and other behavioral strategies (e.g., biofeedback, relaxation) can be effective adjunct or stand-alone treatments for chronic pain, including orofacial pain.[55–61] Referral to such adjunctive treatment can greatly contribute to the physician's ability to address the multiple domains associated with a comprehensive approach to the care for these patients. Table 3.4 depicts the elements

Table 3.4 **ELEMENTS OF COGNITIVE AND BEHAVIORAL THERAPIES FOR CHRONIC PAIN**

COGNITIVE METHODS	BEHAVIORAL METHODS
Socratic questioning and guided discovery	Monitoring pain and activity levels
Keeping thought change records	Activity pacing
Identifying cognitive errors (automatic thoughts)	Relaxation training
Generating rational alternative thoughts	Breathing retraining

Cognitive-behavioral therapy (CBT) for chronic pain combines elements of cognitive therapy and behavioral therapy that are tailored toward increasing mastery over pain, decreasing stress, and improving functional status.

Table 3.5 "EXPRESS" ACRONYM FOR BEHAVIORAL TARGETS

Exercise	There is good evidence supportive of regular, low-impact aerobic land- or pool-based exercise for chronic pain conditions.
Psychiatric comorbidity	Both depression and anxiety disorders are common in chronic pain conditions and contribute significantly to pain and disability.
Regaining function	Functional gains are a more achievable objective as opposed to curing all pain. Set small progressive and measurable goals.
Education	Simply informing a patient where on the Internet they can find reliable information can be a good start.
Sleep	Poor sleep can make pain worse. Counterproductive habits serve to make sleep even more elusive but are often easily remedied.
Stress	Management can include behavioral therapies, biofeedback, coping training, hydrotherapy, and gentle exercise to name just a few.

Reprinted from Hassett AL, Gevirtz RN. Nonpharmacologic treatment for fibromyalgia: patient education, cognitive-behavioral therapy, relaxation techniques, and complementary and alternative medicine. *Rheum Dis Clin North Am*. 2009;35:393–407, with permission from Saunders.

of cognitive therapy and behavioral therapy that are typically combined in CBT for chronic pain.

It can be difficult to take into consideration all the key domains to be addressed when developing a behavioral management program for patients with chronic pain; thus, the acronym "ExPRESS" has been proposed as a helpful tool (Table 3.5).[62] To illustrate how the ExPRESS approach might be used, we address our vignette case from this perspective.

Exercise

Beyond specific exercises for the jaw and face, a more comprehensive program of activity and exercise has been shown to be effective for the treatment of chronic pain in general[55,56,58] and orofacial pain more specifically.[57] Recent reviews indicate that physical activity is associated with improvements in mood and anxiety, physical capacity, and functioning and with a reduction of morbidity and mortality in chronic pain patients.[58] An increased activity program could include physical therapy, gentle stretching, and/or regular low-impact aerobic exercise to improve cardiovascular fitness, manage weight, decrease stress, and improve mood and sleep.

At 92 kg and 186 cm tall, our patient is overweight, and she admitted to engaging in little formal exercise. Initiating a moderate low-impact aerobic exercise regimen could be highly beneficial because she could improve fitness, reduce stress, and lose weight. As a gradual first step, a program of regular brisk walking five times a week for a few minutes a day that increases in duration and intensity was recommended.

To promote long-term adherence to a regular exercise program, identifying an activity that the patient particularly enjoys and can readily access is vital. It is important to emphasize to patients that exercise does not necessarily mean having to go to the gym but can include other activities such as swimming, dancing, yoga, or golf. Furthermore, "exercise" can consist of simply increasing daily activity levels like gardening, house cleaning, and taking the stairs instead of the elevator at work. Slowly increasing these activities of daily living can serve to improve fitness and enhance mood. The "start low and go slow" mantra applies to many aspects of chronic pain management including exercise, medication use, and goal-setting. Last, physical therapy targeting her facial pain directly can be considered if little improvement is observed.

Psychiatric Comorbidity

As previously mentioned, depression and anxiety are extremely common. Our patient reported experiencing problems with thinking and mood that she ascribed to her medications, although this complaint is also consistent with having a central pain disorder.[46,47] The extent of her mood symptoms can be assessed using a medical interview or with a standardized self-report questionnaire such as the Center for Epidemiologic Studies Depression scale (CES-D)[63] or Patient Health Questionnaire (PHQ).[64] Understanding the severity of the mood symptoms informs the decision to address depression as part of your treatment for her or to refer her to a mental health specialist.

In the case of our patient, the mood symptoms were determined to be quite mild and likely to respond to a change in medications (e.g., neuromodulators instead of opioids) and improving her sleep and regular exercise.

Regaining Function

Our patient continues to work, but pain had begun to interfere with her performance. This is consistent with a study that found that 20% of individuals with orofacial pain report that the pain interferes with their daily activities, whereas 10% reported that pain specifically affects their work.[65] A consultation with an occupational therapist could help identify strategies to improve her performance and minimize pain. Reasonable accommodations in her schedule and/or equipment could be adopted. Also, an element of our patient's personality could be undermining her recovery—her obsessive-compulsive behavior. Individuals with obsessive-compulsive behavior tend to be anxious and highly demanding of themselves and those around them. People with perfectionistic behavior are prone to overdoing tasks on days they feel good only to suffer with more pain the next day due to overextension. Instead, regaining function is more likely to occur by setting small obtainable goals over a period of time rather than expecting to get back to "normal" quickly—again, start low and go slow.

We discussed her perfectionism with her, and she agreed to channel her obsessive-compulsive energy into positive activities such as daily walking for exercise, meditation for relaxation, or logging and executing small achievable goals. It was anticipated that improved pain, sleep, and stress would result in improved work performance.

Education

Once a diagnosis is determined, spending time discussing the specifics of the condition and the patient's conceptualization of the problem can be time well spent. Patients all too frequently believe that the medical community has let them down—such is the case with our patient. Endless diagnostic tests, minimal answers, and dismissive attitudes serve as barriers to forming an effective doctor–patient relationship and working together as partners in the patient's recovery.

Because our patient blames previous physicians for "mishandling her pain," she was wary of the assessment and recommendations. A dialog that meshed education about our conceptualization of her condition with a general desire to understand her story went a long way toward building the relationship and enhancing our conceptualization of her illness. Furthermore, explaining that we viewed her as an active partner in the treatment process was empowering for her. We also discussed realistic goals and expectations for treatment overall.

Sleep

Our patient did not mention sleep disturbances until she was asked specifically. She then reported having insomnia 3–4 nights a week, and, when she did sleep, she would awaken feeling unrefreshed. She reported that orofacial pain jarred her awake throughout the night, a phenomenon observed in the literature.[66] She also revealed that she had slept well until the year leading up to her divorce and then her sleep had become less regular. She noted that she became a "clock watcher" and would fret over how many hours of sleep were possible if she fell asleep right away.

Most patients with chronic pain, including those with orofacial pain, have at least some sleep disruption; for others, the sleep disturbance can be quite profound and include chronic insomnia or sleep apnea.[66–69] In response, many individuals engage in a plethora of behaviors that are not conducive to sleep. Such counterproductive behaviors can include clock watching; sleeping in a room that is too light, too hot, or too distracting (TV, cell phone and/or computer nearby); consuming heavy meals or caffeine too close to bedtime; or taking long naps in the afternoon. Some of these minor behavioral issues can be easily addressed with simple suggestions.

We suggested turning the clock around so that it could not be seen from the bed. We also anticipated that regular exercise and stress reduction would translate into better sleep. We discussed that if sleep continued to be a prominent issue, a referral to a sleep specialist and possible CBT for insomnia (CBT-I) would be an appropriate next step.

Stress

A potentially salient aspect of our patient's social history is that she was divorced within the last year. She indicated that her sleep became irregular around that time, and her facial pain began 6 months later. This pattern suggests a role for stress in the etiology and maintenance of her orofacial pain. Yet the debate continues as to whether psychological factors such as depression, anxiety, and stress cause chronic pain or vice versa. Based on the current evidence, it seems likely that, in some cases, psychological distress can cause chronic pain, although somewhat less reliably than other stressors such as physical trauma and infectious disease.[70] In contrast, chronic pain is frequently at the root of psychological stress, in which living with chronic pain becomes a disruptive force affecting every aspect of an individual's life. First and foremost, data suggest that a unidirectional relationship between psychological stress and pain does not exist. These are independent concepts despite being interactive. For example, neuroimaging studies have shown that psychological stress and pain are processed somewhat independently in the brain.[71]

The implications for treatment to decrease stress should be an element of the plan, although attributing the pain solely to stress (blaming the patient) will do little to strengthen the therapeutic alliance.

She had already made the connections among her divorce, stress, and orofacial pain. She was open to beginning a program of regular walking and learning mindfulness meditation, which has been shown to be effective for patients with chronic pain.[72]

In summary, ExPRESS provides the framework from which a comprehensive program can be devised that addresses six critical domains. Intervention can combine pharmacological and nonpharmacological strategies that, ideally, are tailored to a patient's particular needs.

MICROVASCULAR DECOMPRESSION (MVD)

Despite the high initial success rate of medications in alleviating symptoms of TN, over time, the efficacy of medical therapy decreases such that approximately half of all patients ultimately require surgical intervention.[73] The surgical management of TN can be broken down into two types of intervention: MVD and ablative procedures. The decision on which technique to utilize depends on the patient's age and

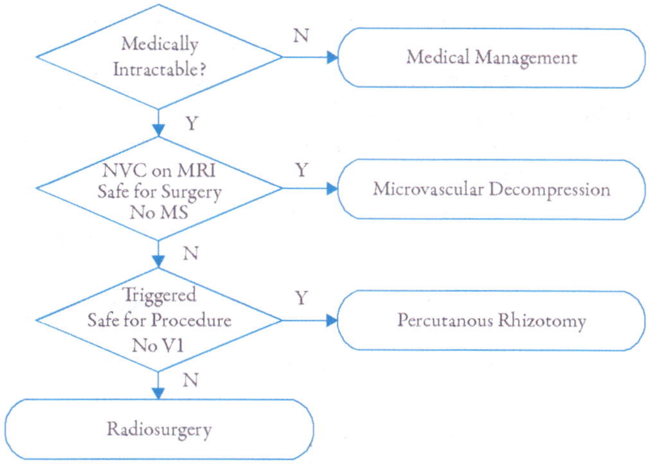

Figure 3.9 Treatment algorithm for trigeminal neuralgia.

comorbidities, anatomy and etiology of pain condition, and the physician's clinical experience (Figure 3.9).

MVD has demonstrated benefit in patients with persistent TN due to vascular compression of the nerve, and it is the standard of care for patients with a clear diagnosis of TN and radiographic findings of neurovascular compression who are refractory to medical management.[74–76] In addition, patients with type 1 TN are more than twice as likely to have long-term pain relief following MVD than are those with type 2 TN.[18] Other predictors of long-term success from MVD include memorable symptom onset, pain triggered by environmental or behavioral stimuli, intact sensorium, relatively short duration of symptoms prior to surgery, single-artery compression of the trigeminal nerve, and complete arterial decompression of the nerve during surgery.[18] The superior cerebellar artery is the most frequent arterial structure to affect the trigeminal nerve. However, venous compression alone or with arterial compression is also possible.

Dandy first described posterior fossa exploration for TN in 1925, at which time he noted vascular compression of the trigeminal nerve in 66 out of 215 patients at the time of surgery.[75] Although Dandy postulated that neurovascular compression was the underlying etiology of TN, he was unable to prove this in the majority of his patients. The binocular microscope allowed for consistent intraoperative identification of neurovascular compression, including vessels too small to be seen with the naked eye.[75] Thus, this surgical technique, which Jannetta popularized and called *microvascular decompression*, was eventually accepted as the standard surgical treatment for TN.[76]

In this procedure, a linear incision is made medial to the mastoid notch, followed by a circular craniotomy large enough to expose the transverse sinus superiorly and the sigmoid sinus laterally. After the bony margins are waxed and hemostasis is obtained, the dura is sharply incised and secured with retraction sutures. At this point, the operating microscope is brought into the field, and, using careful microsurgical technique, the cerebellum is gently retracted medially and dissection is carried out until the arachnoid overlying the junction of the trigeminal nerve and pons is visualized. The arachnoid is opened sharply, and the fifth nerve and adjacent vascular structures are examined. The compression usually appears at the most proximal portion of the nerve, as it exits the pons (Figure 3.10). When the offending vessel is identified and found to be arterial, it is carefully dissected off the neural fibers and held in place by a small piece of Teflon, which is inserted between the vessel and trigeminal nerve at their point of contact. When neural impingement is found to be venous, the vein is cauterized and divided. The wound is then irrigated, hemostasis is obtained, and the dura is closed in a watertight fashion. The bone flap is replaced, and the muscle and skin are closed in sequential layers.[20]

In 1996, Barker et al.[73] published their results from a study tracking 1,185 patients with TN who underwent an MVD over a 20-year period. Patients were excluded from the study if they had a diagnosis of atypical TN (369 patients), symptomatic TN associated with MS (26 patients), or TN associated with aneurysm (one patient) or arteriovenous malformation (five patients).[73] Seventy percent of patients were pain-free without medications 10 years after surgery, and an additional 4% had occasional pain without medications. The annual rate of recurrence was less than 1% at 10 years following surgery. There were very low rates of facial numbness (1%) and dysesthesia (0.3%) postoperatively. The results and complication profile were far better than ablative procedures such as radiofrequency rhizotomy and glycerol rhizolysis, after which facial numbness is an expected side effect. The authors of this study concluded that four factors predicted higher rates of recurrence of TN following surgery (Box 3.4). These included female sex, greater than 8 years of symptoms preoperatively, nerve

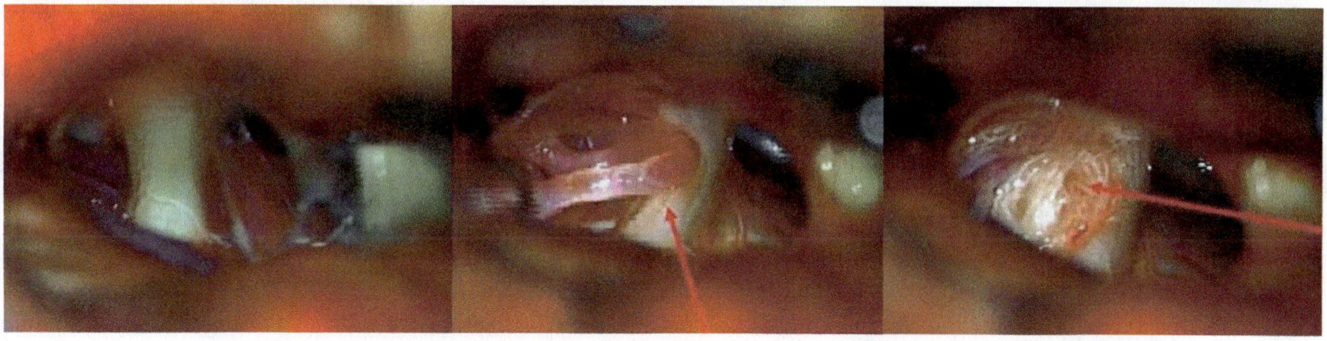

Figure 3.10 Intraoperative views of microvascular decompression. *Left to right:* Intraoperative view of the right trigeminal nerve with ventral compression by the superior cerebellar artery (SCA); intraoperative view of the mobilized SCA; shredded Teflon positioned in between the mobilized SCA and the trigeminal nerve.

Box 3.4 **FACTORS ASSOCIATED WITH HIGHER RECURRENCE RATE OF TRIGEMINAL NEURALGIA AFTER MICROVASCULAR DECOMPRESSION**

Constant pain (rather than episodic, lancinating)

Type 2 TN, rather than type 1 TN

Nerve compression by a vein (rather than artery)

Longer duration of symptoms (>8 years)

Lack of immediate symptom resolution postoperatively

Female Sex

Adapted from Miller J, Magill S, Acar F, Burchiel K. Predictors of long-term success after microvascular decompression for trigeminal neuralgia. *J Neurosurg.* 2009;110:620–626; Barker F, Jannetta P, Bissonette D, Larkins M, Jho H. The long-term outcome of microvascular decompression for trigeminal neuralgia. *N Engl J Med.* 1996;334(17):1077–1083.

compression from a vein rather than an artery, and lack of immediate relief of symptoms postoperatively.[73]

Another study demonstrated that the type of TN (1 or 2) was more predictive of outcome than any other factor, including response to antiepileptics, trigger points, pain-free intervals, and memorable onset of pain. Patients with type 1 TN were more than twice as likely to be pain-free long-term after MVD compared to patients with type 2 TN. There was a trend toward increased responsiveness to MVD in patients who had a shorter duration of preoperative symptoms, a good response to medical therapy, and a history of trigger points, memorable onset of pain, and pain-free intervals. The authors also found that arterial compression was more often associated with type 1 TN and thus slightly predictive of improved outcome; however, this was not statistically significant. Finally, the presence of lancinating pain, as opposed to constant pain, was predictive of improved outcomes both in type 1 and type 2 TN.[18]

As intraoperative brainstem auditory evoked potentials has become more widely available for monitoring associated with the surgery. The most common complication is transient or sometimes permanent CN dysfunction. Manipulation of the trigeminal nerve intraoperatively poses a risk for severe facial numbness or even anesthesia dolorosa, although the latter is more commonly associated with ablative procedures. Injury to the trochlear nerve can result in diplopia, which often resolves over time. The facial nerve is also susceptible to insult during surgery, which may result in a postoperative facial palsy. In contrast to the other CNs, if the cochlear nerve is affected, the deficit is more likely to be a loss of hearing.[20,73] Other complications include intracranial hemorrhage, cerebellar edema secondary to retraction, CSF leak, pseudomeningocele, bacterial meningitis, chemical meningitis, hydrocephalus, infarction of the brainstem, and death.[73]

ABLATIVE PROCEDURES

Given the success of MVD for the treatment of medically refractory TN, other therapeutic interventions are often thought to be second-tier. In contrast to ablative treatments, MVD frequently produces long-term success by correcting the causative agent generating the pain and does so without inducing injury to the nerve. The patients may have permanent resolution of their symptoms and still maintain normal sensation in the distribution of the trigeminal nerve following MVD. However, lesioning procedures serve to treat the symptoms of TN by injuring the nerve. As a result, numbness and paresthesias are expected following these procedures, and the results are short-lived because the nerve recovers over time, thereby necessitating repeated lesioning. It is also important to note that patients with symptoms in the V1 distribution are less suitable candidates for ablation since numbness of the eye affects the blink reflex and may result in significant corneal injury. Thus, these less invasive options are, for the most part, reserved for elderly patients, patients with multiple comorbidities who are poor surgical candidates, and patients with recurrent symptoms after a previous MVD.[10]

The decision of what interventional strategy to utilize depends on the patient's pain distribution, pain characteristics, comorbidities, and operator experience. Blockade of the terminal branches may be an initial starting point if the patient has isolated pain in one or two nerve distributions. These branches include the supraorbital and supratrochlear nerves (ophthalmic division, V1), infraorbital nerve (maxillary division, V2), and mental nerve (maxillary division, V3). If the pain is isolated to one division, maxillary and/or mandibular, then a targeted block of V2 and/or V3 may be indicated. Due to its course of exit from the trigeminal ganglion into the orbit, a peripheral block of the V1 division is not possible. Therefore, generally, if the patient has pain in the V1 division or in more than one other division, interventional strategies targeting the trigeminal (Gasserian) ganglion may be indicated. It should be noted that although blockade of the terminal branches or divisions may be helpful for diagnostic purposes, there are limited studies showing sustained benefit from blockade or neurolytic procedures targeting these structures. Conversely, there is demonstrated benefit with approaches targeting the trigeminal ganglion.

Percutaneous Trigeminal (Gasserian) Ganglion Treatments

Several types of ablative procedures exist for the treatment of TN. A percutaneous transovale approach to the trigeminal (Gasserian) ganglion for ethanol neurolysis was first published by Hartel in 1912.[77] Since that time, glycerol, first described by Hakanson in 1981,[78] has replaced ethanol as the first-choice injectate; however, other techniques utilizing the approach to the trigeminal ganglion have also been described, including retrogasserian radiofrequency ablation (RFA) rhizotomy and balloon compression.

RFA of the Gasserian (Trigeminal) Ganglion

RFA of the Gasserian (trigeminal) ganglion, or thermorhizotomy (TRZ), was originally described by Kirschner in 1932. Kirschner developed the use of an electrocoagulating current to create a well-defined lesion in the Gasserian ganglion that eliminated the spreading phenomenon seen with the injection of chemical substances.[79] The technique was refined and popularized by White and Sweet in 1965[77] and published in 1974.[80] The modifications made by White and Sweet involved the use of a short-acting anesthetic agent, which enabled patients to remain awake for testing during the procedure; electrical stimulation for precision; a radiofrequency current to reliably create a lesion; and temperature monitoring for enhanced control during the ablation.[11]

RFA was originally thought to act through temperature-dependent selective destruction of A-δ and C fibers.[79] It is postulated that action potentials of nociceptive fibers are blocked more easily at lower temperatures than are the larger fibers that carry tactile sensation, namely A-α and A-β fibers. Thus, by using thermocoagulation of the trigeminal rootlets at a temperature ranging from 60°C to 75°C, the activity of the pain fibers can be blocked, while the activity of the tactile fibers remain unaffected.[11] Further studies, however, have suggested that RFA is nonselective in its destruction.[81] Three key steps are involved in RFA: (1) canalization of the trigeminal cistern, (2) stimulation to reproduce the patient's pain, and (3) formation of an adequate lesion.[11]

In a comparative study of ablative procedures for TN, Lopez et al.[82] found that RFA provides the highest rates of early and late complete pain relief compared to glycerol rhizolysis and stereotactic radiosurgery (SRS). Numerous other studies have demonstrated similar efficacy (80–98% high-grade or complete relief)[7,26,74,83,84]; however, a 15–20% symptom recurrence rate can be expected within the first year and 4–65% in studies that track patients up to 13 years. RFA demonstrated better initial success rate and less likelihood of symptom recurrence at 1 year compared with other percutaneous techniques.[83,84] Kanpolat et al., in their series of 1,600 patients who underwent trigeminal ganglion RFA for TN, reported acute pain relief in 97% of patients, although that fell to 92% at 1 year. At 10 and 20 years, the relief rate from the single procedure was 52% and 42%, respectively. However, those patients who underwent multiple procedures had reported pain relief of 94% and 100% at 10 and 20 years after initial treatment.[83] Wu et al.[85] demonstrated similar benefit in their series of 1,860 patients. RFA also has the capability, more so than other ablative procedures, to specifically target individual divisions of the trigeminal nerve.

Patients must be made aware that sensory loss is an expected side effect of the procedure because many studies have demonstrated that greater sensory loss correlates with lower recurrence.[11,86] RFA carries a slightly higher risk of keratitis and anesthesia dolorosa than does MVD or SRS, yet the risk is comparable to that of glycerol rhizolysis.[82] The main anticipated side effect following RFA of the trigeminal ganglion is sensory loss in the distribution of the treated nerve(s) but may also involve corneal anesthesia and masseter weakness. Adverse events related to needle placement for block or RFA lesioning include cheek or retrobulbar hematoma (with exophthalmos), keratitis, meningitis, transient rhinorrhea, intravascular injection, and dural arteriovenous fistulae. Other potential complications related to RFA lesioning include anesthesia dolorosa and hypoesthesia. Anesthesia dolorosa, deafferentation pain, is less common (1–5%) but can be quite severe and disabling. There have been reports of intracranial hemorrhage, stroke, and death following trigeminal ganglion RFA.[26,87,88]

In theory, pulsed radiofrequency (PRF) of the Gasserian ganglion may avoid some of these side effects because it is a neuromodulatory rather than neurodestructive procedure.[81,89] This technique would be expected to have minimal sensory or motor loss or anesthesia dolorosa and potentially even fewer corneal abnormalities. Unfortunately, in clinical practice, the procedure has shown mixed results in terms of efficacy. Van Zundert et al.[90] reported excellent long-term relief (19-month mean follow-up) in 3 of 5 patients, with partial relief in one patient and short-term effect in the other. In contrast, Erdine et al.[91] showed minimal relief with PRF compared with RFA of the Gasserian ganglion, although it should be noted that the authors' reported success with (conventional) RFA was far below the efficacy reported in other studies. At this time, there is not enough supporting evidence to recommend PRF over RFA of the Gasserian ganglion.

Technique of Trigeminal Ganglion RFA

Prior to RFA, the patient often has at least one diagnostic block. The technique for blockade of the trigeminal ganglion is identical to that for RFA except that 0.5–1 mL of local anesthetic is injected once motor stimulation is elicited (and after live contrast injection demonstrates lack of intravascular spread). Complete or significant (>50%) relief is expected prior to proceeding to RFA.

The patient should have an intravenous line established and often requires sedation for the RFA procedure, but preferably not for the diagnostic block. The patient is placed supine with his head within the C-arm. The C-arm is rotated into an ipsilateral oblique submental view to optimize visualization of the foramen ovale, which often projects medially to the mandibular process. After injecting local anesthetic over this area (typically 2 cm lateral to the corner of the mouth), a 22 G, 10 cm (2–5 mm active tip) RFA cannula is advanced toward the foramen ovale under real-time fluoroscopy in the AP submental and then lateral view. A finger should be placed into the oral cavity to prevent and detect oral mucosa penetration. There may be a small egress of CSF once the needle reaches the trigeminal cistern, which indicates that the cannula is in the correct location. However, there may not always be CSF, especially if prior procedures were done. In addition, occasionally CSF is seen when the needle is in an aberrant location, such as the infratemporal subarachnoid space, which may occur if the needle is too deep. Stimulating the nerve is done after the tip of the electrode has been directed into the desired division of the trigeminal nerve. After the needle is inside the foramen ovale (Figure 3.11[23]), motor stimulation should result in muscle twitches of the mastication muscles (V3). If treatment of the V2 or V1 branches is desired, then the needle should be advanced deeper (~2 mm) until the needle tip is visualized over the petrous bone. Then sensory stimulation at 50 Hz should be felt in the painful areas at 0.05–0.1 V. Once appropriate stimulation is attained, and after negative aspiration for heme and CSF, 0.5–1 mL of contrast should be

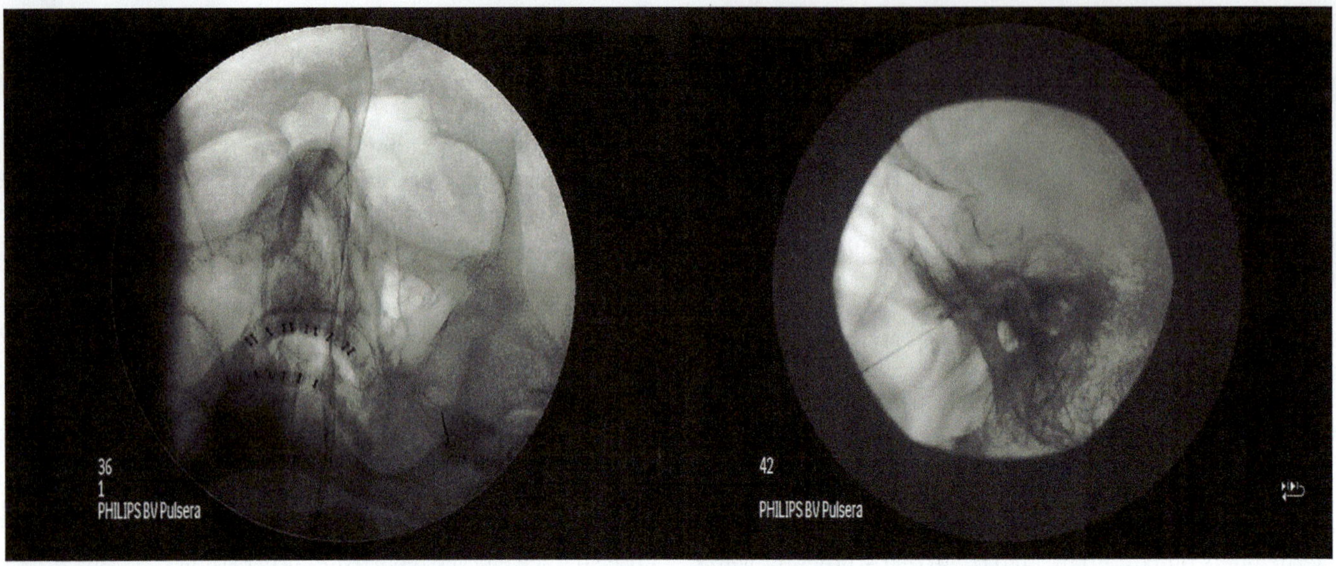

Figure 3.11 Gasserian (trigeminal) ganglion radiofrequency ablation (RFA): *(Left)* Oblique, submental view showing the needle tip inferior to the foramen ovale. *(Right)* Lateral image demonstrating further needle advancement into the foramen ovale. Reprinted with permission from Vorenkamp KE. Interventional procedures for facial pain. *Curr Pain Headache Rep.* 2012;17:308. Epub ahead of print.

injected under-real time fluoroscopy, with digital subtraction angiography (DSA) if possible, to rule out intravascular spread. Then, 1–2 mL of lidocaine or bupivacaine +/- nonparticulate corticosteroid may be injected prior to lesioning. The first lesion is performed at 60°C for 60 seconds, then a second (or even third) lesion is performed for an additional 60–120 seconds at 60–70°C degrees. Finally, it is important to create a lesion that is large enough to damage the pain fibers or else the risk of recurrence is high. Waking up the patient again to test facial sensation helps to gauge the extent of lesioning.[11]

Extracranial peripheral nerve ablation may be considered for patients with more localized pain. This may be performed at the supraorbital notch (V1), infraorbital notch (V2), and the mental foramen (V3). Alternatively, the maxillary (V2) and mandibular (V3) divisions may be blocked more proximally at either the foramen ovale or after first contacting the lateral pterygoid plate via the infrazygomatic approach under fluoroscopic[74] or CT[92] guidance. Recently, this has also been described under ultrasound guidance.[93] There are case reports of patients with TN benefitting from pulsed RF (PRF) treatment to the mental nerve[94] and also V2 PRF combined with topical SPG block and oral medications.[95] Greater occipital nerve blockade with local anesthetic and corticosteroid has also been reported to benefit patients with TN[7], but this is less beneficial in patients with PIFP.[96]

Glycerol Rhizolysis

Retrogasserian glycerol rhizolysis (GR) for the treatment of TN was accidentally discovered in the 1970s while being trialed as a potential vehicle for the delivery of tantalum powder into the Gasserian ganglion. The purpose of delivering tantalum powder, a radiopaque metal dust, into the ganglion was so it could act as a radiographic marker of the ganglion during lesioning procedures with the Leksell γ-knife. However, it was discovered that the injection of tantalum and glycerol eliminated symptoms of TN even before the radiosurgery was performed. In 1981, Hakanson took advantage of these findings and created a formal technique for injecting glycerol into the trigeminal cistern for the treatment of TN.[97]

The technique used for glycerol injection is similar to that of RFA. However, CSF extravasation during needle placement in the trigeminal cistern plays a larger role in GR than in TRZ. Not only is the flow of CSF helpful in confirming that the needle is in the correct location, but it has also been shown to correlate with patient outcome. One study of 4,012 patients who underwent GR for TN found that, among cases with CSF drainage, only 8.58% of patients had recurrence, whereas in the cases without egress of CSF, 31.2% of patients had recurrence.[98] Another difference in the technique of GR is that, following the placement of the needle, patients are moved into a sitting position at which point pure glycerol is slowly injected, with care not to exceed 0.35 mL. The reason this is performed in the sitting position is to minimize the spread of the glycerol into the extracisternal space. Following the procedure, patients should remain seated upright for at least 1 hour.[97]

Short-term pain relief in patients who undergo GR is quite high, ranging from 67% to 97%. In contrast, long-term pain relief is less successful with a 20% average risk of recurrence at 2 years and a 50% average risk of recurrence within 5–10 years.[97] As previously mentioned, the risk of anesthesia dolorosa and keratitis with GR is comparable to that of TRZ, but higher than that of SRS or MVD. Other reported complications include intraprocedural vasovagal events, as well as bleeding, transient masseter weakness, herpes reactivation, aseptic meningitis, and bacterial meningitis.[97]

SRS

SRS for the treatment of TN was first performed in 1951 by Lars Leksell using a modified x-ray tube. Over the next 50 years, radiosurgical devices improved, as did imaging modalities including stereotactic MR and computed tomography (CT), enabling improved visualization of the trigeminal root for treatment planning and implementation.[10] However, many still debated the efficacy and safety of SRS, as well as the optimal dosage of radiation that should be used. In 1996, Kondziolka et al. conducted a multi-institutional study to answer these and other related questions. The study included 50 patients, all with type 1 TN, at five centers; the participants underwent SRS with Leksell γ-knife, using a single 4 mm isocenter at the nerve root entry zone and a target dose ranging from 60 to 90 Gy.[99] The mean patient age was 70 years (ranging from 40 to 87 years), 20 patients were men and 30 were women, 32 patients had prior surgery, and the mean number of previous procedures for each patient was 2.8 (ranging from 1 to 7). The median follow-up period was 18 months (ranging from 11 to 36 months).

The results of the study showed that 58% of patients were pain-free, 36% had good pain control (50–90% relief), and 6% had treatment failure. The median time until pain relief was 1 month, and the responses lasted on average up to 3 years. The study also demonstrated that doses of 70 Gy or greater were associated with a significantly higher rates of pain relief. Six percent of patients had paresthesias and decreased sensation following SRS after receiving doses of 65, 70, and 75 Gy. There were no patients with deafferentation pain or other neurological symptoms.[99] This study was instrumental in demonstrating the efficacy and safety of SRS for the treatment of TN. In fact, comparison studies assessing the long-term outcomes of SRS, TRZ, and GR report that SRS is associated with the lowest rate of complications. These studies also show a long-term pain relief profile that is comparable to that of GR. However, it should be noted that almost two-thirds of SRS patients still require medications for symptom control.[82]

Most recently, a cadaveric study was performed using transcranial magnetic resonance-guided focused ultrasound (MRgFUS) treating the proximal trigeminal nerve at the root entry zone.[100] Although the noninvasive nature of this treatment is promising, further studies are needed to confirm the safety and efficacy of this procedure.

Percutaneous Balloon Compression

Percutaneous balloon compression (PBC) for the treatment of TN was introduced by Sean Mullen in 1983, based on intraoperative techniques used by neurosurgeons since the 1950s.[101] Unlike the other ablative procedures, PBC is typically performed under general anesthesia with the use of fluoroscopy. An incision is made in the cheek, at the same entry point used for TRZ and GR, and a needle is passed through the foramen ovale. A No. 4 Fogarty balloon catheter is then advanced into Meckel's cave, and the balloon is slowly inflated with contrast under fluoroscopic guidance. Ideally, the balloon should appear pear-shaped, indicative of its posterior projection out of Meckel's cave toward the posterior fossa. Balloon compression is maintained for 2–7 minutes. At this point, an episode of bradycardia may be observed, and it is advised to alert the anesthesiologist of the potential need for atropine. The balloon is then slowly deflated, and the catheter is withdrawn along with the needle.[102] Some have advocated the addition of PBC to conventional RFA of the trigeminal ganglion rather than utilizing PBC as a stand-alone procedure.

Outcomes of TN patients following PBC vary widely in the literature. Whereas some studies report success rates comparable to TRZ and GF, other studies report much higher rates of recurrence. There is not enough high-quality data available to effectively compare its outcomes to those of other ablative procedures.[82] With regards to complications, PBC has been associated with neurovascular injury and meningitis more so than other percutaneous procedures, perhaps due to the larger diameter of the cannula used in PBC.[82]

Sphenopalatine (Pterygopalatine) Ganglion Radiofrequency Treatments

Blockade of the SPG, also known as the pterygopalatine ganglion (PPG), can be most reliably accomplished via an infrazygomatic approach under fluoroscopic guidance, Although "blockade" is often performed via transnasal application of local anesthetic (LA) soaked cotton-tipped applicators, this relies upon diffusion (both transmucosal and trans-bony) of the LA and is unpredictable.[103] Similarly, intraoral injection of LA via the greater palatine foramen is a "blind" technique that does not allow verification that the LA injectate has actually reached the SPG.[104]

Technique of SPG RFA

The infrazygomatic approach to the SPG involves aligning the patient so that both mandibles are superimposed on the lateral view. Then, LA is injected into the skin inferior to the zygoma and just anterior to the mandible. Next, a 10 cm RFA cannula (2–5 mm active tip) is advanced toward the PPF under fluoroscopic guidance. If the lateral pterygoid plate is contacted, then the needle is adjusted anterior and cephalad. Once adjusted, the needle is advanced in the AP view and then advanced until positioned just lateral to the lateral nasal wall. Next, sensory stimulation testing is performed at 50 Hz, and needle position is adjusted as needed until stimulation in the root of the nose is attained at less than 0.5 V (Table 3.6[87]). Once satisfactory stimulation is achieved, then contrast is injected under "live" fluoroscopy to confirm there is no intranasal or intravascular spread. Then, 0.5 mL of LA is injected prior to lesioning at 80°C for 60 seconds x 2 lesions.

RFA and PRF of the SPG has demonstrated benefit for cluster headache,[28,103,105] but no controlled studies have been published for PIFP. A retrospective study of PRF of the SPG (PRF-SPG) for 30 patients with chronic facial pain (including "atypical facial pain") demonstrated complete relief in 21%, and 65% experienced good or moderate improvement.[106] Similarly, Varghese[107] reported early relief in 77% of patients undergoing SPG ablation with 6% phenol via a nasal endoscopy-guided approach for facial pain due to head and neck cancers. Neither SPG neurectomy[108] nor radiosurgery[109] provided sustained benefit for patients with PIFP.

Side effects and complications of RFA-SPG are directly related to the close proximity of other nerves and vasculature. Persistent anesthesia, hypoesthesia, or dysesthesia of the palate, maxilla, or posterior pharynx often occurs. Dryness of the

Table 3.6 **DIFFERENT POSSIBLE SCENARIOS OF STIMULATION BEFORE ATTEMPTING RADIOFREQUENCY THERMOCOAGULATION OF THE SPHENOPALATINE GANGLION**

LOCATION OF PARESTHESIA	NERVES STIMULATED	LOCATION OF NEEDLE TIP	ACTION NEEDED
Upper teeth, gums	Maxillary (V2) branches	Superolateral	Redirect caudal and medial
Hard palate	Palatine nerves	Anterior, lateral, caudal	Redirect posteromedial and cephalad
Root of the nose	SPG efferents; posterior lateral nasal nerves	Correct	None

Modified and used with permission from Schmidt-Wilcke T, Hierlmeier S, Leinisch E. Altered regional brain morphology in patients with chronic facial pain. *Headache*. 2010;50(8):1278–1285.

eye, typically temporary, is common due to interruption of the parasympathetic supply. The most common complication is cheek hematoma, which may occur after puncturing the maxillary artery that lies in the PPF. Intravascular injection, epistaxis (if needle is advanced through lateral nasal wall), and infection (particularly if the oral or nasal mucosa are penetrated) are other potential sequelae. Profound reflex bradycardia has been reported during RFA-SPG, likely related to the rich parasympathetic connections to the SPG.[28,74,87,105]

Neurostimulation

Neuromodulation, namely peripheral nerve stimulation (PNS) of the supratrochlear, supraorbital, infraorbital, and occipital nerves, has shown promise for patients with trigeminal autonomic cephalalgias, including cluster headache[110] and other causes of refractory craniofacial pain.[111] PNS for the treatment of TN was first reported by Wall and Sweet in 1967.[111] Since then, there has been resurgence in PNS for the treatment of occipital neuralgia, as well as for the treatment of postherpetic TN and neuropathic trigeminal pain following trauma or surgery. Like other stimulator implants, a trial of stimulation is often initially performed to confirm patient responsiveness, which is defined as a 50% or greater reduction in pain. Neuropsychological testing prior to PNS insertion is also recommended. The primary targets of PNS for facial pain include the branches of the first division of the trigeminal nerve and the greater and lesser occipital nerves.[111] Both SPG stimulation[112] and occipital nerve stimulation[113] have been reported with success for treatment of patients with cluster headache. PNS is a promising technique for investigation in patients with TN and PIFP.

Motor cortex stimulation (MCS) is another potential treatment modality for neuropathic pain. However, the indications for this therapy are primarily limited to patients who suffer from neuropathic pain either secondary to trauma or injury after surgery or due to deafferentation, as seen with intentional destructive lesions of the trigeminal nerve or ganglion.[114] In fact, patients with the most extreme form of deafferentation neuropathic pain, anesthesia dolorosa, are perhaps the most suitable candidates for the procedure. Although some studies report improvement in symptoms by 75–100%, not all patients are responders. Moreover, the effects of MCS have been shown to decrease over time, even with aggressive reprogramming. Other potential complications include postoperative seizures; epidural, subdural, or intracerebral hematomas; and wound infections.[114]

REHABILITATION

Integral to the rehabilitation approaches are several components of the ExPRESS approach outlined under behavioral approaches earlier in this chapter. Specifically, establishment of exercise and functional restoration programs, as well as restoration of a normal sleep cycle, are essential in the management of this patient.

Transcutaneous electric nerve stimulation (TENS) and orthodontic care has also demonstrated benefit for patients with kinesiology (CMS) and electromyography (EMG) verified abnormal facial muscle tone at rest, thus leading the author to conclude: "All patients with PIFP should undergo the CMS-EMG exam."[21]

Clinical Correlate

In the case of the patient from the vignette, the first therapeutic intervention should be to optimize her medications. The patient has not yet had a trial of anticonvulsive therapy.

I would recommend a trial of carbamazepine started at a low dose and then slowly tapered up over the course of one to several weeks to minimize the side effects. I would start the patient at 100 mg one to two times a day and then increase by 100–200 mg every 3 days until significant pain improvement is achieved. Most patients achieve satisfactory relief when taking 400–800 mg/d, but some need higher doses for desired relief. If dosage is greater than 800 mg/d, then it should be divided TID or QID rather than BID.

Simultaneously, the patient should be enrolled in psychological counseling with focus on the ExPRESS[62] approach with a behavioral management program. This will indeed be the framework for working toward her desired wellness, and it can incorporate any pharmacological or interventional strategies.

After remaining on the medication for several months, we can then determine whether the patient has had an appropriate response. The patient's symptoms might be controlled using medication for months or even years. However, when this no longer works to adequately control her symptoms, further intervention should be considered. A good response to medical management is often predictive of the benefit the patient will have from surgery.[18]

For this patient without significant medical comorbidities, MVD may be considered the best interventional approach if her symptoms persist and she has demonstrated vascular compression on imaging studies. If the patient desires a less invasive approach, then a variety of techniques exist with percutaneous RFA of the trigeminal ganglion one of the several options demonstrating good efficacy.

CONCLUSION

Although the differential diagnosis of facial pain is extensive, the most common cause is TN due to vascular compression. Many patients are debilitated by the condition, and a very high percentage of patients with facial pain have coexistent psychiatric conditions, including depression and anxiety. Treatment consists of psychological therapy, pharmacotherapy, and, when symptoms persist, open surgical or a variety of minimally invasive techniques. Carbamazepine is often first-line treatment and is effective in the majority of patients initially; however, this pain improvement may decrease over time. MVD is often the first step for healthy patients with vascular compression when symptoms persist following conservative treatment since MVD is associated with the most sustained symptom-free interval following a single treatment. One of the less invasive techniques is RFA of the trigeminal ganglion, which has documented effectiveness, although it may be accompanied by the side effects of corneal anesthesia and, rarely, deafferentation pain.

REFERENCES

1. Mokri B. Raeder's paratrigeminal syndrome. *Arch Neurol.* 1982;*39*:395–399.
2. Casey K. Role of patient history and physical examination in the diagnosis of trigeminal neuralgia. *Neurosurg Focus.* 2005;*18*(5):E1.
3. Tender G, Walbridge S, Olah Z, et al. Selective ablation of nociceptive neurons for elimination of hyperalgesia and neurogenic inflammation. *Neurosurg Focus.* 2005;*18*(5):E11.
4. Tremont-Lutkats I, Megeff C, Backonja M. Anticonvulsants for neuropathic pain syndromes: mechanisms of action and place in therapy. *Drugs.* 2000;*60*(5):1029–1052.
5. Backonja M-M. Defining neuropathic pain. *Anesth Analg.* 2003;*97*(3):785–790.
6. Hardy D, Rhoton A. Microsurgical relationships of the superior cerebellar artery and the trigeminal nerve. *J Neurosurg.* 1978;*49*:669–678.
7. Rozen TD. Trigeminal neuralgia and glossopharyngeal neuralgia. *Neurol Clin.* 2004; *22*:185–206.
8. Van Kleef M, van Genderen WE, Narouze S, Nurmikko TJ, van Zundert J, Geurts JW, et al.; World Institute of Medicine. 1. Trigeminal neuralgia. *Pain Pract.* 2009;*9*:252–259.
9. Mueller D, Oberman M, Yoon MS, Poitz F, Hansen N, Slomke MA, et al. Prevalence of trigeminal neuralgia and persistent idiopathic facial pain: a population-based study. *Cephalgia.* 2011;*31*(15):1542–1548.
10. Pollock B, Schoelberl K. Prospective comparison of posterior fossa exploration and stereotactic radiosurgery dorsal root entry zone target as primary surgery for patients with idiopathic trigeminal neuralgia. *Neurosurgery.* 2010;*67*:633–639.
11. Morgan C, Tew J. Percutaneous stereotactic rhizotomy in the treatment of intractable facial pain. In: Quinones-Hinojoso A, ed., *Schmidek & Sweet Operative Neurosurgical Techniques: Indications, Methods, and Results.* Vol. *2.* 5th ed. Philadelphia: Elsevier; 2006:1519–1529.
12. Headache Classification Subcommittee of the International Headache Society. The international classification of headache disorders: 2nd ed. *Cephalalgia.* 2004;*24*:8–160.
13. Headache Classification Subcommittee of the International Headache Society. The international classification of headache disorders: 3rd ed. *Cephalalgia.* 2013;*33*(9):629–808.
14. Gronseth G, Cruccu G, Alksne J, Argoff C, Brainin M, Burchiel K, et al. Practice parameter: the diagnostic evaluation and treatment of trigeminal neuralgia (an evidence-based review): report of the Quality Standards subcommittee of the American Academy of Neurology and the European federation of Neurological Societies. *Neurology.* 2008;*71*:1183–1190.
15. Watson JC. From paroxysmal to chronic pain in trigeminal neuralgia-implications of central sensitization. *Neurology.* 2007;*69*:817–818.
16. American Society of Anesthesiology and American Society of Regional Anesthesia and Pain Medicine. Self-assessment module for pain medicine, 2012. http://education.asahq.org/12SAMPM.
17. Eboli P, Stone J, Aydin S, Slavin K. Historical characterization of trigeminal neuralgia. *Neurosurgery.* 2009;*64*(6):1183–1187.
18. Burchiel K. A new classification for facial pain. *Neurosurgery.* 2003;*53*:1164–1167.
19. Miller J, Magill S, Acar F, Burchiel K. Predictors of long-term success after microvascular decompression for trigeminal neuralgia. *J Neurosurg.* 2009;*110*:620–626.
20. Eller J, Raslan A, Burchiel K. Trigeminal neuralgia: definition and classification. *Neurosurg Focus.* 2005;*18*:E3.
21. Lonser R, Apfelbaum R. Neurovascular decompression in surgical disorders of cranial nerves V, VII, IX, and X. In: Quinones-Hinojosa A, ed., *Schmidek & Sweet Operative Neurosurgical Techniques: Indications, Methods, and Results.* Vol. *2.* 5th ed. Philadelphia: Elsevier; 2006:1531–1543.
22. Didier H, Marchetti C, Borromeo G, Tullo V, Bussone G, Santoro F. Persistent idiopathic facial pain: multidisciplinary approach and assumption of comorbidity. *Neurol Sci.* 2010;*31*(Suppl 1):S189–S195.
23. Forsell H, Tenovuo O, Silvoniemi P, Jaaskelainen SK. Differences and similarities between atypical facial pain and trigeminal neuropathic pain. *Neurology.* 2007;*69*:1451–1459.
24. Vorenkamp KE. Interventional procedures for facial pain. *Curr Pain Headache Rep.* 2012;*17*:308. Epub ahead of print.
25. Goadsby P. Trigeminal autonomic cephalalgias. *Continuum.* 2012; *18*(4):883–895.
26. Cornelissen P, van Kleef M, Mekhail N, Day M, van Zundert J. Evidence-based interventional pain medicine according to clinical diagnoses. 3. Persistent idiopathic facial pain. *Pain Pract.* 2009;*9*(6):443–448.
27. Day M. Trigeminal ganglion block and neurolysis. In Manchikanti L, Singh V, eds. *Interventional Techniques in Chronic Non-spinal Pain.* Paducah, KY: ASIPP Publishing; 2009: 213–220.
28. Narouze S, Kapural L, Casanova J, Mekhail N. Sphenopalatine ganglion radiofrequency ablation for the management of chronic cluster headache. *Headache.* 2009; *49*(4):571–577.
29. Devor M, Govrin-Lippmann R, Rappaport H. Mechanism of trigeminal neuralgia: an ultrastructural analysis of trigeminal root specimens obtained during microvascular decompression surgery. *J Neurosurg.* 2002;*96*:532–543.
30. Burchiel K. Abnormal impulse generation in focally demyelinated trigeminal roots. *J Neurosurg.* 1980;*53*:674–683.

31. Miller J, Acar F, Hamilton B, Burchiel K. Preoperative visualization of neurovascular anatomy in trigeminal neuralgia. *J Neurosurg.* 2008;*108*:477–482.
32. Miller J, Acar F, Burchiel K. Classification of trigeminal neuralgia: clinical, therapeutic, and prognostic implications in a series of 144 patients undergoing microvascular decompression. *J Neurosurg.* 2009;*111*:1231–1234.
33. Miller J, Acar F, Hamilton B, Burchiel K. Radiographic evaluation of trigeminal neurovascular compression in patients with and without trigeminal neuralgia. *J Neurosurg.* 2009;*110*: 627–632.
34. Papanastassiou A, Schwartz R, Friedlander R. Chiari I malformation as a cause of trigeminal neuralgia: case report. *Neurosurgery.* 2008;*63*:E614–E615.
35. Kight M, Gatchel RJ, Wesley L. Temporomandibular disorders: evidence for significant overlap with psychopathology. *Health Psychol.* 1999;*18*:177–182.
36. Remich RA, Blasberg B. Psychiatric aspects of atypical facial pain. *J Can Dent Assoc.* 1985;*51*:913–916.
37. Schmidt-Wilcke T, Hierlmeier S, Leinisch E. Altered regional brain morphology in patients with chronic facial pain. *Headache.* 2010;*50*(8):1278–1285.
38. May A. Chronic pain may change the structure of the brain. *Pain.* 2008;*137*:7–15.
39. DaSilva AF, Becerra L, Pendse G, Chizh B, Tully S, Borsook D. Colocalized structural and functional changes in the cortex of patients with trigeminal neuropathic pain. *PLoS ONE.* 2008;*3*:e3396.
40. Mongini F, Ciccone G, Ceccarelli M, Baldi I, Ferrero L. Muscle tenderness in different types of facial pain and its relation to anxiety and depression: a cross-sectional study on 649 patients. *Pain.* 2007;*131*:106–111.
41. Macianskyte D, Januzis G, Kubilius R, Adomaitiene V, Sciupokas A. Associations between chronic pain and depressive symptoms in patients with trigeminal neuralgia. *Medicina* (Kaunas). 2011;*47*:386–392.
42. Hassett AL, Radvanski DC, Buyske S, Savage SV, Sigal LH. Psychiatric comorbidity and other psychological factors in patients with "chronic Lyme disease." *Am J Med.* 2009;*122*:843–850.
43. Arnold LM, Hudson JI, Keck PE, Auchenbach MB, Javaras KN, Hess EV. Comorbidity of fibromyalgia and psychiatric disorders. *J Clin Psychiatry.* 2006;*67*:1219–1225.
44. Dworkin RH, Hetzel RD, Banks SM. Toward a model of the pathogenesis of chronic pain. *Semin Clin Neuropsychiatry.* 1999;*4*:176–185.
45. Aaron LA, Burke MM, Buchwald D. Overlapping conditions among patients with chronic fatigue syndrome, fibromyalgia, and temporomandibular disorder. *Arch Intern Med.* 2000;*160*:221–227.
46. Phillips K, Clauw DJ. Central pain mechanisms in chronic pain states—maybe it is all in their head. *Best Pract Res Clin Rheumatol.* 2011;*25*:141–154.
47. Yunus MB. Fibromyalgia and overlapping disorders: the unifying concept of central sensitivity syndromes. *Semin Arthritis Rheum.* 2007;*36*:339–356.
48. Clauw DJ, Witter J. Pain and rheumatology: thinking outside the joint. *Arthritis Rheum.* 2009;*60*:321–324.
49. Williams DA, Clauw DJ. Understanding fibromyalgia: lessons from the broader pain research community. *J Pain.* 2009;*10*:777–791.
50. Tracey I, Bushnell MC. How neuroimaging studies have challenged us to rethink: is chronic pain a disease? *J Pain.* 2009;*10*:1113–1120.
51. Tolle T, Dukes E, Sadosky A. Patient burden of trigeminal neuralgia: results from a cross-sectional survey of health state impairment and treatment patterns in six European countries. *Pain Pract.* 2006;*6*:153–160.
52. Hickey A, Scrivani S, Bajwa Z. Cranial neuralgias. In: Fishman SM, Ballantyne JC, Rathmell JP, eds. *Bonica's Management of Pain.* 4th ed. Philadelphia: Lippincott Williams & Wilkins; 2010:953–971.
53. Sardella A, Demarosi F, Barbieri C, Lodi G. An up-to-date view on persistent idiopathic facial pain. *Minerva Stomatol.* 2009; *58*:289–299.
54. Medicine Io. *Relieving Pain in America: A Blueprint for Transforming Prevention, Care, Education, and Research.* Washington, DC: National Academy of Sciences; 2011.
55. Hassett AL, Williams DA. Non-pharmacological treatment of chronic widespread musculoskeletal pain. *Best Pract Res Clin Rheumatol.* 2011;*25*:299–309.
56. Hauser W, Klose P, Langhorst J, et al. Efficacy of different types of aerobic exercise in fibromyalgia syndrome: a systematic review and meta-analysis of randomised controlled trials. *Arthritis Res Ther.* *12*:R79.
57. Furto ES, Cleland JA, Whitman JM, Olson KA. Manual physical therapy interventions and exercise for patients with temporomandibular disorders. *Cranio.* 2006;*24*:283–291.
58. Sullivan AB, Scheman J, Venesy D, Davin S. The role of exercise and types of exercise in the rehabilitation of chronic pain: specific or nonspecific benefits. *Curr Pain Headache Rep.* 2012;*16*:153–161.
59. Aggarwal VR, Tickle M, Javidi H, Peters S. Reviewing the evidence: can cognitive behavioral therapy improve outcomes for patients with chronic orofacial pain? *J Orofac Pain.* 2010;*24*:163–171.
60. Bernardy K, Fuber N, Kollner V, Hauser W. Efficacy of cognitive-behavioral therapies in fibromyalgia syndrome—a systematic review and metaanalysis of randomized controlled trials. *J Rheumatol.* 2010;*37*:1991–2005.
61. Rooks DS, Gautam S, Romeling M, et al. Group exercise, education, and combination self-management in women with fibromyalgia: a randomized trial. *Arch Intern Med.* 2007;*167*:2192–2200.
62. Hassett AL, Gevirtz RN. Nonpharmacologic treatment for fibromyalgia: patient education, cognitive-behavioral therapy, relaxation techniques, and complementary and alternative medicine. *Rheum Dis Clin North Am.* 2009;*35*:393–407.
63. Radloff LS. The CES-D scale: a self-report depression scale for research in the general population. *Appl Psychol Meas.* 1977;*1*:385–401.
64. Spitzer RL, Kroenke K, Williams JB. Validation and utility of a self-report version of PRIME-MD: the PHQ primary care study. *JAMA.* 1999;*282*:1737–1744.
65. Wong MC, McMillan AS, Zheng J, Lam CL. The consequences of orofacial pain symptoms: a population-based study in Hong Kong. *Community Dent Oral Epidemiol.* 2008;*36*:417–424.
66. Benoliel R, Eliav E, Sharav Y. Self-reports of pain-related awakenings in persistent orofacial pain patients. *J Orofac Pain.* 2009;*23*:330–338.
67. Kelly GA, Blake C, Power CK, O'Keeffe D, Fullen BM. The association between chronic low back pain and sleep: a systematic review. *Clin J Pain.* 2011;*27*:169–181.
68. Schutz TC, Andersen ML, Silva A, Tufik S. Distinct gender-related sleep pattern in an acute model of TMJ pain. *J Dent Res.* 2009;*88*:471–476.
69. Schutz TC, Andersen ML, Tufik S. The influence of orofacial pain on sleep pattern: a review of theory, animal models and future directions. *Sleep Med.* 2009;*10*:822–828.
70. Hassett AL, Clauw DJ. The role of stress in rheumatic diseases. *Arthritis Res Ther.* 2010;*12*:123.
71. Giesecke T, Gracely RH, Williams DA, Geisser ME, Petzke FW, Clauw DJ. The relationship between depression, clinical pain, and experimental pain in a chronic pain cohort. *Arthritis Rheum.* 2005;*52*:1577–1584.
72. Marchand WR. Mindfulness-based stress reduction, mindfulness-based cognitive therapy, and zen meditation for depression, anxiety, pain, and psychological distress. *J Psychiatr Pract.* 2012;*18*:233–252.
73. Barker F, Jannetta P, Bissonette D, Larkins M, Jho H. The long-term outcome of microvascular decompression for trigeminal neuralgia. *N Engl J Med.* 1996;*334*(17):1077–1083.
74. Narouze, S. Head and neck blocks. In: Huntoon MA, Benzon HT, Narouze S, eds. *Spinal Injections and Peripheral Nerve Blocks: Volume 4: A volume in the interventional and neuromodulatory*

techniques for pain management series by Timothy Deer. Philadelphia : Elsevier-Saunders; 2012:46–57.
75. Jannetta P. Arterial compression of the trigeminal nerve at the pons in patients with trigeminal neuralgia. *J Neurosurg*. 1967;*26*(suppl 1): 159–162.
76. Nurmikko T, Eldridge P. Trigeminal neuralgia. *Br J Anaesth*. 2001;*87*(1):117–132.
77. Racz G, Erdine S. Trigeminal ganglion procedures. In: Raj P, ed., *Textbook of Regional Anesthesia*. Philadelphia: Churchill Livingstone; 2002: 801–808.
78. Loar C. Peripheral nervous system pain. In: Raj P, ed., *Pain Medicine: A Comprehensive Review*. St. Louis, MO: Mosby; 1996:453–460.
79. van Loveren H, Tew J, Keller J, Nurre M. A 10-year experience in the treatment of trigeminal neuralgia: comparison of percutaneous stereotaxic rhizotomy and posterior fossa exploration. *J Neurosurg*. 1982;*57*:757–764.
80. Sweet WH, Wepsic JG. Controlled thermocoagulation of trigeminal ganglion and root for differential destruction of pain fibers. Part I: Trigeminal neuralgia. *J Neurosurg*. 1974;*39*:143–156.
81. Sluijter M, Racz G. Technical aspects of radiofrequency. *Pain Practice*. 2002; *2*(3):195–200.
82. Lopez BC, Hamlyn PJ, Zakrzewska JM. Systematic review of ablative neurosurgical techniques for the treatment of trigeminal neuralgia. *Neurosurgery*. 2004;*54*:973–82. Discussion 982–983.
83. Kanpolat Y, Savas A, Bekar A, Berk C. Percutaneous controlled radiofrequency trigeminal rhizotomy for the treatment of idiopathic trigeminal neuralgia: 25-year experience with 1,600 patients. *Neurosurgery*. 2001;*48*:524–532. Discussion 532–534.
84. Yin W. Radiofrequency Gasserian rhizotomy: the role of RF lesioning in the management of facial pain. *Tech Reg Anesth Pain Manag*. 2004;*8*(1):30–34.
85. Wu CY, Meng FG, Xu SJ, Liu YG, Wang HW. Selective percutaneous radiofrequency thermocoagulation in the treatment of trigeminal neuralgia: report on 1860 cases. *Chin Med J*. 2004;*117*:467–70.
86. Broggi G, Franzini A, Lasio G, Giorgi C, Servello D. Long-term results of percutaneous retrogasserian thermorhizotomy for "essential" trigeminal neuralgia: considerations in 1000 consecutive patients. *Neurosurgery*. 1990;*26*(5):783–787.
87. Narouze S. Complications of head and neck procedures. *Tech Reg Anesth Pain Manag*. 2007;*11*:171–177.
88. Rath GP, Dash HH, Bithal PK, Goyal V. Intracranial hemorrhage after percutaneous radiofrequency trigeminal rhizotomy. *Pain Pract*. 2009;*9*(1):82–84.
89. Van Boxem K, van Eerd M, Brinkhuize T, Patijn J, van Kleef M, van Zundert J. Radiofrequency and pulsed radiofrequency treatment of chronic pain syndromes: the available evidence. *Pain Pract*. 2008;*8*(5):385–393.
90. Van Zundert J, Brabant S, Van de Kelft E, Vercruyssen A, Van Buyten, JP. Pulsed radiofrequency treatment of the Gasserian ganglion in patients with idiopathic trigeminal neuralgia. *Pain*. 2004;*104*:449–452.
91. Erdine S, Ozyalcin NS, Cimen A, Celik M, Talu GK, Disci R. Comparison of pulsed radiofrequency with conventional radiofrequency in the treatment of idiopathic trigeminal neuralgia. *Eur J Pain*. 2007;*11*:309–313.
92. Okuda Y, Okuda K, Shinohara M, Kitajima T. Use of computed tomography for maxillary nerve block in the treatment of trigeminal neuralgia. *Reg Anesth Pain Med*. 2000; *25*(4):417–419.
93. Nader A, Schittekk H, Kendall MC. Lateral pterygoid muscle and maxillary artery are key anatomical landmarks for ultrasound-guided trigeminal nerve block. *Anesthesiol*. 2013;*118*(4):957.
94. Sim SE, Kim YH, Kim YC, Park YO. Pulsed mode radiofrequency lesioning of the mental nerve for the treatment of trigeminal neuralgia. *Reg Anesth Pain Med*. 2007;*32*(5):69.
95. Nguyen M, Wilkes D. Pulsed radiofrequency V2 treatment and intranasal sphenopalatine ganglion block: a combination therapy for atypical trigeminal neuralgia. *Pain Pract*. 2010;*10*(4):370–374.
96. Jurgens TP, Muller P, Seedorf H, Regelsberger J, May A. Occipital nerve block is effective in craniofacial neuralgias but not in idiopathic persistent facial pain. *J Headache Pain*. 2012;*13*(3):199–213.
97. Linderoth B, Hakanson S. Retrogasserian glycerol rhizolysis in trigeminal neuralgia. In: Quinones-Hinojosa A, ed., *Schmidek & Sweet Operative Neurosurgical Techniques: Indications, Methods, and Results*. Vol. 2. 5th ed. Philadelphia: Elsevier; 2006:1498–1512.
98. Chen L, Xu M, Zou Y. Treatment of trigeminal neuralgia with percutaneous glycerol injection into Meckel's Cavity: experience in 4012 patients. *Cell Biochem Biophys*. 2010;*58*:85–89.
99. Kondziolka D, Lunsford L, Flickinger, J, et al. Stereotactic radiosurgery for trigeminal neuralgia: a multiinstitutional study using the gamma unit. *J Neurosurg*. 1996;*84*:940–945.
100. Monteith SJ, Medel R, Kassell NF, Wintermark M, Eames M, Snell J, Zadicario E, Grinfeld J, Sheehan JP, Elias WJ. Transcranial magnetic resonance-guided focused ultrasound surgery for trigeminal neuralgia: a cadaveric and laboratory feasibility study. *J Neurosurg*. 2013;*118*(2):319–328.
101. Brown JA. Percutaneous balloon compression for trigeminal neuralgia. *Clin Neurosurg*. 2009;*56*:73–78.
102. Skirving D, Dan N. A 20-year review of percutaneous balloon compression of the trigeminal ganglion. *J Neurosurg*. 2001;*94*:913–917.
103. Piagkou M, Demsticha T, Troupis T, Vlasis K, Skandalakis P, Makri A, et al. The pterygopalatine ganglion and its role in various pain syndromes: from anatomy to clinical practice. *Pain Pract*. 2011; *12*(5):399–412.
104. Yin W. Sphenopalatine ganglion radiofrequency lesions in the treatment of facial pain. *Tech Reg Anesth Pain Manag*. 2004; *8*(1):25–29.
105. Narouze SN. Role of sphenopalatine ganglion neuroablation in the management of cluster headache. *Curr Pain Headache Rep*. 2010; *14*:160–163.
106. Bayer E, Racz GB, Miles D, Heavner J. Sphenopalatine ganglion pulsed radiofrequency treatment in 30 patients suffering from chronic face and head pain. *Pain Pract*. 2005; *5*:223–227.
107. Varghese BT, Koshy RC, Sebastian P, Joseph E. Combined sphenopalatine ganglion and mandibular nerve, neurolytic block for pain due to advanced head and neck cancer. *Palliat Med*. 2002; *16*:447–448.
108. Cepero R, Miller RH, Bressler KL. Long-term results of sphenopalatine ganglioneurectomy for facial pain. *Am J Otolaryngol*. 1987; *8*:171–174.
109. De Salles AA, Gorgulho A, Golish SR, Medin PM, Malkasian D, Solberg TD, et al. Technical and anatomical aspects of Novalis stereotactic radiosurgery sphenopalatine ganglionectomy. *Int J Radiat Oncol Bio Phys*. 2006;*66*:53–57.
110. Vaisman J, Markley H, Ordia J, Deer T. The treatment of medically intractable trigeminal autonomic cephalgia with supraorbital/supratrochlear stimulation: a retrospective case series. *Neuromodulation*. 2012;*15*(4):374–380.
111. Slavin KV, Colpan ME, Munawar N, Wess C, Nersesyan H. Trigeminal and occipital peripheral nerve stimulation for craniofacial pain: a single-institution experience and review of the literature. *Neurosurg Focus*. 2006;*21*(6):E5.
112. Ansarinia M, Rezai A, Tepper SJ, Steiner CP, Stump J, Stanton-Hicks M, Machado A, Narouze S. Electrical stimulation of sphenopalatine ganglion for acute treatment of cluster headaches. *Headache*. 2010; *50*(7):1164–1174.
113. Burns B, Watkins L, Goadsby PJ. Treatment of medically intractable cluster headache by occipital nerve stimulation: long-term follow-up of eight patients. *Lancet*. 2007;*369*:1099–1106.
114. Henderson J, Lad S. Motor cortex stimulation and neuropathic facial pain. *Neurosurg Focus*. 2006;*21*(6):E6.

4.

CARPAL TUNNEL SYNDROME

Bashar Katirji and Binit J. Shah

CASE PRESENTATION

A 52-year-old right-handed woman had a 2-year history of pain and tingling in both hands, worse on the right. The pain and tingling was triggered by writing, holding a book, or driving. She frequently was awakened at night by the numbness. Shaking the hands tended to relieve the symptoms. She noticed some consistent impairment of dexterity in the right hand. She had no weakness in the hands. There was no numbness or weakness in the legs.

Past medical history is significant for hypertension. She is on hydrochlorothiazide and has no known drug allergy. Social history is significant for being a secretary. She drinks alcohol socially and denies illicit drugs or smoking.

On examination, she has positive Phalen's sign bilaterally. Tinel's sign could not be induced on percussion of the median nerves at the wrist. There was relative hypesthesia bilaterally in the median nerve distribution compared with the ulnar nerve distribution. There was no thenar atrophy or weakness. Deep tendon reflexes are normal throughout. Otherwise, cranial nerve examination, muscle strength, and lower extremity sensation were normal.

QUESTIONS

1. What is the anatomy of the median nerve and carpal tunnel?
2. What is the definition and cause of carpal tunnel syndrome (CTS)?
3. What are the clinical findings in CTS?
4. What are the common and atypical historical features of CTS?
5. What is the differential diagnosis of CTS?
6. What diagnostic studies are necessary for accurate diagnosis?
7. How is CTS managed?:
   a. Rehabilitation and splinting
   b. Pharmacological management
   c. Interventional procedures
   d. Surgical intervention
   e. Behavioral/psychiatric intervention
8. What is the prognosis of CTS?

WHAT IS THE ANATOMY OF THE MEDIAN NERVE AND CARPAL TUNNEL?

The median nerve is a major terminal nerve of the brachial plexus formed by contributions from the lateral and medial cords. The lateral cord component, comprising the C6–C7 fibers, provides sensory fibers to the thumb and thenar eminence (C6), index finger (C6–C7) and middle finger (C7) and motor fibers to the proximal median innervated forearm muscles. The medial cord component, comprising C8–T1 fibers, provides sensory fibers to the lateral half of the ring finger (C8) and motor fibers to the hand and distal median innervated forearm muscles. The median nerve descends with no branches in the arm. In the antecubital fossa, it passes between the two heads of the pronator teres and send muscular branches to the pronator teres, flexor carpi radialis, flexor digitorum sublimis, and palmaris longus muscles. In the proximal forearm, the median nerve gives off the anterior interosseous nerve, which is a pure motor nerve that innervates the flexor pollicis longus, medial head of the flexor digitorum profundus, and the pronator quadratus muscles (Figures 4.1 and 4.2).[1]

The carpal tunnel is a rigid and inelastic channel; its floor and sides are formed by the carpal bones, whereas the roof is made by the transverse carpal ligament that attaches to the scaphoid, trapezoid, and hamate bones.[2] The dimensions of the carpal tunnel are variable, with significant variation between individuals as well as familial differences.[3] The cross-section is approximately 2.0–2.5 cm at its narrowest point in most individuals. The main trunk of the median nerve, along with nine finger flexor tendons, enters the wrist through the carpal tunnel. Before entering the tunnel, the median nerve gives off a cutaneous branch, the palmar

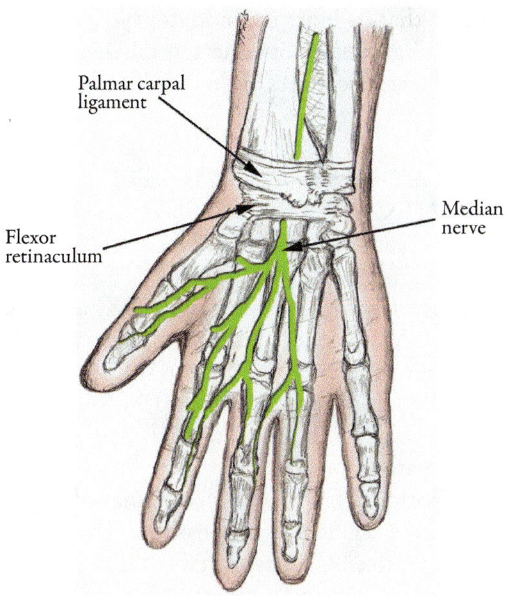

Figure 4.1 Carpal tunnel anatomy. Reprinted with permission from Konik Z, Raghavendra M, Peterson JS. "Carpal Tunnel Steroid Injection."1 Oct. 2012. http://emedicine.medscape.com/article/103333-overview.

cutaneous branch, which does not pass through the carpal tunnel and innervates a small patch of skin over the thenar eminence.

Immediately after exiting the tunnel, the median nerve branches into motor and sensory branches. The motor branch innervates the first and second lumbricals and gives off the recurrent motor branch, which innervates the thenar muscles (abductor pollicis brevis, opponens pollicis, and half of the flexor pollicis brevis). The sensory branch divides into terminal digital sensory branches to innervate three and one-half fingers (thumb, index, middle finger, and lateral half of the ring finger) with the corresponding palm.

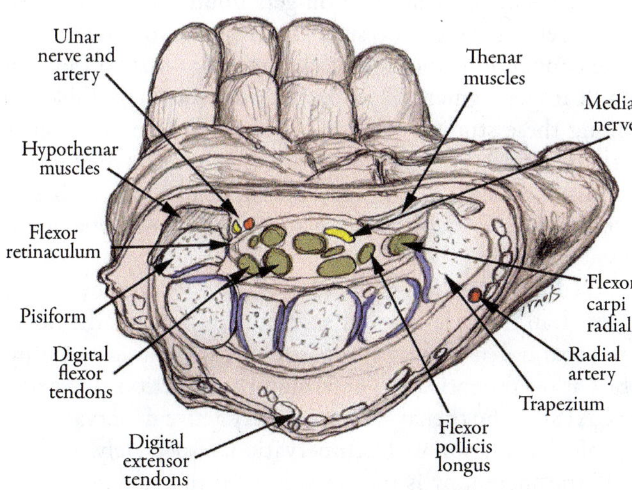

Figure 4.2 Carpal tunnel anatomy, cross-section. Reprinted with permission from Konik Z, Raghavendra M, Peterson JS. "Carpal Tunnel Steroid Injection."1 Oct. 2012. http://emedicine.medscape.com/article/103333-overview.

WHAT IS THE DEFINITION AND CAUSE OF CTS?

CTS is, by definition, median nerve entrapment underneath the transverse carpal ligament.[4] CTS is the most common entrapment neuropathy. It is slightly more common in women (women-to-men ratio 2.2:1).[5] CTS usually involves the dominant hand first. It is most prevalent after 50 years of age, but it may occur in younger patients.[6] The incidence of CTS has significantly increased in the past two decades.[5] Most cases of CTS are idiopathic and possibly related to congenitally small carpal tunnels. Occupations that involve hand-held vibratory tools or prolonged and highly repetitious flexion and extension of the wrist have a higher risk for developing CTS.[7] However, the frequency of CTS in computer and keyboard users is similar to that in the general population.[7,8] Medical conditions associated with a high risk for CTS are pregnancy, rheumatod arthritis, diabetes mellitus, obesity, hypothyroidism, gout, uremia, acromegaly, sarcoidosis, and amyloidosis. These medical comorbidities, particularly rheumatoid arthritis, are most significant in younger patients (<40 years).[6,9,10] The incidence of clinically diagnosed pregnancy-related CTS varies depending on the methods used to detect this syndrome, ranging from 30% to 60% of patients, and the symptoms of CTS persist in more than half of these patients for 1 year after delivery.[11] Anomalous muscles, wrist fractures (Colles's fracture or carpal bone), space-occupying lesions (ganglia, lipoma, schwannoma), crush injury of the hand, or acute tenosynovitis may also compress the median nerve at the carpal tunnel.

WHAT ARE THE CLINICAL FINDINGS IN CTS?

Nocturnal hand paresthesia with or without pain, often awakening the patient from sleep, is the hallmark of CTS and is the most common presenting symptom.[12,13] These paresthesias may also be triggered by wrist activities that require wrist flexion or extension such driving, holding a book, or talking on the phone. In some patients, the symptoms are relieved by shaking or wringing the hands. In more advanced CTS cases, patients become aware of impaired hand dexterity and loss of ability to manipulate objects, and they often drop objects from their affected hands. Fixed sensory loss in one or more median innervated digits (thumb, index finger, or middle finger) or grip weakness are late symptoms of CTS.

Two provocative bedside maneuvers are very useful in confirming the diagnosis of CTS. In Phalen's maneuver, paresthesias into the median innervated digits are reproduced in 1–2 minutes of wrist flexion. This finding is extremely sensitive (positive in 80–90% of cases) and specific, with very few false positives.[14] In Tinel's sign, paresthesias are elicited by tapping over the median nerve at the wrist. This maneuver is less sensitive than Phalen's sign (positive in 50–70% of cases only) and produces up to 30% false positives.[14]

On neurological examination, there is usually hypoesthesia in the median distribution in the hand that may be more prominent in one or more median innervated digits. The tips of fingers tend to be affected early and abnormal two-point discrimination is often more evident before pinprick, touch, or temperature sensations.[13] Thenar sensation remains normal. In advanced cases, weakness and/or atrophy of thenar eminence is evident.

WHAT ARE THE COMMON AND ATYPICAL HISTORICAL FEATURES OF CTS?

Some consistent symptoms common in CTS and do not raise suspicions of other disorders. These include pain that extend proximally from the hand and wrist to the forearm and even shoulder; perception of numbness in all digits rather than median distribution only (lateral fingers); and absence of detectable sensory loss on neurological examination.

In contrast, several other manifestations are not compatible with the diagnosis of CTS and suggest other diagnoses. These include neck pain and radicular pain into the arm or forearm, suggesting cervical radiculopathy; definite numbness over the thenar eminence, suggesting high (proximal) median nerve lesion or brachial plexopathy; or detectable weakness and/or atrophy of hypothenar muscles, finger flexion, or finger extension indicative of a lower cervical radiculopathy or brachial plexopathy.

WHAT IS THE DIFFERENTIAL DIAGNOSIS OF CTS?

CTS should be distinguished from several disorders that may result in similar symptoms. *Cervical radiculopathy,* particularly C6 or C7 radiculopathy, often causes numbness of the thumb, index finger, or middle finger. In contrast to CTS, there are often sensory manifestations above the wrist, radicular pain exacerbated by neck movements, segmental weakness in the arm and forearm, or reflex asymmetry. When bilateral, CTS may mimic *peripheral polyneuropathy,* which may be associated with hand numbness. However, there are often sensory manifestations and/or motor weakness in the legs and distal hyporeflexia or areflexia, especially at the ankles. CTS may be mistaken for *neurogenic thoracic outlet syndrome* because both may be associated with selective thenar atrophy. However, the pain and sensory manifestations in neurogenic thoracic outlet syndrome are along the ring and little fingers and medial aspect of the forearm (C8–T1 distribution). *Cervical myelopathy* may cause hand numbness but is not usually restricted to the median nerve distribution, and other pyramidal manifestations frequently are present. *Transient ischemic attack* may occasionally be difficult to distinguish from CTS when the sensory symptoms are intermittent, occur upon arousal, and are not triggered by use. A *high median mononeuropathy,* a rare condition that includes the pronator syndrome and compression at the ligament of Struthers in the distal arm, is usually associated with weakness of the long finger flexors.

WHAT DIAGNOSTIC STUDIES ARE NECESSARY FOR ACCURATE DIAGNOSIS?

The goals of electrodiagnostic testing (EDX) are to confirm the presence of a distal lesion of the median nerve and exclude other peripheral conditions that may result in similar symptoms, especially peripheral polyneuropathy, C6 or C7 radiculopathy, and, less commonly, brachial plexopathy or high median neuropathy.[15]

In the majority of CTS cases, demyelination is present in the median nerve segment underneath the transverse carpal ligament. In advanced CTS cases, axonal loss occurs. Hence, routine median motor and sensory nerve conduction studies easily demonstrate slowing of median sensory and motor distal latencies across the wrist in moderate or severe cases. The median motor and sensory amplitudes are reduced when axonal loss occurs and, occasionally, with conduction block. It is also essential to study the ulnar motor and sensory nerve to ensure that the abnormalities seen in the median nerve are not present in the ulnar nerves, which may suggest other diagnoses such as a diffuse peripheral polyneuropathy or brachial plexopathy.

In mild cases of CTS (approximately 10–25%), routine median sensory and motor nerve conduction studies are normal or borderline. In these cases, additional more sensitive studies are required to confirm the diagnosis. These studies are the "internal comparison studies." In these nerve conductions studies, the median nerve study is compared to an adjacent nerve of identical length in the same hand, usually the ulnar nerve and, occasionally, the radial nerve. The rationale for these studies is that the slow-conducting segment of the median nerve in CTS usually is very short. Hence, the short segment of demyelination gets diluted when included in a longer nerve segment, such as during the routine median nerve conduction studies that measure the wrist to index or middle finger segments. These studies are shown in Table 4.1. Among these studies, comparing the median motor latency to the second lumbrical and the ulnar motor latency to the interossei muscles is also very useful in patients with suspected severe CTS or in those with underlying generalized polyneuropathy.[16,17]

Needle electromyography (EMG) assesses the severity of the median nerve lesion and excludes C6 or C7 radiculopathy, proximal median neuropathy, or brachial plexopathy. Fibrillation potentials or large motor unit action potentials (MUAPs) in the thenar muscles signify active denervation or chronic denervation with reinnervation, respectively.

Ultrasonography is increasingly used in the diagnosis of CTS. The cross-sectional area of the median nerve at the carpal tunnel inlet is usually significantly increased compared to the distal forearm. This also correlates with the electrodiagnostic and clinical severity of the CTS. However, the

Table 4.1 INTERNAL COMPARISON STUDIES IN THE EVALUATION OF MILD CARPAL TUNNEL SYNDROME (CTS)

STUDY	PALMAR	MEDIAN-ULNAR	2ND LUMBRICAL-INTEROSSEI	MEDIAN-RADIAL
Description	Median-ulnar mixed palmar latency comparison	Median-ulnar sensory latency comparison	Median-ulnar motor latency comparison	Median-radial sensory latency comparison
Fibers evaluated	Mixed (sensory and motor)	Sensory (antidromic)	Motor	Sensory (antidromic)
Technique	Palm stimulation of the median and ulnar nerves, recording at the wrist	Median and ulnar nerves stimulation at the wrist recording ring fingers	Median and ulnar nerves stimulation at the wrist recording 2nd lumbrical and 2nd interossei, respectively (2nd interosseous space)	Median and radial nerves stimulation at the wrist recording thumb
Distance (range)	8 cm	14 cm (11–14 cm)	9 cm (8–10 cm)	10 cm (8–10 cm)
Abnormal values	Median-ulnar peak latency difference ≥0.4 msec	Median-ulnar peak latency difference ≥0.4 msec	Median-ulnar onset latency difference ≥0.5 msec	Median-radial peak latency difference ≥0.4 msec

sensitivity and specificity of ultrasound in the diagnosis of CTS are less than for EDX studies, at 77% and 86%, respectively.[18] Computed tomography (CT) or magnetic resonance imaging (MRI) of the wrist is occasionally performed, mostly in patients with fullness on clinical examination or in those with slowly progressive deficit without intermittent fluctuations. This may detect nerve tumors (e.g., schwannomas, neurofibromas) or ganglion cysts.

HOW IS CTS MANAGED?

REHABILITATION AND SPLINTING

In patients with provoking factors that could have triggered CTS, such as writing, typing, or playing a musical instrument, eliminating these aggravating factors is important. A change in posture or workstation or using a wrist pad on a computer keyboard may improve many of the symptoms. In addition to limiting these provocative factors, a wrist splint is often useful. The splint may be worn only during sleep; the splint keeps the wrist neutral at night and prevents wrist flexion and extension that increases pressure within the carpal tunnel. Splinting is usually indicated in patients with mild to moderate symptoms. However, there is limited evidence on the effectiveness, duration of use, wearing regimen, or splint design in CTS.[19]

PHARMACOLOGICAL MANAGEMENT

Nonsteroidal anti-inflammatory agents, such as ibuprofen or naproxen, are often useful. They help to reduce symptoms by decreasing pain and swelling in the carpal tunnel. A 2–3 week course may offer significant relief. Oral corticosteroids also provide significant relief.[20]

INTERVENTIONAL PROCEDURES

Long-acting corticosteroids, such as 40–80 mg of methylprednisolone (Depo-Medrol) may be injected adjacent to the carpal tunnel to provide good relief.[20] The effect becomes evident within a few days and often last for several weeks or months. Steroid injections are most useful in mild cases or in situations where CTS may be time limited, such as during pregnancy. Local steroid injection is also superior to oral steroid in the treatment of CTS.[20]

Corticosteroids may be only a temporary measure in patients with moderate CTS; repeated injections are possible but often add no benefit to a single injection[21] and carry the risk of damage to the long finger flexor tendons.

SURGICAL INTERVENTION

Surgical carpal tunnel release is recommended for patients who are symptomatic and have failed conservative measures and in patients with severe CTS associated with axonal loss. Open surgical sectioning of the volar carpal ligament or fiberoptic techniques are often successful[22] and are more effective than conservative therapy in treating CTS.[23,24] However, there is no strong evidence that favors one surgical treatment over another, although patients who undergo endoscopic carpal tunnel release return to work or activities of daily living few days earlier than do those receiving open carpal tunnel release.[25,26] Surgery often results in rapid resolution of pain and paresthesias in 80–90% of patients.

BEHAVIORAL/PSYCHIATRIC INTERVENTION

Further history was taken with a specific focus on aggravating factors and repetitive motions. As indicated, the patient is a secretary, spending approximately 90% of her working day at a computer and typing. She has no ergonomic support when using a mouse or keyboard. Her main hobby was reported as TV watching. When asked about other possible factors, the patient is hesitant and embarrassed but does admit to repetitive tapping as well as turning light switches on and off. She states that for the past 30 years she has "had to" engage in either of these behaviors to relieve tension. She is quite aware this is abnormal, hence her hesitancy. While at work, she finds that if not occupied at a computer, she will quickly tap her third digit for what amounts to a total time of 3–4 hours/day. Her preference, however, is for turning light switches on and off. She recognizes the absurdity of the behavior (allowing her to do this only when home) but feels powerless to resist. She estimates she will spend another 1–2 hours daily doing this.

The patient reports classic symptoms of obsessive-compulsive disorder (OCD): she has repetitive behaviors (tapping, light switches) that she feels compelled to perform, they reduce anxiety (in this case she has increased anxiety if she is prevented from completing them), they are time-consuming, and she has insight into the dysfunctional nature of her actions. (For the diagnostic criteria of obsessive-compulsive disorder, see the *Diagnostic and Statistical Manual of Mental Disorders*, 5th edition.)

The hallmark of OCD is either recurrent/persistent thoughts, urges, impulses, or images (obsessions) or repetitive behaviors/mental acts (compulsions). Although either obsessions or compulsions are necessary for diagnosis of OCD, the majority of patients experience both.[27] The 12-month prevalence in the United States is 1.2%,[28,29] making the diagnosis slightly more common than schizophrenia. The mean age of onset is approximately 20 years, and the disorder is more common in females. If left untreated, it has a chronic, lifelong, course and the likelihood of spontaneous remission is rare.[30,31] For those with childhood-onset OCD, however, 40% may experience remission in adulthood.[32]

As in this case, most adult patients are aware of the purposeless nature of their compulsions and often embarrassed by them. The combination of relentless drive to indulge these urges combined with insight leads up to 50% to have suicidal thoughts, and up to 25% have reported a suicidal attempt.[33] In situations where they are unable or unwilling to indulge in the compulsion of choice, they will substitute other behaviors, resuming their preferred behavior when alone or unobserved. Given the often associated shame and embarrassment, OCD symptoms are rarely reported spontaneously, and specific inquiry should be instituted during any standard psychiatric workup, but also in cases where compulsive behavior could be contributing to medical symptoms (e.g., hand gestures causing CTS, overeating leading to obesity, itching leading to rash or dermatologic changes). In addition, there are case reports[34,35] of patients with facial pain who present "obsessed" with their complaints and who have been treated with clomipramine only to see their obsessions and subsequent pain decrease.

There has been some research specifically evaluating pain in patients with OCD. Interestingly, patients with OCD have been found to have higher pain tolerance.[36] This may be because physical pain allows for a distraction from otherwise overwhelming urges and thoughts. In a veteran population with OCD, 24% reported significant pain when evaluated with the SF-36, significantly lower than veterans without OCD (31%).[37] Further support for a diminished pain experience comes from a study that compared 53 patients with OCD to age- and gender-matched controls using the SF-36, Beck Depression Inventory, and Beck Anxiety Inventory. Patients with OCD had lower quality of life ratings in all dimensions *except* for pain.[38] These studies have all included subjects with symptoms or uncontrolled OCD. Therefore, it is unclear if the psychological distress and preoccupation leads to great pain tolerance/less reporting or if, in fact, there is a biological difference.

Pharmacologic therapy is considered first-line treatment for OCD, and the greatest evidence base is for selective serotonin reuptake inhibitors (SSRIs) and the tricyclic antidepressant (TCA) clomipramine. Meta-analysis shows that all SSRIs are more effective than placebo, and no individual SSRI is considered more efficacious than another.[39] When an SSRI is initiated, most often it requires near maximal dosing for best response (e.g. fluoxetine 60–80 mg/d, sertraline 150–200 mg/d, citalopram 40–60 mg/d, escitalopram 20–30 mg/d, paroxetine 40–60 mg/d).

A large body of literature and meta-analysis also shows the efficacy of clomipramine (100–250 mg/d) versus placebo.[40] Direct comparisons between SSRIs and clomipramine have found them to be equal in symptom reduction.[41] Because SSRIs show much greater tolerability, they are typically chosen at treatment initiation. Regardless of which agent is used, about 50% of patients will shows a 20–40% reduction in symptoms.[42,43]

As a TCA, clomipramine is structurally very similar to the agents amitriptyline and nortriptyline, which are used in the treatment of various pain conditions. Therefore, this may be strong consideration in chronic pain patients. Although there are no studies specifically evaluating clomipramine versus SSRIs in patients with OCD and pain, a case report on two patients with OCD and chronic low back pain showed improvement of both with treatment of clomipramine 30–75 mg/d.[44]

Surprisingly, although selective serotonin-norepinephrine reuptake inhibitors (SNRIs; e.g., venlafaxine, duloxetine) are often used interchangeably with SSRIs in the treatment of multiple depressive and anxiety disorders, they are clearly inferior in the treatment of OCD.

Given that most patients will have response rather than remission with monotherapy, augmentation must be considered. Atypical antipsychotics (specifically haloperidol and risperidone) have been found to be efficacious in meta-analysis.[45–48]

Cognitive behavioral therapy (CBT) is perhaps the most efficacious augmenting therapy and, in fact, has shown robust efficacy equal to SSRIs as an independent treatment. There is accumulating evidence that CBT may be more effective than pharmacotherapy for uncomplicated OCD. SSRIs and clomipramine remain first-line treatment strategies due to the extremely high rates of comorbid psychiatric conditions—76% of patients have a lifetime history of another anxiety disorder, and 63% have a mood disorder.[49] Specifically, exposure and response prevention is used. In this method, a patient is made to confront his or her fearful or anxiety provoking situation (exposure) and kept from engaging in his or her escape behavior (preventing the repetitive behavior).

CBT and pharmacotherapy, either alone or more commonly in combination, will reduce symptoms in the majority of patients with OCD. However, despite optimal management, 10% of patients will continue to have severe, refractory symptoms.[50] In these cases, deep brain stimulation (DBS) may be considered. To date approximately 100 patients have received DBS, and it is still considered an experimental treatment. As such, it is beyond the scope of this chapter, but interested readers are referred to recent reviews.[51,52]

After discussing treatment options, our patient elected to begin with pharmacotherapy due to a decreased time commitment for success. For tolerability, an SSRI was considered, and several medications were discussed with the patient. Ultimately, the patient was started on sertraline. We discussed a target dose of 150–200 mg/d, and she was started on 25 mg/d × 1 week, then 50 mg/d × 1 week, then 100 mg/d × 1 week, then 150 mg/d. At 1-month follow-up she had noted no significant benefit (but also no side effects). We discussed that full therapeutic benefit could take up to 12 weeks. Because she was tolerating the medication well, and we anticipated needing near maximal doses, she was also given the option of increasing sertraline to 200 mg/d, which she elected to do. Over the next 2 months, she had a 60% reduction in her symptoms as monitored by the Yale-Brown Obsessive Compulsive Scale. The patient still reported significant tapping and light switch behavior, and she was started in CBT, meeting once a week. Over the next 16 weeks, she continued to have sustained improvement with an easier time resisting her urges to turn on light switches and a decreased number of "flips."

WHAT IS THE PROGNOSIS OF CTS?

The prognosis of CTS is usually very good with either conservative or surgical treatment. Patients with a short duration of CTS symptoms (less than a year) and milder night paresthesias do best with splinting.[53] A comparison between splinting versus surgery suggested that surgery may have a better long-term outcome than splinting.[24] The pain and paresthesias are usually the first symptoms that respond very well to those measures. The recovery of motor or sensory deficits depends on whether the underlying pathology is demyelination, axonal loss, or a combination of both. Remyelination is usually complete within several weeks, but axonal loss recovers slowly over several months. Compared with preoperative values, nerve conduction studies demonstrate improvement in distal latencies, which may lag behind the relief of symptoms. Patients with moderate preoperative EDX abnormalities improve, whereas patients with severe abnormalities have poorer results.[54]

Underlying peripheral polyneuropathy, significant alcohol consumption, male gender, longer disease duration, and cases with significant axonal loss are general factors associated with poorer outcome and incomplete recovery of motor and sensory functions.[54] Poor surgical results may be due to incomplete sectioning of the transverse ligament, surgical damage of the palmar cutaneous branch of the median nerve, scarring within the carpal tunnel, or an incorrect preoperative diagnosis. Surgical re-exploration is sometimes indicated in some cases with poor response to the initial surgical release.[55]

REFERENCES

1. Wertsch JJ, Melvin J. Median nerve anatomy and entrapment syndromes: a review. *Arch Phys Med Rehabil.* 1982;63(12):623–627. Epub 1982/12/01.
2. Rotman MB, Donovan JP. Practical anatomy of the carpal tunnel [published online ahead of print October 10 2002]. *Hand Clin.* 2002;18(2):219–230.
3. Bleecker ML, Bohlman M, Moreland R, Tipton A. Carpal tunnel syndrome: role of carpal canal size [published online ahead of print November 1, 1985]. *Neurol.* 1985;35(11):1599–604.
4. Rosenbaum RB, Ochoa JL. *Carpal tunnel syndrome and other disorders of the median nerve.* 2nd ed. Boston: Butterworth-Heinemann/Elsevier; 2002.
5. Gelfman R, Melton LJ, 3rd, Yawn BP, Wollan PC, Amadio PC, Stevens JC. Long-term trends in carpal tunnel syndrome [published online ahead of print January 1, 2009]. *Neurol.* 2009;72(1):33–41.
6. Becker J, Nora DB, Gomes I, Stringari FF, Seitensus R, Panosso JS, et al. An evaluation of gender, obesity, age and diabetes mellitus as risk factors for carpal tunnel syndrome [published online ahead of print August 10 2002]. *Clin Neurol.* 2002;113(9):1429–1434.
7. Palmer KT, Harris EC, Coggon D. Carpal tunnel syndrome and its relation to occupation: a systematic literature review [published online ahead of print November 4 2006]. *Occup Med* (Lond). 2007;57(1):57–66.
8. Stevens JC, Witt JC, Smith BE, Weaver AL. The frequency of carpal tunnel syndrome in computer users at a medical facility [published online ahead of print June 13 2001]. *Neurol.* 2001;56(11):1568–1570.
9. Tseng CH, Liao CC, Kuo CM, Sung FC, Hsieh DP, Tsai CH. Medical and non-medical correlates of carpal tunnel syndrome in a Taiwan cohort of one million [published online ahead of print June 3 2011]. *Eur J Neurol.* 2012;19(1):91–97.
10. Karpitskaya Y, Novak CB, Mackinnon SE. Prevalence of smoking, obesity, diabetes mellitus, and thyroid disease in patients with carpal tunnel syndrome [published online ahead of print February 2 2002]. *Ann Plast Surg.* 2002;48(3):269–273.
11. Padua L, Di Pasquale A, Pazzaglia C, Liotta GA, Librante A, Mondelli M. Systematic review of pregnancy-related carpal tunnel syndrome [published online ahead of print October 27 2010]. *Musc Nerve.* 2010;42(5):697–702.
12. Uchiyama S, Itsubo T, Nakamura K, Kato H, Yasutomi T, Momose T. Current concepts of carpal tunnel syndrome: pathophysiology, treatment, and evaluation [published online ahead of print February 13 2010]. *J Orth Sci.* 2010;15(1):1–13.
13. Bickel KD. Carpal tunnel syndrome [published online ahead of print February 2 2010]. *J Hand Surg.* 2010;35(1):147–152.
14. Bruske J, Bednarski M, Grzelec H, Zyluk A. The usefulness of the Phalen test and the Hoffmann-Tinel sign in the diagnosis of carpal tunnel syndrome [published online ahead of print June 8 2002]. *Acta Orthop Belg.* 2002;68(2):141–145.
15. Werner RA, Andary M. Electrodiagnostic evaluation of carpal tunnel syndrome [published online ahead of print September 17 2011]. *Musc Nerve.* 2011;44(4):597–607.
16. Boonyapisit K, Katirji B, Shapiro BE, Preston DC. Lumbrical and interossei recording in severe carpal tunnel syndrome [published online ahead of print December 26 2001]. *Musc Nerve.* 2002;25(1):102–105.
17. Ubogu EE, Benatar M. Electrodiagnostic criteria for carpal tunnel syndrome in axonal polyneuropathy [published online ahead of print February 28 2006]. *Musc Nerve.* 2006;33(6):747–52.
18. Fowler JR, Gaughan JP, Ilyas AM. The sensitivity and specificity of ultrasound for the diagnosis of carpal tunnel syndrome: a meta-analysis [published online ahead of print October 22 2010]. *Clin Orthop Rel Res.* 2011;469(4):1089–1094.
19. Page MJ, Massy-Westropp N, O'Connor D, Pitt V. Splinting for carpal tunnel syndrome [published online ahead of print July 13 2012]. *Cochrane Database Syst Rev.* 2012;7:CD010003.
20. Wong SM, Hui AC, Tang A, Ho PC, Hung LK, Wong KS, et al. Local vs systemic corticosteroids in the treatment of carpal tunnel

syndrome [published online ahead of print June 13 2001]. *Neurol.* 2001;56(11):1565–1567.
21. Wong SM, Hui AC, Lo SK, Chiu JH, Poon WF, Wong L. Single vs. two steroid injections for carpal tunnel syndrome: a randomised clinical trial [published online ahead of print December 15 2005]. *Int J Clin Pract.* 2005;59(12):1417–1421.
22. Mirza MA, King ET, Jr., Tanveer S. Palmar uniportal extrabursal endoscopic carpal tunnel release [published online ahead of print February 1 1995]. *Arthroscopy.* 1995;11(1):82–90.
23. Huisstede BM, Randsdorp MS, Coert JH, Glerum S, van Middelkoop M, Koes BW. Carpal tunnel syndrome. Part II: effectiveness of surgical treatments—a systematic review [published online ahead of print July 6 2010]. *Arch Phys Med Rehabil.* 2010;91(7):1005–1024.
24. Gerritsen AA, de Vet HC, Scholten RJ, Bertelsmann FW, de Krom MC, Bouter LM. Splinting vs surgery in the treatment of carpal tunnel syndrome: a randomized controlled trial [published online ahead of print September 7 2002. *JAMA.* 2002;288(10):1245–1251.
25. Mintalucci DJ, Leinberry CF, Jr. Open versus endoscopic carpal tunnel release [published online ahead of print October 3 2012]. *Orthop Clin North Am.* 2012;43(4):431–437.
26. Scholten RJ, Mink van der Molen A, Uitdehaag BM, Bouter LM, de Vet HC. Surgical treatment options for carpal tunnel syndrome [published online ahead of print October 19 2007. *Cochrane Database Syst Rev.* 2007(4):CD003905.
27. Foa EB, Kozak MJ, Goodman WK, et al. DSM-IV field trial: obsessive-compulsive disorder. *Am J Psychiatry.* 1995;152:90.
28. Kessler RC, Chiu WT, Demler O, et al. Prevalence, severity, and comorbidity of 12-month DSM-IV disorders in the National Comorbidity Survey Replication. *Arch Gen Psychiatry.* 2005;62(6):617–627.
29. Ruscio AM, Stein DJ, Chiu WT, Kessler RC. The epidemiology of obsessive-compulsive disorder in the National Comorbidity Survey Replication. *Mol Psychiatry.* 2010;15(1):53–63.
30. Ravizza L, Maina G, Bogetto F. Episodic and chronic obsessive-compulsive disorder. *Depress Anxiety.* 1997;6(4):154–158.
31. Skoog G, Skoog I. A 40-year follow-up of patients with obsessive-compulsive disorder. *Arch Gen Psychiatry.* 1999; 56(2):121–127.
32. Stewart SE, Geller DA, Jenike M, et al. Long-term outcome of pediatric obsessive-compulsive disorder: a meta-analysis and qualitative review of the literature. *Acta Psychiatr Scand.* 2004;110(1):4–13.
33. Torres AR, Ramos-Cerqueira AT, Ferrão YA, et al. Suicidality in obsessive-compulsive disorder: prevalence and relation to symptom dimensions and comorbid conditions. *J Clin Psychiatry.* 2011;72:17.
34. Keyser JJ. Clomipramine for obsessive pain-type syndromes. *Plast Reconstr Surg.* 1992;89:166.
35. Fishbain DA, Trescott J, Cutler B, et al. Do some chronic pain patients with atypical facial pain overvalue and obsess about their pain? *Psychosomatics.* 1993;34:355–359.
36. Hezel DM, Riemann BC, McNally RJ. Emotional distress and pain tolerance in obsessive-compulsive disorder. *J Behav Ther Exp Psychiatry.* 2012;43(4):981–987.
37. Gros DF, Magruder KM, Frueh BC. Obsessive compulsive disorder in veterans in primary care: prevalence and impairment. *Gen Hosp Psychiatry.* 2013;35(1):71–73.
38. Fontenelle IS, Fontenelle LF, Borges MC, et al. Quality of life and symptom dimensions of patients with obsessive-compulsive disorder. *Psychiatry Res.* 2010;179(2):198–203.
39. Soomro GM, Altman D, Rajagopal S, et al. Selective serotonin re-uptake inhibitors (SSRIs) versus placebo for obsessive compulsive disorder (OCD). *Cochrane Database Syst Rev.* 2008;CD001765.
40. Ackerman DL, Greenland S. Multivariate meta-analysis of controlled drug studies for obsessive-compulsive disorder. *J Clin Psychopharmacol.* 2002;22:309.
41. Simpson HB. Pharmacotherapy for obsessive-compulsive disorder. In: Basow DS, ed. UpToDate. Waltham, MA: 2013.
42. Pigott TA, Seay SM. A review of the efficacy of selective serotonin reuptake inhibitors in obsessive-compulsive disorder. A meta-analysis. *J Clin Psychiatry.* 1999;60(2):101–106..
43. Greist JH, Jefferson JW, Kobak KA, et al. Efficacy and tolerability of serotonin transport inhibitors in obsessive-compulsive disorder. A meta analysis. *Arch Gen Psychiatry.* 1995;52:53.
44. Kurokawa K, Tanino R. Effectiveness of clomipramine for obsessive-compulsive symptoms and chronic pain in two patients with schizophrenia. *J Clin Psychopharmacol.* 1997;17(4):329–330.
45. McDougle CJ, Epperson CN, Pelton GH, et al. A double-blind, placebo-controlled study of risperidone addition in serotonin reuptake inhibitor-refractory obsessive-compulsive disorder. *Arch Gen Psychiatry.* 2000;57:794.
46. McDougle CJ, Goodman WK, Leckman JF, et al. Haloperidol addition in fluvoxamine-refractory obsessive-compulsive disorder. A double-blind, placebo-controlled study in patients with and without tics. *Arch Gen Psychiatry.* 1994;51:302.
47. Bloch MH, Landeros-Weisenberger A, Kelmendi B, et al. A systematic review: antipsychotic augmentation with treatment refractory obsessive-compulsive disorder. *Mol Psychiatry.* 2006;11:622.
48. Komossa K, Depping AM, Meyer M, et al. Second-generation antipsychotics for obsessive compulsive disorder. *Cochrane Database Syst Rev.* 2010;CD00841.
49. Ruscio AM, Stien DJ, Chiu WT, et al. The epidemiology of obsessive-compulsive disorder in the National Comorbidity Survey Replication. *Mol Psychiatry.* 2010;15:53.
50. Denys D. Pharmacotherapy of obsessive-compulsive disorder and obsessive-compulsive spectrum disorders. *Psychiatr Clin North Am.* 2006;29:553.
51. de Koning PP, Figee M, van den Munckhof P, et al. Current status of deep brain stimulation for obsessive-compulsive disorder: a clinical review of different targets. *Curr Psychiatry Rep.* 2011;12:274.
52. Blomstedt P, Sjoberg RL, Hansson M, et al. Deep brain stimulation in the treatment of obsessive-compulsive disorder. *World Neurosurg.* 2012 October 5.
53. Gerritsen AA, Korthals-de Bos IB, Laboyrie PM, de Vet HC, Scholten RJ, Bouter LM. Splinting for carpal tunnel syndrome: prognostic indicators of success [published online ahead of print August 23 2003]. *J Neurol Neurosurg Psychiatry.* 2003;74(9):1342–1344.
54. Bland JD. Do nerve conduction studies predict the outcome of carpal tunnel decompression? [published online ahead of print June 19 2001]. Musc Nerve. 2001;24(7):935–940.
55. Steyers CM. Recurrent carpal tunnel syndrome [published online ahead of print October 10 2002]. *Hand Clin.* 2002;18(2):339–345.

SECTION II

MUSCLE, JOINT, AND TENDON PAIN

5.

MYOFASCIAL PAIN SYNDROME

Robert Gerwin

CASE PRESENTATION

A 31-year-old seat-belted woman driving a small car is injured when her vehicle is hit from behind while stopped at a traffic light. She does not experience loss of consciousness. Imaging done in the emergency department shows straightening of the normal cervical lordotic curvature. The emergency department physician diagnoses her as having cervical strain, prescribes acetaminophen and nonsteroidal-anti-inflammatory drugs (NSAIDs), and discharges her home.

Her pain persists with increasing neck pain and stiffness, dizziness, pain when chewing and opening her jaw, and shoulder and low back pain (LBP). She says that pain starts in the neck and shoulders, but she feels it in her head, behind her eyes, and down her arm to her hand. She is referred to a physician at the Interdisciplinary Pain Center.

Past Medical History: Depression.

Review of Symptoms: Noncontributory.

On examination, the patient weighs 58 kg and is 140 cm tall. She is afebrile with normal vital signs. Neurologic examination is within normal limits. The physician finds localized, hardened bands of muscle within the belly of the low back, shoulder, neck, and facial muscles. Palpation of these bands reveals focal areas of hardness that are very tender. Palpation of these focal areas reproduces her pain. Steady pressure on the focal areas for about 5 seconds elicits pain at a distance. Her entire pain complaint is reproduced by stimulation of these trigger points in muscle.

QUESTIONS

1. What is myofascial pain syndrome (MPS)?
2. What is the pathophysiology of myofascial pain?
3. What is the epidemiology of MPS?
4. What are the clinical manifestations of MPS?
5. How is MPS diagnosed?
6. How is MPS managed?
   a. Treatment principles
   b. TPI and deep, dry needling
   c. Manual inactivation of trigger points
   d. Noninvasive, nonmanual treatment techniques
   e. Invasive treatment of myofascial trigger points
   f. Botulinum toxin
   g. Structural and mechanical factors
   h. Restoration of normal function

WHAT IS MPS?

MPS is a condition in which muscle and musculotendinous pain are the primary symptoms. The pain in MPS comes from the *myofascial trigger point*—a small, painful nidus of hardened muscle that sits in a band of contracted muscle within a muscle belly. Like other tissues, the trigger point zone in a muscle is capable of sensitizing the peripheral and central nervous system, resulting in pain referral to distant sites.[1] A small region within the muscle generally harbors multiple trigger points foci that produce local and referred pain. Referred pain is such a common feature of MPS that it can be said to be a hallmark of the syndrome. The taut band in which the trigger point is located is formed by a group of contracted muscle fibers and is readily palpable. The focal hardness within the contracted band may or may not feel nodular. Janet G. Travell (1901–1997) studied the phenomenon of trigger points over much of her career, publishing more than 40 original papers on the subject and co-editing the classic texts on the subject.[1,2] We owe our present awareness of myofascial pain as an important clinical entity to her work and to the incredibly productive later collaboration between Dr. Travell and Dr. David G. Simons.[2] Dr. Travell analyzed the landmark studies of Kellgren[3–5] that described referred pain patterns after injection of hypertonic saline into muscle and other tissues and the subsequent resolution of referred pain by injection of local anesthetic.[4] She applied this knowledge to what were then considered enigmatic clinical syndromes, beginning with noncardiac chest pain that persisted after myocardial infarction.[6] She mapped the referred pain patterns resulting from muscle pain arising in many different areas in the body[6] and described a system of treatment that involved inactivation of the regions of localized muscle soreness through the use of vapocoolant spray and stretch and the injection of procaine, a local anesthetic. She used the term "myofascial" to describe the involvement of both muscle and its covering tissue (the fascia) and "trigger point" to convey the notion that pain initiated at one site in a particular muscle triggered pain felt at a site distant to the point of origin. Andrew Fischer later measured the stiffness of the myofascial taut band with a compliance meter and emphasized the hardness of the discrete band of muscle that harbors the tender trigger point region.[7] In summary, the trigger point is a focus of sensory hyperirritability on a discrete, hyperactive region of muscle. The trigger point is often described by its degree of activity.

A very active trigger point causes spontaneous pain with activation of the muscle and sometimes even at rest. This is called an *active* trigger point. A less active trigger point may be identified by palpation and by its focal hardness on the contracted taut band. It is not painful until stimulated mechanically. This is called a *latent* trigger point. However, the trigger point is a dynamic phenomenon that shifts back and forth between the active and latent states depending on how the muscle is used or rested. There is no term for the underlying manifestation of the trigger point, and it may not be painful in itself. The contracted band develops a locus of painful, further hardened muscle with use or muscle activation, such as typing on a keyboard. Moreover, as it becomes activated, it can activate a painful sensation in a body structure at some distance. The clinical manifestations of MPS, therefore, are the result of local pain, referred pain, and somatic dysfunction caused by motor system dysfunction resulting from the trigger point.

WHAT IS THE PATHOPHYSIOLOGY OF MYOFASCIAL PAIN?

The trigger point is thought to occur after a muscle is contracted supramaximally, whether volitionally or acutely in trauma; is excessively loaded in eccentric contraction; or is repeatedly contracted in low-level, repetitive activity. There are no studies available that describe the development of a trigger point in normal muscle. However, in clinical practice, we see the signs of myofascial trigger points in circumstances that implicate these mechanisms of muscle use that in turn result in the development of trigger points. The common event after any of these activities is a muscle that is overloaded or that is used beyond its capacity.

Muscle that is contracted does not activate all of its muscle fibers at one time. Muscle activation is graduated, with short muscle fibers activated first in non-antigravity muscles and relaxed last.[8] Thus, a set of muscles is repeatedly or supramaximally activated to the point of fatigue and injury. When the muscle is injured in this manner, there is a local accumulation of cytokines and neurotransmitters.[9] The contraction of the muscle causes local capillary constriction, ischemia, and hypoxia.[10] A highly resistive vascular bed causes retrograde flow in diastole in the region near active trigger points,[11] presumably because of greatly contracted muscle in the region of the trigger point.

GENERATION OF THE TAUT BAND

Trigger points appear to form first as taut bands that may be painless but then develop into latent trigger points that become tender as a muscle is activated. This sequence of events is postulated because latent trigger points exist without spontaneous pain, trigger point tenderness does not occur except in association with a taut (contracted, hard) band of muscle, and regions of muscle hardness occur without local or referred pain. Hence, we conclude that muscle hardness or the taut band that occurs in the absence of pain is the first manifestation of abnormality and that the active trigger point is a further stage of trigger point development. However, this sequence of events, as simple as it is, has not been systematically studied and confirmed.

MUSCLE OVERUSE AND MPS

The current hypothesis of trigger point formation is that localized ischemia is associated with the acute development of the trigger point and with its maintenance.[1,10,12] Localized ischemia results from capillary compression resulting from forces generated within the taut band. As a result of capillary compression, blood flow is shunted away from the trigger point[11] creating a zone of hypoxia. In turn, the release of vasodilating substances like calcitonin gene-related peptide (CGRP) and substance P lead to localized noninflammatory edema that further restricts capillary flow.

The Neuromuscular Junction

Trigger points occur only on a myofascial taut band. The initial change in muscle associated with the trigger point is the development of the taut band. There are no studies of this phenomenon, therefore the mechanism of taut band development remains hypothetical. Simons's *integrated hypothesis of the trigger point*,[1] expanded on by Gerwin et al.[10] and by Gerwin[12] postulates that an excess of acetylcholine at the motor endplate—modulated by adrenergic modulation of neurotransmitter release, inhibition of acetylcholine esterase, and other modulating factors like adenosine concentration and by feedback control of neurotransmitter release related to endplate discharge frequency—results in the development of localized muscle contraction, most likely directly under the motor endplate. This is supported by the initial observations by Hubbard and Berkoff[13] of spontaneous low-amplitude electrical activity at the trigger point site, later called "endplate noise" by Simons. Endplate noise is highly localized in muscle and is associated with the motor endplate.[14] This activity is modulated by an α-adrenergic blocking agent[15] and by botulinum toxin,[16] indicating that it is subject to sympathetic nervous system influences dependent on acetylcholine release. Noradrenaline, a sympathetic neurotransmitter, increases endogenous glutamate-mediated excitation and changes glutamatergic activity that is normally subthreshold into a stimulus that can activate the motor neurone.[17] Our understanding of the role of trigger point electrical activity in the development of the trigger point is discussed in detail by Ge et al.[18] Another possible contributing mechanism is postsynaptic ryanodine calcium channel receptor dysfunction that increases intracellular calcium concentrations by leaking calcium into the cytosol from the sarcoplasmic reticulum membrane or through adrenergic-mediated second-messenger systems involving protein kinase C and cyclic AMP that initiates actin-myosin interaction that also increases intracellular calcium concentration.[12] A similar mechanism of trigger point formation was proposed by McPartland and Simons.[19] Endplate noise is significantly inhibited by the calcium channel blocking agent verapamil. Thus, calcium channel activity is important in the generation of trigger point endplate noise.[20] Mense and Simons[21] have also suggested that inhibition of acetylcholine esterase could lead to endplate noise and create contraction knots. However, they were unable to produce contraction knots experimentally.

Peripheral Nerve Alterations in MPS

Peripheral nerve sensitization has been little addressed in MPS. Nevertheless, peripheral nerve sensitization is a consequence of chronic myofascial pain just as it is in other chronic pain syndromes. Some neural manifestations of the myofascial trigger point are clearly related to a spinal reflex, such as the local twitch reflex.[22] Other studies have suggested that a central integration at the spinal cord level in animal trigger point models.[23] Neuromuscular jitter by stimulated single-fiber electromyography (EMG) has a significantly increased mean consecutive difference (jitter) in the trapezius and levator scapulae muscles in subjects with MPS compared to controls.[24] The instability of peripheral endplate function could be related to (1) peripheral motor nerve axonal degeneration and regeneration or (2) motor neuron degeneration with development of collateral reinnervation. Thus, the myofascial trigger point represents a complex peripheral and/or central motor dysfunction, as well as a sensory abnormality with peripheral and/or central hypersensitization.

Hypoxia and Ischemia

The myofascial trigger zone is hypoxic. There is a region of severe oxygen desaturation at the core, surrounded by a region of increased oxygenation, as if the core were ischemic and surrounded by a hyperemic zone.[25]

Biochemistry of the Trigger Point Region

Microdialysis of the trigger point region (not of the intracellular fluid) has elucidated the biochemical characteristics of the trigger point.[9,26] A microdialysis probe placed in the trigger point region of active trigger points is advanced slowly until a twitch response is obtained, signifying that the probe has reached the trigger point zone. Elevations of substance P, CGRP, bradykinin, serotonin (5-HT), and cytokines are found in active trigger point milieu relative to the concentrations of these substances in latent trigger point regions and in normal muscle.[9] As the probe advances toward the trigger point, the concentrations of a number of substances increases until a twitch occurs. The concentration of these substances fell toward the normal range after the twitch, but then slowly rose toward the initial elevated concentrations over 10–15 minutes. The trigger point region pH is low at pH 4–5 compared to a normal pH of 7.4. Increased substance P increases capillary leakage, causes local edema, and potentiates peripheral nociceptor activation. Bradykinin is a nociceptive receptor potentiator. CGRP is active at both sensory receptors and at the neuromuscular junction. Lowered pH implies ischemia. Acetylcholinesterase activity is inhibited at an acidic pH. Increased cytokine levels correlate with local pain.

The concentrations of neurotransmitters and cytokines are elevated at an active trigger point region compared to a distant muscle non-trigger point region. Furthermore, the concentrations of these substances are elevated in distant (gastrocnemius muscle) non-trigger point regions in subjects with active trigger points in the trapezius muscle compared to subjects with latent or absent trigger points.[27] The pH was lower than normal and other analytes, such as substance P and various cytokines, were elevated to a slight but definite degree. Bradykinin was the exception: it was not elevated in the gastrocnemius muscle when there was an active trigger point in the trapezius muscle. This suggests that an active trigger point in one muscle evokes widespread central activation that activates peripheral nociceptors. However, it is also possible that the gastrocnemius muscle in a person with an active trigger point in the trapezius muscle is more likely to have latent trigger points that were unknowingly sampled. The ability to sample the interstitial milieu of the trigger point region has great potential to unravel the mechanism of trigger point nociception.[26]

Trapezius muscle 5-HT and glutamate elevation in women with work-related myalgia correlate directly with pain intensity, whereas lactate and pyruvate increase after low-force exercise significantly more than in controls.[28] Bradykinin and kallidin, potential algesic kinins, are elevated in muscle interstitial fluid of the inferior portion of the trapezius muscle in women with work-related trapezius myalgia (TM), whiplash associated pain (WAP), and controls.[29] Bradykinin and kallidin are increased at rest in TM and WAP and further increase with exercise in study participants more so than in controls. Whiplash associated disorders (WAD) subjects have a lower trapezius pressure pain threshold (PPT) indicating hypersensitivity, and higher interstitial concentrations of interleukin (IL-6) and 5-HT.[30] In the these studies of microdialysis of muscle interstitial fluid, no attempt was made to place the catheter in a trigger point, but the authors noted that, typically, "a brief involuntary muscle contraction and change of resistance were perceived when the needle penetrated the fascia and muscle," thus suggesting that a trigger point local twitch response was elicited. Nonetheless, these studies support the work of Shah et al. and confirm its relevance in clinical muscle pain syndromes. Tissue IL-1 α and β are elevated in the foreleg muscles of rats after 8 weeks of a high-repetition negligible force activity,[31] consistent with trigger point microdialysis findings, but lack the specificity of trigger point localization.

MUSCLE PATHOLOGY

Definitive pathological studies of myofascial trigger points in humans and animals have not been done. Simons and Stolov[32] published a photomicrograph of canine muscle that showed a single fiber with intense sarcomere contraction that Simon later called a "contraction knot." Intense local sarcomere contraction at contraction knots is considered to be the heart of the trigger point. It is thought to be the result of excessive acetylcholine at the motor endplate (Simons's integrated hypothesis of the trigger point).[1:69–78] Such loci of intense sarcomere contraction have not been replicated in a human myofascial trigger point. An attempt to produce contraction knots in rat muscle through inhibition of acetylcholinesterase to increase the concentration of acetylcholine at the motor endplate showed abnormally contracted fibers, torn fibers, and longitudinal stripes.[21] However, "rubber band" morphology appears significantly more frequently in fibromyalgia patients than in myofascial pain patients.[33] Neither the origin of the rubber band morphology nor its relation to contraction knots is clear.

One biopsy study of painful muscle, but without any intention of sampling trigger points, has been published.[34] Of participants, 51.6% had heterogeneous myopathic changes that were mostly nonspecific. The changes included increased fiber size variation, occasional cell necrosis, and some abnormalities of the intermyofibrillar network such as moth-eaten fibers. Specific myopathic changes, occurring in 6.5%, include type I fiber atrophy in 1.6% and type II B fiber atrophy in all 6.5%. Mitochondrial abnormalities were found in 20% of the patients. A third group of 19% had normal muscle. A neurogenic pattern was present in 7%, and 2.4% had a metabolic myopathy. No comment was made in this retrospective study about the presence or absence of myofascial pain.

There is as yet no unequivocal pathological change that is clearly associated with the trigger point. Intense sarcomere contraction at the trigger point zone remains a viable hypothesis but remains to be confirmed pathologically.

CENTRAL PATHWAYS

Myofascial trigger points are associated with central sensitization and hypersensitivity, as is the case with pain generators in other tissues. The mechanisms of central sensitization and expansion of dorsal horn reference zones in acute muscle pain has been extensively studied by Mense and his colleagues.[35] Chemically and mechanically induced muscle pain causes central sensitization in animals. There is no difference in the numbers of dorsal horn neurons in rats with trigger points compared to control animals,[36] indicating that changes occur in individual dorsal horn neurons rather than in the number of neurons when central sensitization occurs.

Referred Pain

Referred pain is the result of sensitization of dorsal horn nociceptive neurons coupled with a convergence of afferent nociceptive fibers on single sensory neurons. Central sensitization is the activation of otherwise ineffective (sometimes called "sleeping") synaptic connections from one afferent nerve fiber to many recipient nociceptive neurons, thereby expanding the receptive fields of any one specific neuron. It occurs through the development of increased synaptic efficacy.[37] Increased synaptic efficiency in the peripheral and central nervous systems is the result of sensitization-induced increase in the synthesis of cell-surface receptors that make activation of the cell much more efficient and that also activate the cell from somatic (muscle) stimulation that ordinarily is outside the nerve cell's receptive field. The dorsal horn neuron generates nociceptive impulses that ascend the spinal cord and brainstem, resulting in activation of the somatosensory cortex. The sensory cortex interprets all input from a dorsal horn neuron as coming from the receptive field of that neuron. The receptive field is expanded when the dorsal horn neuron is sensitized. The expansion of receptive fields that activate specific dorsal horn neurons explains the referred pain patterns seen clinically. In addition, the spread of nociceptive afferent fibers is much more extensive than the one or two segments above and below the level of entry into the dorsal horn described for classical sensory afferent axons, such as those that convey touch sensation. The wider arborization of incoming nociceptive fibers within the spinal cord increases the spatial distribution of sensitized dorsal horn neurons.

The most common referred pain patterns in clinical practice are within the same or adjacent spinal segments as the primary sensory nerve. Thus, trigger points in muscles innervated predominantly by C5 nerve root fibers refer pain largely to the C5 dermatome and myotome, with spread to the overlapping C4- and C6-innervated dermatomes and myotomes. Muscle innervation is relatively constant so that segmental referred pain patterns tend to be relatively constant from one person to another. Pain referral patterns have been mapped and recorded, most extensively by Travell.[1] Others have continued to identify and refine trigger point referral patterns.[38–40] New referred pain patterns have been described for headache.[41]

The segmental spread of referred pain may be bilateral. Referred pain across the body, from right to left or left to right, was noted by Travell for forehead pain caused by trigger points in the clavicular head of the sternocleidomastoid (SCM) muscle.[1:310] Bilateral forearm referred pain from a unilateral trigger point has also been reported in unilateral epicondylalgia.[42] Pain is also referred through the body in a dorsal to ventral and a ventral to dorsal manner, as is referred pain from the pectoralis major or abdominal trigger points.

MUSCLE OVERUSE SYNDROMES

Muscle overuse, a biomechanical form of stress, is one cause of myofascial trigger points. Central to Simons's integrated hypothesis of the trigger point is the concept that trigger points are the result of an energy crisis such as that resulting from muscle overuse. Supramaximal muscle contraction or overloaded eccentric contraction damages muscle and leads to pain, including delayed onset muscle soreness.[43] Repetitive strain is a variant of muscle overload and is thought to have the same effect. A moderate repetition (nine reaches per minute) high force (60% of maximum pulling force) task in rats induces a decrease in motor and nerve function and causes central sensitization with mechanical allodynia.[44] Fixed postures maintained for long periods of time or sustained contraction of muscle, even that associated with emotional stress (anxiety, fear, or depression), also produce muscle overuse. Data are lacking, however, that show that these phenomena actually lead to the development of the trigger point, although this has been postulated.[10]

Sustained low-level muscle contraction, in contrast to supramaximal contraction, has also been implicated in the development of trigger points. The concept is that the earliest recruited and last deactivated motor units are overworked, particularly during prolonged tasks. This concept has been well summarized by Dommerholt et al.[45] Support that this is important in the development of myofascial trigger points comes from the studies of Treaster et al.[46]

The hypothesis that muscle overuse or physical or metabolic stresses lead to muscle dysfunction and pain are based on an underlying assumption, arising from the ischemic, energy-crisis model of the trigger point, that the affected muscle is overworked beyond its capacity to respond without injury.[10] One hypothesis, the *Cinderella hypothesis* postulates the continuous activity of a subset of type I muscle fibers in low-level muscle contraction.[8,47–49] Such continuous activity of one subset of muscle fibers is postulated to lead to muscle fiber overwork, making them vulnerable to damage consistent with the energy crisis model of the trigger point. The finding that type I megafibers are more common in women with trapezius myalgia than in controls[50] supports the concept that type I muscle fibers are overloaded and injured by repetitive, low-load work.[46] Capillary blood supply to the megafibers is poor, suggesting that a local shift to anaerobic metabolism and acidosis has occurred.

Fast-twitch type II muscle fibers are more likely to be recruited and injured with eccentric exercise.[43] Acute muscle overuse in eccentric or supramaximal contraction, in repetitive contractions, or in sustained postural muscle overload causes muscle damage and the local release of neuropeptides, cytokines, and other inflammatory mediators that result in local edema, capillary compression, and energy depletion, as described previously. Muscle sarcomere disorganization occurs with supramaximal and eccentric muscle contraction.[51,52] Muscle pain in vitamin D deficiency is also associated with type II muscle atrophy. Thus, it is likely that when type II muscle fibers are either injured or atrophied and dysfunctional, the remaining type II muscle fibers are overloaded. Atrophy of type II muscle fibers may also lead to overloading of type I muscle fibers, although this has not been demonstrated in this situation. Muscle overload as described can lead to muscle pain through the release of chemical mediators such as neurotransmitters, ions such as protons or potassium, and cytokines, which cause peripheral nociceptors activation. There are no data as yet to directly link these findings to the development of the trigger point, even though these observations are suggestive and intriguing.

Muscle overload results in delayed onset muscle soreness (DOMS),[53] but pain and soreness in DOMS are not necessarily correlated with the structural changes just described. Changes in muscle induced by overuse share the same characteristics as acute muscle injury, repetitive motion-induced pain, and chronic muscle pain.[54] There is no necessary association between postexercise muscle damage, inflammation, and pain.[55] DOMS is an imperfect model for MPS; nevertheless, muscle breakdown caused by acute or chronic muscle overload resulting in local hypoxia and ischemia best fits the picture of MPS, largely based on the time course of pain and the biochemical changes in the trigger point milieu described by Shah et al.[9]

Postural Stresses

Postural stresses are a form of mechanical muscle stress that must be considered as a cause of myofascial trigger point formation and activation. Spondylosis with joint hypomobility results in postural dysfunction associated with neck, trunk, and LBP. Myofascial trigger points are seen in these conditions, but there are few studies that specifically show such an association. The prevalence of myofascial trigger points in the upper trapezius, SCM, and levator scapular muscles in midcervical spine hypomobility did not reach statistical significance, but there is a significant relationship between upper trapezius muscle trigger points and C3–4 hypomobility.[56,57]

Pain Initiation

The current model of myofascial pain is that muscle is damaged by overuse and mechanical or metabolic stress. This model, one that is both based on experimental evidence and is also the most reasonable, posits is that excessive mechanical stress, whether by overuse and excessive mechanical force generated within the muscle or by repetitive, low-effort mechanical activity leading to fatigue and localized areas of excessive mechanical force, creates very localized forces that compress capillaries, veins, and small arterioles and results in multiple small foci of ischemia and hypoxia. Localized ischemia and hypoxia in turn cause leakage of hydrogen ions (H^+), potassium ions, and kinins like bradykinin and several different ILs. Nociceptive peripheral nerve endings are activated. Substance P, 5-HT, and CGRP are also released locally, and antegrade transmission of nociceptive impulses is generated. Glial cells in the form of peripheral nerve Schwann cells are also activated in this process and contribute to the generation of pain and peripheral sensitization, a phenomenon that occurs later in this sequence. More will be said about the role of proton ions and the initiation of pain later.

What is not well understood is the mechanism by which the taut band is generated. However, it is likely that the localized ischemia and hypoxia create localized areas of acidity that inhibits acetylcholinesterase thereby inhibiting the breakdown of acetylcholine. Increased concentrations of

CGRP caused by activation of peripheral sensory nerve endings results in an increase in motor endplate acetylcholine receptors and also causes an increase in the release of acetylcholine from the motor nerve ending. These phenomena together result in localized concentrations of acetylcholine at the motor endplates in the areas of localized ischemia. The means of activation of the sympathetic nervous system, which plays an important role in the taut band, is as yet unknown. The possible role of calcium leakage into the muscle fiber cytosol remains intriguing, but is without supporting experimental evidence.

Models that invoke a neurogenic origin of the trigger point postulate that nerve root compression is the origin of muscle pain or that central sensitization results in secondary development of trigger points. These models do not account for either the EMG phenomena associated with the trigger point or for the decrease or elimination of pain by direct treatment of the trigger point by deep, dry needling or by manual means and hence will no longer be considered in this discussion.

Inflammatory Pain Models

Pain is central to the clinical presentation of myofascial trigger point syndromes and is the major reason that patients seek care. Theories that attempt to account for pain generation in MPS must take into account the apparent lack of overt muscle injury. Few attempts have been made to biopsy trigger points. It is difficult to localize a trigger point in a situation suitable for biopsy, and data are therefore scarce to nonexistent. However, absence of serum creatinine phosphokinase (CPK) elevation in MPS suggests that there is no component of inflammatory myositis in trigger point development. Information available to date suggests that ultrastructural muscle fiber derangement occurs, such as is seen in supramaximal and eccentric muscle contraction, and that significant pathophysiologic biochemical changes occur at the trigger point zone, including localized acidity,[9] but that inflammatory muscle damage that gives rise to an influx of inflammatory cells and that leads to postinflammatory muscle atrophy and fibrosis does not occur in myofascial trigger points.

Acid-Sensing Ion Channels

A model of nociceptive activation of muscle pain in the absence of muscle injury is the acid-sensing ion channel (ASIC), ASIC-3. Asic-3 is found in small sensory neurons that innervate muscle (51% of small muscle afferents).[58] Long-lasting, bilateral hyperalgesia is induced by two intramuscular injections of acidic (pH 4.0) saline given 5 days apart.[59] Muscle pH decreases to pH 6.0 for only 6 minutes in this model. No local inflammatory changes take place. Spinal cord dorsal horn activation, mediated through N-methyl-D-aspartate (NMDA) and glutamate receptor activation, produces widespread hyperalgesia.[60] Phosphorylation of cAMP-responsive element-binding protein (CREB) is increased in the spinal cord.[61] Hyperalgesia is reversed by blockade of NMDA receptors, glutamate receptors, and the cAMP pathway. Furthermore, ASIC-3 knockout mice do not develop central hyperalgesia when challenged with two acidic saline injections.[62] Additionally, acidic buffer injected into the anterior tibial muscle in humans produces mechanical hyperalgesia and referred pain.[63] These experiments, taken together with the observation that the trigger point milieu is acidic, suggest that the rise in proton concentration as a result of ischemia and hypoxia might be enough to initiate pain.

A further complexity in this system is related to nerve growth factor-related neurotrophins, including neurotrophin-3 (NT-3), to which most muscle afferents are responsive. Mice that overexpress NT-3 do not develop hyperalgesia when challenged with acidic saline intramuscular injections. NT-3 injected into muscle prior to the development of hyperalgesia blocks its development but has no effect once hyperalgesia has occurred.[64] Antagonists to ASIC suppress pain induced by carrageenan and eccentric exercise-induced muscle hyperalgesia.[65] ASIC-3 is necessary for the development of central hyperalgesia and chronic widespread pain, and NT-3 prevents central sensitization.[66] Thus, the acid-sensing ion channel system may play an essential, if not dominant, role in the development of trigger point pain.

Serotonergic Mechanisms

There are other potential mechanisms for activation of peripheral nociceptive receptors that involve different chemical mediators and neurotransmitters such as glutamate, bradykinin, and potassium. 5-HT is one neurotransmitter that is elevated in the active trigger point milieu.[9] 5-HT receptors are primarily pronociceptive (pain-promoting) in the periphery, acting directly on afferent nerves and indirectly by release of other mediators (e.g., substance P and glutamate). The 5-HT_{2A} subtype, expressed in CGRP-synthesizing dorsal root ganglion neurons, potentiates peripheral inflammatory pain.[67] 5-HT has both antinociceptive and pronociceptive effects centrally. Centrally, 5-HT activates the descending pain inhibitory system as well as the descending facilitory response. 5-HT peripheral activity in masticatory afferent fibers of the trigeminal nerve is reduced by the 5-HT antagonist tropisetron.[68] 5-HT antagonists block the 5-HT algesic effect when injected into some muscles.[69] Tropisetron and granisetron have produced mixed results when injected into muscle but, on balance, reduce myofascial trigger point pain. Additionally, local injection of 5-HT into muscle reduces pain, further supporting the concept that 5-HT_3 receptor has a peripheral role in mediating pain.[54] These observations have theoretical implications for the generation of pain from trigger points, and they also have therapeutic implications because targeting the actions of 5-HT peripherally and centrally may be effective in modulating trigger point pain syndromes.

CGRP

CGRP is elevated in the trigger point milieu of active trigger points.[9] CGRP is produced in the dorsal root ganglion. It is released from the peripheral terminals of primary sensory afferents and centrally in the spinal cord dorsal horn. It is present in the nerve terminals of nociceptive afferent fibers. CGRP facilitates synaptic plasticity in the spinal dorsal horn,[70] enhances the central release of glutamate and aspartate, and increases neuronal responsiveness to excitatory amino acids (EAA) and to substance P in dorsal horn nociceptive and wide dynamic range neurons. Glutamate activates peripheral EAA receptors and excites and sensitizes muscle afferent fibers.[71] It also acts through second-messenger systems, utilizing protein kinases A and C to initiate and maintain central sensitization.[72]

Spinal Modulation of Pain

Descending facilitation and inhibition of ascending nociceptive impulses modulates pain perception. Tonic, noxious stimulation that induces muscular pain produced by injection of hypertonic saline, as well as cold pressor pain, suppresses descending inhibitory pain controls in humans. The descending pain modulation system is complex, in some cases facilitating rather than inhibiting ascending nociceptive stimuli.

Latent and Active Trigger Points

Trigger points that are spontaneously painful, either with activity or at rest, have been considered active trigger points.[73] Trigger points that are painful only after mechanical stimulation of the trigger point, either by manually strumming or compressing the trigger point or by needling, are considered latent trigger points. The distinction has been made because, at one time, there was a question as to whether latent trigger points were clinically significant in producing either pain or dysfunction. The two differ only in degree of activation but are otherwise similar, and both cause physiologic dysfunction. Most studies of peripheral and central sensitization from trigger points were done with active trigger points, but latent trigger points have been shown to be important in causing sensitization as well. In fact, latent trigger points have been shown to have significant physiologic effects in many respects. They cause increased intramuscular EMG activity in synergistic muscles, potentially overloading these muscle fibers to predispose them to contribute to spatial pain propagation.[74]

WHAT IS THE EPIDEMIOLOGY OF MPS?

A lack of accepted uniform diagnostic criteria for the diagnosis of MPS has made it more difficult to determine the prevalence of MPS than otherwise. In sharp contrast to the situation with fibromyalgia, there have been no community-wide assessments of MPS. Hence, prevalence estimates are extrapolated from data derived from clinics where myofascial pain has been diagnosed. Latent trigger points were reported in about 11% of subjects in Thailand.[75] One study estimated a prevalence rate of myofascial trigger points of 20%.[76] In a university general internal medicine practice, 9% of the total number of a series of 172 patients were found to have myofascial pain.[77] A pain rehabilitation referral center reported that 85% of their patients had MPS.[78] A pain treatment private neurological clinic program known for its interest in MPS reported that 93% of persons with musculoskeletal pain had myofascial trigger points relevant to their pain.[79] Active trigger points were found in more than 75% of Dutch subjects with shoulder pain.[80] Fifty-one percent of patients with cervical radiculopathy had active myofascial trigger points in at least one muscle in the neck and shoulders, whereas none of the healthy controls was found to have active trigger points.[81] However, note that healthy control subjects are selected for the absence of spontaneous pain, part of the definition of active trigger points. There was no difference in the prevalence of latent trigger points between subjects with cervical radiculopathy and healthy controls. MPS was detected in 61% of a series of 41 complex regional pain syndrome subjects.[82] MPS was diagnosed in 67.5% of patients with poststroke central pain syndrome.[83] A study of 243 female sewing machine operators showed a MPS prevalence of 15.2% in neck and shoulder muscles compared to 9.0% among 357 female controls.[84] MPS is also commonly seen in women who have had surgery for breast cancer, whether that surgery is lumpectomy or mastectomy.[85,86] Thus, the conclusion is that myofascial trigger point pain is common in persons with musculoskeletal pain and that workers who are at greater risk for shoulder and neck pain (e.g., computer keyboard operators) or LBP (e.g., manual laborers) are at an increased risk of having active trigger point pain. Myofascial trigger point pain is also a treatable cause of postamputation pain.[87] The other lesson to learn from these reports is that myofascial trigger point pain is a common comorbidity that accompanies many other conditions, and it is more appropriate to consider trigger point pain as comorbidity than to regard it as coming from secondary trigger points. Trigger points may persist after the underlying condition has resolved.

GENDER DIFFERENCES

Sex-related differences are known in a variety of painful conditions, including migraine headache and fibromyalgia. Differential responses to musculoskeletal pain based on gender are known.[88] Days absent from work and expenditures for healthcare are greater for women than men,[89] but that may be the result of different responses to pain in females compared to males, not because pain is more frequent. No difference in muscle pain prevalence was found between men and women, but there were differences in the way women comply with a rehabilitation program. Occupational neck and shoulder pain is more common in women than in men.[90] PPTs are also lower for women, signifying greater hypersensitivity to mechanical stimulation. Injection of hypertonic saline in bilateral trapezius muscles to simulate the real-life bilateral shoulder pain commonly experienced in certain work situations resulted in greater pain inhibition in men than in women 7.5 and 15 minutes after injection. Baseline PPT was lower in women, but the increase in PPT after a second injection of hypertonic saline was much greater in men than in women. The greater increase in PPT in men represents an increased hypoalgesia or increased nociceptive inhibition that is likely to be central. Differences in pain and EMG changes associated with sustained trapezius muscle contractions show that pain-induced changes in motor control strategies differ in men and women. Sustained contraction of the trapezius muscle is more common than other sustained shoulder muscle activation in real-world activities. In this model, pain is induced by injection of hypertonic saline into the trapezius muscle. The root mean square (RMS) and mean power frequency (MPF) computed from EMG signals showed differences between men and women.[91] The RMS slope increased and the MPF slope decreased (less negative) with muscle pain in men but not in women. Glutamate-evoked muscle pain is also greater in women, whereas hypertonic saline-evoked pain is not; and glutamate-evoked afferent discharges are greater in female rats than in males, suggesting that the effect is mediated peripherally.[71,92] One explanation is that there is an increased central sensitization in women, but an alternative explanation is that descending inhibition is weaker in females than in males.

The exact mechanism(s) of gender differences to muscle pain remains to be identified. However, certain effects of sex hormones on pain mechanisms are known. Estradiol modulates NMDA receptor activity in the spinal dorsal horn, increasing the nociceptive response to colorectal distension is rats.[93] Estradiol also modulates the excitability of primary sensory afferent nerves.[94] A role for estrogen in the development of hypersensitization has been considered.[95] In contrast, one study of sex differences in recalled and experimentally induced muscle pain showed no difference between male and female subjects.[96]

HYPERMOBILITY

Hypermobility or ligamentous laxity seems to be a relevant risk factor for the development of MPSs.[97] The mechanism is thought to be the more constant contraction of muscle needed for joint stability that the ligaments are unable to provide. Those persons with recurrent large-joint dislocations or subluxation seem to be at an even higher risk for the development of trigger points.

WHAT ARE THE CLINICAL MANIFESTATIONS OF MPS?

The trigger point has both sensory and motor manifestations. It is comprised of abnormally contracted muscle fibers, collectively called a taut band, and an associated sensation of pain. The taut band is a linear, localized band of muscle that is harder than the surrounding muscle. It is a discrete band, not involving the entire muscle like a cramp or spasm. Muscle containing trigger points has a heterogeneous feel of hard and soft areas, rather than a uniform, homogeneous consistency. The taut band is made up of a group of contracted muscle fibers thought to be the result of multiple foci of intensely contracted sarcomeres located at or near the motor endplate zone. The sensory phenomenon of localized, exquisite pain is always associated with a taut band, and is in fact, always located *in* the taut band. Diagnostically, pain is elicited on physical examination by mechanically stimulating the taut band. Trigger points are categorized as active or latent, depending on whether they are spontaneously painful (an active trigger point) or painful only on palpation or other mechanical stimulation (a latent trigger point).

Additional trigger point characteristics include a *local twitch response* that is elicited by mechanical stimulation. The twitch response is a local contraction of the taut band alone, elicited either manually by strumming or palpation or invasively by intramuscular needle stimulation. A needle-induced twitch is best elicited at the trigger point zone.[22,98,99] The twitch represents a brief (25–250 msec), high-amplitude, polyphasic electrical discharge. A local twitch response elicited by needle stimulation away from the taut band or away from the trigger spot is EMG attenuated. The twitch response is mediated through the spinal cord, requires an intact spinal reflex arc, and is not modulated by supraspinal influences. It is unique to the trigger point, not seen in normal muscle without trigger points, is diagnostic of a trigger point, and yet is not required for the identification of a trigger point.

TRIGGER POINT IDENTIFICATION

Identification of the taut band is now possible with a number of objective techniques. The taut band and the twitch response can be visualized by ultrasound.[100,101] High-resolution ultrasound devices currently available allow visualization of the taut band, are being used in research on the trigger point, and are also being used in clinical practice.[102] Ultrasound imaging is also being used to guide trigger point injections (TPIs)[103] and in quantifying the effect of dry needling on trigger points.[104] Magnetic resonance elastography (MR elastography) is another technique that can differentiate tissues of varying densities. Both MR elastography and ultrasound sonoelastography are useful to define muscle architecture.[105] These techniques allow visualization of the taut band, which is denser than surrounding normal muscle. MR elastography involves the introduction of cyclic waves into the muscle and then using phase contrast imaging to identify tissue distortions. Shear waves travel more rapidly in stiffer tissues and therefore more rapidly in the taut band than in surrounding normal muscle.[106,107]

WEAKNESS

Muscles harboring a trigger point are often weak. Trigger point-associated weakness occurs without atrophy and is neither neuropathic nor myopathic.[1:109] It is usually rapidly reversible immediately on inactivation of the trigger point, suggesting that it is caused by inhibition of muscle activity. A trigger point in one muscle can inhibit effort or contractile force in another muscle, suggesting a role for central motor inhibition rather than simply weakness as a result of pain on movement. There is a paucity of studies looking at the nature of weakness in myofascial pain, however.

RECRUITMENT

Orderly muscle recruitment to produce a specific action is disrupted by latent trigger points in one or more muscles in the relevant functional muscle unit. Orderly recruitment is restored by inactivation of the latent trigger point.[108,109] Likewise, in women with chronic trapezius myalgia with active and latent trigger points, rapid activation of painful and pain-free synergistic muscles is more severely impaired than is the maximal muscle contraction.[50]

RANGE OF MOTION (ROM)

Trigger points impair active and passive ROM. The end range may be painful, but limited ROM may be painless unless the patient is pushed to move beyond comfort. ROM limitation is not a reliable indicator of the presence of a trigger point in persons who are hypermobile because their range can be limited and yet still be within the normal ROM for the general population.

Functional spatial reorganization of muscle occurs in the presence of muscle pain. An active trigger point is one such source of localized muscle pain. Experimental muscle pain induced by injection of hypertonic saline into the trapezius muscle causes a short-term dynamic reorganization of the spatial distribution of muscle activity.[110] Changes in spatial distribution also occur with muscle contraction, and the changes correlate with the duration of contraction.[111] This suggests that a more long-lasting trigger point that is a nociceptive irritant would also cause a functional spatial reorganization of muscle activity, although this has never been studied.

SENSORY CHANGES

The sensory change associated with the trigger point is pain (local, referred) and hypersensitivity. Trigger point pain can be acute or chronic. The trigger point is a *tender focus in muscle*, and the region of tenderness is always located in the taut band. The region of greatest hardness is usually also the region of greatest tenderness. A tender trigger point represents hyperalgesia or allodynia. Pain at the trigger point is due to the release of neuropeptides, cytokines, and inflammatory substances such as substance P, CGRP, IL-1α, and bradykinin (Shah, 2005),9 and of protons that create local acidity, as discussed previously. *Acute muscle pain* models have yielded information about the generation of local and referred pain.[23,36,62,112–117] However, most clinically relevant muscular pain syndromes last far longer than the conditions studied in animals or even in humans studied under laboratory conditions. Therefore, there is great interest in studying longer lasting and chronic pain in humans.

The trigger point is a dynamic, not static, entity, meaning that it can undergo transitions between a nontender taut band to a latent trigger point to an active trigger point and back again. The latent trigger point is hypersensitive to the injection of the known nociceptive activators hypertonic saline and glutamate. In addition, the latent trigger point also has an increased response, with referred pain, to the injection of the non-nociceptive activator isotonic saline, indicating that latent trigger points have both a nociceptive hypersensitivity and a non-nociceptive hypersensitivity (allodynia) not seen in non-trigger point regions.[118] A nontender taut band is not included in trigger point nomenclature, although it is in all likelihood the first, as well as the necessary, component of the trigger point.

A key feature of the trigger point is referred pain, a manifestation of central sensitization. Central sensitization results in a spread of perceived pain to distant and larger areas of the body than just the local tenderness found at the taut band.

ELECTROPHYSIOLOGY OF THE TRIGGER POINT

Spontaneous Electrical Activity (Endplate Noise)

The trigger point in resting muscle had long been considered to be electrically silent. No motor action potential has been associated with the trigger point or the taut band in resting muscle.[9] Hubbard and Berkoff[13] published the first report of persistent, low-amplitude, high-frequency discharges found at the trigger point region in active trigger points. This activity, that initially came to be known as *spontaneous electrical activity* (SEA), is associated with the trigger point region.[1,119] As the electrode is moved away from the trigger zone, the SEA diminishes. Likewise, the SEA diminishes as the needle is placed outside the taut band.[94] A needle placed 1 cm away from the trigger zone and outside the taut band does not display SEA.[13]

HOW IS MPS DIAGNOSED?

DIAGNOSIS

MPS can be diagnosed when there is a history consistent with musculoskeletal pain and a finding of myofascial trigger points that are relevant to the complaint of pain. Diagnosis is not as simple as this sounds because a characteristic feature of myofascial pain is referred pain, often obscuring the origin of the pain. This is particularly so when trigger points form in response to visceral pain or refer pain to the viscera. In practice, trigger points are identified by palpation. Trigger point palpation is a skill that can be learned in a short time, commonly in 2- to 3-day workshops for most clinicians, but it is a skill honed over months and years of practice. The accomplished practitioner can identify subtle changes in muscle that are clinically significant pain generators. Objective means of identifying the myofascial trigger point include MR elastography and the more available high-resolution (HR) ultrasound.

HR ultrasound, still not generally used in clinical practice because of cost and time constraints, is nevertheless being evaluated as a practical means of locating the trigger point taut band for trigger point needling. It remains to be seen whether or not high-resolution ultrasonography will have real clinical utility.

HISTORY

Myofascial pain can present acutely but, if unresolved either spontaneously or with treatment, may evolve into a chronic muscle pain syndrome that can persist for years. MPS may persist long after the initiating cause of pain has resolved. Hence, the history of a remote injury can be relevant.

The nature of myofascial pain is characteristic of all somatic pain. It is dull, deep, aching, and poorly localized, in contrast to well-localized cutaneous pain. It is rarely sharp and stabbing, although acute episodes of stabbing pain can occur, even against a background of chronic pain. It can mimic radicular or visceral pain.

There may be a component of paresthesias or dysesthesias in addition to or instead of pain. Parasthesias such as tingling, when present, are generally in the distribution of the nerve root(s) innervating the muscle harboring the relevant trigger point. In contrast to cutaneous pain, myofascial pain is more likely to cause referred pain. Pain may be experienced as referred to other regions of the body, such as the head, neck, or hip, as referred pain. Importantly, it is the referred pain that may be the presenting complaint. Examples of this include lateral epicondylalgia that may be the result of trigger points in the supraspinatus or extensor carpi radialis longus muscles and pain in the greater trochanter that may be caused by trigger points in the gluteus medius muscle.

Generally speaking, myofascial pain presents as pain, not as sensory paresthesias or numbness. However, trigger points may cause nerve entrapment. In that case, the symptoms of nerve entrapment, including paresthesias, may be the presenting complaint. For example, heel numbness and tingling may be the presenting complaint for trigger points in the piriformis muscle entrapping and compressing the sciatic nerve. In this case, the differential diagnosis would include a lumbosacral radiculopathy. The diagnostic test may be the inactivation of the trigger point to see if that is sufficient to eliminate the symptom. Myofascial pain can also be the presenting symptom for radiculopathy or major joint pain (shoulder or hip). When myofascial pain is the presenting symptom of radiculopathy, it is often acute in onset and may precede neurologic impairments such as weakness or reflex changes by days.

There are certain predisposing factors that make myofascial pain more likely to occur, and the history will suggest their presence. Physical examination and laboratory studies are confirmatory. Some predisposing factors include iron deficiency (most commonly caused by menstrual blood loss in women but also from dietary insufficiency), hypothyroidism, and vitamin D and vitamin B_{12} deficiency. These are discussed later in this chapter. Lyme disease, hypermobility syndromes, and spondylosis also predispose to the development of myofascial pain.

PHYSICAL EXAMINATION

The diagnosis of a MPS can only be made, in the final analysis, by identifying trigger points that reproduce the patient's pain in part or in whole. The rare exception is pain caused by trigger points in the deep paraspinal multifidi muscles, which cannot be palpated in most individuals. The trigger point is felt as a taut band palpable within a muscle. When present in a muscle group, the taut band can almost always be palpated. Trigger point tenderness or pain is always on the taut band, but this can be confusing to those who cannot feel a taut band. Then, the confusion is between fibromyalgia "tender points" and myofascial trigger points. Some taut bands are not painful to palpation but have functional consequences such as limiting the ROM of a body part. The concept of latent trigger points and painless taut bands is discussed earlier, in section "Latent and Active Trigger Points."

Taut Band Palpation

The taut band must be palpated cross-fiber, that is, perpendicular to the direction of the muscle fiber. Muscle fiber direction is not always obvious and is unique to each muscle, as seen in the pectoral muscles, the infraspinatus muscle, and in the gluteal muscles. Knowledge of the fiber direction in individual muscles is of great advantage to the clinician because it permits the differentiation of one muscle palpated through overlying muscle. Examples of this are the palpation of the levator scapulae muscles through the trapezius muscle and palpation of the pectoralis minor muscle through the pectoralis major muscle.

Palpation of a muscle overlying a firm or bony structure is done by flat palpation of the muscle against the underlying structure. Examples of this are palpation of the infraspinatus muscle against the scapula and palpation of the gluteus medius muscle against the ilium. A muscle that can be grasped between the fingers and thumb is examined by pincer palpation, with the muscle between the thumb and the index and long fingers. Once a taut band is identified, the examining fingers move along the band to identify the small region of greatest hardness (the region of least compliance to compression). It is this area that is usually most exquisitely tender, the center or heart of the trigger point. Stimulation of this area induces referred pain. Mechanical stimulation of the trigger point in this area best elicits the local twitch response. The farther away from this area that the taut band is mechanically stimulated, the more attenuated the twitch response becomes, until it cannot be elicited at all.[98,119] The local twitch response generally cannot be elicited when the taut band is stimulated 3 cm or more from this region. The area to be treated specifically by manual trigger point compression or by needling is this area of greatest hardness and greatest tenderness in the taut band—the area variously called the trigger point or the trigger zone.

Eliciting Referred Pain

Compression of the trigger zone for 5–10 seconds can induce referred pain or pain that is at a distance from the point of stimulation. Referred pain represents central activation or central sensitization. It requires a round trip to the spinal cord and back. It does not occur in a second, but takes time to develop. Hence, compression of the trigger point must last for 5–10 seconds in order to be certain that the trigger point can induce referred pain or not.

Once the trigger point is identified, determined to be tender, and referred pain is elicited or not, the patient is asked if the pain or tenderness, local or referred, reproduces or is like all or part of their usual pain. This is a critical part of the examination procedure because the goal is to identify the cause of the patient's pain, and then to relieve it.

Taut Bands

A taut band that is not tender to palpation will not, of course, reproduce pain unless it does so by causing referred pain. Such taut bands will restrict movement because they cannot lengthen fully. Latent trigger points have real and deleterious effects. Lucas[108] has shown that a latent trigger point disrupts the normal sequence of muscle activation. They can activate central effects, such as decreasing the threshold for pain activation distally.[120] They limit muscle lengthening and have a role in activating other trigger points. Hence, a clinical decision has to be made regarding the treatment of nonactive trigger point taut bands, whether latent or not. The decision requires a judgment about whether a taut band is clinically relevant or not. Because that question does not always have an answer, the taut band may be treated more often than not.

ADDITIONAL TRIGGER POINT CHARACTERISTICS

Limited ROM

Limited ROM is due to pain on lengthening a muscle harboring a trigger point and to the limitations imposed by the shortened taut band. ROM testing can be misleading because of the potential multiple causes of limited motion about a joint and because a limited ROM may appear normal in a hypermobile (Ehlers-Danlos syndrome) individual.

Examination of ROM can be a useful clue in determining which muscles harbor trigger points. For example, limited rotation of the head to the left can implicate the left SCM and/or trapezius muscles or the right splenius cervicis and oblique capitis inferior muscles, all muscles that must lengthen to allow this movement. An additional finding of limitation of side bending to the right would focus attention on the left SCM and trapezius muscles that must lengthen to allow this movement.

Weakness

Weakness is often but not always evident in a muscle harboring a trigger point. Weakness in affected muscles is rapidly reversed as the trigger point is inactivated either manually or by needling or laser treatment. It can be a dramatic demonstration of the effectiveness of trigger point inactivation in the clinic.

Autonomic Changes

Vascular dilation and constriction occur as a result of autonomic nervous system activation, resulting in erythema or blanching and warm or cool areas usually in the distribution of the nerve innervating an affected muscle.

Diagnostic Criteria

The question arises as to what exactly is needed to diagnose a trigger point (and thus diagnose myofascial pain). In other words, what are the essential features of the trigger point, and what features, even if unique to the trigger point, are not essential to the diagnosis (Table 5.1)? This question has never really been addressed well. However, the presence of a taut band that is tender and that reproduces the patient's pain complaint in full or in part is a sufficient point on which to base a treatment program. These criteria allow the clinician to select a trigger point for treatment. The proof of efficacy is that treatment based on these criteria alone is sufficient to reduce or eliminate pain. This indeed seems to be the case, although there is no study confirming this.

Is identification of a taut band enough to make a diagnosis? To diagnosis a pain syndrome, one must have pain, so it makes sense that tenderness or pain must be elicited by examination in order to diagnosis a pain syndrome. However, a nontender taut band can be selected for treatment in a patient with trigger point pain syndrome if there is suspicion that it has significant clinical effects.

Reliability of Trigger Point Examination

A number of studies have shown interrater reliability of the physical examination of an MTrP, starting with the paper by Gerwin et al.[121] Subsequent studies were more sophisticated

Table 5.1 **DIAGNOSTIC FEATURES OF MYOFASCIAL TRIGGER POINTS**

Essential characteristics for diagnosis	Taut band Tenderness on taut band
Additional essential feature for treatment	Reproduces all or part of patient's pain
Additional features unique to the trigger point	Local twitch response
Features associated with but not unique to the trigger point	1. Referred pain 2. Weakness 3. Restricted range of motion 4. Autonomic signs (lacrimation, piloerection, vasodilation or constriction)

and showed that clinicians could agree on the identification of the same trigger point, not just the muscle(s) that harbored trigger points. Sciotti et al.[122] showed that examiners could independently identify the same taut band region. Significant interrater agreement of myofascial trigger point palpation of shoulder muscles has also been shown.[123]

A number of reviews have been published questioning the data and purporting to show that physical examination is not reliable. One such review established arbitrary criteria for the identification of trigger points, discounting a number of positive studies that did not include the elements that the authors considered necessary. For example, they discounted studies in which a "nodule" in the taut band was not mentioned. The nodule is a feature they said was mentioned as essential by myofascial pain "experts." In fact, all the experts turned out to be Dr. David Simons, a pioneer in the field. He was referring to the area of tender hardness on the taut band. One has to identify the taut band and to elicit tenderness, but there is no need to identify the region as nodular rather than linear in order to make a diagnosis. The trigger point could simply be described as a sense of swelling, but often all that the palpating finger feels is hardness on the taut band, not a nodularity.

HOW IS MPS MANAGED?

TREATMENT PRINCIPLES

Treatment of trigger point pain syndromes involves trigger point inactivation and restoration of normal body biomechanics to the extent possible. Treatment of the trigger point can help to establish the role of the trigger point in producing a patient's particular pain syndrome, can quickly reduce an acute pain, and can be an integral part of a physical therapy rehabilitation program.

TPI AND DEEP, DRY NEEDLING

TPIs were used by Travell and her students at least since the 1950s if not earlier. There were no studies of its efficacy that meet today's criteria of controlled or randomized studies; however, early examples of the usefulness of TPI date back the late 1930s when Kellgren treated subjects with muscle pain with injections of local anesthetic and showed that their pain and referred pain went away.[4] Travell and Rinsler[6] showed the same result when injecting procaine into chest wall muscle to treat noncardiac chest pain. Since then, TPIs with local anesthetic and with other substances has become a mainstay of MPS treatment. Eliciting a local twitch response results in a better outcome than not eliciting a twitch response. No advantage in clinical outcome has been shown with using or adding any substance other than local anesthetic.[124] Lidocaine is used almost exclusively in the United States since procaine is no longer readily available. Lidocaine 0.25% has the least postinjection soreness compared to other concentrations of lidocaine[125] and is the preferred substance to use in TPIs.

Needling the trigger point without injection of any substance is just as effective in the long run as injecting trigger points with lidocaine.[126] Thus, mechanical stimulation of the trigger point is the effective means of trigger point inactivation, not the injection of local anesthetic. The mechanism remains unknown by which dry needling works. Possibilities include stimulation of local motor nerve axons or stimulation of surrounding muscle fiber surface membranes. What is clinically observed is that trigger point pain and trigger point hardness is best reduced after all local twitch responses are eliminated, whether the trigger point is treated by injection or by dry needling.

A recent review of the effect of deep, dry needling on trigger points in upper quadrant myofascial pain found 246 articles, of which 12 randomized control studies were found and further evaluated.[126] Three studies that compared dry needling to sham or placebo treatment found evidence that dry needling can reduce pain immediately. Two studies showed that dry needling gave relief for up to 4 weeks. Two studies suggested that lidocaine injection may be more effective that deep, dry needling after 4 weeks. The evidence favoring deep, dry needling was considered to be class A evidence.

Randomized, controlled, double-blind studies are difficult because no good control has been devised for injection, although sham needling has been used as a control. Studies with sham needling have shown that deep, dry needing is an effective treatment technique. However, overall, there are few good studies, thus leading to the conclusion that no recommendation for or against TPI or deep, dry needling can be made on the basis of the current literature. Notwithstanding this, deep, dry needling has become a widely used technique that is gaining popularity among physical therapists in particular because there is abundant clinical experience showing that inserting a needle into a trigger point does relieve pain and does facilitate physical therapy, despite the lack of studies. However, it is disputed as to whether the long-term outcome of deep, dry needling is any better than conventional physiotherapy because the results of the two may be similar 1 month after treatment.[127]

Those factors that initiated and maintained the pain need to be identified and corrected in order to sustain the gains made in the therapeutic treatment program (Table 5.2). There are unanswered questions associated with each of these stages

Table 5.2 **THERAPEUTIC MODALITIES FOR TREATMENT OF MYOFASCIAL PAIN**

Trigger point injection	Few good studies; no greater benefit to any injectate than lidocaine; new injectates (like 5-HT agonists and GABA/glycine agonists) are promising, but have few studies to support their use
Trigger point dry needling	Good evidence to support its use
Manual therapies	Good evidence for many manual therapy modalities
Laser therapy	Moderately good evidence to support its use

of treatment. Trigger point inactivation can be accomplished by either noninvasive means or by invasive means (needling or injecting the trigger point). Prophylaxis or prevention of trigger point recurrence can also be accomplished by invasive and noninvasive means.

MANUAL INACTIVATION OF TRIGGER POINTS

Manual inactivation of trigger points includes trigger point compression, spray and stretch, strain/counterstrain, ultrasound, and various forms of muscle stretching. There are few randomized controlled studies of the effectiveness of manual therapy in trigger point inactivation.[128] A limiting factor in assessing manual treatment techniques is the lack of uniform outcome measures. Most studies, but not all, used PPT or an 11-point Likert numerical or visual pain scale. However, some studies used the McGill Short-Form Pain Questionnaire or Quality of Life assessments. ROM has also been used as an outcome measurement of treatment effectiveness. Moreover, some trials evaluate just one manual therapy and others evaluate a combination of manual therapies. The conclusion of Fernandez de las Peñas et al. (2005) was that there was no rigorous evidence that the manual techniques studied have better outcome beyond placebo.[128] The role of manual therapies was neither supported nor refuted by the results of their study. Rickard[129] looked at some manual interventions, but only two of the studies included in the review used typical manual treatments of trigger points used by trained physical therapists (ischemic compression). These two studies demonstrated short-term (immediate) benefit, but had no long-term follow-up. One of the two studies looked at a combination of heat, ROM exercises, inferential current, and myofascial release. The other study looked at ischemic compression.

The mechanism of pain reduction and softening of the taut band by manual therapy remains speculative. Studies of the effectiveness of a commonly used manual technique of trigger point inactivation—trigger point compression—have been few. A novel approach to evaluating the effectiveness of this approach utilized a digital algometer and demonstrated a benefit of manual compression with pain reduction and an increase in PPT.[130]

Trigger point compression (called ischemic compression in Travell and Simons's first edition of *Myofascial Pain and Dysfunction*, but changed to trigger point compression in the second edition)[1] induces a sustained release of lactate in muscle trigger point interstitial fluid.[131] This manual technique may produce a localized stretch on the trigger point taut band. The Moraska study shows that manual trigger point compression does have the capacity to change the biochemical milieu of the trigger point.

Ultrasound therapy and low-level laser therapy are currently being used as noninvasive treatments for trigger point pain. Treatment using either low-level laser or ultrasound or a sham treatment was compared to a control group receiving neither treatment in a randomized controlled trial. Both active treatment groups and placebo treatment groups improved compared to the untreated control groups.[132] The authors concluded that since neither ultrasound nor low-level laser was better than placebo, and because placebo was also better than no treatment, treatment by neither of these two methods could be confirmed to be effective. However, the control group may have not improved compared to the treatment/placebo groups because the treatments and placebo groups had an active treatment whereas the control group had no intervention. Several studies have shown improvement with ultrasound, but these are poor examples because they were unblinded and uncontrolled.

Massage has been used to treat general muscle pain, if not myofascial trigger points specifically. It has long been used, but little scientific evidence exists to support its use.[133] Deep tissue massage reduced mechanical hyperalgesia (lowered PPT) and decreased stretch pain in experimentally induced delayed-onset muscle pain, whereas superficial touch only decreased stretch pain compared to the rest-only control group.[63]

In summary, data are either inadequate or conflicting regarding most manual therapies for the treatment of MPS (evidence level U).

NONINVASIVE, NONMANUAL TREATMENT TECHNIQUES

Treatments in this category include all forms of electrical stimulation, ultrasound, laser, and magnet therapies. Transcutaneous electrical stimulation provides immediate reduction in pain, but its long-term benefit has not been established.[129] Preliminary evidence supported the use of magnetic therapy, but data were very limited and studies were of only moderate quality. Conventional ultrasound is not more effective than placebo in neck and upper back pain based on the limited data available (one high-quality and two lower quality studies). Ultrasound did not improve outcome when combined with massage and exercise (class I study).[134] Ultrasound produced short-term improvement in PPT (class IV study).[135] Ultrasound reduced pain within muscles in the same nerve innervation segment (class I study).[136] PPT values increased (less tenderness) in the infraspinatus muscle when trigger points in the supraspinatus muscle were treated, whereas there was no significant change in the PPT of the ipsilateral gluteus medius muscle (the control muscle) in this randomized, blinded, controlled study. Ultrasound treatment is probably effective in the treatment of trigger points (level B recommendation).

Low-level laser is another noninvasive approach to the inactivation of myofascial trigger points that has created much interest. There have been mixed results in those studies that have been randomized, controlled, and blinded. Earlier studies (class I studies) have shown benefit,[137,138] but a more recent study showed no benefit (class I study).[139] Low-level laser has the level B recommendation of probable effectiveness in the treatment of myofascial trigger point pain.

A randomized, sham-controlled, double-blinded study of the use of a lidocaine 5% patch showed a significant reduction in pain from days 14–28 in patients with upper trapezius pain.[140] The difference between the lidocaine 5% patch and a sham patch was lost after 28 days.

Thioclochicoside is a glycine and γ-aminobutyric acid (GABA) receptor activator that induces muscle relaxation and has analgesic properties with tolerable adverse side effects. It has been shown to reduce myofascial trigger point pain when given topically and when injected intramuscularly into the trigger point.[141] Cervical ROM was also improved after administration of this substance.

Thus, the data supporting recommendations regarding most noninvasive, nonmanual treatments of trigger points are either inadequate or conflicting (level U). Further studies are needed in order to base a treatment recommendation on medical evidence.

INVASIVE TREATMENT OF MYOFASCIAL TRIGGER POINTS

Invasive treatment of myofascial trigger points is generally done either by dry needling or by injection of substances. Deep, dry needling is accomplished by inserting a fine, monopolar needle through the skin into muscle. In general, the needle is guided by the clinician's perception of the trigger point location through palpation. There is now interest in identifying the trigger point for deep, dry needling by high-resolution ultrasound. Deep, dry needling causes transient damage to muscle and nerve. Regeneration of muscle is seen by day 3 and is complete by day 7.[142] Deep, dry needling not only inactivates the local trigger point into which it is inserted, but it also modulates the EMG endplate activity at remote sites via a spinal cord mechanism.[143] In addition, it modulates the biochemical response (endogenous opiates, neurotransmitters, kinins, prostaglandins) associated with hypoxia, inflammation, and pain.[144]

The effectiveness of deep, dry needling has been studied more intensively in recent years because it is increasingly incorporated into clinical practice. Deep, dry needling was considered to be effective in some studies.[145] It is a technique well tolerated and widely used, and it deserves to be evaluated as a treatment of myofascial pain. Dry needling of primary trigger points results in improved ROM and less tenderness at the primary trigger point site and at the site of satellite trigger points in its area of referred pain.[146] Dry needling reduces the shear modulus of the trigger point as seen on ultrasound shear-wave elastography, consistent with reduction in palpable stiffness.[104]

TPI is injection of some form of injectate through a needle inserted into the trigger point. It was reported by Kellgren to be effective in relieving the referred pain from muscle more than 70 years ago.[3,4] The most common material injected is lidocaine. Lidocaine diluted to 0.25% was the most effective concentration associated with the least postinjection soreness.[125] Other substances in addition to lidocaine have been used for injection, most commonly some form of corticosteroid. Cummings and White[124] reviewed 23 papers and found the effect of needling was independent of the material injected. They found no trials of sufficient quality or design to test the efficacy of any needling technique over placebo (level U recommendation). Their conclusion was that direct needling of trigger points appears effective, that in three trials there was no difference between dry needling and injection, and that controlled trials are needed to determine if TPIs are more effective than placebo. An updated review found 15 randomized controlled studies that met their inclusion criteria.[147] However, small sample sizes, deficiencies in reporting, and heterogeneity of the studies precluded a definitive synthesis of the data. TPI appeared to relieve symptoms when it was the sole treatment for whiplash syndrome and for chronic neck, shoulder, and back pain. The authors concluded that there is no clear evidence that TPI is ineffective or beneficial, but that it is a safe procedure in experienced hands (level U). Thiocolchicoside has been shown to be effective both topically and when injected into the trigger point, but there was no placebo control in the one published study (class IV study).[141] A randomized but uncontrolled and unblinded comparison of TPI with lidocaine 0.25%, lidocaine 0.25% plus corticosteroid, and dry needling alone showed that all three treatments were effective in reducing pain, but that only lidocaine plus corticosteroid reduced postinjection sensitivity (level IV study). A single-blinded, randomized controlled study of the effect of dry needling showed that pain was reduced and that ROM and PPT was increased in satellite trigger points, both to a significant degree (level B study).[146] Dry needling was no better than placebo in treating hamstring trigger points in a randomized, controlled double-blinded study.[148] Dry needling increases the PPT in segmentally related muscle, showing that there is a segmental antinociceptive effect in dry needling.[149]

One study compared TPI with lidocaine with dry needling.[150] This study is consistent with current clinical practice because dry needling currently is most commonly done with acupuncture needles. The study demonstrated the effectiveness of both techniques in providing pain relief, better relief of depression with dry needling (!), and improvement in passive ROM with both treatments. Post-treatment soreness was the same in both groups. Local twitch responses were elicited in 97.7% of subjects treated and indicated that the needle placement was in the trigger point zone. An additional study by the same group evaluated peripheral dry needling without and with the addition of dry needling of the multifidi muscles (paraspinal dry needling) in the neck.[151] Although the addition of needling multifidi gave a small statistical advantage, both techniques were effective in relieving pain at 1 month (class III studies). There is, however, a major difficulty in finding appropriate placebo or sham treatments in these controlled studies. Many placebo treatments of myofascial trigger points are active, not inactive, placebos. A prospective, randomized controlled study found that TPI with lidocaine 1% and dry needling were equally effective at producing significant improvement in pain, ROM, and depression up to 12 weeks.[152] Deep, dry needling was found to be more effective than TPI with lidocaine, and both were significantly more effective than sham treatment.[153] There is little evidence to support or negate the use of any injectate over dry needling (level U recommendation).

Attempts to enhance the needle effect on trigger points include electrical stimulation through needles inserted into the myofascial trigger zone (needle electrical intramuscular stimulation [NEIMS]). Visual analog scale rating of pain, PPT, and ROM improved among subjects treated with NEIMS (class III study).[154] The conclusion is that dry needling is probably effective based on available studies (level B recommendation). However, much depends on the outcome measures and the goal of treatment in assessing the treatment benefit. In clinical practice, an immediate reduction in trigger point pain and an improvement in ROM are usually seen with trigger point needling. The benefit lasts from days to a week or 10 days.

Acupuncture trigger point needling is a term used to describe inserting the acupuncture needle into a muscle trigger point. It has been used to treat myofascial trigger points in a manner identical to the dry needling technique described by physical therapists, physicians, and others. It has been shown to be effective in treating chronic neck pain[155] and chronic LBP.[156,157] Blinding using sham needles was effective in these two studies (class I studies). Acupuncture was more effective than dry needling, and both were more effective than sham acupuncture in reducing myofascial trigger point pain (VAS) and ROM.[158] These studies further support the effectiveness of acupuncture and dry needling in treating MPS. However, another systematic review of acupuncture and dry needling (deep needling techniques) concluded that there was only limited evidence from one study showing that deep, dry needling was beneficial compared with standardized care.[159] Some studies were criticized because trigger points were not convincingly the sole cause of pain, although in clinical practice this is often the case. Treatment techniques (depth of insertion of the needle, location of needle placement, duration of needle insertion) varied, and co-treatment varied, all of which reduced the comparability of studies.

A central modulating effect occurs with dry needling of myofascial trigger points. Dry needling of key trigger points diminishes satellite trigger point activity.[146] In this single-blinded, randomized, controlled trial, inactivation of infraspinatus trigger points had a beneficial effect on trigger point manifestations (pain intensity and PPT) in ipsilateral proximal and distal upper extremity muscles (class I study).

The mechanism of action of trigger point needling has never been adequately elucidated. The results of dry needling seem to be about as effective as injection of local anesthetic, suggesting that local anesthetic is not absolutely necessary. Thus, it seems that it is the mechanical action of the needle itself that inactivates the trigger point. Some consideration has been given to disruption of the muscle cell wall by the needle causing alterations of calcium influx into the cytoplasm. This mechanism does not seem credible because disruption of the cell wall on a macroscopic basis would be likely to result in major cell function disruption. Well-documented trigger point inactivation associated with the injection of bupivacaine was significantly reversed with intravenous naloxone (10 mg).[160] This strongly suggests that endogenous opioids are involved in the needle-induced relief of pain and in the reversal of the physical manifestations of the trigger point. There has been no follow-up to this study. Furthermore, there have been no studies of the effect of naloxone on the manual inactivation of the trigger point. Finally, Shah's studies[9] suggests that, as the muscle twitches in response to the needle and then relaxes, capillary and arteriole compression is reversed, and the high concentration of neurotransmitters, cytokines, protons, and ions like potassium are removed over a matter of minutes.

BOTULINUM TOXIN

Botulinum toxin has been used to inactivate trigger points. Theoretically, botulinum toxin should act like a long-lasting TPI if it acts to prevent the development of the trigger point or inactivates it. Botulinum toxin reduced or blocked end-plate noise at the trigger zone in the rabbit.[16] A number of randomized, controlled, double-blind studies have been conducted, but many were small studies or did not utilize appropriate criteria for identification of trigger points. In addition, the variable amounts of toxin have been used in the studies, lack of documentation of injecting precisely at the trigger zone, and lack of intention to treat the entire relevant functional muscle unit may have contributed to the inability to show efficacy.[161] Injection of up to 50 units of botulinum toxin in up to five active trigger points in the neck and shoulders failed to reduce pain more than the placebo control group.[162] Both groups received myofascial release physical therapy, amitriptyline, ibuprofen, and propoxyphene napsylate/APAP, which may have influenced the outcome in this 12-week study.

Treatment of masticatory muscle trigger point pain with botulinum toxin in an open trial showed a mean/median reduction in pain of 57%.[163] However, this was a noncontrolled, nonrandomized, unblinded study.

Some new and interesting substances for TPI are presently being explored, such as bee venom and tropisetron.[164,165] Tropisetron is a 5-HT$_3$ antagonist that has been shown to alleviate pain in myofascial trigger point pain syndromes. It also has a more widespread analgesic effect. It may be the first specific injectate shown to have a positive benefit in the treatment of MTrP pain syndromes.

Baldry's technique of superficial dry needling has never been subjected to adequate study.[166] The needle is inserted 3–4 mm into the subdermal layers of skin over the point of tenderness. Baldry proposes that this technique is effective and less invasive than inserting needles into muscle, and it avoids the potential complications of pneumothorax and other complications of deep needling.

Trigger point dry needling and TPI as presently performed (1) provide immediate relief of pain, (2) are useful diagnostically to see if a particular pain syndrome is myofascial in nature, and (3) are most effective when used to facilitate physical therapy. As the systematic reviews show, there is a need for further studies examining these outcomes.

Interactive neurostimulation was found in one preliminary study to have no effect on pain or PPT at 5 days after treatment compared to sham treatment.[167]

STRUCTURAL AND MECHANICAL FACTORS

Biomechanical factors play a role in the development of myofascial trigger points. Prolonged maintenance of posture may have the same effect as repeated the low-level muscle activation cited earlier. Leg length inequality and scoliosis likewise can produce chronic muscle overuse as compensatory mechanisms. Pelvic torsion can occur as a result of leg-length inequality or cause a pseudo-leg-length inequality. Hypermobility, discussed earlier, is another example of a mechanical dysfunction that causes chronic muscle overuse. Deterioration of the quality of life in hypermobile Ehlers-Danlos patients is mainly associated with pain and fatigue.[168]

RESTORATION OF NORMAL FUNCTION

A multidisciplinary approach to myofascial pain patients is generally considered appropriate. In the case of Ehlers-Danlos patients in particular, attention to dysautonomia, muscle weakness, and lifestyle modifications to prevent joint injury and muscle pain are appropriate.[168] In all patients, attention to sleep disturbances, intestinal malabsorption, depression, and anxiety is necessary to achieve an optimal outcome.

CONCLUSION

MPS is a common cause of pain. It often causes symptoms from pain referred to distal muscle or to viscera. It is readily diagnosed by palpation performed by trained clinicians. The hallmark features are a band of hardened muscle (the taut band), local muscle tenderness on the taut band, and reproduction of the patient's symptoms. Provocative and perpetuating factors should be sought through physical examination, history, and laboratory testing (Box 5.1). Treatment involves elimination of the trigger point, restoration of normal musculoskeletal function, and correction of those amenable provocative and perpetuating factors.

Box 5.1 **PROVOCATIVE FACTORS**

1. Acute supramaximal contraction
2. Eccentric overloaded contraction (like walking downhill)
3. Repetitive low-level contractions (like computer keyboard typing)
4. Prolonged static postures
5. Structural stresses:
   a. Scoliosis
   b. Pelvic torque
   c. Leg-length inequality
6. Other mechanical stresses:
   a. Hypermobility syndrome
7. Medical factors:
   a. Hypothyroidism
   b. Iron deficiency
   c. Vitamin D deficiency
   d. Parasitic infestation
   e. Infection (Lyme disease)
   f. Arthritides
   g. Ehlers-Danlos syndrome, hypermobility type

REFERENCES

1. Simons DG, Travell JG, Simons LS. *Myofascial Pain and Dysfunction: The Trigger Point Manual.* Vol. 1. 2nd ed. Baltimore, MD: Williams & Wilkins; 1999.
2. Travell JG and Simons DG. *Myofascial Pain and Dysfunction: The Trigger Point Manual.* Baltimore, MD: Williams & Wilkins; 1982.
3. Kellgren JH. Observations on referred pain arising from muscle. *Clin Sci.* 1938a;3:175–190.
4. Kellgren JH. A preliminary account of referred pains arising from muscle. *British Med J.* 1938b;1:325–327.
5. Kellgren JH. Deep pain sensibility. *Lancet.* 1949; 1(6562):943–949.
6. Travell JG, Rinzler SH. The myofascial genesis of pain. *Postgrad Med.* 1952;11:425–434.
7. Fischer AA. Tissue compliance meter for objective, quantitative documentation of soft tissue consistency and pathology. *Arch Phys Med Rehabil.* 1987;68:122–125.
8. Hägg GM. The Cinderella hypothesis. In: Johansson H, et al, eds. Chronic Work-related Myalgia. Gävle, Sweden: Gävle University Press; 2003:127–132.
9. Shah JP, Phillips TM, Danoff JV, Gerber LH. An in vitro mircro-analytical technique for measuring the local biochemical milieu of human skeletal muscle. *J Appl Physiol.* 2005;99:1977–1984.
10. Gerwin RD, Dommerholt J, Shah J. An expansion of Simons' integrated hypothesis of trigger point formation. *Curr Pain Headache Rep.* 2004;8:468–475.
11. Sikdar S, Shah JP, Gebreab T, et al. Novel applications of ultrasound technology to visualize and characterize myofascial trigger points and surrounding soft tissue. *Arch Phys Med Rehab.* 2009;90(11):1829–1838.
12. Gerwin RD. The taut band and other mysteries of the trigger point: an examination of the mechanisms relevant to the development and maintenance of the trigger point. *J Musculoskel Pain.* 2008;15(suppl 13):115–121.
13. Hubbard DR, Berkoff GM. Myofascial trigger points show spontaneous needle EMG activity. *Spine.* 1993;18:1803–1807.
14. Simons DG, Hong CZ, Simons LS. Prevalence of spontaneous electrical activity at trigger points and at control sites in rabbit skeletal muscle. *J Musculoskel Pain.* 1995;3(1):35–48.
15. Chen JT, Chen SM, Kuan TS, Chung KC, Hong CZ. Phentolamine effect on the spontaneous electrical activity of active loci in a myofascial trigger spot of rabbit skeletal muscle. *Arch Phys Med Rehab.* 1998;79:790–794.
16. Kuan TS, Chen JT, Chen SM, Chein CH, Hong CZ. Effect of botulinum toxin on endplate noise in myofascial trigger spots of rabbit skeletal muscle. *Am J Phys Med Rehabil.* 2002;81;512–520.
17. Schwarz PB, Yee N, Mir S, Peever JH. Noradrenalin triggers muscle tone by ampliflying glutamate-driven excitation of somatic motoneurons in anaesthetized rats. *J Physiol.* 2008;5787–5802.
18. Ge HY, Fernandez-de-las-Peñas C, Yue SW. Myofascial trigger points: spontaneous electrical activity and its consequences for pain induction and propagation. *Chin Med.* 2011;6:13. doi: 10.11186/1749-8546-6-13.
19. McPartland JM, Simons DG. Myofascial trigger points: translating molecular theory into manual therapy. *J Man Manip Ther.* 2006;232–239.
20. Hou CR, Chung KC, Chen JT, Hong CZ. Effects of a calcium channel blocker on electrical activity in myofascial trigger spots of rabbits. *Am J Phys Med Rehabil.* 2002;81(5):342–349.

21. Mense S, Simons DG, Hoheisel U, Quenzer B. Lesions of rat skeletal muscle after local block of acetylcholinesterase and neuromuscular stimulation. *J Appl Physiol.* 2003;94:2494–2501.
22. Hong CZ. Persistence of local twitch response with loss of conduction to and from the spinal cord. *Arch Phys Med Rehabil.* 1994;7:12–16.
23. Kuan TS, Hong CZ, Chen JT, Chen SM, Chien CH. The spinal cord connections of the myofascial trigger spots. *Eur J Pain.* 2007a;11:624–634.
24. Chang CW, Chen YR, Chang KF. Evidence of neuroaxonal degeneration in myofascial pain syndrome: a study of neuromuscular jitter by axonal microstimulation. *Eur J Pain.* 2008;12:1026–1030.
25. Brückle W, Suckfüll M, Fleckenstein W, Weiss C, Müller W. Tissue pO2 measurement in taut back musculature (m. erector spinae). *Z Rheumatol.* 1990;49(4):208–216.
26. Shah JP, Gilliams EA. Uncovering the biochemical milieu of myofascial trigger points using in vivo microdialysis: an application of muscle pain concepts to myofascial pain syndrome. *J Bodyw Mov Ther.* 2008;12:371–384.
27. Shah J, Danoff JV, Desai MJ, et al. Biochemicals associated with pain and inflammation are elevated in sites near to and remote from active myofascial trigger points. *Arch Phys Med Rehabil.* 2008;89:16–23.
28. Rosendal L, Larsson B, Kristiansen J, et al. Increase in muscle nociceptive substances and anaerobic metabolism in patients with trapezius myalgia. *Pain.* 2004;112:324–334.
29. Gerdle B, Hilgenfeldt U, Larsson B, Kristiansen J, Søgaard K, Rosendal L. Bradykinin and kallidin levels in patients with work-related trapezius myalgia, in patients with whiplash associated pain, and in healthy controls—a microdialysis study of women. *Pain.* 2008a;139:578–587.
30. Gerdle B, Lemming D, Kristiansen J, Larsson B, Peolsson M, Rosendal L. Biochemical alterations in the trapezius muscle of patients with chronic whiplash associated disorders (WAD)—a microdialysis study. *Eur J Pain.* 2008b;12:82–93.
31. Barbe MF, Elliott MB, Abdelmagid SM, Amin M, Popoff SN, Safadi FF, Barr AE. Serum and tissue cytokines and chemokines increase with repetitive upper extremity tasks. *J Orthop Res.* 2008;26:1320–1326.
32. Simons DG, Stolov WC. Microscopic features and transient contraction of palpable bands in canine muscle. *Am J Phys Med.* 1976;55:65–88.
33. Jacobsen S, Bartels EM, Danneskiold-Samsøe B. Single cell morphology of muscle in patients with chronic muscle pain. *Scand J Rheumatol.* 1991;20(5):3336–3343.
34. Filosto et al, N, Tomerlleri G. The role of muscle biopsy in investigating isolated muscle pain. *Neurology.* 2007;68:181–186.
35. Mense S, Gerwin R, eds. *Muscle Pain.* Heidlburg: Springer; 2010.
36. Kuan TS, Hsieh YL, Chen SM, Chen JT, Yen WC, Hong CZ. The myofascial trigger point region: correlation between the degree of irritability and the prevalence of endplate noise. *Am J Phys Med Rehabil.* 2007b;86:183–189.
37. Woolf CJ. Central sensitization: implications for the diagnosis and treatment of pain. *Pain.* 2011;152(3 suppl):S2–S15.
38. Dejung B, Gröbli C, Colla F, Weissmann R. *Triggerpunkt-Therapie.* Bern: Verlag Hans Huber; 2003.
39. Hwang M. Kang YK, Kim DH. Referred pain pattern of the pronator quadratus muscle. *Pain.* 2005a;116: 238–42..
40. Hwang M, Kang JK, Shin JY, Kim DH. Referred pain pattern of the abductor pollicus longus muscle. *Am J Phys Med Rehabil.* 2005b;84:593–597.
41. Fernandez-de-las-Peñas C, Campo MS, Carnero JF, Page JCM. Manual therapies in the myofascial trigger point treatment: a systematic review. *J Bodyw Mov Ther.* 2005a;9:27–35.
42. Fernandez-Carnero J, Fernandez-de-las-Peñas C, Isabel de la Llave-Rincón, Ge HY, Arendt-Nielsen L. Bilateral myofascial trigger points in the forearm muscles in patients with chronic unilateral epicondylalgia: a blinded, controlled study. *Clin J Pain.* 2008;24:802–807.
43. Mizumura K, Taguchi T. Facilitated response of muscle thin-fiber receptors in mechanical hyperalgesia after exercise. In: Graven-Nielsen T, Arendt-Nielsen L, Mense S, eds. *Fundamentals of Musculoskeletal Pain.* Seattle, WA: IASP Press; 2008: 47–49.
44. Elliott MB, Barr AE, Clark BD, Amin M, Amin S, Barbe MF. High force reaching task induces widespread inflammation, increased spinal cord neurochemicals and neuropathic pain. *Neuroscience.* 2009;158:922–931.
45. Dommerholt J, Bron C, Franssen J. Myofascial trigger points: an evidence-informed review. *J Man Manip Ther.* 2006;14:203–221.
46. Treaster D, Marras WS, Burr D, Sheedy JE, Hart D. Myofascial trigger point development from visual and postural stressors during computer work. *J Electromyogr Kinesiol.* 2006;16:115–124.
47. Kitahara T, Schnoz M, Läubli T, Wellig P, Krueger H. Motor-unit activity in the trapezius muscle during rest, while inputting data, and during fast finger tapping. *Eur J Appl Physiol.* 2000;83:181–189.
48. Forsman M, Birch L, Zhang O, Kadefors R. Motor unit recruitment in the trapezius muscle with special reference to coarse arm movements. *J Electromyogr Kinesiol.* 2001;11(3):207–216.
49. Zennaro D, Läubli T, Krebs D, Klipstein A, Krueger H. Continuous and sporadic motor unit activity in the trapezius muscle during prolonged computer work. *J Electromyogr Kinesiol.* 2003;13(2):113–124.
50. Andersen LL, Suetta C, Andersen JL, Kjær M, Sjøgaard G. Increased proportion of megafibers in chronically painful muscles. *Pain.* 2008;139:588–593.
51. Armstrong RB, Oglive RW, Schwane JA. Eccentric exercise-induced injury to rat skeletal muscle. *J Appl Physiol.* 1983;54:80–93.
52. Newham DJ, McPhail G, Mills KR, Edwards RHT. Ultrastructural changes after concentric and eccentric contractions of human muscle. *J Neurol Sci.* 1983;61:109–122.
53. Graven-Nielsen T, Arendt-Nielsen L. Human models and clinical manifestations of musculoskeletal pain and pain-motor interactions. In: Graven-Nielsen T, Arendt-Nielsen L, Mense S, eds. *Fundamentals of Musculoskeletal Pain.* Seattle, WA: IASP Press; 2008:155–187.
54. Ernberg M. Serotonergic receptor involvment in muscle pain and hyperalgesia. In: Graven-Nielsen T, Arendt-Nielsen L, Mense S, eds. *Fundamentals of Musculoskeletal Pain.* Seattle, WA: IASP Press; 2008:139–154.
55. Dannecker EA. Sex-related differences in delayed-onset muscle pain. In: Graven-Nielsen T, Arendt-Nielsen L, Mense S, eds. *Fundamentals of Musculoskeletal Pain.* Seattle, WA: IASP Press; 2008:249–261.
56. Fernandez-de-las-Peñas C, Fernández J, Miangolarra JC. Musculoskeletal disorders in mechanical neck pain: myofascial trigger points versus cervical joint dysfunctions. A clinical study. *J Musculoskelet Pain.* 2005b;13:27–35.
57. Fernandez-de-las-Peñas C, Alonso-Blanco C, Alguacil-Diego IM, Miangolarra-Page JC. Myofascial trigger points and postero-anterior joint hypomobility in the mid-cervical spine in subjects presenting with mechanical neck pain: a pilot study. *J Man Manip Ther.* 2006;14:88–94.
58. Molliver DC, Immke DC, Fierro L, Paré M, Rice FL, McCleskey EW. ASIC3, an acid-sensing ion channel, is expressed in metaboreceptive sensory neurons. *Mol Pain.* 2005;1:35.
59. Sluka K, Kalra A, Moore SA. Unilateral intramuscular injections of acidic saline produce a bilateral, long-lasting hyperalgesia. *Musc Nerve.* 2001; 24:37–46.
60. Skyba DA, King EW, Sluka KA. Effects of NMDA and non-NMDA ionotropic glutamate receptor antagonists on the development and maintenance of hyperalgesia induced by repeated intramuscular injection of acidic saline. *Pain.* 2002;98:69–78.
63. Law LAF, Sluka KA, McMullen, Lee J, Arendt-Nielsen L, Graven-Nielsen T. Acidic buffer induced muscle pain evokes referred pain and mechanical hyperalgesia in humans. *Pain.* 2008;140:254–264.

61. Sluka K. Stimulation of deep somatic tissue with capsaicin produces long-lasting mechanical allodynia and a heat hypoalgesia that depends on early activation of the cAMP pathway. *J Neurosci.* 2002;22:5687–5693.
62. Sluka KA, Price MP, Breese NM, Stucky CL, Wemmie JA, Welsh MJ. Chronic hyperalgesia induced by repeated acid injections in muscle is abolished by the loss of ASIC3, but not by ASIC1. *Pain.* 2003;106:229–239.
64. Gandhi R, Ryals JM, Wright DE. Neurotrophin-3 reverses chronic mechanical hyperalgesia induced by intramuscular acid injection. *J Neurosci.* 2004;24:9405–9413.
65. Fujii Y, Ozaki N, Taguchi T, Mizumura K, Furukawa K, Sugiura Y. TRP channels and ASICs mediate mechanical hyperalgesia in models of inflammatory muscle pain and delayed onset muscle soreness. *Pain.* 2008;140:292–304.
66. DeSantana JM, Sluka KA. Central mechanisms in the maintenance of chronic widespread noninflammatory muscle pain. *Curr Pain Headache Rep.* 2008;12(5):338–343.
67. Okamoto K, Imbe H, Morikawa Y, Itoh M, Sekimoto M, Nemoto K, Senba E. 5-HT2A receptor subtype in the peripheral branch of sensory fibers is involved in the potentiation of inflammatory pain in rats. *Pain.* 2002;99:133–143.
68. Sung D1, Dong X, Ernberg M, Kumar U, Cairns BE. Serotonin (5-HT) excites rat masticatory muscle afferent fibers through activation of peripheral 5-HT3 receptors. *Pain.* 2008;134(1–2):41–50.
69. Christidis N, Kopp S, Ernberg M. The effect on mechanical pain threshold over human muscles by oral administration of granisetron and diclofenac-sodium. *Pain.* 2005;113(3):265–270.
70. Bird GC, Han JS, Fu Y, Adwanikar H, Willis WD, Neugebauer V. Pain-related synaptic plasticity in spinal dorsal horn neurons: role of CGRP. *Mol Pain.* 2006;2:31.
71. Cairns BE, Gambarota G, Svensson P, Arendt-Nielsen L, Berde CB. Glutamate-induced sensitization of rat muscle fibers. *Neuroscience.* 2002;16:105–117.
72. Sun RQ, Tu YJ, Lawand NB, Yan JY, Lin Q, Willis WD. Calcitonin gene-related peptide receptor activation produces PKA and PKC-dependent mechanical hyperalgesia and central sensitization. *J Neurophysiol.* 2004;92:2859–2866.
73. Simons DG, Travell JG. *Myofascial Pain and Dysfunction: The Trigger Point Manual.* (The Lower Extremities) Vol. 2. Baltimore, MD: Williams & Wilkins; 1992.
74. Ge HY, Monterde S, Graven-Nielsen T, Arendt-Nielsen L. Latent myofascial trigger points are associated with an increased intramuscular electromyographic activity during synergistic muscle activation. *J Pain.* 2014;15(2):181–187.
75. Chaiamnuay P, Darmawan J, Muirden KD, Assawatanabodee P. Epidemiology of rheumatic disease in rural Thailand: a WHOILAR COPCORD study. Community Oriented Program for the Control of Rheumatic Disease. *J Rheumatology.* 1998;25:1382–1387.
76. Badley EM, Webster GK, Rasooly I. The impact of musculoskeletal disorders in the population: are they just aches and pains? Findings from the 1990 Ontario Health Survey. *J Rheumatol.* 1995;22:733–739.
77. Skootsky SA, Jaeger B, Oye RK. Prevalence of myofascial pain in general internal medicine practice. *West J Med.* 1989;151:157–160.
78. Fishbain DA, Goldberg M, Meagher BR, Steele R, Rosomoff H. Male and female chronic pain patients categorized by DS-III psychiatric diagnostic criteria. *Pain.* 1986;26:181–197.
79. Gerwin RD. A study of 96 subjects examined both for fibromyalgia and myofascial pain [abstract]. *J Musculoskel Pain.* 1995;3(suppl 1):121.
80. Bron C, Dommerholt J, Stegenga B, Wensing M, Oostendorp RA. High prevalence of shoulder girdle muscles with myofascial trigger points in patients with shoulder pain. *BMC Musculoskelet Disord.* 2011;12:139. doi 10.1186/1471-2474-12-139.
81. San H, Akarimak U, Uludag W. Active myofascial trigger points might be more frequent in patients with cervical radiculopathy. *Eur J Phys Rehabil Med.* 2012;48(2):237–244.
82. Rashiq S, Galer BS. Proximal myofascial dysfunction in complex regional pain syndrome: a retrospective prevalence study. *Clin J Pain.* 1999;15:151–153.
83. Ayres de Oliveira RA, Ciampi de Andrade D, Machado AGG, Teixeira MJ. Central poststroke pain: somatosensory abnormalities and the presence of associated myofascial pain syndrome. *BMC Neurol.* 2012;12:89. doi:10.1186/1471-2377-12-89.
84. Kaergaard A, Andersen JH. Musculoskeletal disorders of the neck and shoulders in female sewing machine operators: prevalence, incidence, and prognosis. *Occup Environ Med.* 2000;57:528–534.
85. Fernández-Lao C, Cantrarero-Villanueva I, Fernández-de-las-Peñas C, Del-Moral-Ávila R, Menjón-Beltrán S, Arroyo-Morales M. Development of active myofascial trigger points in neck and shoulder musculature is similar after lumpectomy or mastectomy for breast cancer. *J Bodyw Mov Ther.* 2012;1 6:183–190.
86. Torres Lacomba M, Mayoral del Moral O, Coperias Zazo JL, Gerwin RD, Goñí AZ. Incidence of myofascial pain syndrome in breast cancer surgery: a prospective study. *Clin J Pain.* 2010;26(4):320–325.
87. Reiestad F, Kulkarni J. Role of myofascial trigger points in post-amputation pain: causation and management. *Prosthet Ortho Int.* 2013;37(2):120–123.
88. Treaster DE, Burr D. Gender differences in prevalence of upper extremity musculoskeletal disorders. *Ergonomics.* 2004;15:495–526.
89. Rollman G, Lautenbacher S. Sex differences in musculoskeletal pain. *Clin J Pain.* 2001;17:20–24.
90. Bergenudd H, Lindgärde F, Nilsson B, Petersson CJ. Shoulder pain in middle age. A study of prevalence and relation to occupational work load and psychosocial factors. *Clin Orthop.* 1988;231:234–238.
91. Ge HY, Arendt-Nielsen L, Farini D, Madeleine P. Gender-specific differences in electromyographic changes and perceived pain induced by experimental muscle pain during sustained contractions of the upper trapezius muscle. *Muscle Nerve.* 2005;32:726–733.
92. Arendt-Nielsen L, Svensson P, Sessle BJ, Cairns BE, Wang K. Interactions between glutamate and capsaicin in inducing muscle pain and sensitization in humans. *Eur J Pain.* 2008;661–670.
93. Tang B, Ji Y, Traub RJ. Estrogen alters spinal NMDA receptor activity via a PKA signaling pathway in a visceral pain model in the rat. *Pain.* 2008;137:540–549.
94. Hucho TB, Dina OA, Kuhn J, Levine JD. Estrogen controls PKCepsilon-dependent mechanical hyperalgesia through direct action on nociceptive neurons. *Eur J Neurosci.* 2006;24:527–534.
95. Isselee H, De Laat A, De Mot B, Lysens R. Pressure-pain threshold variation in temporomandibular disorder myalgia over the course of the menstrual cycle. *J Orofac Pain.* 2002;16:105–117.
96. Dannecker EA, Knoll V, Robinson ME. Sex differences in muscle pain: self-care behaviors and effects on daily activities. *J Pain.* 2008;9:200–209.
97. Nijs J. Generalized joint hypermobility: an issue in fibromyalgia and chronic fatigue syndrome. *J Bodyw Mov Ther.* 2005;9(4):310–317.
98. Hong CZ, Torigoe Y. Electrophysiologic characteristics of localized twitch responses in responsive taut bands of rabbit skeletal muscle. *J Musculoskel Pain.* 1994;2:17–43.
99. Hong CZ, Yu J. Spontaneous electrical activity of rabbit trigger spot after transection of spinal cord and peripheral nerve. *J Musculoskel Pain.* 1998;6:45–58.
100. Gerwin RD, Duranleau D. Ultrasound identification of the myofascial trigger point. *Muscle Nerve.* 1997;20:767–768.
101. Sikdar S, Shah JP, Gilliams E, Gebreab T, Gerber LH. Assessment of myofascial trigger points (MTrPs): a new application of ultrasound imaging and vibration sonoelastography. Proceedings of the 30th Annual International IEEE EMBS Conference; Vancouver, British Columbia, Canada; 2008:5585–5588.
102. Ballyns JJ, Turo D, Otto P, Shah JP, Hammond J, Gebreab T, Gerwber LH, Sikdar S. Office-based elastographic technique for quantifying mechanical properties of skeletal muscle. *J Ultrasound Med.* 2012;31(8):1209–1219.

103. Shankar H, Reddy S. Two- and three-dimensional ultrasound imaging to facilitate detection and targeting of taut bands in myofascial pain syndrome. *Pain Med.* 2012;13(7):971–975.
104. Maher RM, Hayes DM, Shinohara M. Quantification of dry needling and posture effects on myofascial trigger points using ultrasound shear-wave elastography. *Arch Phys Med Rehab.* 2013; 94(11):2146–2150.
105. Debernard L, Robert L, Chadeux F, Bensamoun SR. Characterization of muscle architecture in children and adults using magnetic resonance elastography and ultrasound techniques. *J Biomech.* 2011;44(3):397–401.
106. Chen Q, Bensamoun S, Basford J, Thompson JM, An K-N. Identification and quantification of myofascial taut bands with magnetic resonance elastography. *Arch Phys Med Rehabil.* 2007;88:1658–1661.
107. Chen Q, Basford J, An K-N. Ability of magnetic resonance elastography to assess taut bands. *Clin Biomech.* 2008;23(5):623–629.
108. Lucas KR, Polus BI, Rich PS. Latent myofascial trigger points: their effect on muscle activation and movement efficiency. *J Bodywork Mov Ther.* 2004;8:160–166.
109. Lucas KR, Rich PA, Polus BI. Do latent trigger points affect muscle activation patterns? [abstract]. *J Musculoskel Pain.* 2007;15(suppl 13):30.
110. Madeleine P, Leclerc F, Arendt-Nielsen L, Ravier P, Farina D. Experimental muscle pain changes the spatial distribution of upper trapezius muscle activity during sustained contraction.Clin Neurophysiol. 2006;117:2436–445.
111. Farina D, Leclerc F, Arendt-Nielsen L, Buttelli O, Madeleine P. The change in spatial distribution of upper trapezius muscle activity is correlated to contraction duration. *J Electromyogr Kinesiol.* 2008;18:16–25.
112. Mense S, Hoheisel U. Mechanisms of central nervous hyperexcitability due to activation of muscle nociceptors. In: Graven-Nielsen T, Arendt-Nielsen L, Mense S, eds. *Fundamentals ofMusculoskeletal Pain.* Seattle, WA: IASP Press; 2008: 61–73.
113. Mense S. Nociception from skeletal muscle in relation to clinical muscle pain. *Pain.* 1993;54(3):241–289.
114. Graven-Nielsen T, Mense S. The peripheral apparatus of muscle pain: evidence from animal and human studies. *Clin J Pain.* 2001;17:2–10.
115. Hoheisel U, Reinohl J, Unger T, Mense S. Acidic pH and capsaicin activate mechanosensitive group IV muscle receptors in the rat. *Pain.* 2004;110:149–157.
116. Lambertz D, Hoheisel U, Mense S. Influence of a chronic myositis on rat spinal field potentials evoked by TTX-resistant unmyelinated skin and muscle afferents. *Eur J Pain.* 2008;12:686–695.
117. Taguchi T, Hoheisel U, Mense S. Dorsal horn neurons having input from low back structures in rats. *Pain.* 2008;138:119–129.
118. Li LT, Ge HY, Yue SW, Arendt-Nielsen L. Nociceptive and non-nociceptive hypersensitivity at latent myofascial trigger points. *Clin J Pain.* 2009;25:132–137.
119. Hong CZ, Simons DG. Pathophysiologic and electrophysiologic mechanisms of myofascial trigger points. *Arch Phys Med Rehabil.* 1998;79:863–872.
120. Xu YM, Ge HY, Arendt-Nielsen L. Sustained nociceptive mechanical stimulation of latent myofascial trigger point induces central sensitization in healthy subjects. *J Pain.* 2010;11(2):1348–1355.
121. Gerwin RD, Shannon S, Hong CZ, Hubbard, Gevirtz R. Interrater reliability in myofascial trigger point examination. *Pain.* 1997;69:65–73.
122. Sciotti VM, Mittak VL, DiCarco L, et al. Clinical precision of myofascial trigger point location in the trapezius muscle. *Pain.* 2001;93:259–266.
123. Bron C, Franssen J, Wensing M, Oostgendorp RA-B. Interrater reliability of palpation of myofascial trigger points in three shoulder muscles. *J Man Manip Ther.* 2007;15:203–215.
124. Cummings TM, White AR. Needling therapies in the management of myofascial trigger point pain: a systematic review. *Arch Phys Med Rehabil.* 2001;82:986–992.
125. Iwama H, Ohmori S, Kaneko T, Watanabe K. Water-diluted local anesthetic for trigger-point injection in chronic myofascial pain syndrome: evaluation of types of local anesthetic and concentrations in water. *Reg Anesth Pain Med.* 2001;26:333–336.
126. Kietrys DM, Palombaro KM, Azzaretto E, Hubler R, Sschaller B, Schussel JM, Tucker M. Effectiveness of dry needling for upper quadrant myofascial pain: a systematic review and meta-analysis. *J Orthop Sports Phys Ther.* 2013;43(9):620–634.
127. Raygani SM, Bayat M, Bahrami MH, Raeissadat SA, Kargozar E. Comparison of dry needling and physiotherapy in treatment of myofascial pain syndrome [published online ahead of print December 19 2013]. Clin Rheumatol. 2013;33(6):859–864.
128. Fernandez-de-las-Peñas C, Palonecque del Cerro L, Fernandez Carnero J. Manual treatment of post-whiplash injury. *J Bodywork Movement Ther.* 2005c;9:109–119.
129. Rickard LD. The effectiveness of non-invasive treatments for active myofascial trigger point pain: a systematic review of the literature. *Int J Osteopath Med.* 2006; 9:120–136.
130. Fryer G, Hodgson L. The effect of manual pressure release on myofascial trigger points in the upper trapezius muscle. *J Bodyw Mov Ther.* 2005;9:248–255.
131. Moraska AF, Hickner RC, Kohrt WM, Brewer A. Changes in blood flow and cellular metabolism at a myofascial trigger point with trigger point release (ischemic compression): a proof-of-principle pilot study. *Arch Phys MNed Rehabili.* 2013;94(1):196–200.
132. Manca A, Limonta E, Pilurzi G, De Natale ER, Mercante B, Deriu F. Ultrasound and laser as stand-alone therapies for myofascial trigger points: a randomized, double-blind, placebo [published online ahead of print January 2 2014]. *Physiother Res Int.* 2014. doi: 10 1022/pri 1580.
133. Furlan AD, Brosseau L, Imamura M, Irvin E. Massage for low-back pain: a systematic review with the framework of the Cochrane Collaboration Back Review Group. *Spine.* 2002;27:1896–1910.
134. Gam AN, Warming S, Larsen LH, et al. Treatment of myofascial trigger-points with ultrasound combined with massage and exercise—a randomized controlled trial. *Pain.* 1998;77:73–79.
135. Srbely JZ, Dickey JP. Randomized controlled study of the antinociceptive effect of ultrasound on trigger point sensitivity: novel applications in myofascial therapy. *Clin Rehabil.* 2007;21:411–417.
136. Srbely JZ, Dickey JP, Lowerison M, Edwards AM, Nolet PS, Wong LL. Stimulation of myofascial trigger points with ultrasound induces segmental antinociceptive effects: a randomized controlled study. *Pain.* 2008;139:260–266.
137. Ilbuldu E, Cakmak A, Disci R, Aydin R. Comparison of laser, dry needling and placebo laser treatments in myofascial pain syndrome. *Photomed Laser Surg.* 2004;22:306–311.
138. Gur A, Sarac AJ, Cevik R, Altindag O, Sarac S. Efficacy of 904 nm gallium arsenide low level laser therapy in the management of chronic myofascial pain in the neck: a double-blind and randomized-controlled trial. *Lasers Surg Med.* 2004;35:229–235.
139. Dundar U, Evcik D, Samli F, Pusak H, Kavuncu V. The effect of gallium arsenide aluminum laser therapy in the management of cervical myofascial pain syndrome: a double blind, placebo-controlled study. *Clin Rheumatol.* 2007;26:930–934.
140. Lin YC, Kuan TS, Hsieh PC, Yen WU, Chang WC, Chen SM. Therapeutic effects of lidocaine patch on myofascial pain syndrome of the upper trapezius: a randomized, double-blind, placebo-controlled study. *Am J Phys Med Rehabil.* 2012;91:871–882.
141. Ketenci A, Basat H, Esmailzadeh S. The efficacy of topical thiocolchicoside (Muscoril®) in the treatment of acute cervical myofascial pain syndrome: a single-blind, randomize, prospective, phase IV clinical study. *AĞRI.* 2009;21:95–103.
142. Domingo A, Mayoral O, Monterde S, Santafé MM. Neuromuscular damage and repair after dry needling in mice. *Evid Based*

Complement Alternat Med. 2013; Article ID 260806. http://dx.Doi/org/10.1155/2013/260806.

143. Hsieh YL, Chou LW, Joe YS, Hong CZ. Spinal cord mechanism involving the remote effects of dry needling on the irritability of myofascial trigger spots in rabbit skeletal muscle. *Arch Phys Med Rehab.* 2011;92(7):1098–1105.
144. Hsieh YL, Yang SA, Yang CC, Chou LW. Dry needling at myofascial trigger points of rabbit skeletal muscles modulates the biochemical associated with pain, inflammation, and hypoxia. *Evid Based Complement Alternat Med.* 2012: article ID 432165. doi: 10.1155/2012/342165.
145. Dommerholt J, Mayoral del Moral O, Gröbli C. Trigger point dry needling. *J Man Manip Ther.* 2006b;14:E70–E87.
146. Hsieh YL, Kao MJ, Kuan TS, Chen SM, Shen JT, Hong CZ. Dry needling to a key myofascial trigger point may reduce the irritability of satellite MTrPs. *Am J Phys Med Rehabil.* 2007;86:397–403.
147. Scott NA, Guo B, Barton PM, Gerwin RD. Trigger point injections for chronic non-malignant musculoskeletal pain: a systematic review. *Pain Med.* 2009;10:54–69.
148. Huguenin L, Brukner PD, McCrory P, Smith P, Wajsweiner H, Bennell K. Effect of dry needling of gluteal muscles on straight leg raise: a randomized, placebo controlled, double blind trial. *Br U Sports Med.* 2005;39(2):84–90.
149. Srbelly JZ, Dickey JP, Lee D, Lowerison M. Dry needle stimulation of myofascial trigger points evokes segmental anti-nociceptive effects. *J Rehabil Med.* 2010;42(5):483–488.
150. Ga H, Ko HJ, Choi JH, Kim CH. Intramuscular and nerve root stimulation vs lidocaine injection of trigger points in myofascial pain syndrome. *J Rehabil Med.* 2007a;39:374–378.
151. Ga H, Choi JH, Yoon HY. Dry needling of trigger points with and without paraspinal needling in myofascial pain syndromes in elderly patients. *J Altern Compl Med.* 2007b;13:617–623.
152. Ay S, Evcik D, Tur BS. Comparison of injection methods in myofascial pain syndrome: a randomized controlled trial. *Clin Rheumatol.* 2010;29(1):19–23.
153. Couto C, de Souza IC, Torres IL, Fregni F, Caumo W. Paraspinal stimulation combined with trigger point needling and needle rotation for the treatment of myofascial pain: a randomized sham-controlled clinical trial. *Clin J Pain.* 2014;30(3):214–223.
154. Lee SH, Chen CC, Lee CS, Lin TC, Chan RC. Effects of needle electrical intramuscular stimulation on shoulder and cervical myofascial pain syndrome and microcirculation. *J Chin Med Assoc.* 2008;71:200–206.
155 Itoh K, Katsumi Y, Hirota S, Kitakoji H. Randomized trial of trigger point acupuncture compared with other acupuncture for treatment of chronic neck pain. *Compl Ther Med.* 2007;15:172–179.
156. Itoh K, Katsumi Y, Kitakoji H. Trigger point acupuncture treatment of chronic low back pain in elderly patients—a blinded RCT. *Acupunct Med.* 2004;22:170–177.
157. Itoh K, Katsumi Y, Hirota S, Kitakoji H. Effects of trigger point acupuncture on chronic low back pain in elderly patients—a sham-controlled randomized trial. *Acupunct Med.* 2006;24:5–12.
158. Irnich D, Behrens N, Gleditsch JM, Stör W, Schreiber MA, Schöps P, Vickers AJ, Beyer A. Immediate effects of dry needling and acupuncture at distant points in chronic neck pain: results of a randomized, double-blind, sham-controlled crossover trial. *Pain.* 2002;99:83–89.
159. Tough EA, White AR, Cummings TM, Richards SH, Campbell JL. Acupuncture and dry needling in the management of myofascial trigger point pain: a systematic review and meta-analysis of randomized controlled trials [published online ahead of print]. *Eur J Pain.* 2008.
160. Fine PG, Milano R, Hare BD. The effects of myofascial trigger point injections are naloxone reversible. *Pain.* 1988;32:15–20.
161. Ho KY, Tan KH.Botulinum toxin A for myofascial trigger point injection: a qualitative systematic review. Eur J Pain. 2007 Jul;11(5):519–527.
162. Ferrante FM, Bearn L, Rothrock R, King L. Evidence against trigger point injection technique for the treatment of cervicothoracic myofascial pain with botulinum toxin type A *Anesthesiology.* 2005;103:377–383.
163. Sidebottom AJ, Patel AA, Amin J. Botulinum injection for the management of myofascial pain in the masticatory muscles. A prospective outcome study. *Brit J Oral Maxillofac Surg.* 2013;51(3):199–205.
164. Statz T, Müller W. Treatment of chronic low back pain with tropisetron. *Scand J Rheumatol.* (suppl). 2004;(119):76–78.
165. Müller W, Fiebich BL, Stratz T. New treatment options using 5-HT3 receptor antagonists in rheumatic diseases. *Curr Top Med Chem.* 2006;6:2035–2042.
166. Baldry P. Management of myofascial trigger point pain. *Acupunct Med.* 2002;20:2–10.
167. Schabrun SM, Cannan A, Mullens R, et al. The effect of interactive neurostimulation on myofascial trigger points associated with mechanical neck pain: a preliminary randomized, sham-controlled trial. *J Altern Complement Med.* 2012; 18:946–952.
168. Castori M, Morlino S, Celletti C, et al. Management of pain and fatigue in the joint hypermobility syndrome (a.d.a. Ehlers-Danlos syndrome, hypermobility type): principles and proposal for a multidisciplinary approach [published online ahead of print July 11 2012]. *Am J Med Genet A.* 2012; doi: 10.10.1002/ajmg.a.335483.

6.

PAIN OF RHEUMATOLOGICAL DISEASE

David G. Borenstein, Philip R. Appel, and Joseph Signorino

CASE PRESENTATION

A 29-year-old corporate lawyer complains of worsening low back pain (LBP) of 6 months' duration. He reports prior episodes of LBP managed ineffectively with over- the-counter ibuprofen. The most recent episode has been protracted, with persistent morning stiffness and with modest response to persistent nonsteroidal therapy. The pain is a constant aching with referred pain to the buttocks. He denies weakness, falling, or bowel/bladder/sexual dysfunction. Activity improves pain, whereas immobility exacerbates stiffness and pain. He reports significant workplace stress with 80+-hour work weeks. Furthermore, he is in the midst of a contentious divorce. He is referred to the Interdisciplinary Pain Medicine clinic for further evaluation and management.

Past medical history is positive for an episode of uveitis.

Social history is as above.

Review of systems is significant for morning stiffness.

Physical examination demonstrates an anxious male who weighs 90 kg and is 190 cm tall. His vital signs are normal. Skin examination is normal. Neurological examination is unremarkable. Reflexes are 2+ and symmetrical. Special tests for nerve root tension signs are negative. Musculoskeletal examination demonstrates 5/5 strength in all myotomes tested. His peripheral skeleton has no sign of inflamed joints. The range of motion of the axial is limited in all directions including the lumbar, thoracic, and cervical spine.

Radiographic examination demonstrates bilateral sacroiliitis, squaring of vertebral bodies, with early syndesmophyte formation.

Laboratory examination demonstrates elevated erythrocyte sedimentation rate, positive HLA-B27, and negative rheumatoid factor.

QUESTIONS

1. What are the clinical manifestations of ankylosing spondylitis (AS)?
2. How is AS diagnosed?
3. Are there any specific diagnostic modalities that may be helpful?
4. What is the differential diagnosis for this patient?
5. What are the characteristics of pain in acute and chronic rheumatologic disease?
6. How is this clinical situation managed?
   a. Pharmacological choices
   b. Physical therapy examination and management
   c. Psychiatric interventions
   d. Investigational biologic therapies

WHAT ARE THE CLINICAL MANIFESTATIONS OF AS?

AS is a chronic inflammatory disease characterized by a variable course that may affect any portion of the axial skeleton from the sacroiliac (SI) joints to the cervical spine. This disease is characterized by axial skeletal arthritis, the presence of a tissue factor on host cells (human leukocyte antigen [HLA]-B27), and the absence of rheumatoid factor in serum (seronegative); it is the classic form of the spondyloarthritides.

AS is a disease of the synovial and cartilaginous joints of the axial skeleton, including SI joints, spinal apophyseal joints, costovertebral joints, the atlantoaxial joint, and the symphysis pubis. The large peripheral joints (hips, shoulders, knees, elbows, and ankles) are also affected in about a third of patients. The inflammatory process is characterized by chondritis (inflammation of cartilage) or osteitis (inflammation of bone) at the junction of the cartilage and bone in the spine. As opposed to rheumatoid arthritis, which is associated with bone lysis, the inflammation of AS is characterized by ankylosis of joints and ossification of ligaments surrounding the vertebrae (syndesmophytes) and other musculotendinous structures, such as the pelvis and heels.

Enthesitis is another form of musculoskeletal inflammation characteristic of the spondyloarthridites.[1] An *enthesis* is a dynamic structure undergoing constant modification in response to applied stress. This area is a target for inflammation. Although entheses are primarily affected in the spondyloarthritides, inflammation of these structures is insufficient to explain all the alterations that occur in joints (SI). Synovitis plays an important role as well. However, synovitis may be a secondary event after initiation with an enthesitis.[2]

CLINICAL CHARACTERISTICS

The usual presentation of a patient with AS is a man whose age may range from teen years to about 40 who develops intermittent dull LBP. The onset of morning stiffness is slowly progressive measured in months to years. Back pain, which occurs throughout the disease in 90–95% of patients, is greatest in the morning and reappears with periods of inactivity during the day. Patients will describe increasing difficulty arising from chairs after being seated for varying lengths of time. Pain and lumbar stiffness may make sleeping through the night difficult. Individuals will awaken at night and find it necessary to leave bed and move about for a few minutes before returning to sleep. Fatigue can be a major symptom.3,4

Back pain associated with AS improves with exercise. The first location of disease involvement is variable, but most have pain in the lumbosacral region. In a small number, peripheral joints (hips, knees, and shoulders) are initially involved. Less common is an initial presentation of acute iritis (eye inflammation), heel pain, or Achilles tendonitis. On occasion, back pain may be severe in association with radiation into the lower extremities, mimicking acute lumbar disc herniation. These patients have symptoms related to contraction of the piriformis muscle deep in the buttock. This symptom complex of radicular pain is referred to as *pseudo-sciatica*. The neurological examination is helpful in differentiating pseudo-sciatica related to sciatic nerve compression from single nerve root compression. Nerve root compression results in sensory, motor, and reflex changes related to a single nerve root (L5 distribution) for example. Pseudo-sciatica causes vague symptoms in a wider distribution related to more than one nerve root level.

The usual AS patient has a moderate degree of intermittent aching pain localized to the lumbosacral area. Paraspinal musculoskeletal spasm may also contribute to the discomfort. With progression of the disease, pain develops in the thoracic and cervical spine and costovertebral joints.

Flattening of the lumbar spine and loss of normal lordosis are consistent with spinal involvement. Thoracic spine disease causes decreased motion at the costovertebral joints, reduced chest expansion, and impaired pulmonary function. In a vast majority of patients, the initial symptoms are back pain; back stiffness; thigh, hip, or groin pain; and sciatica. Pain in peripheral joints is the initial complaint in a small minority of patients, with a smaller number presenting with chest pain or generalized aches.

Cervical spine disease occurs less frequently than lumbosacral involvement in AS and at a later time in the course of the illness. Cervical spine involvement may be more common as an initial area of disease in women. Studies of large groups of AS patients report cervical spine involvement to range from none to about half. The primary symptom of cervical spine disease is neck stiffness and pain. Patients may develop intermittent episodes of torticollis. Involvement of the cervical spine causes flexion of the neck, making it difficult to look straight ahead.

Peripheral joint arthritis (hips, knees, ankles, shoulders, and elbows) occurs in 30% of patients within the first 10 years of disease. In regard to dysfunction, hip disease is the most frequent limiting factor rather than spinal stiffness.

Ankylosis may also occur in cartilaginous joints, such as the symphysis pubis, sternomanubrial, and costosternal joints. Erosions of the plantar surface of the calcaneus at the attachment of the plantar fascia result in an enthesitis. This inflammation causes a fasciitis and periosteal reaction, which causes heel pain and the formation of heel spurs. Achilles tendinitis is another enthesitis associated with heel pain and AS.

AS is more than a skeletal disease. It is a systemic, inflammatory illness associated with a variety of nonarticular abnormalities. In particular, those with peripheral joint manifestations are at risk of constitutional manifestations including fever, fatigue, and weight loss. Iritis or uveitis may be the presenting complaint of 25% of the patients with spondylitis and is present in up to 40% of patients over the course of the disease. Patients with disease durations of 30 years or longer may develop heart involvement. Aorta and aortic valve disease may be more common in AS patients with peripheral arthritis. Other cardiac features include pericarditis, tachycardia, and other conduction defects. Cardiac conduction disturbances include bradyarrhythmias most commonly. The aorta is modified by a fibrosing process that results in widening and thickening of the aorta. The associated most serious cardiac abnormality is proximal aortitis, which results in aortic valve insufficiency, heart failure, and death. Prosthetic valve replacement may forestall cardiac deterioration. Involvement of the thoracic spine results in diminished chest expansion. Severely kyphotic individuals have pulmonary involvement manifested by decreased chest expansion, limited lung capacity, and apical fibrosis.

PHYSICAL EXAMINATION

A careful musculoskeletal examination is helpful in identifying the early findings of limitation of motion of the axial skeleton, which is especially noticeable with lateral bending and hyperextension. Percussion over the SI joints elicits pain in most circumstances. Distraction of the pelvic wings anteriorly and posteriorly places stress on the SI joints and is associated with LBP.

Measurements of spinal motion, including Schober's test (lumbar spine motion), lateral bending of the lumbosacral spine, occiput to wall (cervical spine motion), and chest expansion (costovertebral joint motion) are important in ascertaining limitations of motion and following the progression of the disease. Finger-to-floor measurements are more closely associated with hip motion than with back mobility. Rotation of the thoracic spine should be checked with the patient seated because this position fixes the pelvis, thus limiting pelvic rotation. Chest expansion is measured at the fourth intercostal space in men and below the breasts in women. Patients raise their hands over their head and are asked to take a deep inspiration. Normal expansion is at least 2.5 cm. Cervical spine evaluation includes measurement of all planes of motion. An important component of the evaluation is palpation of the paraspinous muscles. These muscles are frequently contracted in response to the inflammatory disease in the associated apophyseal joints. These muscles are tense and tender on palpation. Tight muscles result in limitation of spinal motion.

Evaluation of peripheral joints is appropriate. Careful hip examination is necessary to determine the potential loss of function involved with simultaneous arthritis of the back and hip. The movement of the shoulders should be completed to document loss of ranges of motion (ROM). Examination of the eyes, heart, lungs, and nervous system may uncover unsuspected extra-articular disease, such as uveitis, arrhythmias, bradycardia, aortic valve murmurs, or apical fibrotic rales.

EPIDEMIOLOGY

AS affects 1–2% of the white population, a number equal to the prevalence for rheumatoid arthritis. A strikingly high association between HLA-B27 and AS has been demonstrated. HLA-B27 is present in more than 90% of white patients with AS compared with a frequency of 7–8% in a normal white population. In North American whites, with a prevalence of HLA-B27 of 7%, the frequency of AS is 0.2%.5 A positive family history of AS or related spondyloarthropathy increases the risk to as high as 30% among the HLA-B27–positive first-degree relatives, as compared with HLA-B27–positive control subjects (1–4%).6

The male-to-female ratio is reported in the range of 3:1. However, women tend to be less symptomatic and develop less severe disease.[7] Women may also present more often with cervical spine disease with minimal lumbar spine symptoms. Therefore, the overall pattern of illness may be similar in men and women.[8]

The patient has classic symptoms and signs compatible with a diagnosis of ankylosing spondylitis (AS). He has prolonged morning stiffness and pain over the sacroiliac and lumbar spine region. He also has a history of uveitis. His physical examination reveals limitation of motion in the lumbar, thoracic, and cervical spine.

HOW IS AS DIAGNOSED?

DIAGNOSIS

Two sets of diagnostic criteria exist for AS. The *Rome clinical criteria*, used in research studies of AS, include bilateral sacroiliitis on radiologic examination and LBP for more than 3 months that is not relieved by rest, pain in the thoracic spine, limited motion in the lumbar spine, and limited chest expansion or iritis. When these criteria proved to lack sensitivity in identifying patients with spondylitis, the Rome criteria were modified at a New York symposium in 1966 (Box 6.1). These criteria included a grading system for radiographs of the SI joints in addition to limited spine motion, chest expansion, and back pain.9 A diagnosis of AS is confirmed with the presence of one clinical and one radiographic parameter. Although these criteria are used mostly for studies of patient populations, they are helpful in the clinical setting because they list disease characteristics useful in differentiating inflammatory spine disease from mechanical back disorders (Figure 6.1).

Box 6.1 DIAGNOSTIC CRITERIA FOR ANKYLOSING SPONDYLITIS

Rome Criteria

A. Clinical criteria:
   1. Low back pain and stiffness for more than 3 months not relieved by rest
   2. Pain and stiffness in the thoracic region
   3. Limited motion in the lumbar spine
   4. Limited chest expansion
   5. History of evidence of iritis or its sequelae

B. Radiologic criterion:
   1. Radiograph showing bilateral sacroiliac changes characteristic of ankylosing spondylitis

Diagnosis: Criterion B + 1 clinical criterion *or* four clinical criteria in absence of radiologic sacroiliitis

New York Criteria

A. Clinical criteria:
   1. Limitation of motion of the lumbar spine in anterior flexion, lateral flexion, and extension
   2. History of or presence of pain at the dorsolumbar junction or in the lumbar spine
   3. Limitation of chest expansion to 1 inch or less

B. Radiologic criteria (sacroiliitis)

Grade 3: unequivocal abnormality, moderate or advanced sacroiliitis with one or more erosions, sclerosis, widening, narrowing, or partial ankylosis

Grade 4: severe abnormality, total ankylosis

Diagnosis:

Definite grade 3–4 bilateral sacroiliitis + 1 clinical criterion

Grade 3–4 unilateral or grade 2 bilateral sacroiliitis with clinical criterion 1 or 2 and 3

Probable grade 3–4 bilateral sacroiliitis alone

Although spondyloarthritis is a common inflammatory musculoskeletal disorder, this group of illnesses is frequently overlooked by nonrheumatologists.[10] A delay in diagnosis from the onset of symptoms and referral to a rheumatologist ranges from 6 months to 20 years. Individuals who are misdiagnosed by primary care physicians have mild to moderate disease, with atypical presentations, and are women.[11]

One of the problems resulting in a delay in diagnosis was the requirement for radiographic sacroiliitis that necessitated

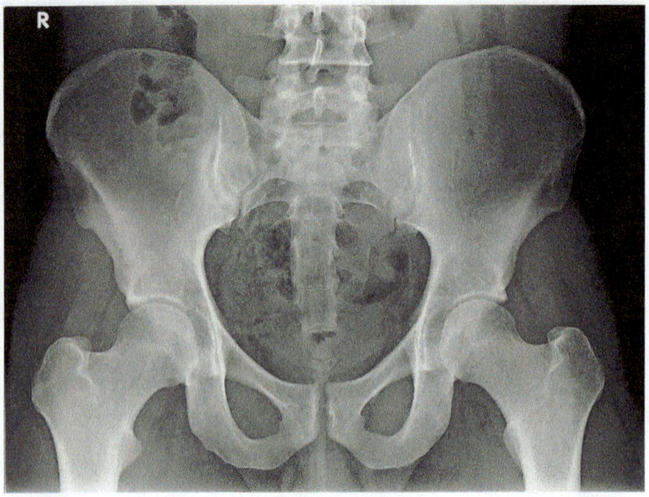

Figure 6.1 A 24-year-old man with low back pain and stiffness. Anteroposterior view of the pelvis reveals bilateral "pseudo-widening" of the sacroiliac joints with reactive iliac wing sclerosis. Symphysis pubis has erosions with reactive sclerosis. His hip joints are normal.

the presence of structural damage that occurred as a consequence of prolonged inflammation. In an attempt to diagnose the illness at an earlier stage before structural damage, the Assessment of Spondyloarthritis International Society (ASAS) published classification criteria for axial spondyloarthritis.[12] A diagnosis of spondyloarthritis requires the presence of inflammatory back pain (IBP). IBP is defined as the presence of four of the following five characteristics (back pain for longer than 3 months in duration in association with age of onset of less than 40 years, no improvement with rest, improvement with exercise, insidious onset, and nocturnal pain). In addition to IBP, one additional feature plus sacroiliitis on magnetic resonance imaging (MRI) or two additional features and sacroiliitis on radiographs need to be present. Spondyloarthritis features include axial and/or peripheral arthritis, heel enthesitis, iritis, dactylitis, psoriasis, inflammatory bowel disease, good response to nonsteroidal anti-inflammatory drugs, positive family history for spondyloarthritis, HLA-B27, or elevated C-reactive protein (CRP).

Another diagnostic classification system was proposed by the European Spondyloarthritides Study Group (ESSG) for the identification of the different forms of spondyloarthritis.[13] The criteria were based on a study of 140 spondyloarthritis patients and 1,829 controls from seven different European countries. The ESSG criteria have specificity of 87% and sensitivity of 86% for the diagnosis of spondyloarthritis. A patient is classified as having spondyloarthritis if they have one of two entry criteria plus one additional parameter. ESSG entry criteria include inflammatory back pain (four of five criteria: onset of back pain before age 45 years, persistence for a minimum of 3 months, improvement with exercise, presence of morning stiffness, and insidious onset) or asymmetrical synovitis. Asymmetrical synovitis is found predominantly in the lower extremities manifested by joint effusions, soft tissue swelling, warmth over a joint, reduction in both passive and active movement, and worsening with inactivity. Additional ESSG parameters include the presence of psoriasis, inflammatory bowel disease, urethritis, cervicitis, or acute diarrhea within 1 month before the onset of arthritis; alternating buttock pain; enthesopathy; and positive family history for spondylarthritis.

ARE THERE ANY SPECIFIC DIAGNOSTIC MODALITIES THAT MAY BE HELPFUL?

LABORATORY DATA

Laboratory results are nonspecific and add little to the diagnosis of AS. Only 15% of patients have mild anemia. The erythrocyte sedimentation rate (ESR) is increased in 80% of patients with active disease. Patients with normal sedimentation rates with active arthritis may have elevated levels of CRP.14 Rheumatoid factor and antinuclear antibody are characteristically absent. Histocompatibility testing (for HLA) is positive in 90% of AS patients but is also present in an increased percentage of patients with other spondyloarthritis (reactive arthritis, psoriatic spondylitis, and spondylitis with inflammatory bowel disease). It is not a diagnostic test for AS. HLA testing may be most useful in the young patient with early disease for whom the differential diagnosis may be narrowed by the presence of HLA-B27.

RADIOGRAPHIC EVALUATION

A number of imaging techniques are potentially useful in identifying structural alterations of the musculoskeletal system at different stages of spondyloarthritis. Knowing the capabilities of each technique can help the clinician choose the most appropriate imaging technique for the individual with IBP. Characteristic changes of AS in the SI joints and lumbosacral spine are helpful in making a diagnosis but may be difficult to determine in the early stages of the disease. The areas of the skeleton most frequently affected include the SI, apophyseal, discovertebral, and costovertebral joints.

The disease affects the SI joints initially and then appears in the upper lumbar and thoracolumbar areas. Subsequently, in ascending order, the lower lumbar, thoracic, and cervical spine are involved. The radiographic progression of disease may be halted at any stage, although sacroiliitis alone is a rare finding except in some women with spondylitis or in men in the early stage of disease.

Plain Radiographs

Evaluation of the SI joints is difficult on conventional anteroposterior supine view of the pelvis because of bony overlap and the oblique orientation of the joint. Ferguson's view of the pelvis (X-ray tube tilted 15–30 degrees in a cephalad direction) provides a useful view of the anterior portion of the joint, the initial area of inflammation in sacroiliitis. Radiographic evaluation of the SI joints is based on five observations: (1) distribution, (2) subchondral mineralization, (3) cystic or erosive bony change, (4) joint width, and (5) osteophyte formation. The symmetry of involvement must be compared with the same areas of the joint (superior-fibrous, inferior-synovial) and to the iliac (thinner cartilage) and sacral (thicker cartilage) sides of the joint.

Sacroiliitis is a bilateral, symmetrical process in AS. During the next stage, the articular space becomes "pseudo-widened" secondary to joint surface erosions. With continued inflammation, the area of sclerosis widens and is joined by proliferative bony changes that cross the joint space. In the final stages of sacroiliitis, complete ankylosis with total obliteration of the joint space occurs (Figure 6.2). Ligamentous structures surrounding the SI joint may also calcify. The radiographic changes associated with sacroiliitis may be graded from 0 (normal) to 5 (complete ankylosis) (see Table 6.1).

In the lumbar spine, osteitis affecting the anterior corners of vertebral bodies is an early finding. The inflammation associated with osteitis results in loss of the normal concavity of the anterior vertebral surface resulting in a "squared" body.

While osteopenia of the bony structures appears, calcification of outer portions of the intervertebral disc and ligamentous structures emerges. Thin, vertically oriented calcifications of the annulus fibrosus and anterior and posterior longitudinal ligaments are termed *syndesmophytes. Bamboo spine* is the term used to describe the spine of a patient with AS with extensive syndesmophytes encasing the axial skeleton.

The apophyseal joints are also affected in the illness. As the disease progresses, fusion of the apophyseal joints occurs. Radiographs of the spine may demonstrate the loss of joint space and complete fusion of the joints. Cervical spine ankylosis may be particularly severe. Complete obliteration of articular spaces between the posterior elements of C2 through C7 results in a column of solid bone. Patients with complete ankylosis of the apophyseal joints and syndesmophytes may develop extensive bony resorption of the anterior surface of the lower cervical vertebrae late in the course of the illness. Bone under the ligaments connecting the spinous processes may also be eroded in the setting of apophyseal joint ankylosis (Figure 6.3).

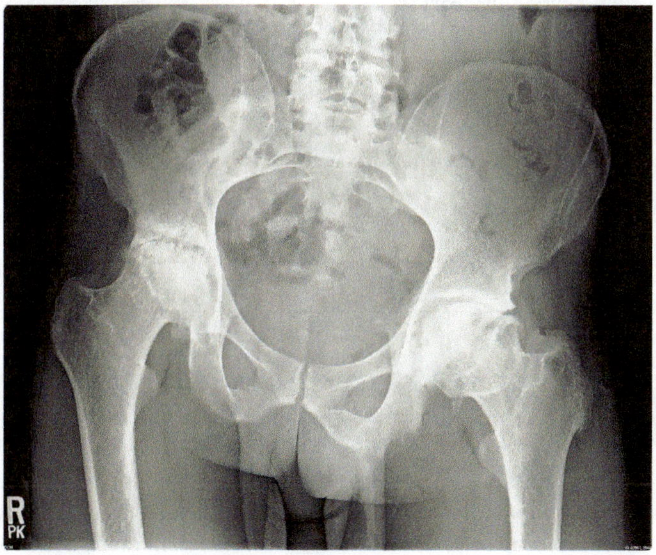

Figure 6.2 A 28-year-old man with 10 years of ankylosing spondylitis. Anteroposterior view of the pelvis demonstrates bilateral fusion of the sacroiliac joints with severe narrowing of the right hip and subchondral cysts.

Table 6.1 SACROILIITIS PLAIN RADIOGRAPHIC GRADES

GRADE	CRITERIA
0	Normal: sharp joint margins, normal joint width
1	Suspicious changes: radiologist is uncertain whether grade 2 changes are present
2	Definite early changes: pseudo-widening with erosion or sclerosis on both sides of the joint
3	Unequivocal abnormality: erosions, sclerosis, widening, narrowing, or partial ankylosis
4	Severe abnormalities: narrowed joint space, ankylosis
5	Ankylosis of joints with regression of surrounding sclerosis

The C1–C2 joints may become eroded and subluxed. Synovial tissue around the dens may cause erosion of the odontoid process. Further damage of the surrounding ligaments results in instability that is measured by the movement of the odontoid process from the posterior aspect of the atlas with flexion and extension views of the cervical spine. Widening of the space is indicative of a dynamic subluxation. No movement of the distance between the atlas and axis suggests a fixed subluxation. In addition to atlantoaxial subluxation, migration of the odontoid into the foramen magnum and rotary subluxation may occur. Subaxial subluxation is more characteristic of rheumatoid arthritis than AS.

Bone Scintigraphy (Bone Scan)

Bone scintigraphy has the capability of identifying tissues that are inflamed prior to the development of structural changes. The limiting factor is that scintigraphy is not differentiating among the various causes of inflammatory disorders of the spine,[15] therefore it has marginal additional benefit. Bone scan has been used primarily for evaluation of sacroiliitis. Scintigraphic testing can demonstrate increased activity over the SI joints in early disease before radiographic changes appear in other spinal joints.[16]

Computed Tomography (CT)

CT scan detects erosions on both sides of the joint that are frequently missed by plain radiographs.[17] CT scan is reserved for patients with grade 0 or 1 plain radiographic changes in whom a diagnosis of spondyloarthritis is suspected.[18]

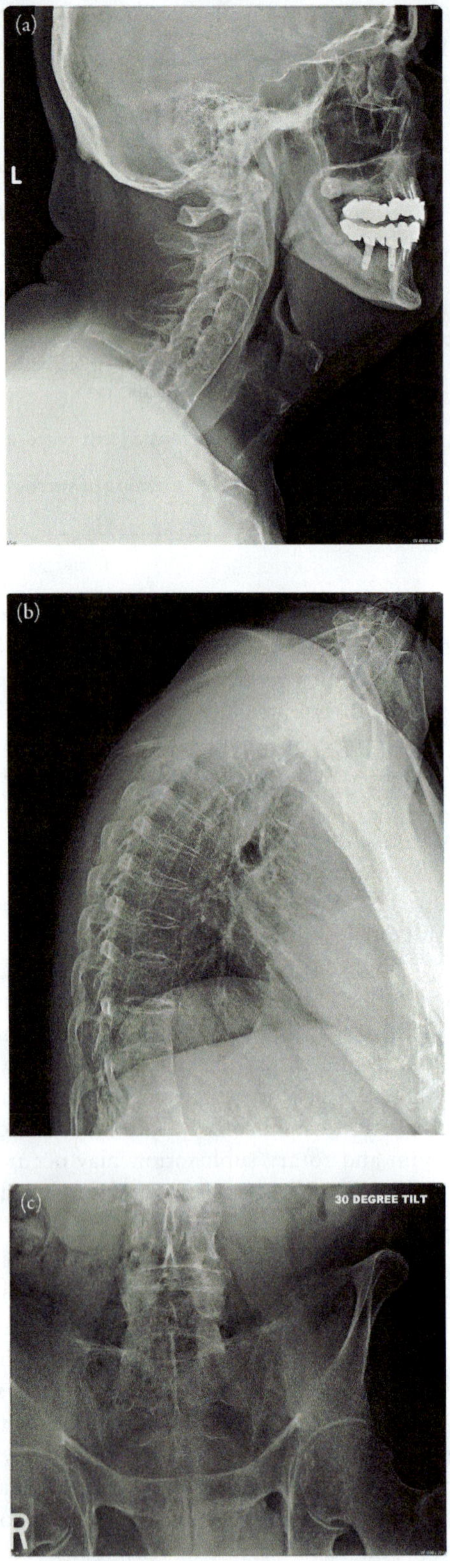

Figure 6.3 (A) A 69-year-old man with 43-year history of ankylosing spondylitis. Lateral view of the cervical spine with thin anterior syndesmophytes from C3 to C7, with fusion of the apophyseal joints. (B) Lateral view of the thoracic spine reveals thin anterior syndesmophytes with preservation of the disc spaces. Fusion of the apophyseal joints is present. (C) Ferguson view of pelvis reveals bilateral fusion of the sacroiliac joints

However, CT scan is unable to detect acute inflammatory changes in bone marrow. The amount of radiation exposure is significantly increased with CT compared to all the other diagnostic radiographic techniques.

Magnetic Resonance (MR)

MR is more sensitive than plain radiography in detecting modifications of the axial skeleton associated with spondyloarthritis. MR with fat saturation or contrast medium–enhanced images is able to detect early inflammatory lesions in the SI joints and the lumbar spine.[19] Bone marrow edema is associated with the early inflammatory lesions of AS. These are visible at a time when plain radiographs are normal in individuals with AS. T1-weighted MR images can visualize sclerosis and erosions of the SI joints. MR is a good choice for young women with suspected sacroiliitis as a means of decreasing radiographic exposure to the ovaries. Debate remains in the literature about the appropriate use of this expensive radiographic technique for the usual diagnosis of spondyloarthritis.[20,21] At this time, MR evaluation of the SI joints and axial skeleton is not required to diagnosis or to follow the progress of AS.

Ultrasound

Power Doppler ultrasound is another imaging technique reported to be effective as an imaging technique to identify enthesitis.[22] A limitation of the technique is a consensus on the ultrasound characteristics of enthesitis. Overlap exists between different forms of enthesitis, both inflammatory and mechanical. This noninvasive imaging technique shows promise but has not been included in diagnostic schema at this time.

From a diagnostic and clinical perspective, plain radiographs normally provide adequate information at a reasonable cost. Plain radiographs remain the usual radiographic technique used for the diagnosis of AS.

> The patient meets the diagnostic and classification criteria for a diagnosis of AS by New York, ESSG, and ASAS criteria. He has inflammatory back pain (starting before age 40, morning stiffness, and more than 3 months' duration of symptoms, improved by activity and aggravated by inactivity) He also has radiographic evidence of sacroiliitis. He is HLA-B27 positive and has a history of iritis.

WHAT IS THE DIFFERENTIAL DIAGNOSIS FOR THIS PATIENT?

The differential diagnosis of spinal pain includes other forms of spondyloarthritis, acute herniated intervertebral disc, and diffuse idiopathic skeletal hyperostosis. Characteristics of these specific diseases are listed in Table 6.2.

Table 6.2 DIFFERENTIAL DIAGNOSIS OF ANKYLOSING SPONDYLITIS

	ANKYLOSING SPONDYLITIS	REACTIVE SYNDROME	PSORIATIC ARTHRITIS	ENTEROPATHIC ARTHRITIS	HERNIATED NUCLEUS PULPOSUS
Sex	Male	=	=	=	=
Age at Onset	15–40	Any age	30–40	15–45	20–40
Presentation	Back pain	GI, GU Infection	Extremity arthritis Psoriasis Back pain	Abdominal pain	Radicular pain
Sacroiliitis	Symmetrical	Symmetrical	Asymmetrical	Symmetrical	–
Axial Skeleton	+	±	±	+	–
Peripheral Joints	Lower	Lower	Upper	Lower	–
Enthesopathy	+	±	+	–	–
ESR	Elevated	Elevated	Elevated	Elevated	Normal
Rheumatoid Factor	–	–	–	–	–
HLA-B27	90%	90%	60%	50%	8%
Course	Continuous	Self-limited	Continuous	Continuous	Episodic or continuous
Therapy	NSAIDs TNF	NSAIDs Antibiotics	NSAIDs Methotrexate	NSAIDs Corticosteroids	NSAIDs Epidural corticosteroids
Disability	Hip		Lower extremity	Lower extremity	Neurologic dysfunction

GI, gastrointestinal; GU, genitourinary; ESR, erythrocyte sedimentation rate; NSAIDs, nonsteroidal anti-inflammatory drugs; TNF, tumor necrosis factor.

PSORIATIC ARTHRITIS (PSA)

Patients with psoriasis who develop a characteristic pattern of joint disease have PsA.23 About 12 million individuals have psoriasis in the United States. The prevalence of psoriasis is 1–3% of the US population. PsA is characterized by heterogeneity. Why individual patients develop one form of PsA versus another is unknown. Some of the psoriatic phenotypes are influenced by local factors like repeated trauma. Classic PsA is described as involving distal interphalangeal (DIP) joints and associated nail disease alone.24 This pattern occurs in 5% of patients. The most common form of the disease, affecting 70% of patients with PsA, is an asymmetrical oligoarthritis; a few large or small joints are involved. Dactylitis, diffuse swelling of a digit, is most closely associated with this form of the disease. Skin activity and joint symptoms do not correlate, and patients with little skin activity may experience continued joint pain and stiffness. Psoriatic spondyloarthritis is found in 25–70% of patients with PsA. Patients who develop axial skeletal disease, sacroiliitis, or spondylitis are usually men who have the onset of psoriasis later in life. They also have a longer duration of disease. HLA-B27 is more common in individuals with axial disease along with iritis. SI involvement may be unilateral or bilateral. Symmetrical involvement, from side to side, and severity of disease predominates over asymmetrical disease. Percussion over the SI joints can elicit symptoms over the affected side. Patients may develop spondylitis in the absence of sacroiliitis, and this has maximal tenderness with percussion over the spine above the sacrum. Sacroiliitis may occur without spondylitis. Spinal disease progression occurs in a random rather than orderly fashion, ascending the spine as commonly noted in AS. In the cervical spine, limitation of motion is a primary manifestation of neck involvement. Spondylitis on radiographs is characterized by asymmetrical involvement of the vertebral bodies and nonmarginal syndesmophytes. Joint ankylosis occurs less commonly than in AS. Cervical spine disease may occur in the absence of sacroiliitis or lumbar spondylitis. This makes for a higher prevalence of cervical spine disease in PsA patients compared to AS patients. Alterations in the cervical spine include joint space sclerosis and narrowing and anterior ligamentous calcification.

REACTIVE ARTHRITIS (REA)

Reactive arthritis is a disease associated with an infectious agent causing an aseptic inflammation in joints and other organs.25 This disorder has been associated with the triad of urethritis (inflammation of the lower urinary tract), arthritis, and conjunctivitis formerly referred to as *Reiter syndrome*, a form of reactive arthritis. ReA is the most common cause of arthritis in young men and primarily affects the lower extremity joints and the low back. Involvement of the cervical spine is rare. The disease results from the interaction of an environmental factor, usually a specific infection, and a genetically predisposed host (HLA–B27+). Approximately 1% of patients with the common infection nongonococcal urethritis develop the syndrome. Others suggest that between 2% and 3% of individuals with nonspecific urethritis develop ReA. The syndrome develops in 0.2–15% of all patients with enteric infections secondary to *Shigella, Salmonella, Campylobacter*, and *Yersinia*. The male-to-female ratio in venereal infection is in the range of 10:1, and the ratio is 1:1 in large outbreaks secondary to enteric infection. ReA is associated with HLA-B27 in 60–80% of individuals. The classic picture of the patient with reactive arthritis is a young man about 25 years old who develops urethritis and a mild conjunctivitis followed by the onset of a predominantly lower extremity oligoarthritis.26 The conjunctivitis is usually mild and is manifested by an erythema (redness) and crusting of the lids. Arthritis may occur 1–3 weeks after the initial infection. In many patients, arthritis is the only manifestation of disease.27 Back pain is a frequent symptom of patients with reactive arthritis. During the acute course between 31% and 92% of the patients may develop pain in the lumbosacral region. Occasionally, the pain will radiate into the posterior thighs but rarely below the knees; it may be unilateral. This finding corresponds to the asymmetrical involvement of the SI joints and contrasts to the symmetrical involvement of AS.28 Spondylitis affecting the lumbar, thoracic, and cervical spine occurs less commonly than sacroiliitis, with up to 23% of patients with severe disease showing such involvement.29 Neck pain is an uncommon symptom of patients with ReA. Constitutional symptoms occur in about one-third of patients and are characterized by fever, anorexia, weight loss, and fatigue.

On examination, men tend to have involvement in the knees, ankles, and feet, and women have more upper extremity disease. Percussion tenderness over the SI joints may be unilateral, correlating with asymmetrical involvement in ReA. The mobility of the lumbosacral and cervical spine should be measured in all planes of motion. Evaluation for enthesopathy, heel pain, or Achilles tendon tenderness is also required.

SI involvement may mimic AS (symmetrical disease) or may be asymmetrical in severity of joint changes. Unilateral SI disease occurs early in the disease process. Variable amounts of sclerosis are associated with erosions. Widening of the joint (erosion), then narrowing (fusion), is the progression of radiographic changes. Fusion of the joints occurs less frequently than in AS. Sacroiliitis may be detected in 5–10% of individuals early in the illness and in up to 60% in prolonged illness. Spondylitis is discontinuous in its involvement of the axial skeleton (skip lesions) and is characterized by nonmarginal bony bridging of vertebral bodies. These vertebral hyperostoses are markedly thickened compared with the thin syndesmophytes of AS. Cervical spine disease is associated with hyperostoses at the anteroinferior corners of one or more cervical vertebrae.

Laboratory results are nonspecific. These include anemia, a leukocytosis, and elevation of ESR. HLA-B27 is found in about 80% of patients but is not essential for the diagnosis. Detection of bacterial antigens is also helpful in identifying the putative organism but is also not essential for the diagnosis.[30]

The course of the illness is unpredictable. Thirty percent to 40% of patients have a self-limited illness lasting 3 months to 1 year. Another 30–50% develop a relapsing pattern of illness with periods of complete remission. The final 10–25% develop chronic, unremitting disease associated with significant disability.

ENTEROPATHIC ARTHRITIS

Ulcerative colitis (UC) and Crohn disease (CD) are inflammatory bowel diseases. UC is limited to the colon; CD may involve any part of the gastrointestinal tract. Inflammation of the gut results in numerous gastrointestinal symptoms, including abdominal pain, fever, and weight loss. These inflammatory diseases are also associated with extraintestinal manifestations, including arthritis. Articular involvement in inflammatory bowel disease includes both peripheral and axial skeleton joints. Peripheral arthritis is generally nondeforming and follows the activity of the underlying bowel disease.31 Axial skeleton disease is similar to AS and follows a course independent of activity of bowel inflammation.

Symptomatic UC usually occurs from 25 to 45 years of age, and the disease is more common among women than men. CD occurs in all races and is distributed worldwide. In the United States, the annual incidence of the disease is 4 per 100,000 people. The disease appears most often from 15 to 35 years of age. Men and women are equally affected. The frequency of peripheral arthritis is 11% in UC and 20% in CD. Spondylitis occurs in 3–4% of both diseases, and radiographic sacroiliitis occurs in 10%.

Axial arthritis of inflammatory bowel disease may be a hereditary accompaniment of the disease and not a manifestation of the activity of bowel disease itself. Both non–HLA-related factors and HLA-B27 may play a role.

The early symptoms of UC are frequent bowel movements with blood or mucus. Mild disease is associated with some abdominal pain and a few bowel movements per day. Severe disease is characterized by fatigue, weight loss, fever, and extracolonic involvement. CD is frequently an indolent illness characterized by generalized fatigue, mild nonbloody diarrhea, anorexia, weight loss, and cramping lower abdominal pain. Patients may have symptoms for years before the diagnosis is made.

Joint involvement in inflammatory bowel disease is divided into two forms: peripheral and spondyloarthritis. Axial skeleton involvement in UC and CD is similar. Spondylitis antedates bowel disease in about one-third of patients. This interval may be as long as 10–20 years. Seventy percent are HLA-B27 positive, 68% have radiographic changes of spondylitis, and 25% have iritis. The spondylitis of inflammatory bowel disease has a course totally independent of that of the bowel disease. The clinical and radiographic findings are similar to those of AS, including involvement of shoulders and hips.

Patients with spondyloarthritis may have decreased motion of the spine in all planes and percussion tenderness over the SI joints. In rare circumstances, chest expansion is diminished. Patients with more extensive disease have limitation of motion of the cervical spine. Occiput-to-wall measurements document the immobility of the entire axial skeleton, including the cervical spine.

The radiographic changes of spondylitis in inflammatory bowel disease are indistinguishable from those with classic AS. Findings include squaring of vertebral bodies, erosions, widening and fusion of the SI joints, symmetrical involvement of SI joints, and marginal syndesmophytes involving the lumbar, thoracic, or cervical spine.

The factors that help make the diagnosis of enteropathic spondyloarthropathy are the pattern of peripheral arthritis if present (upper extremity disease is uncommon in AS and ReA; bilateral ankle arthritis is uncommon in psoriatic disease), erythema nodosum, and iritis.

HERNIATED INTERVERTEBRAL DISC (HID)

An HID occurs in individuals most commonly between 30 and 40 years of age. This is a time when discs contain a normal amount of gel in the nucleus pulposus but the outer layer (annulus) starts to deteriorate. The crisscross of the fibers is broken, and the contained nucleus pulposus escapes. A disc protrusion or bulging occurs when the escaped gel remains within the annulus. A disc extrusion or herniation occurs when the gel escapes outside the outer portions of the annulus. Herniated discs may be painless unless they contact spinal nerves in the neural foramen or the canal. The body attempts to remove the tissue with an inflammatory response. Sciatica (leg pain) occurs when the spinal nerve is inflamed. This symptom is associated with dysfunction in the corresponding nerve root. Nerve dysfunction is associated with progressive loss of reflex, sensory, and motor function. Pseudo-sciatica related to sacroiliitis and reflex contraction of the piriformis muscle can be confused with radiculopathy related to disc herniation. The absence of specific neurologic deficits with pseudo-sciatica helps differentiate these disorders.

Individuals with a disc disruption may have mild back pain on the side of the herniation but have a greater degree of leg pain. The pain is deep and sharp, and it may be accompanied with a "pins and needles" tingling sensation. The pain may vary in intensity but can severe enough to cause immobility. The affected leg may feel weak. Pain is increased with sitting, driving, coughing, or having a bowel movement because these activities increase pressure in the herniated disc.

A plain radiograph will not identify the location of a herniated disc. MR is able to pinpoint the area of disc extrusion that corroborates the findings on physical examination. MR can also identify if bone marrow edema is present in the SI joints suggesting sacroiliitis as the cause of "radicular" symptoms.

It is important to make the appropriate diagnosis for individuals with back and leg pain. Spinal surgery is not beneficial to AS patients who do not require the procedure. The injury to the spine resulting from surgery can increase the inflammatory response, resulting in the potential for more rapidly advancing disease.

DIFFUSE IDIOPATHIC SKELETAL HYPEROSTOSIS (DISH)

DISH is another disease that may occur in the setting of spondylitis. DISH and AS can occur in the same individual. Patients with AS and DISH should be easily differentiated by careful radiographic evaluation.32 DISH is an illness associated with spinal pain and stiffness and extensive calcification of spinal and extraspinal structures (Figure 6.4). Stiffness may occur in the absence of pain. In a majority, back pain occurs in the thoracolumbar region as an initial complaint. DISH occurs in older men predominantly. The stance of the individual may be similar to that of a patient with AS.33 Physical examination reveals little in the form of percussion tenderness. Motion is mildly limited. DISH is a radiographic diagnosis. Three characteristics of DISH in the axial skeleton include flowing calcification along the anterolateral aspect of four continuous vertebral bodies, preservation of intervertebral disc height, and absence of apophyseal joint bony ankylosis and SI joint sclerosis, erosion, or fusion. DISH may cause bony alterations of the SI joints.34 CT of the SI joints differentiates the hyperostotic joint changes from those associated with joint erosion and fusion. Also of note is the occurrence of fracture in patients with DISH as well as in those with AS. The convergence of two common diseases in the same host, a middle-aged man, is likely. AS and DISH of the cervical spine can occur simultaneously.

The patient has radiographic evidence of bilateral sacroiliitis. Additional radiographic evaluation of the axial skeleton is warranted to determine the extent of thoracic and cervical spine involvement. The extent of radiographic changes can identify the reasons if he does not respond to appropriate therapy.

WHAT ARE THE CHARACTERISTICS OF PAIN IN ACUTE AND CHRONIC RHEUMATOLOGICAL DISEASE?

The nerve supply to components of the musculoskeletal system plays a significant role in the kind and distribution of pain experienced by patients with rheumatic diseases. Nerves that supply joints with sensory sensation frequently supply surrounding skin, muscle, and bones. There is an overlap of innervation, with several nerves supplying a single joint. Terminal branches of myelinated and unmyelinated fibers are distributed through the periosteum and synovium. The joint capsule is richly supplied with sensory innervation. Sensory innervation to the joints includes nociceptors surrounding blood vessels and near the surface of synovial cells and mechanoreceptors in the joint capsule. In addition, unmyelinated C nerve fibers of the posterior primary rami of multiple spinal segments supply these musculoskeletal

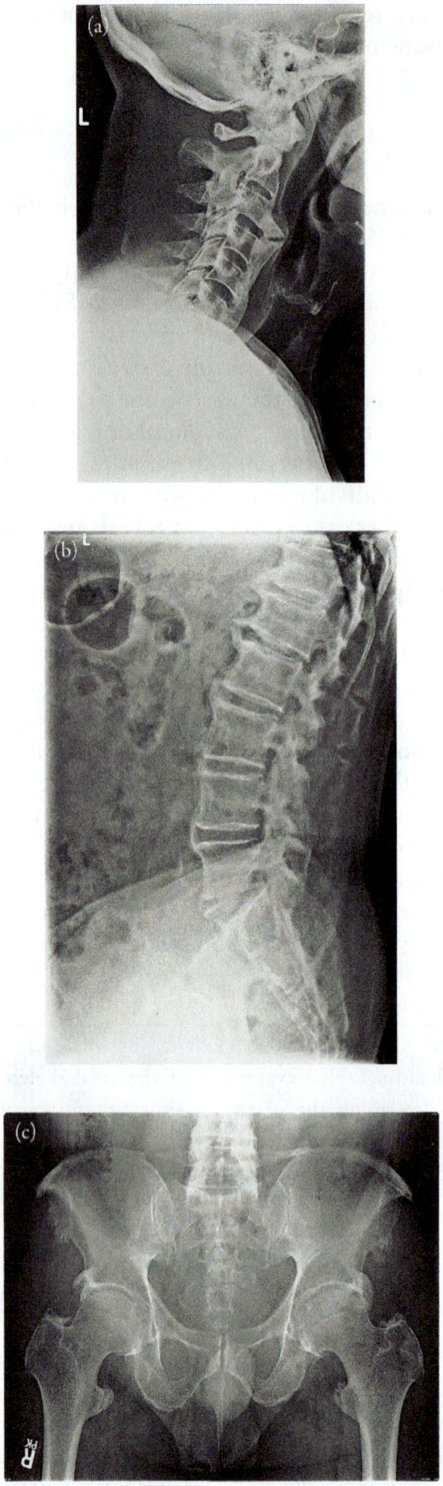

Figure 6.4 (A) A 58-year-old man with increasing spinal stiffness over the past 6 years. Lateral view of the cervical spine reveals large anterior horizontally oriented osteophytes at multiple cervical levels. Large osteophyte at C4 is impinging on the esophagus. (B) Lateral view of the lumbar spine reveals large, thick anterior osteophytes with nonfused apophyseal joints. (C) Anteroposterior view reveals normal sacroiliac joints.

structures. The consequence of this anatomy is the difficulty of patients describing the exact location for the sources of their pain. For example, because of the distribution of motor and sensory nerves, patients with articular and ligamentous disease may develop reflex muscle spasm on both sides of the spine and cutaneous hyperesthesia over the same areas.

The interaction of peripheral inflammatory cells, neuropeptides, and chemical mediators of inflammation is complex. Peripheral nociceptors are stimulated by inflammatory mediators, like prostaglandins, released during tissues damage. Excitation of nociceptors stimulates the peripheral release of neuropeptides like substance P and calcitonin gene-related peptide. Other sensitizing factors include interleukin-1 (IL-1), neutrophil-chemotactic peptides, and nerve growth factor-derived octapeptide. Immune cells activated by damage also produce proinflammatory cytokines (IL-1, IL-6, and tumor necrosis factor [TNF]-α) that activate peripheral nerves.

The sensory pain system involves specific tracts through the peripheral nerves to the dorsal horn, spinothalamic tract, and the cerebral cortex. All of these components have associated neuroanatomy and neuropeptides that mediate the sensory, affective, and cognitive responses to tissue damage or the threat of tissue damage. An increasing number of nociceptive receptors and channels have been identified that mediate different components of acute tissue damage. For example, capsaicin/vanilloid receptor, transient receptor potential vanilloid 1, responds to noxious heat, acidic pH, and capsaicin. Molecular channels such as tetrodotoxin (TTX)-resistant (Nav1.8 and 1.9) and TTX-sensitive (Nav1.9) sodium channels have profound effects on the up- or down-regulation of pain, respectively.

Genetic haplotypes may also play a significant role in the perception of pain.[35] For example, catechol-O-methyltransferase (COMT) may play a significant role in human pain perception. Observations regarding the role of COMT are notable because of the relevance to human pain perception. Zubieta et al. showed that the COMT val158met polymorphism in humans may influence differential pain sensitivity, working in part by modulating the endogenous μ-opioid system.[36] In investigations of this polymorphism, haplotype analyses identified three subsets of individuals based on four single nucleotide polymorphisms (SNPs) termed low pain sensitive (LPS), average pain sensitive (APS), and high pain sensitive (HPS) groups.[37] These studies indicated that the subgroups are highly predictive of pain sensitivity on a variety of different experimental pain tasks. Moreover, in a prospective 3-year study of 240 individuals who were pain free at baseline, the development of temporomandibular joint disorder (TMD), was three times as likely in HPS individuals as in APS and LPS individuals.[38]

Studies in animals provide further evidence for the influence of COMT on pain. In rats, animals with the LPS haplotype produced much higher levels of COMT enzymatic activity when compared with the APS or HPS haplotypes, and inhibition of COMT in the rat results in a profound increase in pain sensitivity. Finally, molecular studies have provided a biochemical basis for these differences because these synonymously coding SNPs, when combined into haplotypes, each led to a different RNA structure with markedly different activity.[38]

A study applying information about COMT haplotypes to clinical situations using a large OA database found a very weak association between the degree of OA of the knee or hip and pain.[39] These authors noted that those individuals with the 158-Met COMT variant had an almost three times higher risk for hip pain as compared to the ValVal-genotype. Female carriers drove this effect. Women with the 158-Val allele were 4.9 times more likely to have pain, although in both genotype groups radiographic damage to the hip was present. This sex difference is notable because expression of COMT is inducible by estrogen and may contribute to certain "phenotypic" characteristics that differ in women and men, including pain sensitivity.[39]

Pain associated with rheumatic diseases is difficult to simply categorize. Damage to specific tissues results in pain of varying qualities. The Pain Management Task Force of the American College of Rheumatology recently published a classification of rheumatic disease pain syndromes (see Box 6.2).[40]

Deep somatic pain is the category most commonly associated with disorders of the axial skeleton. Mechanical or inflammatory disorders that disrupt the vertebral column, paraspinous muscles, and associated ligaments, tendons, and fascia result in pain. Acute injuries are associated with sudden-onset of sharp stabs of pain at the moment of damage, followed by a dull ache that may persist for weeks, along with tenderness on palpation and associated muscle contraction. The initial pain originates in the unmyelinated nerve fibers that are stimulated by the mechanical disruption of the tendons, blood vessels, or fascial sheaths of muscles. The prolonged aching pain is a result of nerve endings being stimulated by chemical mediators associated with the healing inflammatory response.

In regard to AS, inflammatory disorders can cause joint pain. These diseases of the axial skeleton joints cause the production of joint swelling along with release of inflammatory mediators that are irritating to nociceptors in the fibrous joint capsule. Structural changes to the synovium and articular cartilage may not be associated with pain because these tissues contain no free nerve fiber endings. The clinical correlate of this anatomic circumstance is the lack of relationship between the extent of structural joint damage on radiographic evaluation of the spinal column and the severity of pain.

Other sources of deep somatic pain are ligaments, tendons, and fascia surrounding and attaching to the spine. Entheses, the attachments of tendons and ligaments to bones, are a primary locus of inflammation in spondyloarthritis. Ligaments of the spine play an essential role in the static posture of the axial skeleton. In its normal configuration, ligaments stretch to their normal length to support the spine without excessive muscular contraction. Pain is generated in nociceptors of ligaments if they are placed under mechanical stress caused by a variety of circumstances. In response to inflammation in joints or entheses, associated muscles may undergo tonic contraction or spasm. Tonic contraction results in increased metabolic activity and the production of chemical mediators that may stimulate unmyelinated nerve fibers.

Acute rheumatic disease pain is frequently related to rapid-onset inflammatory conditions. These are most frequently seen with crystal-induced and infectious disorders.

Box 6.2 **CLASSIFICATION OF RHEUMATIC DISEASE PAIN SYNDROMES**

1. Superficial somatic (skin subcutaneous tissue):
   Autoimmune conditions (vasculitis, systemic lupus erythematosus) with pain arising from the skin
2. Deep somatic (muscles, periosteum, ligaments, joints, vessels):
   Noninflammatory and inflammatory conditions of the peripheral joints
   Osteoarthritis
   Rheumatoid arthritis
      Spondyloarthritis (e.g., ankylosing spondylitis, psoriatic arthritis)
      Crystal-induced disorders, including urate gout, calcium crystal-induced arthritis (e.g., pseudogout, calcium phosphate arthritis, hydroxyapatite disease)
   Degenerative and inflammatory conditions of the tendons and ligaments and bursae (e.g., rotator cuff disorders, diabetic arthropathy)
   Degenerative and inflammatory conditions of the spine
      Spondylosis of the cervical, thoracic, and lumbar spine including facet syndrome
      Postsurgical pain syndromes (e.g., failed back syndrome)
   Metabolic and other bone disease
   Osteoporosis of all forms:
   Osteomalacia
   Paget's disease of bone and related secondary osteoarthritis.
   Avascular necrosis of bone
3. Radicular (spinal nerve roots):
   Lumbar spinal stenosis, lateral recess impingement, disc compression
4. Neurogenic/central (peripheral/central nervous system):
   Neurogenic neuropathic conditions of the extremities.
   Causalgia/complex regional pain syndrome, type II
   Thoracic outlet syndrome
   Entrapment neuropathies
   Other peripheral neuropathies
   Pain conditions related to central sensitization
   Fibromyalgia:
   Myofascial pain syndrome
   Reflex sympathetic dystrophy syndrome/complex regional pain syndrome, type I

Acute pain is generated by activation of high-threshold nociceptors.

Chronic rheumatic disease pain is associated with a wide variety of noninflammatory and inflammatory disorders such as OA and spondyloarthritis, respectively. In these individuals, deep somatic pain is the category causing the predominance of their symptoms. However, the generation of pain mediators in these respective groups is different. In OA, pain is generated in joints because of deterioration of joint structures that results in local inflammation. Spondyloarthritis is an inflammatory disease that causes systemic inflammation associated with a different set of immune mediators. In either circumstance, despite the potential for a different mechanism, the replacement of the destroyed joint, whether caused by noninflammatory or inflammatory diseases, is associated with almost immediate resolution of chronic pain. In the setting of chronic musculoskeletal disease, the absence of direct damage to the nervous system suggests that plastic remodeling of the nervous system has not occurred. Removal of the musculoskeletal pain source has the potential to resolve severe pain almost entirely. The challenge is to modify the "unplasticized" nervous system without the need for joint replacement.

The patient has pain characteristics most likely associated with chronic inflammatory disease.

HOW IS THIS CLINICAL SITUATION MANAGED?

The goals of therapy for AS, as with other forms of inflammatory arthritis, are to control pain and stiffness, reduce inflammation, maintain function, and prevent deformity with avoidance of undue toxicity41A. Patients require a comprehensive program of education, physiotherapy, medications, and other measures. Patients are taught proper posture and mobilizing and breathing exercises to prevent the tendency to stoop forward and lose chest motion. The importance of a firm upright chair for sitting and a hard mattress with no pillows for sleeping is stressed.

Patients are encouraged to participate in a home exercise program, but supervision from a physical therapist has the potential to result in a better outcome.41

PHARMACOLOGICAL CHOICES

Nonsteroidal Anti-inflammatory Drugs (NSAIDs)

Medications to control pain and inflammation are useful to the patient with AS. NSAIDs possess antipyretic, analgesic, and anti-inflammatory characteristics. They are anti-inflammatory and analgesic when given long-term in larger doses. NSAIDs currently available for the treatment of spinal disorders are listed in Table 6.3. NSAIDs are effective at decreasing pain and improving movement and are the only therapy necessary for most. About 80% of AS patients report decreased pain and relief of stiffness with NSAIDs.42 Increasing evidence in the literature shows the inhibition of calcification of the spine with the use of consistent, prolonged NSAID dosing.43 No specific NSAID is preferred, although indomethacin has been shown to be effective in a wide range of patients when tolerated.44

Cyclo-oxygenase Inhibitors

Cyclo-oxygenase-2 (COX-2) inhibitors are a class of NSAIDs that have efficacy equal to COX-1 inhibitors (aspirin, naproxen) with less gastrointestinal toxicity (see Table 6.3). The cardiovascular risk associated with these agents is an active area of research. Therefore, exclusive use of COX-2 inhibitors should be considered for individuals with increased risks of gastrointestinal bleeding. COX-2 inhibitors are effective in OA and rheumatoid arthritis. AS patients are reported to be responsive to celecoxib, a COX-2 inhibitor, in a 6-week controlled study.45

Muscle Relaxants

Patients with acute AS may develop severe muscle spasm with associated limited motion that may hinder their return to normal daily activities. In these patients, the addition of a muscle relaxant to an NSAID helps decrease muscle pain and muscle spasm and improve back motion. Muscle relaxants, such as cyclobenzaprine, at low dosage levels (5–10 mg/d) are helpful while limiting possible drug toxicity. The sleepiness associated with muscle relaxants with long half-lives can be limited by giving the medication 2 hours before bedtime.

Corticosteroids

Systemic corticosteroids are rarely needed and are ineffective for the spinal articular disease of AS. For the occasional patient with continued joint symptoms receiving maximum doses of NSAIDs, adding small doses of corticosteroids (5 mg/d prednisone) may prove useful. Larger doses of corticosteroids cause appreciably more toxicity without an increased benefit. Injection of corticosteroids in SI joints have the potential to help decrease back pain in patients who may otherwise not be responsive to systemic therapies.46

Disease-Modifying Agents (DMARDs)

DMARDs are agents that work more slowly than NSAIDs but have the capability of modifying the progression of disease. In AS, sulfasalazine is the agent most closely associated with benefit for the peripheral arthritis of AS. This drug is most effective for arthritis of the knees, ankles, and root joints.[47]

The initial dose is 500 mg once a day to document tolerability; tolerability is enhanced with the enteric-coated form of the drug. The dose is gradually increased to 1,500 mg twice a day. The most common toxicities include nausea, dizziness, headache, and rash. Individuals with sulfonamide sensitivities are unable to tolerate sulfasalazine.

Other DMARDs include methotrexate and leflunomide. Although these agents have been shown to be effective for rheumatoid arthritis, they are ineffective in the treatment of axial or nonaxial spondyloarthritis.[48,49] In addition, the combination of methotrexate along with a TNF antagonist does not increase the benefit or decrease the risk of adverse effects compared with the TNF alone.[50]

Anti–TNF Inhibitors

An inflammatory cytokine, TNF-α, is associated with the inflammatory process that results in the phenotypic expression of AS. Anti-TNF therapies are available in the form of infliximab, etanercept, adalimumab, and golimumab, which inhibit the inflammatory effects of TNF.

Table 6.3 NONSTEROIDAL ANTI-INFLAMMATORY DRUGS (PARTIAL LIST)

DRUG (CHEMICAL CLASS)	TRADE NAME	SIZE (MG)	MAXIMUM DOSE (MG/D)	FREQUENCY (×/D)
Salicylates				
Aspirin	Bayer	81, 325	5,200	4–6
Enteric-coated	Ecotrin	325	5,200	4–6
Substituted Salicylates				
Diflunisal	Dolobid	250/500	1,500	2–3
Salsalate	Disalcid	500/750	3,000	2
Choline magnesium trisalicylate	Trilisate	500/750	3,000	2
Propionic Acid				
Ibuprofen	Motrin	200, 400,	4,800	4–6
Naproxen	Naprelan	375, 500	1,500	2–3
Ketoprofen	Orudis	25, 50, 75	300	3–4
Extended release	Oruvail	200	200	1
Flubiprofen	Ansaid	50, 100	300	2–3
Oxaprozin	Daypro	600	1,800	1–2
Pyrole Acetic Acid				
Sulindac	Clinoril	150, 200	450	2–3
Tolectin	Tolectin	200, 400	1,600	4
Indomethacin	Indocin	25, 50, 75	225	1–3
Benzeneacetic Acid				
Diclofenac sodium	Voltaren	25, 50, 75, 100SR	225	2–3
Diclofenac/misoprostol	Arthrotec	50/75	225	2–3
Oxicam				
Piroxicam	Feldene	10, 20	20	1
Meloxicam	Mobic	7.5, 15	15	1
Pyranocarboxylic Acid				
Etodolac	Lodine	200, 300, 400XL, 500XL	1,600	2–4
Fenemate				
Meclofenemate	Meclomen	50, 100	400	4
Pyrrolopyrrole				
Ketorolac	Toradol	10	40	4
Naphthylalkanone				
Nabumetone	Relafen	500, 750	2,000	2
Cyclooxygenase-2 Inhibitors				
Celecoxib	Celebrex	100, 200, 400	800	2

Infliximab is a chimeric mouse-human monoclonal anti-TNF-α antibody. The drug may be used at 3 mg/kg, 5 mg/kg, or up to 10 mg/kg. The 5 mg/kg dose is the usual dose for spondyloarthritis. Infusions are given at different intervals ranging from 4 to 8 weeks. Infusion of intravenous infliximab in a dose of 5 mg/kg was studied in 357 AS patients in a placebo-controlled trial over a 24-week period. Infliximab resulted in improvement in axial symptoms and signs, enthesitis, and peripheral arthritis.51 Open-label extension of studies for as long as 54 weeks have documented persistent improvement with infliximab infusions at 6-week intervals.52

Etanercept is a recombinant form of the p73 TNF receptor fusion protein. Etanercept 50 mg is administered by subcutaneous injection once a week or 25 mg twice a week. Currently, etanercept is delivered in auto-filled syringes or in a self-injector pen. In a placebo-controlled, 4-month study of 40 AS patients taking 25 mg of etanercept, 80% of patients on the active drug experienced an improvement in morning stiffness, enthesitis, quality of life, ESR, or CRP.53 A large study of 277 AS patients evaluated etanercept 25 mg twice a week versus placebo over a 12-week period. Etanercept patients had significant improvement in clinical symptoms.54 A subgroup of these patients had MR evaluations that demonstrated decreased spinal inflammation.55 The sustained benefit of etanercept has been documented in clinical trials.56

Adalimumab is a humanized anti-TNF-α monoclonal antibody. Adalimumab 40 mg is administered by subcutaneous injection once every 2 weeks.57 The medicine is delivered by a self-injector pen. In a study of 315 AS patients, adalimumab was associated with a greater number of individuals who achieved a clinically significant improvement in their axial arthritis at the end of 12 weeks.58 At the end of this 2-year study, 71% of those who remained on adalimumab had a 50% improvement in clinical symptoms including fatigue, morning stiffness, and spinal pain.

Golimumab is a human anti-TNF-α monoclonal antibody. Golimumab 50 mg is injected subcutaneously once every 4 weeks. A study of 356 AS patients randomly assigned to 50 mg, 100 mg, or placebo injections every 4 weeks demonstrated clinical improvement at 14 weeks for those in the golimumab groups compared to placebo.59

The efficacy of the TNF-α therapies shows no benefit of one particular agent compared to another. The use of specific agents in individuals is based on personal preference related to infusion versus injections and the frequency of dosing.

The ASAS has published new management guidelines that include nonpharmacologic and pharmacologic therapies for spondyloarthritis.60,61 NSAIDs remain the first-line therapy for spondyloarthritis. They should be used for a month. If no response occurs, TNF-α antibody therapy should be considered.

Toxicities associated with the use of TNF-α therapies include the activation of latent tuberculosis. TNF-α therapies are associated with an increased risk of bacterial and viral infections. The degree of the increased risk for malignancy above that associated with the underlying disorders is being investigated.

PHYSICAL THERAPY EXAMINATION AND MANAGEMENT

Physical therapy is a beneficial component of patient care for individuals with AS by maintaining and improving function, mobility, fitness, and global health. Physical therapy interventions play a pivotal role in the prevention and early management of axial and peripheral deformities associated with the natural progression of AS.[62] Performing regular exercise can improve function despite no change in disease activity.[63] Patients with a confirmed or suspected diagnosis of AS may benefit from physical therapy when pain, decreased cardiovascular endurance and muscle performance, loss of function, fatigue, and diminished muscle flexibility are present. The physical therapist can address a knowledge deficit in symptomatology self-management and on the natural disease process. Because disease activity and severity varies considerably among individual patients with AS, physical therapists must create specific exercise programs to address each patient's impairments and functional goals.[64]

Examination

Physical therapists are increasingly treating individuals through direct access. As a result, physical therapists need to immediately determine if patients are safe to treat or are safe to treat with a concurrent referral to another healthcare practitioner, or they must refer the patient to a physician prior to proceeding with physical therapy management. When a patient presents to physical therapy with a either new or gradually worsening pain in the low back, SI joints, hips, knees, and/or heels in the absence of injury, along with associated systemic signs and symptoms, the therapist must recognize that the patient's symptoms may not be mechanical in nature. Therapists should evaluate and discuss these "red flag" findings with the appropriate medical professional including internal, rheumatology, or orthopedic medicine, if not previously addressed. It is important to make this distinction because serious consequences can ensue with treatment of individuals without accurate disease process knowledge. For example, a fused osteopenic spine is at risk for fracture, and the clinician must use caution when attempting to mobilize an ankylosed or fusing spine.[65]

Collecting the patient's social history will assist the clinician in developing patient-centered care and goals. The history should include the magnitude of family and social support, current and previous activity levels, limited activities of daily living (ADLs), recreational activities, work description, and previously modified activities to accommodate the symptoms.

The initial subjective intake examination will help identify if generalized joint stiffness is present that is worse in the morning.[66] Exercises or regular movement alleviates this stiffness but worsens with inactivity. A patient may report a deep and dull pain to describe a diffuse or nonspecific pain in the lower back and SI joint.

The clinician assesses cognition to determine the patient's motivation level and learning abilities. Certain patient populations may require a screen for depression-like symptoms. Depression is common with a chronic disease diagnosis such as AS, particularly given the natural progression of the pathology and early onset age. If a patient presents with depression along with AS, a multidisciplinary treatment approach could potentially maximize the patient's outcome.[67]

Physical therapists can screen for depression using the reliable two-question depression-screening test developed by Arroll et al.[68] The first question is "During the past month have you often been bothered by feeling down, depressed, or hopeless?" The second question is, "During the last month have you often been bothered by little interest or pleasure in doing things?" The sensitivity and specificity for the presence of depression is 97% and 67%, respectively, if the patient answers "yes" to both questions. Answering "yes" to both the questions indicates the need for a referral to a mental health specialist.

The patient requires a neurological screen to both the upper and lower extremities to assess for the possibility of upper motor neuron (UMN) changes and/or any nerve root compression. The clinician should assess deep tendon reflexes, myotomes, and dermatomes for any limitations. The Hoffman test for the upper extremity can assess for UMN changes, which consists of "flicking" the patient's middle fingernail with the clinician's fingernail. A positive test results in twitching in the thumb and second finger. Additionally, the clonus and Babinski test to the lower extremities will test for UMN involvement anywhere within the spinal cord.

Active ROM measurements to the lumbar spine must be collected with the patient standing for standard testing. Lumbar ROM can be measured with a bubble inclinometer by placing the measurement tool on L1 while the patient flexes fully with knees straight and without upper extremity involvement. The same is repeated with the inclinometer on L5. The two measurements are then subtracted to identify the active ROM in the lumbar spine. This same process can be used to measure thoracic ROM with the bubble inclinometer placed on T1 and T12. Thoracic rotation should be observed and objectively measured with the use of rotational percentages in the seated position. However, the reliability of this method is limited. Both active and passive ROM measurements should be taken in the spine, shoulders, hips, knees, and ankle when limitations are noted. Pain intensity in any direction can be collected using the numerical pain rating scale (NPRS) with zero being no pain and 10 being the worst imaginable pain.

Assessing posture in standing can help the clinician identify forward head positioning, protracted scapulae, rounded shoulders, increased thoracic kyphosis, diminished lumbar lordosis, and other various postural abnormalities that may be associated with AS.

Physical therapists should assess spinal mobility and paraspinal muscles to identify limitations. Posterior to anterior mobilizations test joint mobility in the lumbar, thoracic, and cervical spine along with the SI joint. Both lower and upper extremity joints may be screened if active ROM is limited in any joint. A lack of spinal mobility is the hallmark sign of AS.

Special tests help assess spinal mobility. These tests include the Schober's test, fingertip-to-floor distance, tragus-to-wall distance, and cervical rotation tests.[63,69,70] These mobility measures have adequate levels of reliability and validity,[69] and spinal mobility limitations may be one of the earliest predictors to prognosis.[71] The Thomas test assesses muscle length changes.[63]

The Schober's test assesses spinal flexion. The patient is instructed to stand erect with the heels together and markings are made over the spine 5 cm below and 10 cm above the lumbosacral junction; these landmarks are found by drawing a horizontal line between the posterosuperior iliac spines.[69] The patient is asked to bend forward and the distance between the two marks is noted with a tape measure. Normal change in the distance between the two markings is greater than or equal to 5 cm and indicates normal spinal mobility.[69] A measurement of less than 5 cm indicates lumbar hypomobility and restriction.[63,69] The change between the upper and lower markings correlates with anterior flexion measured radiologically.[63]

The fingertip-to-floor test measures both hip and spine ROM. The patient bends maximally forward reaching toward his or her toes with the fingertips extended while maintaining heel contact. The distance between the right middle finger and the floor is measured with measuring tape. The larger the distance, the greater mobility and ROM restrictions.[69]

The tragus-to-wall distance test measures cervical and thoracic posture, which has been correlated with radiographic changes.[69] The patient stands with both heels and buttock against the wall along with chin retraction and extended knees. The distance between the right tragus and the wall is measured with a measuring tape. The larger the distance measured reflects progressive forward head posture and cervicothoracic kyphosis.[69]

The cervical rotation test measures cervical rotational ROM. Begin by measuring the distance between the nose and the acromioclavicular joint (ACJ) with the head in a neutral position. Then measure the distance between the nose and ACJ with the patient's head maximally rotated to the right. Calculate the difference between the two measurements and then repeat the process with left rotation. The smaller the differences between the neutral and ipsilateral measurement, the greater restriction in the rotational ROM. The distance between the tip of the nose and the ACJ is collected with a tape measure.

The Thomas test assesses the hip flexor muscle length, which is a commonly shortened muscle group in people with AS. This test is performed by placing the patient supine at the end of the examination table with both knees pulled toward his or her chest. The patient is then instructed to lower one leg. A positive test consists of the femur resting above zero degrees of hip ROM, or the neutral position. This indicates limited hip flexor muscle length. Any identified positive tests can assist the physical therapist with providing appropriate treatments.

A preliminary clinical prediction rule (CPR) can help clinicians identify which patients with AS are most likely to benefit in the short term from specific exercise programs.[70] In one study, patients completed three self-reported measures including the Bath Ankylosing Spondylitis Functional Index (BASFI), the Bath Ankylosing Spondylitis Disease Activity Index (BASDAI), and the Short-Form 36 (SF-36). This prospective cohort study identified three variables to predict success: physical role of greater than 37 (SF-36 measure), bodily pain of greater than 27 (SF-36 measure), and BASDAI of greater than 3. The positive likelihood ratio was 11.2 (95% confidence interval, 1.7–76.0) when two of the three variables are present. This means that patients who meet two out of the three variables are 11.2 times more likely to respond to a specific exercise program. The post-test success probability increased to 91% when two variables were present. Although CPRs help to determine which interventions may be most beneficial, the clinician is urged to always integrate clinical reasoning and patient values when creating treatment plans. In addition, caution should be used because future validation studies are required.

Collecting as much objective information as possible can assist the clinician in developing an all-encompassing treatment program to maximize the patient's potential for a successful outcome. A thorough physical examination with objective data early in the disease process can help monitor for disease progression.

Interventions

Recent research has identified the benefits of specific exercise recommendations along with medication management for people with AS.[72] Exercise is a commonly suggested intervention for AS, but little is actually known regarding the long-term outcomes. Exercise can improve pain, stiffness, and function when performed for at least 30 minutes a day, for 5 days a week.[63] The disease progression stage must be considered when prescribing and developing a treatment plan.

An exercise program developed by a physical therapist is based on the impairments found during the initial assessment. The effectiveness of exercise provided by a physical therapist has been evaluated and found effective in patients with AS.[73] In addition to exercise, physical therapy interventions often include manual therapy, aerobic conditioning, pain reducing modalities, education, and activity modification, not only to decrease symptoms but also to maximize function and decrease disease progression rates.

A referral to physical therapy early in the disease progression can be more beneficial than later in the disease course in order to educate the patient on exercises and activity modifications to prevent or slow the onset of structural changes.

Therapeutic Exercises

The Cochrane Musculoskeletal Group recognized that supervised physiotherapeutic exercises were better than home exercises in improving pain, stiffness, spinal mobility, and overall well-being in the AS population.[74] A 2008 review performed by the Cochrane Review found low-quality evidence for exercise programs compared with no intervention and moderate evidence for supervised group physiotherapy compared with individualized home programs.[75]

Flexibility exercises biased toward spinal extension along with postural reeducation will promote erect posture over time as the disease progresses. Stretching tight muscles, such as the pectorals and hip flexors, can help prevent the forward flexed posture associated with AS. The patient should avoid aggressive stretching because this can lead to muscle strains or ankylosing joint fractures. Some cues to prevent overstretching would be intolerable pain in the muscle being stretched, altered body positioning from the instructed approach, or if muscle soreness persists after stretch cessation. A 5- to 10-minute warm-up prior to stretching should be incorporated to minimize any potential for a muscle injury while stretching.

Lumbar and lower extremity stabilization exercises are prescribed for specifically weak muscle groups. Strengthening of the trunk extensors is important to maximize the spine in a properly aligned and functionally appropriate extension-biased posture. Simple prone lying is a method to encourage spinal extension, but it must be repeated daily.

Limitations to the cardiovascular and pulmonary systems can occur with progressive cervicothoracic kyphosis along with compensatory forward head positioning. Breathing patterns and techniques can be taught for the patient to perform throughout activities to help maintain chest expansion and improve oxygen saturation.[63] Pursed lip breathing during exercise participation and high-performance activities should be taught. The stair-step breathing technique can be performed regularly to maintain chest expansion and prevent atelectasis. This technique consists of the patient taking a deep inhalation breath and holding it for 5 seconds. The patient then takes a short inhalation breath to further expand the chest wall and holds that breath for another 5 seconds. This can be performed 3–5 times before the patient fully exhales.

A forward head posture is also associated with other pathologies such as headaches, neck pain, TMJ dysfunction and a variety of shoulder pathologies including but not limited to impingement.[76] Self-mobilization extension exercises for the thoracic spine with a foam roller and prone scapular stabilization activities can diminish kyphosis progression. The foam roller can also be used for lumbar stabilization exercises with the patient lying lengthwise on the roller with the entire spine on the roller. With the transversus abdominis contracted and the spine remaining in contact with the roller, the patient can march the lower extremities in an alternating pattern. Active ROM exercises in the prone, sitting, or standing positions can encourage spinal extension. One activity that minimizes flexion is a lumbar stabilization exercise in the quadruped position with alternation upper and lower extremities. Prone lying while alternating upper extremity flexion and lower extremity extension also minimizes any flexion forces and promotes extension.

Aerobic conditioning activities, such as the use of a recumbent bike, stationary bike, or walking program, can help to maintain cardiovascular health and respiratory function. Deep breathing techniques are taught to assist with maintaining chest wall expansion to limit future respiratory restrictions. Facedown swimming positions should be avoided to prevent flexion bias positioning during repeated activity. Backstroke swimming will encourage spinal extension and may be more beneficial.

Manual Therapy

Manual therapy can be beneficial at reducing or eliminating joint and soft tissue restrictions associated with AS and promote decreased pain and improved function. Joint mobilization techniques can improve the patient's spinal mobility and relieve symptoms. Manual treatments are specific to spinal areas that are identified as hypomobile during the examination.[77] Caution should be applied during treatment. A sound clinical understanding of the AS spinal condition is imperative to prevent possible injury during treatment. In addition to interventions directed specifically at the spine, therapists should also address other lumbopelvic, thoracic, hip, knee, ankle, and foot restrictions to facilitate improved gait and function. Further research is needed to identify the effects of manual techniques.

Education

Education is one of the most important interventions physical therapists can provide. Physical therapists have the opportunity to spend a greater amount of time with a patient to allow for patient-centered education. Education should include information on natural disease progression, prognosis, breathing techniques, posture, proper lifting techniques, weight management, avoidance of flexion-based activities, and the importance of quality and consistent exercise.

Proper lifting body mechanics training is important to prevent future injury or fracture to the osteopenic and fused spinal vertebrae. Proper lifting includes bending the knees, keeping the lifted object close to the body, and moving the feet to avoid spinal rotation. In combination, these will prevent flexion-biased forces to the spine.

Workstation ergonomic handouts should be provided to instruct the patient on proper seated positioning. The computer screen height should be at or slightly below eye level, elbows resting at 90 degrees, feet flat on the floor, and the body positioned close to the desk to avoid scapular protraction. The patient should minimize sitting time because this position encourages spinal flexion. Frequent standing rest breaks every 30–60 minutes will readjust the sitting posture. An ergonomic chair with the use of a lumbar roll can help modify spinal flexion throughout a workday. A standing desk, although expensive, does encourage extension bias throughout the workday.

The risk of overexercising must be highlighted. Rigorous exercise can exacerbate symptoms. Signs and symptoms indicating an inflammatory exacerbation must be explained so that the patient can recognize the signs early in the flare-up. An exacerbation of symptoms may indicate both a need to return to physical therapy and a follow-up with the physician to initiate NSAID treatment.

Weight management is recommended to minimize stress on the weight-bearing joints and the cardiovascular system. Participation in high-contact sports, such as football, water skiing, and the like should be avoided.[63] Each person with AS will need to recognize personal limitations and safe activity participation levels. Low-impact aerobic exercise with a bias toward extension and rotation must be stressed. Regular lifelong exercise directed by a physical therapist is essential for maintaining overall wellness, safety, and function in people with AS.[78]

Follow-Up and Physical Therapy Goals

Duration and frequency of follow-up physical therapy visits is determined by the evaluating physical therapist at the time of the examination. Depending on the acuity, chronicity, limitation in function, and disease progression, treatment duration could range anywhere from 2–4 weeks to 8–12 weeks. Visit frequency during an episode of care is determined by the treating physical therapist based on the information collected at the initial examination. Typically, visit frequency will increase as the number of identified impairments increases. A person's overall function tends to diminish with the increased number of impairments. Exacerbation and remission periods are common throughout the course of AS. A patient may be referred to physical therapy more than once if an exacerbation occurs and/or if the patient's presentation changes.

Physical therapy outcome goals are influenced by disease progression. Physical therapy interventions are based on the patient's individualized goals, the physical therapist's clinical decision making, and the available research.

The patient is appropriate for a physical therapy referral given the new diagnosis and limited ROM into all directions including the lumbar, thoracic, and cervical spine. Physical therapy management needs to include an evaluation, extension-bias activities, lumbar and postural strengthening, manual therapy, gentle stretching, and education on disease progression, activity modifications, and workstation ergonomics.

PSYCHOLOGICAL INTERVENTION

In 1977, the psychiatrist George Engle outlined his biopsychosocial model of disease and pointed out that "psychological and social factors are not only sequelae but also determinants of the biological state of the individual" and that "an individual's ongoing psychosocial status influences behavioral choices such as adherence to medical treatment, exercise, nutrition, and social contact, which, in turn, have an impact on the disease process."[79:162] The impact of AS on psychological health has been studied, and it is not uncommon for patients to respond in anxious or depressed ways.[80] Baysal et al.[80:795] reported that "the psychological status had close interaction with disease activity and quality of life in patients with AS." Martindale et al.[81] also found that AS disease status scores correlated significantly with anxiety, depression, internality, and health status, and they also said that healthcare providers should take into account the psychological health of the patient. In fact, Brionez et al.[82] found that psychological variables contributed significantly to the variance in BASFI scores and stated that psychological health should be examined and accounted for when assessing functional status in AS patients.

The effectiveness of psychological interventions with patients with rheumatologic conditions and diseases has also been demonstrated by several authors.[83–85] Research has also shown that decreasing suffering impacts rheumatologic pain outcomes and increases functionality.[86] Research has also shown the prevalence of work disability and its psychological impact among patients with AS and "the impact of pain, fatigue, and progressive disability on the individual's life style, career, family, and social life are likely to be long-term and far-reaching."[87:424]

When treating patients with persistent pain from a behavioral medicine perspective, it is not enough to look at reduction of pain but also to address how the person is suffering and in what way he may be disabled. In our case study patient, we can infer that the combination of a divorce plus workplace stress, extended periods of limited movement (given his 80-plus hour work week), and persistent pain from his condition create "the perfect storm." All of this will impact his mental abilities, which are needed to address and respond to pain.

In general, the overall treatment goals for this patient consist of (1) learning to live and thrive in spite of pain, (2) learning to find meaning in the life being lived, and (3) finding ways of expressing himself in a healthy fashion. Clearly, he will have to learn how to increase self-awareness for pacing during the workday to avoid holding postures for extended periods of time. He will have to learn how to juggle the anxieties of an intense work environment, the dissolution of a marriage, and persistent pain. It will be important to determine what he thinks about his life and whether he finds meaning in the life that he is living.

Treatment planning consists of five elements. The first is restoration of homeostasis, which includes sleep hygiene and the maintenance of physical and mental health. Sleep is a critical element in chronic pain management because most self-regulation interventions require attention and concentration, and fatigue arising from lack of sleep interferes with these abilities. Even the use of distraction requires adequate alertness and an ability to maintain focus. Nutrition and the development of a balanced meal plan also should be a patient goal.

Foremost among behavioral interventions is assessment of our patient's psychological state. "Research has demonstrated the importance of psychological factors in coping, quality of life, and disability in chronic pain."[88:678] Is he responding in anxious, depressed, or angry ways? If he is, he will have to be taught how to think about his condition in ways that do not trigger his autonomic nervous system. In addition, he will have to be evaluated and treated for psychological comorbidities such as the presence of anxiety, depression, or other mental conditions (including personality disorders) that may contribute to his experience of suffering.

> Few individuals have images of themselves as disabled. When an individual is disabled, there are many emotional and intellectual struggles that emerge, including development of an evolving self-image as having a disabled body in an able-bodied world. It is the image of the broken self, the self no longer able to do for oneself and that is dependent upon others, the self that no longer fits into the image of pre-disability life, that engenders suffering and anxiety.[89:291]

When considering the nature of the suffering response, adjuvant medications to deal with the somato-affective component of the pain can help attenuate the overall experience of pain. In this case, prescribing an antidepressant with a strong anxiolytic component may be advisable.

The second focus of treatment is *self-regulation training*, which refers to the teaching of techniques and strategies for regulation of experience in the sensory, affective, cognitive, and conative realms. In the sensory realm, our patient would be taught skills to achieve states of physical and mental relaxation, as well as techniques for influencing awareness of pain, such as hypnoanalgesic techniques and mindfulness meditation. He would also be taught strategies for influencing his emotional state through development of self-awareness of somato-affective states and the internal dialogues producing those somato-affective states. He would be taught to examine his internal dialogue for its veracity, its temporal qualities (whether it might be anxious speculation about the future, sad remembrances of the past, or focused on the present moment), and whether it is helpful and positive in nature. The conative realm refers to striving, whether it is internal through the use of imagination or external through impulsive behavior. An examination of what he is striving for and whether those impulses support health and well-being are critical. As a prelude, however, we would begin with a psychoeducational approach to help him understand the difference between pain, suffering, and disability, as well as understand what the pain generators peculiar to his condition are. An important educational item for him will be understanding the impact of stress on pain, how pain management requires cognitive resources, and how those resources are limited when he responds to external stressors.[88] Assessing how he is coping with his divorce and its impact will also have to be addressed. Particularly as Sarno[90] pointed out, our patient will have to learn how the suppression of anger intensifies back pain.

The third focus is the *fostering of hope*, facilitating our patient's belief in his ability to respond to his medical condition and pain, and, most importantly, facilitating the patient in switching his goals from pain relief to alleviation of suffering. When an individual learns that he can influence his experience of pain, whether through physical means, pharmacotherapy, or psychological means, it increases his sense of self-mastery and efficacy and contributes to a feeling of confidence. If our patient were focused on a goal of pain elimination, chances are he would never experience total success. However, he can learn how to not suffer in response to the pain and experience success in a different way. Helping him understand that he is responsible for the hands-on management of his pain under the direction of his physician is critical. Just as the individual with diabetes is responsible for proper blood testing, administration of insulin, and adherence to nutritional guidelines, so must the patient with persistent pain learn to be responsible for managing his condition as well.

The fourth focus is *threshold management*, helping our patient understand how to pace himself, conserve energy, and build stamina and endurance. Many individuals believe that they should pace activity by monitoring pain and stopping what they are doing when the pain increases. Paradoxically, this increases the sensitization process and lowers the threshold. The only effective way to pace is to pay attention to time and change pacing or activity before the pain intensifies. This requires developing self-awareness, establishing a baseline of tolerance, and then increasing the time interval by 10% every 7–10 days. So, we would help our patient figure out how long he could sit or stand comfortably before there is an increase in pain and then maintain that time interval; when the time limit has been reached, he will need to change that activity (musculoskeletal demands), such as getting up from sitting and stretching or going for a walk. After 7–10 days, he could increase his sitting time by 10%. In any event, we know, given his condition, that he has to learn how to vary the biomechanical demands on his body and avoid extended periods of holding patterns and immobility.

The fifth focus of treatment concerns the arena of *performance enhancement*, helping the patient identify life goals, work tasks, and activities of daily living that he wants to engage in and helping him problem-solve how to accomplish them. Sometimes this is through making accommodations, using assistive devices, or maintaining and adhering to his exercise regimen program. An ergonomic assessment of his workstation may be helpful in maintaining neutral postures and providing good postural alignment. Given how much writing an attorney does, it would be very useful to ensure that he is dictating with a wireless headset so that he can stand while working or even to get a flexible workstation desk that can accommodate standing as well as sitting. In addition, our patient can be taught mental practice techniques [91] to assist with flexibility and increased range of motion.

INVESTIGATIONAL BIOLOGIC THERAPIES

A number of different immune targets are being investigated for the therapy of spondyloarthritis, including B cells, T cells, and IL-6.92 These therapies have included rituximab in patients who have failed TNF-α therapy and those naïve to TNFs. TNF-α naïve AS patients show as good a response to rituximab as that seen with initial TNF-α therapy. Individuals who have failed TNF-α therapy seem nonresponsive to rituximab in these investagations.93

Abatacept is a T-cell modulator CTLA-4 immunoglobulin that selectively dampens the CD80/86:CD28 costimulatory signal required for complete T-cell activation. It is approved for the treatment of rheumatoid arthritis. Clinical trials investigating the efficacy of this agent in TNF-α naïve and failure patients have shown a benefit similar to placebo.94

Tocilizumab is a monoclonal antibody to IL-6 receptor. IL-6 is a cytokine with multiple functions regulating a number of immune responses and inflammation. Case reports have suggested the potential for benefit.95 Clinical trials are under way to determine the potential benefit of this biologic therapy in AS.

REFERENCES

1. Braun J, Khan MA, Siepper J. Enthesitis and ankylosis in spondyloarthropathy: what is the target of the immune response? *Ann Rheum Dis.* 2000;59:985–994.
2. McGonagle D, Gibbon W, Emery P. Classification of inflammatory arthritis by enthesitis. *Lancet.* 1998;352:1137–1140.
3. Van Tubergen A, Coenen J, Landewe R, Spoorenberg A, Chonis A, Boonen A, van der Linden s, van der Heijde D. Assessment of fatigue in patients with ankylosing spondylitis: a psychometric analysis. *Arthritis Rheum.* 47:8–16.
4. Dagfinrud H, Vollestad NK, Loge JH, Kvein TK, Mengshoel AM. Fatigue inpatients with ankylosing spondylitis: a comparison with the general population and associations with clinical and self-reported measure. *Arthritis Rheum.* 2005;53:5–11.
5. Helmick CG, Felson DT, Lawrence RC, et al. Estimates of the prevalence of arthritis and other rheumatic conditions in the United States. Part 1. *Arthritis Rheum.* 2008;58:15–25.
6. Reveille JD, Ball EJ, Khan MA. HLA-B27 and genetic predisposing factors in spondyloarthropathies. *Curr Opin Rheumatol.* 2001;13:265–272.
7. Lee W, Reveille JD, David JC Jr, Learch TJ, Ward MM, Weisman MH. Are there gender differences in severity of ankylosing spondylitis? Results from the PSOAS cohort. *Ann Rheum Dis.* 2007;66:633–638.
8. Gran JT, Ostensen M. Spondyloarthritides in females. *Ballieres Clin Rheumatol.* 1998;12:695–715.
9. Bennett PH, Wood PHN, eds. Population studies of the rheumatic diseases: proceedings of the 3rd International Symposium, New York; 1966. Amsterdam: Excerpta Medica; 456.
10. Braun A, Saracbasi E, Grika J, Schnitker J, Braun J. Identifying patients with axial spondyloarthritis in primary care: how useful are items indicative of inflammatory back pain? *Ann Rheum Dis.* 2011;70:1782–1787.
11. Boyer GS, Templin DW, Bowler A, et al. A comparison of patients with spondyloarthropathy seen in specialty clinics with those identified in a communitywide epidemiologic study. *Arch Intern Med.* 1997;157:2111–2117.
12. Rudwaleit M, van der Heijde D, Landewe R, et al. The development of Assessment of Spondyloarthritis International Society classification criteria for axial spondyloarthritis (part II): validation and final selection. *Ann Rheum Dis.* 2009;68:777–783.
13. Dougados M, van der Linden S, Juhlin R, et al. The European Spondyloarthropathy Study Group preliminary criteria for the classification of spondyloarthropathy. *Arthritis Rheum.* 1991;34:1218–1227.
14. Spoorenberg A, van der Heijde D, de Klerk E, et al. Relative value of erythrocyte sedimentation rate and C-reactive protein in assessment of disease activity in ankylosing spondylitis. *J Rheumatol.* 1999;26:980–984.
15. Esdaile JM, Rosenthall L, Terkeltaub R, Kloiber R. Prospective evaluation of sacroiliac scintigraphy in chronic inflammatory back pain. *Arthritis Rheum.* 1980;23:998–1003.
16. Russell AS, Lentle BC, Percy JS. Investigation of sacroiliac disease: comparative evaluation of radiological and radionuclide techniques. *J Rheumatol.* 1975;2:45–51.
17. Forrester DM. Imaging of the sacroiliac joint. *Radiol Clin North Am.* 1990;28:1055–1072.
18. Kozin F, Carrera GF, Ryan LM, Foley D, Lawson T. Computed tomography in the diagnosis of sacroiliitis. *Arthritis Rheum.* 1981;24:1479–1485.
19. Oostveen J, Prevo R, den Boer J, van de Laar M. Early detection of sacroiliitis on magnetic resonance imaging and subsequent development of sacroiliitis on plain radiography. A prospective, longitudinal study. *J Rheumatol.* 1999;26:1953–1958.
20. van der Heijde D, Rudwaleit M, Landewe RBM, Sieper J. Justification for including MRI as a tool in the diagnosis of axial SpA. *Nat Rev Rheumatol.* 2010;6:670–672.
21. De Ryce L, Maas M, Tak PP, Baeten D. MRI-tis in the early diagnosis of axial SpA: issues and limitations. *Nat Rev Rheumatol.* 2010;6:666–669.
22. D'Agostino MA. Role of ultrasound in the diagnostic work-up of spondyloarthritis. *Curr Opin Rheumatol.* 2012;24:375–379.

23. Cohen MR, Reda DJ, Clegg DO. Baseline relationships between psoriasis and psoriatic arthritis: analysis of 221 patients with active psoriatic arthritis. *J Rheumatol.* 1999;26:1752–1756.
24. Gladman DD. Psoraitic arthritis. *Rheum Dis Clin North Am.* 1998;24:829–844.
25. Sieper J. Disease mechanisms in reactive arthritis. *Curr Rheumatol Rep.* 2004;6:110–116.
26. Carron P, van Praet L, Ven den Bosch F. Peripheral manifestations in spondyloarthritis: relevance for diagnosis, classification and follow-up. *Curr Opin Rheumatol.* 2012;24:370–374.
27. Arnett FC, McClusky E, Schacter BZ, Lordon RE: Incomplete Reiter's Syndrome: Discriminatory features and HLA-W27 in diagnosis. Ann Intern Med. 1976;84:8–12.
28. Russell AS, Davis P, Percy JS, Lentle GC. The sacroiliitis of acute Reiter's syndrome. *J Rheumatol.* 1977;4:293–296.
29. Good AE. Reiter's syndrome: long-term follow-up in relation to development of ankylosing spondylitis. *Ann Rheum Dis.* 1979;38:39–45.
30. Sieper J, Rudawaleit M, Braun J, van der Heijde D. Diagnosing reactive arthritis: role of clinical setting in the value of serologic and microbiologic assays. *Arthritis Rheum.* 2002;46:319–327.
31. Orchard TR, Wordsworth BP, Jewell DP. Peripheral arthropathies in inflammatory bowel disease: their articular distribution and natural history. *Gut.* 1998;42:387–391.
32. Yagan R, Khan MA. Confusion of roentgenographic differential diagnosis of ankylosing hyperostosis (Forestier's disease) and ankylosing spondylitis. *Spine St Art Rev.* 1990;4:561–572.
33. Olivieri I, D'Angelo S, Cutro MS, et al. Diffuse idiopathic skeletal hyperostosis may give the typical postural abnormalities of advanced ankylosing spondylitis. *Rheumatol.* 2007;46:1709–1711.
34. Durback MA, Edelstein G, Schumacher HR Jr. Abnormalities of the sacroiliac joints in diffuse idiopathic skeletal hyperostosis: demonstration by computed tomography. *J Rheumatol.* 1988;15:1506–1511.
35. Diatchenko L, Slade GD, Nackley AG, et al. Genetic basis for individual variations in pain perception and the development of a chronic pain condition. *HumMolGenet.* 2005;14(1):135–143.
36. Zubieta JK, Heitzeg MM, Smith YR, et al. COMT val158met genotype affects mu-opioid neurotransmitter responses to a pain stressor. *Science.* 2003;299(5610):1240–1243.
37. Diatchenko L, Nackley AG, Slade GD, et al. Catechol-O-methyltransferase gene polymorphisms are associated with multiple pain-evoking stimuli. *Pain.* 2006;125(3):216–224.
38. Nackley AG, Shabalina SA, Tchivileva IE, et al. Human catechol-O-methyltransferase haplotypes modulate protein expression by altering mRNA secondary structure. *Science.* 2006;314(5807):1930–1933.
39. van Meurs JB, Uitterlinden AG, Stolk L, et al. A functional polymorphism in the catechol-O-methyltransferase gene is associated with osteoarthritis-related pain. *Arthritis Rheum.* 2009;60(2):628–629.
40. American College of Rheumatology Pain Management Task Force. Report of the American College of Rheumatology Pain Management Task Force. *Arthritis Care Res.* 2010;62:590–599.
40a. Van Tubergen AM, Landewe RBM. Tools for monitoring spondylitis in clinical practice. Nat Rev Rheumatol 2009;5:608–615
41. Passalent LA, Soever LJ, O'Shea FD, Inman RD. Exercise in ankylosing spondylitis: discrepancies between recommendations and reality. *J Rheumatol.* 2010;37:835–841.
42. Song IH, Poddubnyy DA, Rudwaleit M, Sieper J. Benefits and risks of ankylosing spondylitis treatment with nonsteroidal anti-inflammatory drugs. *Arthritis Rheum.* 2008;58:929–938.
43. Wanders A, van de Heijde D, Landewe R, Behier JM, Calin A, Olivieri I, Zeidler H, Dougados M. Nonsteroidal anti-inflammatory drugs reduce radiographic progression in patients with ankylosing spondylitis: a randomized clinical trial. *Arthritis Rheum.* 52:1756–1765.
44. Calin A, Elswood J. A prospective nationwide cross-sectional study of NSAID usage in 1331 patients with ankylosing spondylitis. *J Rheumatol.* 1990;17:801–803.
45. Dougados M, Behier JM, Jolchine I, et al. Efficacy of celecoxib, a cyclooxygenase-2–specific inhibitor, in the treatment of ankylosing spondylitis: a six-week controlled study with comparison against placebo and against a conventional nonsteroidal anti-inflammatory drug. *Arthritis Rheum.* 2001;44:180–185.
46. Maugars Y, Mathis C, Berthelot JM, Charlier C, Prost A. Assessment of the efficacy of sacroiliac corticosteroid injections in spondyloarthropathies: a double-blind study. *Br J Rheumatol.* 1996;35:767–770.
47. Chen J, Liu C. Is sulfazalazine effective in ankylosing spondylitis? A systematic review of randomized controlled trials. *J Rheumatol.* 2006;33:722–731.
48. Gonzalez-Lopez L, Garcia-Gonzalez A, Vazquez-Del-Merado M, Munoz-Valle JF, Gamez-Nava JL. Efficacy of methotrexate in ankylosing spondylitis: a randomized, double-blind, placebo controlled trial. *J Rheumatol.* 2004;31:1568–1574.
49. Haibel H, Rudwaleit M, Braun J, Sieper J. Six months open label trial of leflunomide in active ankylosing spondylitis. *Ann Rheum Dis.* 2005;64:124–126.
50. Marzo-Ortega H, McGonagle D, Jarrett S, et al. Infliximab in combination with methotrexate and Infliximab in patients with ankylosing spondylitis: a clinical and imaging study. *Ann Rheum Dis.* 2005;64:1568–1575.
51. van der Heijde D, Dijkmans B, Geusens P, et al. Efficacy and safety of infliximab in patients with ankylosing spondylitis: results of a randomized placebo-controlled trial (ASSERT). *Arthritis Rheum.* 2005;52:582–591.
52. Brandt J, Sieper J, Braun J. Infliximab in the treatment of active and severe ankylosing spondylitis. *Clin Exp Rheumatol.* 2002;20(suppl 28): S106–S110.
53. Gorman JD, Sack KE, David JC Jr. Treatment of ankylosing spondylitis by inhibition of tumor necrosis factor alpha. *N Engl J Med.* 2002;346:1349–1356.
54. Davis JC Jr, Van der Heijde D, Braun J, et al. Recombinant human tumor necrosis factor receptor (etanercept) for treating ankylosing spondylitis: a randomized, controlled trial. *Arthritis Rheum.* 2003;48:3230–236.
55. Baraliakos X, David J, Tsuji W, Braun J. Magnetic resonance imaging examinations of the spine in patients with ankylosing spondylitis before and after therapy with the tumor necrosis factor alpha receptor fusion protein etanercept. *Arthritis Rhum.* 2005;52:1216–1223.
56. Davis JC Jr, Van der Heijde D, Braun J, et al. Efficacy and safety of up to 192 weeks of etanercept therapy in patients with ankylosing spondylitis. *Ann Rheum Dis.* 2008;67:346–352.
57. van der Heijde D, Kivitz A, Schiff M, et al. Efficacy and safety of adalimumab in the patients with ankylosing spondylitis: results of a multicenter, randomized placebo-controlled trial. *Arthritis Rheum.* 2006;54:2136–2146.
58. van der Heijde D, Schiff MH, Sieper J, et al. Adalimumab effectiveness for the treatment of ankylosing spondylitis is maintained for up to 2 years long-term results from the ATLAS trial. *Ann Rheum Dis.* 2009;68:922–929.
59. Inman RD, Davis JC Jr, van der Heijde D, et al. Efficacy and safety of golimumab in patients with ankylosing spondylitis: results of a randomized, double-blind, placebo-controlled, phase III trial. *Arthritis Rheum.* 2008;58:3402–3412.
60. Braun J, van den Berg R, Baraliakos X. 2010 update of the ASAS/Eular recommendations for the management of ankylosing spondylitis. *Ann Rheum Dis.* 2011;70:896–904.
61. van der Heijde D, Sieper J, Maksymowych WP, et al. 2010 Update of the international ASAS recommendations for the use of anti-TNF agents in patients with axial spondyloarthritis. *Ann Rheum Dis.* 2011;70:905–908.
62. Gyurcsik Z, Andras A, Bodnar N, Szekanecz, Szanto S. Improvement in pain intensity, spine stiffness, and mobility during a controlled individualized physiotherapy program in ankylosing spondylitis. *Rheum International.* 2012;32(12):3931–3936.
63. Goodman C, Fuller K, Boissonnault W. Pathology: *Implications for the Physical Therapist.* 2nd Ed. WB Saunders; 2002.
64. Spoorenberg A, van Tubergen A, Landewe R, et al. Measuring disease activity in ankylosing spondylitis: patient and physician have different perspectives. *Rheumatology (Oxford).* 2005;44:789–795.

65. Imboden J, Hellmann DB, Stone JH. Section II rheumatoid arthritis and spondyloarthropathies. In: *Current Rheumatology Diagnosis and Treatment.* Vol. Chapter 18: *Spondyloarthropathies.* 1st ed. McGraw-Hill; 2004.
66. Ince G, Sarpel T, Durgun B, Erdogan S. Effects of a multimodal exercise program for people with ankylosing spondylitis. *Phys Ther.* 2006 Jul;86(7):924–35.
67. Middleton P, Pollard H. Are chronic low back pain outcomes improved with co-management of concurrent depression? *Chiropr Osteopat.* 2005;13:8.
68. Arroll B, Khin N, Kerse N. Screening for depression in primary care with two verbally asked questions: cross sectional study. *BMJ.* 2003 Nov 15;327(7424):1144–1146.
69. Haywood K, Garrat A, Jordan K, Dziedzic K, Dawes P. Spinal mobility in ankylosing spondylitis: reliability, validity and responsiveness. *J Rhematol.* 2004;43:750–757.
70. Cleland J, Alonso-Blanco C, Fernandex-de-las-Penas C. Preliminary clinical prediction rule for identifying patients with ankylosing spondylitis who are likely to respond to an exercise program: a pilot study. *Am J Phys Med Rehabil.* 2009;88:445–454.
71. Braun J, Pincus T. Mortality, course of disease, and prognosis of patients with ankylosing spondylitis. *Clin Exp Rheumatol.* 2002;20(suppl 28):S16–S22.
72. Braun J, van den Berg R, Baraliakos X, et al. 2010 update of the ASAS/EULAR recommendations for the management of ankylosing spondylitis. *Ann Rheum Dis.* 2011;70:896–904.
73. Wang C, Chiang P, Lee H, Wei J. The effectiveness of exercise therapy for ankylosing spondylitis: a review. *Int J Rheum Dis.* 2009;12(3):207–210.
74. Dagfinrud H, Mengshoel AM, Hagen KB, Loge JH, Kvien TK. Health status of patients with ankylosing spondylitis: a comparison with the general population. *Ann Rheum Dis.* 2004 Dec;63(12):1605–1610.
75. Dagfinrud H, Kvien T, Hagen K. Physiotherapy interventions for ankylosing spondylitis. *Cochrane Database Syst Rev.* 2008:23:CD002822.
76. Jordan C, Rhon D. Differential diagnosis and management of ankylosing spondylitis masked as adhesive capsulitis: a resident's case problem. *J Orthop Sports Phys Ther.* 2012;42(10):842–852.
77. Dagfinrud H, Kvien T, Hagen K. The Cochrane review of physiotherapy interventions for ankylosing spondylitis. *J Rhematol.* 2005;32:1899–1906.
78. Ozgocmen S, Akgul O, Altay Z, et al. Expert opinion and key recommendations for the physical therapy and rehabilitation of patients with ankylosing spondylitis. *Int J Rheum Dis.* 2012;15(3)229–238.
79. Broderick JE. Mind-body medicine in rheumatologic disease. *Rheum Dis Clin N Am.*, 2000;26(1);161–176.
80. Baysal Ö, Durmuş B, Ersoy Y, et al. Relationship between psychological status and disease activity and quality of life in ankylosing spondylitis. *Rheumatol Int.* 2011;31(6):795–800.
81. Martindale J, Smith J, Sutton CJ, Grennan D, Goodacre L, Goodacre JA. Disease and psychological status in ankylosing spondylitis. *Rheumatology.* 2006;45(10):1288–1293.
82. Brionez TF, Assassi S, Reveille JD, et al. Psychological correlates of self-reported functional limitation in patients with ankylosing spondylitis. *Arthritis Res Ther.* 2009;11(6).
83. Bradley LA, Young LD, Anderson KO, et al. Effects of psychological therapy on pain behavior of rheumatoid arthritis patients. treatment outcome and six-month followup. *Arthritis Rheum.* 1987;30(10):1105–1114.
84. Bradley LA, Alberts KR. Psychological and behavioral approaches to pain management for patients with rheumatic disease. *Rheum Dis Clin N Am.* 1999;25(1):215–232.
85. Keefe FJ, Abernethy AP, Campbell L. Psychological approaches to understanding and treating disease-related pain. *Annu Rev Psychol.* 2005;56:601–630.
86. Lin EH, Katon W, Von Korff M, et al. Effect of improving depression care on pain and functional outcomes among older adults with arthritis. *JAMA.* 2003;290(18):2428–2429.
87. Barlow JH, Wright CC, Williams B, Keat A. Work disability among people with ankylosing spondylitis. *Arthritis Care Res.* 2001;45(5):424–429.
88. Turk DC, Okifuji A. Psychological factors in chronic pain: evolution and revolution. *J Consult Clin Psychol.* 2002 Jun;70(3):678–690.
89. Appel PR, Bleiberg J. Evaluation and treatment of anxiety in neuromuscular rehabilitation. In: Mostofsky DI, Barlow DH, eds. *The Management of Stress and Anxiety in Medical Disorders.* Needham Heights: Simon & Schuster; 2000.
90. Sarno JE. *Healing Back Pain: The Mind-Body Connection.* New York: Warner Books; 1991.
91. Appel PR. Performance enhancement in physical medicine and rehabilitation. *Am J Clin Hypnosis.* 1992;35(1):11–19.
92. Song IH, Poddubnyy D. New treatment targets in ankylosing targets in ankylosing spondylitis and other spondyloarthritides. *Curr Opin Rheumatol.* 2011;23:346–351.
93. Song IH, Heldmann F, Rudwaleit M, Listing J, Appel H, Sieper J. Different responses to rituximab in tumor necrosis factor blocker-naïve patients with active ankylosing spondylitis and in patients in whom tumor necrosis factor blockers have failed: a twenty four-week clinical trial. *Arthritis Rheum.* 2010;62:1290–1297.
94. Olivieri I, D'Angelo S, Mennillo GA, Pistome G, Scarano E, Padula A. Abatacept in spondyloarthritis refractory to tumor necrosis factor alpha inhibition. *Ann Rheum Dis.* 2009; 68:151–152.
95. Henes JC, Horger M, Guenaydin I, Kanz L, Koetter I. Mixed response to tocilizumab for ankylosing spondylitis. *Ann Rheum Dis.* 2010;69:2217–2218.

7.

TENDINOPATHIES

Troy Henning and Jeanne M. Lackamp

CASE PRESENTATION

A 21-year-old collegiate wrestler presents with right antecubital pain worsening over 2 months. The pain initially began while performing close-grip resisted curl-ups for the first time. Training-related activities are painful, particularly extreme shoulder internal rotation and elbow flexion. Prior treatment with ibuprofen 800 mg three times daily with meals resulted in no significant improvement. The patient demonstrates a high level of anxiety because he is concerned about his athletic scholarship and about an upcoming international tournament in Europe. He also finds that when he is stressed, such as before an upcoming examination, his pain severity worsens. He is referred to the Interdisciplinary Pain Medicine Clinic for further evaluation.

Past medical/surgical history is noncontributory.

Radiographic analysis: negative for fracture or other pathology of humerus and elbow

ROS is noncontributory.

Physical examination reveals a well-developed muscular male in no apparent distress. He weighs 72 kg and is 173 cm tall. Neurological examination demonstrates intact sensation to all dermatomes tested. Musculoskeletal examination demonstrates full strength in all myotomes tested with the exception of mild weakness of right elbow flexion: right elbow flexion with forearm supinated 4/5, elbow flexion with forearm in neutral 4/5, elbow flexion with forearm pronated 5/5 with slight pain, supination 4/5 and painful. Reflexes are +2 symmetrical at the biceps, brachioradialis, and triceps. Special testing is negative for Speed's and Yergason's tests. Hook's test reveals an intact distal biceps tendon. Palpation at the right biceps distal insertion at the radial tuberosity and at the antecubital fossa is positive.

QUESTIONS

1. What is the differential diagnosis for this patient?
2. What is the epidemiology of tendinopathies?
3. What is the anatomy of a tendon?
4. What is the pathophysiology of tendinopathies?
5. What are the clinical manifestations of distal biceps tendonitis pain, and how is it diagnosed?
6. How would this clinical situation be managed?
   a. Eccentric loading
   b. Glycerin trinitrite
   c. Tendon needle tenotomy/fenestration with or without the use of autologous blood or platelet-rich plasma tissue graft
7. What is the long-term prognosis?
8. How does psychological state effect the development and presentation of physical symptoms?

WHAT IS THE DIFFERENTIAL DIAGNOSIS FOR THIS PATIENT?

The differential diagnosis for this patient includes distal biceps tendinopathy, bicipital radial bursitis, distal brachialis strain, and elbow joint synovitis. Given the demographics of the patient, mechanism of injury, absence of significant past medical history, and physical examination findings, his injury is most consistent with distal biceps tendinopathy.

WHAT IS THE EPIDEMIOLOGY OF TENDINOPATHIES?

Tendon disorders account for 7% of all U.S. physician office visits annually.[1] Most commonly, these involve the rotator cuff, wrist flexor/extensor tendons, patella, and Achilles tendons.[2] Among athletic injuries, tendinopathy accounts for 30% of running-related injuries, 40% of elbow injuries in tennis players, and 32% and 45% of patellar tendon injuries in basketball and volleyball players, respectively.[1]

Traditionally, tendonitis has been used as a descriptive term for a primary tendon disorder. However, numerous histologic studies have revealed a paucity of inflammatory cells within diseased tendons. Current histologic studies reveal degenerative changes within the involved tendon. As a result, tendinosis is the currently preferred histologic term, whereas tendinopathy is used clinically.[2]

WHAT IS THE ANATOMY OF A TENDON?

Tendons are composed of multiple collagen fiber bundles. Each bundle is composed of progressively smaller groupings of collagen fibrils. The bundles are encased in an endotendon, and the entire tendon is wrapped in an epitendon. Tendons that curve around bony structures usually have a synovial-lined sheath (tenosynovial sheath), whereas others have only a paratendon layer. These layers serve to protect the tendon from frictional forces.

Collagen fibrils are composed of type 1 collagen (able to withstand high tensile forces) and elastin (provides flexibility). Water, proteoglycans, and glycoproteins form the ground substance. Within this matrix, tenocytes and tenoblasts can be found. Tenoblasts are immature spindle-shaped cells that eventually form tenocytes.[2]

The metabolic activity of tendons is much lower than that of muscle tissue. Additionally, some tendons have areas of hypovascularity or watershed regions making them potentially more prone to injury and portend a longer healing time.[2]

WHAT IS THE PATHOPHYSIOLOGY OF TENDINOPATHIES?

The pathophysiology of tendinopathies in humans is not well understood. What little is known is based mostly on extrapolations from experimental animal models and a few human studies. Some animal models support the notion of an early inflammatory response with acute tendon loading, whereas, with a more gradual loading model, only degenerative changes are found.[3] Alfredson's group performed microdialysis of human Achilles tendons in subjects with chronic tendinopathy. They found no difference in the prostaglandin E2(PGE2) levels in the diseased tendons versus normal tendons.[4]

Based on this information, Abate et al. proposed the *Iceberg Theory* to help explain the potential sequences involved in the development of tendinopathies. As shown in Figure 7.1,[2] The bottom of the iceberg represents the normal physiology of the tendons. Under normal cyclical loading conditions, tendons undergo periods of breakdown and repair, maintaining normal health within the tendon. If the tendon is overwhelmed with repetitive stress or exposed to local hyperthermic conditions during periods of strenuous exercise, microinjury of the tendon can occur. This leads to the overproduction of matrix metalloproteinases (MMP-3). MMP-3 leads to the breakdown of the tendon extracellular matrix and production of inflammatory cytokines platelet-derived growth factor (PDGF), leukotrienes, PGE2, and endothelial growth factor that continue to promote tissue injury. At the same time, hypoxia within the tendon stimulates the production of vascular endothelial growth factor (VEGF) that promotes neoangiogenesis. This process potentially weakens the tendon and leads to more tissue injury. Free nerve endings accompany the ingrowth of the blood vessels, which is paralleled with increased levels of glutamate, substance P, and calcitonin gene-related peptide (nerve pain transmitters). At some point after this step, the patient may become symptomatic and present to the office for evaluation. The later part of this theory can be used to help develop a treatment approach that will be discussed later in this chapter.

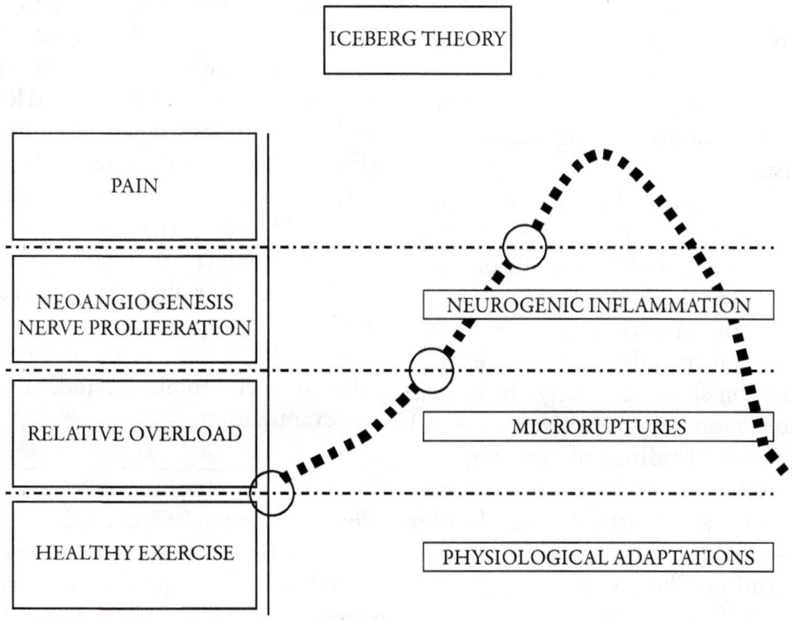

Figure 7.1 The Iceberg Theory of potential sequences in the development of tendinopathies. Reprinted with permission from Abate M, Gravare-Silbernagel K, Siljeholm C, et al. Pathogenesis of tendinopathies: inflammation or degeneration? *Arthritis Res Ther.* 2009;11(3):235.

WHAT ARE THE CLINICAL MANIFESTATIONS OF DISTAL BICEPS TENDONITIS PAIN, AND HOW IS IT DIAGNOSED?

Patients will typically report an insidious onset of discomfort around the region of the involved tendon. The interviewer should elicit information about activities that may have led to the injury. Specifically, inquiries should be made about sudden changes in activity level such as starting a new job, home project, sport, or activity. If the patient is an athlete, did he or she have a sudden change or escalation in the training program? Patients who work on an assembly line or who perform heavy manual labor should be questioned about the amount of maintenance exercise performed.

Pain will often be reported along or just distal to the tendon. Elicitation of pain with palpation of the involved tendon or activation and stretching of the associated muscle is common. Differentiating pain related to the tendon compared to the adjacent joint can be difficult at times. In general, painful articular structures should be provoked with passive movement of the joint while taking care to not stretch the adjacent tendons.

Our patient presents with a classic clinical presentation for tendinopathy. He likely injured the distal biceps tendon as a result of the sudden overstressing of the tendon with a new biceps curl exercise. The location of his pain, tenderness to palpation of the tendon, and ability to reproduce his pain with provocative maneuvers are all consistent with distal biceps tendinopathy. Although the Hook test may reproduce his pain, a firm end feel with lateralization of the tendon would help to confirm that at least some portion of the tendon remains intact.

RADIOGRAPHIC EVALUATION: PLAIN FILMS, ULTRASOUND, MRI

Radiographic evaluation of tendon injuries can include plain film imaging, ultrasound and/or magnetic resonance imaging (MRI). Several factors may play a role in which study(s) is ordered, including availability of the imaging modality and patient-specific characteristics.

Ultrasound is quickly becoming the study of choice for assessing soft-tissue structures of the musculoskeletal system. It has three times the spatial resolution of MRI (150 vs. 450 microns), can be performed around prosthetic joints without concern for artifacts, has virtually no contraindications, and can include a dynamic examination of the involved tendon(s). Additionally, diagnostic ultrasound is considerably more cost effective compared to MRI. Hallmark ultrasound findings of tendinopathy include a thickened heterogeneous or hypoechoic tendon (Figure 7.2). Enthesophytes and cortical irregularities maybe seen. Split or partial thickness tears of the tendon are not uncommon and may be associated with adjacent joint or bursa effusion. Doppler imaging may reveal neovascularization.

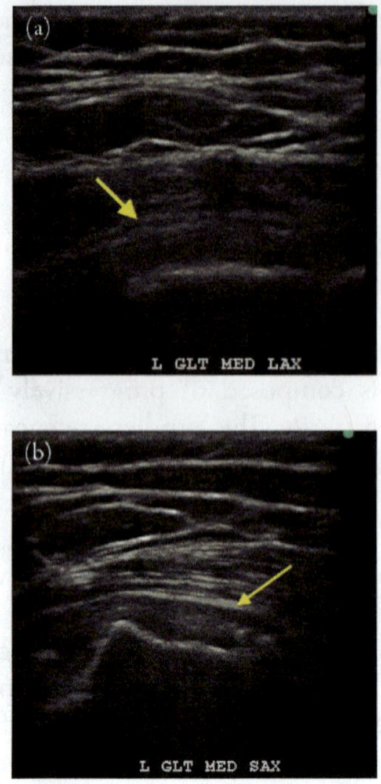

Figure 7.2 Ultrasound images of distal biceps tendinopathy. A: Long axis view of the distal biceps tendon. Top, superficial; left, distal; right, proximal; bottom, deep. Yellow arrows point to biceps tendon.

A potential limitation of ultrasound in the United States at this time includes the limited availability of qualified ultrasonographers. Fortunately, many physicians in a variety of fields (radiology, physiatry, family medicine, rheumatology, orthopedics, and others) are being trained to perform diagnostic scans of the musculoskeletal system. Also, ultrasound is not capable of adequately assessing intra-articular structures at this time.

If there is suspicion of an intra-articular process, a MRI maybe more appropriate. Obese patients may have too much adipose tissue overlying the region in question because adipose tissue attenuates the ultrasound signal making it more difficult to adequately assess for tendon abnormalities. Hallmark findings of tendinopathy on MRI include increased intra- and peritendinous signal intensity on fluid sensitive images (Figure 7.3). Fraying or tears along with enthesophytes and cortical irregularity may be present.

MRI has been the modality of choice for most providers in the assessment of tendinopathies. Potential limitations of this modality include presence of implanted electronic devices or metallic shrapnel in the body, risks of light sedation needed for claustrophobic patients, artifacts created by adjacent metal implants, and, last, the cost associated with the examination.

Diagnostic sonography of the distal biceps tendon and anterior elbow joint would help to confirm the diagnosis and help determine if activity restrictions are warranted. In our patient's case, distal biceps tendinopathy is confirmed with an absence of tendon tear (Figures 7.2 and 7.3). Given the absence of a tear and the upcoming European competition, he can participate in training and events as tolerated, with heavy workout stress of the biceps limited to certain maneuvers. Presence of a tendon tear increases the risk of tendon rupture and would limit his training intensity and potentially jeopardize his ability to compete effectively. As can be seen from Figure 7.3, MRI of the tendon makes it more difficult to detect the presence/absence of tendon tear. Ultrasound in this case clearly has an advantage.

HOW WOULD THIS CLINICAL SITUATION BE MANAGED?

Effective treatment of tendinopathies generally should be tailored to each patient. Identifying causative factors during the history and physical examination of the patient is key to developing strategies to help the patient correct modifiable risk factors. Generally, younger, more active patients develop tendon injuries as a result of rapid progression of a training program or due to lack of maintenance strengthening exercises. Older individuals or those with repetitive stress injuries need to make adjustments to work volume and postural/biomechanical corrections and to engage in maintenance strength and conditioning programs. Education on modifying other risk factors, including smoking cessation and better management of systemic disease processes such as diabetes and obesity, is also important in creating an environment to help foster both tendon healing and prevention of future injury.

Traditionally, rehabilitation of tendinopathies has included the use of relative rest from offending activity, modalities, and splinting/ambulatory aides for modification of pain and inflammation followed by the introduction of a gentle strengthening/flexibility program.

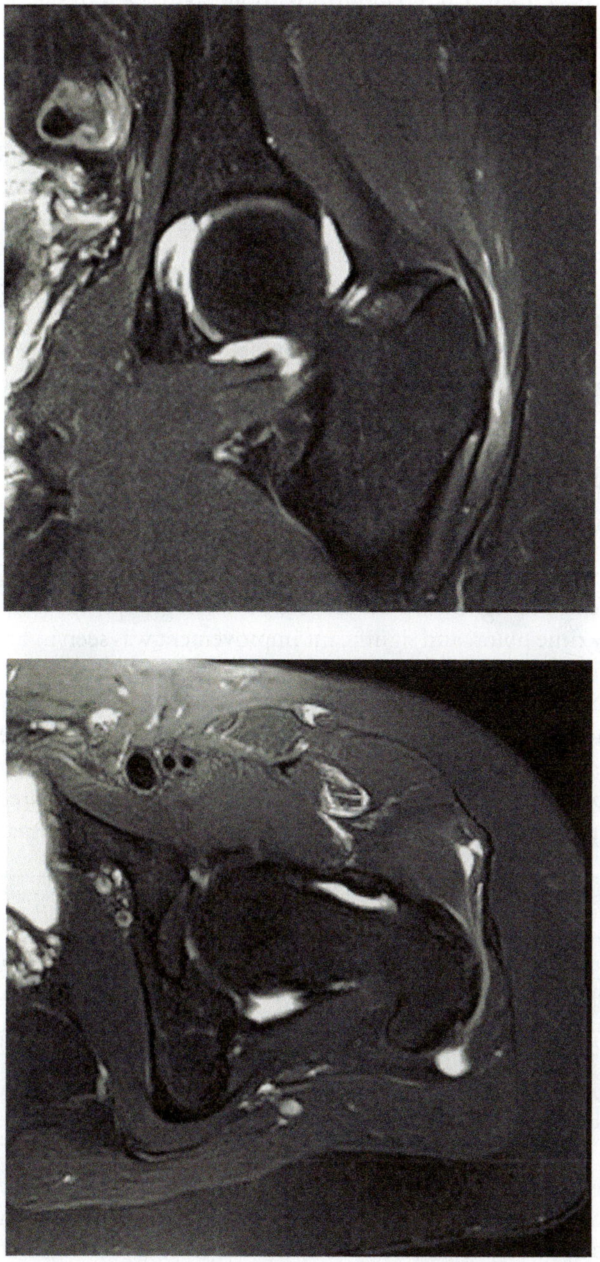

Figure 7.3 Correlative magnetic resonance image (sagittal PD) of the same distal biceps tendinopathy. Top, superficial; left, distal; right, proximal; bottom, deep.

ECCENTRIC LOADING

More recent literature supports the gradual introduction of a progressive eccentric-based strengthening program.[5,6] Eccentric strengthening involves a muscle contraction in which the origin and insertion are allowed to separate in a controlled fashion. Eccentric contractions allow for more motor units to be activated; as a result, more force is generated and spread along the musculoskeletal unit (bone/tendon/muscle). Eccentric exercise training was originally described by Stanish and Curwin in 1986 for the treatment of tendinopathy about the Achilles tendon.[7] Alfredson et al. then repopularized this program in several studies related to the treatment of Achilles and patellar tendinopathy. In 1988, Alfredon's group compared a progressive eccentric loading exercise program to a traditional nonoperative group for the treatment of mid-portion Achilles tendinopathy in athletes.[8] After 12 weeks of treatment, all the eccentrically trained subjects had a significant reduction in pain and were able to return to a preinjury level of activity. All subjects in the control group went on to have surgery. Eccentric exercise treatment has shown promise in other areas such as the knee[9] and elbow.[10]

Our patient should initially minimize undue stressing of the distal biceps tendon outside of eccentric loading in a controlled fashion. He should continue to maintain his strength and cardiovascular conditioning in preparation for his upcoming competition. He can continue to spar but may need to reduce the intensity of exposure based on pain levels and exacerbation of his symptoms. Consultation with sports psychology can help the athlete manage stress related to injury and time away from the sport. Sports psychologists are integral members of the sports medicine team at most major universities.

GLYCERIN TRINITRITE

Topical glyceryl trinitrite patches can be used to help with modulation of pain and to potentially enhance healing of the tendon. Murrell et al. studied the role of nitric oxide synthase in the healing of rat tendons. They discovered that blocking the synthase enzyme led to impaired healing and reduced strength of the tendon. Reactivating the enzyme led to normalization of the tendons.[11] Other studies have assessed the effects of topical nitroglycerin on the effects of tendinopathies in a variety of regions about the body.[12–14] A 5 mg/d sustained release topical glyceryl trinitrate patch cut into ¼ size (delivering 1.25 mg over 24 hours) is applied over the painful tendon and changed daily. One long-term study assessing use for noninsertional Achilles tendinopathy showed sustained pain relief through 3 years.[12] However, a 5-year follow-up study assessing treatment effect for lateral elbow tendinopathy only showed significant pain reduction up to 6 months.[13] Typical side effects can include headaches or hypotension.[14] One should use caution when considering use in patients already using nitroglycerin or phosphodiesterase inhibitors for other disease processes.

A trial of topical glyceryl trinitrate in this patient is warranted. It is simple to use and can be quite effective at modulating pain. He should stop use of nonsteroidal anti-inflammatories (NSAIDs) because we know this is not an inflammatory condition; additionally, NSAIDs may interfere with the healing process.

TENDON NEEDLE TENOTOMY/ FENESTRATION WITH OR WITHOUT THE USE OF AUTOLOGOUS BLOOD OR PLATELET-RICH PLASMA TISSUE GRAFT

Treatment of resistant cases may involve the use of needle tenotomy or fenestration with or without blood components (autologous whole blood or platelet-rich plasma [PRP]). Needle tenotomy, or fenestration, involves repeated needling of the diseased portion of the tendon along its long axis, including the enthesis and enthesophytes. Typically a 22–18 gauge needle is used for the procedure after the area has been adequately anesthetized through either a local tissue block or regional nerve block.[15,16] The needle is passed through the diseased portion of the tendon enough times to cause a softening effect of the tissue. Most of the literature supporting the use of these methods comes from case reports or series with small subject numbers.[5,15,16]

McShane et al. reported an initial case series assessing the effectiveness of needle fenestration along with corticosteroid injection for patients with persistent lateral elbow tendinopathy. At an average of 28 months post treatment, 63.6% of the patients reported excellent relief of pain symptoms. A follow-up study omitted the use of corticosteroid injection along with the fenestration; at an average follow-up of 22 months, 57.7% of the patients reported excellent pain relief.[16]PRP tissue grafts have been proposed as a treatment modality that can be used either alone or in conjunction with needle tenotomy. PRP has been theorized to help promote healing of bone and soft-tissue injuries including tendinopathies. A concentrated load of autologous platelets is delivered into the injured tissue with the intention of activating nearby fibroblasts, tenocytes, and other cellular components needed to normalize the tendon through exposure to supraphysiologic loads of transforming growth factor-β (TGF-β), PDGF, insulin-like growth factor (IGF-I), and epithelial growth factor (EGF).[17–19]

Thanasas et al, compared PRP versus autologous whole blood injections for the treatment of lateral elbow tendinopathy.[20] Only the assessors were blinded in this study. Primary outcome measures included change in visual analog scale (VAS) and Liverpool elbow score. A total of 28 patients were randomized to receive either a 3 mL injection of PRP or 3 mL of whole blood into the common wrist extensor tendon group. Both cohorts performed an eccentric loading exercise program after the injections. At 6 weeks postinjection, there was a significant difference in the VAS favoring PRP treatment. However, both groups revealed continued reductions in the VAS at 3 and 6 months without significant differences between the groups at these later time points. The Liverpool elbow score improved in both groups at all time points without differences between groups.

Mishra et al. compared nonguided buffered PRP grafting to nonguided injection of bupivacaine (control group) for the treatment of elbow tendinopathy. Analysis of this study is limited due to 60% of the control group subjects dropping out of the study at 8 weeks. The PRP group was followed for an average of 2 years post treatment. At final follow-up, these subjects reported a 93% reduction in pain level.[21]

De Vos et al. performed a double-blind, randomized controlled trial comparing PRP to normal saline injections for the treatment of chronic mid-portion Achilles tendinopathy.[22] Fifty-four patients were equally randomized with 100% follow-up of both groups. Again, both cohorts performed an eccentric loading exercise program after the injections. The primary outcome measure, Victorian Institute of Sports Assessment-Achilles (VISA-A), was assessed at 6, 12, and 24 weeks. No significant differences between groups was seen at any time point, and significant improvement was seen in both groups at 24 weeks.

At this time, it is still unclear whether adding autologous whole blood or PRP provides any additional benefit over needle tenotomy alone. In this author's opinion, these techniques should be utilized only after a patient has not demonstrated a response to a progressive 3-month eccentric exercise program.

> Tendon fenestration and/or autologous blood or PRP tissue grafting maybe an option for this patient if his pain persists beyond the sports season or if he has to refrain from competition for a prolonged period of time. These procedures can cause a flare up of symptoms (up to 8 weeks in this author's experience). Ability to participate in training and sports maybe significantly limited during this period of time. Additionally, the tendon maybe weakened by this treatment.

To date, there are no studies assessing the effect these procedures have on tendon strength. Post-treatment protocols that limit activity level or utilize splinting to protect the tendon are based solely on clinical judgment and vary considerably by practitioner. Outside of these interventions, surgery is not warranted for subacute (the patient in this chapter's case presentation) cases of tendinopathy. Surgery may be followed by a prolonged convalescent period to allow the tendon to heal. Additionally, surgery or major trauma about the elbow places the patient at risk for joint contracture. Given these risk factors, surgery should be reserved for those cases where complete disruption of the tendon has occurred.

WHAT IS THE LONG-TERM PROGNOSIS?

Tendon injuries are a very common reason for patients to seek medical care. Tendonitis has traditionally been used as the diagnostic term; however, this implies the presence of an inflammatory process. Recent evidence supports the notion that repetitive microtrauma leads to degenerative changes within the tendon. As a result, tendinopathy or tendinosis are the preferred clinical terms. Clinical suspicion of tendinopathy can be confirmed with either diagnostic ultrasound or MRI. Management typically involves modification of activities to prevent ongoing injury in concert with a progressive eccentric loading exercise program. Interventional techniques such as tenotomy with or without autologous blood or PRP injections can be performed if patients do not respond to the exercise prescription.

HOW DOES PSYCHOLOGICAL STATE EFFECT THE DEVELOPMENT AND PRESENTATION OF PHYSICAL SYMPTOMS?

Further discussion with the patient and review of referring medical records shows that he has been described as quiet and compliant. He has been seen by his PCP for the past 3 years, and usually for a variety of mild-moderate musculoskeletal complaints. Largely these were given nonspecific diagnoses and have always been attributed to the patient's involvement with athletic competition. Many times these complaints would precede important, stressful events for the patient (final exams, match against the rival school, etc.). Usual treatment course has involved NSAIDs +/– physical therapy and the complaints have resolved over time, even though it is unclear if the interventions were useful.

OVERVIEW

> In the days of the Malleus, if the physician could find no evidence of natural illness, he was expected to find evidence of witchcraft; today, if he cannot diagnose organic illness, he is expected to diagnose mental illness.
>
> —THOMAS SZASZ, *The Manufacture of Madness (1997)*

The terms "somatic," "somatoform," and "somatization" all share the ancient Greek root *soma*—that is, the *body* of a being (www.merriam-webster.com). Patients who are focused on bodily sensations are commonly labeled as "somatizers," and patients with frequent somatic complaints present challenges in every field of medicine. Patients with verified or established medical illnesses are unlikely to be referred to as somatizers until or unless their worries extend beyond (subjective) clinician expectations. Conversely, patients who do not have established medical illnesses, yet persist in reporting physical symptoms, are more quickly labeled as somatizers.

Patients with somatic complaints may report poorly characterized physical symptoms that are difficult to detect, tricky to treat, and changeable over time. They may have had multiple medical tests completed, but have not received satisfactory answers regarding the etiology of their physical problems. They often have tried multiple treatments with limited success. Patients are desperate for answers, and desperate for relief of their presenting symptoms. Clinicians caring for these patients may experience anxiety, frustration, and helplessness, and may recommend psychiatric consultation referrals).

Current Concepts Regarding Somatization

Somatizing, or the process of focusing on physical symptoms, is a common patient characteristic. It is not a simple one, however, and clinicians have struggled for centuries to describe, understand, and treat it. Patients with somatic issues are seen throughout all medical practices throughout the world, and our taxonomy is far from standardized. Articles written about somatic-spectrum issues and treatments have mind-boggling variability, so it is difficult to identify a coherent set of guidelines for clinical diagnosis and management. A further complicating factor is that there are, obviously, no research papers that utilize our latest criteria and diagnoses (see below). Thus, current evaluation, management, and recommendation strategies are predicated upon past diagnostic categories. It remains to be seen how closely the new diagnoses will match up with earlier ones and how effective previously-used treatment strategies will be.

Modern ideas of somatic-spectrum illness are built upon the rather simplistic models of the past—from the works of Sydenham, Briquet, Reynold, and Charcot, all of whom commented on "hysteria" as a medical issue; Steckel who cited neurosis and anxiety as leading to organic/somatic symptoms; and Freud and Breur who drew further connections between emotional stress and physical symptoms.[23,24] Important concepts now seen in somatization literature include "medically unexplained symptoms," "somatosensory amplification," and "illness behavior."[23]

"Medically unexplained symptoms" (sometimes abbreviated as MUS) long were the cornerstones of diagnosing somatic-spectrum illnesses. This diagnostic feature previously set somatic complaints apart from other psychiatric or medical issues. Unfortunately, this term reinforces so-called mind-body dualism; that is, if there wasn't a physical problem identified, the patient must have a mental problem.[23,25] There also was the implication of certitude. While deeming something "unexplained" was difficult to prove, once a symptom was labeled "medically unexplained" some clinicians ceased their quest for additional information, pertinent clinical signs/symptoms, or treatment options to the despair and frustration of their patients.[23,25] One author cautions, "functional somatic symptoms are best considered as a working hypothesis based on probability rather than a definitive diagnosis."[26] It is based on these concerns, and others, that the requirement for symptoms to be "medically unexplained" has been removed from the most recent edition of the DSM.

"Somatosensory amplification," or a heightened sense of body sensations, is described in somatic patient populations. Patients are acutely aware of bodily feelings, they preferentially identify and focus on "weak or infrequent bodily sensations," and they react more dramatically to these sensations than nonsomatic peers.[23]

Finally, "illness behavior" is the patient's inability to perceive, evaluate, or act in an expected manner given the information provided by medical clinicians.[23] There are several common tasks undertaken by people who are medically ill, as detailed by Groves and Muskin. First, they have to accurately acknowledge their illness. Second, they have to achieve "regressive dependency" on others to assist in their care. And finally, they have to resume normal function and activities when they recover (if applicable).[27] The challenge faced by providers who treat somatic patients is that patients may fail to navigate these domains in what is judged to be an appropriate way. They may identify illness where there is none, and they may lack the ability to follow clinician recommendations based on presence or absence of disease. They may achieve regressive dependency, but then fail to resume expected function once evaluation or treatment is completed.

Clinicians now recognize that there are many etiological factors that contribute to patient reports of medical symptoms. One comprehensive review of somatization cited elements such as pathophysiology (physiological, psychological, and interpersonal); genetic factors; developmental factors (starting in childhood via personal experience or observation); cognitive theories; personality characteristics (particularly introspection and negativity); abuse histories; sociocultural factors (now recognized as more universal than previously thought); gender issues; and iatrogenesis.[23] Added to these can be personal and family or friend expectations and reactions to illness, and (in some cases) secondary gains or benefits.[28] Thus, somatic disorder etiologies include *factors that would play a role in any other medical or psychiatric diagnosis*. Somatic complaints, therefore, should be seen as a complex interplay of all possible etiologies, and not as one simple causal link between emotional distress and physical symptoms.

An element of somatic complaints that distinguishes them from some other psychiatric diagnoses is their heavy prevalence in general medical arenas, even more than in psychiatric clinics. While it is commonly known that many patients with general psychiatric issues such as anxiety and depression seek treatment from primary care physicians, somatic disorder patients also are seen by primary care physicians and by a host of other specialists. Articles about somatic issues span all medical specialties from general medicine, to obstetrics, to neurology, to pain management, and so on. It is by the very nature of their physical symptoms that these patients commonly find themselves visiting multiple clinicians prior to, or instead of, seeing a psychiatrist. This should not be surprising—after all, any one of us concerned about a physical symptom would seek the care of a primary care or other "physical" health provider, not a mental health provider.[29] Typically, it is only when physicians fail to identify physical conditions to correlate with reported physical symptoms that referrals to mental health providers and discussion of psychiatric issues emerge.

Notably, many patients with somatic-spectrum illnesses decline offers of psychiatric treatment[30] and may (mis)interpret such referrals as meaning that their providers "disbelieve their symptoms, think that the patient has made them up or view them as weak or selfish individuals who are to blame for their symptoms."[26] Thus, primary care physicians and other medical specialists find themselves in a two-pronged battle: evaluating and referring the patient appropriately while navigating the patient's reactions to said evaluations and referrals.

Frustration among Clinicians

In a classic 1978 article, Groves describes the struggles that physicians have with treating various types of "hateful patients," that is, "patients whom most physicians dread."[31] These are not strictly somatizing patients, but one can readily identify characteristics of somatically preoccupied patients in Groves's "dependent clingers" and "manipulative help-rejecters." Dependent clingers are described as patients who conceptualize themselves as being constantly in need of treatment. These patients relentlessly seek medical treatment, to the exhaustion and frustration of their providers. In contrast, manipulative help-rejecters also may conceptualize themselves as ill but "they appear to feel that no regimen will help."[31] These patients continue to deny relief or cure, despite all efforts on the part of their physicians—in fact, "their pessimism and tenacious nay-saying appear to increase in direct proportion to the physician's efforts and enthusiasm."[31] Clinicians readily identify these two contrasting types of patients as similarly frustrating and exhausting, and often present with somatic symptoms.

Many papers have addressed the issue of provider frustration in caring for somatic patients. Providers find these patients to be challenging, not only because of the refractory nature of their symptoms but also because of the complexities of the patient interaction.[30] Some authors note that providers "often feel blamed for their poor results in managing patients with mental illness and also feel that they are unable to do so and have emphasised the sense of frustration, anger and powerlessness in the face of patients with persisting somatising symptoms."[32] Providers can feel ill-unequipped to manage these patients, which can lead to over-testing and over-treating, since they worry about missing a physical illness. Further, general practitioners or other medical specialists often hesitate to diagnose psychiatric issues, as they perceive them as outside their scope of practice.[33]

One study looking at high utilizer patients (those in the top decile of outpatient visits) noted that many patients had high scores for anxiety, depression, and somatization. Over one-third of these patients were seen as "frustrating" to their physicians.[34] In comparing "frustrating," "typical," and "satisfying" patient groups, physician determination of disease severity was similar among three groups of patients. However, the group of "frustrating" patients rated their own health less positively, reported more somatic problems and disability, and also utilized more medical services.[34] This highlights the important role of patient perceptions and interpretations of their sickness, and the tendency for these patients to continue pursuing medical care when they conceive themselves as ill.

DSM CLASSIFICATIONS

History of Somatic-Spectrum Disorders Described in the Diganostic and Statistical Manual

As recently as the DSM-II in 1968 and the ICD-9 in 1977, labels existed such as "Hysterical Neurosis," "Hypochondriacal Neurosis," "Psychalgia," and "Other Neurotic Disorders: Somatization Disorder, Briquet's Disorder."[24,28,35] It was not until 1980 that the DSM-III included a category for "Somatoform Disorders." Here, somatoform disorders were distinguished from other disorders thought to be under voluntary control and gained traction as formal diagnoses apart from simple "neurosis."[24,35]

Few changes were made to DSM-III criteria through the DSM-III-R and DSM-IV-TR iterations, though the addition of "Undifferentiated Somatoform Disorder" in DSM-IV was notable.[24,28,35] The DSM-IV criteria were criticized for several reasons. First, Somatization Disorder criteria were judged to be so strict that virtually no patients fully met criteria for this diagnosis.[36,37] Second, Undifferentiated Somatoform Disorder criteria were felt to be too lenient or vague, and therefore this diagnosis also was rarely used.[37] Finally, these diagnoses were identified as clumsy for nonpsychiatrists to use effectively in their daily practice.

DSM-5 Classification

With the unveiling of the DSM-5 in May 2013, clinicians were faced with new diagnostic entities and changes to existing disorders. Previous diagnoses of Somatization Disorder, Undifferentiated Somatoform Disorder, Conversion Disorder, Pain Disorder, Hypochondriasis, and Body Dysmorphic Disorder were replaced and changed to fit into the new category of "Somatic Symptom and Related Disorders." New diagnostic entities include Somatic Symptom Disorder, Illness Anxiety Disorder, Conversion Disorder (eliminating the requirement for an inciting trigger or precipitating stressor and replacing it with specifiers), Psychological Factors Affecting Other Medical Conditions, Factitious Disorder (which now has a new place in the realm of somatic symptom diagnoses), and Other Specified Somatic Symptom and Related Disorder. Goals included making the diagnoses more accessible and understandable for nonpsychiatric providers (eg, primary care providers, pain management providers, and the like); reducing the mind-body dualism associated with the concept of "medically unexplained symptoms"; and acknowledging that there are many reasons for patients to report (and worry about) physical symptoms.[38] Of particular importance is the emphasis on patient suffering regardless of the etiology of the patient's symptoms. To quote the DSM-5 text "the individual's suffering is authentic, whether or not it is medically explained."

GENERAL INFORMATION

Somatic symptoms, as previously described, are difficult to define and quantify. One has only to read articles about somatizing in primary care to find that data are plentiful yet inconsistent. Whereas nonspecific physical symptoms might affect up to 10% of the population, prevalence in medical arenas is variable.[39] Authors quote prevalence rates of medically unexplained symptoms in primary care anywhere from 3% to 74%.[26,30,39–44] Notably, there is a distinction between the number (or percentage) of patients versus the number (or percentage) of visits. In healthcare utilization data, it is recognized that relatively small numbers of somatizing patients may account for a relatively high number of visits.[26,44]

Regardless of specific nomenclature, somatic symptoms without physical health correlations are more disabling than symptoms from physical illness or other psychiatric illnesses.[29] Additionally, the more numerous the somatic complaints, the more dire the outcomes; having more somatic symptoms is associated with worse health status, risk of negative treatment effects, and iatrogenic sequelae.[44,45] Finally, according to one author, more than 90% of primary care patients reporting multiple somatic complaints continue to have symptoms up to 5 years later.[33] This may dovetail into studies describing higher rates of somatization symptoms, somatization syndromes, and hypochondriacal features seen as patients age.[46]

Of the six current somatic-spectrum diagnoses in the DSM-5, we will briefly review the first two: Somatic Symptom Disorder and Illness Anxiety Disorder. Readers may refer to the text of the new DSM-5 for further details.

Somatic Symptom Disorder

At its core, this new diagnostic entity focuses on distressing somatic symptoms that affect the quality of life. It is easy to see that this can include physical symptoms with or without physical illness diagnoses, physical symptoms related to other primary psychiatric illnesses, and physical symptoms related to other factors.

Furthermore, in a pattern that is all too familiar to clinicians patients may show and over-concern or rumination regarding somatic symptoms, which result in bothersome thoughts about the severity of illness, high levels of anxiety about symptoms, and inordinate time spent on these issues. Where the DSM-IV had a diagnostic entity specifically for patients who reported pain (Pain Disorder), the DSM-5 subsumes these patients under Somatic Symptom Disorder, with the specifier "with predominant pain." Other specifiers allow clinicians to describe the duration and severity of symptoms. Of note, in this new diagnostic scheme patients can in fact have a medical diagnosis, but their perception of symptoms and preoccupation exceeds what would be expected by their treating providers.

The prevalence of Somatic Symptom Disorder may be roughly 5%–7% in a general adult population[33] and, as in Somatization Disorder of the past, more females than males may meet criteria for this disorder.

Illness Anxiety Disorder

Most patients previously diagnosed with Hypochondriasis actually would be diagnosed with Somatic Symptom Disorder in the new DSM. However, if patients lack (or have only mild) physical symptoms but instead have prominent worry about having or acquiring an illness, they would qualify for the new diagnostic entity Illness Anxiety Disorder. Patients with this disorder are preoccupied with the thought of having or getting an illness as opposed to being preoccupied by physical symptoms per se. Like the new diagnosis of Somatic Symptom Disorder, patients can have diagnoses of medical issues. However, their worry and preoccupation is deemed out of proportion to the condition and would be judged by most providers as clearly excessive.

The prevalence of Illness Anxiety Disorder may approach 10% in a general adult population.[46,47] Contrary to Somatic Symptom Disorder, but similar to Hypochondriasis of the past, this disorder is thought to have similar prevalence in males and females. Additionally, Illness Anxiety Disorder may vary over time, may have a transient element in up to one-third of patients, and may be more prevalent as individuals age.

COMMON COMORBIDITIES

> After all, general practice can be characterised as the art of unraveling the medically unexplained.
>
> —WILLIAMS AND JOHNSON *2011*

Patient admitted increased stressors in his life since the unexpected death of his mother 6 months prior. Since that loss, patient reports feeling "alone" with limited family support. He describes his mood as down, adding "but I always try to smile." He does endorse occasional tearfulness, some trouble sleeping, variable interest and energy, and variable appetite with preserved weight. He denies psychosis or any suicidal thinking and does endorse brightening of mood in response to positive events (eg, socializing with family and friends, weight lifting). Patient endorses anxiety and worries about many things (including health and schoolwork).

Regarding his pain, patient states that he first noticed a similar pain several months before his mother died. This has progressed and worsened over time, despite repeated treatments. (Of note, he states that his mother was diagnosed with fibromyalgia and had issues with diffuse pain.)

Common Medical Issues

Somatizing patients can pose a particular challenge in the realm of pain management. Literature reviews reveal that many patients diagnosed with somatoform disorders (including former diagnoses such as Somatization Disorder, Somatoform Disorder Not Otherwise Specified, and Pain Disorder) have pain complaints as their main concern. Indeed, "among multiple somatoform symptoms, pain symptoms are very frequent, and somatoform pain disorders account for a major part of somatoform disorders in the general population."[48]

Researchers recognize that somatization and hypochondriasis are associated with chronic pain.[49] Degree of pain informs the presence of somatization and hypochondriasis, and pain treatment helps improve somatization and hypochondriasis in some patients.[49] Common areas of pain found to be comorbid with somatization include low back pain (LBP), other musculoskeletal pain, abdominal pain, and headaches. Many physicians cite LBP as particularly challenging to evaluate and treat. Some authors note LBP is "ranked first as a cause of disability and inability to work" and "the most prevalent form of chronic musculoskeletal pain worldwide."[50] They assert that there is higher frequency and severity of somatization, depression, and anxiety in patients with LBP versus those without, and that these patients have overall increased psychological distress and lower quality of life.[50]

It is important to remember that many somatic complaints can be subsumed under Somatic Symptom Disorder, not simply pain. As noted earlier, the DSM-IV criteria for full Somatization Disorder were very complicated. These included four pain symptoms, two gastrointestinal symptoms, one sexual symptom, and one pseudoneurological symptom. Our new DSM-5 diagnosis of Somatic Symptom Disorder does not require such a laundry list of symptoms. The specifier for pain hints at the fact that pain is a central theme for many somatic-spectrum patients, but the reader is cautioned to remember that pain is not the only complaint for many patients who tend to focus on physical health issues.

Healthcare Utilization

So-called high utilizer patients are challenging to study because the criteria for labeling someone as a "high utilizer" vary among researchers. Many papers note that patients with somatic diagnoses tend to have more medical visits than peers without somatic diagnoses, though this remains difficult to quantify. Nonetheless, many authors note that "clinically significant somatization" is extremely costly in the United States. As of 2009, estimated cost of care for these patients approached $100 billion annually.[30]

Some of this costly care is received through general medical physicians, but patients with unexplained somatic complaints are noted to have increased medical use related to specialist referrals, as compared to nonsomatic peers.[51] Other areas of care (including inpatient care, emergency department care, and diagnostic testing) have shown inconclusive results.[51] With regard to psychiatric treatment, authors note that MUS patients have "significantly elevated rates of medical, but not mental health, outpatient visits."[44] This relates to the concept that patients with somatic symptoms preferentially seek somatic care, not psychiatric care, since they believe they are medically ill. Simply put, somatizing patients "characteristically deny any psychosocial influences on their symptoms, resist psychiatric referral, remain unreassured following a negative examination, and are often refractory to palliative and supportive medical management."[44]

One challenge is that in certain cases, patients who report multiple somatic symptoms eventually will be diagnosed with actual (there read, "real") somatic disease. According to one article, "up to 10% of symptoms initially judged by general practitioners to be functional somatic symptoms will manifest later to have been the first presentation of organic disease."[26] This is a sobering reminder for clinicians. While it is important to avoid catastrophizing unsubstantiated physical complaints, medical science is imperfect. Sometimes, the only road to the truth is through time.

Psychiatric Comorbidities

Somatic symptoms are described in countless writings on depression and anxiety. While clinicians may not be able to clearly delineate which issues emerge first (somatic issues or mental illness) they can be sure of one universal truth: patients with somatic complaints experience mental illness and patients with mental illness experience somatic symptoms.

It is recognized that all types of somatic symptoms are associated with anxiety and depression, whether or not the symptoms are explained by actual physical illness.[28] Further, the number of symptoms can predict comorbidity: the more somatic symptoms a patient has, the more likely he or she is to also have co-occurring psychopathology, notably depression and/or anxiety.[29,45] Similarly, patients with depression are more likely to report physical symptoms to their providers.[23] Further, anxiety symptoms (with their obvious physical components, including tachycardia, tachypnea, tremulousness, diaphoresis) both increase the likelihood of reporting somatic illness and themselves can be mistaken for physical illness by both patients and physicians.[23] From a safety standpoint, patients with medically unexplained symptoms, particularly those who have unexplained pain, are at a higher lifetime risk of suicide.[39]

Somatization can be associated with other psychiatric illnesses, including psychotic illnesses (physical symptoms might emanate from medication side effects or even psychotic misinterpretation of bodily sensations); personality disorders; and substance use disorders (patients may have somatic sensations during use or withdrawal from a substance, and patients with chronic pain are at risk of addiction as well as over- and under-treatment with controlled substances).[23,39,52] The importance of identifying substance use disorders in the somatically focused population cannot be overstated, and is a topic well-deserving of its own chapter.

One author reminds us not to over-attribute physical complaints in psychiatrically ill patients:

> Physical symptoms of a patient who has a serious mental illness must not be considered less important than (or derivative of) his or her psychiatric symptoms or interpreted as somatization. People with mental illness have more general medical comorbidities and die, usually from medical diseases, at a much earlier age than the general population. In particular, physical symptoms of persons with serious mental illness may result from untreated physical illness, especially because many persons with serious mental illness... lack access to primary care. Such symptoms may also result from psychotropic medication side effects."[29]

TREATMENTS

Past medical treatments have included various NSAIDS, tramadol, physical therapy, and osteopathic manipulation. It is unclear how long the patient continued these medications and how useful they were in resolving the patients pain versus the natural history of his illness. The patient reported a long-standing history of diffuse anxiety sympotoms but has never been prescribed psychiatric medication.

Central Tenets of Managing Somatoform Spectrum Patients

The prevailing wisdom recommends that somatizing patients should be managed with well-coordinated care plans including frequent follow-up visits; limitation of unnecessary testing and treatments (to minimize iatrogenic harm); and clear, direct communication not only with the patient but also with other physicians who are contributing to their care.[23,43] Of course, in the real world, these plans may be challenging to put into place. Many patients come to treatment with limited records from other providers, limited understanding of the procedures and past treatment trials that have occurred, and limited ability to provide their clinicians with a complete picture of their medical history.

Who Should Manage Treatments?

Clinicians typically feel most comfortable managing patients who report clear, concise symptoms, and who respond quickly and thoroughly to treatment. When symptoms are variable and/or treatment response is incomplete, clinicians commonly reach out for assistance. This can be in the form of a consultation, request for comanagement of the patient, or (in dire straits) even transfer of care.

"Stepped (or progressive) care," "collaborative care," and "coordinated care" can be important in these cases.[39] Unfortunately, just as diagnoses are inconsistent, the terms for these treatment modalities are far from standardized. In some stepped care programs, treatment is offered based on severity of the illness, beginning with care by one primary care physician (PCP), and extending to integrated care with other providers as severity increases.[39] In other cases, stepped care refers to the gradual progression in treatment of pain (from simple medications to more complex, controlled substances and possibly utilizing several medications).[30] Another conceptualization of stepped care is the incorporation of regularly scheduled appointments with the same provider with regular, but decreasing, frequency.[26] Collaborative care highlights the importance of cooperation among all members of the medical team caring for the patient; coordinated care emphasizes that the patient's PCP is the care team leader.[39]

Recognizing that clinicians often refer patients for second opinions or consultations, we should be mindful that communication is of utmost importance. This is true in all steps of care: first, with patients during initial and follow-up visits; second, with patients when sending them for other consultations (particularly important when referring patients for psychiatric or psychological treatment to which they may be opposed); and finally with consulting providers who will need a thorough yet unbiased account of patients' history of present illness.

Ideally, treatment of patients with somatic issues includes some or all of the following: regularly scheduled appointments; documentation about origin of symptoms; establishment of treatment goals; restriction of examinations to the most crucial ones; control of specialist referrals and organization of care; management of the patient by one primary physician; reassurance; identification and mediation of psychosocial stressors; avoidance of ambiguous information about physical findings; avoidance of unnecessary testing; avoidance of unnecessary treatments; avoidance of mind-body dualism; sincerity and consistency; multidisciplinary approaches; and use of psychiatric referrals when needed.[43] So-called unfavorable physician behavior includes "either/or" dualistic models; poor cooperation among clinicians; overtesting/overdiagnosing/overtreating patients; communication flaws (including promoting anxiety, failing to clarify diagnosis, failing to address patient concerns, and not involving patients in their evaluation/treatment); inadequate or unstructured treatment planning; and utilizing treatments (medications, other referrals, work excuses) in a hasty or poorly considered manner.[39]

Studies of interventions with specialized clinical staff including mental health workers, counselors, and specially trained nurses have revealed some positive findings.[41,53,54] Unfortunately, it is unlikely that the average outpatient clinical practice could incorporate elaborate treatment modalities into routine clinical practice. However, in the era of quality improvement projects and emphasis on outcomes-based practice patterns, additional studies may lend credence (and funding) to some of thes ideas.

Pharmacological Treatments

Antidepressants of various classes might be helpful for somatically focused patients. Among antidepressants, selective serotonin reuptake inhibitor (SSRI) and serotonin norepinephrine reuptake inhibitor (SNRI) medications are fairly well tolerated and accessible for many patients.[23] Tricyclic antidepressants (TCA) also are popular for use in certain chronic pain patients. However, PCPs and pain management specialists are reminded to evaluate patients carefully for suicidal ideation, as all antidepressants can be fatal in overdose.[55] The classic question regarding antidepressants is whether these medications treat an underlying depression or anxiety disorder or a fundamental part of a somatic-spectrum illness.[23] According to Kroenke, "it seems the effect of CBT [cognitive behavioral theory] and antidepressants on somatic symptoms is not entirely mediated through reduction of depression and psychological distress... On the other hand, depression and anxiety frequently co-occur in patients with functional somatic syndromes as well as somatoform disorders, and some studies have suggested that somatic symptoms may improve to a lesser degree than emotional symptoms."[30] Additionally, patients may view psychiatric medications negatively and thus may decline offers to start such interventions.

There is some evidence that combining antidepressants and antipsychotics might confer an advantage to patients regarding their report of somatic symptoms and anxiety symptoms.[56] Caution should be applied, given the potential for side effects including metabolic syndrome with second-generation antipsychotic medications, which then can cause additional medical complications.

Psychotherapeutic Treatments

Overall, CBT has been deemed effective for multiple somatic-spectrum illnesses.[30] Recall, however, that much like psychiatric medications, many patients with somatic-spectrum illnesses decline psychiatric or mental health referrals for therapy.

In one study of "multisomatoform disorder" patients were randomized to either 12 sessions of psychodynamic interpersonal psychotherapy or several sessions of "enhanced medical care."[53] The authors found that patients who participated in the psychotherapy experience reported an increased physical quality of life but did not report less depression, anxiety, or healthcare utilization than the other cohort of patients.[53] There are several interesting elements of this study: first, that quality of life might not have a direct link to symptoms and/or healthcare utilization; and second, that psychotherapy (not increasing medical care per se) had more impact on quality of life. This should encourage physicians not to simply increase medical testing and treatments, hoping to improve their patients' outcomes.

Other Therapeutic Options

Activity

Out of creativity, or desperation, many authors consider alternative treatment modalities to help patients with medically mysterious symptoms. With regard to pain specifically, Hennings notes "physical inactivity is of relevance in the development and maintenance of depressive and somatoform disorders. As a possible intervention, regular moderate exercise can reduce depressive, somatoform, and pain-related symptoms and lead to an increase of function in chronic pain and functional somatic symptoms."[48] Indeed, in many studies of multidisciplinary therapies, even modest activity helped pain and psychopathology for patients with depression, pain, and multiple somatoform symptoms.[48]

Acupuncture

One study of somatic patients with medically unexplained symptoms looked at acupuncture as a novel, albeit not new, therapeutic intervention. These patients had 8 or more physician visits each year, and thus were targeted as relatively high utilizers of medical care. Patients responded positively to the 12-session acupuncture experience, citing increased psychological well-being and improved energy levels. While it is unclear how this would translate to other patient populations, the study was encouraging.[57]

"Psychophysiological" Treatment

Psychophysiological treatment, including progressive muscle relaxation, surface electromyographic biofeedback, and heart rate variability feedback, targets the central nervous system.[54] These modalities may be appealing to somatically focused patients because they are perceived as more "medical" (ie, less psychological) than CBT or psychiatric medications. Further, training in these techniques gives patient a measure of control over their symptoms, something which many somatic patients feel they are lacking.[54]

Reassurance

Patients with somatic complaints typically do not respond as robustly to reassurance as their clinicians would wish. Clinical studies have revealed that some somatic patients may be reassured, but later their health-related anxiety recurs. One possible exception is in the realm of Conversion Disorder, where some studies noted a better response to reassurance.[51]

Watchful Waiting

Recommendations for watchful waiting are sometimes spurned by patients who are eager for action and information, or by clinicians who may share a sense of urgency and desire for conclusive answers. In fact, in one study that promoted the concept of watchful waiting, the reduction in laboratory testing at follow-up visits might have been "due to the fact that not many patients returned." Are we to assume that the patients all got better, or perhaps went elsewhere for treatment?[42] In many cases, the more convinced patients are of their medical symptoms, the less likely they will be to adopt a "wait-and-see" attitude to treatment.

Additional Concepts

The clinician is reminded to consider culture as an important variable for both symptom reporting and treatment planning. This is no less true in somatic-spectrum disorders than in any other part of psychiatric practice. Indeed, as noted by Rief et al., "somatic symptoms may be an index of disease, an idiomatic expression of distress, or a form of social protest, etc."[46] Engaging patients in a discussion of their symptoms within their cultural context is an important step toward understanding patients' interpretation of their health status, and a critical part of treatment planning in which patient participation is required.

Satisfaction?

After reviewing studies that focused on satisfaction in somatic patients, it has been found that "overall, no particular type of somatoform disorder patient was more or less likely to be satisfied with their medical care."[51] This can be interpreted in two ways: Pessimistically, one could interpret this to mean that treatment options confer few differential benefits because these patients remain refractory to treatment and perpetually displeased. However, optimism is called for as immense room for improvement exists in the evaluation, treatment, and outcomes of these patients in need.

CONCLUSIONS

Our patient was relieved to have a "treatable" diagnosis and was complaint with all recommendations. After the patient discussed his stressors, he was able to recognize that his pain seemed to flare up after the passing of his mother and, in fact, past events were related to life stressors as well. A careful psychiatric evaluation revealed some increased somatic focus as well as nonspecific heightened anxiety symptoms that did not meet specific anxiety disorder diagnositic criteria. A plan of care was established for the patient to be seen monthly in the pain medicine clinic. In addition, every other month while at the pain center he would "check in" with the psychiatrist to see how things were progressing. Psychiatric medication was deferred at this time, given the patient's willingness to discuss emotional issues, optimism, and compliance with care.

Patients who report physical symptoms not borne out by, or beyond expectation for, medical illness can be taxing for any medical care provider. These patients have comorbidities in various realms of psychiatric and medical illness, and they pose diagnostic and management challenges. It is important to remember that the *patients* are suffering during these encounters; not just the clinicians who feel burdened by such patients. Managing these patients with clear expectations, appropriate caution, and genuine caring, while mindfully engaging other specialists and consultants as needed, can be a rewarding and successful endeavor for patients and clinicians alike.

REFERENCES

1. Skjong CC, Meininger AK, Ho SSW. Tendinopathy treatment: where is the evidence? *CSM*. 2012;31(2):329–350.
2. Abate M, Gravare-Silbernagel K, Siljeholm C, et al. Pathogenesis of tendinopathies: inflammation or degeneration? *Arthritis Res Ther*. 2009;11(3):235.
3. Xu Y, Murrell GAC. The basic science of tendinopathy. *Clin Orthop Relat Res*. 2008;466(7):1528–1538.
4. Alfredson H, Forsgren S, Thorsen K, Lorentzon R. In vivo microdialysis and immunohistochemical analyses of tendon tissue demonstrated high amounts of free glutamate and glutamate NMDARl receptors, but no signs of inflammation, in Jumper's knee. *J. Orthop. Res*. 2001;19:881–886.
5. Finnoff JT, Fowler SP, Lai JK, et al. Treatment of chronic tendinopathy with ultrasound-guided needle tenotomy and platelet-rich plasma injection. *PMRJ*. 2011;3(10):900–911.
6. van der Plas A, de Jonge S, De Vos RJ, et al. A 5-year follow-up study of Alfredson's heel-drop exercise programme in chronic midportion Achilles tendinopathy. *British Journal of Sports Medicine*. 2012 Mar;46(3):214–8.
7. Stanish WD, Rubinovich RM, Curwin S. Eccentric exercise in chronic tendinitis. *Clin Orthop Relat Res*. 1986;208:65–68.
8. Alfredson H, Pietila T, Jonsson P, Lorentzon R. Heavy-load eccentric calf muscle training for the treatment of chronic Achilles tendinosis. *Am Journal of Sports Medicine*. 1998;26(3):360–366.
9. Jonsson P, Wahlström P, Öhberg L, Alfredson H. Eccentric training in chronic painful impingement syndrome of the shoulder: results of a pilot study. *Knee Surg Sports Traumatol Arthrosc*. 2005;14(1):76–81.

10. Stasinopoulos D. An exercise programme for the management of lateral elbow tendinopathy. *British Journal of Sports Medicine.* 2005;39(12):944–947.
11. Murrell GA, Szabo C, Hannafin J, et al. Modulation of tendon healing by nitric oxide. *Inflammatory Research.* 1997;46:19–27.
12. Paoloni JA, Murrell GA. Three-year followup study of topical glyceryl trinitrate treatment of chronic noninsertional Achilles tendinopathy. *Foot Ankle Int.* 2007:1064–1068.
13. McCallum SD, Paoloni JA, Murrell GA. Five-year prospective comparison study of topical glyceryl trinitrate treatment of chronic lateral epicondylosis at the elbow. *British Journal of Sports Medicine.* 2011;45(5):416–420.
14. Berrazueta J, Losada A, Poveda J, et al. Successful treatment of shoulder pain syndrome due to supraspinatus tendinitis with transdermal nitroglycerin. A double blind study. *Pain.* 1996;66:63–67.
15. Housner J, Jacobson J, Misko R. Sonographically guided percutaneous needle tenotomy for the treatment of chronic tendinosis. *J Ultrasound Med.* 2009;(28):1187–1192.
16. McShane J, Shah V, Nazarian L. Sonographically guided percutaneous needle tenotomy for treatment of common extensor tendinosis in the elbow. *J Ultrasound Med.* 2008;27:1137–1144.
17. Leitner GC, Gruber R, Neumuller J, et al. Platelet content and growth factor release in platelet-rich plasma: a comparison of four different systems. *Vox Sang.* 2006;91(2):135–139.
18. Sampson S, Gerhardt M, Mandelbaum B. Platelet rich plasma injection grafts for musculoskeletal injuries: a review. *Curr Rev Musculoskelet Med.* 2008;1(3-4):165–174.
19. Paoloni JA, De Vos RJ, Hamilton B, Murrell GAC, Orchard J. Platelet-rich plasma treatment for ligament and tendon injuries. *Clin J Sports Med.* 2011;21:37–45.
20. Thanasas C, Papadimitrou G, Charalambidis C, Paraskevopoulos I, Papanikolaou A. Platelet-rich plasma versus autologous whole blood for the treatment of chronic lateral elbow epicondylitis: a randomized controlled clinical trial. *Am J Sports Med.* 2011;39(10):2130–2134.
21. Mishra A, Pavelko T. Treatment of chronic elbow tendinosis with buffered platelet-rich plasma. *Am J Sports Med.* 2006;34(11):1774–1778.
22. De Vos RJ, Weir A, van Schie HTM, et al. Platelet-rich plasma injection for chronic Achilles tendinopathy. *JAMA.* 2010;303(2):144–149.
23. Abbey SE, Wulsin L, Levenson JL. Somatization and somatoform disorders. In: JL Levenson, ed. *Textbook of Psychosomatic Medicine: Psychiatric Care of the Medically Ill.* 2d ed.. Arlington, VA: American Psychiatric Publishing, Inc.; 2011:261–289.
24. Kallivayalil RA, Punnoose VP. Understanding and managing somatoform disorders: making sense of non-sense. *Indian J Psychiatry.* 2010; 52(suppl1):S240–S245.
25. Williams AC, Johnson M. Persistent pain: not a medically unexplained symptom. *Br J Gen Pract.* 2011 Oct;61(591):638–639. doi: 10.3399.
26. Morriss R. Role of mental health professionals in the management of functional somatic symptoms in primary care. *Br J of Psychiatry.* 2012; 200:444–445.
27. Groves MS, Muskin PR. Psychological responses to illness. In: JL LEvenson, ed. *Textbook of Psychosomatic Medicine: Psychiatric Care of the Medically Ill.* 2d ed. Arlington, VA: American Psychiatric Publishing, Inc.; 2011:45–67.
28. Mayou R, Kirmayer LJ, Simon G, Kroenke K, Sharpe M. Somatoform disorders: time for a new approach in DSM-V. *Am J Psychiatry.* 2005; 162(5):847–855.
29. Minsky S, Etz RS, Gara M, Escobar JI. Service use among patients with serious mental illnesses who presented with physical symptoms at intake. *Psych Services.* 2011; 62(10):1146–1151.
30. Kroenke K. Efficacy of treatment for somatoform disorders: a review of randomized controlled trials. *FOCUS The Journal of Lifelong Learning in Psychiatry.* 2009; VII(3):414–423.
31. Groves JE. Taking care of the hateful patient. *NEJM.* 1978; 298(16):883–887.
32. Aiarzaguena JM, Gaminde I, Grandes G, Salazar A, Alonso I, Sanchez A. Somatisation in primary care: experiences of primary care physicians involved in a training program and in a randomised controlled trial. *BMC Family Practice.* 2009; 10:73.
33. Rief W, Mewes R, Martin A, Glaesmer H, Brahler E. Evaluating new proposals for the psychiatric classification of patients with multiple somatic symptoms. *Psychosomatic Medicine.* 2011; 73:760–768.
34. Lin EH, Katon W, Von Korff M, Bush T, Lipscomb P, Russo J, Wagner E. Frustrating patients. *J of Gen Internal Medicine.* 1991; 6(3):241–246.
35. Yutzu S, Parish B. Somatoform disorders. In: RE Hales, SC Yudofsky, GO Gabbard, eds. *American Psychiatric Publishing Textbook of Psychiatry.* 5th ed. Arlington VA: American Psychiatric Publishing, Inc.; 2008.
36. Frances A. The new somatic symptom disorder in DSM-5 risks mislabeling many people as mentally ill. *BMJ.* 2013; 346:f1580–f1581.
37. Frances A. DSM-5 somatic symptom disorder. *J Nerv and Mental Dis.* 2013; 201(6):530–531.
38. Moran M. The ninth chapter in DSM-5 contains disorders of disproportionate response to somatic symptoms. *Psychiatric News.* 2013; 48(5):7.
39. Schaefert R, Hausteiner-Weihle C, Hauser W, Ronel J, Herrmann M, Henningsen P. Non-specific, functional, and somatoform bodily complaints. *Deutsches Arzteblatt International.* 2012; 109(47):803–813.
40. Zonneveld LN, van't Spijker A, Passchier J, van Busschbach JJ, Duivenvoorden HJ. The effectiveness of a training for patients with unexplained physical symptoms: protocol of a cognitive behavioral group training and randomized controlled trial. *BMC Public Health.* 2009; 9:251.
41. Smith RC, Gardiner JC, Zhehui L, Schooley S, Lamerato L, Rost K. Primary care physicians treat somatization. *J Gen Intern Med.* 2009; 24(7):829–32.
42. van Bokhoven MA, Koch H, van der Weijden T, Weekers-Muyres A, Bindels P, Grol R, Dinant GJ. The effect of watchful waiting compared to immediate test ordering instructions on general practitioners' blood test ordering behaviour for patients with unexplained complaints; a randomized clinical trial. *Implementation Science.* 2012; 7:29.
43. Lopez-Garcia-Franco A, del-Cura-Gonzalez I, Caballero-Martinez L, et al. Effectiveness of a cognitive behavioral intervention in patients with medically unexplained symptoms: cluster randomized trial. *BMC Family Practice.* 2012; 13:35.
44. Barksy AJ, Ettner SL, Horsky J, Bates DW. Resource utilization of patients with hypochondriacal health anxiety and somatization. *Medical Care.* 2001; 39(7):705–715.
45. Creed FH, Davies I, Jackson J, et al. The epidemiology of multiple somatic symptoms. *J Psychosom Res.* 2012; 72(4):311–371.
46. Rief W, Hessel A, Braehler E. Somatization symptoms and hypochondriacal features in the general population. *Psychosomatic Medicine.* 2001: 63:595–602.
47. Noyes R, Carney CP, Hillis SL, Jones LE, Langbehn DR. *Psychosomatics.* 2005; 46(6):529–39.
48. Hennings A, Schwarz MJ, Riemer S, Stapf TM, Selberdinger VB, Rief W. The influence of physical activity on pain thresholds in patients with depression and multiple somatoform symptoms. *Clin J Pain.* 2012; 28(9):782–789.
49. Fishbain DA, Lewis JE, Gao J, Cole B, Steele Rosomoff R. Is chronic pain associated with somatization/hypochondriasis? An evidence-based structured review. *Pain Pract.* 2009; 9(6):449–467.
50. Bener A, Verjee M, Dafeeah EE, et al. Psychological factors: anxiety, depression, and somatization symptoms in low back pain patients. *J Pain Res.* 2013; 6:95–101.
51. Puri PR, Dimsdale JE. Healthcare utilization and poor reassurance: potential predictors of somatoform disorders. *Psychiatr Clin North Am.* 2011; 34(3):525–544.
52. Clark MR. Pain. In: JL LEvenson, ed. *Textbook of Psychosomatic Medicine: Psychiatric Care of the Medically Ill.* 2d ed. Arlington, VA: American Psychiatric Publishing, Inc.; 2011:901–927.

53. Sattel H, Lahmann C, Gundel H, et al. Brief psychodynamic interpersonal psychotherapy for patients with multisomatoform disorder: a randomised controlled trial. *Br J Psychiatry*. 2012; 200(1):60–7.
54. Katsamanis M, Lehrer PM, Escobar JI, Gara MA, Kotay A, Liu R. Psychophysiologic treatment for patients with medically unexplained symptoms: a randomized controlled trial. *Psychosomatics*. 2011; 52(3):218–229.
55. Kerr GW, McGuffie AC, Wilkie S. Tricyclic antidepressant overdose: a review. *Em Med J*. 2001; 18:236–241.
56. Huang M, Luo B, Hu J, et al. Combination of citalopram plus paliperidone is better than citalopram alone in the treatment of somatoform disorder: results of a 6-week randomized study. *International Clinical Psychopharmacology*. 2012: 27(3):151–158.
57. Rugg S, Paterson C, Britten N, Bridges J, Griffiths P. Traditional acupuncture for people with medically unexplained symptoms: a longitudinal qualitative study of patients' experiences. *Br J of General Practice*. 2011; 61(587):e306–e315.

SECTION III

SPINE AND RELATED DISORDERS

8.

DISCOGENIC PAIN

Irina L. Melnik, Richard Derby, Binit J. Shah, and Jason Eubanks

CASE PRESENTATION

A 30-year-old secretary presents with the complaint of low back and buttock pain for the past 6 months. There is no radiation of the pain to the lower extremities. The pain occurs mostly with sitting but is also worsened with standing and physical activity. Pain is relieved by lying down. There is no weakness or changes in bowel/bladder/sexual function observed. A course of physical therapy, nonsteroidal anti-inflammatories, and muscle relaxant did not result in noticeable improvement. The patient is referred to the Interdisciplinary Back Pain clinic for further evaluation and management.

Past Medical History is otherwise negative

Social History: History of one pack per day smoking for 11 years; social alcohol consumption is reported; no illicit drug use

Review of systems is otherwise negative

On examination, the patient weighs 74 kg and is 151 cm tall. She is sitting comfortably. Detailed neurologic examination reveals normal sensory and motor function, and reflexes are symmetric and 2+. The lower lumbar spine is tender to deep palpation over the midline. Flexion of the lumbar spine is limited by pain to 15 degrees; extension occurs to 15 degrees with minimal discomfort.

A magnetic resonance image (MRI) of the lumbar spine was obtained and was reported normal with the exception of a mild degeneration of the L4–L5 disc without evidence of disc protrusion. A high-intensity zone (HIZ)/annular fissure is also noted at that level.

QUESTIONS

1. What are potential pain generators in this case, and what is the likely diagnosis?
2. How is the diagnosis confirmed?
3. What is the incidence and prevalence of discogenic back pain?
4. What is the natural history of discogenic back pain?
5. What are the clinical manifestations of discogenic back pain?
6. How is discogenic back pain managed?
    a. Interventional procedures
    b. Psychiatric interventions
    c. Surgical options
7. What is the long-term prognosis for discogenic back pain?

WHAT ARE POTENTIAL PAIN GENERATORS IN THIS CASE, AND WHAT IS THE LIKELY DIAGNOSIS?

Low back pain (LBP) is a very common and complex disease of the spine, and it is one of the leading causes of chronic pain. It has profound effect on individual morbidity as well as on a society as a whole, given its substantial socioeconomic burden.

Many factors contribute to the complex nature of this condition. These include the complexity of the spine as an anatomic structure, with numerous potential pain generators within the spine that may cause symptoms similar in distribution and character. Additional factors may include confounding psychosocial issues, the subjective nature of pain itself, and the limitations of available diagnostic tools.

Targeting specific pain generators through precision diagnostic methods is the first step toward appropriate and effective treatments of spinal pain.[1]

Among common structures that are known to produce LBP are elements of anterior column (vertebral bodies, intervertebral disc [IVD]), middle column (nerve roots, ligaments of the spine, dura, and neural elements), and posterior column (facet joints, sacroiliac (SI) joints, soft tissue, etc.). Each one of those structures, if injured, could present with a specific complex of symptoms or could mimic symptoms similar to other painful structures within the spine.

Despite this complexity, specific tissue pain generators can be hypothesized based on history, physical examination, imaging studies, and response to directed treatment. Given the fact that these tests have been shown to have low specificity and sensitivity for diagnosing chronic benign spinal pain, interventional spinal procedures have been developed over the past few decades as the new diagnostic reference standards.

These interventional injection procedures can be used to test the hypothesis that pain is related to a structural abnormality hypothesized by clinical and imaging findings by systematically excluding various tissue causes of axial back pain.[1,2]

As reported, if one uses interventional diagnosis with precision fluoroscopically guided procedures as a reference standard for identifying pain, one can arrive at a diagnosis, identifying pain generators in approximately 70–80% of cases.[3,4]

Discogenic pain is defined as pain originating from the IVD itself.[5,6] It is nonradicular and may occur in the absence of spinal deformity, instability, and signs of neuronal tension.[7] Although the external outline of the disc may remain intact, there are many pathologic processes, including annular tears, degeneration, endplate injury, and inflammation, that can cause sensitization and stimulate nociceptors within the disc itself independent of nerve root involvement. The concept of discogenic pain was initially introduced by Inman and Saunders as early as 1947.[8] This notion was not fully accepted at the time because some believed that discs had no nerve supply. In 1959, Malinsky[9] demonstrated a variety of nerve endings in the outer third to outer half of the annulus fibrosus in cadaveric discs of various ages. In 1980, this finding was confirmed by Yoshizawa and colleagues who studied material obtained at surgical operations.[10]

Fernstrom in 1969 was first to use the term *discogenic pain* when he found the association between annulus stimulation and back pain perception during in vivo studies.[11] Crock[12] in 1970, defined the term *internal disc disruption* to describe unremitting lumbar spinal pain that lasted longer than 4 months, was unresponsive to conservative care, and could be reproduced with discography.

Dissection studies and histological studies using classical techniques established that nerve endings occurred throughout the outer third of the annulus fibrosus and that the source of these endings were branches of the sinuvertebral nerves, the gray rami communicantes, and the lumbar vertebral rami.[9,10,13,14] These studies were extended by histochemical studies in human and animal material to show that nerves in discs contain peptides such as calcitonin gene-related peptide (CGRP), vasoactive intestinal polypeptide (VIP), and substance P, which are characteristic of nociceptive nerve fibers.[15–17] In addition, the work of Takahashi and Nakamura[18,19] over the past decade has demonstrated involvement of the sympathetic chain in the complex network of nerves surrounding disc tissue via afferent pathways to upper lumbar dorsal root ganglion neurons.

In a diseased disc, pain may be generated from deep within its own tissue, beyond the outer third of the annulus, with pain-carrying nerve fibers extending deep inward into the middle annulus and even into the nucleus. This has been observed in degenerative discs and has been linked to the discogenic back pain,[20,21] peripheral sensitization, and resultant amplification of the pain response through the secretion of pro-inflammatory mediators, including substance P. The degenerating disc continues to produce inflammatory cytokines, including tumor necrosis factor-α (TNF-α), nitric oxide, and matrix metalloproteinases (MMPs).[22]

An increased number of mechanoreceptors and pain-producing neurons have also been confirmed clinically and experimentally in the discs of patients with chronic discogenic pain by Roberts and others.[23]

Given the somatosensory and autonomic neural innervations and the peripheral sensitization and amplification mechanisms impacting the pain response, it is understandable why the etiology and ultimate presentation of discogenic pain is so complex.[24]

Further clinical research by Nachemson, Bogduk, April, Derby, and others has helped further define the importance of this complex pain generator over the past four decades.

In our patient's case, she has been complaining of axial back and buttock pain, without radicular component, with preserved lower-extremity strength and sensation. MRI was significant for degenerative changes of the L4–L5 disc with the presence of an annular tear. This would exclude nerve root impingement syndrome and spinal canal stenosis, in addition to other rare disorders of the spine. Clinical suspicion at this stage would include facet joint-mediated pain, discogenic pain syndrome, and SI joint pain syndrome.

HOW IS THE DIAGNOSIS CONFIRMED?

Often discogenic back pain is a diagnosis of exclusion made when other areas of the spine have been ruled out as potential causes of pain. As a result of the complexity of this condition, no single test or intervention can accurately establish the diagnosis of discogenic pain. Rather, a comprehensive and systematic investigation is recommended, starting with obtaining a targeted history, physical examination, imaging tests, establishment of clear differential diagnoses, performance of diagnostic and therapeutic interventions, and, ultimately, for selected individuals, a discography procedure to confirm the diagnosis.

In establishing a diagnosis of discogenic pain, it is important to remember not to rely on imaging studies; they may be misleading in identifying the diseased symptomatic disc because anatomical criteria often do not correlate with pain.

Once the differential diagnosis is narrowed, the spinal causes of pain may be explored systematically following evidence-based algorithmic patterns. History, physical examination, imaging, and electrodiagnostic studies have been shown to have a higher degree of sensitivity and specificity in identification of radiculopathy, with a very favorable risk-benefit profile for treatment as opposed to chronic benign spinal pain. Therefore identification and treatment of radicular symptoms is the first step in the management of spinal pain. Next, attention is given to possible somatic causes of spine pain related to structures of posterior column, including facet joints and the SI joint. As previously mentioned, other potential sources of pain in the axial region should also be identified because they may mimic discogenic back pain.

Only when radicular and somatic causes have been ruled out or treated is attention focused on discogenic pain. This approach allows the clinician to select a population of patients with the highest pretest probability of discogenic pain, thus leading to a high level of success. This approach also ensures that more conservative, lower risk, and less expensive modalities appropriate to the care of the patient are used first.[25]

Advance imaging studies are recommended, most commonly MRI, not only for diagnostic purposes, but also for screening for rare and unsuspected serious conditions that may cause back pain, such as tumors, infections, and metabolic disorders.[26]

When a discogenic origin of back pain is suspected, the patient maybe a candidate for a confirmatory diagnostic discography procedure. Discography is utilized when the patient is considered a candidate for more invasive treatment, such as interventional or surgical procedures. If discography findings will not affect treatment, it should not be performed. Discography is an invasive diagnostic procedure not intended to be an initial screening examination, although it is particularly useful in challenging or inconclusive cases.[27] Discography is a provocative test that attempts to mimic physiologic disc loads and evoke the patient's pain by increasing intradiscal pressure with an injection of contrast médium (Figure 8.1). Increased intradiscal pressure is thought to stimulate annular nerve endings, sensitized nociceptors, or pathologically innervated annular fissures. Discography was introduced in 1940s to diagnose herniation and internal annular disc disruption of the lumbar IVD. Discography combined with post-discography computed tomography (CT) scan remains the most accurate method of detailing internal disc disruption and disc morphology (Figure 8.2).[28] Pain assessment is the most important information obtained from discography; if the patient's pain intensity, location, and character are similar to or the same as the patient's clinical symptoms, then the criteria for concordant pain are satisfied.

The single purpose of discography is to obtain useful clinical information. The test endeavors to confirm or refute the hypothesis that a particular disc is a source of the patient's familiar pain. Because it is a provocation test, disc stimulation is liable to false-positive results; however, a recent meta-analysis of asymptomatic subjects demonstrated that a false-positive rate of less than 10% can be obtained[29] if the discographer adheres to International Spine Intervention Society (ISIS) /International Association for the Study of Pain (IASP) operational standards and interpretation criteria: pain 7/10 or greater, concordant pain, pressure of less than 50 psi a.o., a grade 3 or higher annular tear, a volume limit of 3.5 mL or less, and the presence of a negative control disc.[30,31]

Because abnormal disc morphology alone is not diagnostic, as shown on CT and MRI scans of subjects asymptomatic of LBP,[32] the prime indication for discography is to help to distinguish which disc is symptomatic. A parallel application is to identify asymptomatic discs. When a single disc is found to be symptomatic in the presence of adjacent asymptomatic discs, focused surgical therapy can be entertained. Patients with symptomatic or abnormal discs at multiple levels constitute a greater surgical challenge.

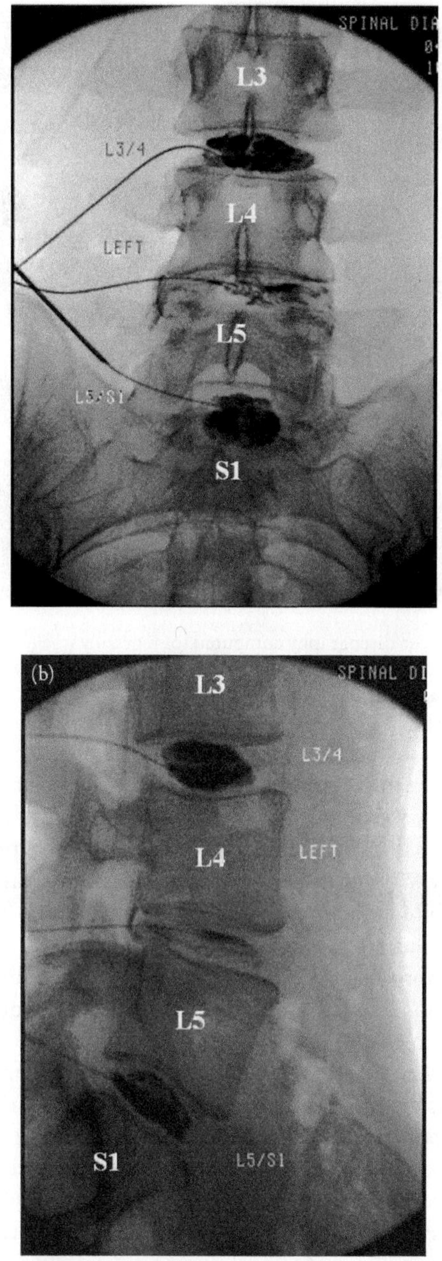

Figure 8.1 Diagnostic provocative discography procedure, demonstrating an abnormal pattern of contrast material spread within L4–L5 disc and suggestive of contained disc protrusion with annular tear. Normal pattern of contrast distribution is seen within the other two control discs, L3–L4 and L5–S1. Fluoroscopic AP (A) and lateral (B) images.

Identification of "negative discs" in response to a disc stimulation—thus limiting the number of levels requiring surgical intervention or a need for interventional disc procedures altogether—is another important value that discography may provide.

On the basis of CT-discography findings, a new concept arose: that of annular disruption. Saches et al.[33] developed the Dallas discogram scale, grading between 0 to 4 the extent of annulus fibrosus disruption; later, Aprill and Bogduk[34] elaborated this classification further. Subsequently, Vanharanta et al.[6] found that pain reproduction on discography correlated

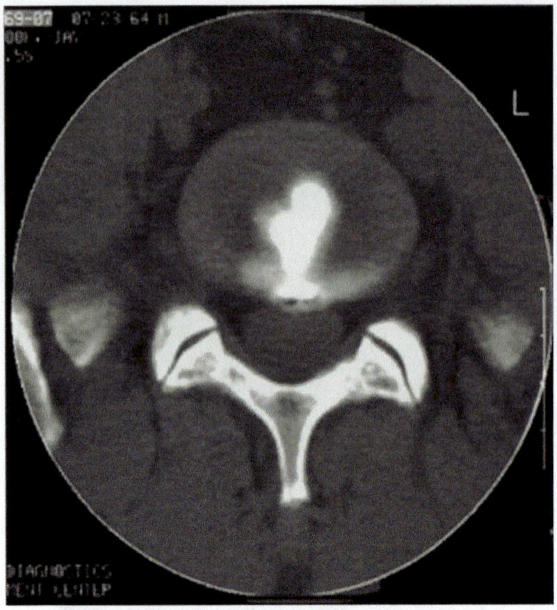

Figure 8.2 Post-discography computed tomography image demonstrating contrast material spread within a contained posterior intradiscal annular tear. Axial view.

with the extent of annular disruption. Grade 0 and grade 1 disruptions were rarely painful, but 75% of grade 3 disruptions were associated with exact or similar pain reproduction; conversely, 77% of discs with exact or similar pain reproduction exhibited grade 3 annular disruptions. These findings, in turn, correlated with the disruption of nerve endings in the annulus fibrosus, thus providing firm correlation between innervations of a structure, pain reproduction from it, and a demonstrable anatomic lesion.[26]

However, the diagnostic power of discography remains controversial.[35] As a provocative test, it has been criticized for having a potentially high false-positive rate.[36] The reasons for this can occur due to technical errors, neurophysiologic phenomena, or psychosocial factors.[26]

Correct technical performance is paramount to the accuracy of the discography results and has been underestimated over the past decades, thus leading to questionable medical outcomes and important legal implications. Discography without strict standards for pressure, volume, speed of injection controls, and limits is unsupportable. Dynamic and static pressures, volumes, and pain responses must be gathered and documented using a consistent and reproducible technique, preferably using a controlled injection syringe with digital pressure readout rather than manual pressurization.[37] It was shown that speed-sensitive dynamic pressure is more liable to provoke a positive pain response, thus requiring a slow injection rate (0.05–0.1 mL/sec) that most accurately reflects the pressures transferred to the outer annulus.[37] Many of the reported false-positive responses occurred at pressures of 50 psi a.o. or greater. In addition, provocation response should not be accepted as positive unless it can be confirmed by a repeat pressurization and pain does not decrease by more than 50% over 30 seconds. Transient pain provocation may occur when an asymptomatic fissure opens or a thin membrane sealing the outer annulus ruptures during disc pressurization.

Central hyperalgesia also must be taken into account as a physiological phenomenon when the perception of stimuli from a receptive field is facilitated by ongoing nociceptive activity arising from adjacent or nearby but separate receptive fields. In this regard, formal studies have shown that in patients with no history and no symptoms of back pain, but with a painful donor site on the iliac crest, disc stimulation can evoke back pain,[38] thus producing a false-positive response.

Concerns have been raised regarding psychologic comorbidity and psychosocial factors as significant confounding factors in patients undergoing discography, questioning the results of discography in patients with chronic pain or somatization disorders other than back pain.[38] Evidence indicates that patients with chronic or chronic intermittent LBP respond similarly to disc stimulation as do asymptomatic volunteers undergoing discography, as was shown by Derby in a prospective controlled study of patients with grade 3 disc tears.[39] Shin also confirmed that a majority of patients with grade 4 tears could distinguish between "positive" and "negative" discs by magnitude of pain response, thus casting doubt on the argument that a majority of patients with chronic pain undergoing discography would overreport pain.[40]

In addition, a randomized controlled trial (RCT) comparing the discography results of 25 patients with and without somatization disorder found no significant difference in positive responses between groups.[41] There was also no difference in positive responses in patients with depression and/or general anxiety disorder. This calls into question the results of a limited Carragee study of six somatization patients in which only four of the six were able to complete their discography test because of pain.[36] Derby et al.[42] reported the Distress and Risk Assessment Method (DRAM) scores of 81 patients undergoing discography: 15% (12/81) were normal, 52% (42/81) were at risk, and 33% (27/81) were abnormal (distressed, depressive, or somatic). The positive rates of discography were not statistically significant by subgroup ($p > 0.05$). In patients with chronic LBP, no correlation was found between presenting DRAM score and discography result.

A recent meta-analysis of studies of asymptomatic subjects undergoing discography obtained a specificity of 0.94 (95% CI 0.89–0.98) or a false-positive rate of 6%.[29] This critical examination of most studies in the literature since the 1960s showed that an acceptably low false-positive rate can be achieved when strict ISIS/IASP standards for a positive discography are utilized, as listed earlier.

Another recent concern raised by Carragee et al.[43] is a long-term risk that discography, as an invasive test, can potentially cause damage to punctured discs over time and result in accelerated disc degeneration. The authors showed a 21% increase in the degree of disc degeneration using small-gauge needles and an increase in the number of new disc herniations of all types in the discography versus control group over 10 years. These results require attention and further investigation. It is important to determine what proportion of those degenerative discs can be attributed to discography rather than to the expected natural history of accelerated degeneration in this small cohort of patients with known cervical disc disease. Those patients might be already genetically predisposed to accelerated disc degeneration and multilevel spondylosis compared to the normal population, as was shown in a well-designed twin study, in which 74% of degenerative findings at the lower lumbar levels were accounted for by heritability.[44]

Even though the diagnostic power of discography remains controversial, it is a relatively safe and sensitive test for identifying painful discs, and it may predict surgery-related outcomes. In a multicenter surgical and nonsurgical outcome study after pressure-controlled discography, Derby et al.[45] stated that precise prospective categorization of positive discographic diagnoses may predict treatment outcomes, surgical or otherwise, thereby greatly facilitating therapeutic decision making. Technical challenges, potential complications, and interpretation mistakes can be avoided with proper selection of patients, including those with a favorable psychological profile, use of sterile technique, intravenous and intradiscal antibiotics, judicious use of sedation, and good technical training for practitioners.[46]

In addition to provocative discography, there are alternative confirmatory procedures that have been developed over the past years; these include analgesic discography and functional analgesic discography. Analgesic discography involves injection of analgesic drugs into the suspected painful disc in hope of relieving the patient's back pain related to a specific disc(s) level(s). It represents a "diagnosis by exclusion" approach. Typically, one disc at a time can be reliably tested. Functional analgesic discography is similar to analgesic discography test and involves insertion of intradiscal catheter(s) that allows physicians to isolate the source of LBP by selectively anesthetizing suspected disc(s) while the patient performs activities that typically generate and reproduce his or her pain (Figure 8.3). These tests might be biased toward false-negative results. It is likely that, in contrast to provocative discography, analgesic discography has a low sensitivity. However, the value of analgesic discography is its robust specificity.[47–50]

In the presence of MRI findings suggestive of a single-level disc disease, with degenerative changes at the L4–L5 disc without disc protrusion, and the presence of a HIZ/annular tear, our patient is a good candidate for a provocative or analgesic discography provided that she has a favorable psychological profile. Some discographers obtain a brief psychometric test such as the Distress and Risk Assessment Method (DRAM) to assess if the patient has a normal, at risk, distressed depressive, or distressed somatic profile.[42]

Additional indications and inclusion criteria include failed conservative treatment for LBP of probable spinal origin, ongoing pain for greater than 4 months, other common pain generators have been ruled out (e.g., facet joint and SI joint mediated pain), symptoms are severe enough to consider surgery or percutaneous interventions, surgery is planned and the surgeon desires an assessment of the adjacent disc levels, the patient is capable of understanding the nature of the technique and can participate in the subjective interpretation, and both patient and physician need to know the source of pain to guide further treatments. Contraindications include inability to assess patient response during the procedure or lack of cooperation, coagulopathy (INR >1.5 or platelets <50,000/mm), known localized or systemic infection, and pregnancy (to prevent fetal radiation exposure).

WHAT IS THE INCIDENCE AND PREVALENCE OF DISCOGENIC BACK PAIN?

LBP is one of the most common medical problems in developed countries. It occurs in diverse groups of the population, has many possible etiologies, and is one of the major causes

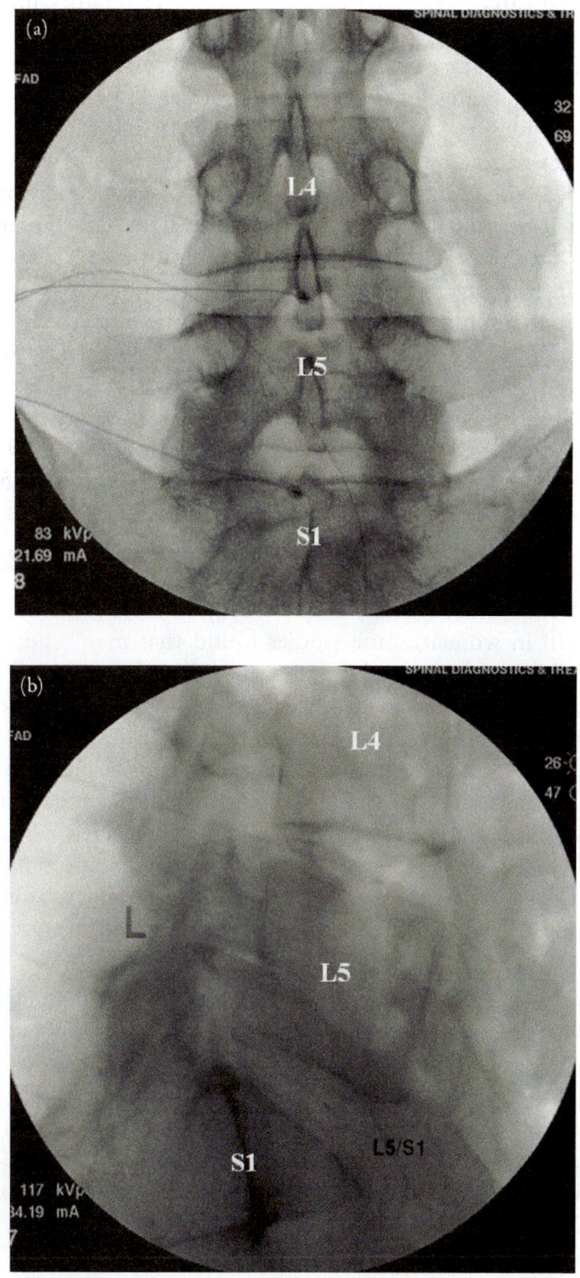

Figure 8.3 Functional anesthetic discography procedure demonstrating intradiscal positioning of the catheters in the center of L4–L5 and L5–S1 discs. A. Central positioning of the catheters with contrast-inflated "anchoring" balloon tips. AP view. B. Catheter positioning in the middle of the nucleus before inflating the tips. Lateral fluoroscopic view.

of disability in industrial countries with important clinical, social, economic, and public health problem impacts affecting the population indiscriminately.

Discogenic LBP is considered to be one of the most common causes of chronic LBP, accounting for approximately 26–39% of its incidence.[51,52]

LBP is a widely prevalent condition. At some time in their lives, an estimated 65–80% of the population will suffer from LBP.[53] Spinal pain disorders account for a tremendous cost both in lost productivity and medical care, with 890 million physician office visits a year related to back pain in the United States, accounting for one of the top two reasons person seek medical care, superseded only at times by respiratory infections.[54,55] It has been estimated that 1% of the population is disabled by back pain. It is the leading cause of disability in the United States for the population under 45 years old and the second most prevalent cause for those 45–65 years old.[56]

Back pain accounts for approximately one-fourth of workers compensation claims in the United States. Construction workers (in males) and nurses aides (in females) had the highest prevalence rates, of 22.6% and 18.8%, respectively. In a 2003 study in the United States, back pain was the second most common pain condition resulting in lost time from work after headache.[57]

Yearly direct healthcare costs associated with back pain in the United States was estimated \$85.9 billion in 2005.[58] Multiple studies have shown an incidence of recurrent or chronic LBP at 3, 6, and 12 months to range from 35% to 79%. Frequent or persistent LBP also has been shown at around 15% in numerous evaluations. Age-related LBP studies show that 12% of children or adolescents suffer persistent back pain, in contrast to 15% of adults and as high as 27% of the elderly.[59]

Although many studies reported higher rates of incidence of LBP in women, some studies found that men reported more LBP at the time of the interview than did women.[60]

There have been many challenges in the accurate collection of epidemiologic data due lack of standardized methods, absence of clear definitions and durations, and the presence of other variables that at times make it difficult to compare statistics across studies. One of the main steps to evidence-based medicine in the treatment of spine pain is the collection of valid, consistent epidemiologic data. This will serve as the foundation on which to build rational treatment in the future.[61]

> Based on the epidemiologic data, our patient is the classic example of a young female patient who developed a chronic discogenic back pain. Her age and gender are in line with those who are most commonly affected. Women tend to have a higher incidence of back pain, as discussed earlier. It is not known from her history if she is currently on disability for her back pain condition, but, if she is, it could also be in line with the most common cause of disability in the United States for the population under 45 years of age.

WHAT IS THE NATURAL HISTORY OF DISCOGENIC BACK PAIN?

The natural history of LBP and its prognosis can often be determined by and distinguished on the base of its temporality. Even though the incidence of LBP in industrial societies is very high, the majority of common LBP episodes are trivial, often beginning with minor aches and pains in the lower spine that can occur without reason or shortly after an unusually heavy bout of physical activity and resolve within a few days without a need for any intervention.[62]

The prognosis for a single episode of back pain is excellent, with 90–95% of acute episodes resolving fully. Resolution of symptoms usually occurs within 3 months. In other instances of LBP, it can present with more severe, debilitating symptoms, including muscle spasms precipitated by movement, and pain in the low back that may radiate into the buttocks and is usually worse with sitting. The sudden appearance of one or more of those symptoms can be frightening and can severely impact a patient's activities of daily living.

Those patients who do not recover endure significant costs in disability and medical care. It is becoming evident that there is a significant recurrence rate for acute back pain with an associated progression to chronic pain.[61]

People whose symptoms last less than 6 weeks are generally categorized as having "acute LBP," progressing to "subacute LBP" if symptoms last 6–12 weeks, and to "chronic LBP" if symptoms persist beyond 12 weeks. Further gradation has been suggested for those with long-standing symptoms that disappeared for a period of time and reappeared, which can be categorized as "recurrent" or "episodic" LBP.[63]

The prognosis for LBP is generally favorable for those with recent symptoms and less favorable for those with long-standing symptoms, although this demarcation of patients into those with acute, subacute, or chronic LBP has not been reliable in predicting patient outcomes. Both the severity and duration of symptoms vary from episode to episode, and some episodes may overlap each other, thus making this temporal gradation inaccurate. The perception that acute LBP goes away rapidly without returning has been proved false, as well as the perception that chronic back pain of more than 3 months' duration might be incurable. Currently, LBP is considered a recurrent disorder that can occur at any time in a person's life and fluctuates between a status of no pain/mild pain and pain that reaches a point at which it interferes with activities of normal living or becomes debilitating.[64]

> Given her 6-month history, she is currently in the category of patients suffering "chronic LBP." She has also failed conservative treatment, including a course of physical therapy (PT), NSAIDs, and muscle relaxant. In this case, her prognosis might not be as favorable, and she may need more advanced care including interventional diagnostic and treatment procedures.

WHAT ARE THE CLINICAL MANIFESTATIONS OF DISCOGENIC BACK PAIN?

History, physical examination, and imaging studies have limited specificity for discogenic back pain. At the same time, they can provide important information that can help to navigate a diagnostic algorithmic process and, most importantly, can help to rule out and screen for potentially serious and rare spinal disorders, so-called *red flags*.

Overall, several categories of red flags described in clinical practice guidelines (CPGs) have been associated with potentially serious medical conditions, including spinal cancer, cauda equina syndrome, spinal fracture, and spinal infection. Those requiring immediate attention include recent trauma with a history of osteoporosis, unexplained weight loss, history of cancer, fever, pain worse at night, bowel and bladder dysfunction, gait abnormalities, and saddle numbness.[65]

The history should look for symptoms that tend to be more associated with discogenic pain, including persistent LBP that worsens with axial loading; pain that is increased with sitting, flexion, coughing, sneezing, or activities that increase intradiscal pressure such as straining; and improvement with recumbency. During history taking, it is important to screen for signs of nondiscogenic pain. Although the signs taken in isolation are nor very valuable, together with the physical examination and diagnostic testing they can prove helpful at ruling out facet or SI joint-mediated pain and other causes.[1]

On physical examination, in the absence of neural compromise, the neurological examination of patients with discogenic LBP is usually normal. The most common presentation is axial back pain reproduction associated with decreased range of motion of the spine, especially with flexion. Palpation usually reveals midline tenderness near the affected segments. Muscle spasm in the paravertebral region is common.

Two additional examinations have been utilized and are proposed to be more specific for detection of discogenic pain: centralization phenomenon and the bony vibration test. Hancock et al., in a systematic review of tests designed to identify the disc as a pain generator, concluded that centralization was the only clinical feature associated with a discogenic pain etiology. The test involves repeated flexion-extension or side bending maneuvers of the spine while observing a subjective report of migration of pain toward the midline of the spine or centralization. This pain pattern is thought to arise because of the central location of the disc, which is perceived as midline pain when stressed, compared to facet and SI joint pain, which tend to cause more lateral pain. The specificity of this test has been reported to range from 70% to 100% with a sensitivity of 64%.[66] However, the utilization value of this test is very low because the time and training required for proper performance of this test limits its usefulness. The bony vibration test involves applying a blunt electric vibrator over the spinous process of the vertebra at the suspected segment. If the patient reports pain, it suggests discogenic LBP. The sensitivity and specificity of this test are controversial, and studies are considered to be inconclusive, possibly due to questionable patient selection.[67] Nonetheless, both tests should be used in combination with other clinical tests to make the diagnosis of discogenic LBP.

Electromyographic diagostic (EMG) testing is an extension of the history and physical examination. Although EMG does not diagnose discogenic LBP, it can be useful in identifying radiculopathy and in differentiating referred pain from radicular pain in nondiscogenic cases of LBP. Unfortunately, its sensitivity was shown to be limited.[68]

Imaging studies used in evaluation of painful spinal disorders may include plain radiographs, MRI, CT, nuclear medicine scans, myelography, single-proton emission computed tomography (SPECT), and others. It is well established that imaging should only be performed when severe or progressive neurological deficits are present, serious underlying systemic disease is suspected, or the patient has a disease or impairment that may require interventional treatment. The lack of utility of imaging in the acute setting was also illustrated by Carragee and colleagues.[69] Imaging in patients who present with acute LBP is not routinely indicated, except in the presence of red flag features, which have been described previously.

When indicated, imaging can provide important information that can be used in the algorithmic process of diagnostic decision making and prior to a selection of appropriate treatment procedures. Plain radiographs, including dynamic imaging of the spine with flexion and extension views in the upright weight-bearing position, may help detect segmental spinal instability that may preclude the patient from percutaneous disc treatment procedures and shift the care toward surgical intervention. Low-grade degenerative spondylolisthesis without instability does not automatically preclude patients from percutaneous treatment options but may have a negative prognostic impact. Imaging findings that potentially predict discogenic pain may include loss of disc space height, endplate sclerosis, vertebral osteophytes, and vacuum phenomenon (nitrogen gas) within the disc. The disadvantages of plain radiographs are their limited ability to provide information about the integrity of the discs and significant radiation exposure.

The most commonly used imaging test of choice for painful spinal disorders is MRI, given that it provides high degree of spatial resolution and the best soft-tissue contrast of all the imaging modalities. Several findings detected on MRI may signal discogenic pain: low signal intensity of the disc on T2 weighting, a HIZ (also called an *annular fissure*), alterations in disc contour (bulges, protrusions, extrusions), loss of disc height, and changes in the sub-endplate marrow (Modic changes).[70]

MRI findings of low signal intensity or "black disc" on T2 weighting associated with disc degeneration with reduced water content is poorly correlated with discogenic pain.[25] A study of healthy discs showed that 17% of the discs had low-intensity signals and concluded that this finding had close to 100% sensitivity but very low specificity for discogenic LBP.[71,72]

The MRI hallmark of internal disc disruption is the HIZ. The HIZ is associated with annular fissures; however, the correlation of the HIZ with discogenic LBP is controversial. The HIZ is thought to result from inflammation caused by annular disruption, which leads to stimulation of pain fibers and possibility to the disc being a source of pain. The correlation of the HIZ to discogenic pain has a sensitivity that ranges from 81% to 92.5%, a specificity that ranges from 26.7% to 89%, and a positive predictive value (PPV) that ranges from 87% to 90%, as reported by Aprill and Bogduk.[34] Although there is evidence that supports the predictive value of the HIZ for discogenic pain, HIZ is present in a large number of asymptomatic discs, with incidence ranging from 25% to 39%, thus putting into question its predictive value for discogenic pain.[73]

The functional unity of the disc and the cartilaginous endplate is manifest in signal changes within the endplate and adjacent subchondral marrow that accompany disc degeneration. These endplate changes are classified as Modic I–III changes. Multiple studies have shown a strong correlation between Modic changes, particularly type I, chronic LBP and positive discography.[74,75] Modic I changes, known as the inflammatory phase, are characterized by low signal intensity on T1-weighted and high signal intensity on T2-weighted imaging. Modic changes appear to have a high sensitivity but low specificity for discogenic pain.[72]

Patients with a single-level minimal to moderate degenerative disc, good disc height preservation, and minimal to no evidence of stenotic lesion are ideal candidates for provocative discography and potential percutaneous disc treatments.

Patients with three or more levels of degenerative discs, sequestered or extruded discs, 60% or greater loss of disc height, severe degenerative changes, and high-grade stenotic lesions are poor candidates for percutaneous disc treatments. In these situations, discography is not routinely recommended but may be appropriate in individual cases to help determine potential treatment options.

Before proceeding with examination of individual imaging findings, we must first consider the gold standard dilemma. There is no surgical or pathological marker of a painful IVD. The most restrictive golden standard for a painful disc is a concordant response to manometrically controlled provocative discography with nonpainful control levels as defined by the practice guidelines of the ISIS.[76]

The patient's history indicates that she has been experiencing axial low back and buttock pain that is worst with sitting, aggravated by flexion, and relieved by recumbence. These are the common findings in patients with discogenic back pain. Her neurologic examination was intact, supporting absence of spinal neuronal element involvement, including radiculopathy. MRI of the lumbar spine shows L4–L5 mild degeneration with the presence of HIZ/annular fissure. It is possible to hypothesize that her L4–L5 disc is the source of her LBP symptoms. As was discussed earlier, the correlation of the HIZ to discogenic pain is high. Because this patient has symptomatic back pain, and her history, physical examination, and imaging findings combined point toward a probable discogenic origin of her pain, she would be a good candidate for provocative discography testing and, if positive, for a percutaneous disc treatment.

HOW IS DISCOGENIC BACK PAIN MANAGED?

INTERVENTIONAL PROCEDURES

Percutaneous minimally invasive interventional procedures for the treatment of discogenic back pain have become increasingly available over the past few decades as an alternative to surgical treatment, which remains challenging and controversial.

The development of nonsurgical interventions, based on current understanding of the pathophysiology of discogenic back pain, has several general therapeutic goals: restoration or mitigation of abnormal nociception resulting from post-injury neo-innervation and neovascularization of posterior annular tears, resolution or normalization of abnormal nucleoannular pro-inflammatory and anabolic-catabolic biochemical balance, and restoration of lost mechanical and hydraulic function and the annular integrity of abnormal IVDs.

Interventional therapeutic procedures discussed in this chapter include intradiscal electrothermal therapies and intradiscal therapeutic injections as the most common or emerging forms of treatment of axial nonradicular discogenic back pain.

Intradiscal thermal therapies encompass a group of interventions that deliver heat energy to the IVD with the goal of reducing discogenic pain by a variety of proposed mechanisms, including shrinking subannular disc protrusions, destroying nociceptors, sealing annular tears by collagen modification, and stimulating a healing response.[77,78] The original intradiscal thermal therapies delivered heat to the nucleus using the same radiofrequency device used in lumbar medial branch neurotomy (LMBN). Subsequently, the more widely used intradiscal electrothermal therapy (IDET) procedure used a catheter inserted into the nucleus and advanced circumferentially to the outer annulus (Figure 8.4). A later modification of the device used the same catheter technique but a shorter active heating length using radiofrequency rather than electrothermal energy to heat the adjacent annulus. This procedure is also called *intradiscal electrothermal annuloplasty* (IDEA) or *intradiscal thermal annuloplasty* (IDTA). The heat

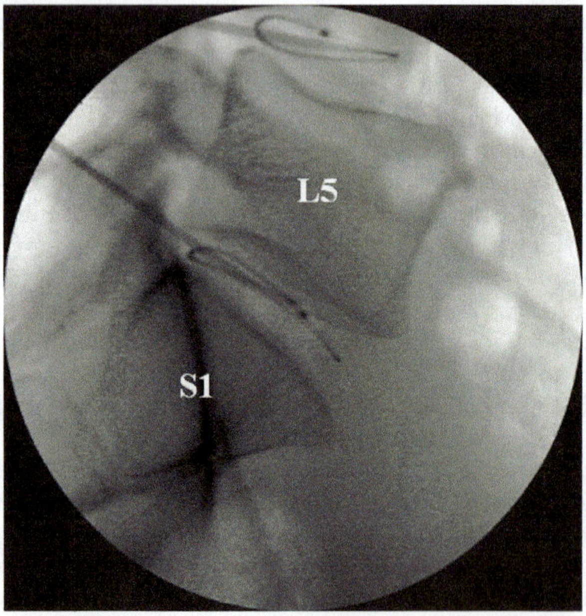

Figure 8.4 Intradiscal electrothermal therapy (IDET) procedure, with intradiscal placement of the thermal coil advanced circumferentially to the outer annulus inside the L4–L5 and L5–S1 discs. Lateral fluoroscopic view.

delivered with IDET can be generated through a variety of means, including electrocautery, thermal cautery, laser, and radiofrequency energy (RFE). IDET using RFE may also be termed *intradiscal radiofrequency treatment* or *intradiscal radiofrequency thermocoagulation* (IRFT). Other devices also use radiofrequency energy targeting the outer annulus using an electrode passed through an introducer needle inserted into the outer posterior lateral annulus and passed across the posterior annulus. The most recent advance in intradiscal thermal treatments is the *cooled bipolar RFE* or *intradiscal biacuplasty* (IDB) procedure, where a radio frequency probe is actively cooled using circulating water pumped through a cannula. IDB uses a bipolar system that includes two cooled RFE electrodes placed on the posterolateral sides of the annulus fibrosus portion of the IVD. Cooled RFE electrodes are thought to increase the lesion size and facilitate ablation when compared with standard RFE electrodes, whereas the linear placement of the two electrodes makes the procedure less complicated. Cooling is thought to facilitate a more uniform heating profile across the disc annulus between two bilateral introducer needles placed in the outer annulus while sparing adjacent tissue and concentrating heating energy on the posterior wall.[79] Most of these procedures, if performed correctly by a well-trained practitioner, are considered to be well tolerated and have a small number of serious complications reported.

Tissue modulation, including shrinkage, denaturation, and structural changes to collagen fibers in the annulus as well as denervation of ingrown nociceptors by neuroablation, has been the proposed explanation for the mechanisms of action, but scientific evidence to support this is lacking.[80] There is conflicting evidence of thermal healing response post-IDET, with no data to support sealing of annular tears that might lead to pain reduction. A few studies report that IDET does not reach therapeutic temperatures throughout the posterior annulus, and some studies show no change in HIZs on MRI imaging following the IDET procedure. The majority of studies on minimally invasive intradiscal therapies in recent years were pilot trials or they enrolled patients in a prospective manner but lacked randomization and blinding, thus adversely influencing the interpretation of clinical efficacy by third-party payers and critics.

Four published RCTs have assessed intradiscal heating treatments for chronic LBP and generally reported mixed results. Freeman and colleagues[81] showed no statistically significant differences in pain or function for either the treatment or the sham group compared with baseline and no differences in pain or function between the two groups.

Pauza and colleagues[82] performed an RCT in patients with painful disc disruption identified by pressure-controlled lumbar discography. After 6 months, more people in the IDET group experienced pain relief than those in the placebo group (statistical significance not reported). The IDET group experienced statistically significant improvements in pain on one score (VAS) but not on another (SF-36 Bodily Pain) versus the placebo group. Similarly, the IDET group experienced statistically significant improvements in function on one score (ODI) but not on another (SF-36 Physical Function) versus the placebo group.

Barendse and colleagues[83] performed an RCT in patients with chronic LBP with no reported difference between sham and treatment groups. Lau and colleagues[84] showed in their RCT that, after 12 months, patients in the IDET group experienced pain relief, yet no statistically significant differences in pain were observed between the IDET and sham control groups.

Multiple observational studies have shown optimistic results, especially when strict patient selection criteria and provocation discography with pressure manometry were used prior to IDET.

A study by Derby and colleagues reported positive response rates of 73% when the catheter position was optimal, but only 16.5% in patients with a fair catheter placement.[85] Saal and colleagues reported a positive response rate in 80% of participants, decreases in SF-36 bodily pain of 59–78%, and average decreases in VAS of 62–72%.[86,87] Despite early published optimistic results similar to those of Saal and colleagues, Derby's study reported that approximately one-third of his IDET-treated patients were much better, one-third were slightly better, and one-third were the same or worse. In addition, his patients had on average only a 1.84/10 (18%) decrease in VAS. Since then, prospective and retrospective case series have reported a dichotomy of results.[85]

The clinical results of five observational prospective studies on patients with chronic LBP treated with biacuplasty by Kapural and Bogduk showed fairly positive outcomes, including on patients who previously had failed discectomy procedures.[88–91]

When comparing published IDET studies, differences in outcomes are thought to be related to variability of patient selection, the number of disc levels degenerated on MRI, recruitment of workers compensation patients, and involvement of industry sponsors in the studies.

Overall, although the evidence for IDET is conflicting, it weakly supports the method of heating the outer annulus using the catheter technique in well-selected patients. A controlled but nonrandomized study showed superiority of IDET over continued conservative care, and almost all retrospective and prospective observational studies report positive results for IDET, although the magnitude of the treatment effect is not large.

A randomized placebo-controlled trial of biacuplasty in highly selected patients with discogenic pain was published with 6-month results. Of 1,894 screened, 64 were enrolled and randomized to intradiscal biacuplasty or sham. Compared to sham, the intradiscal biacuplasty group had significantly improved pain scores and functional and disability outcomes at 6 months.[92] However, results of the 1-year follow-up failed to show persistent statistically significant effect (data presented at the Cleveland Clinic Symposium, Sarasota, Florida, February, 2013).

Minimally invasive nuclear decompression (or nucleoplasty) is a procedure in which a probe is inserted transcutaneously through a catheter into the nucleus of an injured, herniated, but contained disc, and a form of radiofrequency termed *coblation* is targeted at a portion of the nucleus to eliminate it. The main indication for this procedure is radicular pain due to a discogenic pathology. A scientific literature search found insufficient evidence supporting nucleoplasty, due to a lack of RCTs.[93] There are several observational studies supporting the use of nucleoplasty as an intervention for radicular pain and a few studies supporting its use for chronic LBP. However, few systematic review studies endorse the technique for radicular pain, and none endorse the technique for chronic LBP.[94] For this reason, the nucleoplasty procedure is not reviewed in this chapter.

In addition to electrothermal intradiscal therapies, the injection of substances that could either decompress, denervate, or perhaps even restore disc cartilaginous tissue has been and continues to be an area of active investigation.

Historically, percutaneous disc decompression began in 1963 with the development of chemonucleolysis using chymopapain (Chymodiactin).[95] Most literature addressing the efficacy of this treatment assesses radicular rather than axial back pain, with April in 1992 demonstrating that whereas chemical decompression of the disc for the treatment of extremity pain is effective, improvement in axial pain is inconsistent. Chymopapain was withdrawn from clinical practice due to frequent allergic reactions and reports of rare fatal anaphylactic reactions.

Since that time, various investigators have considered a variety of substances for intradiscal injections that lyse or denature protein, including collagenase, ethanol, osmic acid, phenol, and 50% dextrose. Additional substances, such as ozone and methylene blue, have been used for the purposes of chemical oxidation or denaturing of potential nociceptive structures within the disc, including neurolysis.[96]

An intradiscal absolute ethanol injection study was published by Riquelme and colleagues[97] and reported "total improvement of symptoms" in 97.5% of cases (118 total patients). Two patients continued to have LBP, and the failure rate was 0.84% (1 case). It is unclear whether the patients had a diagnosis of discogenic pain because most of the patients treated had sciatica. Avoidance of spread into the epidural space or onto the dural surface prompted the use of a gel carrier, ethylcellulose, reported by Theron and associates for lumbar and cervical discs, with around a 90% success rate.[98] The results are encouraging, but additional clinical studies will be necessary to determine the proper place of this relatively inexpensive and reportedly safe treatment.

Intradiscal ozone treatment has been popularized in Italy and is slowly spreading to other European countries and India. The majority of scientific literature addressed herniated nucleus pulposus and radicular pain using concentrations of 27 mcg/mL, with better outcomes observed by concomitant infiltration of the nerve root with local anesthetic and steroids with a goal of decompressing disc herniations and reducing peridiscal inflammation. Gallucci and his colleagues showed some evidence that the procedure may be effective in reducing leg pain in a randomized double-blinded trial.[99] Some studies report 78% improvement at 6 months.[100] The therapeutic effect is presumably associated with the formation of peroxide and oxidative injury, although the exact mechanism of action is still debated. Potential serious complications, including gaseous emboli formation and adjacent tissue injury with catalase and superoxide dismutase, as well as development of basilar stroke, epidural abscess, and sepsis have been reported.[101]

Use of methylene blue as a neurotoxic substance that might reduce nitric oxide synthesis in the IVD was reported by Peng.[102] In his RCT of 72 patients, he reported relief of back pain in 91% of cases.[103]

Even though methylene blue is considered neurotoxic in both intrathecal and epidural applications, no complications were reported. These impressive outcomes are still awaiting duplication by other researchers before worldwide adoption of this novel and seemingly simple technique.

Treatment of painful advanced internal lumbar disc derangement with intradiscal injection of hypertonic 50% dextrose was reported by Miller and colleagues. Their practice audit showed favorable results achieved with bi-weekly disc injections of this neurolytic and cytotoxic substance. Each patient was injected an average of 3.5 times. Overall, 43.4% of patients fell into the sustained improvement group with an average improvement in numeric pain scores of 71% comparing pre-treatment and 18-month measurements.[104]

Intradiscal steroids have been tried since 1956, with a reported 60% permanent relief of symptoms at 8 months, as reported by Feffer. Even though, theoretically, steroids should reduce inflammatory intradiscal pain, subsequent RCTs and other observational studies evaluating patients with LBP have not shown substantiated effectiveness.[105] In addition, Aoki reported that methylprednisolone acetate and its vehicle polyethylene glycol caused degeneration and primary calcifications in discs. However, more rational selection (e.g., patients with evidence of endplate and adjacent bone inflammation; Modic I changes) showed more favorable outcomes, although with short duration of overall pain relief.[106]

Similarly, an anti-inflammatory approach using an antagonist of TNF-α (etanercept), has not proved useful in the treatment of discogenic pain.[107]

A biochemical treatment approach, including attempts at restoring disc matrix by inducing proteoglycan synthesis, have been pioneered by Eek.[108] He developed a disc restorative solution (DRS) containing chondroitin sulfate, glucosamine, dextrose, carboxycellulose, and a cephalosporin antibiotic that is injected at 2-month intervals, for a total of three injections, to modulate discogenic back pain and to "nourish" disc tissue (Figure 8.5). Derby and colleagues[109] published results of a prospective trial of DRS versus IDET. They reported weak evidence that, compared to IDET, DRS was more effective in reducing axial pain. DRS is currently in continued development. Recent in vitro cell cultures showed a very significant decrease in several inflammatory cytokines and decreased apoptosis compared to controls. Animal study results are currently pending.

In the category of regenerative injection treatments, recent developments have been made using intradiscal platelet rich plasma (PRP) and stem cell injections. PRP has been gaining popularity in the treatment of a variety of musculoskeletal disorders. The exact mechanism of action is not clearly understood, but a combination of factors, including the activity of multiple cytokines, growth factors, and a small fraction of captured blood-circulating adult autologous stem cells within the PRP, have been suggested to be responsible for tissue

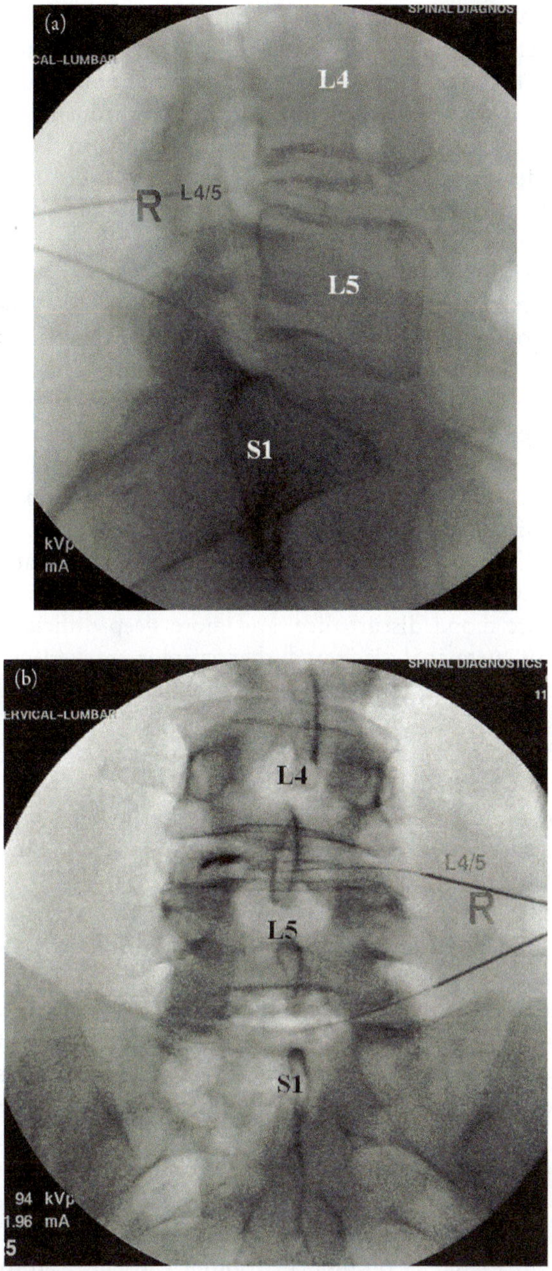

Figure 8.5 Therapeutic percutaneous intradiscal injection of disc restorative solution (DRS). Fluoroscopic images demonstrating needle positioning in the center of the L4–L5 and L5–S1 discs with small amount of contrast material injected at the L4–L5 level, with the outline of the contained posterior disc protrusion with annular tear. Lateral and AP views (A,B).

healing, regeneration, and anti-inflammatory activity. Ex vivo culture study results suggest the possible beneficial effect of intradiscal PRP injection in the treatment of discogenic back pain, although the main factors behind this effect remain unstudied.[110] A randomized clinical trial of intradiscal PRP was initiated in 2009, with early promising results recently presented by Lutz at the annual ISIS meeting in 2012. Final results are pending at the time of this writing.

Injection of mesenchymal stem cells (MSCs), harvested from a disc, bone marrow, or knee and grown in culture before implantation, has been demonstrated to have good viability in animal models.[111] Issues relevant to successful human therapeutic application include identification of optimal tissue source, ease of cellular harvesting, choice of implantation carrier, and assurance of clinically significant long-term viability of cellular transplants in the harsh disc nucleus avascular environment. Research must also quantify the potential for malignant transformation of transplanted MSCs.[112]

In the category of biologic disc repair are some members of the transforming growth factor superfamily, which includes the bone morphogenic protein (BMP) family and BMP-7 (also called osteogenic protein [OP]-1). Intradiscal injections of these substances have demonstrated stimulation of collagen and production of proteoglycan, as well as the proliferation of nuclear cells, evidenced by annular healing and even restoration of disc height.

OP-1 injection into a degenerated disc induced disc height restoration, with improvement of the MRI images of the damaged disc and resolution of histochemical abnormalities, as was shown by Masuda[113] in the rabbit annular puncture model. This study gives evidence that biological repair or regeneration is feasible by injecting growth factors into the degenerated disc. Potentially, these substances may reduce inflammation and improve the weight-bearing capacity of the nucleus. Currently, the cost of BMP and injectable growth factors remains a concern.

In addition, various intradiscal "filler substances" are currently under development for the treatment of discogenic back pain. Although many of these will be used as carriers of more exotic genetic and growth-promoting substances, the filler substances themselves may have a role in promoting a healing response by "sealing" annular tears and perhaps temporarily providing nuclear weight-bearing support and thus potentially lowering outer annular loads. As an example, fibrin sealer has long been used for a similar function in neurological, dermatologic, and ophthalmologic surgery. Fibrin has been shown to improve cell proliferation and matrix production in vitro by Sha'ban et al.[114]

Human use of injectable fibrin sealants produced by mixing fibrinogen and thrombin solutions in a needle mounted on a Y-connector that combines two syringes in one system has been reported by Derby and Talu[115] following IDET and nucleoplasty procedures and as a stand-alone treatment by Yin and colleagues.[116] Greater than 50% reduction in both back and leg pain was demonstrated at 12 weeks. A single case of discitis was the only reported complication in the clinical series reported by Yin and Pauza. A multicenter, randomized, controlled phase III trial began in 2009 and is under way in the United States.

Nuclear bulking techniques have been described by Taylor, Salvatierra, and associates, whereas procedures using other filler substances that can be injected through narrow-gauge needles into the discs are under development. For example, Arteseal is a combination of bovine collagen mixed with very small polymethyl-methacrylate (PMMA) spheres; it is used under the skin to remove facial wrinkles. The size of the spheres is such that they are not reabsorbed. Fibroblasts attach to the spheres and gradually replace the bovine collagen with newly created fibrous tissue.

Some of the these emerging technologies are capable of addressing multiple pathophysiologic factors responsible for the development of discogenic LBP and preventing or reversing degenerative disc disease, but their use will require much further research and development prior to incorporation into routine clinical practice.

Given her relatively young age, minimally invasive percutaneous procedures would be recommended as a first choice before considering surgical treatment. Assuming that she has positive findings on provocative (or other types of) discography, with a single-level disc disease, she could be a good candidate for several percutaneous treatment options as discussed earlier. Unfortunately, many of these procedures are not routinely covered by third-party payers and are considered "experimental." Injection of biological disc restorative substances (such as DRS) or PRP seems to be fairly simple and low-risk treatment option for her as a first step. Alternatively, IDET or intradiscal radiofrequency biaculoplasty could also be good options if choosing electrothermocoagulation types of treatment.

PSYCHIATRIC INTERVENTIONS

As noted, the patient does report a history of smoking 1 ppd × 11 years. Like many smokers, she reports that this began with recreational or occasional use but quickly progressed to daily smoking, escalating to her current level within 9 months of onset. Further education and smoking cessation counseling was provided to the patient. She reports that she has often thought about quitting and even attempted "cold turkey" in the past but has been unsuccessful. In particular, she felt a strong need to smoke upon waking, which she feels derailed the process. She admits that she did not intend to become a chronic smoker and, upon discussion, is well aware of the negative effects smoking has on her health. She is interested in attempting to stop smoking at this time.

Cigarette smoking is the single leading preventable cause of mortality. In the United States, 57% of adults are never smokers, 22% are former smokers, and 21% are current smokers.[117] Of these, 80% are daily smokers. Rates are similar between males and females but vary by ethnicity. Nicotine dependence is significantly greater among Native Americans and Alaskan natives and significantly lower in Asian Americans and Hispanics compared to Caucasians and African Americans.[118] Smoking is responsible for approximately 30% of all cancer deaths, and 21% of all U.S. deaths can be attributed to the effects of smoking.[119] The average smoker dies 10 years earlier than a comparable nonsmoker. Those who stop smoking by age 30 can restore 9 years of life expectancy and even those who stop at age 60 can restore 3 years.[120] This proves that it is never too late for a patient to benefit from smoking cessation. In fact, many patients are willing to quit, and there are multiple pharmacologic options available to help them.

Very different from other substances of abuse (e.g., alcohol), 70% of smokers will say they want to quit, and more than 40% report trying to quit in the past year.[121] Even in motivated individuals, the long-term success after one quit attempt is low with only about 5% sustaining abstinence at 1 year. With clinician-directed treatment, however, quit rates can increase dramatically to 25–33%.[121,122] The primary barriers to cessation are the addictive properties of nicotine and the behavioral component/oral gratification from the act of smoking itself. Nicotine causes physical and psychological dependence, tolerance, and subsequent well-documented withdrawal. Withdrawal symptoms include dysphoria, irritability, anxiety, restlessness, and weight gain and may begin to occur within hours of last use.

Every patient who uses tobacco products should undergo—at the minimum—brief counseling and assessment of readiness to quit. One structured, time-efficient method applicable in daily office use is the "5 A's" developed by Fiore et al. (see Table 8.1). In pain patients, a personalized message is easily given due to the strong, well-documented evidence of the effects of smoking on pain and outcomes. Among patients with pain, smokers experience greater pain than do nonsmokers.[123] Compared to nonsmokers, smokers have great pain intensity on BPI, greater pain interference with general activity, more mood disturbance, and more sleep difficulties.[124] A 2010 meta-analysis found that current smokers have a higher prevalence of chronic and disabling LBP.[125] Therefore, in addition to the proven cardiovascular and pulmonary benefits, *smoking cessation should be considered both an active and preventive treatment of pain.*

First-line agents for smoking cessation include nicotine replacement, bupropion, or varenicline, with combination treatment providing even greater quit rates. The U.S. Public Health Service does not recommend any one agent above another, but patient characteristics can often guide the choice. When there is concern about potential drug-drug interactions or with patients with particularly strong cravings for an early morning cigarette, a nicotine transdermal patch +/– nicotine gum may be an excellent choice. In patients with associated depressive features or with strong concern about weight gain, bupropion is preferred. It is also the agent of choice in schizophrenia because nicotine replacement appears to be less effective in this population.[126] It has long been believed that antidepressant medication (such as bupropion) has a destabilizing effect on bipolar disorder and may lead to the development of manic/hypomanic episodes. More recent data have rejected this notion, including a 2011 systematic review and meta-analysis that found that selective serotonin reuptake inhibitors (SSRIs), serotonin norepinephrine reuptake inhibitors (SNRIs), and bupropion are not associated with an increased switch rate. Varenicline[127] may provide slightly higher quit rates, but it has been associated with destabilizing previously well-controlled mental illness, as well as with suicidal behavior (attempts and completion) in those with no history of mental illness.

Direct nicotine replacement is most successfully utilized by combining a long-acting form (nicotine transdermal patch) with a short-acting form (nicotine lozenge, gum, or nasal spray). The patch will prevent development of nicotine withdrawal while the short-acting form can be used to combat cravings. All available nicotine replacement products are superior to placebo and approximately double quit rates,[122] although there is no evidence for superiority of one product

Table 8.1 **THE 5 A'S**

INTERVENTION	TECHNIQUE
Ask	Ask every patient about tobacco use
Advise	Strongly urge user to quit in a clear, strong, personalized manner • Clear: "I think it is important for you to quit smoking now, and I can help you." "Cutting down while you are ill is not enough." • Strong: "As your clinician, I need you to know that quitting smoking is the most important thing you can do to protect your health now and in the future. The clinic staff and I will help you." • Personalized: Tie tobacco use to current health/illness and/or to its social and economic costs, motivation level/ readiness to quit, and/or the impact of tobacco use on children and others in the household.
Assess	Determine the patient's willingness to quit smoking within the next 30 days: • If the patient is willing to make a quit attempt at this time, provide assistance. • If the patient will participate in an intensive treatment, deliver such a treatment or refer to an intensive intervention. • If the patient clearly states he or she is unwilling to make a quit attempt at this time, provide a motivational intervention. • If the patient is a member of a special population (e.g., adolescent, pregnant smoker), provide additional information specific to that population.
Assist	Provide aid for the patient to quit.
Arrange	Schedule follow-up contact, either in person or by telephone. Follow-up contact should occur soon after the quit date, preferably during the first week. Congratulate success during each follow-up.

From Fiore MC, Jaen C, Baker T, et al. Treating tobacco use and dependence: 2008 update. Clinical Practice Guideline. Rockville, MD: US Department of Health and Human Services. Public Health Service. 2008.

over another. When initiating nicotine replacement, the goal should be use for 2–3 months before beginning discontinuation. The strength of transdermal patch to use is based on the patient's consumption of cigarettes. One cigarettes contains approximately 1 mg of nicotine. Therefore, a patient who smokes 1 ppd can be started on a 21 mg/24-hour patch. Those who smoke ½ ppd should begin on a 14 mg/24-hour patch, and a 7 mg/24-hour patch can be used in those who smoke less. Two commonly occurring side effects with the patch include application site reactions and insomnia/vivid dreams. The former can be addressed by rotating the site and the latter by taking the patch off at night. For those who do remove the patch nightly, strong cravings should be anticipated the next morning and appropriate use of a short-acting agent made available.

One of the substantial difficulties in estimating total nicotine exposure through smoking is the variability in patient puffing and depth of inhalation. Use of short-acting nicotine gum (available in 2 mg and 4 mg strength) can aid with this. One piece of gum can be chewed every 1–2 hours, for example. Interestingly, there is a specific method to chewing the gum (very different than conventional chewing gum). If the gum is chewed too rapidly, nicotine release is rapid and is in fact swallowed rather than absorbed through the mucosa. This leads to nausea and stomach upset. Therefore, it must be chewed slowly and regularly over the course of 30 minutes. Given this, many patients prefer the nicotine lozenge (also in 2 mg and 4 mg strengths). It dissolves over the course of 30 minutes and there are no special instructions regarding use. Nicotine nasal spray is also available and is the quickest acting agent (10 minutes vs. 20–30 minutes for gum/lozenge). Patients may use up to 10 sprays/hour (maximum 80/day). Although the rapid onset of action more closely approximates smoked cigarettes, this form has the most side effects including nasal irritation that persists in more than 80% of patients.[128]

Buproprion is an antidepressant medication that works by enhancing the release of norepinephrine and dopamine. It currently is available in immediate release (IR), sustained release (SR), and extended release (XL). Because all formulations are generic, bupropion XL is the formulation of choice because it allows once-daily dosing and has an improved tolerability profile. The majority of efficacy studies utilized 150–300 mg of bupropion SR dosing, and an equivalent dose of XL formulation is appropriate. Meta-analysis shows that bupropion doubles quit rates compared to placebo (23% vs. 12%).[129] Bupropion should be started 2–3 weeks before the established quit date at 150 mg PO every morning. If well tolerated, strong consideration should be given to increasing the dose to 300 mg PO every morning by week 3 because there is some evidence that this higher dose may be more effective. Treatment should continue for 6–12 weeks after quit date.

Varenicline is the most recently FDA-approved medication for smoking cessation. It is a partial agonist at the $\alpha 4\beta$ subunit of the nicotinic receptor. It had dual actions in promoting cessation: stimulation of the nicotinic receptor, which reduces withdrawal symptoms, and blocking nicotine binding, which reduces the reinforcing aspects of cigarette smoking. There is accumulating evidence that varenicline is the most effective available treatment. A meta-analysis found that varenicline 1 mg BID tripled quit rates (33%) compared to placebo.[122] Three trials compared bupropion 300 mg/d versus varenicline 1 mg BID, and the latter was produced higher quit rates at 13 and 52 weeks.[130–132] Like bupropion, varenicline should be started before the quit date. Patients should begin 1 week before quitting at 0.5 mg daily for 3 days, then increase to 0.5 mg BID for 4 days. Starting at day 8, the dose is increased to 1 mg BID maintenance dosing for 11 weeks (12 weeks total treatment time).

The most serious side effects from varenicline include psychiatric disturbances and cardiovascular effects. There have been numerous case reports of new-onset mood symptoms, suicidal ideation, and even completed suicides. A pooled analysis of 10 RCTs, however, found no association between varenicline and psychiatric issues.[133] The FDA released an advisory in 2011 that varenicline may increase the risk of cardiovascular events in patients with a history of cardiovascular disease.[134] Two subsequent 2012 meta-analyses found no increased rate of cardiovascular events comparing varenicline to placebo.[135] Curiously, there has also been found an association between varenicline use and increased rates of motor vehicle accidents and falls.[136] It is unclear what this mechanism of action may be and whether varenicline has synergistic or potentiating effects with medications commonly prescribed to pain patients (opioids, benzodiazepines).

Other options include nortriptyline, clonidine, and alternative therapies (acupuncture, hypnosis, aversive therapy, financial incentives). Nortriptyline 75–100 mg/d doubles quit rates (OR = 2.1) with efficacy greater than bupropion.[137] A Cochrane meta-analysis also concluded that nortriptyline is an efficacious agent but did not show any benefit to combining nortriptyline + nicotine replacement.[138] Nortriptyline has significantly higher side effects and drop-out rates due to intolerability, which relegates it to a second-line agent. Clonidine has also been found to increase quit rates, but not to the extent of nortriptyline or other first-line agents. Use is limited by a dose-dependent increase in side effects.[138] Both oral and transdermal preparations aid with smoking cessation. Therapy can be started at 0.1 mg PO BID or 0.1 mg transdermally and increased up to 0.75 mg/d orally and 0.3 mg/d transdermally.

The use of acupuncture for smoking cessation is growing; however, the data do not support its efficacy. One meta-analysis comparing acupuncture versus sham acupuncture versus placebo found no difference in abstinent rates.[139] Even in cases where it has shown benefit, it is less effective than nicotine replacement.[140] Aversive therapy uses classical conditioning to associate smoking with a negative physical sensation. In this case, the patient is instructed to rapidly increase the amount smoked in the hope that nausea and vomiting from associated nicotine toxicity will lead to abstinence. Although some patients will report rapid and dramatic results from this method, a meta-analysis of 25 trials was not able to support this method.[141] *Contingency management* offers incentives or rewards to encourage specific behavioral goals (in this case smoking cessation). In illicit substance use, it is the most effective psychosocial intervention.[142] For smoking, the results have been less positive. One randomized trial among 878 smokes gave financial rewards of up to $750 for smoking cessation; at 12 months, the success rate was 15% versus 5% in a standard intervention group.[143] Not only was this less effective than nicotine replacement, it also introduces the ethical dilemma of rewarding patients for what they should be doing anyway. Hypnosis, both through self-hypnosis (audio) and therapist-directed means, has been used for decades in smoking cessation. Although popular as a self-guided or "drug-free" way to achieve abstinence, a Cochrane review found insufficient data to support hypnotherapy.[144]

Even though every reduction in smoking should be congratulated, the goal should be complete cessation. Consistent benefits (e.g., in cardiovascular risk) do not occur unless there is cessation.[145] Even smokers who decrease tobacco use by 50% had no improvement in mortality.[146,147] This lack of benefit may be due to compensatory behaviors by smokers, such as increased puffs, volume, or duration.[148]

The patient's daily use, unsuccessful efforts to cut down, smoking for a longer period than intended, craving, tolerance, withdrawal, and continued use despite awareness of negative health consequences meet criteria for severe tobacco use disorder (for the diagnostic criteria of Tobacco Use Disorder, see the *Diagnostic and Statistical Manual of Mental Disorders*, 5th edition). After discussing treatment options, the decision is made to begin bupropion XL. This is started at 150 mg, and a quit date is set for 3 weeks. After 1 week, the patient calls and complains of persistent insomnia since starting the medication. Rather than rotate to another first-line agent, given that the patient suffers from chronic pain and reports sleep disturbance from it, the decision is made to initiate nortriptyline. She is started at 25 mg QHS and instructed to increase her dose by 25 mg every 3 days to a goal dose of 100 mg/d. She is scheduled for follow-up in 2 weeks. When the patient is seen in the office, she is tolerating the medication well and reports improved sleep. She is ready to quit smoking, and a nicotine transdermal patch 21 mg/24- hours s added to the nortriptyline. When the patient is next seen in 4 weeks, she has been smoke free and also notes that the nortriptyline has begun to help with her LBP. She is congratulated on her efforts, nortriptyline 100 mg QHS is continued, and she is decreased to a 14 mg/24-hour transdermal patch.

SURGICAL OPTIONS

Surgical management of symptomatic disc disease remains a controversial topic.[149–154] In theory, removal of the degenerative, symptomatic disc through fusion or a motion-sparing procedure can eliminate the pain generator and lead to better clinical outcomes in patients with intractable LBP. Arthrodesis and motion-sparing technology represent two surgical options available to the patient with persistent, discogenic LBP who has failed nonoperative management.

Arthrodesis focuses on removing the provocative motion of the symptomatic disc. This surgery often entails removing the disc itself. Arthrodesis can be achieved with or without instrumentation and interbody techniques, from an anterior or posterior approach. Although instrumentation and interbody techniques improve fusion rates, it is unclear whether this translates into meaningful clinical differences.[149] It is also unclear whether fusion for discogenic LBP is superior to a focused nonoperative treatment program. The widely quoted Swedish Lumbar Spine Study Group found surgery to provide superior outcomes when compared to standard nonoperative care.[150] A more recent meta-analysis of five RCTs found improvement in Owestery Disability Index (ODI) scores of 7.39 points in favor of fusion over nonoperative treatment. However, it is uncertain whether this translates into significant clinical differences.[151] However, a similar, but smaller study with long-term follow-up (11.4 years) found no significant difference over a focused nonoperative treatment program.[152]

Motion-sparing technology arose out of an effort to mitigate the potential for adjacent segment disease in lumbar fusion patients. Total disc arthroplasty (TDA) replaces the symptomatic disc with a motion preserving device. Numerous studies have evaluated the efficacy of TDA and, in general, found TDA to be a reasonable alternative to fusion.[153] Because LBP can emanate from so many sources, there is a whole list of contraindications to TDA, ranging from stenosis to facet arthrosis and chronic steroid use.[153] Reoperation on a patient with a failed TDA can have grave consequences, including a significantly higher incidence of vascular injuries (16.7%) than in the primary implantation setting (3.4%).

Although this patient has a single-level, symptomatic disc and has failed a trial of therapy and NSAIDs, she is not currently a good surgical candidate. The patient is a current smoker. Smoking has been shown to be a predictor of poorer outcome in lumbar fusion surgery.[154] This young woman is also obese (BMI 32.5) and therefore not a good candidate for motion-preserving techniques.[153] Our patient would be best served by a focused nonoperative management program stressing the importance of nicotine cessation, weight reduction, and cognitive-behavioral therapy.

WHAT IS THE LONG-TERM PROGNOSIS FOR DISCOGENIC BACK PAIN?

The occurrence of LBP is statistically very high, with an estimated lifetime prevalence of 65–80% regardless of age, sex, or country, and this rate varies only slightly among occupations. Any pathological change of the structures in the lumbar spine can become a pain generator. Beyond more specific problems like nerve compression or structural disease of the vertebrae, discogenic pain is a major cause of chronic LBP. Among a population of chronic LBP patients, 39% had an internal disc disruption, confirmed by concordant pain on provocative discography tests and indicative of the discogenic origin of their pain.[51,52] Disc degeneration is considered to be one of the primary events, in addition to endplate pathology, that subsequently and in a cascading manner may lead to a secondary deterioration of the other structures of the spine, including facets, ligaments, and muscles. Studies have shown that the majority of patients who suddenly develop LBP will quickly improve on their own regardless of the care received.[155] In these prospective studies, patients have reported that their symptoms improved markedly within several weeks. Based on these relatively short-term observations, the assumption was made that symptoms would disappear entirely within, at most, a few months. However, this assumption was subsequently challenged by other epidemiologists who found it difficult to reconcile this theoretically favorable prognosis with the presence of a substantial number of patients who still reported symptoms many years after their original studies. They hypothesized that by truncating the length of the follow-up, these studies failed to observe the true pattern of waxing and waning symptoms. Although symptoms often do recede within a few months, the follow-up periods were often too short to capture the longer term recurrences and exacerbations of symptoms that were common with LBP.

Currently, LBP can be considered a recurrent disorder that can occur at any time in a person's life and that fluctuates between a status of no pain or mild pain and pain that reaches a point at which it interferes with activities of normal living or becomes debilitating.[64]

Chronic unremitting LBP is one of the most challenging conditions to treat. Some portions of this patient population have improvement in their functional level and achieve symptomatic improvement with a comprehensive nonoperative treatment program. However, a substantial number of patients are unresponsive to aggressive nonoperative interventions and have shown to have a low probability of spontaneous resolution.[156,157] As a result, they are faced with the choice of living with the pain and functional limitations or undergoing chronic pain management or more invasive treatments. Surgical and percutaneous minimally invasive procedures might be helpful, but are all associated with limitations related to the morbidity of the procedure, perioperative complications, failed interventions, increased probability of repeat treatments, and poor outcomes. Relying on published literature, there is no magic bullet and no treatment that stands head and shoulders above the rest for treatment of chronic LBP related to painful internal disc disruption with mild protrusion. Newer treatments in development are aimed at restoring disc tissue, disc height, and biomechanical function of the disc. These include biological therapies, novel surgical interventions, stem cell treatments, and gene therapy. They all provide hope for the successful management of chronic discogenic back pain, although a critical evidence-based approach will be necessary to adequately demonstrate their positive outcome and safety. Currently, it is felt that adequate physical exercise, avoidance of smoking, and minimization of harmful loads on the spine are the only known ways of preventing painful disc disease.[158]

A few factors may contribute to a less favorable prognosis for this patient, including the chronicity of her symptoms and the presence of confounding factors. She smokes, she is obese according to BMI calculations, and she failed to respond to conservative treatment. Assuming that she had positive findings on provocative or other type of discography, has only one-level disc disease, and that she is relatively young, she could have a positive outcome following one of the interventional percutaneous treatment procedures. If not, she might need to consider surgical treatment after she completes specific lifestyle modifications, including cessation of smoking and weight loss.

REFERENCES

1. Derby R, Wolfer L. Targeting pain generators. In: Herkowitz HN, Garfin SR, Eismont FJ, Bell GR, Balderston RA, eds. *Rothman-Simeone: The Spine.* Philadelphia: Elsevier Saunders; 2011:246–279.

2. Wetzel FT. Chronic benign cervical pain syndromes. Surgical considerations. *Spine.* 1992;17:S367–S374.
3. Manchikanti L, Pampati V, Rivera J, Fellows B, Beyer C, Damron K. Role of facet joints in chronic low back pain in the elderly: a controlled comparative prevalence study. *Pain Practice.* 2001a;1:332–337.
4. Yin W, Bogduk N. The nature of neck pain in a private pain clinic in the United States. *Pain Med.* 2008;9:196–203.
5. Mooney V. Presidential address. International Society for the Study of the Lumbar Spine. Dallas, 1986. Where is the pain coming from? *Spine.* 1987;12:754–759.
6. Vanharanta H, Sachs BL, Spivey MA, et al. The relationship of pain provocation to lumbar disc deterioration as seen by CT/discography. *Spine.* 1987;12:295–298.
7. Smith SE, Darden BV, Rhyne AL, Wood KE. Outcome of unoperated discogram-positive low back pain. *Spine.* 1995;20:1997–2000.
8. Inman VT, Saunders JB. Anatomicophysiological aspects of injuries to the intervertebral disc. *Journal of Bone and Joint Surgery* (American Volume). 1947;29:461–475.
9. Malinsky J. The ontogenetic development of nerve terminations in the intervertebral discs of man. (Histology of intervertebral discs, 11th communication). *Acta Anat* (Basel). 1959;38:96–113.
10. Yoshizawa H, O'Brien JP, Smith WT, Trumper M. The neuropathology of intervertebral discs removed for low-back pain. *J Pathol.* 1980;132:95–104.
11. Fernstrom U. A discographical study of ruptured lumbar intervertebral discs. *Eur J Surg Suppl.* 1960:1–60.
12. Crock HV. A reappraisal of intervertebral disc lesions. *Med J Aust.* 1970;1:983–989.
13. Bogduk N, Tynan W, Wilson AS. The nerve supply to the human lumbar intervertebral discs. *J Anat.* 1981;132:39–56.
14. Groen GJ, Baljet B, Drukker J. Nerves and nerve plexuses of the human vertebral column. *Am J Anat.* 1990;188:282–296.
15. Konttinen YT, Gronblad M, Antti-Poika I, et al. Neuroimmunohistochemical analysis of peridiscal nociceptive neural elements. *Spine* (Phila Pa 1976). 1990;15:383–386.
16. Korkala O, Grönblad M, Liesi P, Karaharju E. Immunohistochemical demonstration of nociceptors in the ligamentous structures of the lumbar spine. *Spine.* 1985;10:156–157.
17. Weinstein J, Claverie W, Gibson S. The pain of discography. *Spine* (Phila Pa 1976). 1988;13:1344–1348.
18. Nakamura SI, Takahashi K, Takahashi Y, Yamagata M, Moriya H. The afferent pathways of discogenic low-back pain. Evaluation of L2 spinal nerve infiltration. *J Bone Joint Surg Br.* 1996;78:606–612.
19. Takahashi K, Aoki Y, Ohtori S. Resolving discogenic pain. *Eur Spine J.* 2008;17:428–431.
20. Brisby H. Pathology and possible mechanisms of nervous system response to disc degeneration. *J Bone Joint Surg Am.* 2006;88:68–71.
21. Freemont AJ, Peacock TE, Goupille P, Hoyland JA, O'Brien J, Jayson MI. Nerve ingrowth into diseased intervertebral disc in chronic back pain. *Lancet.* 1997;350:178–181.
22. Podichetty VK. The aging spine: the role of inflammatory mediators in intervertebral disc degeneration. *Cell Mol Biol* (Noisy-le-grand). 2007;53:4–18.
23. Roberts S, Eisenstein SM, Menage J, Evans EH, Ashton IK. Mechanoreceptors in intervertebral discs. Morphology, distribution, and neuropeptides. *Spine.* 1995;20:2645–2651.
24. Calodney A, Buchalter J. Epidemiology and etiology of discogenic pain: how big is the problem? In: Kapural L, Kim P, Deer TR, eds. *Diagnosis, Management, and Treatment of Discogenic Pain.* Vol. 3. Philadelphia: Elsevier, Saunders; 2012:1–13.
25. Ahadian, FM, Wallace MS. Estabilshing the diagnosis of discogenic back pain: an evidence-based algorithmic approach. In: Kapural L, Kim P, eds. *Diagnosis, Management, and Treatment of Discogenic Pain.* Vol. 3. Philadelphia: Elsevier, Saunders; 2012:14–28.
26. Bogduk, N. *Practice Guidelines for Spinal Diagnostic and Treatment Prodedures.* San Francisco: International Spine Intervention Society; 2004a.
27. Derby R, Lee S-H, Chen Y Discograms: cervical,thoracic, and lumbar. *Tech Reg Anesth Pain Manag.* 2005;9:97–105.
28. Guyer RD, Ohnmeiss DD. Lumbar discography. Position statement from the North American Spine Society Diagnostic and Therapeutic Committee. *Spine.* 1995;20:2048–2059.
29. Wolfer LR, Derby R, Lee J-E, Lee S-H. Systematic review of lumbar provocation discography in asymptomatic subjects with a meta-analysis of false-positive rates. *Pain Physician.* 2008;11:513–538.
30. Bogduk, N. Proposed discography standards [newsletter]. *International Spinal Injection Society.* 1994;1(1):10–13.
31. Derby, R. A second proposal for discography standards. *International Spinal Injection Society.* 1994;2(2):108–122.
32. Jensen MC, Brant-Zawadzki MN, Obuchowski N, Modic MT, Malkasian D, Ross JS. Magnetic resonance imaging of the lumbar spine in people without back pain. *N Engl J Med.* 1994;331:69–73.
33. Sachs BL, Vanharanta H, Spivey MA, et al. Dallas discogram description. A new classification of CT/discography in low-back disorders. *Spine.* 1987;12:287–294.
34. Aprill C, Bogduk N. High-intensity zone: a diagnostic sign of painful lumbar disc on magnetic resonance imaging. *Br J Radiol.* 1992;65:361–369.
35. Carragee EJ. Prevalence and clinical features of internal disk disruption in patients with chronic low back pain. *Spine.* 1996; 21:776–777.
36. Carragee EJ, Tanner CM, Khurana S, et al. The rates of false-positive lumbar discography in select patients without low back symptoms. *Spine.* 2000b;25:1373–1380.
37. Derby R, Guyer R, Lee SH, Seo KS, Chen Y. The rational use and limitations of provocative discography. *International Spine Intervention Society 13th Annual meeting in NY* [ISIS newsletter]. 2004;5:6–20.
38. Carragee EJ, Tanner CM, Yang B, Brito JL, Truong T. False-positive findings on lumbar discography. Reliability of subjective concordance assessment during provocative disc injection. *Spine.* 1999;24:2542–2547.
39. Derby R, Kim BJ, Lee SH, Chen Y, Seo KS, Aprill C. Comparison of discographic findings in asymptomatic subject discs and the negative discs of chronic LBP patients: can discography distinguish asymptomatic discs among morphologically abnormal discs? *Spine J.* 2005a;5:389–394.
40. Shin D, Kim H, Jung J, Sin D, Lee J. Diagnostic relevance of pressure-controlled discography. *J Korean Med Sci.* 2006;21:911–916.
41. Manchikanti L, Singh V, Pampati V, et al. Provocative discography in low back pain patients with or without somatization disorder: a randomized prospective evaluation. *Pain Physician.* 2001c;4:227–239.
42. Derby R, Lee S-H, Chen Y, et al. The influence of psychologic factors on diskography in patients with chronic axial low back pain. *Arch Phys Med Rehabil.* 2008a;89:1300–1304.
43. Carragee EJ, Don AS, Hurwitz EL, Cuellar JM, Carrino J, Herzog R. Does discography cause accelerated progression of degeneration changes in the lumbar disc: a ten-year matched cohort study. *Spine* (Phila Pa 1976). 2009;13:2338–2345.
44. Derby R, Wolfer L, Summers J. Does discography cause accelerated progression of degeneration in the lumbar spine. *SpineLine.* Mar/April 2010b:26–30.
45. Derby R, Howard MW, Grant JM, Lettice JJ, Van Peteghem PK, Ryan DP. The ability of pressure-controlled discography to predict surgical and nonsurgical outcomes. *Spine.* 1999;24:364–371.
46. Melnik I, Derby R. Provocative Discography, AAPM (American Academy of Pain Medicine) Textbook of Pain Medicine-Interventional Section. In process.
47. Derby R, Aprill CN, Lee JE, Depalma MJ, Baker RM. Comparison of four different analgesic discogram protocols comparing the incidence of reported pain relief following local anesthetic injection into concordantly painful lumbar intervertebral discs. *Pain Med.* 2012a;13:1547–1553.
48. Derby R, Baker RM, Wolfer L. Analgesic discography. In: Kakpural L, Kim P, Deer TR, eds. *Interventional and Neuromodulatory Techniques for Pain Management: Diagnosis, Treatment, and*

Evaluation of Discogenic Pain. Vol. 3. Philadelphia: Elsevier Saunders; 2012c:65–74.
49. Derby R, Lee J-E, Lee S-H. Analgesic discography: effect of adding a local anesthetic to routine lumbar provocation discography. *Pain Med*. 2010a;11:1335–1342.
50. Derby R, Wolfer LR, Chen Y. Analgesic discography: can analgesic tesing identify a painful disc? *SpineLine*. Nov/Dec 2008b:17–24.
51. Manchikanti L, Singh V, Pampati V, et al. Evaluation of the relative contributions of various structures in chronic low back pain. *Pain Physician*. 2001b;4:308–316.
52. Schwarzer AC, Aprill CN, Derby R, Fortin J, Kine G, Bogduk N. The prevalence and clinical features of internal disc disruption in patients with chronic low back pain. *Spine*. 1995;20:1878–1883.
53. Manchikanti L. Epidemiology of low back pain. *Pain Physician*. 2000;3:167–192.
54. Deyo RA, Mirza SK, Martin BI. Back pain prevalence and visit rates: estimates from U.S. national surveys, 2002. *Spine*. 2006;31:2724–2727.
55. Hart LG, Deyo RA, Cherkin DC. Physician office visits for low back pain. Frequency, clinical evaluation, and treatment patterns from a U.S. national survey. *Spine*. 1995;20:11–19.
56. Frank JW, Brooker AS, DeMaio SE, et al. Disability resulting from occupational low back pain. Part II: What do we know about secondary prevention? A review of the scientific evidence on prevention after disability begins. *Spine*. 1996;21:2918–2929.
57. Stewart WF, Ricci JA, Chee E, Morganstein D, Lipton R. Lost productive time and cost due to common pain conditions in the US workforce. *JAMA*. 2003;290:2443–2454.
58. Martin BI, Deyo RA, Mirza SK, et al. Expenditures and health status among adults with back and neck problems. *JAMA*. 2008;299:656–664.
59. Wood P, Bradley E. Back pain in the community. *Clin Rheum Dis*. 1980;6:3–11.
60. Nagi S, Riley L, Newby L. Social epidemiology of back pain in a general population. *J Chronic Disc*. 1973;26.
61. Lenrow D. Epidemiology. In: Slipman CW, Derby R, Simeone FA, Mayer TG, eds. *Interventional Spine: An Algorithmic Approach*. Philadelphia: Saunders Elsevier; 2008:9–15.
62. Bogduk, N. Evidence-based clinical guidelines for the management of acute low back pain. Submitted to the Medical Health and Research Concil of Australia; 1999.
63. Chiodo AE, Alvarez DJ, Graziano GP, et al. *Acute Low Back Pain: Guidlelines for Clinical Care*. Ann Arbor: University of Michigan Health System; 2010:1–14.
64. Dagenais S, Haldeman S. Evidence-based management of low back pain. In: Dagenais S, Haldeman S, eds. *Evidence-Based Management of Low Back Pain*. St. Louis, MO: Elsevier Mosby; 2012:1–12.
65. Dagenais S, Tricco AC, Haldeman S. Synthesis of recommendations for the assessment and management of low back pain from recent clinical practice guidelines. *Spine J*. 2010;10:514–529.
66. Berthelot JM, Delecrin J, Maugars Y, Passuti N. Contribution of centralization phenomenon to the diagnosis, prognosis, and treatment of diskogenic low back pain. *Joint Bone Spine*. 2007;74:319–323.
67. Yrjämä M, Tervonen O, Kurunlahti M, Vanharanta H. Bony vibration stimulation test combined with magnetic resonance imaging. Can discography be replaced? *Spine*. 1997;22:808–813.
68. Dillingham TR. Electrodiagnostic approach to patients with suspected radiculopathy. *Phys Med Rehabil Clin N Am*. 2002;13:567–588.
69. Carragee E, Alamin T, Cheng I, Franklin T, van den Haak E, Hurwitz E. Are first-time episodes of serious LBP associated with new MRI findings? *Spine J*. 2006;6:624–635.
70. Hancock MJ, Maher CG, Latimer J, et al. Systematic review of tests to identify the disc, SIJ or facet joint as the source of low back pain. *Eur Spine J*. 2007;16:1539–1550.
71. Collins CD, Stack JP, O'Connell DJ, et al. The role of discography in lumbar disc disease: a comparative study of magnetic resonance imaging and discography. *ClinRadiol*. 1990;42:252–257.
72. Zhang YG, Guo TM, Guo X, Wu SX. Clinical diagnosis for discogenic low back pain. *Int J Biol Sci*. 2009;5:647–658.
73. Carragee EJ, Paragioudakis SJ, Khurana S. 2000 Volvo Award winner in clinical studies: lumbar high-intensity zone and discography in subjects without low back problems. *Spine* (Phila Pa 1976). 2000a:25:2987–2992.
74. Braithwaite I, White J, Saifuddin A, Renton P, Taylor BA. Vertebral end-plate (Modic) changes on lumbar spine MRI: correlation with pain reproduction at lumbar discography. *Eur Spine J*. 1998;7:363–368.
75. Kjaer P, Korsholm L, Bendix T, Sorensen JS, Leboeuf-Yde C. Modic changes and their associations with clinical findings. *Eur Spine J*. 2006;15:1312–1319.
76. Bogduk, N. 2004b. Practice guidelines: spinal diagnostic and treatment procedures. In: Bogduk N, ed. *Lumbar Disc Stimulation* (Provocation Discography). San Francisco: International Spine Intervention Society; 2004b:20–46.
77. Biyani A, Andersson GBJ, Chaudhary H, An HS. Intradiscal electrothermal therapy: a treatment option in patients with internal disc disruption. *Spine*. 2003;28:S8–S14.
78. Chou LH, Lew HL, Coelho PC, Slipman CW. Intradiscal electrothermal annuloplasty. *Am J Phys Med Rehabil*. 2005;84:538–549.
79. Derby R, Baker RM, Melnik I, Lee JE, Lee CH, Anderson PA. Intradiscal thermal therapies. In: Dagenais S, Haldeman S, eds. *Evidence-Based Management of Low Back Pain*. St. Louis, MO: Elsevier Mosby; 2012b:364–388.
80. Helm S, Hayek SM, Benyamin RM, Manchikanti L. Systematic review of the effectiveness of thermal annular procedures in treating discogenic low back pain. *Pain Physician*. 2009;12:207–232.
81. Freeman BJ, Fraser RD, Cain CM, Hall DJ, Chapple DC. A randomized, double-blind, controlled trial: intradiscal electrothermal therapy versus placebo for the treatment of chronic discogenic low back pain. *Spine*. 2005;30:2369–2377; discussion 2378.
82. Pauza KJ, Howell S, Dreyfuss P, Peloza JH, Dawson K, Bogduk N. A randomized, placebo-controlled trial of intradiscal electrothermal therapy for the treatment of discogenic low back pain. *Spine J*. 2004;4:27–35.
83. Barendse GA, van Den Berg SG, Kessels, AH, Weber WE, van Kleef M. Randomized controlled trial of percutaneous intradiscal radiofrequency thermocoagulation for chronic discogenic back pain: lack of effect from a 90-second 70 C lesion. *Spine*. 2001;26:287–292.
84. Lau P, Mercer S, Govind J, Bogduk N. The surgical anatomy of lumbar medial branch neurotomy (facet denervation). *Pain Med*. 2004;5:289–298.
85. Derby R, Eek B, Chen Y, O'Neill C, Ryan D. Intradiscal electrothermal annuloplasty (IDET): a novel approach for treating chronic discogenic back pain. *Neuromodulation*. 2000;3:82–88.
86. Saal JA, Saal JS. Intradiscal electrothermal treatment for chronic discogenic low back pain: a prospective outcome study with minimum 1-year follow-up. *Spine*. 2000;25:2622–2627.
87. Saal JA, Saal JS. Intradiscal electrothermal treatment for chronic discogenic low back pain: prospective outcome study with a minimum 2-year follow-up. *Spine* (Phila Pa 1976). 2002;27:966–973; discussion 973–964.
88. Bogduk N, Lau P, Gowaily K,Bailey B. A pilot audit of radiofrequency biacuplasty for back pain due to internal disc disruption. In *International Spine Intervention Society(ISIS)*, 16th annual scientific meeting. Las Vegas, NV; 2008:184–185.
89. Kapural L. Intervertebral disk cooled bipolar radiofrequency (intradiskal biacuplasty) for the treatment oflumbar diskogenic pain: a 12-month follow-up of the pilot study. *Pain Med*. 2008;9:407–408.
90. Kapural L, Cata JP, Narouze S. Successful treatment of lumbar discogenic pain using intradiscal biacuplasty in previously discectomized disc. *Pain Pract*. 2009;9:130–134.
91. Kapural L, Mekhail N. Novel intradiscal biacuplasty (IDB) for the treatment of lumbar discogenic pain. *Pain Pract*. 2007;7:130–134.
92. Kapural L, Vrooman B, Sarwar S, et al. A randomized, placebo-controlled trial of transdiscal radiofrequency, biacuplasty for treatment of discogenic lower back pain. *Pain Med*. 2013; 14(3):362–373.

93. Chou R, Atlas SJ, Stanos SP, Rosenquist RW. Nonsurgical interventional therapies for low back pain: a review of the evidence for an American Pain Society clinical practice guideline. *Spine* (Phila Pa 1976). 2009;34:1078–1093.
94. Manchikanti L, Derby R, Benyamin RM, Helm S, Hirsch JA. A systematic review of mechanical lumbar disc decompression with nucleoplasty. *Pain Physician*. 2009;12:561–572.
95. Smith, L. Enzyme dissolution of the nucleus pulposus in humans. *JAMA*. 1964;187:137–140.
96. Shioda M. [Intradiscal injection of hypertonic saline, phenol-glycerin and osmic acid for the treatment of lumbar disc herniation: an experimental study]. *Nihon Seikeigeka Gakkai zasshi*. 1995;69:964–976.
97. Riquelme C, Musacchio M, Mont'Alverne F, Tournade A. Chemonucleolysis of lumbar disc herniation with ethanol. *J Neuroradiol*. 2001;28:219–229.
98. Theron J, Cuellar H, Sola T, Guimaraens L, Casasco A, Courtheoux P. Percutaneous treatment of cervical disk hernias using gelified ethanol. *Am J Neuroradiol*. 2010;31:1454–1456.
99. Gallucci M, Limbucci N, Zugaro L, et al. Sciatica: treatment with intradiscal and intraforaminal injections of steroid and oxygen-ozone versus steroid only. *Radiology*. 2007;242:907–913.
100. Andreula, CF, Simonetti L, De Santis F, Agati R, Ricci R, Leonardi M. Minimally invasive oxygen-ozone therapy for lumbar disk herniation. *Am J Neuroradiol*. 24:996–1000.
101. Corea F, Amici S, Murgia N, Tambasco N. A case of vertebrobasilar stroke during oxygen-ozone therapy. *J Stroke Cerebrovasc Dis*. 2004;13:259–261.
102. Peng B, Zhang Y, Hou S, Wu W, Fu X. Intradiscal methylene blue injection for the treatment of chronic discogenic low back pain. *Eur Spine J*. 2007;16:33–38.
103. Peng B, Pang X, Wu Y, Zhao C, Song X. A randomized placebo-controlled trial of intradiscal methylene blue injection for the treatment of chronic discogenic low back pain. *Pain*. 2010;149:124–129.
104. Miller M, Mathews R, Reeves KD. Treatment of painful advanced internal lumbar disc derangement with intradiscal injection of hypertonic dextrose. *Pain Physician*. 2006;9:115–121.
105. Khot A, Bowditch M, Powell J, Sharp D. The use of intradiscal steroid therapy for lumbar spinal discogenic pain: a randomized controlled trial. *Spine*. 2004;29:833–836.
106. Fayad F, Lefevre-Colau MM, Rannou F, et al. Relation of inflammatory modic changes to intradiscal steroid injection outcome in chronic low back pain. *Eur Spin J*. 2007;16:925–931.
107. Cohen SP, Wenzell D, Hurley RW, et al. A double-blind, placebo-controlled, dose-response pilot study evaluating intradiscal etanercept in patients with chronic discogenic low back pain or lumbosacral radiculopathy. *Anesthesiology*. 2007;107:99–105.
108. Klein RG, Eek BC, O'Neill CW, Elin C, Mooney V, Derby RR. Biochemical injection treatment for discogenic low back pain: a pilot study. *Spine J*. 2003;3:220–226.
109. Derby R, Eek B, Lee S-H, Seo KS, Kim B-J. Comparison of intradiscal restorative injections and intradiscal electrothermal treatment (IDET) in the treatment of low back pain. *Pain Physician*. 2004;7:63–66.
110. Chen WH, Liu HY, Lo WC, et al. Intervertebral disc regeneration in an ex vivo culture system using mesenchymal stem cells and platelet-rich plasma. *Biomaterials*. 2009;30:5523–5533.
111. Wuertz K, Godburn K, Neidlinger-Wilke C, Urban J, Iatridis JC. Behavior of mesenchymal stem cells in the chemical microenvironment of the intervertebral disc. *Spine*. 2008;33:1843–1849.
112. Petersohn JD. Discogenic pain: intradiscal therapeutic injections and use of intradiscal biologic agents. In: Kapural L, Kim P, eds. *Diagnosis, Management, and Treatment of Discogenic Pain*. Vol. 3. Philadelphia: Elsevier, Saunders;2012:75–79.
113. Masuda K, Aota Y, Muehleman C, et al. A novel rabbit model of mild, reproducible disc degeneration by an anulus needle puncture: correlation between the degree of disc injury and radiological and histological appearances of disc degeneration. *Spine* (Phila Pa 1976). 2005;30:5–14.
114. Sha'ban M, Yoon SJ, Ko YK, et al. Fibrin promotes proliferation and matrix production of intervertebral disc cells cultured in three-dimensional poly(lactic-co-glycolic acid) scaffold. *J Biomater Sci Polym Ed*. 2008;19:1219–1237.
115. Derby R, Talu G, Kazala K, Chen Y. Injection of fibrin sealant into discs following IDET and nucleoplasty early outcome in six cases. *International Spine Intervention Society*. 2005b;5:12–19.
116. Yin W, et al. Intradiscal injection of fibrin sealant for the treatment of symptomatic internal disc disruption: results of a prospective multicenter IDE pilot study with 6-month follow-up. *Pain Med*. 2009;10:955.
117. Centers for Disease Control and Prevention. Vital signs: current cigarette smoking among adults aged ≥18 years—United States, 2005–2010. *Morb Mortal Wkly Rep*. 2011;60(35):1207–1211.
118. Grant BF, Hasin DS, Chou SP, et al. Nicotine dependence and psychiatric disorders in the United States: results from the national epidemiologic survey on alcohol and related conditions. *Arch Gen Psychiatry*. 2004;61(11):1107–1115.
119. Peto R, Lopez AD, Boreham J, et al. *Mortality from Smoking in Developed Countries 1950–2000* (Rev.). Oxford: Oxford University Press; 2006.
120. IARC. *Reversal of Risk after Quitting Smoking*. Lyon, France: IARC Handbooks for Cancer Prevention, Tobacco Control; 2007:11.
121. Rigotti NA. Clinical practice. Treatment of tobacco use and dependence. *N Engl J Med*. 2002;346:506.
122. Fiore MC, Jaen CR, Baker TB, et al. Treating tobacco use and dependence: 2008 update. US Department of Health and Human Services; 2008. Available at: www.surgeongeneral.gov/tobacco/treating_tobacco_use08.pdf
123. Eriksen WB, Brage S, Bruusgaard D. Does smoking aggravate musculoskeletal pain? *Scand J Rheum*. 1997;26:49–54.
124. Weingarten TN, Moeschler SM, Ptaszynski AE, et al. An assessment of the association between smoking status, pain intensity, and functional interference in patients with chronic pain. *Pain Phys*. 2008;11:5:643–653.
125. Shiri R, Karppinen J, Leino-Arjas P, et al. The association between smoking and low back pain: a meta-analysis. *Am J Med*. 2010;123(1):87;e7–e35.
126. 1. Tsoi DT, Porwal M, Webster AC. Interventions for smoking cessation and reduction in individuals with schizophrenia. *Cochrane Database Syst Rev*. 2010;CD007253.
127. Sidor MM, MacQueen GM. Antidepressants for the acute treatment of bipolar depression: a systematic review and meta-analysis. *J Clin Psychiatry*. 2011;72(2);156–167.
128. Nicotrol NS. Product Information. Available at: /www.nicotrol.com.
129. Hughes JR, Stead LF, Lancaster T. Antidepressants for smoking cessation. *Cochrane Database Syst Rev*. 2007;CD000031.
130. Gonzales D, Rennard SI, Nides M, et al. Varenicline, an alpha-4beta2 nicotinic acetylcholine receptor partial agonist, vs sustained-release bupropion and placebo for smoking cessation: a randomized controlled trial. *JAMA*. 2006;296:47.
131. Jorenby DE, Hays JT, Rigotti NA, et al. Efficacy of varenicline, an alpha4beta2 nicotinic acetylcholine receptor partial agonist, vs placebo or sustained-release bupropion for smoking cessation: a randomized controlled trial. *JAMA*. 2006;296:56.
132. Nides M, Oncken C, Gonzales D, et al. Smoking cessation with varenicline, a selective alpha4beta2 nicotinic receptor partial agonist: results from a 7-week, randomized, placebo- and bupropion-controlled trial with 1-year follow-up. *Arch Intern Med*. 2006;166:1561.
133. Tonstad S, Davies S, Flammer M, et al. Psychiatric adverse events in randomized, double-blind, placebo-controlled clinical trials of varenicline: a pooled analysis. *Drug Saf*. 2010;33:289. Available at: www.fda.gov/Drugs/DrugSafety/ucm259161.htm

134. http://www.fda.gov/Drugs/DrugSafety/ucm259161.htm
135. Prochaska JJ, Hilton JF. Risk of cardiovascular serious adverse events associated with varenicline use for tobacco cessation: systematic review and meta-analysis. *Br Med J.* 2012;344:e2856. Available at: www.fda.gov/Drugs/DrugSafety/ucm330367.htm
136. www.ismp.org/docs/vareniclineStudy.asp
137. Hughes JR, Stead LF, Lancaster T. Nortriptyline for smoking cessation: a review. *Nicotine Tob Res.* 2005;7(4):491–499.
138. Cahill K, Stevens S, Perera R, Lancaster T. Pharmacological interventions for smoking cessation: an overview and network meta-analysis. *Cochrane Database of Systematic Rev.* 2013:CD009329. doi: 10.1002/14651858.CD009329.pub2
139. White AR, Rampes H, Liu JP, et al. Acupuncture and related interventions for smoking cessation. *Cochrane Database Syst Rev.* 2011:CD000009.
140. Tahiri M, Mottillo S, Joseph L, et al. Alternative smoking cessation aids: a meta-analysis of randomized controlled trials. *Am J Med.* 2012;125:576.
141. Hajek P, Stead LF. Aversive smoking for smoking cessation. *Cochrane Database Syst Rev.* 2004:CD000546.
142. Dutra L, Stathopoulou G, Basden SL, et al. A meta-analytic review of psychosocial interventions for substance use disorders. *Am J Psychiatry.* 2008;165:179–187.
143. Volpp KG, Troxel AB, Pauly MV, et al. A randomized, controlled trial of financial incentives for smoking cessation. *N Engl J Med.* 2009;360:699.
144. Barnes J, Dong CY, McRobbie H, et al. Hypnotherapy for smoking cessation. *Cochrane Database Syst Rev.* 2010:CD001008.
145. Office of the Surgeon General. Cardiovascular diseases. In: *A Report of the Surgeon General: How Tobacco Smoke Causes Disease.* US Department of Health and Human Services; 2011. Available at: www.surgeongeneral.gov/library/tobaccosmoke/report/chapter6.pdf. Accessed December 6, 2011.
146. Tverdal A, Bjartveit K. Health consequences of reduced daily cigarette consumption. *Tob Control.* 2006;15:472.
147. Godtfredsen NS, Holst C, Prescott E, et al. Smoking reduction, smoking cessation, and mortality: a 16-year follow-up of 19,732 men and women from The Copenhagen Centre for Prospective Population Studies. *Am J Epidemiol.* 2002;156:994.
148. Rennard SI, Rigotti NA, Daughton DM. Overview of smoking cessation management in adults. In: Basow DS, ed. *UpToDate.* Waltham, MA: UpToDate; 2013.
149. Fritzell P, Hagg O, Jonsson, Nordwall A. Swedish Lumbar Spine Study Group. Chronic low back pain: a comparison of three surgical techniques. *Spine.* 2002;27:1131–1141.
150. Fritzell P, Hagg O, Jonsson, Nordwall A. Lumbar fusion versus nonsurgical treatment for chronic low back pain: a multicenter randomized controlled trial from the Swedish Lumbar Spine Study Group. *Spine.* 2001;26:2521–2532.
151. Bydon M, De la Garza-Ramos R, Macki M, Baker A, Gokaslan AK, Bydon A. Lumbar fusion versus non-operative management for treatment of discogenic low back pain: a systematic review and meta-analysis of randomized controlled trials. *J Spinal Disord Tech.* 2014.
152. Mannion AF, Brox JI, Fairbank JC. Comparison of spinal fusion and nonoperative treatment in patients with chronic low back pain: a long-term follow-up of three randomized controlled trials. *Spine J,* 2013;(11):1438–1448.
153. Madigan L, Vaccaro A, Spector L, Milam R. Management of symptomatic lumbar degenerative disk disease. *J Am Acad Orthop Surg.* 2009;17:102–111.
154. LaCaille RA, DeBerard MS, Masters KS, Colledge AL, Bacon W. Presurgical biopsychological factors predict multidimensional patient: outcomes of interbody cage lumbar fusion. *Spine J.* 2005;5:71–78.
155. Coste J, Delecoeuillerie G, Cohen de Lara A, Le Parc JM, Paolaggi JB. Clinical course and prognostic factors in acute low back pain: an inception cohort study in primary care practice. *Br Med J* (BMJ.com). 1994;308:577–580.
156. McCoy CE, Selby D, Henderson R, Handal J, Peloza J, Wolf C. Patients avoiding surgery. Pathology and one-year life status follow-up. *Spine.* 1991;16:S198–200.
157. Von Korff M. Studying the natural history of back pain. *Spine.* 1994;19:2041S–2046S.
158. Hurri H, Karppinen J. Discogenic pain. *Pain.* 2004;112:225–228.

9.

LUMBAR FACET PAIN

Michael Gofeld, James P. Robinson, John G. Hanlon, and Binit J. Shah

CASE PRESENTATION

A recently retired 65-year-old male presents with paravertebral axial low back pain (LBP) of 6 months' duration. His pain is worse in the morning and is worsened with standing and twisting/turning, relieved with recumbency. The pain is described as an intermittent and deep aching with a vague discomfort noted in the buttocks bilaterally. There is no history of recent trauma. He denies weakness, falling, or bowel/bladder/sexual dysfunction. The patient has tried over-the-counter (OTC) pain relievers including ibuprofen and acetaminophen. The patient is referred to the Interdisciplinary Pain Clinic for further evaluation and management.

Past medical history is significant for osteoarthritis, post-traumatic stress disorder (PTSD), and hypertension.

Past surgical history is significant for left total knee replacement 1 year ago.

Review of systems is significant for anxiety and weight gain (10 lbs/1 year).

Physical examination demonstrates an obese man who weighs 105 kg and is 165 cm tall. His vital signs are stable. Neurological examination reveals intact sensation in all dermatomes. Musculoskeletal examination demonstrates 5/5 strength in all myotomes tested. Reflexes are +2 symmetrical and equal. Special testing is negative for nerve root tension signs with straight leg and Slump testing. Lumbar range of motion is limited in extension. Rotation-extension maneuvers are painful to the left. Palpation reveals paravertebral tenderness on the left lower segments on manual examination.

Magnetic resonance imaging (MRI) demonstrates multilevel spondylosis with facet hypertrophy particularly at left L5–S1, less than 3 mm of spondylolisthesis at L4–L5, mild degenerative disc changes, and bulges in the lumbar spine without significant nerve root impingement. Stable 3 mm anterolisthesis of L4 on L5 is noted with multilevel spondylosis and left L5–S1 facet arthrosis on standing flexion-extension radiographs.

QUESTIONS

1. What is the differential diagnosis?
2. Are there any further diagnostic modalities that may be helpful?
3. What is the etiology and prevalence of lumbar facet pain?
4. What is the prevalence of facet pain in patients with prior lumbar surgery?
5. What are the clinical manifestations of lumbar facet pain, and how is it diagnosed?
6. How is lumbar facet pain managed?
   a. Rehabilitation
   b. Pharmacological management
   c. Interventional procedures
   d. Psychiatric interventions
   e. Surgery
7. What is the long-term prognosis?

WHAT IS THE DIFFERENTIAL DIAGNOSIS?

To help better organize the differential diagnosis and address spinal pain, many clinicians divide spinal pain into three categories: mechanical, nonmechanical, and referred or visceral spinal pain. Mechanical pain is by far the most common etiology and often results from benign degenerative conditions afflicting the various spinal structures. Nonmechanical pain is rare and often the result of something more sinister. Last, visceral or referred spinal pain originates from structures outside the spine and is referred to the low back, neck, or dorsal spine. Visceral and referred pain are also less prevalent than mechanical pain and can often be distinguished from pain of spinal etiology by their lack of spinal stiffness and the pain-free range of spinal movements.

When assessing a patient with LBP, it is essential for the clinician to be open-minded and to avoid the pitfalls of early diagnostic closure. The importance of remaining diagnostically curious is twofold. First, a patient's pain may be the result of multiple factors, and, if all components of chronic pain are not recognized and addressed, the likelihood of choosing the appropriate management and achieving a clinically successful outcome diminishes. Second, and most importantly, as mentioned earlier, seemingly benign pain in the back can originate not only from components of the spinal column itself but can also arise from other nonspinal structures or nerve elements.

In this patient, most of the sinister etiologies, including neoplasm, infections, inflammatory spinal disorders, or fractures, can be ruled out based on the careful history, physical examination, and imaging that was conducted and obtained. For completeness, the generally agreed upon red flags for back pain are listed in Box 9.1. Although this patient's pain started after age 50, the 6-month duration of his symptomatology and lack of other ominous features suggests a less serious etiology. Furthermore, the patient has no history of trauma, has negative constitutional symptoms for systemic illness, and the pain is relieved by recumbency.

Referred pain is an even less probable diagnosis for this patient, but, for instance, nephrolithiasis can sometimes mimic lumbar spinal pain.

Although much less likely in this particular case, catastrophic pathology such as growing abdominal aortic aneurysm should always be considered, especially if the presentation is vague or atypical.

In addition to the search for a structural etiology for a patient's pain, a complete patient assessment should include an exploration of social and psychological factors that may influence the patient's pain. Although the history of anxiety in this clinical case patient should not be overlooked, this comorbidity should not be cause for the clinicians to discount the possibility of underlying structural or mechanical problems that may also be amenable to treatment.

Based on the history, physical examination, and imaging, this patient's pain is most likely mechanical. The components of the spinal column that could be contributing to his pain include facet joints, intervertebral discs, paraspinal muscles and ligaments, periosteum, and sacroiliac joint, as well as all of the neural elements associated with them. It is possible that this patient has more than one pain generator, and, as such, each of these causes could exist in isolation or simultaneously. The wide interneuronal convergence within the spinal cord makes topographic localization of spinal pain vague or even misleading.[1] Although the imaging in this case does not demonstrate disc herniation or nerve root compression, there are certainly signs of spondylosis, including facet hypertrophy and arthropathy as well as spondylolisthesis and degenerative disc changes and bulges. Each of these degenerative findings could potentially be contributing to this patient's pain. Accordingly, pain of myofascial origin and sacroiliac joint pain (discussed elsewhere in this book) must also be recognized as a possible but less likely sources of pain based on the patient's presentation.

Box 9.1 BACK PAIN RED FLAGS

"Red Flags" in Clinical Evaluation of a Patient

Age <20 or >50
Symptoms of less than 3 months' duration
History of trauma
Presence of constitutional symptoms
Presence of systemic illness
Unrelenting pain
Presence of cauda equina syndrome

In this particular case, there are many clues in the patient's history that help narrow down the differential diagnosis for his pain. Comprehensive history, musculoskeletal and neurological examinations, as well as the imaging findings, are consistent with facet joint contribution to the patient's pain. This notwithstanding, it is important to recognize that there is no history, physical examination, or imaging finding that, in isolation or combination, has sufficient sensitivity and specificity to make the diagnosis of lumbar facet pain.[2–4]

The discussion thus far would seem to lead inexorably to the conclusion that our patient has LBP that is caused by a single abnormality—a facet arthropathy on the left side at the L4–L5 level. In addressing this issue, it is worth considering the kind of evidence that is needed to diagnose a facet arthropathy and, once this diagnosis is suspected, the methods that might be used to confirm it. It should be noted that LBP thought to arise from facet origin does not have any characteristic antecedent to its pathogenesis. Thus, the search for an etiologic agent (e.g., a microbe) or event (e.g., falling from a height) is invariably unsuccessful. Also, there is no characteristic tissue pathology that grounds the diagnosis. As such, in contrast to patients with pneumococcal pneumonia or cirrhosis of the liver, analysis of a tissue sample by a pathologist does nothing to rule in or rule out the diagnosis of facet-mediated pain. Moreover, whereas in principle advanced imaging such as computed tomography (CT) or MRI scans might be viewed as proxies to pathology in a living patient, the correlation between abnormalities on these scans and clinical symptoms is modest at best.[5,6]

In the absence of a gold standard to diagnose facet arthropathy, a variety of diagnoses might be proposed to explain the present patient's symptoms, often guided by the clinician's specialty bias. Some orthopedically oriented physicians would argue that although facet joints might well be one of the sources of pain in a patient like ours, a more plausible analysis of his symptoms would be that he has "motion segment disease," in which all three joints of the three-joint complex at every segment of the lumbar spine are contributing to pain.[7] Others would argue for the importance of myofascial pain or muscle dysfunction as a major driver of the patient's symptoms.[8,9] Chiropractors would probably offer a diagnosis of spinal subluxation; osteopaths might attribute his symptoms to a facilitated segment.

Diagnoses of facet arthropathy, segmental motion disturbance, muscle dysfunction, subluxation, and facilitated segment seem to be utterly different ways of construing our patient's symptoms, but they do have something in common—they explain the patient's symptoms in terms of a peripheral pathology of some kind. But even this seemingly obvious attribution can be challenged. In particular, there is evidence that persistent LBP can reflect primarily alterations in the way in which a person's nervous system processes incoming sensory information, rather than normal processing of continued nociceptive input from a damaged spinal structure. Alterations in nervous system functioning have been identified at the level of the peripheral neuron,[10] the spinal cord,[11,12] and the brain.[13]

As discussed by Robinson and Apkarian,[14] several different specific models of altered nervous system in chronic pain have been developed. The common thread among the different models is that they all reject the hypothesis that chronic pain is mediated in a straightforward way by ongoing peripheral damage that generates nociceptive signals that are processed in a "normal" way. Some models are best described as physiological models because they identify structural and functional alterations in the central nervous system (CNS) of organisms exposed to painful stimuli and postulate that these alterations form the basis of the altered pain sensations (or pain behaviors when animals are studied) that can be observed in organisms with chronic pain.[15] Other models propose that the experiences of chronic LBP patients cannot be understood fully in terms of ongoing nociception, but rather attribute the dissociation between pain experience and nociception to a variety of psychological processes.[16] Examples include models that explain persistent pain on the basis of depression[17] or fear of reinjury[18] on the part of patients. Although such models are typically not couched in the language of physiology, it is plausible to assume that processes that researchers describe as psychological involve changes in CNS structure or function. Thus, Robinson and Apkarian included them in the broad category of models that attribute chronic pain to altered CNS functioning.[14]

Given the logical distinction between pain that is driven by ongoing nociception from a damaged spinal structure and pain that is driven largely by altered CNS functioning, an obvious question arises: How can a clinician determine which kind of process is dominant in an individual patient with LBP? Unfortunately, there is no definite answer to this question in clinical settings, in large part because there is no gold standard for identifying altered CNS functioning in humans.

A clinician should strongly consider the possibility of altered CNS functioning when a patient describes multiple pains, rather than just the LBP that may represent the chief complaint.[19] Although widespread pain can be the product of nociception (in conditions such as rheumatoid arthritis), it is also a hallmark of fibromyalgia and other disorders in which altered CNS functioning is thought to be dominant. Other hints of altered CNS functioning include reports by patients that their pain is extremely severe (10/10 intensity), is getting worse rather than better over time, has caused enormous emotional distress, or has caused severe disability in work activities and activities of daily living.

This chapter reviews the prevalence and diagnosis of facet pain. Emphasis will be given to understanding the importance of psychosocial factors in a patient's pain, suffering, and response to treatment. It will also highlight the appropriate use of *medial branch blocks* (MBB) as a diagnostic tool that prognosticates response to treatment for this type of pain with medial branch neurotomy, also known as *medial branch radiofrequency ablation* (RFA).

ARE THERE ANY FURTHER DIAGNOSTIC MODALITIES THAT MAY BE HELPFUL?

Whereas any diagnostic modality has the theoretical possibility of revealing "degenerative" or "abnormal" findings in this patient's anatomy, it is important to refrain from indiscriminate investigations and imaging of LBP. Spinal imaging, in particular, is sensitive but not very specific. Multiple studies have demonstrated that similar abnormalities may be seen in symptomatic and asymptomatic individuals.[20,21] This lack of specificity can lead to inappropriate diagnosis and poor treatment outcomes. In response, the United States Agency for Healthcare Policy and Research (AHCPR) published some of the first guidelines almost 20 years ago to help clinicians decrease their reliance and high use of spinal imaging.[22]

In animal research on altered CNS functioning, invasive procedures such as implantation of microelectrodes in the dorsal horn of the spinal cord are frequently used.[11,12] In human research, altered nervous system functioning is inferred on the basis of various self-report measures (e.g., Tampa Scale of Kinesiophobia[23]), behavioral indicators (Conditioned Pain Modulation, wind up[24,25]), or imaging with functional MRI.[26] In clinical settings, fewer assessment tools are available, and there is no tool that serves as a gold standard for identifying altered CNS function. However, a clinician who has a high index of suspicion that altered CNS functioning can play a major role in a patient's pain should consider several tools that at least bear on the likelihood that this is occurring in a specific patient. These can be divided into three groups—historical information, self-report measures, and physical findings.

In the case at hand, this patient has already had an MRI and X-rays to investigate structural abnormalities. There is clear evidence that imaging findings of facet pathology such as arthropathy are poorly correlated with a patient's response to diagnostic lumbar MBB or RFA of the lumbar facet joints.[27] It should also be noted that disc degeneration, as seen in this patient's MRI, almost always precedes the development of degeneration in facet joints, especially with increasing age.[28]

Overall, diagnostic imaging will tend to overestimate the prevalence of facet pathology, and, based on CT scanning, the prevalence of facet pathology by imaging ranges anywhere from 40% to 85%, increasing as people age.[29] Although one study showed that the presence of facet joint degeneration or hypertrophy was weakly correlated with response to MBB, it did not show a correlation with response to treatment by RFA.[30]

CT scans certainly show more detailed bony anatomy than MRIs, albeit at the expense of soft-tissue clarity, which is better delineated by MRI.[31] However, in this particular case, there are no findings on the MRI that suggest bony pathology beyond spondylosis, and, as such, further imaging with CT or plain films is not warranted. Similar to what has been shown for MRI studies, there are no imaging features on CT that have been shown to be diagnostic or predictive of response to treatment.[4] Conversely, uncontrolled studies have found that patients with active inflammatory processes demonstrated by positive single proton emission computed tomography (SPECT) scan may obtain intermediate relief from intra-articular steroid injections.[1]

Bone scintigraphy can be useful for detecting biochemical osseous processes. However, in this case, the absence of findings that suggest either spinal osteomyelitis, neoplasm, or an old fracture should all dissuade the clinician from ordering this test.

Similarly, there is no role for electrodiagnostic studies such as electromyography (EMG), nerve conduction studies (NCV), or evoked potentials. These studies are useful in localizing pathologic nerve lesions and determining the extent of neural injury, but they do not have a role in this case due to the absence of neurologic symptoms.

Other potential diagnostic tests such as a complete blood count (CBC), erythrocyte sedimentation rate (ESR), C-reactive protein (CRP), rheumatoid factor (Rh-factor) are useful tests in the appropriate patient. They have the greatest utility when the history, physical, and/or imaging is suggestive of tumors, infections, or rheumatological disorders or other forms of connective tissue ailments.

Due to a nonspecific nature of the clinical picture and imaging studies, reductionism is considered a practical paradigm for precise anatomical and functional diagnosis of localized chronic LBP. Medial branch and intra-articular facet blocks are commonly performed procedures for diagnosis and prognostication in patients with suspected facetogenic pain.[32–34] The merits and limitations of these blocks are discussed later in this chapter.

MENTAL HEALTH SCREENING IN MANAGEMENT OF SPINAL PAIN

There is a possibility that altered CNS function is playing a role in the patient's pain. More specifically, because the case presentation mentions anxiety, psychiatrists are likely to consider both DSM-5 anxiety diagnoses (e.g., panic disorder, PTSD) and also anxiety problems that may or may not fit DSM-5 categories but do contribute to the severity and duration of LBP. In particular, fear of pain/reinjury should be assessed because there is evidence that people with this type of fear are relatively likely to be severely impacted by their back problems.[18]

WHAT IS THE ETIOLOGY AND PREVALENCE OF LUMBAR FACET PAIN?

Pain originating from the lumbar facet joints has been long recognized as a common cause of LBP in the adult population. The syndrome was first described by Golthwaite in 1911, but it is Gormley who is generally credited with coining the actual term "facet syndrome" some 20 years later.[35,36]

Facet joint pain can result from an acute trauma, but, most commonly, it is the result of repetitive stress and wear and tear that lead to the inflammatory cascade responsible for the pain. It is believed that inflammation causes fluid accumulation and swelling that leads to joint capsular stretch and the clinical manifestations of facetogenic pain.[37]

It is helpful to understand the prevalence of lumbar facet pain before attempting to make the diagnosis in any population. This allows more accurate interpretation of tests based on the pre-test probability. Unfortunately, the prevalence of facet pain in patients with or without prior lumbar surgery is difficult to determine and varies widely depending on the literature and operational definitions. Part of this challenge stems from the limitations of history, physical examination, and imaging findings to make the diagnosis. Moreover, because the most accepted method to diagnose facet pain is via a diagnostic block, the ability to directly determine incidence in the general population is greatly reduced.[3]

In 1994, Schwarzer and colleagues helped to initially establish the prevalence of lumbar zygapophysial joint pain. Among younger workers who suffered from chronic LBP, they determined the prevalence of facet joint pain to be around 15%.[38] They subsequently determined the incidence of facet joint pain to be approximately 40% in older noninjured rheumatology patients.[4] A systematic review examining the prevalence of chronic lumbar facet joint pain among patients with chronic LBP without disc displacement or radiculitis was found to be 31%.[39] A review by Van Kleef and colleagues noted that the highly variable prevalence rates that exist in the literature are heavily dependent on the diagnostic criteria and selection methods. They concluded that, based on studies that were done on well-selected patient populations, the estimated prevalence ranged between 5% and 15% of those individuals with axial LBP.[36] Other reports have also suggested that the prevalence of lumbar facet pain is likely in the range of 10–15%. In nearly every study, increasing prevalence rates with age were noted due to the prominent role that arthritis plays as a cause of facetogenic pain.[40,41] It should, however, be noted that many studies have excluded patients with radicular symptomatology despite our current understanding that facet arthropathy can be the underlying cause of neuroforaminal stenosis.[40,42]

WHAT IS THE PREVALENCE OF FACET PAIN IN PATIENTS WITH PRIOR LUMBAR SURGERY?

What role, if any, does the history of prior lumbar laminectomy have on this patient's scenario? (A detailed review of failed back surgery syndrome can be found in Chapter 13.) Multiple studies have looked at the incidence of lumbar facet pain post spine surgery. Manchikanti et al. performed what they described as a randomized, controlled comparative evaluation of lumbar facet pain in post-lumbar laminectomy patients with a comparative nonsurgical group who also had persistent pain. They reported a prevalence of 44% in the nonsurgical group compared to 32% in the postsurgical patients.[43] This same group also performed a prospective study of consecutive patients to determine the prevalence of facet joint pain in post-spine surgery patients who were experiencing recurrent pain. This study included patients who had undergone various kinds of lumbar spine surgery and reported a prevalence of 16%. Notably, prevalence of facet joint pain was not significantly different among patients who had undergone one surgery versus multiple spine surgeries.[44]

A prospective cohort study to evaluate the reasons for persistent pain following a variety of approaches for surgical lumbar nerve root decompression was able to determine the cause of residual pain in the majority of cases. Among those who underwent microdiscectomy, the incidence of facet joint pain was found to be 23.1%. The rates of radicular pain caused by epidural scar and pain of myofascial origin were 12.3% and 26.1%, respectively. Among patients who underwent nucleoplasty, the rate of facet joint pain was 16.9%.[45] In a retrospective study of the predictors of facet joint pain after lumbar disc surgery, Steib et al. found that 8.4% of patients developed clinically evident painful facet joint syndrome.[46]

The accelerated and increased degenerative changes at levels adjacent to a spinal fusion are well understood. Specifically, after facetectomy, the load on the vestigial facet is reduced, peak pressure is increased, and adjacent joints bear increased stress. These mechanical realities must be considered in evaluating facet-related pain in a patient post spinal fusion.[47–49]

WHAT ARE THE CLINICAL MANIFESTATIONS OF LUMBAR FACET PAIN, AND HOW IS IT DIAGNOSED?

The nomenclature of what we have been describing as facet joint pain is confusing for a variety of reasons. First, the ubiquitous term "facet joint" is a neologism coined in the 1970s to describe what had previously been called the zygapophysial joint (or Z-joint for short).[35] Furthermore, subsequent neologisms such as "lumbar facet syndrome" and "facet loading" that were coined from a small retrospective study have become pervasive in the literature,[50] despite the fact that larger, well-designed studies have been unable to validate these findings.[1,51] Last, despite the fact that MBBs are routinely described as diagnostic, they actually serve more of a prognostic role, enabling the selection of patients who might respond to RFA treatment.

Although the clinical manifestations of lumbar facet pain can be quite vague and hard to differentiate from other spinal sources of pain, the clinician can obtain some clues from the patient's history. Lumbar facet joint-mediated pain tends to present as a progressive pain rather than an acute process. Revel and others suggested features that increase the likelihood of zygapophysial joint pain. These include age greater than 65; pain relieved by recumbency; absence of pain aggravation by coughing, forward flexion, or rising from flexion, and, accordingly, absence of aggravation by hyperextension or extension rotation.[2]

In a seminal paper, Waddell and colleagues identified five "nonorganic" signs that can be assessed reliably during an examination of the lumbar spine.[52] Subsequent research has supported the conclusion that patients with nonorganic signs are very apprehensive.[53,54] When physicians identify nonorganic signs, they should strongly consider the possibility that the pain complaints of their patient are heavily influenced by altered nervous system functioning. There is good evidence that widespread hyperalgesia, as measured by reduced pressure pain threshold, is a marker of altered CNS functioning.[55–56]

Reports of the patient's pain referral pattern can also be helpful. Although most studies demonstrate a significant variability in the referral pattern, as a general rule, the upper lumbar facet joints tend to refer pain into the flank, hip, and upper lateral thigh in comparison to the lower lumbar facet joints, where the pain may be experienced in the posterolateral thigh and occasionally as far distally as the calf (Figure 9.1).[57,58] Because referred pain, as far as the leg and foot, has been relieved by anesthetizing the facet joints, somatic referred pain into the lower limb should not be considered a contraindication for lumbar MBB.

Perhaps the most useful physical examination finding is tenderness to palpation in the paraspinal regions. This has been shown to be a predictor of treatment success in two large,

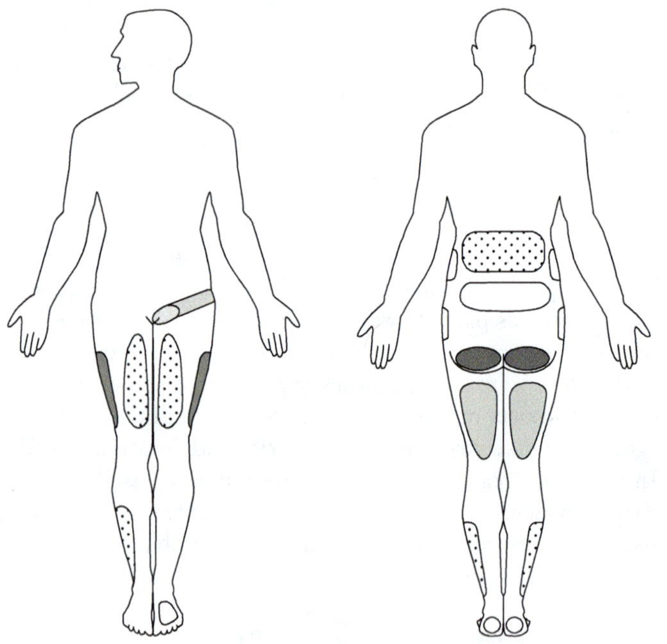

Figure 9.1 Pain referral patterns from the lumbar facet joints. Reprinted with permission from Cohen SP, Raja SN. Pathogenesis, diagnosis and the treatment of zygapophysial (facet) joint pain. *Anesthesiology* 2007;3:591–614.

retrospective studies.[27,59] However, one must recognize that this finding is certainly not diagnostic or pathognomonic.

It is the lack of diagnostic specificity, outlined here, that led clinicians to increasingly turn to lumbar MBB and intra-articular facet blocks to aid with diagnosis and patient management.[32–34]

Lumbar MBBs are used to determine if the patient's pain is originating from one or more of the medial branches and will therefore be relieved with RFA of these branches. Because the facet joints are supplied by the medial branches of the dorsal rami (and the L5 dorsal ramus itself for the L5–S1 facet joint), it is believed that if these medial branches are blocked in isolation and the pain resolves, it is prima facie evidence that this joint is the patient's pain generator. Dreyfuss et al. demonstrated the specificity of the method[60] and helped elucidate the clinical manifestations of facet pain by provoking pain in healthy volunteers (using capsular distention or direct stimulation of the medial branch), as well as by investigating pain patterns in patients whose pain was relieved by diagnostic block.[61] Soon thereafter, methodologically sound clinical trials of lumbar facet RFA proved the efficacy of the treatment and that lasting relief can be achieved with medial branch neurotomy.[62,63]

Although the concept of MBB as a diagnostic or prognostic tool is very appealing, these blocks are certainly not a diagnostic panacea because both technical and anatomic limitations affect their ability to aid the clinician in making a diagnosis. The main areas of contention regarding these procedures include the optimal volume of local anesthetic necessary to avoid false-positive blocks, the percentage of pain relief necessary to declare a block as positive, and how many (true) positive blocks must be completed to make the diagnosis. Changes to any of these cutoff thresholds will lead to changes in the incidence of false-positive and false-negative blocks, both of which can lead to suboptimal or inappropriate patient management.[58,61,64]

The volume of local anesthetic is important because studies have shown that with larger volumes the anatomical specificity is lost and one can therefore no longer be sure if the pain relief obtained is a result of MBB made in isolation or due to other nearby pain generators having been inadvertently anesthetized. Most authors now recommend a volume of no more than 0.5 mL for a lumbar MBB.[32, 58]

The exact percentage of pain relief required to categorize the block as positive is also controversial. Although some groups suggest that a positive block must entail near complete pain relief (i.e., >80%), others have suggested that 50% pain relief is sufficient to designate a block as positive.[32,40,65] Retrospective analyses have failed to find a difference in results between these two cutoffs for a positive block.[58] Most recently, in an attempt to determine the optimal threshold for diagnostic lumbar facet blocks, Cohen et al. performed a prospective correlational study and demonstrated that there were no significant differences in RFA outcomes based on any MBB pain relief of greater than 50%. They also reported a trend whereby those patients who obtained less than 50% pain relief subsequently reported poor outcomes. They concluded that employing more stringent selection criteria (than 50% pain relief in response to diagnostic blocks) for lumbar facet RFA is likely to result in withholding a beneficial procedure from a substantial number of patients without improving success rates.[66]

The debate regarding the number of blocks necessary to rule in or rule out the facet joint as the pain generator for any specific patient extends beyond clinical evidence because one must also consider cost-effectiveness and pragmatic realities in addition to block specificity. Certainly, by requiring two positive blocks, the rate of false-positive results will decrease and the efficacy of the treatment will improve. On the other hand, this approach entails an increased overall cost, procedural risks, and radiation exposure, as well as an amplified rate of false negatives that results in denying an appropriate treatment to patients who may benefit. Accordingly, individual factors like the need for the patient to repeatedly stop anticoagulants or travel large distances are reasonable pragmatic concerns that some but not all clinicians believe should shape clinical decision making.[32,58,67,68]

Regardless of the criteria applied, once a patient is deemed to have had a positive response to MBB(s), the diagnosis of lumbar facet pain is generally applied and the patient can be considered for treatment.

HOW IS LUMBAR FACET PAIN MANAGED?

As outlined from the preceding multiple perspectives described, the treatment of lumbar facet joint pain ideally consists of a multimodal approach comprising conservative therapy, medical management, procedural interventions, and psychotherapy if warranted. Because there are no clinical studies specifically assessing pharmacotherapy or noninterventional treatment for lumbar facet pain, we must extrapolate from the numerous studies evaluating conservative treatment for axial LBP.

REHABILITATION

Three important aspects that should be addressed in the course of rehabilitation are obesity, deconditioning and weakness, and sleep hygiene.

Obesity

An important comorbid condition is this patient's obesity (body mass index [BMI] = 38.5).

There is evidence that obesity is associated with increased incidence and prevalence of LBP,[69–71] although one systematic review found that the association between obesity and LBP is only modest.[72] There is also evidence that obese patients are less likely than those of normal weight to benefit from at least some kinds of treatment for LBP.[73] However, this association does not mean that patients can improve their chance of successful treatment outcome by losing weight. Some research has shown that, in limited circumstances, weight loss can lead to clinical improvement among LBP patients.[74–76] But this research has not involved randomized controlled trials and, for the most part, has been limited to morbidly obese people treated with bariatric surgery. Given the difficulty of obtaining compliance with weight loss programs and the uncertainty about whether a successful weight loss program would help a patient like this, it is probably better to focus on weight loss in conjunction with an exercise program and other wellness behaviors rather than to focus on weight loss in isolation.

Physiatrists may address this patient's obesity either directly or indirectly. They might discuss it with him as an aspect of his condition that needs specific, targeted treatment. This treatment could, in principle, take a variety of forms, including referral to a nutritionist, recommendation that the patient join a support group such as Weight Watchers, or, conceivably, referral to a bariatric surgeon. Alternatively, physiatrists might frame the patient's obesity as a component of a broader pattern of deconditioning. From this perspective, it would be reasonable to refer him to an exercise program and hope that he would lose weight as he progressed in the program and became more physically active.

Deconditioning and Weakness

There is evidence that patients with LBP are physically inactive relative to healthy controls. In fact, most of the items on standard tools for assessing LBP patients—including the Roland-Morris Disability Questionnaire and the Oswestry Disability Index—focus on activity limitations that patients experience because of their back pain.[77]

Also, LBP patients have less strength in core muscles,[78] and have abnormal kinesiologic patterns of activation of core muscles as they go through daily activities.[79] These problems presumably reflect a combination of deconditioning[80] and inhibition due to pain or fear of pain. They rationalize the emphasis that physiatrists place on physical therapy as a treatment. A few issues related to physical therapy need emphasis. First, the type of therapy found to be effective in treating LBP is exercise therapy—passive therapies do not appear to be helpful.[81,82] Second, the bulk of evidence supports the conclusion that specific types of exercise therapy (e.g., McKenzie exercises vs. spine stabilization vs. Pilates vs. general conditioning) yield similar results.[83,84] Thus, although physical therapy needs to focus on exercise, there is quite a bit of latitude in the specific exercise program a therapist establishes for an LBP patient. Third, an effective exercise program leads not only to improvement in a patient's physical functioning but also to improved psychological functioning.[85] For example, it is reasonable to anticipate that if this patient learns that he can perform activities that he previously thought were impossible, he would experience an increase in his confidence that he can manage his back pain. Research to date suggests that improvement in patients' psychological state (measured, for example, by changes on the Chronic Pain Self-Efficacy Scale[86]) is more closely related to their functional recovery than improvement in their physical capacities.[85,87] Finally, a physical therapy program that stresses exercise should be viewed as a means to an end rather than an end in itself. Such a program is likely to have long-lasting benefit only if the patient incorporates what he has learned during the program and translates this knowledge to a self-directed exercise program after the formal physical therapy program has ended.

A physiatrist would almost certainly recommend a physical therapy program that emphasized core strengthening and spine stabilization. As noted earlier, research does not provide a clear basis for choosing one kind of exercise program over another. But common sense would dictate that in a patient suspected of having a painful facet arthropathy, it would be prudent to avoid exercises that load the facet joints unduly. Thus, for example, a neutral spine program would be preferable to a McKenzie program.

Sleep Impairment

Informal observation strongly suggests that patients with chronic LBP have difficulty sleeping and typically attribute their disturbed sleep to their pain. This observation is consistent with research on the connection between sleep disturbance and LBP. A recent review on this subject concluded that "Consistent evidence found that CLBP was associated with greater sleep disturbance; reduced sleep duration and sleep quality; increased time taken to fall asleep; poor day-time function; and greater sleep dissatisfaction and distress."[88]

It is likely that the two problems interact with each other. Thus, as commonly described by patients, pain may cause sleep interference. However, there is good evidence that poor quality sleep can intensify the aversive experiences of chronic pain patients with a wide range of conditions.[89] These data indicate that, at the very least, the physician should ascertain whether the patient is having sleep impairment. If this is found, a number of strategies to improve his sleep might be considered.

PHARMACOLOGICAL MANAGEMENT

No conservative treatment has been specifically evaluated for lumbar facet pain.[35] Whereas pharmacotherapy—especially if carried out over an extended period of time—has only modest benefits for axial spinal pain,[90] a physiatrist would probably consider a few different pharmacologic options. The most obvious choice would be a nonsteroidal anti-inflammatory drug (NSAID). There is evidence that these are effective agents in patients with LBP.[90] They are recommended for LBP patients in general and, more specifically, for elderly ones.[91] But because elderly patients are at higher risk than younger patients for adverse effects of NSAIDs, a decision about these drugs probably is best made with input from the patient's family physician. Opioids represent another pharmaceutical choice.[92] Although the trend toward a liberal use of opioids in the United States during the past 20 years[93] has been challenged, there may be some evidence for their efficacy in chronic LBP,[92] and some patients report significant benefits from them. The main problem is the lack of long-term effectiveness data. In addition, the lack of proof of sustained functional improvements, as well as their safety concerns, must all be considered before a trial of opioids is initiated.[94–95] A third choice would be an antidepressant such as a tricyclic antidepressant or one of the newer agents such as duloxetine, a selective serotonin norepinephrine reuptake inhibitor (SNRI). Although systematic reviews have not found evidence that antidepressants help unselected patients with LBP,[90,96] there are reasons to believe that they could help targeted symptoms in this patient. Antidepressants have been shown to be modestly effective for spinal pain.[97,98] However, duloxetine has been found helpful in chronic musculoskeletal painful conditions and is FDA approved for this indication.[99–101] Specifically, some antidepressants are helpful in treating sleep impairment. Second, patients with chronic pain often have an associated mood disorder or anxiety disorder. Antidepressants could help these types of emotional dysfunction. Third, it is possible for a patient who has undergone prior lumbar decompressive surgery to have neuropathic pain as one contributor to his overall problem. Some antidepressants have been shown to be effective in relieving this kind of pain.[102]

A fourth category of medication to be considered is an anticonvulsant such as gabapentin.[103,104] Anticonvulsants are effective in the treatment of neuropathic pain and have been shown to be somewhat beneficial for patients with failed back surgery syndrome.[105–107]

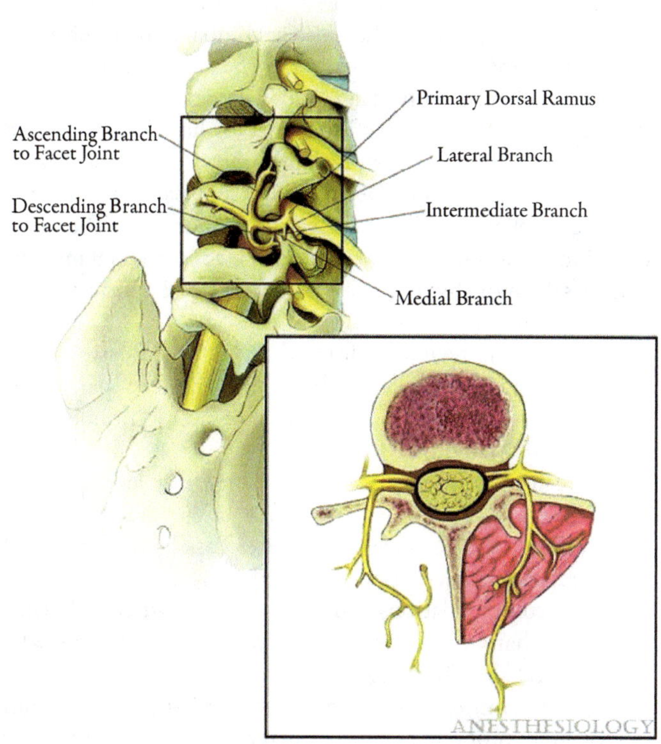

Figure 9.2 Anatomy of the lumbar facet joint. Reprinted with permission from Cohen SP, Raja SN. Pathogenesis, diagnosis and the treatment of zygapophysial (facet) joint pain. *Anesthesiology* 2007;106(3):591–614.

INTERVENTIONAL PROCEDURES

Interventional procedures for facetogenic pain are primarily in the form of radiofrequency denervation of the medial branch or intra-articular local anesthetic and steroid.

The exact details of medial branch denervation are beyond the scope of this chapter and described elsewhere,[68] but a general description is warranted. The medial branch of the dorsal rami wraps around the lateral neck of the superior articular process at the junction of the transverse process (Figure 9.2). This provides a fluoroscopically identifiable target to place a radiofrequency cannula parallel to the nerve and produce a thermal lesion to the medial branch (Figure 9.3). Although the duration of relief from RFA varies widely between studies, most studies have demonstrated relief ranging between 6 and 12 months. This procedure can be repeated thereafter, and there is some evidence to suggest that with the repeat denervation the length of sustained relief is increased.[108]

Although these blocks have traditionally been performed under radiologic guidance with X-ray or CT imaging, the use of ultrasound for pain medicine procedures, including potential applications in the management of lumbar facet pain, is very appealing.[109] An anatomic study using ultrasound guidance for lumbar facet joint injection with fluoroscopic validation has been successfully performed.[110] There remains a paucity of evidence in the literature regarding the validity of performing lumbar MBBs with ultrasound.

Intra-articular steroid injections are also frequently performed; however, the evidence for this is less robust than for medial branch RFA. Two well-designed studies have shown no sustained benefit.[111,112] Part of the challenges in evaluating intra-articular facet injections are likely related to the technical challenges associated with this block and the high incidence of inadvertent spread of local anesthetic and/or steroid. It must be noted that, despite the frequent interchanging

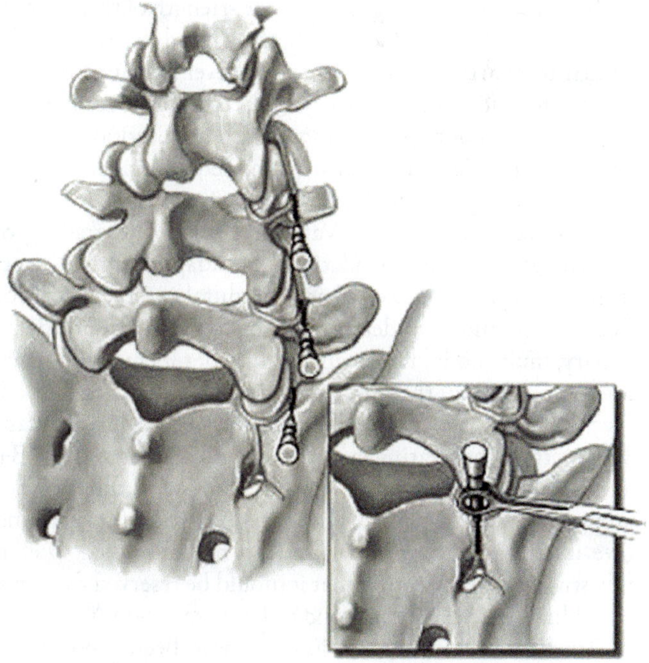

Figure 9.3 Cannula placed parallel to the third and fourth medial branch and the L5 dorsal rami (insert of S1). Reprinted with permission from Gofeld M, Faclier G. Radiofrequency denervation of the lumbar zygapophysial joints—targeting the best practice. *Pain Med.* 2008;9:204–211.

of these two techniques by some authors, there are no randomized crossover studies to allow direct comparison or definitive conclusions about the relative merits of each procedure.

The evidence supporting fluoroscopically guided facet diagnostic and therapeutic interventions has been evaluated in a variety of ways. A relatively large prospective clinical audit by Gofeld et al. found that almost 70% of patients reported good to excellent results after a 6-month follow-up. The mean duration of pain relief among the entire cohort was 9 months and was 12 months in those who maintained good to excellent results for at least 6 months.[113]

A systematic review performed in 2007 by Boswell et al. found moderate evidence for short- and long-term pain relief of lumbar facet pain with intra-articular facet joint injections as well as MBB and RFA.[114]

More recent systematic reviews have been less favorable toward intra-articular injections. Datta et al. graded evidence according to the U.S. Preventive Services Task Force (USPSTF) for therapeutic interventions,[115] and then graded the strength of their recommendations as described by Guyatt et al.[116] They concluded that, overall, lumbar facet joint nerve blocks are safe, valid, and reliable. They rated the strength of evidence for diagnostic facet joints techniques to be level I or II-1 (evidence from one or more properly conducted diagnostic accuracy study of adequate size). Of note, they determined a false positive rate of 30% with a single diagnostic block. Their systematic review found that, for therapeutic facet joint interventions (local anesthetic with or without steroid), the strength of evidence was slightly lower (level II-1or II-2) and graded the strength of their recommendation to be 1B or C (strong recommendation based on moderate or low-quality evidence, respectively). For facet RFA, they also reported the strength of the evidence to be II-2 or II-3 and gave a similar grading to the strength of their recommendation (1B or 1C). Conversely, they found the evidence for lumbar intra-articular injections to be level III (limited) with the recommendation of 2C (very weak recommendation or recommendation not to provide intra-articular injections).

Another review of literature compiled as "evidence-based interventional pain medicine according to clinical diagnosis" has been published by Van Kleef et al. The grading of the strength of recommendations was adapted from Guyatt et al.[116,117] They suggested that procedural interventions for facet pain should be undertaken in the context of a multidisciplinary, multimodal treatment regime that includes pharmacotherapy, physical therapy, regular exercise, and, if indicated, psychotherapy. They concluded that RFA is the current standard method for treating facetogenic pain and rated it as 1B+ recommendation (strongly positive). They found the evidence supporting intra-articular corticosteroids to be limited and gave it a 2B± recommendation (can be considered, preferably study-related), stating that it should be reserved for those individuals who do not respond to RFA treatment.[36]

To date, very few complications have been reported in the medical literature when lumbar medial branch RFA has been performed according to current procedural guidelines (including motor stimulation). The most common complication is a neuritis that occurs in fewer than 5% of procedures and can be further reduced by the concurrent injection of steroids or pentoxifylline.[118] Although serious complications of weakness and numbness in the lower leg have been reported in medicolegal proceedings, these have occurred when RFA was performed under general anesthesia.[68]

PSYCHIATRIC INTERVENTIONS

The patient reports service in the U.S. Army when he was drafted into the military. He served time in the infantry and was stationed in Vietnam where he saw extensive combat operations. Upon return from the war, he struggled with alcoholism for years because he self-medicated with alcohol. Only after he had maintained sobriety for 2 years and continued to struggle with irritability and nightmares did he see a psychiatrist who diagnosed him with PTSD, chronic pain, and alcohol use disorder in remission.

PTSD is characterized by an exposure to trauma and subsequent development of a constellation of symptoms including intrusive symptoms, avoidance of trauma-related memories, negative alterations in mood, and hyperarousal (for the diagnostic criteria of PTSD, see the *Diagnostic and Statistical Manual of Mental Disorders*, 5th edition). Essentially, the mind tries to make sense of and master a traumatic experience by reliving it on both conscious and unconscious levels.

Trauma is an unfortunately common experience, with 50–80% of people experiencing it at some point in their lives.[119] Thankfully, the majority of people exposed will *not* develop PTSD. The lifetime prevalence of PTSD is approximately 9%.[120] Most people who develop PTSD will show symptoms within 3 months of the trauma; however, up to 25% display no symptoms until after 6 months.[121] A history of low socioeconomic status, physical/sexual abuse, lower intelligence, or minority status are risk factors for development of PTSD after a trauma.[122–124] Positive social support (healthy relationships with family and friends) is a protective factor.[125,126] PTSD is more common among females than males, and this is partly due to females' greater exposure to traumatic events in the form of rape and interpersonal violence.[127] Intimate partner violence (IPV) is a particularly malicious trauma because 25–65% of female IPV victims develop PTSD. Even after adjusting for exposure to traumatic events, however, women are four times more likely to develop PTSD than men. Although rape is ten times more common among women than men, the incidence of PTSD after rape is higher in men than women (65% vs. 46%). Conversely, rates of PTSD are lower in men than women after molestation (12% vs. 27%) and physical assault (2% vs. 21%).[128] PTSD rates are also high in patients who are refugees or from areas of military conflict, about 31%.[129] The rates of PTSD in those deployed to combat zones in Iraq and Afghanistan is 13–20%, which is similar to the prevalence of PTSD after intensive care unit (ICU) stay.[130]

The rate of PTSD among chronic pain patients is both tremendous and bidirectional. Up to 50% of patients with chronic pain report PTSD symptoms,[131–134] and up to 80% of patients with PTSD have chronic pain.[135,136] One study in a tertiary pain center found that when specifically assessed

70% of men and 65% of women reported a history of abuse and, compared to Caucasians, African Americans had significantly more childhood physical abuse.[137]

In addition to the complexity of treating PTSD by itself, comorbid mental illness is the rule: 16% have another mental disorder, 17% have two, and 50% have three or more.[127] Suicidal thoughts occur in 1% of the general population, but in up to 40% of those with PTSD, and 19% have attempted suicide.[138] Although chronic pain patients have very high rates of current and past substance use, this is even higher in those with PTSD. Comorbid substance use disorders occur in 65% in those with PTSD.[139,140]

With such high rates of PTSD, substance abuse, and comorbid psychiatric illness, all patients with chronic pain should be screened. This can either be done through a thorough social history that asks for any history of physical abuse, sexual abuse, or military experience. A more thorough screen can be accomplished through the use of the PTSD checklist, which has been validated in both civilian and military populations.[141–143] If positive, the patient should be referred to a psychiatrist for further evaluation and treatment.

Treatment

There are currently six clinical treatment guidelines for PTSD, and of these four recommend selective serotonin reuptake inhibitors (SSRIs)/SNRIs as first-line monotherapy.[144] Nefazodone has also been found to be as effective as sertraline, but is recommended as a second-line agent due to rare hepatotoxicity. Although there has been an increase in the use of atypical antipsychotics (e.g., risperidone, quetiapine, olanzapine, aripiprazole), there is very little evidence for efficacy. Benzodiazepines are specifically *not recommended* because they may aggravate the fear response and have a high risk for abuse. Also, although bupropion is FDA approved and is of benefit in the treatment of depression, it has no efficacy in PTSD. A wide variety of anticonvulsants (valproate, tiagabine, lamotrigine) have been tried and not found to be efficacious.[145–148] Interestingly, the antiepileptic topiramate has been shown to be effective for a broad spectrum of PTSD symptoms in three randomized, controlled trials.[149–151] The Agency for Healthcare Research and Quality has found it to be as effective as sertraline, paroxetine, and venlafaxine, making it the only non-SSRI/SNRI with such positive findings.[152]

Several trauma-focused cognitive behavioral therapy (CBT) approaches have been found to be equivalent or superior to pharmacotherapy, including exposure therapy, cognitive processing therapy, and eye movement desensitization and reprocessing (EMDR). A meta-analysis of 26 PTSD psychotherapy studies found that of patients who completed treatment, 67% no longer met criteria for PTSD and 54% reported significant clinical improvement.[153] The more widespread use of therapy for PTSD has been limited by a lack of trained clinicians (outside the Veterans Affairs [VA] system), insurance coverage, and the time commitment required for fruitful therapy.

Due to multiple negative past experiences with the VA system, the patient reports his PTSD is managed by his internist. He is treated with a combination of quetiapine (Seroquel) 300 mg PO QHS and alprazolam (Xanax) 1 mg BID PRN for anxiety. He reports the medication has been minimally helpful for sleep, but otherwise he continues to experience moderate to severe levels of distress. After discussion with the patient, several changes were made. His Seroquel was decreased to 200 mg QHS for the first night, then to 100 mg QHS for the second night, then discontinued. He was educated regarding the addictive potential of alprazolam and general lack of benefit and agreed with discontinuation. Given the difficulty that many patients have with discontinuing this medication, it was switched to clonazepam 0.5 mg BID for 1 week, then to 0.5 mg QHS for 1 week, then 0.25 mg QHS for 1 week, then discontinued. Concurrently, he was started on sertraline 50 mg/d and trazodone 50–100 mg QHS for sleep. The patient was also strongly encouraged to initiate VA services in order to take advantage of trauma-focused CBT.

The key features of all the treatments recommended to our case study patient are that they attempt to address multiple contributors to the pain, and they focus on promoting functional improvement. The treatments can easily be combined with the interventional procedures described earlier. In this kind of combined treatment, an important question of sequencing of therapeutic interventions arises. For example, would it be better for him to undergo MBBs with possible facet neurotomy first, or would it be better to have him get started in a broader rehabilitation program first? It should be noted that there is no systematic research that addresses the issue of optimum sequencing of therapies in this clinical setting.

SURGERY

There is no convincing evidence to support surgery for lumbar spondylosis generally or lumbar facet pain specifically, and, as such, surgery is not recommended as a treatment for facetogenic pain.[40,48] Regardless, surgery or minimally invasive facet fusion is occasionally attempted to treat spondylosis or lumbar facet pain.[154] It should also be recognized that in the process of some surgeries such as spinal fusions, surgeons may purposefully or inadvertently transect the medial branches during their placement of pedicle screws and, in doing so, could theoretically provide some pain relief but at the expense of further degenerative changes at adjacent levels, including further facet arthropathy.

WHAT IS THE LONG-TERM PROGNOSIS?

Although this chapter cautioned earlier against premature diagnostic closure and overemphasis on the role of psychological factors, it must be stated that these comorbidities do predict a poorer response to treatment, and, as such, our case study patient's comprehensive assessment and care should optimally be delivered within a multidisciplinary clinic in order to maximize his chances of functional improvement and a decrease in pain intensity.[27]

CONCLUSION

A significant portion of spinal pain can be attributed to the facet joints, especially in the elderly. That notwithstanding, for each patient the relative contribution of nociception directly from the affected joint compared to the contribution of CNS processing alterations must be considered. Once this full clinical picture is understood, the treatment of lumbar facet joint pain ideally consists of a multimodal approach comprising conservative therapy, medical management, procedural interventions, and possibly psychiatric therapy when indicated. Although diagnosis of this clinical entity remains challenging, prognostic blocks are currently the best method for selecting patients who may benefit from RFA of their medial branches. As outlined in this chapter, further research is necessary to improve our ability to diagnose and optimally treat patients with facet joint pain. Accordingly, rigorous evaluation of the role of pharmacotherapy and other noninterventional or behavioral treatments for lumbar facet pain is also needed.

REFERENCES

1. Cohen SP, Raja SN. Pathogenesis, diagnosis and the treatment of zygapophysial (facet) joint pain. *Anesthesiology.* 2007;3:591–614.
2. Revel M, Poiraudeau S, Auleley GR, et al. Capacity of the clinical picture to characterize low back pain relieved by facet joint anesthesia: proposed criteria to identify patients with painful facet joints. *Spine.* 1998;23:1972–1976.
3. Dreyfuss PH, Dreyer SJ. Lumbar zygapophysial (facet) joint injections. *Spine J.* 2003;3:50S–59S.
4. Schwarzer A, Wang S, Bogduk N, McNaught P, Laurent R. Prevalence and clinical features of lumbar zygapophysial joint pain: a study in an Australian population with chronic low back pain. *Ann Rheum. Dis.* 1995;54:100–106.
5. Chou R, Deyo RA, Jarvik JG. Appropriate use of lumbar imaging for evaluation of low back pain. *Radiol Clin North Am.* 2012;50:569–585.
6. van Tulder MW, Assendelft WJ, Koes BW, Bouter LM. Spinal radiographic findings and nonspecific low back pain. A systematic review of observational studies. *Spine.* 1997;22:427–434.
7. Yong-Hing K, Kirkaldy-Willis WH. The pathophysiology of degenerative disease of the lumbar spine. *Orthop Clin North Am.* 1983;14:491–504.
8. D'hooge R, Hodges P, Tsao H, Hall L, Macdonald D, Danneels L. Altered trunk muscle coordination during rapid trunk flexion in people in remission of recurrent low back pain. *J Electromyogr Kinesiol.* 2013;23:173–181.
9. Borg-Stein J, Simons DG. Focused review: myofascial pain. *Arch Phys Med Rehabil.* 2002;83:S40–S49.
10. Fornasari D. Pain mechanisms in patients with chronic pain. *Clin Drug Investig.* 2012;32(suppl 1):45–52.
11. Fitzgerald M, Woolf CJ. The time course and specificity of the changes in the behavioural and dorsal horn cell responses to noxious stimuli following peripheral nerve capsaicin treatment in the rat. *Neuroscience.* 1982;7:2051–2056.
12. Woolf CJ. Evidence for a central component of post-injury pain hypersensitivity. *Nature.* 1983;306:686–688.
13. Saab CY. Pain-related changes in the brain: diagnostic and therapeutic potentials. *Trends Neurosci.* 2012;35:629–637.
14. Robinson JP, Apkarian AV. Low back pain. In: Mayer EA, Bushnell MC, eds. *Functional Pain Syndromes: Presentation and Pathophysiology.* Seattle, WA: IASP Press; 2009:3–53.
15. Baliki MN, Petre B, Torbey S, et al. Corticostriatal functional connectivity predicts transition to chronic back pain. *Nat Neurosci.* 2012;15:1117–1119.
16. Ramond A, Bouton C, Richard I, et al. Psychosocial risk factors for chronic low back pain in primary care—a systematic review. *Fam Pract.* 2011;28:12–21.
17. Hoy D, Brooks P, Blyth F, Buchbinder R. The epidemiology of low back pain. *Best Pract Res Clin Rheumatol.* 2010;24:769–781.
18. Leeuw M, Goossens ME, Linton SJ, et al. The fear-avoidance model of musculoskeletal pain: current state of scientific evidence. *J Behav Med.* 2007;30:77–94.
19. Croft P, Dunn KM, Von Korff M. Chronic pain syndromes: you can't have one without another. *Pain.* 2007;131:237–238.
20. Borenstein D, O'Mara J, Boden S. The value of magnetic resonance imaging of the lumbar spine to predict low-back pain in asymptomatic subjects. a seven year follow-up study. *J Bone Joint Surg* (Am). 2001;83:A:1306–1311.
21. Jensen M, Brant-Zawadzki M, Obuchowski N. Magnetic resonance imaging of the lumbar spine in people without back pain. *New Engl J Med.* 1994;331:69–73.
22. Bigos S, Bowyer O, Braen G. Acute low back problems in adults. AHCPR Clinical practice guideline, Quick reference guide number 14. Rockville, MD: Agency for Health Care Policy and Research; 1994; No. 95-0643.
23. Burwinkle T, Robinson JP, Turk DC. Fear of movement: factor structure of the Tampa scale of kinesophobia in patients with fibromyalgia syndrome. *J Pain.* 2005;6:384–391.
24. Staud R. Abnormal endogenous pain modulation is a shared characteristic of many chronic pain conditions. *Expert Rev Neurother.* 2012;12:577–585.
25. Yarnitsky D. Conditioned pain modulation (the diffuse noxious inhibitory control-like effect): its relevance for acute and chronic pain states. *Curr Opin Anaesthesiol.* 2010;23:611–615.
26. Baliki MN, Chialvo DR, Geha PY, et al. Chronic pain and the emotional brain: specific brain activity associated with spontaneous fluctuations of intensity of chronic back pain. *J Neurosci.* 2006;26:12165–12173.
27. Cohen SP, Hurley RW, Christo PJ, Winkley J, Mohiuddin MM, Stojanovic MP. Clinical predictors of success and failure for lumbar facet radiofrequency denervation. *Clin J. Pain.* 200;23:45–52.
28. Suri P, Miyakoshi A, Hunter DJ, et al. Does lumbar spinal degeneration begin with the anterior structures? A study of the observed epidemiology in a community-based population. *BMC Musculoskelet Disord.* 2011;12:1–7.
29. Murtagh FR. Computed tomography and fluoroscopy guided anesthesia and steroid injection in facet syndrome. *Spine.* 1988;13:686–689.
30. Stojanovic MP, Sethee J, Mohiuddin M, et al. MRI analysis of the lumbar spine: can it predict response to diagnostic and therapeutic facet procedures? *Clin J. Pain.* 2010;26:110–115.
31. Deen H. Diagnosis and management of lumbar disc disease. *Mayo Clin Proc.* 1996;71:283–287.
32. Bogduk N. International Spinal Injection Society guidelines for the performance of spinal injection procedures. Part 1. Zygapophysial joint blocks. *Clin J Pain.* 1995;13:285–302.
33. Dreyfuss PH, Dreyer SJ. Lumbar zygapophysial (facet) joint injections. *Spine J.* 2003;3:50S–59S.
34. Marks RC, Houston T, Thulbourne T. Facet joint injection and facet nerve block: a randomised comparison in 86 patients with chronic low back pain. *Pain.* 1992;49:325–328.
35. Bogduk N. Evidence-informed management of chronic low back pain with facet injections and radiofrequency neurotomy. *Spine J.* 2008;8:56–64.

36. Van Kleef M, Vanelderen P, Zundert J Van, Mekhail N. Evidence based medicine 12. pain originating from the lumbar facet joints. *Pain Pract.* 2010;10:459–469.
37. Igarashi A, Kikuchi S, Konno S. Correlation between inflammatory cytokines released from the lumbar facet joint tissue and symptoms in degenerative lumbar spinal disorders. *J Orthop Sci.* 2007;12:154–160.
38. Schwarzer A, Aprill C, Derby R, Fortin J, Kine G, Bogduk N. Clinical features of patients with pain stemming from the lumbar zygapophysial joints. Is the lumbar facet syndrome a clinical entity? *Spine.* 1994;19:1132–1137.
39. Datta S, Lee M, Falco FJE, Bryce DA, Hayek SM. Systematic assessment of diagnostic accuracy and therapeutic utility of lumbar facet joint interventions. *Pain Physician.* 2009;12:437–460.
40. Brummett CM, Cohen SP. Facet syndrome: facet joint injections, medial branch blocks and radiofrequency denervation. In: Benzon HT, Raja SN, Liu SS, Fishman SM, Cohen SP, eds. *Essentials of Pain Medicine.* 3rd ed. Philadelphia: Elsevier Saunders; 2011:322–329.
41. Manchikanti L, Boswell MV, Singh V, Pampati V, Damron KS, Beyer CD. Prevalence of facet joint pain in chronic spinal pain of cervical, thoracic, and lumbar regions. *BMC Musculoskel Disord.* 2004;5:15.
42. Oudenhoven R. Lumbar monoradiculopathy due to unilateral facet hypertrophy. *Neurosurgery.* 1982;11:726–727.
43. Manchikanti L, Pampati V, Baha AG, Fellows B, Damron KS, Barnhill RC. Contribution of facet joints to chronic low back pain in postlumbar laminectomy syndrome : a controlled comparative prevalence evaluation. *Pain Physician.* 2001; 4:175–180.
44. Manchikanti L, Manchukonda R, Pampati V, Damron KS, McManus CD. Prevalence of facet joint pain in chronic low back pain in postsurgical patients by controlled comparative local anesthetic blocks. *Arch Phys Med Rehab.* 2007;88:449–455.
45. Bokov A, Isrelov A, Skorodumov A, Aleynik A, Simonov A, Mlyavykh S. An analysis of reasons for failed back surgery syndrome and partial results after different types of surgical lumbar nerve root decompression. *Pain Physician.* 2011;14:545–557.
46. Steib K, Proescholdt M, Brawanski A, Lange M, Schlaier J, Schebesch K-M. Predictors of facet joint syndrome after lumbar disc surgery. *J Clin Neurosci.* 2012;19:418–422.
47. Lee CK. Accelerated degeneration of the segment adjacent to a lumbar fusion. *Spine.* 1988;13:375–377.
48. Deyo RA, Nachemson A, Mirza SK. Spinal-fusion surgery—the case for restraint. *N Engl J Med.* 2004;350:722–726.
49. Schofferman J, Reynolds J, Herzog R, Covington E, Dreyfuss P, O'Neill C. Failed back surgery: etiology and diagnostic evaluation. *Spine.* 2003;3:400–403.
50. Helbig T, Lee CK. The lumbar facet syndrome. *Spine.* 1988;13:61–64.
51. Cohen SP, Stojanovic MP, Crooks M, Kim P, Schmidt RK, Shields CH, et al. Lumbar zygapophysial (facet) joint radiofrequency denervation success as a function of pain relief during diagnostic medial branch blocks: a multicenter analysis. *Spine J.* 2008;8:498–504.
52. Waddell G, McCulloch JA, Kummel E, Venner RM. Nonorganic physical signs in low-back pain. *Spine.* 1980;5:117–125.
53. Apeldoorn AT, Ostelo RW, Fritz JM, et al. The cross-sectional construct validity of the Waddell score. *Clin J Pain.* 2012;28:309–317.
54. Manchikanti L, Fellows B, Singh V, Pampati V. Correlates of non-physiological behavior in patients with chronic low back pain. *Pain Physician.* 2003;6:159–166.
55. Neziri AY, Curatolo M, Limacher, et al. Ranking of parameters of pain hypersensitivity according to their discriminative ability in chronic low back pain. *Pain.* 2012;153:2083–2091.
56. Arendt-Nielsen L, Fernández-de-Las-Peñas C, Graven-Nielsen T. Basic aspects of musculoskeletal pain: from acute to chronic pain. *J Man Manip Ther.* 2011;19:186–193.
57. McCall I, Park W, O'Brien J. Induced pain referral from posterior elements in normal subjects. *Spine.* 1979;4:441–446.
58. Cohen SP, Huang JHY, Brummett C. Facet joint pain—advances in patient selection and treatment. *Nat Rev Rheum.* 2013;9:101–116.
59. Cohen SP, Bajwa ZH, Kraemer JJ, Dragovich A, Williams KA, Stream J, et al. Factors predicting success and failure for cervical facet radiofrequency denervation: a multi-center analysis. *Reg Anes Pain Med.* 2007;32:495–503.
60. Dreyfuss P, Schwarzer A, Lau P. Specificity of lumbar medial branch and L5 dorsal ramus blocks. *Spine* 1997;22:895–902.
61. Kaplan N, Dreyfuss P, Halbrook B, Bogduk N. The ability of lumbar medial branch blocks to anesthetize the zygapophysial joint. A physiologic challenge. *Spine.* 1998;23:1847–1852.
62. Van Kleef M, Barendse G, Kessels A, Voets HM, Weber WE, De Lange S. Randomized trial of radiofrequency lumbar facet denervation for chronic low back pain. *Spine.* 1999;24:1937–1942.
63. Dreyfuss P, Halbrook B, Pauza K, Joshi a, McLarty J, Bogduk N. Efficacy and validity of radiofrequency neurotomy for chronic lumbar zygapophysial joint pain. *Spine.* 2000;25:1270–1277.
64. Lord SM, Barnsley L, Bogduk N. The utility of comparative local anesthetic blocks versus placebo-controlled blocks for the diagnosis of cervical zygapophysial joint pain. *Clin J Pain.* 1995;11:208–213.
65. Manchikanti L, Pampati V, Fellows B, CE B. Prevalence of lumbar facet joint pain in chronic low back pain. *Pain Physician.* 1999;2:59–64.
66. Cohen SP, Strassels SA, Kurihara C, Griffith SR, Goff B, Guthmiller K, et al. Establishing an optimal "cutoff" threshold for diagnostic lumbar facet blocks. *Clin J Pain.* 2013;29:382–391.
67. Van Zundert J, Vanelderen P, Kessels A, Van Kleef M. Radiofrequency treatment of facet-related pain: evidence and controversies. *Curr Pain Headache Rep.* 2012; 16:19–25.
68. International Spine Intervention Society. Lumbar Medial Branch Block and Percutaneous Radiofrequency Lumbar Medial Branch Neurotomy. In: Bogduk N, ed. *International Spine Intervention Society. Practice Guidelines: Spinal Doagnostic and Treatment Procedures.* 2nd ed. San Francisco, CA: International Spine Intervention Society; 2004:47–65, 188–218.
69. Shiri R, Solovieva S, Husgafvel-Pursiainen K, et al. The role of obesity and physical activity in non-specific and radiating low back pain: the Young Finns study. *Semin Arthritis Rheum.* 2012;42:640–650.
70. Briggs MS, Givens DL, Schmitt LC, Taylor CA. Relations of C-reactive protein and obesity to the prevalence and the odds of reporting low back pain. *Arch Phys Med Rehabil.* 2013;94:745–752.
71. Zhao I, Bogossian F, Turner C. The effects of shift work and interaction between shift work and overweight/obesity on low back pain in nurses: results from a longitudinal study. *J Occup Environ Med.* 2012;54:820–825.
72. Leboeuf-Yde C. Body weight and low back pain. A systematic literature review of 56 journal articles reporting on 65 epidemiologic studies. *Spine.* 2000;25:226–237.
73. Rihn JA, Kurd M, Hilibrand AS, et al. The influence of obesity on the outcome of treatment of lumbar disc herniation: analysis of the Spine Patient Outcomes Research Trial (SPORT). *J Bone Joint Surg Am.* 2013;95:1–8.
74. Roffey DM, Ashdown LC, Dornan HD, et al. Pilot evaluation of a multidisciplinary medically supervised, nonsurgical weight loss program on the severity of low back pain in obese adults. *Spine J.* 2011;11:197–204.
75. Lidar Z, Behrbalk E, Regev GJ, et al. Intervertebral disc height changes after weight reduction in morbidly obese patients and its effect on quality of life and radicular and low back pain. *Spine.* 2012;37:1947–1952.
76. Vincent HK, Ben-David K, Conrad BP, Lamb KM, Seay AN, Vincent KR. Rapid changes in gait, musculoskeletal pain, and quality of life after bariatric surgery. *Surg Obes Relat Dis.* 2012;8:346–354.
77. Smeets R, Köke A, Lin CW, Ferreira M, Demoulin C. Measures of function in low back pain/disorders: Low Back Pain Rating Scale (LBPRS), Oswestry Disability Index (ODI), Progressive Isoinertial Lifting Evaluation (PILE), Quebec Back Pain Disability Scale (QBPDS), and Roland-Morris Disability Questionnaire (RDQ). *Arthritis Care Res.* 2011;63:S158–S173.

78. Fryer G, Morris T, Gibbons P. Paraspinal muscles and intervertebral dysfunction: part two. *J Manipulative Physiol Ther.* 2004;27:348–357.
79. D'hooge R, Hodges P, Tsao H, et al. Altered trunk muscle coordination during rapid trunk flexion in people in remission of recurrent low back pain. *J Electromyogr Kinesiol.* 2013;23:173–181.
80. Verbunt JA, Seelen HA, Vlaeyen JW, et al. Disuse and deconditioning in chronic low back pain: concepts and hypotheses on contributing mechanisms. *Eur J Pain.* 2003;7:9–21.
81. Philadelphia panel evidence-based clinical practice guidelines on selected Rehabilitation interventions for low back pain. *Phys Ther.* 2001;81:1641–1674.
82. Taylor NF, et al. Therapeutic Exercise in physiotherapy practice is beneficial: a summary of systematic reviews 2002–2005. *Australian Journal of Physiotherapy,* 2007;53:7–16.
83. Cairns MC, Foster N E, Wright C. Randomized controlled trial of specific spinal stabilization exercises and conventional physiotherapy for recurrent low back pain. *Spine.* 2006;31:E670–E681.
84. Koumantakis GA, Watson PJ, Oldham JA. Trunk muscle stabilization training plus general exercise versus general exercise only: randomized controlled trial of patients with recurrent low back pain. *Phys Ther.* 2005;85:209–225.
85. Wessels T, van Tulder M, Sigl T, et al. What predicts outcome in non-operative treatments of chronic low back pain? A systematic review. *Eur Spine J.* 2006;15:1633–1644.
86. Anderson KO, Dowds BN, Pelletz RE, Edwards WT, Peeters-Asdourian C. Development and initial validation of a scale to measure self-efficacy beliefs in patients with chronic pain. *Pain.* 1995;63:77–84.
87. Steiger F, Wirth B, de Bruin ED, Mannion AF. Is a positive clinical outcome after exercise therapy for chronic non-specific low back pain contingent upon a corresponding improvement in the targeted aspect(s) of performance? A systematic review. *Eur Spine J.* 2012;21:575–598.
88. Kelly GA, Blake C, Power CK, O'Keeffe D, Fullen BM. The association between chronic low back pain and sleep: a systematic review. *Clin J Pain.* 2011;27:169–181.
89. Okifuji A, Hare BD. Do sleep disorders contribute to pain sensitivity? *Curr Rheumatol Rep.* 2011;13:528–534.
90. White AP, Arnold PM, Norvell DC, Ecker E, Fehlings MG. Pharmacologic management of chronic low back pain: synthesis of the evidence. *Spine.* 2001;36:S131–S143.
91. Davis MP, Srivastava M. Demographics, assessment and management of pain in the elderly. *Drugs Aging.* 2003;20:23–57.
92 Chaparro LE, Furlan AD, Deshpande A, Mailis-Gagnon A, Atlas S, Turk DC. Opioids compared to placebo or other treatments for chronic low-back pain. *Cochrane Database Syst Rev.* 2013;8:CD004959. doi: 10.1002/14651858.CD004959.pub4.
93. Ballantyne JC. Is lack of evidence the problem? *J Pain.* 2010;9:830–832.
94. Ballantyne J. "Safe and effective when used as directed": the case of chronic use of opioid analgesics. *J Med Toxicol.* 2012;8:417–423.
95. Schofferman J, Mazanec D. Evidence-informed management of chronic low back pain with opioid analgesics. *Spine.* 2008;8:185–194.
96. Urquhart DM, Hoving JL, Assendelft WW, Roland M, van Tulder MW. Antidepressants for non-specific low back pain. *Cochrane Database Syst Rev.* 2008;(1):CD001703. doi: 10.1002/14651858. CD001703.pub3.
97. Schnitzer T, Ferraro A, Hunsche E, Kong S. A comprehensive review of clinical trials on the efficacy and safety of drugs for the treatment of low back pain. *J Pain Symptom Manage.* 2004;28:72–95.
98. White AP, Arnold PM, Norvell DC, Ecker E, Fehlings MG. Pharmacologic management of chronic low back pain: synthesis of the evidence. *Spine.* 2011;36:S131–S143.
99. Skljarevski V, Zhang S, Desaiah D, Alaka KJ, Palacios S, Miazgowski T, Patrick K. Duloxetine versus placebo in patients with chronic low back pain: a 12-week, fixed-dose, randomized, double-blind trial. *J Pain.* 2010;11(12):1282–1290.
100. Skljarevski V, Desaiah D, Liu-Seifert H, Zhang Q, Chappell AS, Detke MJ, Iyengar S, Atkinson JH, Backonja M. Efficacy and safety of duloxetine in patients with chronic low back pain. *Spine* (Phila Pa 1976). 2010;35(13):E578–585.
101. Skljarevski V, Ossanna M, Liu-Seifert H, et al. A double-blind, randomized trial of duloxetine versus placebo in the management of chronic lowback pain. *Eur J Neurol.* 2009;16(9):1041–1048.
102. Dharmshaktu P, Tayal V, Kalra BS. Efficacy of antidepressants as analgesics: a review. *J Clin Pharmacol.* 2012;52:6–17.
103. Spallone V, Lacerenza M, Rossi A, Sicuteri R, Marchettini P. Painful diabetic polyneuropathy: approach to diagnosis and management. *Clin J Pain.* 2012;28:726–743.
104. Edelsberg JS, Lord C, Oster G. Systematic review and meta-analysis of efficacy, safety, and tolerability data from randomized controlled trials of drugs used to treat postherpetic neuralgia. *Ann Pharmacother.* 2011;45:1483–1490.
105. Zencirci B. Analgesic efficacy of oral gabapentin added to standard epidural corticosteroids in patients with failed back surgery. *Clin Pharmacol.* 2010;2:207–211.
106. Wu YT, Lai MH, Lu SC, Chang ST. Beneficial response to gabapentin portraying with interval change of brain SPECT imaging in a case with failed back surgery syndrome. *J Clin Pharm Ther.* 2011;36:525–528.
107. Mens J. The use of medication in low back pain. *Best Pract Res Clin Rheumatol.* 2005;19:609–621.
108. Gofeld M, Faclier G. Radiofrequency denervation of the lumbar zygapophysial joints—targeting the best practice. *Pain Med.* 2008;9:204–211.
109. Gofeld M. Ultrasonography in pain medicine: a critical review. *Pain pract.* 2008;8:226–240.
110. Gofeld M, Bristow SJ, Chiu S. Ultrasound-guided injection of lumbar zygapophyseal joints: an anatomic study with fluoroscopy validation. *Reg Anes Pain Med.* 2012;37:228–231.
111. Barnsley L, Lord S, Wallis B, Bogduk N. Lack of effect of intraarticular corticosteroids for chronic pain in the cervical zygapophyseal joints. *N Engl J Med.* 1994;330:1047–1050.
112. Carette S, Marcoux S, Truchon R, et al. A controlled trial of corticosteroid injections into facet joints for chronic low back pain. *New Engl J Med.* 1991;325:1002–1007.
113. Gofeld M, Jitendra J, Faclier G. Radiofrequency denervation of the lumbar zygapophysial joints: 10-year prospective clinical audit. *Pain Physician.* 2007;10:291–300.
114. Boswell M V, Colson JD, Sehgal N, Dunbar EE, Epter R. A systematic review of therapeutic facet joint interventions in chronic spinal pain. *Pain Physician.* 2007;10:229–253.
115. Berg A, Allan J. Introducing the third U.S. Preventive Services Task Force. *Am J Prev Med.* 2001;20:S3–S4.
116. Guyatt G, Gutterman D, Baumann M. et al. Grading strength of recommendations and quality of evidence in clinical guidelines: report from an American College of Chest Physicians Task Force. *Chest.* 2006;129:174–181.
117. Van Kleef M, Mekhail N, Van Zundert J. Evidence based guidelines for interventional pain medicine according to clinical diagnoses. *Pain Pract.* 2009;9:247–251.
118. Dobrogowski J, Wrzosek A, Wordliczek J. Radiofrequency denervation with or without addition of pentoxifylline or methylprednisolone for chronic lumbar zygapophysial joint pain. *Pharmacol. Rep.* 2005;57:475–480.
119. Aupperle RL, Allard CB, Grimes EM, et al. Dorsolateral prefrontal cortex activation during emotional anticipation and neuropsychological performance in posttraumatic stress disorder. *Arch Gen Psychiatry.* 2012;69(4):360–371.
120. Kessler RC, Berglund P, Demler O, et al. Lifetime prevalence and age-of-onset distributions of DSM-IV disorders in the National Comorbidity Survey Replication. *Arch Gen Psychiatry.* 2005;62(6):593–602.
121. Smid GE, Mooren TT, van der Mast RC, et al. Delayed posttraumatic stress disorder: systematic review, meta-analysis, and meta-regression analysis of prospective studies. *J Clin Psychiatry.* 2009;70:1572.

122. Binder EB, Bradley RG, Liu W, et al. Association of FKBP5 polymorphisms and childhood abuse with risk of posttraumatic stress disorder symptoms in adults. *JAMA.* 2008;299(11):1291–1305.
123. Cougle JR, Resnick H, Kilpatrick DG. Does exposure to interpersonal violence increase risk of PTSD following subsequent exposure? *Behav Res Ther.* 2009;47(12):1012–1017.
124. Smith TC, Wingard DL, Ryan MA, et al. Prior assault and posttraumatic stress disorder after combat deployment. *Epidemiology.* 2008;19(3):505–512.
125. Breslau N. The epidemiology of trauma, PTSD, and other posttrauma disorders. *Trauma Violence Abuse.* 2009;10(3):198–210.
126. Vogt DS, King DW, King LA. Risk pathways for PTSD: making sense of the literature. In: *Handbook of PTSD: Science and Practice.* Friedman MJ, Keane TM, Resick PA, eds. New York: Guilford; 2007:99–115.
127. Kessler RC, Sonnega A, Bromet E, et al. PTSD in the National Comorbidity Survey. *Arch Gen Psychiatry.* 199552(12):1048–1060.
128. Vieweg WV, Julius DA, Fernandez A, et al. Posttraumatic stress disorder: clinical features, pathophysiology, and treatment. *Am J Med.* 2006;119:383.
129. Steel Z, Chey T, Silove D, et al. Association of torture and other potentially traumatic events with mental health outcomes among populations exposed to mass conflict and displacement: a systematic review and meta-analysis. *JAMA.* 2009;302:537.
130. Davydow DS, Gifford JM, Desai SV, et al. Posttraumatic stress disorder in general intensive care unit survivors: a systematic review. *Gen Hosp Psychiatry.* 2008;30:421.
131. Amir M, Kaplan Z, Neumann L, et al. Posttraumatic stress disorder, tenderness and fibromyalgia. *J Psychosom Res.* 1997; 42:607–613.
132. Asmundson GJ, Norton GR, Allerdings MD, et al. Posttraumatic stress disorder and work-related injury. *J Anxiety Disord.* 198;12:57–69.
133. Benedikt RA, Kolb LC. Preliminary findings on chronic pain and posttraumatic stress disorder. *Am J Psychiatry.* 1986;143:908–910.
134. Engel Jr CC, Lie X, McCarthy BD, et al. Relationship of physical symptoms to posttraumatic stress disorder among veterans seeking care for gulf war related health concerns. *Psychosom Med.* 2000;62:739–745.
135. Beckham JC, Braxton LE, Kudler HS, Feldman ME, Lytle BL, Palmer S. Minnesota multiphasic personality inventory profiles of Vietnam combat veterans with posttraumatic stress disorder and their children. *J Clin Psychol.* 1997;53:847–852.
136. Sharp TJ, Harvey AG. Chronic pain and posttraumatic stress disorder: mutual maintenance. *Clin Psychol Rev.* 2001; 12:857–877.
137. Hart-Johnson T, Green CR. The impact of sexual or physical abuse history on pain-related outcomes among blacks and whites with chronic pain: gender influence. *Pain Med.* 2012;13;229–242.
138. Cougle JR, Keough ME, Riccardi CJ, et al. Anxiety disorders and suicidality in the national comorbidity survey-replication. *J Psychiatr Res.* 2009;43:825–829.
139. Krystal JH, Rosenheck RA, Cramer JA, et al. Veterans Affairs cooperative study No. 504 Group. Adjunctive risperidone treatment for anti-depressant-resistant symptoms of chronic military service-related PTSD: a randomized trial. *JAMA.* 2011; 306(5):493–502.
140. Pietrzak RH, Goldstein RB, Southwick SM, et al. Prevalence and axis I comorbidity of full and partial posttraumatic stress disorder in the United States: results from wave 2 of the National Epidemiologic Survey on Alcohol and Related Conditions. *J Anxiety Disord.* 2011;25(3):456–465.
141. Weathers FW, Huska JA, Keane TM. *The PTSD Checklist Civilian Version* (PCL-C). Boston, MA: National Center for PTSD (Boston Veterans Affairs Medical Center);1991.
142. Blanchard EB, Jones-Alexander J, Buckley TC, Forneris CA. Psychometric properties of the PTSD Checklist (PCL). *Behav Res Ther.* 1996;34:669.
143. Andrykowski MA, Cordova MJ, Studts JL, Miller TW. Posttraumatic stress disorder after treatment for breast cancer: prevalence of diagnosis and use of the PTSD Checklist-Civilian Version (PCL-C) as a screening instrument. *J Consult Clin Psychol.* 1998;66:586.
144. Friedman MJ. PTSD: pharmacotherapeutic approaches. *Focus.* 2013;11(3):315–320.
145. Davis LL, Davidson JRT, Ward LC, et al. Divalproex in the treatment of posttraumatic stress disorder: a randomized, double-blind, placebo-controlled trial in a veteran population. *J Clin Psychopharmacol.* 2008;28:84–88.
146. Hamner MB, Faldowski RA, Robert S, et al. A preliminary controlled trial of divalproex in posttraumatic stress disorder. *Ann Clin Psychiatry.* 2009;21:89–94.
147. Hertzberg MA, Butterfield MI, Feldman ME, et al. A preliminary study of lamotrigine for the treatment of posttraumatic stress disorder. *Biol Psychiatry.* 1999;45:1226–1229.
148. Davidson JR, Brady KT, Mellman TA, et al. The efficacy and tolerability of tiagabine in adult patients with post-traumatic stress disorder. *J Clin Psychopharmacol.* 2007;27:85–88.
149. Akuchekian SH, Amanat S. Comparison of topiramate and placebo in the treatment of posttraumatic stress disorder: a randomized, double-blind study. *J Res med Sci.* 2004;5:240–244.
150. Tucker P, Trautman RP, Wyatt DB, et al. Efficacy and safety of topiramate monotherapy in civilian posttraumatic stress disorder: a randomized, double-blind, placebo-controlled study. *J Clin Psychiatry* 2007;68:201–206.
151. Yeh MSL, Mari JJ, Costa MCP, et al. A double-blind randomized controlled trial to study the efficacy of topiramate in a civilian sample of PTSD. *CNS Neurosci Ther.* 2011;17:305–310.
152. Jonas DE, Cusack K, Forneris CA, et al. Psychological and pharmacological treatments for adults with Posttraumatic Stress Disorder(PTSD) [Comparative Effectiveness Reviews, No. 92]. Rockville, MD: Agency for Healthcare Research and Quality; 2013.
153. Bradley R, Greene J, Russ E, et al. A multidimensional meta-analysis of psychotherapy for PTSD. *Am J Psychiatry.* 2005;162:214–227.
154. Gibson JN, Waddell G. Surgery for degenerative lumbar spondylosis: updated Cochrane Review. *Spine.* 2005;30:2312–2320.

10.

SACROILIAC JOINT PAIN

Samuel L. Holmes, Steven P. Cohen, Michael-Flynn L. Cullen,

Christopher D. Kenny, Harold J. Wain, and S. Avery Davis

CASE PRESENTATION

A 29-year-old paratrooper presents with right-sided lower back pain of 3 months' duration. The pain started spontaneously following a training session where he sustained a particularly hard parachute landing. The pain is described as intermittent, aching, and sharp with occasional referral to the back of the thigh. He denies weakness, falling, or bowel/bladder/sexual dysfunction. The pain is made worse by changing position and getting in and out of a truck. It is somewhat improved with massage and tramadol 100 mg taken every 6 hours. Initial field management with rest, analgesics, and osteopathic manipulation was not helpful. The patient is referred to the Interdisciplinary Back Pain clinic for further evaluation and management.

Past medical history is significant for chronic knee and back pain.

Social history is significant for social alcohol use.

Review of systems is negative aside from the finding of right-sided low back pain (LBP) radiating to the back of the thigh.

On examination, the patient weighs 82 kg and is 186 cm tall. His lower extremities' neurologic examination including sensory, motor, and reflexes is normal. When asked to point with one finger to the point of maximal pain, he points near the right posterior superior iliac spine (PSIS) with good reproducibility on multiple occasions. Musculoskeletal examination reveals tenderness over the lateral aspect of the right sacrum. Flexion, abduction, and external rotation of the right hip reproduces the pain, as does sacral compression and distraction testing.

Magnetic resonance imaging (MRI) of the lumbar spine reveals normal findings.

QUESTIONS

1. What are potential causes of the patient's symptoms?
2. What is the prevalence and incidence and prevalence of sacroiliac (SI) joint pain and related disability?
3. What is the pathophysiology of SI joint pain?
4. What is the natural history and long-term prognosis of SI joint pain?
5. How is a definite diagnosis of SI joint pain made?
6. How is SI joint pain managed?

WHAT ARE POTENTIAL CAUSES OF THE PATIENT'S SYMPTOMS?

DIFFERENTIAL DIAGNOSES

The broad differential for LBP is quite extensive. It can be helpful to separate potential sources into two broad categories: mechanical and nonmechanical syndromes (Box 10.1).[1,2]

The differential diagnosis in this chapter's clinical case can be narrowed based on the patient's history, physical examination, and imaging findings. His occupation as a paratrooper entails repetitive high axial forces that stress the kinetic chain from his back through his lower extremities. He has experienced a potential inciting event with a particularly hard parachute landing with resultant unilateral lower back pain radiating to the back of his thigh, which is exacerbated by shifting weight and rising from a seated position. He does not endorse red flag symptoms for neurological compromise, his examination is negative for neurological findings one would expect to be associated with a radiculopathy, and he does not present with signs or symptoms of infection or systemic disorders. Pain is localized to the SI joint region by patient report, and he endorses sacral sulcus tenderness. He demonstrates three positive tests that localize symptoms to the SI joint: Patrick-FABER, sacral compression, and distraction testing. A normal MRI study helps to rule out readily identifiable structural pathology. Lack of SI joint imaging findings should not discourage the diagnosis of SI joint dysfunction, which is suspected in this case. These findings will be expanded on throughout the chapter.

Box 10.1 **DIFFERENTIAL DIAGNOSIS FOR LOWER BACK PAIN**

Mechanical Syndromes

- SI joint dysfunction
- Disc/facet motion segment degeneration
- Myofascial pain and syndromes
- Discogenic pain
- Radiculopathy due to structural impingement
- Axial or radicular pain related to a biochemical or inflammatory reaction to injury
- Motion segment or vertebral osseous fractures
- Spondylosis with or without central or lateral canal stenosis
- Macroinstability/microinstability of the spine with/without radiographic hypermobility or evidence of subluxation
- Piriformis syndrome
- Iliotibial band syndrome
- Trochanteric bursitis

Nonmechanical Syndromes

NEUROLOGIC SYNDROMES

- Myelopathy or myelitis related to intrinsic/extrinsic structural or vascular processes
- Lumbosacral plexopathy (e.g., diabetes, vasculitis, malignancy)
- Acute, subacute, or chronic polyneuropathy (e.g., acute and chronic inflammatory demyelinating polyneuropathy, diabetes)
- Mononeuropathy, including causalgia (e.g., trauma, diabetes)
- Myopathy, including myositis and various metabolic conditions
- Spinal segmental, lumbopelvic, or generalized dystonia

SYSTEMIC DISORDERS

- Primary or metastatic neoplasms
- Infection (e.g., osseous, discal, or epidural)
- Inflammatory spondyloarthropathy
- Metabolic bone diseases (e.g., osteoporosis)
- Vascular disorders (e.g., atherosclerosis, vasculitis)

REFERRED PAIN

- Gastrointestinal disorders (e.g., pancreatitis, pancreatic cancer, cholecystitis)
- Cardiorespiratory disorders (e.g., pericarditis, pleuritis, pneumonia)
- Disorders of the ribs or sternum
- Genitourinary disorders (e.g., nephrolithiasis, prostatitis, pyelonephritis, endometriosis, ectopic pregnancy)
- Thoracic or abdominal aortic aneurysms
- Hip disorders (e.g., injury, inflammation, degeneration of the joint/tendons/bursae/ligaments)

Adapted from Wheeler AH et al. Low back pain and sciatica. *Medscape* 2013.

WHAT IS THE PREVALENCE AND INCIDENCE OF SI JOINT PAIN AND RELATED DISABILITY?

PREVALENCE

The overall prevalence of SI joint pain is generally reported as a subgroup of chronic LBP and ranges between 13% and 32%. The variability in evidence-based prevalence is partially attributed to the selectivity of patients recruited and the diagnostic standard. The patient populations in which the prevalence of SI joint pain is reported include chronic LBP, pregnancy, and inflammatory sacroiliitis. Diagnostic standards utilized include examination maneuvers, positive response to therapy, radiographs, and SI joint injections (Table 10.1).[3–9]

DISABILITY

The economic impact of nonspecific LBP reaches into billions of dollars annually, considering the cost of medical care, time lost from work, disability payments, productivity loss, staff retraining, and litigation expenses. It will cause approximately 25 million Americans to lose 1 or more days from work a year. More than 5 million people are disabled from LBP. Generally, increasing time missed from work is associated with lower return to work expectations. After 6 months away from work, the return-to-work rate is approximately 50%; at 1 year it declines to 25%, and at 2 years, the return-to-work rate approaches zero.[10] Slightly more than 1% of adults in the United States are permanently disabled by back pain, and another 1% are temporarily disabled.[11]

Both the cost and incidence of patients disabled by LBP has increased during the past 30 years. The two most commonly cited factors are the increasing societal acceptance of back pain as a reason to become disabled and changes in the social system that financially rewards patients with back pain.[12]

According to the 2012 Council for Disability Awareness long-term disability claims review, 30% of claims in the United States are related to a diagnosis in the general category of Musculoskeletal/Connective Tissue. Back pain is one of the most common diagnoses within these claims.[13]

A systemic review determined common risk factors for disability to include recurrence, chronicity, non-return to work, low level of job satisfaction, poor general health, occupational physical demands, and socioprofessional factors.[14]

WHAT IS THE PATHOPHYSIOLOGY OF SI JOINT PAIN?

ANATOMY

The SI joint is of significant functional importance in its role of supporting the upper body and transmitting forces via the ileum to the lower extremities and vice versa while enabling

Table 10.1 **PREVALENCE OF SACROILIAC (SI) JOINT PAIN IN PATIENTS WITH LOW BACK PAIN**

AUTHORS	SUBJECTS	DIAGNOSTIC CRITERIA	PREVALENCE
Bernard et al. 1987[5]	Chronic LBP N = 1,293	Examination and response to therapy or SI joint injection	22.5%
Sembrano et al 2009[6]	Chronic LBP referrals N = 348	Examination and response to therapy or injection	14.5% (10% with nonspecific cause)
Swartzer et al. 1995[7]	Chronic LBP maximally below L5-S1 N = 43	Positive response to single SI joint block	13–30%
Maigne et al. 1996[8]	Suspected SI joint mediated pain based on examination and provocative maneuvers N = 54	Double SI blocks	18.5%
Irwin et al. 2007[9]	Referred patients with complaint of low back or SI joint pain N = 158	Double SI blocks	26.6%
Liliang et al. 2011[163]	Prior lumbar and lumbosacral fusion. 52 had suspected SI joint pain based on examination. N= 130	Double SI blocks	16.2%
O'Shea et al.[4] 2010	Chronic low back pain referred for radiographs N = 315	AP pelvis and/or lumbar radiographs	31.7%

Adapted from Cohen SP et al. Sacroiliac joint pain: a comprehensive review of epidemiology, diagnosis and treatment. *Expert Rev Neurother.* 2013 Jan;13(1):99–116.

movement of the pelvis about the axis of the sacrum. It is a true diarthrodial synovial joint approximated by a fibrous capsule at the anterior one-third of its articular surface. It is considered the largest axial joint in the body and is estimated to be approximately 17.5 cm^2 although there is great variability in dimensions within and among individuals.[15,16]

The posterior portion of the joint is a fibrocartilage syndesmosis reinforced by powerful ligamentous attachments. These ligaments include the anterior SI ligament, dorsal SI ligament, sacrospinous ligament, sacrotuberous ligament, and interosseus ligaments, with the latter considered to be the strongest.[15,17] The wedged C-shape and orientation of the sacrum as it is seated between the ilia acts in concert with these ligaments to stabilize the joint. Weight translated from the body through the SI joint tends to force the cephalad aspect of the sacrum inferior and anterior, exerting greater tension on the interosseous and posterior SI ligaments and resulting in firmer apposition of the sacrum within the ilea. The articular surfaces of the SI joint also have many complimentary ridges and grooves rather than the typical smooth joint surfaces found elsewhere. This attribute tends to reinforce and enhance stability via minimization of movement (Figure 10.1).[18]

The innervation of the SI joint is poorly understood and remains a topic of debate. Recent literature suggests that lateral branches of the S1–S3 dorsal rami compose the major innervation to the posterior SI joint with some suggestion that dorsal rami components as extensive as L3–S4 may contribute in many individuals.[15] The innervation of the anterior joint is likewise uncertain, with recent literature indicating contributions from different combinations of the ventral rami of L2–S2[18] and older literature suggesting possible contributions from the obturator and superior gluteal nerves.[19]

BIOMECHANICS

The SI joint is thought to have three linear (translational) axes of movement in the transverse, longitudinal, and sagittal planes with angular (rotational) components of each essentially creating six degrees of freedom. Sacral flexion and extension generally occur at the second sacral segment. Nutation applied to sacral kinematics indicates sacral base movement anteroinferior in relation to the ileum during lumbosacral extension, and counternutation indicates sacral base movement posterosuperior during lumbosacral flexion.[18] The functional effect of the SI joint's overall anatomical relationships is to limit this motion in all planes of movement (i.e., prevent excess translation and rotation). Some studies have estimated mean rotation ranging between 1 and 12 degrees, and mean translation ranging between 3 and16 mm.[20] In females, there is increased ligamentous laxity and joint mobility that allows for parturition. Joint motion decreases with age and degenerative changes, usually occurring earlier in males around the fourth decade of life compared to the fifth decade for females. Ultimately, there is minimal movement about the healthy SI joint in serving its primary functional role as a support structure. Although it is believed that increased SI joint motion can lead to pain, the results of studies examining this relationship have been mixed.

Similar to other joints, SI joint function is kinetically interdependent with adjacent joints. The spine transmits forces to the SI joint via the lumbosacral joint. Force is then transmitted through the ilea to the hip joints and femurs. The symphysis pubis plays an important role in maintaining the ring structure integrity of the pelvis in order to appropriately transmit forces through the above joints and related

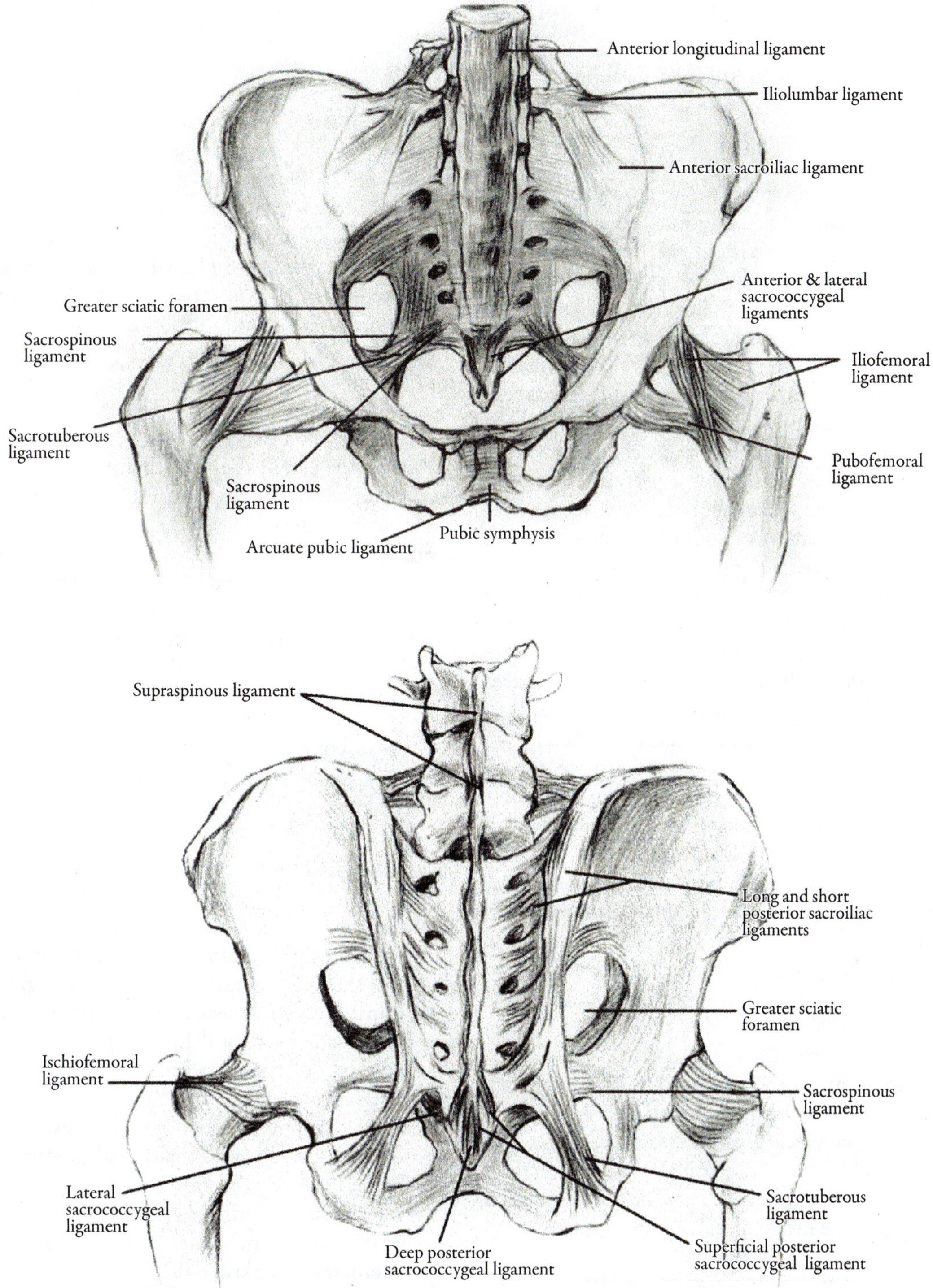

Figure 10.1 Bony and ligamentous anatomy of the sacroiliac joint. Reprinted with permission from Cohen SP. Sacroiliac joint pain: a comprehensive review of anatomy, diagnosis, and treatment. *Anesth Analg.* 2005 Nov;101(5):1440–1453.

structures. Alterations in the function of any of these structures will impact the SI joint.

The joint and supporting structures are further acted upon by a network of muscles and fascia. The piriformis muscle originates from the anterior surface of the sacrum and inserts on the greater trochanter as part of the external rotator group of the hip. The gluteus maximus originates from the lateral surface of the ilium, the posterior SI and sacrotuberous ligaments, and the posterior surface of the sacrum, and it inserts on the iliotibial band and gluteal tuberosity of the femur to function as the primary hip extensor while also externally rotating the hip. Additional myofascial structures functionally impacting the SI joint due to close anatomical associations include the gluteus minimus and medius, biceps femoris, iliopsoas, iliacus, abdominals, latissimus dorsi, quadrates lumborum, erector spinae, and thoracolumbar fascia.

PATHOPHYSIOLOGY

Because the SI joint primarily functions to limit motion while transmitting and dispersing truncal loads through the lower extremities via its anatomical relationships, injury and production of pain generally result from a failure of these stabilizing mechanisms and an alteration of these anatomical relationships. Excessive axial load and rotation can result in destabilizing compressive and torsional shearing forces that may injure the associated myofascial structures impacting the SI joint , especially when these forces are high velocity, repetitive, and asymmetrical. Maladaptive compensatory biomechanics can also lead to injury or further exacerbate SI joint dysfunction once injury has occurred. Common pathways to pain include capsular or synovial disruption, capsular and ligamentous tension, hypomobility or hypermobility, abnormal joint mechanics, microfractures or macrofractures, chondromalacia, soft-tissue injury, and inflammation.[15] Nociceptors have been histologically demonstrated throughout the joint capsule, ligaments, and subchondral bone, suggesting that injury to any of these joint and supporting structures may produce pain.[21,22] It is often useful to consider two broad differential diagnosis categories of SI joint pain generators: intra-articular versus extra-articular. Intra-articular sources include inflammation, arthritis, infection, and malignancy. Extra-articular sources are more common and include enthesopathy, fractures, ligamentous injuries, and myofascial components (Box 10.2).[15]

Multiple risk factors exist that may predispose the SI joint to insidious onset of dysfunction. True and apparent leg length discrepancy,[23] gait abnormalities,[24] prolonged vigorous exercise,[25] scoliosis,[26] and spinal fusion to the sacrum[27] can all increase forces about the SI joint and lead to dysfunction. Additional factors associated with lumbar spine surgery, such as SI ligament weakening and/or surgical violation of the joint cavity during iliac graft bone harvest[28] and postsurgical hypermobility,[29] have also been implicated in SI joint pathology. General risk factors shared with lower back pain include smoking, poor physical condition, psychosocial pathology, transitional anatomy and other anatomical abnormalities, positive family history, and occupational lifting.

The numerous physiological changes associated with childbearing may result in SI joint pathology. Pregnancy associated weight gain, exaggerated lordotic posture, hormone-induced ligamental laxity, and the mechanical trauma associated with parturition all predispose women to SI joint pain. Increased estrogen and relaxin in the first trimester and peripartum periods soften the symphysis pubis and SI joint ligaments resulting in reports of sprains and SI subluxation.[30–32]

There are multiple and varied etiologies associated with SI joint pain. Seronegative and HLA-B27-associated spondyloarthropathies produce prominent inflammation at one or both SI joints.[33] Infectious-related sources of SI joint pain include the autoimmune response to infection in reactive arthritis associated with HLA-B27 carriers, reactive arthritis associated with HIV-positive individuals, and rare pyogenic infections.[34] Malignancy has been reported to mimic sacroiliitis and cause SI joint pain as well.[35] Biomechanical mechanisms of injury and dysfunction include bracing of the legs in a motor vehicle accident,[36] falls,[36] athletic injuries,[37] prolonged lifting and bending,[38] and torsional strain.[38] A retrospective study of 54 patients with injection-confirmed SI joint pain identified trauma as the cause in 44% of cases and cumulative effects of repetitive stress in 21% of the cases; 35% were deemed to be idiopathic. Of the 24 patients citing trauma as the source of pain, 13 were associated with motor vehicle accidents, six with falls onto the buttock, and three with childbirth.[36] Another study reported a 58% association of trauma with SI joint pain based on clinical examination findings.[5]

Box 10.2 CAUSES OF INTRA-ARTICULAR VS. EXTRA-ARTICULAR SI JOINT PAIN

INTRA-ARTICULAR PAIN	EXTRA-ARTICULAR PAIN
Arthritis	Ligamentous injury
Spondyloarthropathy	Bone fractures
Malignancies	Malignancies
Trauma	Myofascial pain
Infection	Enthesopathy
Cystic disease	Trauma
	Pregnancy

Adapted from Cohen SP et al. Sacroiliac joint pain: a comprehensive review of epidemiology, diagnosis and treatment. *Expert Rev Neurother.* 2013 Jan;13(1):99–116.

WHAT IS THE NATURAL HISTORY AND LONG-TERM PROGNOSIS OF SI JOINT PAIN?

Although some studies have examined the natural history of inflammatory spondyloarthritides and pregnancy-related SI joint pain, studies that assess the long-term natural history of untreated SI joint pain are lacking. Physiologically, the SI joint will show degenerative changes on imaging regardless of symptoms. One study assessed SI joint computed tomography (CT) scans in 95 healthy asymptomatic volunteers aged 21–86 years and found radiologic evidence of degenerative changes as early as in the 20s. By age 50, there was 100% CT evidence of SI joint degenerative changes, with greater progression in females versus males and parous versus nulliparous women.[39] Although this was not clinically correlated, it suggests a natural history of senescent SI joint pathological degeneration that may impact prognosis.

Overall, the prognosis of SI joint pain is favorable in terms of disability. Prognosis of SI joint pain is difficult to address due to multiple etiologies, varying clinical presentations, and lack of long-term studies evaluating different treatments. Negative prognostic variables include older age, lower education levels, unskilled work, high intensity of pain, low index of mobility, and a high number of positive pain tests. Discussing prognosis with patients experiencing SI joint pain should therefore be individualized.

Reportedly, more than 90% of patients with inflammatory spondyloarthritis will continue to function independently.[40] In pregnancy, during which a significant percentage of women suffer SI joint pain, 5–9% will continue to experience SI joint pain for as long as 2 years postpartum.[41,42]

HOW IS A DEFINITE DIAGNOSIS OF SI JOINT PAIN MADE?

BACKGROUND

The diagnosis and management of SI pain was first described in 1905 by Goldthwaite and Osgood, and this diagnosis survived as a predominant etiology for lower back pain until a paper in 1936 by Mixter and Barr in the *New England Journal of Medicine* questioned its legitimacy.[43–45] Mixter and Barr's cadaveric research showed prominent intervertebral pathology exhibited by prolapsed nucleus pulposus. Consequently, SI joint pathology became relatively dismissed as an important contributing diagnosis despite a study published four years after Mixter and Barr's paper that showed promise in treating lumbago by injecting the SI joint with provicaine.[46,47] In 1956, Norman and May became the first physicians to fluoroscopically inject the SI joint.[48] Yet it wasn't until the work of Fortin et al.,[49,50] Schwarzer et al., and Maigne et al. in the 1990s that the objective data necessary to regain the subsequent acceptance of SI joint dysfunction as a progenitor of LBP was established.

In 1998, Broadhurst and Bond published a sensitivity range of 77–87% when three provocative SI joint maneuvers were deemed positive.[51] Although the general consensus seems to be that neither history nor physical examination are able to definitively diagnosis the SI joint as a pain generator, using a combination of historical and examination features can increase the clinician's suspicion enough to enter the diagnosis within the working differential. Since 1994, the diagnosis of SI pain has been established by the International Association for the Study of Pain (IASP) as meeting the criteria of a positive Fortin finger test, pain relieved by SI joint injection, and at least three positive provocative tests on physical examination (Box 10.3).[52,53] However, a more recent systemic review in 2009 concluded that clinicians should exercise caution because there is no gold standard in the diagnosis of SI joint pain.[54]

HISTORY OF ILLNESS, CLINICAL MANIFESTATIONS

Patients with SI joint dysfunction will typically present with unilateral (4:1 vs. bilateral)[16] pain that is below the belt line and is exacerbated by transitional activities such as rising from a seated position, getting out of a car, getting out of bed in the morning, and ascending stairs.[55,56] They may describe hearing a popping, cracking, or clicking sound and experiencing groin or posterolateral thigh pain.[57]

Box 10.3 IASP CRITERIA FOR SI PAIN

- Positive Fortin finger test, i.e. pain located within 1 cm inferior-medial to the PSIS
- Pain that is relieved by injection of the SI joint
- At least three positive provocative pain tests (0.82 for sensitivity, 0.88 for specificity, 0.86 for positive predictive value of a test, and 0.84 for negative predictive value)

Landmarks and pain patterns for SI joint pain and those of lumbar zygapophyseal joint mediated pain are shown in Figures 10.2–10.4.

Retrospective analyses have shown that 44–58% of patients with SI joint dysfunction will have a history of trauma (e.g., motor vehicle accidents, falls, postpartum, sports injury, and fracture).[5,36] SI joint pain has been shown to be more prevalent in pregnant women and athletes involved in sports that require unilateral loading or prolonged sitting (martial arts, ballet, rowing).[58–60] An increased prevalence rate has also been associated with sports-related cumulative repetitive force injuries (e.g., weight lifting, running, rowing, cross-country skiing; see Box 10.4; Table 10.2).

INSPECTION

Seeking to identify a simple, reproducible, and accurate diagnostic tool for SI joint dysfunction, Fortin published a study in 1997 describing the "Fortin finger test," in which the patient points to the SI joint as the source of his or her LBP.[61] The test is considered positive if the patient points to within 1cm inferomedial of the PSIS on at least two consecutive trials. The interrater reliability was found to be 100% in his original research. Although the Fortin finger test is sometimes considered to be one of the most reliable clinical examination findings for SI joint pain, there have been no attempts made to validate the findings of his study.

In addition to having the patient identify the principal area of pain, other areas of the low back should be visually inspected. The skin overlying the SI joint can be revealing for dermatological etiologies of lumbago (soft-tissue infections, zoster, soft tissue masses, skin changes concerning for autoimmune arthritic conditions). Assessment for lumbar lordosis may assist with recognition of underlying sacral misalignment. Quantification begins with the assessment

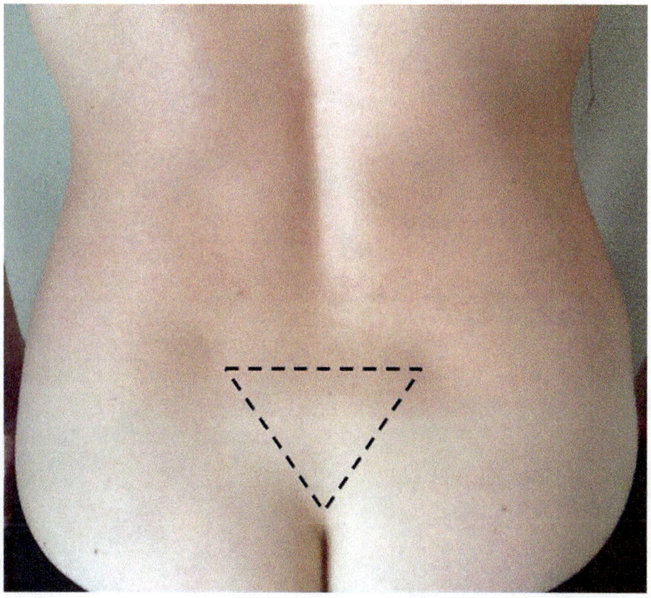

Figure 10.2 Surface landmarks of the sacroiliac joint: the presacral dimples indicate the PSIS and form the base of the sacral triangle. The sacral sulci are formed by the junction of the sacrum and ilium and are palpated just medial to the presacral dimples bilaterally.

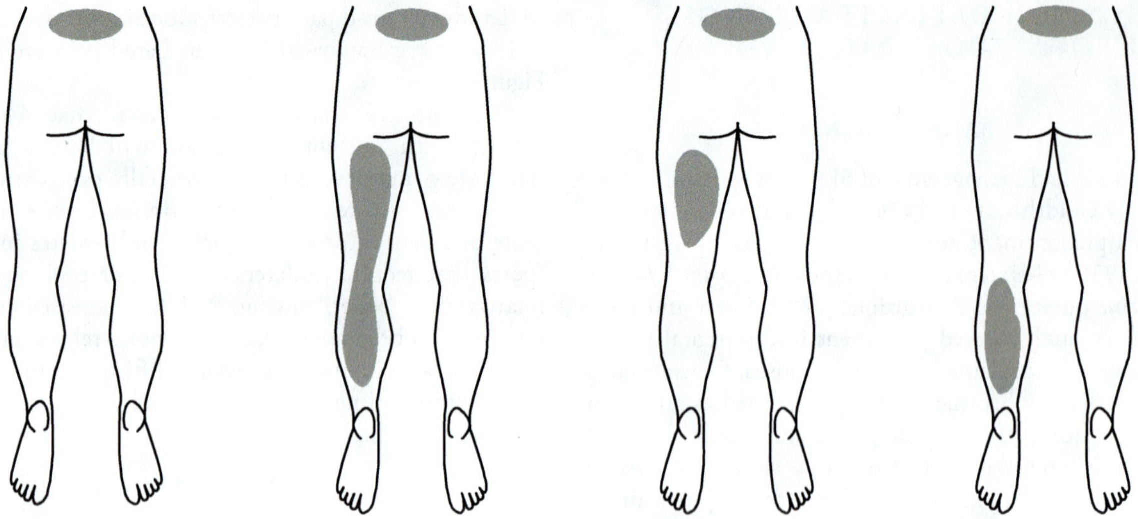

Figure 10.3 Pain referral patterns for lumbar zygapophyseal joint dysfunction.

Box 10.4 **KEY CLINICAL FEATURES AND ASSOCIATIONS OF SI JOINT PAIN**

- Unilateral pain below belt line
- Pain with transitional activities
  - Rising from seated position
  - Standing after prolonged periods of sitting
  - Getting out of bed in the morning
  - Ascending stairs
- Referred pain patterns
  - Groin
  - Gluteal region
  - Posterolateral thigh
- Predisposing factors
  - Occupational lifting
  - Leg length discrepancy
  - Gait abnormalities
  - Scoliosis
  - Previous spine surgery, especially fusion to the sacrum
  - Smoking
  - Poor physical condition
  - Positive family history
  - Inflammatory arthritis
  - Older age
  - Pregnancy
- Inciting event
  - Trauma
  - MVC
  - Falls
  - Postpartum
- Athletic activities
  - Weight lifting
  - Running
  - Rowing
  - Cross-country skiing
  - Martial arts
  - Ballet

of symmetry of the iliac crests, anterior superior iliac spine (ASIS), PSIS, ischial tuberosities, gluteal folds, greater trochanters, sacral sulci, inferior lateral angles, and pubic tubercles (Figure 10.2). Measurement of leg length is essential when examining patients with suspected SI joint dysfunction. Leg length discrepancy (LLD) can be measured by the examiner utilizing a tape measure using either of two techniques, with the first being associated with greater reliability: (1) *apparent leg length* is the measurement from the umbilicus to the medial malleolus on each side, and discrepancies may result from scoliosis, hip abnormalities, or pelvic obliquity; (2) true leg length is the measurement from the ASIS or greater trochanter to the medial malleolus,[62] and discrepancies may result from trauma, rheumatoid arthritis, and cerebral palsy. Both measurements are limited by rotation, leg circumference, body habitus, and difficulty palpating bony landmarks. Clinicians can order radiologic studies to corroborate and obtain a more precise measurement of LLD. LLDs of at least 20 mm (3/4")[63] are considered clinically significant and a potential cause of SI joint pain. LLD should therefore be corrected and reassessed prior to or concurrent with entertaining other treatments.

PALPATION

During this portion of the examination, the clinician attempts to isolate where the patient is experiencing his or her pain. Once the clinician is able to localize the patient's pain, he or she can compare this pattern with known referral maps of common etiologies of LBP (Figures 10.3 and 10.4).[64] Assessment for any masses and underlying structural or soft-tissue abnormalities should constitute part of the screening examination but may prove difficult in patients with a large body habitus. If the patient points to his sacral sulcus (positive Fortin finger sign) and demonstrates sacral tenderness on examination, the diagnosis of SI joint dysfunction is considered probable, and the clinician should perform special provocative tests, and/or consider diagnostic injections.[16,49,50,65]

Table 10.2 EVIDENCE-BASED FINDINGS SUGGESTIVE OF SACROILIAC (SI) JOINT PAIN

STUDY	PATIENTS	FINDING
Fortin[49,50]	10 volunteers and 16 patients with SI joint pain	Point of maximum discomfort within 10 cm caudal & 3 cm lateral to PSIS
Murakami et al.[128]	38 patients responders to periarticular injections	Point of maximum discomfort within 3 cm from PSIS
Schwarzer et al.[7]	43 patients with axial LBP	Radiation to groin
Dreyfuss et al.[89]	85 patients with axial LBP	None
Slipman et al.[90]	50 patients with axial LBP	94% had buttock, 72% lumbar, 28% lower leg, and 14% groin pain
Van der Wurff et al.[68]	60 patients with axial LBP	None
Jung et al.[64]	160 patients with SI joint arthropathies	Buttock pain alone, extending into posterolateral thigh, or into groin
Laslett et al.[91]	48 patients with axial LBP	Noncentralization or peripheralization of pain
DePalma et al.[164]	127 responders to IA SI joint blocks	Lateral midline pain
Young et al.[55]	102 patients with non-radicular LBP	Pain rising from sitting, non-midline pain below L5
Liliang et al.[163]	130 patients evaluated for SI joint pain after fusion	Unilateral pain, ≥3 provocative maneuvers, postoperative pain different from preoperative pain
Ostgaard et al.[165]	855 pregnant women	Pain in the pubic symphysis
LaPlante et al.[166]	153 patients with axial LBP	None

IA, Intra-articular; PSIS, Posterior superior iliac spine; LBP, Low back pain

Adapted from Cohen SP et al. Sacroiliac joint pain: a comprehensive review of epidemiology, diagnosis and treatment. *Expert Rev Neurother.* 2013 Jan;13(1):99–116.

RANGE OF MOTION

Range of motion (ROM) testing for the SI joint encompasses the clinician examining (1) the back ROM (flexion, extension, lateral, and rotational), (2) hip ROM (flexion, extension, internal and external rotation), and (3) knee ROM. Any areas of pain should be recognized and treated. These baseline measurements can help the clinician reassess in subsequent examinations any progress obtained from the prescribed interventions.

MUSCLE TESTING

A detailed muscular examination is not required when the clinician suspects SI dysfunction. However, establishing symmetric myotomal distribution of strength should be a priority when ruling out other spinal etiologies for LBP. Additionally, the clinician should assess the flexibility of the iliopsoas, quadriceps, and hamstring muscles because these may contribute to pelvic and SI joint misalignment.

NEUROVASCULAR TESTING

Particular emphasis should be placed on ruling out radicular symptoms because the two diagnoses share significant overlap. A detailed neurological assessment that includes sensory testing, motor testing, and assessment of deep tendon reflexes will assist the clinician in establishing SI joint dysfunction as the likely etiology of LBP.

SPECIAL TESTS

Special tests include provocative and mobility/alignment maneuvers. Provocative maneuvers include distraction/gapping, compression, Patrick's/FABER test, thigh thrust, Gaenslen's test, resisted abduction, Yeoman's test, and Gillet's or the Stork test. Mobility/alignment maneuvers include standing flexion or Vorlauf's test. Multiple studies have assessed the predictive power of provocative maneuvers. Individual provocative maneuvers alone generally lack sufficient sensitivity and/or specificity; however, multiple studies have demonstrated that, in combination, three or more positive provocative maneuvers yield sensitivities ranging from 77% to 94% and specificities ranging from 57% to 100% (Table 10.3).[66–68] Study design bias has called into question the validity of some of these studies; nevertheless, a sensitivity and specificity of approximately 80% is generally accepted for a combination of three or more provocative maneuvers. Due to decreased reliability among examiners and lack of studies demonstrating a correlation between positive tests and response to injections, mobility and alignment maneuvers are not widely utilized.[15]

SI joint special tests are described in Figures 10.5 through 10.13, with the first five representing the best evidence-based provocative maneuvers.[51,54,68]

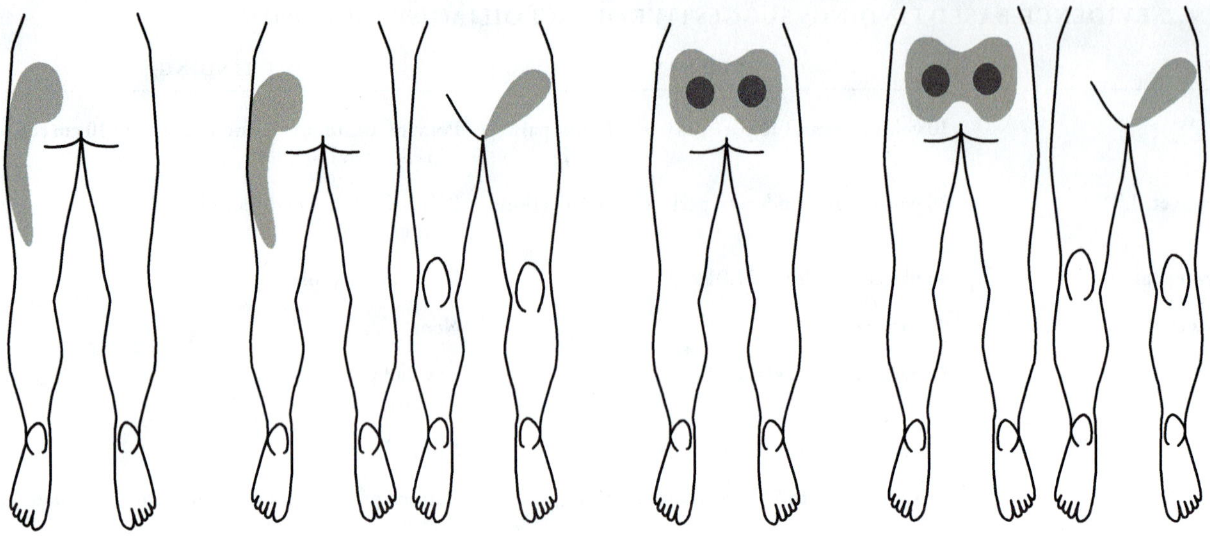

Figure 10.4 Pain referral patters for sacroiliac joint dysfunction.

Table 10.3 **PREDICTIVE VALUE OF PROVOCATIVE MANEUVERS REPRODUCING SACROILIAC JOINT SYMPTOMS**

STUDY	SENSITIVITY	SPECIFICITY	POSITIVE PROVOCATIVE MANEUVERS
Van Der Wurff et al.[68]	85%	79%	3 of 5
Stanford et al.[167]	82%	57%	3 of 6
Laslett et al.[91]	94%	78%	3 of 6
Young et al.[55]	Phi coefficient 0.6, effect size 0.36	Not reported	3 of 5
Broadhurst and Bond[51]	Range of 77–87% for each test	100% for each test	3
Slipman et al.[65]	Not reported	Positive predictive value 60%	3 of 6

Adapted from Cohen SP et al. Sacroiliac joint pain: a comprehensive review of epidemiology, diagnosis and treatment. *Expert Rev Neurother.* 2013 Jan;13(1):99–116.

DIAGNOSTIC INJECTIONS

Diagnostic injections of the SI joint are generally considered the reference standard for identifying the SI joint as a source of a patient's pain.[8,17,52,56,72,73] The SI joints are richly innervated and have been shown to be capable of being a source of LBP and referred pain in the lower extremity.[15,16,44,74–88] Blockade of nociceptive impulses via intra-, extra-articular, or combination injections, typically employ local anesthetic, with or without corticosteroids, to identify a painful SI joint. Pain relief that lasts at least as long as the duration of action of the anesthetic is considered a positive response.[7,89,90]

Diagnostic injection techniques including single injections, placebo-controlled injections, and comparative injections are generally done under fluoroscopic guidance. Comparative injections are also known as "double blocks" and employ two different local anesthetics with different durations of action administered in random order. A positive response occurs when a person experiences significant pain relief with both blocks but longer pain relief with the longer

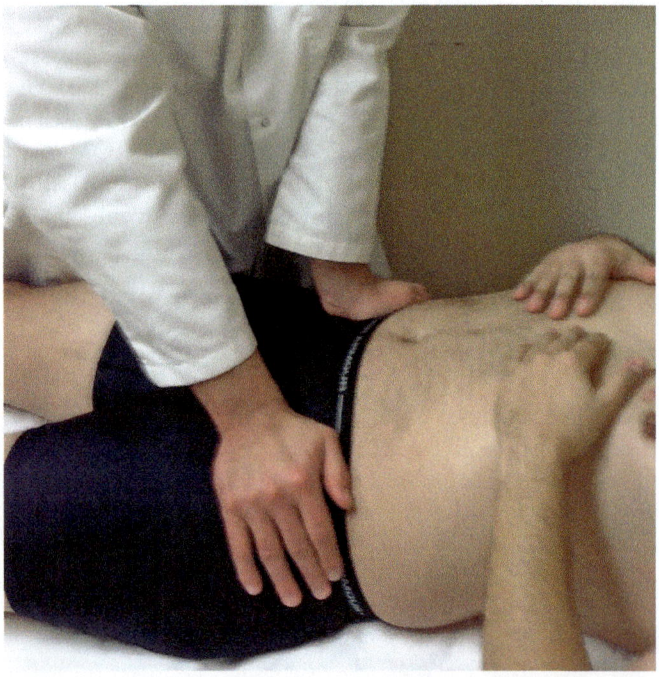

Figure 10.5 **Distraction or Gapping Test:** The patient lies in the supine position and the clinician places one hand over the left ASIS and their other hand over the right ASIS. The clinician then applies pressure attempting to separate the ASISs. A positive test is indicated by pain in the sacroiliac joint region.

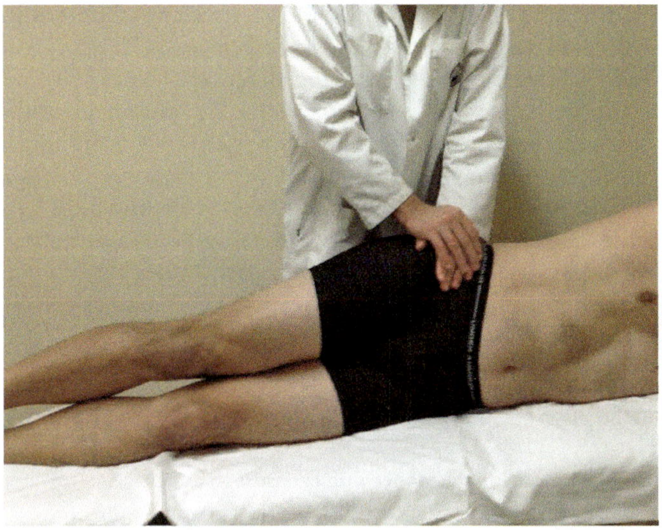

Figure 10.6 **Compression Test:** The patient lies on his side and the clinician places both hands over the lateral aspect of the pelvis and applies downward pressure. A positive test is indicated by pain in the sacroiliac joint region.

acting local anesthetic, consistent with the drugs' pharmacodynamics. This approach has been advocated to reduce the false-positive rate associated with use of single blocks but has not been validated (Table 10.4).[9,73,91–93]

Many authors have, however, identified multiple confounding factors that may complicate the interpretation of these procedures.[15] The surrounding anatomy, placebo response of the patient, the validity of the chosen imaging modality, and the technical expertise of the clinician can all influence the reported sensitivity and specificity of these blocks. One study compared both provocative SI maneuvers and SI joint blocks

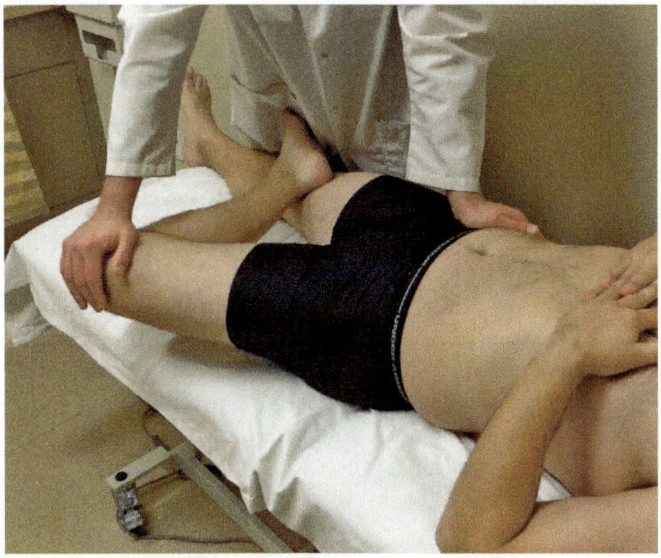

Figure 10.7 **Patrick's or FABER (Flexion Abduction External Rotation) Test:** The patient lies in the supine position. The clinician has the patient flex one hip, followed by abduction and external rotation. This is accomplished by placing the patient's heel over the contralateral knee, then applying downward pressure with one hand over the knee and the other hand over the ASIS. A positive test is indicated by pain in the sacroiliac joint region.[51]

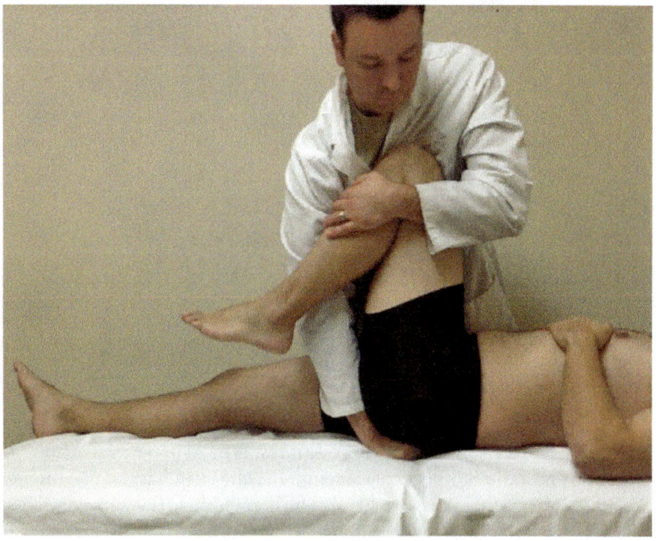

Figure 10.8 **Thigh Thrust Test:** The patient lies supine and flexes the hip to 90 degrees, as well as the knee. The clinician rotates the patient to face him, places his hand over the contralateral sacroiliac joint, then rotates the patient back to the supine position. Next, the clinician places the bent knee in the center of his chest and applies downward continuous force through the femur. The clinician should try to maintain a neutral position and avoid excessive adduction or abduction. A positive test is indicated by pain in the sacroiliac joint region.

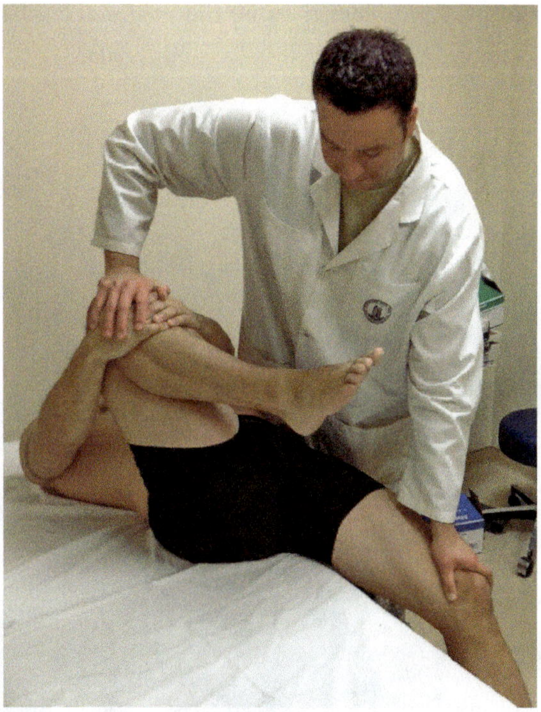

Figure 10.9 **Gaenslen's Test:** The patient lies in the supine position and slides to the edge of the examination table so that one leg is freely hanging off the edge. The patient then brings his contralateral knee into his chest and holds it. The clinician then applies downward pressure to both knees. A positive test is indicated by pain in the sacroiliac joint region.[51]

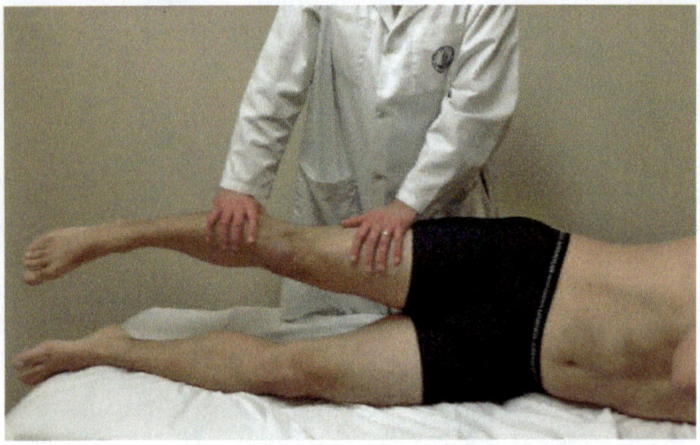

Figure 10.10 **Resisted Abduction:** This test is ideal in patients who are status post hip or knee replacement. The clinician has the patient lie on his unaffected side with his legs fully extended. The patient then abducts the leg 30 degrees. The clinician applies downward force to the patient's leg while the patient applies opposing lateral resistance. This effectively stresses the cephalic portion of the sacroiliac joint. A positive test is indicated by pain in the sacroiliac joint region.[51]

and concluded that neither were reliable for diagnosing of SI joint pain.[94] Despite these shortcomings, the reference standard for diagnosis remains low-volume anesthetic blocks.

DIAGNOSTIC IMAGING

Numerous published studies have analyzed the ability of varying imaging modalities to diagnose SI joint dysfunction. CT, considered to be the gold standard imaging modality for identifying bony pathology, is a fast and readily accessible option for most clinicians. One study estimated the sensitivity and specificity of CT at 57.5% and 69%, respectively, utilizing diagnostic blocks as the reference standard.[95] Investigations of radionucleotide bone scanning have revealed low sensitivities ranging between 13% and 46.1%, with relatively high specificities (89.5–100%), thus rendering them poor screening tools.[96,97] MRI has a reported sensitivity exceeding 90% in detecting early spondyloarthropathic SI joint pathologies but has not been shown helpful in identifying noninflammatory conditions (Boxes 10.5 and 10.6).[98]

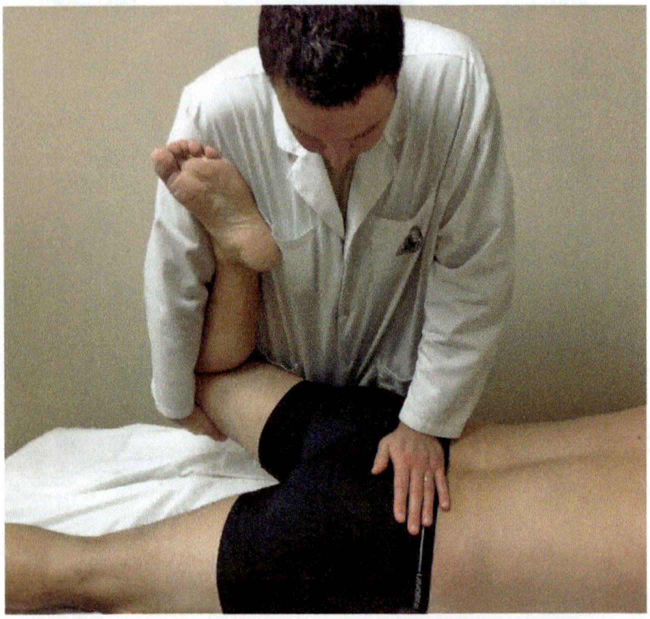

Figure 10.11 **Yeoman's Test:** The clinician places the patient in the prone position. The clinician then raises the ipsilateral knee to a maximally flexed position and extends the thigh while holding the pelvis in place with the opposite hand over the SI joint. The clinician then applies continuous downward force through the sacroiliac joint. A positive test is indicated by pain in the sacroiliac joint region.

Reviewing the findings suggesting SI joint dysfunction in our patient:

- Occupation as paratrooper with exposure to repetitive high axial forces
- Inciting event of a particularly hard parachute landing
- Unilateral right-sided LBP below belt line of 3 months' duration
- Pain exacerbated by shifting weight and rising from a seated position
- Pain referral pattern to posterolateral thigh
- PE findings suggestive of SI joint dysfunction:
  - Positive Fortin finger test
  - Sacral sulcus tenderness
  - Three positive provocative maneuvers:
    - Patrick-FABER
    - Sacral compression
    - Distraction testing

Lack of SI joint findings on his MRI should not discourage the diagnosis of SI joint dysfunction because MRI is best for identifying acute and inflammatory etiologies that this patient may not exhibit.

HOW IS SI JOINT PAIN MANAGED?

Similar to most disorders, the management of SI joint pain is best approached along a spectrum ranging from initial conservative treatment to more invasive procedures. Eliminating neurological sources such as radiculopathy and referring patients with rheumatoid arthritis and spondyloarthropathies to rheumatology for the consideration of disease-modulating agents are essential first steps. The multiple means by which to address SI joint dysfunction include initiating conservative therapies and rehabilitation, addressing psychosocial factors, employing complementary and alternative techniques, and beginning interventional procedures.

PHARMACOLOGICAL MANAGEMENT

Pharmacotherapeutic approaches to SI joint dysfunction are similar to treatment for other musculoskeletal disorders. Oral analgesics such as acetaminophen can be effective for pain alone. Oral #nonsteroidal anti-inflammatory drugs (NSAIDs) may be employed to decrease acute inflammation

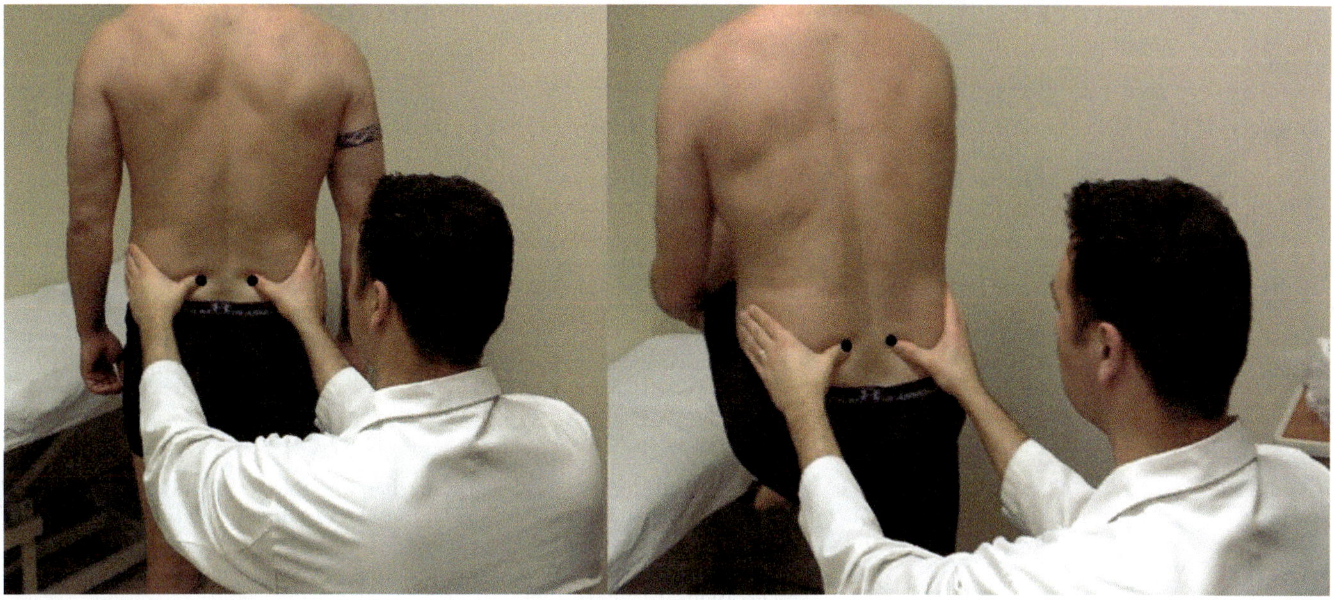

Figure 10.12 **Gillet or Stork Test:** The patient places his feet 12 inches apart and stands facing away from the examiner. The examiner then locates and positions his index finger over the posterior superior edge of the hemipelvis. Next the examiner locates and places his thumbs over the PSISs. The examiner asks the patient to raise one knee toward the chest. Normally, the ipsilateral PSIS should rotate inferiorly. The examiner observes the relationship in orientation of each thumb. The test is positive if either thumb overlying the PSIS fails to move or is displaced significantly more compared to the contralateral side. Although this was long thought to indicate pelvic misalignment, recent evidence suggests asymmetry is indicative of sacroiliac joint pain and not mobility.[69–71]

while also addressing pain. NSAIDs and acetaminophen are sometimes combined to reduce side effects and enhance analgesia. Topical NSAIDs and lidocaine may provide some relief, although there is a lack of controlled trials demonstrating benefit. Muscle relaxants, benzodiazepines, and occasionally short-acting opioids have been used in the acute phase. However, concerns regarding dependence, tolerance, multiple additional side effects, and a lack of documented long-term efficacy limit their utility.

Chronic SI joint pain is challenging to address pharmacotherapeutically, with minimal evidence available to guide management. Antidepressants (serotonin norepinephrine reuptake inhibitors [SNRIs], tricyclic antidepressants [TCAs]), antiseizure agents, and antiarrhythmic agents have been advocated but are generally considered to be more effective for neuropathic pain than nociceptive pain.

More abundant evidence exists for pharmacotherapeutic management of spondyloarthropathies. The applicability of

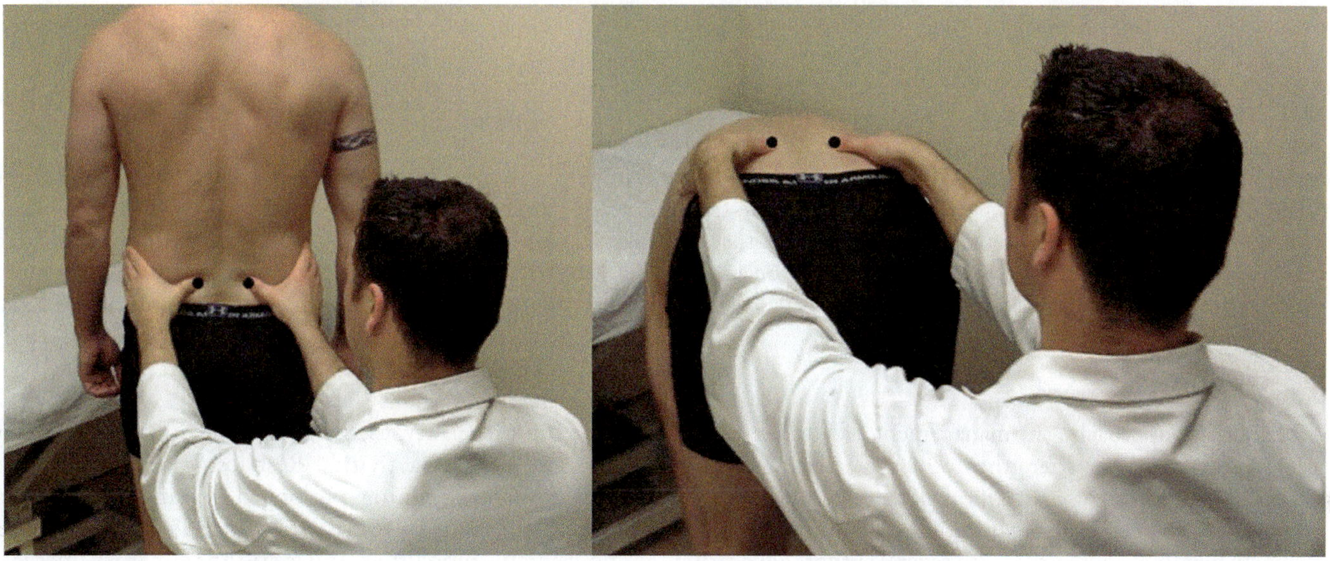

Figure 10.13 **Standing Flexion Test or Vorlauf Test:** Palpation of the pelvis includes assessing the alignment of the right hemipelvis in comparison to the left hemipelvis by performing the standing forward flexion test with the patient. The examiner's thumbs are placed at the PSIS, and the patient is asked to flex fully forward at the waist. The thumbs should remain level in standing and flexed positions. If one thumb moves further cephalad than the other, this indicates possible underlying articular restriction between the ilium and sacrum on the affected side.

Table 10.4 **PREVALENCE RATES OF SACROILIAC JOINT PAIN ASSESSED BY DIAGNOSTIC INJECTIONS**

STUDY	SUBJECTS	TECHNIQUE	DIAGNOSTIC CRITERIA	RESULTS
Maigne et al.[8]	54 patients with chronic unilateral LBP with or without radiation to posterior thigh	Intra-articular blocks using 2 mL of lidocaine and bupivacaine on separate occasions. Authors avoided anesthetizing periarticular ligaments.	>75% pain relief, with the bupivacaine block lasting >2 hours	Prevalence rate 18.5%; false-positive rate 17%
Manchikanti et al.[73]	20 patients with chronic LBP without neurological deficits	Intra-articular blocks with unspecified volume of lidocaine and bupivacaine on separate occasions.	Not noted	Prevalence rate 10%; false-positive rate 20%
Irwin et al.[9]	158 patients with chronic LBP with or without lower extremity pain.	Intra-articular blocks with 2 mL of lidocaine and 2 mL bupivacaine and steroid on separate occasions.	>70% pain relief, with the bupivacaine block lasting >4 hours	Prevalence rate 27%; false-positive rate 43%
Laslett et al.[91]	48 patients with buttock pain, with or without lumbar or lower extremity symptoms, without signs of nerve root compression	Intra-articular blocks with <1.5 mL of lidocaine + steroid and bupivacaine on separate occasions.	>80% pain relief with lidocaine and bupivacaine	Prevalence rate 26%; false-positive rate 0%
van der Wurff et al.[68]	60 patients with chronic LBP below L5 with or without lower extremity symptoms, without neurological symptoms.	Intra-articular blocks with 2 mL lidocaine and bupivacaine on separate occasions.	>50% pain relief with lidocaine and bupivacaine, with the bupivacaine block lasting >4 hours	Prevalence rate 45% False-positive rate 12%
Liliang et al.[163]	52 patients with previous spine fusion and pain below L5	Intra-articular blocks with 2 mL of lidocaine or bupivacaine + steroid on separate occasions.	>75% pain relief lasting 1–4 hours; those who had 1 positive and 1 negative block underwent 3rd injection	Prevalence rate 40%. 27% false-positive rate

LBP, Low back pain; L, Lumbar

Adapted from Cohen SP et al. Sacroiliac joint pain: a comprehensive review of epidemiology, diagnosis and treatment. *Expert Rev Neurother.* 2013 Jan;13(1):99–116.

this data to SI joint dysfunction remains limited due to systemic factors associated with spondyloarthropathies and outcome measures that do not address SI joint pain specifically. Overall, these therapies are not often employed in the management of SI joint dysfunction without a spondyloarthropathy component and are best addressed via consultation and/or referral to rheumatology.[15]

CONSERVATIVE MANAGEMENT

Conservative approaches to management of SI dysfunction tend to focus on core strengthening and flexibility training in order to address biomechanical deficits and enhance SI joint stability. Temporal organization of treatment options can help maximize outcomes, with several authors advocating a three-phase approach: acute phase (1–3 days post inciting event), recovery phase (3 days to 8 weeks), and maintenance phase (>8 weeks).[56,57,75]

ACUTE-PHASE TREATMENT

Acute-phase treatments are best applied when a specific inciting event is identifiable within a 1- to 3-day window. As previously mentioned, SI joint pain is often associated with trauma or a specific activity that produces symptoms. These inciting events commonly involve compressive axial loading and rotational forces, such as those experienced by the patient in this case scenario. These forces can be especially deleterious when they are repetitive, asymmetrical, and of high intensity, as is typically encountered in many sports and exercise activities. Restricting single-leg stance activities such as running, prolonged walking, skating, and step aerobics helps to rest the SI joint in the acute phase. Cold therapy modalities and anti-inflammatory medications help mitigate acute inflammation, edema, pain, and muscle spasms.[99] Addressing muscle strength and stiffness asymmetries with muscle energy techniques should begin

Box 10.5 IMAGING AND DIAGNOSIS

MRI
- Study of choice; STIR and contrast-enhanced superior; 85% sensitive for active sacroiliitis

CT Scan
- Good for already established bone changes; does not detect inflammation
- 58% sensitive and 69% specific in identifying symptomatic joint

Bone Scans
- Low sensitivity, high specificity (>90%)

X-rays
- Very low sensitivity, high specificity

Ultrasound
- May be used to detect posterior ligamentous pathology; may be used in pregnancy

CT, computed tomography; STIR, short TI inversion recovery magnetic resonance image

Adapted from Cohen SP et al. Sacroiliac joint pain: a comprehensive review of epidemiology, diagnosis and treatment. *Expert Rev Neurother.* 2013 Jan;13(1):99–116.

as early as possible within pain-free limits. Care should be taken with these mobilization techniques in the pregnant patient due to the hypermobility associated with hormonal-induced ligament laxity. The patient is ready to advance to the recovery phase once adequate pain control is achieved.

RECOVERY-PHASE TREATMENT

The focus of treatment in the recovery phase is rehabilitation and correction of biomechanical deficits. Predisposing factors such as leg length discrepancy and gait abnormalities should be corrected. Muscle imbalances that impact the pelvic ring and SI joint mobility must first be addressed via length and flexibility training. These muscles include the erector spinae, iliopsoas, rectus femoris, hip abductors including the tensor fascia late, hip adductors, quadratus lumborum, and deep hip external rotators including the obturator internus and piriformis muscles.[100] Once length and flexibility are restored, muscle strength training is added to the regimen. Closed kinetic chain exercises are preferred early with a progression to multiplanar exercises as tolerated. Evidence is mixed regarding the use of orthoses such as SI joint belts, with some cadaveric studies reporting benefit by reducing SI joint rotation but no clear benefit demonstrated in peripartum females.[101,102] Benefit may also be associated with proprioceptive feedback encouraging proper biomechanics. The belt should be secured across the sacral base posteriorly and inferior to the ASIS anteriorly. It should be worn during walking and standing activities at a minimum, with some additional reported benefit when used during sedentary activities.[57] Functional and anatomical length discrepancies may be addressed with heel lifts; however, caution should be exercised when correcting functional LLDs past the recovery phase because these deficits should be addressed in the long-term by muscle rebalancing. The patient is ready to advance to maintenance phase treatment once pain, inflammation, and functional joint and myofascial dysfunction have been mitigated and a return to 75% of preinjury strength and flexibility is demonstrated. At this stage, normal activities of daily living, including walking, should not exacerbate symptoms.

Box 10.6 KEY DIAGNOSTIC FINDINGS IN SI DYSFUNCTION

Positive Fortin finger test

Three or more positive provocative maneuvers on physical examination

Positive diagnostic injection

+/− findings on imaging

MAINTENANCE-PHASE TREATMENT

The focus of the maintenance phase is the retraining of multiple muscle groups to act in a coordinated fashion to promote and maintain proper biomechanics and prevent reinjury. This is accomplished by lumbopelvic stabilization, proprioceptive reeducation, plyometrics, and exercise- and sports-specific training. Lumbopelvic stabilization is essential for pelvic and SI joint load transfer and may be enhanced through core strengthening and coordination. Inner core muscles include the transverse abdominis, deep fibers of the multifidus, diaphragm, and levator ani. The outer core muscles include the oblique abdominals, latissimus dorsi, erector spinae, biceps femoris, hip adductors and adductors, and the gluteus maximus, medius, and minimus. In a functional pelvis, the inner core muscles activate prior to the initiation of movement in order to stabilize the pelvic ring for load transfer. The outer core muscles activate secondarily to further enhance stabilization. The development of motor planning strategies through core strengthening and coordination training should emphasize inner to outer core activation, which limits shearing forces that produce and exacerbate SI joint dysfunction.[103,104] Appropriate ergonomic strategies for the home, leisure, and work environments are essential to maintain proper pelvic and SI joint biomechanics. Return to play and full activity should be done under close monitoring once the patient is pain-free without medication. The muscle balance, flexibility, and strength strategies established via the three phases of conservative management should be maintained to prevent reinjury. Most patients with SI joint dysfunction will benefit from conservative management, with one study reporting functional improvement in 95% of patients following physical therapy at 2-year follow-up.[105]

MANUAL MEDICINE

There is a growing body of evidence that manipulation techniques including manual therapy, osteopathic manual treatment, and chiropractic adjustments reduce SI joint pain and improve function. Specific techniques and methodology vary but generally fall within two categories: non-impulse-based and impulse-based therapies. Non-impulse-based therapies involve low-velocity, low-amplitude practices such as trigger point therapies and muscle energy techniques.[56] Impulse-based therapies involve high-velocity and either high- or low-amplitude SI joint and lumbar thrusts.[106] The vast majority of evidence supporting joint manipulation focuses on the impulse-based therapies. Neurophysiological studies have suggested that the positive effect of impulse-based joint manipulation is a consequence of stressing forces applied to periarticular structures, which activate high-threshold muscle and joint mechanoreceptors. This in turn results in postmanipulation muscle relaxation and reflex inhibition of pain receptors at the segmental level.[107] Improved muscle tone has been demonstrated in the hamstrings, quadriceps, and abdominal musculature following manipulation.[108–110] Additional studies have linked benefit to the correction of bony asymmetries.[111,112] Disparities exist concerning the evidence for bony asymmetry correction, with one study employing roentgen stereophotogrammetric analysis and concluding that manipulation did not alter the position of the SI joint.[113] Treatment frequency and duration have varied from study to study, with impulse-based therapies typically applied three times per week for 2–5 weeks. Improved pain and function have been reported in the majority of patients and persist anywhere from 2 weeks to 2 year postintervention.[16,114–116] Despite the conflicting and anecdotal evidence, the favorable risk-benefit profile with noninvasive manipulation performed by trained professionals makes this treatment a viable alternative in the management of SI joint dysfunction.

PROLOTHERAPY

Prolotherapy (aka. proliferative therapy) involves the injection of otherwise nonpharmacological and nonactive irritant solutions such as dextrose and platelet rich plasma into the body, usually around tendons or ligaments, in an attempt to strengthen connective tissue and relieve musculoskeletal pain. It is hypothesized to work by initiating an inflammatory process that results in proliferative phase healing via enhanced blood flow and accelerated tissue repair. Multiple procedures are advocated at 4- to 6-week intervals to allow completion of the proliferative phase healing cycle prior to repeat treatment to further strengthen connective tissue in the affected area. NSAIDs are avoided during prolotherapy treatment in order to allow the inflammatory process necessary for proliferative healing.

Unfortunately, prolotherapy suffers from a paucity of evidence-based studies. One randomized study evaluating prolotherapy for injection-confirmed SI joint pain reported promising results when comparing intra-articular dextrose to steroid injections. Although positive short-term outcomes were observed with both groups at 2 weeks, 58.7% of patients who received prolotherapy continued to experience a positive outcome at 15 months post-treatment versus 10.2% in the intra-articular steroid group.[117] An observational study reported similarly promising results with success rates of 76%, 76%, and 32%, at 3-, 12-, and 24-month follow-up visits, respectively.[118] The current lack of placebo-controlled studies evaluating prolotherapy in the treatment of SI joint pain warrants caution when interpreting these findings; however, the potential benefit and relatively low risk of the procedure make it a viable option in the treatment of SI joint pain.

PSYCHOSOCIAL MANAGEMENT

Pain in general is a complex subjective experience that is predisposed not only by physiological parameters but by affective, cognitive, and behavioral components. Rating scales are often used to measure the severity of pain, but they, too, are influenced by contextual circumstances, diseased state distress, anxiety, past memories, cultural background, medications, and even environmental stimuli. Psychiatric disorders such as somatoform spectrum, mood, and anxiety disorders affect pain responses. Personality disorders and traits also frequently contribute to the maintenance and presentation of pain responses. Although not discussed as much in recent literature, psychological defenses are also relevant to recognize in the presentation of symptoms. Inherent in this population of pain patients are those who are drug seekers.

Multiple studies have demonstrated increased rates of psychiatric disorders in patients with LBP and work-related musculoskeletal disability.[119] One study found the rate to be 64% compared to 15% in the general population.[120] Depression is most common, whereas other psychiatric comorbidities include substance abuse and anxiety disorders.[121] Interestingly, many of these individuals experience psychiatric symptoms prior to the onset of LBP, and 60% of patients with depression report pain symptoms at the time of diagnoses.[122] One study employing the Beck Depression Inventory (BDI) identified a unique pattern of symptomatology in chronic LBP.[123] Severity of depression was found to increase the degree of somatic difficulties such as sleep disturbance, work disturbance, work inhibition, and anergia. The authors advocated the BDI as a means to discern psychosocial and physiologic components of pain and further guide therapy.

Untreated psychiatric diagnoses and self-reported pain and disability have also been linked to a negative effect on LBP treatment outcomes.[14,124] Social factors such as job satisfaction, return-to-work issues, secondary gain, catastrophizing, poor role models, co-dependent behavior, inadequate coping mechanisms, and attitudes, beliefs, and expectations are associated with a negative prognosis for LBP.[125]

To extract the psychiatric and psychological components contributing to a patient's response of pain, a thorough biopsychosocial evaluation is recommended. This evaluation addresses the issues just mentioned and facilitates the use of psychotropic medication as necessary, in addition to assisting the primary team in developing strategies to help the patient cope more effectively with his or her discomfort. When a patient presents with chronic pain regardless of the etiology, her functioning is disrupted and she is suffering. Even those who have a need to embellish their symptoms or are drug seeking may have an element of distress and/or may be suffering.

Treatment of these patients from a psychiatric-psychological basis is an important aspect of their care and helps to limit prolonged pain disability. Types of treatment include psychopharmacology, cognitive behavioral therapy, hypnosis, relaxation training, family therapy, and traditional psychotherapy. All can be excellent adjuncts to the primary treatment team.

INTERVENTIONAL TREATMENT

Extra- and Intra-articular Steroid Injections

Nociceptive innervation in the SI joint capsule, surrounding ligaments, and subchondral bone has been demonstrated histologically.[21,22] Intra-articular injections employ injecting anesthetic and steroid into the true diarthrodial inferior portion of the joint, whereas extra-articular injections are generally made into the surrounding SI joint ligaments. Comparative studies suggest greater efficacy for extra-articular[126–128] or combination extra- and intra-articular steroid injections[129] than for intra-articular injections alone. Although the evidence supporting intra-articular injections is weaker than that for extra-articular injections, it still augurs in favor of an effect.[130–134]

Radiofrequency Denervation

Radiofrequency (RF) lesioning of the branches of the primary dorsal rami innervating the facet and SI joints has been used since the 1970s to treat spinal pain.[135] For SI joint pain, RF denervation has been employed for more than 10 years with uniformly positive results. Studies indicate that the best candidates for SI joint denervation are those who experienced effective short-term relief with SI joint blocks and those with pain arising from the posterior joint because these nerves are the most amenable to lesioning. One study assessing RF denervation found that multisite lateral branch blocks inhibited perceived pain from ligamentous probing in 70% of cases; however, 86% of these individuals retained the ability to perceive capsular distension.[136] These findings suggest that lateral branch RF denervation may be more effective in alleviating extra-articular SI joint pain than intra-articular joint pain. By extension, this also suggests that lateral branch and/or extra-articular blocks may better predict positive response to RF denervation than intra-articular blocks, although this contention has not been critically evaluated.

Appropriate patient selection is essential to RF denervation treatment success. Factors affecting poor response to interventional treatment failure can be divided into three main categories: poor patient selection, inaccurate diagnosis, and technical treatment failures (Box 10.7). Few studies have specifically examined the factors impacting SI joint RF denervation success. Some studies have found an association between greater disease burden (higher preprocedure pain scores, regular opioid use) and older age with RF treatment failure.[137,138] A plausible explanation for why younger patients may experience higher success rates is that they are more likely to have extra-articular SI joint pathology (i.e., ligaments), with pain-generating structures innervated by the lateral branches lesioned with RF treatment.

Box 10.7 **FACTORS AFFECTING POOR RESPONSE TO RF DENERVATION**

PATIENT SELECTION	INACCURATE DIAGNOSIS	TECHNICAL FAILURE
Extensive disease burden Secondary gain Social factors High-dose opioid therapy Older age Coexisting psychiatric illness	False-positive block Ventral or intra-articular SI joint pain Coexisting pain generators	Poor lesion placement Procedural complication

Adapted from Cohen SP et al. Sacroiliac joint pain: a comprehensive review of epidemiology, diagnosis and treatment. *Expert Rev Neurother.* 2013 Jan;13(1):99–116.

Adapted from Cohen SP et al. SI joint pain: a comprehensive review of epidemiology, diagnosis and treatment. Expert Rev Neurother. 2013 Jan;13(1):99–116.

Conventional RF

In conventional RF, heat generated from a high-frequency alternating current is employed for denervation. Single RF probes are fluoroscopically guided to the anticipated lateral branch locations, usually just lateral to the S1, S2, and S3 foraminal rims, and RF ablation is conducted. Multiple uncontrolled studies have reported excellent success rates using conventional RF lesioning.[139–141] However, no controlled studies have been published evaluating conventional RF denervation. The main limitation to conventional RF is that the lesions are smaller (approximately 3–4 mm in diameter), resulting in a higher likelihood of missing the nociceptive input of the lateral branches, which cannot be visualized with imaging techniques and demonstrate high anatomical variability. As a result, it is necessary to create multiple lesions around each foramen in order to adequately interrupt nociceptive input. Local anesthetic is commonly employed and has been shown to enhance lesion diameter by approximately 50%, likely due to fluid modulation amplification. Local anesthetic also has the added benefit of reducing procedure-related pain.[142]

Bipolar RF

Bipolar RF employs a second electrode in close proximity to the first. This allows current to flow between the two electrodes to create a continuous strip lesion. Studies indicate that optimal lesions occur when the electrodes are placed 6–24 mm apart.[143–146] Bipolar RF denervation is appealing in its ability to maximize lesion size and theoretically interrupt all nociceptive input without the requirement for multiple discrete lesions, as is necessary with conventional RF.

Cooled RF Ablation

Cooled RF is a newer technique compared to conventional RF and was adapted from techniques used to treat tumors and cardiac arrhythmias.[147–150] The primary distinguishing feature of cooled RF is the employment of internally cooled, large-bore electrodes to create lesions. The irrigation-cooled electrodes allow the targeted tissues to slowly heat to neuroablative temperatures while minimizing temperature increases and collateral damage to adjacent tissue. This technique therefore promotes greater lesion expansion with substantially increased lesion diameter, depth, and area, resulting in an increased likelihood of successful neurotomy and pain resolution. Disadvantages of cooled RF include greater expense, longer lesioning time, and larger electrode size (and thus increased risk of bleeding, nerve damage, and procedure-related pain). The larger lesion sizes are also more likely to affect proximal, superficial branches, leading to a higher incidence of cutaneous paresthesias.

Multiple studies including two placebo-controlled trials have reported benefit from cooled ablation, with positive outcomes reported in 47–64% of individuals and with benefit lasting up to 9 months.[151–153] Two studies comparing cooled and conventional RF ablation reported conflicting results, with one study indicating better outcomes with cooled RF and the other indicating no significant advantage for cooled over conventional RF.[137,154] Inherent flaws in these studies include nonrandomization, nonstandardization of patients and techniques, and unblinded personnel.

Complications of RF Ablation

Serious complications from SI joint RF denervation are unusual. Postprocedure numbness and tingling occur in up to 20% of individuals and are believed to be related to damage of cutaneous sensory branches. Generally, this is not considered troublesome by most patients. One study supported a reduced incidence of neuritis with prophylactic administration of steroids during lumbar facet joint denervation, although this has not been formally studied for SI joint pain.[142] Bleeding and infection are low-incidence risks associated with any percutaneous procedure. Misplaced electrodes can result in damage to sacral spinal nerves that causes bowel or bladder incontinence, sexual dysfunction, worsening pain, or lower extremity weakness. A summary of RF ablations studies is included in Table 10.5.[155]

OTHER TREATMENTS

Neuromodulation

Spinal cord and peripheral nerve stimulation are widely considered to be more effective for neuropathic than nociceptive pain. Evidence supporting neuromodulation for SI joint pain currently includes only case reports, with one investigator reporting good results with S3 stimulation[156] and another report touting benefit for S1 stimulation.[157]

Surgical Intervention for SI Joint Pain

For many, surgical intervention is considered an option for those patients whose symptoms are unresponsive to more conservative management. Most studies assessing surgical treatment involve fusion of the SI joint. In the postfracture and dislocation population, studies include relatively small cohorts of patients and do not detail clinical/functional outcome measures.[158,159] Studies assessing interventions for nontraumatic SI joint pain include slightly larger patient populations and provide more relevant outcome measures; however, the results are not necessarily encouraging, with 50–82% indicating no benefit and/or dissatisfaction and high reoperation rates.[160–162] Caveats to these studies include disparate inclusion criteria and the technical challenges associated with achieving complete fusion in SI joints. Surgical study designs are inherently challenged by confounding factors such as an inability to blind patients and a variability in operative technique. Whereas surgery is clearly indicated for fractures or dislocations involving the SI joints, its applicability in SI joint degenerative disease appears less clear and is best reserved for recalcitrant cases.

CONCLUSION

SI joint pain is an underappreciated source of LBP that affects between 13% and 32% of individuals with chronic LBP. Predisposing factors for SI joint pain include true and apparent LLD, gait abnormalities, scoliosis, previous spine surgery, smoking, poor physical condition, positive family history, inflammatory arthritis, older age, and pregnancy. Compared with facet-mediated and discogenic LBP, individuals with SI joint pain are more likely to report a specific inciting event and to experience unilateral pain below L5 that is made worse with transitional activities such as rising from a seated position. Owing in part to its size and heterogeneity, the pain referral patterns of the SI joint are extremely variable and often include radiation to the buttocks or posterolateral thigh and sometimes even to the lower leg. Although no single physical sign or historical symptom can reliably identify a painful SI joint, studies suggest that a battery of three or more provocation tests are good indicators of SI joint pathology and can predict response to diagnostic blocks to further confirm the diagnosis. Treatment of SI joint pain is best addressed in an interdisciplinary manner and along a spectrum from conservative management to more invasive procedures (Box 10.8). A host of tools exist along this spectrum including conservative therapies and rehabilitation (activity modification, pharmacotherapy, physical therapy), addressing psychosocial factors (mood disorders, work- and family-related stressors), employing complementary and alternative techniques (manipulation, prolotherapy), and minimally invasive interventional procedures (extra- and intra-articular corticosteroid injections, RF nerve ablation). Last, surgical fusion of the SI joint is an option that may be considered for debilitating symptoms unresponsive to less invasive treatment.

Table 10.5 STUDIES ASSESSING RADIOFREQUENCY (RF) DENERVATION

STUDY	DESIGN	# OF PATIENTS	CUTOFF THRESHOLD	NERVES TARGETED	RF TECHNIQUE	FOLLOW-UP	SUCCESS RATE
Ferrante et al.[146]	Retrospective	33	Not noted	Intra-articular	Leapfrog Bipolar	6 months	36%
Gevargez et al.[168]	Prospective, observational	38	Not noted	CT = guided, L5 + SI ligaments	Conventional	3 months	66%
Cohen et al.[169]	Retrospective	9	80% for SI, 50% for LBB	L4–S3/4	Conventional	9 months	89%
Yin et al.[140]	Retrospective	14	70%	L5, S1, +/- S2 and S3	Conventional	6 months	64%
Buijs et al.[141]	Observational	38	50%	L4–S3 or S1–S3	Conventional	4 months	67%
Burnham and Yasui[170]	Prospective, observational	9	50%	L5–S3	Bipolar leapfrog	12 months	89%
Hagiwara et al.[171]	Prospective, observational	22	75%	L4–S2	Pulsed	>10 weeks	55%
Kapural et al.[152]	Retrospective	26	50%	L5–S3	Cooled	3–4 months	69%
Cohen et al.[172]	Randomized, controlled	28	50%	L4–S3	Cooled	1–6 months	57%
Karaman et al.[173]	Prospective, observational	15	75%	L5–S3	Cooled	6 months	80%
Speldewinde[174]	Prospective, observational	20	80%	L5–S3	Conventional	>2 months	80%
Patel et al.[151]	Randomized, controlled	51	75% for lateral branch blocks	L5–S3	Cooled	9 months	59%
Cheng et al.[154]	Retrospective	88	50%	L4–S3	Cooled, Conventional	> 6 months	50–60% at 6 months; 40% at 9 months
Stelzer et al.[155]	Retrospective	105	50%	L5–S3	Cooled	4–12 months	79% at 4–6 months; 7% at >12 months

Box 10.8 THE INTERDISCIPLINARY TREATMENT PARADIGM FOR SI JOINT DYSFUNCTION

- Conservative therapies and rehabilitation
  - Activity modification
  - Pharmacotherapy
  - Physical therapy
- Psychosocial factors
  - Mood disorders
  - Work- and family-related stressors
- Complementary and alternative techniques
  - Manipulation
  - Prolotherapy
- Interventional procedures
  - Extra- and intra-articular corticosteroid injections
  - Radiofrequency nerve ablation
  - Neuromodulation
- Surgical SI joint fusion

After referral to the Interdisciplinary Back Pain Clinic for further evaluation and management, a diagnostic SI joint injection is performed. Our case study patient reports initial reproduction of symptoms followed by relief for the duration of the anesthetic, further suggesting SI joint dysfunction as the source of his pain.

A pain psychologist interviews the patient and identifies occupational and home life stressors. Together, they develop coping strategies to address these stressors.

Physical medicine, physical therapy, and interventional pain management teams meet with the patient and outline a treatment plan:

1. Modify activity to avoid high-impact single leg stance activities. Duty restrictions to limit running and parachuting are emplaced.
2. Physical therapy for core strengthening, muscle rebalancing, and stabilization training is initiated.

3. A trial of combination extra- and intra-articular corticosteroid injection is performed. The patient is given a pain diary to follow symptoms over time.
4. Potential future treatments, including RF ablation or prolotherapy, are discussed. The patient decides he would like to learn more about each in the interim, and educational information sources are provided.
5. Follow-up is scheduled with the Interdisciplinary Back Pain Clinic in 4–6 weeks.

REFERENCES

1. Wheeler AH, Murrey DB. Spinal pain: pathogenesis, evolutionary mechanisms, and management. In: Pappagallo M, ed. *The Neurological Basis of Pain*. New York: McGraw-Hill; 2005:421–452.
2. Argoff CE, Wheeler AH. Backonja MM, eds. Spinal and radicular pain syndromes. *Neurologic Clinics*. 1998:833–845.
3. Simopoulos TT, Manchikanti L, Singh V, et al. A systematic evaluation of prevalence and diagnostic accuracy of sacroiliac joint interventions [review]. *Pain Physician*. 2012;15(3):E305–E344. PubMed PMID: 22622915.
4. O'Shea FD, Boyle E, Salonen DC, et al. Inflammatory and degenerative sacroiliac joint disease in a primary back pain cohort. *Arthritis Care Res* (Hoboken). 2010;62(4):447–454. PubMed PMID: 20391497.
5. Bernard TN Jr, Kirkaldy-Willis WH. Recognizing specific characteristics of nonspecific low back pain. *Clin Orthop Relat Res*. 1987;(217):266–280. PubMed PMID: 2951048.
6. Sembrano JN, Polly DW Jr. How often is low back pain not coming from the back? *Spine* (Phila Pa 1976). 2009;34(1):E27–E32. PubMed PMID: 19127145.
7. Schwarzer AC, Aprill CN, Bogduk N. The sacroiliac joint in chronic low back pain. *Spine* (Phila Pa 1976). 1995;20(1):31–37. PubMed PMID: 7709277.
8. Maigne JY, Aivaliklis A, Pfefer F. Results of sacroiliac joint double block and value of sacroiliac pain provocation tests in 54 patients with low back pain. *Spine* (Phila Pa 1976). 1996;21(16):1889–1892. PubMed PMID: 8875721.
9. Irwin RW, Watson T, Minick RP, Ambrosius WT. Age, body mass index, and gender differences in sacroiliac joint pathology. *Am J Phys Med Rehabil*. 2007; 86:37–44. PubMed PMID: 17304687.
10. Cuccurullo SJ. *Physical Medicine and Rehabilitation Board Review*. 2nd ed. New York: Demos Medical Publishing; 2010.
11. Nachemson AL, Waddell G, Norlund AI. Epidemiology of neck and low back pain. In: Nachemson AL, Jonsson E, eds. *Neck and Back Pain: The Scientific Evidence of Causes, Diagnosis, and Treatment*. Philadelphia: Lippincott Williams & Wilkins; 2000:165–188.
12. Waddell G, Waddell H. A review of social influences on neck and back pain and disability. In: Nachemson AL, Jonsson E, eds. *Neck and Back Pain: The Scientific Evidence of Causes, Diagnosis, And Treatment*. Philadelphia: Lippincott Williams & Wilkins; 2000: 13–55.
13. http://disabilitycanhappen.org/
14. Fayad F, Lefevre-Colau MM, Poiraudeau S, et al. Chronicity, recurrence, and return to work in low back pain: common prognostic factors [review, French]. *Ann Readapt Med Phys*. 2004;47(4):179–189. PubMed PMID: 15130717.
15. Cohen SP. Sacroiliac joint pain: a comprehensive review of anatomy, diagnosis, and treatment [review]. *Anesth Analg*. 2005;101(5):1440–1453. PubMed PMID: 16244008.
16. Bernard TN Jr. The sacroiliac joint syndrome: pathophysiology, diagnosis, and management. In: Frymoyer JW, ed. *The Adult Spine. Principles and Practice*. New York: Raven; 1991:2107–2130.
17. Goode A, Hegedus EJ, Sizer P, Brismee JM, Linberg A, Cook CE. Three-dimensional movements of the sacroiliac joint: a systematic review of the literature and assessment of clinical utility. *J Man Manip Ther*. 2008;16(1):25–38. PubMed PMID: 19119382; PubMed Central PMCID: PMC2565072.
18. Forst SL, Wheeler MT, Fortin JD, Vilensky JA. The sacroiliac joint: anatomy, physiology and clinical significance [review]. *Pain Physician*. 2006;9(1):61–67. PubMed PMID: 16700283.
19. Pitkin HC, Pheasant HC. Sacrarthrogenic telalgia I: a study of referred pain. *J Bone Joint Surg*. 1936;18:111–133.
20. Walker JM. The sacroiliac joint: a critical review. *Phys Ther*. 1992;72(12):903–916. PubMed PMID: 1454866.
21. Szadek KM, Hoogland PV, Zuurmond WW, de Lange JJ, Perez RS. Nociceptive nerve fibers in the sacroiliac joint in humans. *Reg Anesth Pain Med*. 2008;33(1):36–43.
22. Szadek KM, Hoogland PV, Zuurmond WW, De Lange JJ, Perez RS. Possible nociceptive structures in the sacroiliac joint cartilage: an immunohistochemical study. *Clin Anat*. 2010;23(2):192–198. PubMed PMID: 20014392.
23. Schuit D, McPoil TG, Mulesa P. Incidence of sacroiliac joint malalignment in leg length discrepancies. *J Am Podiatr Med Assoc*. 1989;79(8):380–383. PubMed PMID: 2810074.
24. Herzog W, Conway PJ. Gait analysis of sacroiliac joint patients. *J Manipulative Physiol Ther*. 1994;17(2):124–127. PubMed PMID: 8169541.
25. Marymont JV, Lynch MA, Henning CE. Exercise-related stress reaction of the sacroiliac joint. An unusual cause of low back pain in athletes. *Am J Sports Med*. 1986;14(4):320–323. PubMed PMID: 2942046.
26. Schoenberger M, Hellmich K. Sacroiliac dislocation and scoliosis [German]. *Hippokrates*. 1964;35:476–479. PubMed PMID: 14237984.
27. Katz V, Schofferman J, Reynolds J. The sacroiliac joint: a potential cause of pain after lumbar fusion to the sacrum. *J Spinal Disord Tech*. 2003;16(1):96–99. PubMed PMID: 12571491.
28. Ebraheim NA, Elgafy H, Semaan HB. Computed tomographic findings in patients with persistent sacroiliac pain after posterior iliac graft harvesting. *Spine* (Phila Pa 1976). 2000;25(16):2047–2051. PubMed PMID: 10954635.
29. Frymoyer JW, Hanley E, Howe J, Kuhlmann D, Matteri R. Disc excision and spine fusion in the management of lumbar disc disease. A minimum ten-year followup. *Spine* (Phila Pa 1976). 1978;3(1):1–6. PubMed PMID: 644389.
30. Albert H, Godskesen M, Westergaard J. Prognosis in four syndromes of pregnancy-related pelvic pain. *Acta Obstet Gynecol Scand*. 2001;80(6):505–510. PubMed PMID: 11380285.
31. Berg G, Hammar M, Möller-Nielsen J, Lindén U, Thorblad J. Low back pain during pregnancy. *Obstet Gynecol*. 1988;71(1):71–75. PubMed PMID: 2962023.
32. Daly JM, Frame PS, Rapoza PA. Sacroiliac subluxation: a common, treatable cause of low-back pain in pregnancy. *Fam Pract Res J*. 1991;11(2):149–159. PubMed PMID: 1829312.
33. Bollow M, Braun J, Hamm B. Sacroiliitis: the key symptom of spondyloarthropathies. 1. The clinical aspects [review, German]. *Rofo*. 1997;166(2):95–100. PubMed PMID: 9116265.
34. Dunn EJ, Bryan DM, Nugent JT, Robinson RA. Pyogenic infections of the sacro-iliac joint. *Clin Orthop Relat Res*. 1976;(118):113–117. PubMed PMID: 954263.
35. Humphrey SM, Inman RD. Metastatic adenocarcinoma mimicking unilateral sacroiliitis. *J Rheumatol*. 1995;22(5):970–972. PubMed PMID: 8587091.
36. Chou LH, Slipman CW, Bhagia SM, et al. Inciting events initiating injection-proven sacroiliac joint syndrome. *Pain Med*. 2004;5(1):26–32. PubMed PMID: 14996234.
37. Baquie P, Brukner P. Injuries presenting to an Australian sports medicine centre: a 12-month study. *Clin J Sport Med*. 1997;7(1):28–31. PubMed PMID: 9117522.

38. LeBlanc KE. Sacroiliac sprain: an overlooked cause of back pain [review]. *Am Fam Physician*. 1992;46(5):1459–63. Review. PubMed PMID: 1442464.
39. Shibata Y, Shirai Y, Miyamoto M. The aging process in the sacroiliac joint: helical computed tomography analysis. *J Orthop Sci*. 2002;7(1):12–18. PubMed PMID: 11819126.
40. Carette S, Graham D, Little H, Rubenstein J, Rosen P. The natural disease course of ankylosing spondylitis. *Arthritis Rheum*. 1983;26(2):186–190. PubMed PMID: 6600615.
41. Kristiansson P, Svärdsudd K, von Schoultz B. Back pain during pregnancy: a prospective study. *Spine* (Phila Pa 1976). 1996;21(6):702–709. PubMed PMID: 8882692.
42. Larsen EC, Wilken-Jensen C, Hansen A, et al. Symptom-giving pelvic girdle relaxation in pregnancy. I: Prevalence and risk factors. *Acta Obstet Gynecol Scand*. 1999 ;78(2):105–110. PubMed PMID: 10023871.
43. Goldthwait GE, Osgood RB. A consideration of the pelvic articulations from an anatomical, pathological, and clinical standpoint. *Boston Med Surg J*. 1905;152: 593–601.
44. Slipman CW, Whyte WS 2nd, Chow DW, Chou L, Lenrow D, Ellen M. Sacroiliac joint syndrome. *Pain Physician*. 2001;4(2):143–152. PubMed PMID: 16902687.
45. Mixter WJ, Barr JS. Rupture of the intervertebral disc with involvement of the spinal canal. *N Engl J Med*. 1934;211:210–215.
46. Bogduk N, McGuirk B, eds. Causes and sources of chronic low back pain. In: *Medical Management of Acute and Chronic Low Back pain. An Evidence-Based Approach: Pain Research and Clinical Management*. Vol. 13. Amsterdam: Elsevier Science BV; 2002:115–126.
47. Haldeman K, Soto-Hall R. The diagnosis and treatment of sacro-iliac conditions involving injection of procaine (Novocain). *J Bone Joint Surg*. 1938;3:675–685.
48. Norman GF, May A. Sacroiliac conditions simulating intervertebral disc syndrome. *West J Surg Obstet Gynecol*. 1956;64(8):461–462. PubMed PMID:13353013.
49. Fortin JD, Dwyer AP, West S, Pier J. Sacroiliac joint: pain referral maps upon applying a new injection/arthrography technique. Part I: Asymptomatic volunteers. *Spine* (Phila Pa 1976). 1994;19(13):1475–1482. PubMed PMID: 7939978.
50. Fortin JD, Aprill CN, Ponthieux B, Pier J. Sacroiliac joint: pain referral maps upon applying a new injection/arthrography technique. Part II: Clinical evaluation. *Spine* (Phila Pa 1976). 1994;19(13):1483–1489. PubMed PMID: 7939979.
51. Broadhurst NA, Bond MJ. Pain provocation tests for the assessment of sacroiliac joint dysfunction. *J Spinal Disord*. 1998;11(4):341–345. PubMed PMID:9726305.
52. Merskey H, Bogduk N. *Classification of Chronic Pain: Descriptions of Chronic Pain Syndromes and Definitions of Pain Terms*. Seattle, WA: IASP Press; 1994:190–191.
53. Cibulka MT, Koldehoff R. Clinical usefulness of a cluster of sacroiliac joint tests in patients with and without low back pain. *J Orthop Sports Phys Ther*. 1999;29(2):83–89; discussion 90–2. PubMed PMID: 10322583.
54. Szadek KM, van der Wurff P, van Tulder MW, Zuurmond WW, Perez RS. Diagnostic validity of criteria for sacroiliac joint pain: a systematic review [published online ahead of print December 19 2008]. *J Pain*. 2009;10(4):354–368. PubMed PMID: 19101212.
55. Young S, Aprill C, Laslett M. Correlation of clinical examination characteristics with three sources of chronic low back pain. *Spine J*. 2003;3(6):460–465. PubMed PMID: 14609690.
56. Zelle BA, Gruen GS, Brown S, George S. Sacroiliac joint dysfunction: evaluation and management [review]. *Clin J Pain*. 2005;21(5):446–455. PubMed PMID: 16093751.
57. Prather H, Hunt D. Conservative management of low back pain, part I. Sacroiliac joint pain [review]. *Dis Mon*. 2004;50(12):670–683. PubMed PMID: 15767995.
58. Brolinson PG, Kozar AJ, Cibor G. Sacroiliac joint dysfunction in athletes [review]. *Curr Sports Med Rep*. 2003;2(1):47–56. PubMed PMID: 12831676.
59. Ross J. Is the sacroiliac joint mobile and how should it be treated? *Br J Sports Med*. 2000;34(3):226. PubMed PMID: 10854029; PubMed Central PMCID: PMC1763263.
60. Dietrichs E. Anatomy of the pelvic joints—a review. *Scand J Rheumatol Suppl*. 1991;88:4–6. PubMed PMID: 2011709.
61. Fortin JD, Falco FJ. The Fortin finger test: an indicator of sacroiliac pain. *Am J Orthop*. 1997;26(7):477–480. PubMed PMID: 9247654.
62. Sabharwal S, Kumar A. Methods for assessing leg length discrepancy [published online ahead of print October 4 2008]. *Clin Orthop Relat Res*. 2008;466(12):2910–2922. PubMed PMID: 18836788; PubMed Central PMCID: PMC2628227.
63. Knutson GA. Anatomic and functional leg-length inequality: a review and recommendation for clinical decision-making. Part I, anatomic leg-length inequality: prevalence, magnitude, effects and clinical significance. *Chiropr Osteopat*. 2005;13:11. PubMed PMID: 16026625; PubMed Central PMCID: PMC1232860.
64. Jung JH, Kim HI, Shin DA, et al. Usefulness of pain distribution pattern assessment in decision-making for the patients with lumbar zygapophyseal and sacroiliac joint arthropathy. *J Korean Med Sci*. 2007;22(6):1048–1054. PubMed PMID: 18162721; PubMed Central PMCID: PMC2694630.
65. Slipman CW, Sterenfeld EB, Chou LH, Herzog R, Vresilovic E. The predictive value of provocative sacroiliac joint stress maneuvers in the diagnosis of sacroiliac joint syndrome. *Arch Phys Med Rehabil*. 1998;79(3):288–292. PubMed PMID: 9523780.
66. Laslett M, Aprill CN, McDonald B, Young SB. Diagnosis of sacroiliac joint pain: validity of individual provocation tests and composites of tests. *Man Ther*. 2005;10(3):207–218. PubMed PMID: 16038856.
67. Laslett M, Aprill CN, McDonald B. Provocation sacroiliac joint tests have validity in the diagnosis of sacroiliac joint pain. *Arch Phys Med Rehabil*. 2006;87(6):874; author reply 874–75. PubMed PMID: 16731225.
68. van der Wurff P, Buijs EJ, Groen GJ. A multitest regimen of pain provocation tests as an aid to reduce unnecessary minimally invasive sacroiliac joint procedures. *Arch Phys Med Rehabil*. 2006;87(1):10–14. PubMed PMID: 16401431.
69. Buyruk HM, Snijders CJ, Vleeming A, Laméris JS, Holland WP, Stam HJ. The measurements of sacroiliac joint stiffness with colour Doppler imaging: a study on healthy subjects. *Eur J Radiol*. 1995;21(2):117–121. PubMed PMID: 8850505.
70. Sturesson B, Selvik G, Udén A. Movements of the sacroiliac joints. A roentgen stereophotogrammetric analysis. *Spine* (Phila Pa 1976). 1989;14(2):162–165.PubMed PMID: 2922636.
71. Damen L, Buyruk HM, Güler-Uysal F, Lotgering FK, Snijders CJ, Stam HJ. The prognostic value of asymmetric laxity of the sacroiliac joints in pregnancy-related pelvic pain. *Spine* (Phila Pa 1976). 2002;27(24):2820–2824. PubMed PMID: 12486354.
72. Bogduk N. Sacroiliac joint blocks. In: *Practice Guidelines for Spinal Diagnostic and Treatment Procedures*. 1st ed. San Francisco: International Spine Intervention Society; 2004:66–86.
73. Manchikanti L, Singh V, Pampati V, et al. Evaluation of the relative contributions of various structures in chronic low back pain. *Pain Physician*. 2001;4(4):308–316. Erratum in: *Pain Physician*. 2002;5(1):114. PubMed PMID: 16902676.
74. McKenzie-Brown AM, Shah RV, Sehgal N, Everett CR. A systematic review of sacroiliac joint interventions. *Pain Physician*. 2005;8(1):115–125. PubMed PMID: 16850049.
75. Foley BS, Buschbacher RM. Sacroiliac joint pain: anatomy, biomechanics, diagnosis, and treatment. *Am J Phys Med Rehabil*. 2006;85(12):997–1006.Review. PubMed PMID: 17117004.
76. Hansen HC, Helm S 2nd. Sacroiliac joint pain and dysfunction. *Pain Physician*. 2003;6(2):179–189. PubMed PMID: 16883378.
77. Boswell MV, Shah RV, Everett CR, et al. Interventional techniques in the management of chronic spinal pain: evidence-based practice guidelines. *Pain Physician*. 2005;8(1):1–47. PubMed PMID: 16850041.
78. Murata Y, Takahashi K, Yamagata M, Takahashi Y, Shimada Y, Moriya H. Origin and pathway of sensory nerve fibers to the

ventral and dorsal sides of the sacroiliac joint in rats. *J Orthop Res.* 2001;19(3):379–383. PubMed PMID: 11398849.
79. Fortin JD, Kissling RO, O'Connor BL, Vilensky JA. Sacroiliac joint innervation and pain [review]. *Am J Orthop.* 1999;28(12):687–690. PubMed PMID: 10614759.
80. Grob KR, Neuhuber WL, Kissling RO. Innervation of the sacroiliac joint of thehuman [German]. *Z Rheumatol.* 1995;54(2):117–122. PubMed PMID: 7793158.
81. Ikeda R. Innervation of the sacroiliac joint. Macroscopical and histological studies [Japanese]. *Nihon Ika Daigaku Zasshi.* 1991;58(5):587–596. PubMed PMID: 1744230.
82. Vilensky JA, O'Connor BL, Fortin JD, et al. Histologic analysis of neural elements in the human sacroiliac joint. *Spine* (Phila Pa 1976). 2002;27(11):1202–1207. PubMed PMID: 12045518.
83. Sakamoto N, Yamashita T, Takebayashi T, Sekine M, Ishii S. An electrophysiologic study of mechanoreceptors in the sacroiliac joint and adjacent tissues. *Spine* (Phila Pa 1976). 2001;26(20):E468–E471. PubMed PMID: 11598526.
84. Solonen KA. The sacroiliac joint in the light of anatomical, roentgenological and clinical studies. *Acta Orthop Scand Suppl.* 1957;27:1–127. PubMed PMID: 13478452.
85. Minaki Y, Yamashita T, Ishii S. An electrophysiological study on the mechanoreceptors in the lumbar spine and adjacent tissues. *Neurol Orthop.* 1996; 20:23–35.
86. Manchikanti L, Boswell MV, Singh V, Hansen HC. Sacroiliac joint pain: should physicians be blocking lateral branches, medial branches, dorsal rami, or ventral rami? *Reg Anesth Pain Med.* 2003;28(5):488–490; author reply 490–491. PubMed PMID: 14556149.
87. Yamashita T, Cavanaugh JM, el-Bohy AA, Getchell TV, King AI. Mechanosensitive afferent units in the lumbar facet joint. *J Bone Joint Surg Am.* 1990;72(6):865–670. PubMed PMID: 2365719.
88. Yamashita T, Minaki Y, Oota I, Yokogushi K, Ishii S. Mechanosensitive afferent units in the lumbar intervertebral disc and adjacent muscle. *Spine* (Phila Pa 1976). 1993;18(15):2252–2256. PubMed PMID: 8278841.
89. Dreyfuss P, Michaelsen M, Pauza K, McLarty J, Bogduk N. The value of medical history and physical examination in diagnosing sacroiliac joint pain. *Spine* (Phila Pa 1976). 1996;21(22):2594–2602. PubMed PMID: 8961447.
90. Slipman CW, Jackson HB, Lipetz JS, Chan KT, Lenrow D, Vresilovic EJ. Sacroiliac joint pain referral zones. *Arch Phys Med Rehabil.* 2000;81(3):334–338. PubMed PMID: 10724079.
91. Laslett M, Young SB, Aprill CN, McDonald B. Diagnosing painful sacroiliac joints: a validity study of a McKenzie evaluation and sacroiliac provocation tests. *Aust J Physiother.* 2003;49(2):89–97. PubMed PMID: 12775204.
92. van der Wurff P, Buijs EJ, Groen GJ. Intensity mapping of pain referral areas in sacroiliac joint pain patients. *J Manipulative Physiol Ther.* 2006;29(3):190–195. PubMed PMID: 16584942.
93. Maigne JY, Planchon CA. Sacroiliac joint pain after lumbar fusion. A study with anesthetic blocks [published online ahead of print March 11 2005]. *Eur Spine J.* 2005;14(7):654–658. PubMed PMID: 15761709.
94. Berthelot JM, Labat JJ, Le Goff B, Gouin F, Maugars Y. Provocative sacroiliac joint maneuvers and sacroiliac joint block are unreliable for diagnosing sacroiliac joint pain [review]. *Joint Bone Spine.* 2006;73(1):17–23. PubMed PMID: 16461204.
95. Elgafy H, Semaan HB, Ebraheim NA, Coombs RJ. Computed tomography findings in patients with sacroiliac pain. *Clin. Orthop. Relat. Res.* 2001;382:112–118. PubMed PMID: 11153977.
96. Maigne JY, Boulahdour H, Chatellier G. Value of quantitative radionuclide bone scanning in the diagnosis of sacroiliac joint syndrome in 32 patients with low back pain. *Eur Spine J.* 1998;7(4):328–331. PubMed PMID: 9765042.
97. Slipman CW, Sterenfeld EB, Chou LH, Herzog R, Vresilovic E. The value of radionuclide imaging in the diagnosis of sacroiliac joint syndrome. *Spine.* 1996;21(19):2251–2254. PubMed PMID: 8902970.
98. Puhakka K, Jurik A, Schiøttz-Christensen B, et al. MRI abnormalities of sacroiliac joints in early spondylarthropathy: a 1-year follow-up study. *Scand J Rheumatol.* 2004;33(5): 332–338. PubMed PMID: 15513683.
99. Herring SA. Rehabilitation of muscle injuries. *Med Sci Sports Exerc.* 1990;22(4):453–456. PubMed PMID: 2402205.
100. DonTigny RL. Function and pathomechanics of the sacroiliac joint. A review. *Phys Ther.* 1985;65(1):35–44. PubMed PMID: 3155567.
101. Vleeming A, Buyruk HM, Stoeckart R, Karamursel S, Snijders CJ. An integrated therapy for peripartum pelvic instability: a study of the biomechanical effects of pelvic belts. *Am J Obstet Gynecol.* 1992;166(4):1243–1247. PubMed PMID: 1566778.
102. Nilsson-Wikmar L, Holm K, Oijerstedt R, Harms-Ringdahl K. Effect of three different physical therapy treatments on pain and activity in pregnant women with pelvic girdle pain: a randomized clinical trial with 3, 6, and 12 months follow-up postpartum. *Spine* (Phila Pa 1976). 2005;30(8):850–856. PubMed PMID: 15834325.
103. Bergmark A. Stability of the lumbar spine. A study in mechanical engineering [review]. *Acta Orthop Scand Suppl.* 1989;230:1–54. PubMed PMID: 2658468.
104. Hodges PW, Butler JE, McKenzie DK, Gandevia SC. Contraction of the human diaphragm during rapid postural adjustments. *J Physiol.* 1997;505 (Pt 2):539–548. PubMed PMID: 9423192; PubMed Central PMCID: PMC1160083.
105. Sasso RC, Ahmad RI, Butler JE, Reimers DL. Sacroiliac joint dysfunction: a long-term follow-up study. *Orthopedics.* 2001;24(5):457–460. PubMed PMID: 11379994.
106. Kamali F, Shokri E. The effect of two manipulative therapy techniques and their outcome in patients with sacroiliac joint syndrome. *J Bodyw Mov Ther.* 2012;16(1):29–35. Epub 2011 Mar 11. PubMed PMID: 22196424.
107. Murphy BA, Dawson NJ, Slack JR. Sacroiliac joint manipulation decreases the H-reflex. *Electromyogr Clin Neurophysiol.* 1995;35(2):87–94. PubMed PMID: 7781578.
108. Cibulka MT, Rose SJ, Delitto A, Sinacore DR. Hamstring muscle strain treated by mobilizing the sacroiliac joint. *Phys Ther.* 1986;66(8):1220–1223. PubMed PMID: 3737692.
109. Suter E, McMorland G, Herzog W, Bray R. Decrease in quadriceps inhibition after sacroiliac joint manipulation in patients with anterior knee pain. *J Manipulative Physiol Ther.* 1999;22(3):149–153. PubMed PMID: 10220713.
110. Marshall P, Murphy B. The effect of sacroiliac joint manipulation on feed-forward activation times of the deep abdominal musculature. *J Manipulative Physiol Ther.* 2006;29(3):196–202. PubMed PMID: 16584943.
111. Childs JD, Piva SR, Erhard RE. Immediate improvements in side-to-side weight bearing and iliac crest symmetry after manipulation in patients with low back pain. *J Manipulative Physiol Ther.* 2004;27(5):306–313. PubMed PMID: 15195038.
112. Cibulka MT, Delitto A, Koldehoff RM. Changes in innominate tilt after manipulation of the sacroiliac joint in patients with low back pain. An experimental study. *Phys Ther.* 1988;68(9):1359–1363. PubMed PMID: 2971233.
113. Tullberg T, Blomberg S, Branth B, Johnsson R. Manipulation does not alter the position of the sacroiliac joint. A roentgen stereophotogrammetric analysis. *Spine* (Phila Pa 1976). 1998;23(10):1124–1128; discussion 1129. PubMed PMID: 9615363.
114. Flynn T, Fritz J, Whitman J, et al. A clinical prediction rule for classifying patients with low back pain who demonstrate short-term improvement with spinal manipulation. *Spine* (Phila Pa 1976). 2002;27(24):2835–2843. PubMed PMID: 12486357.
115. Herzog W, Nigg BM, Read LJ. Quantifying the effects of spinal manipulations on gait using patients with low back pain. *J Manipulative Physiol Ther.* 1988;11(3):151–157. PubMed PMID: 2969026.
116. Osterbauer PJ, De Boer KF, Widmaier R, Petermann E, Fuhr AW. Treatment and biomechanical assessment of patients with

chronic sacroiliac joint syndrome. *J Manipulative Physiol Ther.* 1993;16(2):82–90. PubMed PMID: 8445358.
117. Kim WM, Lee HG, Jeong CW, Kim CM, Yoon MH. A randomized controlled trial of intra-articular prolotherapy versus steroid injection for sacroiliac joint pain. *J Altern Complement Med.* 2010;16(12):1285–1290. PubMed PMID: 21138388.
118. Cusi M, Saunders J, Hungerford B, Wisbey-Roth T, Lucas P, Wilson S. The use of prolotherapy in the sacroiliac joint [published online ahead of print April 9 2008]. *Br J Sports Med.* 2010;44(2):100–104. PubMed PMID: 18400878.
119. Dersh J, Polatin PB, Gatchel RJ. Chronic pain and psychopathology: research findings and theoretical considerations [review]. *Psychosom Med.* 2002;64(5):773–786. PubMed PMID: 12271108.
120. Dersh J, Gatchel RJ, Polatin P, Mayer T. Prevalence of psychiatric disorders in patients with chronic work-related musculoskeletal pain disability. *J Occup Environ Med.* 2002;44(5):459–468. PubMed PMID: 12024691.
121. Polatin PB, Kinney RK, Gatchel RJ, Lillo E, Mayer TG. Psychiatric illness and chronic low-back pain. The mind and the spine—which goes first? *Spine* (Phila Pa 1976). 1993;18(1):66–71. PubMed PMID: 8434327.
122. Lipowski ZJ. Somatization and depression [review]. *Psychosomatics.* 1990;31(1):13–21. PubMed PMID: 2405448.
123. Wesley AL, Gatchel RJ, Garofalo JP, Polatin PB. Toward more accurate use of the Beck Depression Inventory with chronic back pain patients. *Clin J Pain.* 1999;15(2):117–121. PubMed PMID: 10382925.
124. Gatchel RJ, Polatin PB, Kinney RK. Predicting outcome of chronic back pain using clinical predictors of psychopathology: a prospective analysis. *Health Psychol.* 1995;14(5):415–420. PubMed PMID: 7498112.
125. Seres JL. Evaluating the complex chronic pain patient [review]. *Neurosurg Clin N Am.* 2003;14(3):339–352. PubMed PMID: 14567136.
126. Luukkainen R, Nissilä M, Asikainen E, et al. Periarticular corticosteroid treatment of the sacroiliac joint in patients with seronegative spondylarthropathy. *Clin Exp Rheumatol.* 1999;17(1):88–90. PubMed PMID: 10084038.
127. Luukkainen RK, Wennerstrand PV, Kautiainen HH, Sanila MT, Asikainen EL. Efficacy of periarticular corticosteroid treatment of the sacroiliac joint in non-spondylarthropathic patients with chronic low back pain in the region of the sacroiliac joint. *Clin Exp Rheumatol.* 2002;20(1):52–54. PubMed PMID: 11892709.
128. Murakami E, Tanaka Y, Aizawa T, Ishizuka M, Kokubun S. Effect of periarticular and intraarticular lidocaine injections for sacroiliac joint pain: prospective comparative study [published online ahead of print May 31 2007]. *J Orthop Sci.* 2007;12(3):274–280. PubMed PMID: 17530380.
129. Borowsky CD, Fagen G. Sources of sacroiliac region pain: insights gained from a study comparing standard intra-articular injection with a technique combining intra- and peri-articular injection. *Arch Phys Med Rehabil.* 2008;89(11):2048–2056. PubMed PMID: 18996232.
130. Fischer T, Biedermann T, Hermann KG, et al. Sacroiliitis in children with spondyloarthropathy: therapeutic effect of CT-guided intra-articular corticosteroid injection [German]. *Rofo.* 2003;175(6):814–821. PubMed PMID: 12811695.
131. Hanly JG, Mitchell M, MacMillan L, Mosher D, Sutton E. Efficacy of sacroiliac corticosteroid injections in patients with inflammatory spondyloarthropathy: results of a 6 month controlled study. *J Rheumatol.* 2000;27(3):719–722. PubMed PMID: 10743815.
132. Maugars Y, Mathis C, Berthelot JM, Charlier C, Prost A. Assessment of the efficacy of sacroiliac corticosteroid injections in spondyloarthropathies: a double-blind study. *Br J Rheumatol.* 1996;35(8):767–770. PubMed PMID: 8761190.
133. Sadreddini S, Noshad H, Molaeefard M, Ardalan MR, Ghojazadeh M, Shakouri SK. Unguided sacroiliac injection: effect on refractory buttock pain in patients with spondyloarthropathies [published online ahead of print February 13 2009]. *Presse Med.* 2009;38(5):710–716. PubMed PMID: 19217752.
134. Rosenberg JM, Quint TJ, de Rosayro AM. Computerized tomographic localization of clinically-guided sacroiliac joint injections. *Clin J Pain.* 2000;16(1):18–21. PubMed PMID: 10741814.
135. Shealy CN. Percutaneous radiofrequency denervation of spinal facets. Treatment for chronic back pain and sciatica. *J Neurosurg.* 1975;43(4):448–451. PubMed PMID: 125787.
136. Dreyfuss P, Henning T, Malladi N, Goldstein B, Bogduk N. The ability of multi-site, multi-depth sacral lateral branch blocks to anesthetize the sacroiliac joint complex. *Pain Med.* 2009;10(4):679–688. PubMed PMID: 19638143.
137. Cohen SP, Strassels SA, Kurihara C, et al. Outcome predictors for sacroiliac joint (lateral branch) radiofrequency denervation. *Reg Anesth Pain Med.* 2009;34(3):206–214. PubMed PMID: 19587617.
138. Cohen SP, Hurley RW, Christo PJ, Winkley J, Mohiuddin MM, Stojanovic MP. Clinical predictors of success and failure for lumbar facet radiofrequency denervation. *Clin J Pain.* 2007;23(1):45–52. PubMed PMID: 17277644.
139. Aydin SM, Gharibo CG, Mehnert M, Stitik TP. The role of radiofrequency ablation for sacroiliac joint pain: a meta-analysis. *PM R.* 2010;2(9):842–851. PubMed PMID: 20869684.
140. Yin W, Willard F, Carreiro J, Dreyfuss P. Sensory stimulation-guided sacroiliac joint radiofrequency neurotomy: technique based on neuroanatomy of the dorsal sacral plexus. *Spine* (Phila Pa 1976). 2003;28(20):2419–2425. PubMed PMID: 14560094.
141. Buijs E, Kamphuis E, Groen G. Radiofrequency treatment of sacroiliac joint-related pain aimed at the first three sacral dorsal rami: a minimal approach. *The Pain Clinic.* 2004;16(2):139–46.
142. Dobrogowski J, Wrzosek A, Wordliczek J. Radiofrequency denervation with or without addition of pentoxifylline or methylprednisolone for chronic lumbar zygapophysial joint pain. *Pharmacol Rep.* 2005;57(4):475–480. PubMed PMID: 16129914.
143. Pino CA, Hoeft MA, Hofsess C, Rathmell JP. Morphologic analysis of bipolar radiofrequency lesions: implications for treatment of the sacroiliac joint. *Reg Anesth Pain Med.* 2005;30(4):335–338. PubMed PMID: 16032584.
144. Kang SS, Park JC, Yoon YJ, Shin KM. Morphologic analysis of water-cooled bipolar radiofrequency lesions on egg white in vitro [published online ahead of print June 28 1012]. *Korean J Pain.* 2012;25(3):151–154. PubMed PMID: 22787544; PubMed Central PMCID: PMC3389318.
145. Cosman ER Jr, Gonzalez CD. Bipolar radiofrequency lesion geometry: implications for palisade treatment of sacroiliac joint pain. *Pain Pract.* 2011;11(1):3–22. doi: 10.1111/j.1533-2500.2010.00400.x. PubMed PMID: 20602716.
146. Ferrante FM, King LF, Roche EA, et al. Radiofrequency sacroiliac joint denervation for sacroiliac syndrome. *Reg Anesth Pain Med.* 2001;26(2):137–142. PubMed PMID: 11251137.
147. Lorentzen T. A cooled needle electrode for radiofrequency tissue ablation: thermodynamic aspects of improved performance compared with conventional needle design. *Acad Radiol.* 1996;3(7):556–563. PubMed PMID: 8796717.
148. Solbiati L, Goldberg SN, Ierace T, et al. Hepatic metastases: percutaneous radio-frequency ablation with cooled-tip electrodes. *Radiology.* 1997;205(2):367–373. PubMed PMID: 9356616.
149. Goldberg SN, Gazelle GS, Solbiati L, Rittman WJ, Mueller PR. Radiofrequency tissue ablation: increased lesion diameter with a perfusion electrode. *Acad Radiol.* 1996;3(8):636–644. PubMed PMID: 8796727.
150. Delacretaz E, Stevenson WG, Winters GL, et al. Ablation of ventricular tachycardia with a saline-cooled radiofrequency catheter: anatomic and histologic characteristics of the lesions in humans. *J Cardiovasc Electrophysiol.* 1999;10(6):860–865. PubMed PMID: 10376924.
151. Patel N, Gross A, Brown L, Gekht G. A randomized, placebo-controlled study to assess the efficacy of lateral branch neurotomy for chronic sacroiliac joint pain [published online ahead of

print February 2 2012]. *Pain Med.* 2012;13(3):383–398. doi: 10.1111/j.1526-4637.2012.01328.x. PubMed PMID: 22299761.

152. Kapural L, Nageeb F, Kapural M, Cata JP, Narouze S, Mekhail N. Cooled radiofrequency system for the treatment of chronic pain from sacroiliitis: the first case-series. *Pain Pract.* 2008;8(5):348–354. PubMed PMID: 18844853.
153. Cohen SP, Hurley RW, Buckenmaier CC 3rd, Kurihara C, Morlando B, Dragovich A. Randomized placebo-controlled study evaluating lateral branch radiofrequency denervation for sacroiliac joint pain. *Anesthesiology.* 2008;109(2):279–288. PubMed PMID: 18648237; PubMed Central PMCID: PMC2666931.
154. Cheng J, Pope JE, Dalton JE, Cheng O, Bensitel A. Comparative outcomes of cooled versus traditional radiofrequency ablation of the lateral branches for sacroiliac joint pain [published online ahead of print June 7 2012]. *Clin J Pain.* PubMed PMID: 22688606.
155. Stelzer W, Aiglesberger M, Stelzer D, Stelzer V. Use of cooled radiofrequency lateral branch neurotomy for the treatment of sacroiliac joint-mediated low back pain: a large case series [published online ahead of print December 28 2012]. *Pain Med.* 2013;14(1):29–35. doi: 10.1111/pme.12014. PubMed PMID: 23279364.
156. Calvillo O, Esses SI, Ponder C, D'Agostino C, Tanhui E. Neuroaugmentation in the management of sacroiliac joint pain. Report of two cases. *Spine* (Phila Pa 1976). 1998;23(9):1069–1072. PubMed PMID: 9589549.
157. Kim YH, Moon DE. Sacral nerve stimulation for the treatment of sacroiliac joint dysfunction: a case report. *Neuromodulation.* 2010;13(4):306–310. doi: 10.1111/j.1525-1403.2009.00270.x. PubMed PMID: 21992888.
158. Dabezies EJ, Millet CW, Murphy CP, Acker JH, Robicheaux RE, D'Ambrosia RD. Stabilization of sacroiliac joint disruption with threaded compression rods. *Clin Orthop Relat Res.* 1989;(246):165–171. PubMed PMID: 2766606.
159. Simpson LA, Waddell JP, Leighton RK, Kellam JF, Tile M. Anterior approach and stabilization of the disrupted sacroiliac joint. *J Trauma.* 1987;27(12):1332–1339. PubMed PMID: 3694724.
160. Waisbrod H, Krainick JU, Gerbershagen HU. Sacroiliac joint arthrodesis for chronic lower back pain. *Arch Orthop Trauma Surg.* 1987;106(4):238–240. PubMed PMID: 2956935.
161. Buchowski JM, Kebaish KM, Sinkov V, Cohen DB, Sieber AN, Kostuik JP. Functional and radiographic outcome of sacroiliac arthrodesis for the disorders of the sacroiliac joint. *Spine J.* 2005;5(5):520–528; discussion 529. PubMed PMID: 16153580.
162. Schütz U, Grob D. Poor outcome following bilateral sacroiliac joint fusion for degenerative sacroiliac joint syndrome. *Acta Orthop Belg.* 2006;72(3):296–308. PubMed PMID: 16889141.
163. Liliang PC, Lu K, Liang CL, Tsai YD, Wang KW, Chen HJ. Sacroiliac joint pain after lumbar and lumbosacral fusion: findings using dual sacroiliac joint blocks. *Pain Med.* 2011;91(4):1283–1285.
164. DePalma MJ, Ketchum JM, Trussell BS, Saullo TR, Slipman CW. Does the location of low back pain predict its source? *P M R.* 2011;3(1):33–39.
165. Ostgaard H, Andersson G, Karlsson K. Prevalence of back pain in pregnancy. *Spine.* 1991;16(5):549–552.
166. Laplante BL, Ketchum JM, Saullo TR, DePalma MJ. Multivariable analysis of the relationship between pain referral patterns and the source of chronic low back pain. *Pain Physician.* 2012;15(2):171–178.
167. Stanford G, Burnham RS. Is it useful to repeat sacroiliac joint provocative tests post-block? *Pain Med.* 2010;11(12):1774–1776.
168. Gevargez A, Groenemeyer D, Schirp S, Braun M. CT-guided ercutaneous radiofrequencydenervation of the sacroiliac joint. *Eur. Radiol.* 2002;12(6):1360–1365.
169. Cohen SP, Abdi S. Lateral branch blocks as a treatment for sacroiliac joint pain: a pilot study. *Reg. Anesth. Pain Med.* 2003;28(2):113–119.
170. Burnham RS, Yasui Y. An alternate method of radiofrequency neurotomy of the sacroiliac joint: a pilot study of the effect on pain, function, and satisfaction. *Reg. Anesth. Pain Med.* 2007;32(1):12–19.
171. Hagiwara S, Iwasaka H, Takeshima N, Noguchi T. Mechanisms of analgesic action of pulsed radiofrequency on adjuvant-induced pain in the rat: roles of descending adrenergic and serotonergic systems. *Euro. Jour. Pain.* 2009;13(3): 249–252.
172. Cohen SP, Hurley RW, Buckenmaier III CC, Kurihara C, Morlando B, Dragovich A. Randomized placebo-controlled study evaluating lateral branch radiofrequency denervation for sacroiliac joint pain. Anesthesiology. 2008;109(2):279–288.
173. Karaman H, Kavak GÖ, Tüfek A, et al. Cooled radiofrequency application for treatment of sacroiliac joint pain. *Acta Neurochir.* 2011;153(7):1461–1468.
174. Speldewinde GC. Outcomes of percutaneous zygapophysial and sacroiliac joint neurotomy in a community setting. *Pain Med.* 2011;12(2):209–218.

11.

LUMBAR SPINAL STENOSIS

John D. Markman and Kiran Nandigam

CASE PRESENTATION

A 72-year-old woman experiences severe pain in her anterior thighs and knees when standing and walking. Her initial symptoms began approximately 2 years earlier with onset of lower back pain radiating to the right leg, as well as paresthesias in the dorsum of the right foot. At that time, there was no antecedent trauma or infectious prodrome. The pain was described as shooting and exacerbated with walking, twisting, and lifting. At the onset of her symptoms, the patient managed her pain with exercise and the use of analgesic medication (ibuprofen 1,600 mg/d). There was no associated weakness in the lower extremities, lateralized reflex deficit, or change in her bowel or bladder habits during this time period.

Her initial magnetic resonance imaging (MRI) study demonstrated moderate stenosis at the L3–L4 segment in the setting of facet hypertrophy and lateral recess stenosis at L3–L4 affecting the traversing L4 nerve root (Figure 11.1). In addition to the initial conservative treatments with nonsteroidal anti-inflammatory drugs (NSAIDs), physical therapy, and activity moderation, she underwent epidural steroid injection for this flare of radicular pain 3 months after its onset. This initial treatment was sufficient in managing her pain and symptoms. Her pain was reduced to the 1–2/10 level in the right leg with standing and walking at the 5-month time point. She resumed walking through the mall for 40 minutes three times per week.

Two years later, the patient returns for evaluation. Her pain has increased gradually over the past 5 months, and her walking tolerance is dramatically reduced. She is no longer able to tolerate walking for more than "a few minutes" before needing to sit down. With frustration, she states "I just can't walk any distance anymore." The pain radiating to her legs has changed from the initial pattern. It is now bilateral. She also describes cramping discomfort in her legs—buttocks and calves—at night. She denies any progressive weakness or sensory deficit in her legs. There has been no change in her bowel or bladder habit or new constitutional symptoms. An MRI is taken (Figure 11.2). She undergoes a pair of repeat epidural steroid injections through both the interlaminar and transforaminal approaches, but these do not reduce her pain significantly or improve her walking tolerance as they had previously (Figure 11.3).

Past medical history is notable for hyperlipidemia, hypothyroidism, migraine headache, osteopenia, restless legs syndrome, and a right supraspinatus tendon complete tear.

Past surgical history: Bilateral eye surgery as a child, hysterectomy at age 31.

Allergies include amitriptyline HCl, Lipitor, Lovastatin, Lunesta, Pravastatin, and Simvastatin.

Current medications include aspirin, calcium + vitamin D, Crestor, Levoxyl, loratadine, multivitamins, and omeprazole.

Examination highlights: Alert and oriented senior with broad stable affect discussing her inability to walk long distances. There is no manifest pain behavior such as grimacing, groaning, or slowed movements. Cranial nerve examination is normal. Neck is supple with negative Lhermitte's sign. Tone is normal in the upper and lower extremities. Reflexes are 2+ and symmetric at the C5, C6, C7; there is no Hoffman's sign. Range of motion is full at the lumbar spine. There is no tenderness on palpation of the spinous processes. There is no focal tenderness over the sacroiliac joints or greater trochanteric bursae. Pain is evoked with prolonged standing in extensor posture. There is altered sensation in the right L4 dermatome as compared with the left. There is no focal weakness of the iliopsoas, quad, tibialis anterior, or the extensor hallucis longus (EHL). Reflexes are 2+ at the L4 and 1+ at the S1. Toes are downgoing. Gait is narrow-based, steady, and mildly antalgic. Decreased vibratory sensation distally; joint position sense is preserved at the great toe bilaterally. Distal pulses are 2+, and feet are well perfused. There is no lower extremity edema. No warm joints or joint effusions noted on examination.

The patient is referred for surgical evaluation for possible decompression after MRI is repeated because of the increase in segmental stenosis, worsened symptoms of neurogenic claudication, and lack of benefit from epidural steroid injections. She is considered to be a reasonable surgical candidate based on the tight correlation of her imaging findings and symptom pattern. She met with her surgical team on multiple occasions to discuss this option. The progressive reduction in her ability to exercise was a major factor in her decision. Her candidacy for surgical decompression is not compromised by major comorbid medical conditions. Definitive anatomic treatment for this syndrome with decompressive laminectomy, foraminotomies, and posterior fixation/fusion is planned.

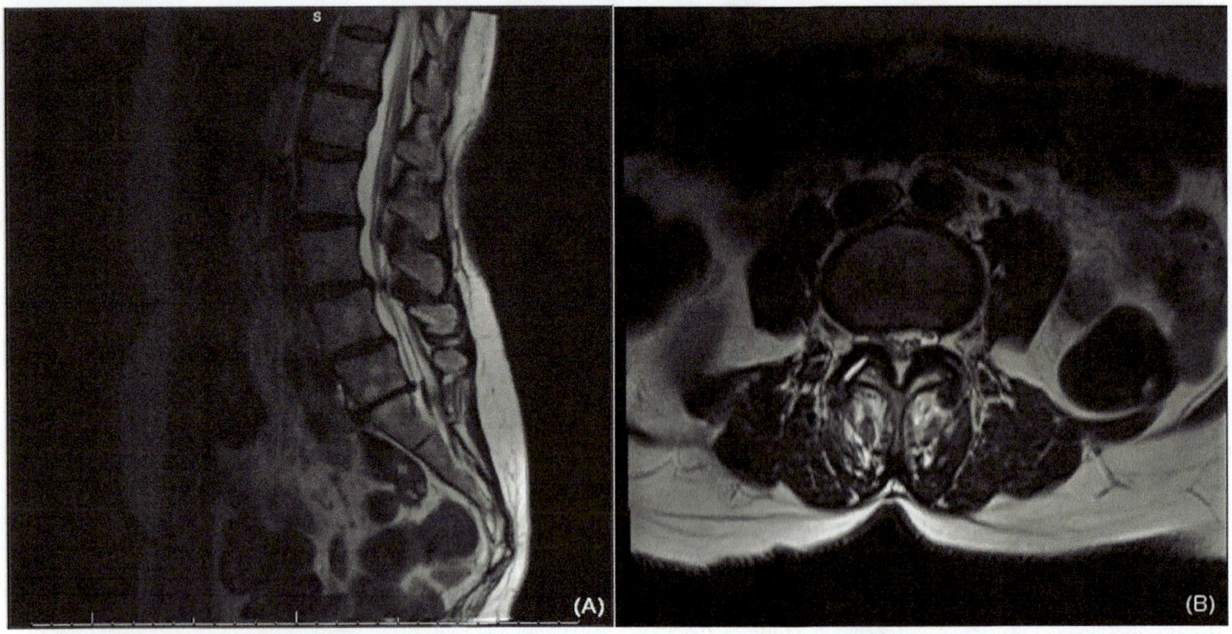

Figure 11.1 Patient initial lumbar imaging. Magnetic resonance image showing T2-weighted images of spinal stenosis. (A) Sagittal view of patient. Posterior disc bulge/osteophyte complex at L2–L3. Superimposed posterior disc bulge at L3–L4 with moderate bilateral facet and ligamentum flavum hypertrophic degenerative changes. (B) Axial image of L3 segment.

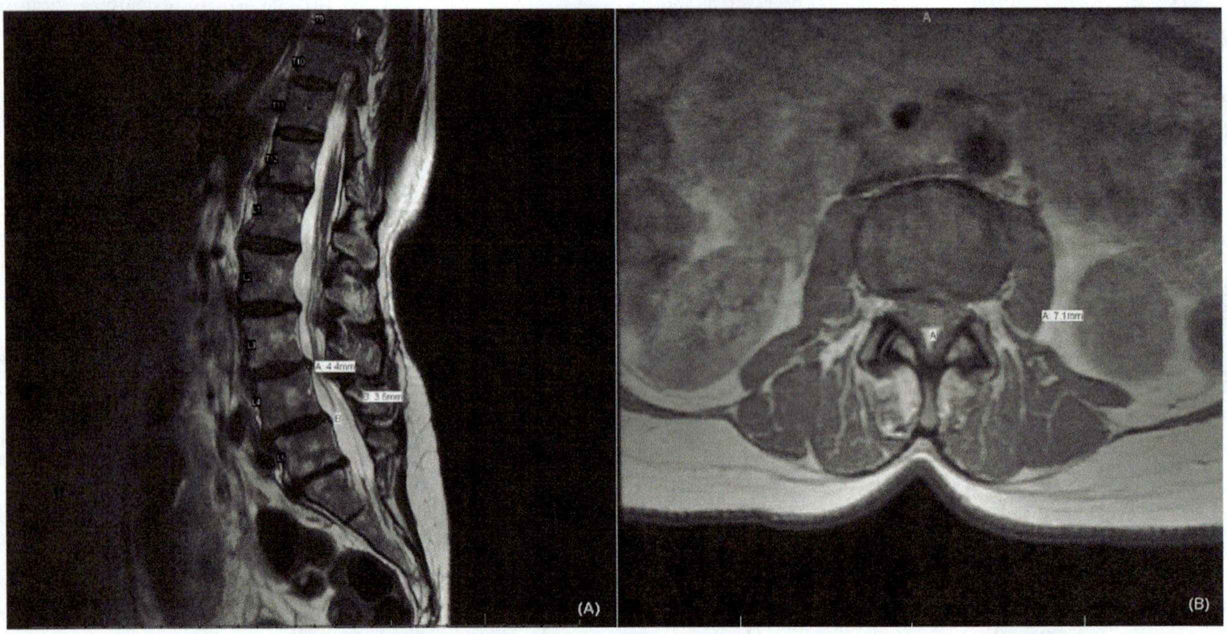

Figure 11.2 Patient follow-up imaging presurgery. Magnetic resonance imaging showing T2-weighted images of spinal stenosis. (A) Sagittal view of patient. Posterior disc osteophyte complex at L2–L3 with 2 mm anterolisthesis. Marked spinal canal narrowing. 4 mm anterolisthesis L3 over L4 with marked spinal canal narrowing. (B) Axial image of L3 segment.

QUESTIONS

1. What defines lumbar spinal stenosis (LSS) and neurogenic intermittent claudication (NIC)?
2. How is the epidemiology of LSS changing?
3. What is the underlying pain mechanism of LSS and NIC?
4. What is the natural history of LSS?
5. What are the clinical manifestations of LSS, and what are the key indications for diagnosis?
6. Is LSS a relentlessly progressive condition?
7. How is LSS managed?
    a. Nonsurgical approaches
    b. Surgical approaches
8. How will treatment for this condition evolve over the coming decade?

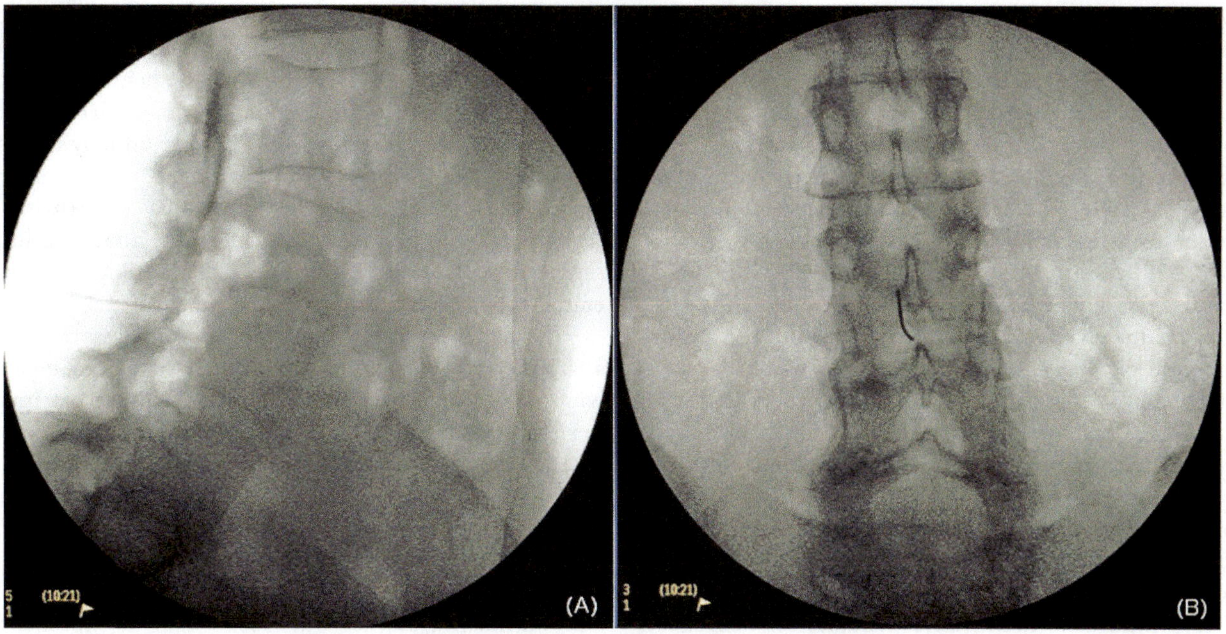

Figure 11.3 Patient epidural injection imaging. Interlaminar lumbar epidural steroid injection at level L3 using 20-gauge Tuohy needle with Depo-Medrol and saline. Contrast visible up to T12. (A) Lateral view of injection. (B) PA view of needle at L3.

WHAT DEFINES LSS AND NIC?

The distinctive pattern of pain in the lower back and legs commonly described as a "heaviness" or "deep aching" brought on by standing or walking readily distinguishes neurogenic claudication associated with LSS from other chronic LBP syndromes. This episodic pain problem is typically induced by erect postures and remits with lumbar flexion. The evoked low back and leg symptoms associated with lumbar stenosis are characteristically "intermittent" to the extent that they are predictably eased with sitting or lying down. NIC is a major cause of impaired mobility and loss of independence in seniors.[1]

NIC is the hallmark of the clinical syndrome of LSS, but patients with narrowed spinal segments are at increased risk for bouts of radicular pain as well.

HOW IS THE EPIDEMIOLOGY OF LSS CHANGING?

The advent of axial imaging technologies has increased the sensitivity of diagnostic testing for LSS over the past three decades.[2] In his 1954 landmark paper, the Dutch surgeon Henk Verbiest correlated progressively worsening leg pain and impairment of motor function experienced upon standing and walking with a narrowed spinal canal.[3] Pain with walking, so-called claudication, was presumed to be to be caused by peripheral vascular disease involving the aortoiliac system until Verbiest demonstrated that such a symptom pattern could be reliably alleviated with resection of the spinal laminae.[4] The relatively young age of symptom onset in the patients in Verbiest's initial series of seven patients, ranging between 37 and 67 years, contrasts with the epidemiology most commonly associated with the diagnosis of LSS today. At that time, life expectancy in the United States was only 68.2 years, whereas today it is 83.[5] The cumulative degenerative osteoarthritic processes, loss of paraspinal muscle tone, and vascular changes during these additional 15 years of life span are thought to contribute to a marked increase in symptomatic lumbar stenosis. Recent epidemiological studies support an accelerating demographic shift, with most patients seeking treatment for symptomatic LSS being over the age of 60 at the time of diagnosis.[6]

Approximately 1.2 million physician office visits annually in the United States are attributed to symptoms of LSS.[7] Pain, NIC in particular, is the predominant symptom pattern leading to evaluation and treatment.[8] For this chronic pain problem, approximately 89,000 laminectomy procedures were performed in the United States in 2009.[9] The prevalence of degenerative LSS and associated cost is expected to soar as the number of persons aged 60 years or older quadruples to approximately 2 billion worldwide in the year 2050.[10]

A recent prospective study compared 345 individuals to determine associations between demographic factors and physical characteristics for patients with degenerative LSS.[11] The study found that females who were significantly heavier and shorter than average were more prone to develop spinal stenosis. Additionally, males who performed heavy manual labor and/or had diabetes mellitus and females who were primarily housekeepers were more likely to develop LSS.

A cross-sectional study of 1,862 community-dwelling individuals who were diagnosed with LSS showed a clear trend of prevalence gradually increasing with age.[12] Less than 10% of the population was younger than 50; approximately 15% of the population with LSS were aged 55–64. Twenty percent of the population was identified as aged 65–69, and the female population's prevalence increased to 45–50% for ages 70 and older, whereas the prevalence of LSS in males remained approximately 20–30%.

As life expectancy is extended, patients will seek more treatment for recurrent symptoms of neurogenic claudication in the years following initial surgical treatment.[13] The benefit of lumbar laminectomy has consistently been shown to wane over time. The benefit from repeat decompression is inferior to initial procedures across multiple studies.[13,14] Based on 2007 estimated life expectancies, approximately one-third of patients who undergo laminectomy will experience approximately 10 years of recurrent neurogenic claudication following their initial decompression. Further surgical decompression of the spinal canal is a more complex proposition and is associated with greater perioperative risk.[15] The risk is further elevated because subsequent decompressive procedures are more likely to require instrumentation to prevent the long-term sequelae of spinal instability.[16,17]

The rapidly growing population of patients for whom the risk of surgery may outweigh the benefit highlights the need to develop innovative noninvasive therapies for neurogenic claudication. Older patients with impaired mobility are less likely to live independently. Reduced activity tolerance further exacerbates many comorbid conditions that affect elderly patients, such as obesity and diabetes.[18]

WHAT IS THE UNDERLYING PAIN MECHANISM OF LSS AND NIC?

Spinal stenosis is defined as a narrowing of the spinal canal caused by degeneration of osseous and intraspinal soft tissues.[19] Disc degeneration, facet joint capsule hypertrophy, infolding of the ligamentum flavum, and osteophyte formation culminate in a reduction in the volume of the spinal canal in the acquired or degenerative type of LSS.[20] Spinal stenosis broadly refers to any site of narrowing in the central canal, lateral recess, or intervertebral foramen. In the elderly, these subtypes frequently occur together, as in the patient vignette presented in this chapter.[21] Older patients with congenitally narrow canals, thickened laminae, and short pedicles are at increased risk for acquired stenosis and may be expected to seek care for NIC at a younger age.

> Our patient suffers from the acquired form of stenosis. Age-related degeneration of spinal structures associated with the upright posture required for bipedal locomotion is, by far, the most common form of acquired stenosis.

Reduction in the height of the lumbar disc with normal aging figures prominently in segmental narrowing of the lateral recess and central canal. Age-related desiccation of the nucleus pulposus and resultant buckling of the dorsal annulus are most common at the L3 through L5 spinal levels.[22] Loss of disc competency increases biomechanical stress on the facet joints. Hypertrophy of the facet joints due to synovial overgrowth and subchondral bone formation observed in this patient's initial and follow-up MRI encroaches on the lateral aspect of the central canal (Figures 11.2 and 11.3, respectively). Progressive change in the angle and contour of these joints endows the canal with the classic trefoil form seen in the most severe cases. The loss of disc height also reduces tension on the elastic ligamentum flavum, which brings about inward buckling of the ligament. Diverse underlying disease processes may promote development of acquired lumbar stenosis, including Paget disease and rheumatoid arthritis. The realignment—stable or dynamic—of one anatomic lumbar segment in relation to adjacent levels in the context of degenerative spondylolisthesis is another important cause.[23]

The development of clinical symptoms associated with anatomic narrowing is critically related to posture in patients with LSS. Biomechanical studies have shown that forward flexion increases the cross-sectional area of the neural foramen by 12% on average. Lumbar extension narrows the canal and lateral recesses by an additional 15% over a neutral posture.[24] For this reason, our patient's symptoms are alleviated with the seated position and exacerbated by standing. Eighty percent of the population has degenerative changes in the spine evident on imaging studies, but most remain asymptomatic.[6,25] Multiple factors, in addition to posture and segmental narrowing, appear to separate mild from moderate to severe symptoms. The number of stenotic levels and effects of recurrent dynamic loading appear to influence the intensity of pain and extent of activity limitation with standing and walking.[26] Acknowledgment of the lack of sensitivity and specificity of static images in the recumbent position has led to the development of functional concepts of potential space such as spinal reserve capacity.[27]

The preeminence of surgical treatments that address canal stenosis has emphasized the precision of anatomic measurement. The concept of the transverse area of the dural sac has supplanted measurement of the anteroposterior diameter championed by Verbiest during the era of myelography, when a distance of less than 10 mm was equated with *absolute* stenosis.[28] The borderline minimum canal area between moderate and severe symptoms (e.g., inability to walk ≥500 meters) has consistently been shown in animal models and retrospective series to be in the 70 mm^2 range.[29] Lateral recess and neuroforaminal stenosis giving rise to unilateral symptom patterns have undergone far less systematic study; an anteroposterior dimension of less than 4 mm in the lateral recess is a threshold frequently cited as a critical level by experts.[30]

NEUROVASCULAR DYSFUNCTION

LSS and NIC have characteristic vascular and neuropathologic changes. MRI studies often provide rich detail of serpiginous dilation of the epidural venous plexus. Cadaveric studies reveal constriction of the nerve roots and hypertrophy of the pia arachnoid.[31] Watanabe described a characteristic reduction in number, collapse, and grossly visible congestion of veins proximal to the stenotic level. Large-caliber fiber dropout empty axons and varying degrees of demyelination are revealed with histological examination and scanning electron microscopy. Pia arachnoid adhesions, interstitial fibrosis, and thick-walled veins are present on nerve section, as are arteriovenous anastomoses. The clinical significance of the adhesive pia arachnoiditis may impede normal cerebrospinal fluid (CSF) flow and compromise cauda equina homeostasis.

> The absence of allodynia and hyperalgesia on our patient's clinical examination likely reflects the relative sparing of the dorsal root ganglion in this type of cauda equina injury and dysfunction but does not necessarily make a neuropathic pain mechanism less likely.

The episodic painful symptoms of mild to moderate NIC may be the consequence of endoneural edema; swelling in a constricted environment may produce mild levels of ischemia or arterial engorgement or further impairment of CSF diffusion of metabolites.[32] Only those cases of stenosis with severe cauda equina compression demonstrate the pathoanatomic finding of Wallerian degeneration.[33] Because treatments have focused on decompression of non-neural structures, less is known about the clinical significance of the vascular and neural changes. The neuroanatomic changes identified so far have been linked to the chronic inflammatory consequences of episodic neuroischemia presented in the next section.

PATHOPHYSIOLOGY OF NIC

Narrowing of the spinal canal in many does not equate to pain and would not explain the waxing and waning course of symptoms associated with relatively stable lumbar stenosis. For example, the patient in our vignette experienced symptoms of a subacute L4 radiculitis in her initial presentation despite having moderate stenosis; this may be explained by lateral recess stenosis at L3–L4 with compression of the L4 traversing nerve root. A compelling account of the pathophysiology must at once account for the many patients with stenosis who experience no pain or highly variable pain intensity despite an unchanged anatomic environment.[25] Increases in pressure applied to the cauda equina induce neurophysiologic and local hemodynamic alterations.[34,35] The complex relationship among recurrent inadequate blood flow, compromised metabolic status of the nerve roots, modulating inflammatory cell effects on the blood–nerve barrier, and the pain of NIC is unresolved.

Microcirculatory Derangement

Multiple lines of evidence establish the importance of diminished flow of CSF and arterial and venous blood in the pathophysiology of neurogenic intermittent claudication.[36] Elevated intraspinal pressures reduce the flow of CSF and may account for some the episodic symptoms our patient describes in her legs. Up to 58% of nerve root tissue nutrients are supplied by the CSF in porcine models.[37] The relatively thin epineurium and perineurium of the cauda equine dangling in the canal bathed in spinal fluid with their fenestrated outer layers enable this source of nutrition. Cauda equina metabolism appears to be critically dependent on CSF flow. It has been proposed that hypertrophic thickening of the pia arachnoid is the sine qua non of claudication pathology; however, tissue sampling is not a feasible way to confirm this hypothesis in our patient.[31] An adhesive pia arachnoiditis at the most stenotic L3–L4 level likely impairs diffusion of CSF; impaired permeability coupled with compromised CSF flow may provoke a localized hypometabolic state in the nerve root(s) at this segment. It is possible that mechanical compression may overwhelm these pathophysiological processes after a critical threshold of intraspinal pressure.

Microvascular arterial insufficiency of the nerve roots has been invoked to explain the spectrum of reversible symptoms in NIC.[39,40] Endothelial dysfunction that compromises neural metabolism of the cauda equina may provide a more compelling account of what is clinically observed in patients with a syndrome of NIC. That model would explain why this escalating pain does not culminate with infarction and irreversible deficits indicative of a cauda equine syndrome. An experimental constriction injury model in adult dogs characterized breakdown of the blood–nerve barrier. These investigators detected intraradicular edema with gadolinium-enhanced imaging.[41] Nerve root macrophage invasion coupled with increased vascular permeability appears to provoke an inflammatory neuritis.[42] The pathogenesis of NIC may be attributable to macrophage generation of interleukin (IL-1), tumor necrosis factor (TNF), and other mediators of the inflammatory process.[43] To the extent that administration of epidural steroids suppresses these pathways, reduction in pain intensity may be achieved.

WHAT IS THE NATURAL HISTORY OF LSS?

The insidious onset of neurogenic claudication in the setting of lumbar stenosis in the patient featured in the opening vignette is common. This moment in the clinical course is commonly heralded by a long history of recurrent episodes of central LBP.[44] A recent longitudinal, prospective, controlled cohort study of patients who declined or deferred decompressive surgery upheld the claim that LSS is not associated with relentlessly progressive neurologic deficit.[45] The authors concluded that the natural history of lumbar stenosis is characterized by fluctuation in symptom severity; there is a medium-term tendency toward modest improvement in patients who do not elect to undergo surgery. In his landmark study, Johnsson compared the course of 19 surgically untreated patients with myelographically defined LSS for a mean duration of 4 years. Eighty percent of these patients endorsed symptom patterns consistent with NIC. Severe neurologic deterioration was not identified in the untreated patients; nearly 60% of these patients were unchanged from the standpoint of symptom severity.[46]

The natural history of this condition is understood through the prospective, long-term observational studies made by Amundsen and colleagues and the Maine Lumbar Spine Study.[47] At 4 years, Amundsen found superior outcomes in a greater number of surgically treated patients, but the results of delayed surgery in patients in the conservative management group who crossed over were equivalent. Atlas

Table 11.1 NATURAL HISTORY OF LUMBAR SPINAL STENOSIS

ONSET	CLINICAL FEATURES	EXAMINATION FINDINGS	COURSE
• 25% of patients undergoing surgery have symptoms for 10 years • 50% have symptoms for over 2 years • 50% recall the initial symptom as back pain	• Nondermatomal bilateral lower extremity pain with exertion • 75% report relief with forward bending when standing • 13% of patients with stenosis have radicular pain	• Thigh pain following 30 seconds of lumbar extension ($p = 0.002$)[1] • Stooped posture • Wide-based gait • Abnormal Romberg	• Degenerative condition with a tendency for exacerbations and remissions • 15–45% report spontaneous improvement • 15–30% worsen significantly • 15% report stable symptoms

Adapted from Katz JN. *Arthritis and Rheumatism.* 1995;38:1236–1241; Atlas SJ, Deyo RA, Keller RB, et al. The Maine lumbar spine study, Part III: 1 year outcomes of surgical and nonsurgical management of lumbar spinal stenosis. *Spine* 1996;21:1787–1795; Swezey, RL. Outcomes for lumbar stenosis: A 5 year follow up study. *J Clin Rheumatol.* 1996;2:129–134; Johnsson K-E, Rosen I, Uden A. The natural course of lumbar spinal stenosis. *Clin Ortho Related Res.* 1992;279:82–86.

et al. found no difference in LBP relief, predominant symptom improvement, and current symptoms among those initially receiving conservative or surgical treatment at 8- to 10-year follow-up. Leg pain relief and back pain-related function as measured by the modified Roland Morris disability scale favored those managed surgically at the outset. In summary, the syndrome of LSS is characterized by periodic exacerbations and remittances (Table 11.1).[48]

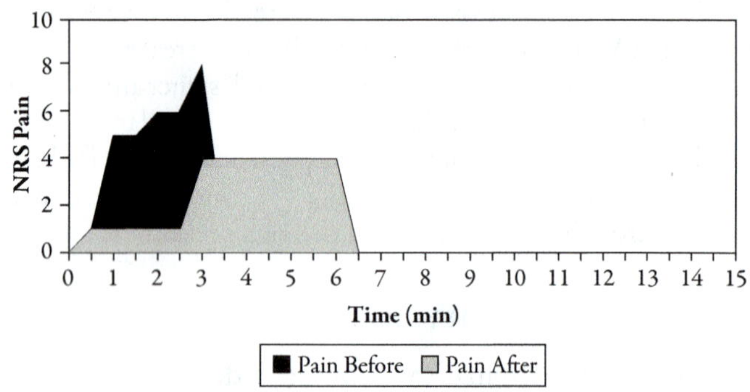

Figure 11.4 Numeric rating scale of patient pain pre- and postinjection. Patient walking on treadmill pre- and postinjection. The black area represents pain level prior to injection, reaching a maximum pain of 8/10 at 3 minutes and the walk ending at 3.5 minutes. The gray area represents pain level postinjection, reaching a maximum pain of 4/10 at 3 minutes and the walk ending at 6.5 minutes.

WHAT ARE THE CLINICAL MANIFESTATIONS OF LSS, AND WHAT ARE THE KEY INDICATIONS FOR DIAGNOSIS?

Increased utilization of axial imaging has produced a sharp increase in the diagnosis of LSS, but these technological refinements still do not differentiate symptomatic from asymptomatic patients. For this reason, it is essential to obtain a thorough history, perform a neurological examination, conduct functional testing, and place anatomic imaging results in a clinical context (Figure 11.4).

> The patient in our vignette describes rapidly declining walking tolerance. This adverse consequence of stenosis was having a negative impact on her physical and emotional health. She was unable to exercise and felt that her independence was being compromised.

Older age, severe lower extremity pain, and absence of pain when seated are the historical features most strongly associated (likelihood ratio ≥2) with the diagnosis of LSS in a group of 93 patients from three different specialty clinics.[44] Physical examination findings most closely associated with this diagnosis were a gait with widened base, abnormal Romberg test result, thigh pain following 30 seconds of lumbar extension, and neuromuscular deficits. The quality of the pain is classically described as dull or aching and characterized as "heaviness."

Because degenerative changes in multiple spinal structures are uniformly found in the elderly, the primary role of imaging in this population with chronic symptoms is to rule out other causes of pain, ensure the safety of interventional treatments, and plan surgical treatment. Imaging obtained in the supine position may underestimate stenosis that would be apparent in an upright, weight-bearing position; for this reason, some advocate myelographic images in the symptomatic standing posture or upright MRI.[49] Imaging acute, nonspecific LBP frequently yields diagnoses of LSS lacking clinical relevance and puts the patient at risk for unnecessary treatment.[50] If narrowing of the canal is observed and surgery is considered, computed tomography (CT) combined with myelography (CTM) will provide the most sensitive picture of posture-dependent anatomic targets; however, the benefit of added detail is counterbalanced by the risks of an invasive procedure and radiation exposure. In CTM, myelography is first performed with the patient in flexed and extended standing postures.[51]

Because the degree of narrowing observed in imaging often does not correlate to the severity of symptoms, functional testing is an essential supplement to imaging in patients with induced symptoms with standing and walking. Treadmill testing has repeatedly been shown to be a safe, easy, and reliable method of assessing a patient's disease severity and response to treatment.[52,53] The unique clinical phenomenology of neurogenic claudication lends itself to objective measure because of its direct impact on the duration of standing and walking tolerance. The value of an endpoint that links pain intensity and function is clear to the patient who times his medication dose to enable a walk from his parked car to a store. The capacity to assess dose-dependent responses to therapy over time is also critical to the task of adapting treadmill-based methods to the evaluation of novel treatments. The incorporation of baseline treadmill testing will allow for more precise treatment matching for surgical therapies and ultimately guide dose titration of emerging therapeutics.

DIFFERENTIAL DIAGNOSIS

Although NIC associated with LSS is a common condition, other etiologies may create a similar symptom pattern, especially in the elderly, and should be considered. One benefit of MRI is that it screens for nondegenerative causes of pain such as a tumor, infection, and vascular causes in circumstances where risk factors or so-called red flags are present. These are rare causes of spinal pain but may be life-threatening and not respond to decompression or epidural steroids. Clinical evaluation should exclude aortic aneurysm, visceral diseases such as pyelonephritis, and systemic inflammatory conditions including polymyalgia rheumatica. The differential diagnosis includes vascular claudication that will not be affected by posture and is less likely if peripheral pulses are palpable (Table 11.2). Vascular claudication may coexist with NIC and should be ruled out with flow studies if there is clinical suspicion. Far more often, the diagnostic challenge is parsing the low back and leg pain of lumbar stenosis from other mechanical causes of pain localizing to soft tissues, joints, and bony sources. Herniated lumbar disc with corresponding level radiculitis and peripheral neuropathy are common considerations. As in this patient's case, neuroforaminal stenosis/lateral recess stenosis predisposed her to a bout of radiculitis 2 years earlier. An acute lumbar disc extrusion typically has a distinctive temporal pattern marked by rapid onset of symptoms and other examination features, such as pain elicited with straight leg raise testing; radiculitis may occur in the absence of disc mechanical compression. Inflammation associated with facet-mediated pain is typically associated with axial-predominant symptoms. Because postures such as standing and walking require lumbar extension that loads the facet joint, pain evoked by a mechanical syndrome can overlap with LSS and mimic the distribution and pattern of symptom provocation. Osteoporotic compression fractures have a distinctive pattern of symptom onset (i.e., rapid), commonly cause pain in the seated and supine position, and have a distinctive set of imaging correlates. NIC and osteoporotic compression fractures may coexist when there is concurrent stenosis at the symptomatic level caused by an associated change in canal dimensions due to a retropulsed bone fragment. Electrophysiological techniques such as the tibial F-wave are rarely useful in distinguishing between LSS and peripheral neuropathy in cases where multiple neuropathic syndromes exist unless performed in the rested and symptomatic states. NIC is the key distinguishing feature of lumbar stenosis (Table 11.3). Case reports of pain provoked by extension and exertion that remits with rest has been reported in cases of tumors of the conus medullaris and cauda equina, benign cystic lesions, and vascular malformations, but these instances are exceptional.

IS LSS A RELENTLESSLY PROGRESSIVE CONDITION?

LSS is the leading indication for lumbar surgery in the United States for persons older than 65 years of age.[54] Treatment approaches for lumbar stenosis target the distinctive pain of NIC. As in our patient vignette, worsening activity interference with standing and walking and escalating pain intensity compel patients to seek care. The decision to pursue treatment for a fluctuating symptom pattern is highly personalized. Change in societal beliefs about the experience of pain, expectations for function, and the goal of independent living beyond the seventh decade of life are preferences that drive increased utilization of all treatments for chronic LBP.[55]

Table 11.2 NEUROGENIC CLAUDICATION VERSUS VASCULAR CLAUDICATION

	NEUROGENIC	VASCULAR
Pathology	Mechanical and/or ischemic	Ischemic
Type of Pain	Radicular (present or absent)	Cramping (continuous)
Relief for pain	Adjustment of posture or sitting	Rest
Location of pain	Sciatic/Lumbosacral	Exercised muscles
Diagnostic Tool	Magnetic resonance imaging (MRI), computerized tomography (CT), and/or myelogram	Aortography
Pulsation	Normal; no apparent bruit	Decreased; may present with arterial bruit
Motor deficit	Variable; may be exacerbated by walking	Not common

Reprinted with permission from Binder DK, Schmidt MH, Weinstein PR. Lumbar spinal stenosis. *Semin Neurol.* 2002 Jun;22(2):157–166.

Table 11.3 CARDINAL FEATURES OF NEUROGENIC INTERMITTENT CLAUDICATION

Anatomic Distribution	**Lumbar and legs**
Temporal Pattern	**Fluctuating with periodic exacerbations**
Key Exacerbating Factor	**Standing and walking**
Key Alleviating Factor	**Postures that reduce the lumbar lordosis**

Increased reliance on diagnostic imaging by primary care and specialty providers alike is another powerful driver of surging demand for treatment.[56]

There is wide variation in the rates of utilization of different diagnostic and treatment methods. The surgical literature focusing on decompressive laminectomy provides the vast majority of evidence related to outcomes of LSS treatment. There is a robust evidence base supporting the efficacy of laminectomy, but there is little consensus about optimal timing, advantages of newer techniques and technologies, durability of functional improvement, and benefit of surgery compared with nonsurgical approaches. There is a major gap in understanding with respect to the controlled evaluation of conservative management.[57,58]

HOW IS LSS MANAGED?

NONSURGICAL APPROACHES

In elderly patients at risk for perioperative complications and in those with mild to moderate symptom severity, surgical treatment is often not preferred.[63] In these groups of patients and the substantial number of patients with neurogenic claudication that recurs years after surgery, conservative treatment may be more appropriate.[47,60] The most common intervention for this problem is self-directed activity modification. Many patients control their experience of pain by curtailing time spent standing or the distances walked.

The other ubiquitous patient-initiated strategy to control pain is forward flexion at the lumbar spine. Patients experiencing NIC often unconsciously modify their posture to mitigate symptoms; others classically report extended walking tolerance when adapting to an activity, such as when leaning on a shopping cart. Using a walker or walking stick promotes this postural adjustment; such appliances are likely the most common solution for NIC. Shared decision making is of paramount importance because even the most advanced cases of LSS are so rarely associated with irreversible neurologic deficit. Decision making in cervical and thoracic stenosis levels where the spinal cord may be compressed must weigh the prospect of irreversible neurological deficit differently. At these spinal levels, surgical decompression frequently spares permanent neurologic deficit such as a weakness, spasticity, or loss of bladder control.

Studies of nonoperative treatment for LSS advocate exercise regimens that improve range of motion (e.g., reduce hamstring tightness) and include strengthening, general stretching, the McKenzie method of passive end-range stretching exercises, and conventional physical therapy modalities. Although there is robust evidence that exercise appears to increase the rate of return to normal activities in patients with persistent LBP, virtually none of these studies focuses on study populations with LSS or the symptom pattern of NIC.[61] Exercises that strengthen the abdominal core muscles (e.g., recti) and promote mobility of the lumbar paraspinal muscles may offer benefit because they can help stabilize the lumbar spine and minimize lordosis.[62] Cardiovascular conditioning can be beneficial by promoting weight loss because heavier patients may be at increased risk for degenerative changes leading to stenosis.[63] Several studies of conservative or nonoperative treatment with a variety of physical therapy approaches described a majority (~70%) of patients who perceived no worsening of their symptoms and a far smaller number (~15%) who reported improvement.[61] In Simotas's study, the surgical groups tended to report greater reduction in leg pain intensity and improved activity tolerance, but nearly a third of conservatively managed patients in one cohort study reported no pain or minimal pain at 36 months. McGregor's meta-analysis included 373 patients from three studies and determined that patients following a specific active rehabilitation program once or twice weekly, starting 6–12 weeks postsurgery, had reduced back pain and improved ability to carry on with their everyday tasks, both in a 6-month and 1-year follow-up.[64]

There is scant evidence supporting the use of oral analgesics for the symptom pattern of NIC. There is no double-blind, placebo-controlled trial of an oral analgesic medication for neurogenic claudication. There is a single, unblinded drug trial specifically targeting this condition with gabapentin. In that study, 55 patients were randomized to conservative management with corset and NSAIDs or gabapentin (max 2,400 mg/d) in addition to conservative therapy over the course of 4 months. The patients in the gabapentin group demonstrated a statistically significant increase in walking distance and a decrease in the intensity of low back and leg pain (visual analog scale [VAS] scale) upon movement. The results of this trial have not been replicated and should be interpreted with caution because of the enhanced placebo effect expected with lack of blinding. Porter reported 11 patients with improved walking tolerance associated with calcitonin 100 units administered four times per week for 4 weeks.[65] This polypeptide hormone secreted by the parafollicular cells of the thyroid was thought to possess both analgesic and anti-inflammatory properties, in addition to its role in the promotion of osteoclastic bone resorption that accounts for its efficacy in Paget disease. A large well-designed double-blind, randomized, placebo-controlled trial of a nasal spray formulation did not demonstrate improvement in pain or walking time to first pain. Additional nonrandomized studies have reported an improvement in pain scores, but, in a second randomized, well-designed study, the benefit compared with placebo did not reach statistical significance.[66]

Anti-inflammatory therapy with NSAIDs and more selective cyclo-oxygenase (COX-2) inhibitors have analgesic benefit compared with placebo in the minimally detectable range for chronic LBP.[67] There are no trials available to be included in this meta-analysis using the neurogenic claudication study population. There is evidence supporting the use of opioids for chronic LBP,[60] but their analgesic benefit in NIC is unstudied (Table 11.4).

Lumbar epidural steroid injections are commonly administered for the treatment of NIC in LSS.[72,73] The rationale for this treatment is reduction of the intraradicular edema and inflammatory cell infiltration associated with the pain of NIC.[41] Tomkins-Lane objectively measured the physical activity of 17 patients who received epidural steroid injections; by 1 week postinjection, more than 50% of subjects demonstrated increased total activity as well as increased maximum continuous activity; however, neither value was statistically significant.[74] A recent study compared pain relief from CT-guided lumbar epidural steroid injection among 47 patients who were graded into different severities of LSS. The study found that the grade of LSS severity had no effect on the degree of pain relief associated with the injection, with 77.6% patients reporting improvement after 8 weeks.[75] Delport described the outcomes of epidural steroid injection in a retrospective review of 140 patients. One-third experienced relief for greater than 2 months, and more than 50% of patients demonstrated an improvement in walking tolerance.[76] One recent study was unable to determine the critical spinal canal dimensions, as measured by CT scanning, that would be more predictive of a response to interlaminar epidural steroid injection.[77] A second retrospective study showed reduction in pain intensity that correlated with the number of stenotic levels and degree of stenosis except in patients with greater than three levels of involvement and MRI findings rated as severe.[78] There are no prospective, placebo-controlled studies evaluating the use of epidural steroid injection specifically for spinal stenosis. This therapy is often considered a second-tier conservative approach to managing NIC in patients who wish to avoid surgery.

SURGICAL APPROACHES

Dating to its original conception as a disease caused by bony anatomic changes, clinical study of lumbar stenosis has emphasized surgical treatment. Decompressive laminectomy aims to afford pain relief, improve mobility, preserve neural tissue, and prevent worsening of clinical deficits if present. There are multiple surgical techniques in widespread use, ranging from multilevel decompressive laminectomies, unilateral decompressive hemilaminectomy, and multilevel laminotomy with a fenestrating technique that preserves the interspinous ligaments. The technique typically involves excision of the ligamentum flavum and partial removal of the laminae; medial facetectomies and foraminotomies are often performed as well.

Surgical treatment is still considered the most effective treatment modality in patients with symptomatic lumbar stenosis and NIC.[7] As seen in Table 11.5, patients of one study were capable of walking for a longer period of time and had delayed onset of symptoms following surgical treatment. Turner's attempted meta-analysis from 1991, which included 74 studies of laminectomy, found good to excellent outcomes at long-term follow-up of 64%. The rates of successful surgical outcomes vary widely.[7,79] The authors' critique of the surgical literature described heterogeneity with regard to patient population, patient selection, and outcome measures. Since that time, several prospective, long-term, observational follow-up studies attempting to evaluate conservative versus surgical treatment have been completed. Weinstein's Spine Patient Outcomes Research Trial (SPORT) enrolled 654 patients who were separated into either a randomized or an observational cohort.[80] After 2 years, 67% of patients who were randomly assigned to surgery underwent surgery, whereas 43% of patients randomly assigned for nonsurgical treatment also

Table 11.4 **LOWER BACK PAIN DRUG TRIALS DUE TO NEUROGENIC CLAUDICATION**

AUTHOR	YEAR	DRUG	OUTCOME	# PATIENTS
Eskola et al.[68]	1992	Calcitonin (subcutaneous)[a]	Calcitonin > Placebo	39
Podichetty et al.[58]	2004	Calcitonin (nasal)[a]	Calcitonin = Placebo	47
Tafazal et al.[69]	2007	Calcitonin (nasal)[a]	Calcitonin = Placebo	37
Yaksi et al.[70]	2007	Gabapentin + conservative management vs. conservative management alone	Gabapentin > Conservative Management	55[b]
Matsudaira et al.[71]	2009	Limaprost vs. Etodolac	Limaprost > Etodolac	66[b]
Waikakul et al.[72]	2000	Methylcobalamin vs. Control	Methylcobalamin > Control	152

[a]As compared to placebo

[b]Open label

Reprinted with permission from Tran de QH, Duong S, Finlayson RJ. Lumbar spinal stenosis: a brief review of the nonsurgical management. *Can J Anaesth.* 2010 Jul;57(7):694–703.

Table 11.5 **VALIDITY OF TREADMILL TESTING**

	TIME TO FIRST SYMPTOMS (MINS)		TOTAL AMBULATION TIME (MINS)	
	Mean	Median	Mean	Median
Preoperative	1.82	0.58	6.91	5.22
Post Operative	11.93	15.0	13.26	15.0

Reprinted with permission from Deen, HG, Zimmerman RS, Lyons MK, et al. Use of the exercise treadmill to measure baseline functional status and surgical outcome in patients with severe lumbar spinal stenosis. *Spine* 1998; 23(2):244–248.

Note: The data listed are from a study designed to determine the validity of treadmill testing as an objective measure of pain levels for patients with lumbar spinal stenosis. Postoperative values were 3 months postoperation.

underwent surgery. Although there was a high level of nonadherence between the cohorts, intention-to-treat analysis of the randomized cohort showed a significant positive effect due to surgery in improving bodily pain. There was no difference between the surgical and nonsurgical patients for physical function or on the Oswestry Disability Index.

Surgery has been repeatedly shown to improve short-term outcomes, but long-term outcomes are less favorable as compared with other approaches.[14,81] The Maine Lumbar Spine Study found that for patients with persistent radicular leg pain, radiologic signs of stenosis, nerve root compression, and no previous back surgery, outcomes are superior with surgery than with conservative care.[13] The consensus emerging from this body of research is that deferring surgical intervention does not preclude a favorable outcome at a later date.

A recent cohort study of long-term outcome of laminectomy in octogenarians (average age at time of surgery 82.2) with follow-up at 1.5 years resulted in an improvement in back-related functional status (Oswestry Disability Index) consistent with results in younger age groups and reduction in pain intensity and use of opioid and NSAID analgesics.[17] The authors cited the low complication rate in this small group (i.e., perioperative delirium in three patients and persistent bladder dysfunction in one patient) as support for the use of this treatment in older patents. As in other age groups, one-third of patients remained dissatisfied with their surgical outcome.

Depression has a relatively high prevalence (36% in one cohort, $n = 3{,}801$) in patients with LSS and has been associated with higher pain intensity, worsened functional status, and poorer surgical outcomes.[82] Although conservative treatment is the first choice of treatment in LSS, surgery is indicated for patients who do not experience sufficient relief.[83] A recent prospective observational study determined that patients who have had poorer surgical outcomes are associated with greater depression. The study evaluated the outcome of surgery with the Oswetry Disability Index, VAS pain assessment, and self-reported walking capacity, and depressive symptoms were assessed with the Beck Depression Inventory. Based on a 5-year follow-up of 62 patients, a correlation existed between a high depressive burden with higher Oswestry Disability Index scores. The most common cause of poor outcomes relates to poor selection of patients; however, clear data on which patients are the best candidates for this surgery are lacking.[79,84] Coexisting cardiovascular morbidity and scoliosis also predict poorer patient rating of outcome. Longer baseline walking tolerance, higher self-rated health, higher income, reduced coexisting disease, and pronounced central stenosis predict a more favorable outcome.[85]

Using a shared decision-making model, patients should be counseled that the likelihood of benefit from laminectomy will likely be limited in the case of multilevel stenosis; functional gains may also be reduced in the context of a coexisting musculoskeletal disorder. One commonly cited liability specific to laminectomy is compromise of the structure of the lumbar motion segment that in turn may lead to further degeneration, excessive or abnormal motion, or deformity. Lumbar fusion was thought to have the benefit of providing definitive stabilization along with decompression. Since the introduction of new fusion technologies, the Washington State registry has found a 32% greater likelihood of reoperation after the first year postoperatively following an initial fusion compared to decompression alone for the indication of LSS.[86] A 2-year follow-up study involving 5,390 patients compared the outcome of patients who received decompressive surgery only versus patients who had decompressive surgery with fusion.[87] Using the National Swedish Registry for Spine Surgery as a database, the authors found no significant difference in patient satisfaction between the two treatment groups for any of the outcome measures—thus, the addition of fusion to decompression was not associated with an improved outcome in this cohort.

A retrospective analysis using national administrative data found that surgical management of patients with LSS and scoliosis increased from 2004 to 2009.[9] The rate of decompression decreased from 58.5% of 94,011 patients in 2004 to 49.2% of 102,107 in 2009. Fusion rates have increased from 21.5% to 31.2%, whereas complex fusions occurred at the same frequency of 6.7%. The use of interbody devices increased from 28.5% to 45.1%. As of 2009, 26.2% of the patients with LSS without instability had a spinal fusion procedure; 82.7% of LSS patients with spondylolisthesis and 67.6% of patients with coexisting scoliosis had a spinal fusion procedure.

Interspinous process spacers are a relatively new class of implantable devices that have recently received FDA approval in the United States. This device introduces a relative kyphosis at the level of insertion, reducing extension while allowing flexion.[88] Various designs ranging from static spacers to dynamic (i.e., spring-like) are surgically inserted between adjacent spinous processes at the culprit level. This type of approach was first tried in the 1950s but fell out of favor because of a tendency of the device to become displaced over time.[89] The first approved device in this class, the X-STOP, has an indication for mild to moderate NIC on the basis of a multicenter, prospective randomized trial with 191 patients.[90] Many features of the study design and the use of the NIC as an endpoint represent significant advances in the evaluation of treatments for LSS. At 2 years, there was a significant improvement in symptoms and function as compared with epidural steroid injection and conservative therapy. One important limitation is the use of a single epidural steroid injection in most patients as a comparator when the half -life of the injected anti-inflammatory medication is relatively short-lived. The authors compared the outcomes of the X-STOP placement to Katz's study of laminectomy but highlighted the higher risk of complication for laminectomy (12.6% from the Turner meta-analysis). Interspinous process spacers require smaller exposure, local anesthesia, and less time than laminectomy but at a significantly higher cost. The challenge of identifying the culprit level of stenosis that correlates with symptoms is more crucial than ever with the use of spacers because there is not the flexibility to extend resection as in the case of laminectomy. Implantation of such devices may prove to be a safer option for elderly patients than the traditional, more invasive procedures but longer term follow-up is needed.

Another study compared 498 patients who received interspinous devices to a matched laminectomy patient to determine which procedure was more effective in terms of costs and recovery.[91] The laminectomy cohort had a longer length of stay (2.5 days vs. 1.6 days, $p < .0001$) and index hospitalization, and 90-day complications were higher in the laminectomy cohort. However, the interspinous device cohort had significantly higher reoperation rates at a 1-year follow-up (12.6% vs 5.8%, $p = .026$) and incurred higher cumulative costs in that period ($39,173 vs. $35,324, $p = .289$). A randomized controlled trial of 159 patients compared the success rate of interspinous device patients to standard bony decompression.[92] The study found that only 63% of interspinous device patients were determined to be successful, based on a disorder-specific functional score obtained by the Zurich Claudication Questionnaire, versus a 72% success rate with conventional decompression. There was no difference of disability detected between the two groups, but the study also found that repeat surgery was substantially higher at 29% for the interspinous group as compared to the conventional group at 6.8%.

A recent study has suggested that minimally invasive surgery through endoscopic laminotomy and foraminotomy may be beneficial in treating patients in comparison to open decompression surgery.[93] The use of minimally invasive surgery is believed to be beneficial due to short operative time, low operative complication rate, minimally estimated blood loss, and reduced pain and disability level in contrast to open decompression surgery.

HOW WILL TREATMENT FOR THIS CONDITION EVOLVE OVER THE COMING DECADE?

The patient vignette underscores the unmet clinical need for nonsurgical therapies for NIC, the primary symptom of LSS for which patients seek treatment.

Neuro Animal models have revealed key insights into the underlying pain mechanisms of NIC and validated a host of therapeutic targets that may be amenable to medical treatment. The adaptation of treadmill-based clinical trial methodologies, developed to assess surgical outcomes, provide compelling endpoints to assess the efficacy of novel therapies. The regulatory pathway for therapies targeting NIC has been opened with the recent approval of a novel class of spinal devices. A new generation of nonsurgical therapies for the treatment of LSS and NIC will offer the possibility of improved mobility and independence throughout the life span.

REFERENCES

1. Weiner DK. Office management of chronic pain in the elderly. *Am J Med.* 2007;20(4):306–315.
2. Bennett, G. Neuropathic pain: an overview. In: Borsook D, ed. *Molecular Neurobiology of Pain, Progress in Pain Research and Management.* Vol. 9. Seattle, WA: IASP Press; 1997.
3. Verbiest H. A radicular syndrome from developmental narrowing of the lumbar vertebral canal. *J Bone Joint Surg Am.* 1954;36*B*(2):230–237.
4. Sugar O. Jean-Francois Bouley. *Spine.* 1994;19:346–349.
5. National Center for Health Statistics. *Health, United States, 2006: With Chartbook on Trends in the Health of Americans.* Hyattsville, MD: US Dept. of Health and Human Services, Centers for Disease Control and Prevention; 2006.
6. Kauffman C, Garfin SR. Spinal stenosis: pathophysiology and symptom complex update 1999. *Semin Spine Surg.* 1999; 11(3):209–214.
7. Knowledge Enterprises. *The Ortho FactBook.* 5th ed.; Chagrin Falls, OH: Author; 2005.
8. Turner JA, Ersek M, Herron L, Deyo R. Surgery for lumbar spinal stenosis: attempted meta-analysis of the literature. *Spine.* 1992;17:1–8.
9. Bae HW, Rajaee SS, Kanim LE. Nationwide trends in the surgical management of lumbar spinal stenosis. *Spine.* 2013;38(11):916–926.
10. *An Aging World 2001.* U.S. Department of Commerce, UN Department of Public Information, DP/2264; March 2002.
11. Abbas J, Hamoud K, May H, et al. Socioeconomic and physical characteristics of individuals with degenerative lumbar spinal stenosis. *Spine.* 2013;38(9):E554–E561.
12. Otani K, Kikuchi S, Yabuki S, et al. Lumbar spinal stenosis has a negative impact on quality of life compared with other comorbidities: an epidemiological cross-sectional study of 1862 community-dwelling individuals. *Sci World J.* 2013;Article ID 590652:1–9.
13. Atlas SJ, Keller RB, Wu YA, Deyo RA, Singer DE. Long-term outcomes of surgical and nonsurgical management of lumbar spinal stenosis: 8–10 year results from the Maine lumbar spine study. *Spine.* 2005;300:936–943.
14. Postacchini F. Spine update surgical management of lumbar spinal stenosis. *Spine.* 1999;24:1043–1047.
15. Katz JN, Stucki G, Lipson SJ, et al. Predictors of surgical outcome in degenerative lumbar spinal stenosis. *Spine.* 1999;24:2229–2233.

16. Deyo RA, Ciol MA, Cherkin DC, et al. Lumbar spine fusion: a cohort study of complications, reoperations, and resource use of the Medicare population. *Spine.* 1993;18:1463–1470.
17. Galiano K, Obwegeser AA, Gabl MV, et al. Long-term outcome of laminectomy for spinal stenosis in octogenarians. *Spine.* 2005;30(3):332–335.
18. Loureiroa ML, Nayga RM. Obesity, weight loss, and physician's advice. *Soc Sci Med.* 2006;62(10):2458–2468.
19. Porter RW. Spinal stenosis and neurogenic claudication. *Spine.* 1996;21:2046–2052
20. Andersson GBJ. Surgical aspects on lateral spinal stenosis: indications and principles. *Acta Orthop Scand.* 1993;64(Supp 251):74–75.
21. Onel D, Hidayet S, Cigdem D. Lumbar spinal stenosis: clinical/radiologic therapeutic evaluation in 145 patients. *Spine.* 1993;18:291–298.
22. Lewin, T. Osteoarthritis in lumbar synovial joints. A morphologic study. *Acta Orthop Scand Suppl.* 1964;73:1–112.
23. Akuthota V, Lento P, Sowa G. Pathogenesis of lumbar spinal stenosis pain: why does an asymptomatic stenotic patient flare? *Phys Med Rehabil Clin N Am.* 2003;14:17–28.
24. Inufusa A, An HS, Lim TH, Hasegawa T, Haughton VM, Nowicki BH. Anatomic changes of the spinal canal and intervertebral foramen associated with flexion-extension movement. *Spine.* 1996;21(21):2412–2420.
25. Boden SD, Davis DO, Dina TS, Patronas NJ, Wiesel SW. Abnormal magnetic-resonance scans of the lumbar spine asymptomatic subjects. *J Bone Joint Surg Am.* 1990;72:403–408.
26. Johnson KE, Rosen I, Uden A. The natural course of lumbar spinal stenosis. *Clin Orthop Rel Res.* 1992;279:82–86.
27. Weisz GM, Lee, P. Spinal canal stenosis. *Clin Ortho Rel Res.* 1983;178:134–140.
28. Verbiest H. Neurogenic intermittent claudication in cases with absolute and relative stenosis of the lumbar vertebral canal (ASLC and RSLC), in cases with narrow lumbar intervertebral foramina, and in cases with both entities. *Clin Neurosurg.* 1973;20:204–214.
29. Ogikubo O, Forsberg L, Hanson T. The relationship between the cross-sectional area of the cauda equina and the preoperative symptom of central lumbar spinal stenosis. *Spine.* 2007;32:1423–1428.
30. Eisenstein S. Lumbar vertebral canal morphometry for computerized tomography in spinal stenosis. *Spine.* 1983;8:187–191.
31. Watanabe R, Parke WW. Vascular and neural pathology of lumbosacral spinal stenosis. *J Neurosurg.* 1986;64:64–70.
32. Sekiguchi M, Konno S, Anzai H, et al. Nerve vasculature changes induced by serotonin under chronic cauda equina compression. *Spine.* 2002;27:1634–1639.
33. Powell HC, Myers RR. Pathology of experimental nerve compression. *Lab Invest.* 1986;139:28–38.
34. Blau JN, Logue V. Intermittent claudication of the cauda equina: an unusual syndrome resulting from central protrusion of a lumbar intervertebral disc. *Lancet.* 1961;1:1081–1086.
35. Rydevik B, Brown M, Lundborg G. Pathoanatomy and pathophysiology of nerve root compression. *Spine.* 1984;9:7–15.
36. Rydevik B. Neurophysiology of cauda equina compression. *Acta Orthop Scand.* 1993;64(Supp 255):52–55.
37. Olmarker K, Rydevik B, Hansson T, Holm S. Compression-induced changes of the nutritional supply to the porcine cauda equine. *J Spinal Dis.* 1990;3:25–29.
38. Watanabe R, Parke WW. Vascular and neural pathology of lumbosacral spinal stenosis. *J Neurosurg.* 1986;64:64–70.
39. Takahashi K, Olmareker K, Holms S, et al. Double –level cauda equina compression: an experimental study with continuous monitoring of intraneural blood flow in the porcine cauda equina. *J Orthop Res.* 1993;11(1):104–109.
40. Rydevik BL, Pedowitz RA, Hargens AR, et al. Effects of acute, graded compression on spinal nerve root function and structure: an experimental study of the pig cauda equina. *Spine.* 1991; 16(5):487–493.
41. Kobayashi S, Uchida K, Takeno K, et al. Imaging of cauda equina edema in lumbar canal stenosis by using gadolinium enhanced MR imaging: experimental constriction injury. *Am J Neuroradiol.* 2006;27:346–353.
42. Kobayashi S, Baba H, Uchida K, et al. Localization and changes of intraneural inflammatory cytokines and inducible-nitric oxide induced by mechanical compression. *J Ortho Pres.* 2005;23:771–778.
43. Sekiguchi M, Kikuchi S, Myers RR. Experimental spinal stenosis. *Spine.* 2004;29(10):1105–1111.
44. Katz JN, Dalgas M, Stucki G, et al. Degenerative lumbar spinal stenosis: diagnostic value of the history and physical examination. *Arthritis Rheum.* 1995;38(9):1236–1341.
45. Haig, AJ, Tong HC, Yamakawa KSJ, et al. Predictors of pain and function in persons with spinal stenosis, low back pain, and no back pain. *Spine.* 2006;31(5):2950–2957.
46. Johnsson KE, Uden A, Rosen I. The effect of decompression on the natural course of spinal stenosis: a comparison of surgically treated and untreated patients. *Spine.* 1991;16:615–619.
47. Amundsen T, Weber H, Nordal H, et al. Lumbar spinal stenosis: conservative or surgical management. *Spine.* 2000;25:1424–1436.
48. Atlas SJ, Keller RB, Robson D, et al. Surgical and nonsurgical management of lumbar spinal stenosis. Four-year outcomes from the Maine Lumbar Spine Study. *Spine.* 2000;25:556–562.
49. Saint-Louis LA. Lumbar spinal stenosis assessment with computed tomography, magnetic resonance imaging, and myelography. *Clin Orthop Rel Res.* 2001;384:122–136.
50. Jinkins JR. MR evaluation of stenosis involving the neural foramina, lateral recesses, and central canal of the lumbosacral spine. *MRI Clin North Am.* 1999;7(3):493–511.
51. Willen J, Danielsson B, Gaulitz A, et al. Dynamic effects on the lumbar spinal canal. *Spine.* 1997;24:2698–2976.
52. Tenhula J, Lenke LG, Bridwell KH, et al. Prospective functional evaluation of the surgical treatment of neurogenic claudication in patients with lumbar spinal stenosis. *J Spinal Disord.* 2000;13(4):276–282.
53. Deen GH, Zimmerman RS, Lyons MK, et al. Test-retest reproducibility of the exercise treadmill examination in lumbar spinal stenosis. *Mayo Clin Proc.* 2000;75(10):1002–1007.
54. Taylor VM, Deyo RA, Cherkin DC, Kreuter W. Low back pain hospitalization: recent US trends and regional variations. *Spine.* 1994;19:1207–1211.
55. Friedly J, Chan L, Deyo R. Increases in lumbosacral injection in the Medicare population. *Spine.* 2007;32(16):1754–1760.
56. Ciol M, Deyo R, Howell E, Kreif S. An assessment of surgery for spinal stenosis: time trends, geographic variations, complications, and reoperations. *J Am Geriatr Soc.* 1996;44:285–290.
57. Vogt M, Kwoh C, Cope D, Osial T, Culyba M, Starz T. Analgesic usage for low back pain: impact on health care costs and service use. *Spine.* 2005;9:1075–1081.
58. Podichetty V, Segal A, Lieber M, Mazanec D. Effectiveness of salmon calcitonin nasal spray in the treatment of lumbar canal stenosis: a double-blind, randomized, placebo-controlled, parallel group trial. *Spine.* 2004;29:2343–2349.
59. Deyo RA. Back surgery—who needs it? *N Engl J Med.* 2007;356(22);2239–2243.
60 . Simotas AC, Dorey FJ, Hansraj KK, et al. Nonoperative treatment for lumbar spinal stenosis: clinical and outcome results and a 3-year survivorship analysis. *Spine.* 2000;25(2):197–204.
61. Van Tulder MW, Malmivaara A, Esmail R, Koes BW. Exercise therapy for low back pain. *Cochrane Database Syst Rev.* 2000;2:CD000335.
62. Nagler W, Hausen HS. Conservative management of lumbar spinal stenosis: identifying patients likely to do well without surgery. *Postgrad Med J.* 1998:103(4):69–88.
63. US Dept. of Health and Human Services Agency for Healthcare Research and Quality. Treatment of degenerative lumbar spinal stenosis: summary. *Evidence Report/Technology Assessment.* 2001;32:1–5.
64. McGregor AH, Probyn K, Cro S, et al. Rehabilitation following surgery for lumbar spinal stenosis. *Cochrane Collab.* 2013;12:1–54.

65. Porter RW, Hibbert C.Calcitonin treatment for neurogenic claudication. *Spine*. 1983;8:585–592.
66. Porter RW, Miller CG. Neurogenic claudication and root claudication treated with calcitonin: a double-blind trial. *Spine*. 1988;13:1061–1064.
67. van Tulder MW, Scholten RJ, Koes BW, Deyo RA. Nonsteroidal anti-inflammatory drugs for low back pain: a systematic review within the framework of the Cochrane Collaboration Back Review Group. *Spine*. 2000;25:2501–2513.
68. Eskola A, Pohjolainen T, Alaranta H, Soini J, Tallroth K, Slätis P. Calcitonin treatment in lumbar spinal stenosis: a randomized, placebo-controlled, double-blind, cross-over study with one-year follow-up. *Calcif Tissue Int*. 1992 May;50(5):400–403.
69. Tafazal SI, Ng L, Sell P. Randomised placebo-controlled trial on the effectiveness of nasal salmon calcitonin in the treatment of lumbar spinal stenosis. *Eur Spine J*. 2007 Feb;16(2):207–212. Epub 2006 Jul 25.
70. Yaksi A, Ozgonennel L, Ozgonenel B. The efficiency of gabapentin therapy in patients with lumbar spinal stenosis. *Spine (Phila Pa 1976)*. 2007 Apr 20;32(9):939–942.
71. Matsudaira K, Seichi A, Kunogi J, et al. The efficacy of prostaglandin E1 derivative in patients with lumbar spinal stenosis. *Spine (Phila Pa 1976)*. 2009 Jan 15;34(2):115–120.
72. Waikakul W, Waikakul S. Methylcobalamin as an adjuvant medication in conservative treatment of lumbar spinal stenosis. *J Med Assoc Thai*. 2000 Aug;83(8):825–831.
72. Cummins J, Lurie JD, Tosteson TD, et al. Descriptive epidemiology and prior healthcare utilization of patients in the spine patient outcomes research trials three observational cohorts. *Spine*. 2006 31;7:806–814.
73. Rydevik BL, Cohen DB, Kostuik JP. Spine epidural steroids for patients with spinal stenosis. *Spine*. 1997;22:2313–2317.
74. Tomkins-Lane CC, Conway J, Helper C, Haig AJ. Changes in objectively measured physical activity (performance) after epidural steroid injection for lumbar spinal stenosis. *Arch Phys Med Rehabil*. 2012;93:2008–2014.
75. Park CH, Lee SH. Correlation between severity of lumbar spinal stenosis and lumbar epidural steroid injection. *Pain Med*. 2014;;15:556–561.
76. Delport EG, Cucuzella AR, Marley JK, et al. Treatment of lumbar spinal stenosis with epidural steroid injections: a retrospective outcome study. *Arch Phys Med Rehab*. 2004;85:479–484.
77. Campbell MJ, Carron LY, Glassman SD, McGinnis MD, Elmlinger BS. Correlation of spinal canal dimensions to efficacy of epidural steroid injection in spinal stenosis. *J Spinal Disord Tech*. 2007;20:168–171.
78. Kapural L, Mekhail N, Bena J, et al. Value of the magnetic resonance imaging in patients with painful lumbar spinal stenosis undergoing lumbar epidural steroid injections. *Clin J Pain*. 2007;23:571–575.
79. Katz JN, Lipson ST, Larson MG, et al. The outcome of decompressive laminectomy for degenerative lumbar stenosis. *J Bone Joint Surg*. 1991;73-A:809–816.
80. Weinstein JN, Tosteson TD, Lurie JD, et al. Surgical versus nonsurgical therapy for lumbar spinal stenosis. *N Engl J Med*. 2008;358:794–810.
81. Weinstein JN, Lurie JD, Tosteson TD, et al. Surgical versus nonsurgical treatment for lumbar degenerative spondylolisthesis. *N Engl J Med*. 2007;356(22):2257–2270.
82. Herron L, Turner J, Clancy S. et al. The differential utility of the Minnesota multiphasic personality inventory: a predictor of outcome in lumbar laminectomy for disc herniation versus spinal stenosis. *Spine*. 1986;11:847–850.
83. Pakarinen M, Vanhanen S, Sinikallio S, Aalto T, Lehto SM, Airaksinen O, Viinamäki H, Depressive burden is associated with a poorer surgical outcome among lumbar spinal stenosis patients: a 5-year follow-up study. *Spine J*. 2014;doi: 10.1016/j.spinee.2014.01.047.
84. Deen HG, Zimmerman RS, Lyons MK, et al. Analysis of early failures after lumbar decompressive laminectomy for spinal stenosis. *Mayo Clin Proc*.1995;70(1):33–36.
85. Aalto, TJ, Malmivaara A, Kovacs F, et al. Preoperative predictors for postoperative clinical outcome in lumbar spinal stenosis: systemic review. *Spine*. 2006;31: E648–E663.
86. Martin BI, Mirza SK, Comstock BA, et al. Reoperation rates following lumbar spine surgery and the influence of spinal fusion procedures. *Spine*. 2007;32:382–387.
87. Försth P, Michaëlsson K, Sandén B. Does fusion improve the outcome after decompressive surgery for lumbar spinal stenosis? *Bone Joint J*. 2013;95-B:960–965.
88. Lindsey DP, Swanson KE, Fuchs P, et al. The effects of an interspinous implant on the kinematics of the instrumented and adjacent levels in the lumbar spine. *Spine*. 2003;28:2192–2197.
89. Bono CM, Vaccaro AR. Interspinous process devices in the lumbar spine. *J Spinal Disord Tech*. 2007;20:255–261.
90. Zucherman JF, Hsu KY, Hartjen CA, et al. A multicenter, prospective, randomized trial evaluating the X STOP interspinous process decompression system for the treatment of neurogenic intermittent claudication: two-year follow-up results. *Spine*. 30(12):1351–1358.
91. Patil CG, Sarmiento JM, Ugiliweneza B, et al. Interspinous device versus laminectomy for lumbar spinal stenosis: a comparative effectiveness study. *Spine J*. 2013;13:01501–01505.
92. Moojen WA, Arts MP, Jacobs WCH, et al. Interspinous process device versus standard conventional surgical decompression for lumbar spinal stenosis: randomized controlled trial. *Br Med J*. 2013;347:f6415. doi: 10.1136/bmj.f6415.
93. Polikandriotis JA, Hudak EM, Perry MW. Minimally invasive surgery through endoscopic laminotomy and foraminotomy for the treatment of lumbar spinal stenosis. *J Orthop*. 2013;10:13–16.

12.

LUMBAR DISC DISPLACEMENT

Mehul J. Desai, Jeffrey D. Petersohn, Joseph O'Brien, Mathew Cyriac, and Chili Lati

CASE PRESENTATION

A 34-year-old man presents with 3 weeks of low back and left leg pain. The pain started at home following a recent move in which he was lifting boxes. The pain is described as a constant aching with a shooting sensation radiating to the outside of his left leg to the ankle with an occasional feeling of numbness. He denies weakness, falling, or bowel/bladder/sexual dysfunction. The pain is made worse by lifting and physical activity. An Urgent Care physician diagnosed him with lumbar sprain and prescribed oxycodone/acetaminophen 5/325 PO q4h as well as cyclobenzaprine 10 mg PO q6h. He does note some relief of pain with oxycodone and rest. The patient is referred to the Interdisciplinary Spine Pain clinic for further evaluation and management.

Past medical history is significant for heartburn treated with over-the-counter omeprazole.

Review of systems is otherwise negative.

On examination, the patient weighs 92 kg and is 186 cm tall. He is afebrile with normal vital signs. His neurologic examination shows decreased sensation to pinprick in the web-space between the left first toe and second toe, and he has difficulty with long toe extension. His lower lumbar spine is tender to deep palpation. Special testing is positive for straight leg and slump tests on the left.

A magnetic resonance image (MRI) of the lumbar spine reveals a large left paracentral disc extrusion at L4–L5.

QUESTIONS

1. What causes back pain and radicular pain secondary to disc herniation?
2. What is the incidence of disc herniation and related disability?
3. What are the clinical manifestations of lumbar disc displacement, how is it diagnosed, and what other entities are entertained in the differential diagnosis?
4. How is disc herniation managed?
    a. Rehabilitation
    b. LDD classification
    c. Physical therapy assessment
    d. Pharmacological management
    e. Interventional limits of the medical literature
    f. Other minimally invasive interventions
    g. Surgery

WHAT CAUSES BACK PAIN AND RADICULAR PAIN SECONDARY TO DISC HERNIATION?

Multiple studies have demonstrated the occurrence of radiographic abnormalities in the lumbar spine in asymptomatic individuals.[1,2] The clinician's approach to the disc herniation with radiculopathy must attempt to balance the known pathophysiology of pain generation while reconciling the physical examination and radiographic findings with technical considerations for treatment. Following Mixter and Barr's landmark publication in 1934, direct mechanical compression or irritation of the nerve root by a herniated disc has often been viewed as the sole etiology of pain in lumbar disc herniation with radiculopathy.[3] Although most patients do obtain resolution of pain without the necessity for surgery, some patients fail to obtain the expected pain relief following surgical excision of the putatively offending disc fragment. Accordingly, this simple mechanistic view has been superseded by a more complex pathophysiology in which inflammatory mediators produce a final common pathway of neural hyperirritability accompanied by enhanced neural pain processing at the dorsal root ganglion and perhaps within the central nervous system (CNS) as well. We have also begun to understand that one of the common presentations of symptomatic lumbar internal disc disruption is a persistent or recurrent radiculopathy, also without evidence of neural compression.

Kuslich first showed that application of nucleus pulposus extract to a nerve root initiated mechanical sensitivity of the nerve root at the time of surgery.[4] Cuellar further demonstrated that increases in epidural cytokines and neuropeptides such as interleukin (IL-6), tumor necrosis factor-α

(TNF-α) and interferon-γ (IFN-γ) follow specific exposure to the nucleus pulposus and that this might be prevented by co-application of a soluble IFN-γ antibody.[5] IL-6 has been experimentally shown by Murata to initiate apoptosis in the dorsal root ganglia (DRG).[6] Removal or suppression of the effects of these mediators forms the rational basis of the interventionist's most common therapeutic approach: administration of epidural steroid injections (ESI). ESI are typically performed following a period of unsuccessful conservative treatment. Because IL-6 may exert some of its effects via the cyclo-oxygenase system, which can be modulated by nonsteroidal anti-inflammatory drugs (NSAIDs) or steroids, oral agents of one or both of these classes are typically part of a conservative care regimen, although a recent systematic review showed little evidence of clinical success to support this practice.[7] Whereas TNF-α is a major initiator of disc nuclear catabolism, a recent clinical trial showed the TNF-α antagonist, etanercept in epidural application was markedly inferior to either epidural steroid or saline.[8] Epidural lavage with detection of a fibronectin-aggrecan aggregate may be useful in determining which patients will likely benefit from ESIs[9]; this technique, however, is not yet available for routine incorporation in clinical practice.

WHAT IS THE INCIDENCE OF DISC HERNIATION AND RELATED DISABILITY?

Disc herniation is a common cause of low back pain (LBP) disorders.[10–12] Within the literature, the prevalence of disc herniation varies considerably, ranging from 0% to 47% in asymptomatic and symptomatic patients.[13]

The annual prevalence of lumbosacral radiculopathy defined as LBP and leg pain traveling below the knee varies from 9.9% to 25%.[14] The most important risk factors for the development include being male, obesity, smoking, history of lumbago, anxiety and depression, work that requires lengthy periods of standing and bending forward, heavy manual labor, lifting heavy objects, and being exposed to vibration.[15]

> Our patient has multiple risk factors. Pain completely or partially resolves in 60% of patients within 12 weeks of onset; however, 30% of patients will continue to complain of pain at 1 year following onset.[16] In those under 50 years of age, herniated disc is the most common cause of lumbosacral radiculopathy.[17]

WHAT ARE THE CLINICAL MANIFESTATIONS OF LUMBAR DISC DISPLACEMENT, HOW IS IT DIAGNOSED, AND WHAT OTHER ENTITIES ARE ENTERTAINED IN THE DIFFERENTIAL DIAGNOSIS?

Typically, patients experience radiating pain that may be described as sharp, dull, piercing, throbbing, or burning. Forward flexion, sitting, bending, or Valsalva maneuvers may also exacerbate symptoms by transiently increasing posterior annular pressure.[15,17] Lumbar extension may worsen pain if there is compromise of the spinal canal or foraminal space by the herniated disc. Additionally, dermatomal paresthesias are often reported. Nondermatomal pain is more likely to be referred pain from other structures such as the sacroiliac joint or facet joints.

DEFINITIONS

Prior to further extrapolating this section, it may be worthwhile to pause to clarify the nomenclature. The common nomenclature interchanges sciatica, radicular pain, and radiculopathy. The International Association for the Study of Pain (IASP) classification guidelines define radicular pain as "that which arises in a limb or trunk wall caused by ectopic activation of nociceptive afferent fibers in a spinal nerve or its roots or other neuropathic mechanisms... [resulting from] lesions that directly compromise the dorsal root ganglion mechanically or indirectly compromise the spinal nerve and its roots by causing ischemia or inflammation of the axons."[18] By contrast, radiculopathy is defined as "objective loss of sensory and/or motor function as a results of conduction block in axons of a spinal nerve or its roots... [as a result of] any lesion that causes conduction block of axons of a spinal nerve or its roots either directly by mechanical compression of the axons or indirectly by compromising their blood supply and nutrition."[18] Radiculopathy and radicular pain are differentiated by the presence of objective neurological signs (numbness, weakness, positive electrodiagnostic testing [EDX]) due to conduction block versus symptoms caused by ectopic impulse generation.[18] They may coexist and may be caused by the same lesion. The IASP suggests that sciatica is a term that should be abandoned; it is often indiscriminately misused to describe symptoms attributed to the sciatic nerve and/or S1 nerve root.[18]

Diagnosis of radiculopathy based on positive nerve tension tests generally requires reproduction of concordant extremity pain with the nerve stretching maneuver. Neither buttock pain nor focal medial proximal calf pain on straight leg raise or sitting root maneuver ("slump" test) nor point-tenderness in the medial calf support a diagnosis of radiculopathy pain, although practitioners often wrongly report these as positive "radiculopathic" findings.[5,19,20] Unfortunately, positive nerve tension tests are only 70% sensitive, making a purely clinical diagnosis of radiculopathy challenging.

In the clinical case presented, a lateral disc herniation at L4–L5 appears to be the likely source of pain present in the left L5 nerve root distribution and resulting in objective sensory loss in the left L5 dermatome and weakness in the left L5 myotome—truly meeting the criteria for radiculopathy. The goal of this section is to briefly discuss pathophysiology and anatomy as they affect decisions for treatment, with a subsequent discussion of technical considerations and risks relevant to the choice of procedural treatment by the physician.

IMAGING FOR DIAGNOSIS

Estimation of the anatomic disc level causing pathology by history and physical examination only with subsequent non-image-guided ESI might be used to treat herniated nucleus pulposus (HNP) with radiculopathy as a cost-saving strategy, but due to lowered efficacy, this approach should likely be abandoned where imaging technology is readily available. Superior clinical outcomes are routinely obtained using MRI (or CT) to identify the anatomically compromised disc structure(s) followed by subsequent performance of ESI under image guidance. The substantial prevalence of asymptomatic disc herniation and bulges requires the physician to correlate any anatomic disc abnormality seen on CT or MRI imaging with the clinical presentation prior to considering intervention (e.g., a L2–L3 HNP is unlikely to be the source of L5 dermatomal distribution manifesting as lateral calf pain). As well, it is unreasonable to impugn a right-sided disc herniation as the source of a left sided radicular pain process. Central disc herniation, however, may in reality be more prominent to either left or right side, and the interventionist should consider reviewing imaging studies personally prior to deciding on the most appropriate intervention. Disc herniation, depending on the resolution of the imaging study as well as the thinness, number, placement, and orientation of the axial and sagittal imaging sections, may be ill-described due to poor imaging technique. Motion artifact can significantly compromise the quality of the study as well. It is the opinion of the authors that common imaging practices such as using 3.5–4 mm thick slices with three to five slices per disc level, especially if the slices are not aligned with the disc axis, are often insensitive for subtle details of anatomy including focal disc protrusions, small extrusions, or foraminal disc herniations that are often clinically relevant as sources of pain.

Imaging should be routinely obtained in 1.5 Tesla (or greater) closed MRI units or in 1.2 Tesla open MRI units, where possible. Due to markedly inferior spatial resolution, 0.3T open MRI units should be entirely abandoned for contemporary spinal imaging. As well, midfield 0.5–0.6 Tesla open MRI scans lack the diagnostic detail of studies performed on higher power MRI machines, relying on mathematical interpolative algorithms to approximate the more granular signal data obtained in high-field MRI machines. In the supine position used for MRI scan, patients are typically positioned with hips and knees flexed, which, by slightly flexing the lumbar spine, opens the vertebral canal and neural foramina. Some midfield 0.6T open MRI machines are capable of scanning the patient in standing, lumbar-flexed, or extended postures, which may be helpful when a supine scan is nondiagnostic. The flexed and extended images are more sensitive for changes in foraminal dimension, but the incidence of detected disc herniation pathology not seen on supine scan is rare overall.[21,22] In studying patients with symptomatic disc herniation and radiculopathy, Weishaupt noted that 6 of 36 patients could not complete the postural MRI due to pain, suggesting that although this modality may be sensitive, it may not be clinically feasible.[22] Zou studied 553 patients in a 0.6 Tesla open MRI to report statistically significant greater sensitivity of flexion-extension MRI views as compared with supine-only imaging for detection of small HNP of less than 5 mm in size (19% of patients with 1–3 mm HNP showed enlargement of HNP with flexion-extension view; 13% with 4–5 mm HNP demonstrated similar findings); however, an unspecified portion of the patient population had LBP without radiculopathy.[23] Although there may be a potential role for flexion-extension MRI sequences, the routine diagnostic utility of flexion-extension MRI sequences is far from proved and may not outweigh the less adequate image resolution delivered by these machines. In the case presented here, there is no doubt as to the presence of a disc herniation.

Whereas MRI is the generally preferred axial imaging modality due to lack of ionizing radiation, CT scanning can be used for patients with implanted devices such as cardiac pacemakers, defibrillators, some spinal cord or deep brain stimulators and metallic aneurysm clips, or bare metal stents or for severely claustrophobic patients. Newer high-resolution CT scanners using 16 or 64 detectors or newer panel detectors offer substantially improved imaging, including enhanced soft-tissue resolution, as compared with older devices.

Electromyography and nerve conduction studies known in combination as EDX are commonly utilized in the evaluation of lower extremity pain resulting from lumbar herniated disc. EDX demonstrate various strengths in diagnosing radiculopathy, including:[24]

1. Corroborating structural changes noted on MRI with physiologic abnormalities in the nerve root
2. Determining the most likely affected level and correlation between imaging and clinical symptoms
3. Investigating physiologic evidence of noncompressive radiculopathies
4. Assessing prognosis regarding axonal loss
5. Investigating other neurologic symptoms

EDX are very specific and rarely false positive, particularly when strict criteria for diagnosis are utilized. On the other hand, sensitivity is not high. Furthermore, some studies suggest interoperator variability; in one study, diagnosis agreement was only achieved 46.9% of the time.[25]

There are circumstances where clinical radiculopathy is present with an absence of findings on electrodiagnostic studies. Some limitations of EDX include:[24]

1. Inability to detect pure sensory radiculopathies; in these cases the site of nerve injury is proximal to the DRG resulting in normal sensory nerve conduction studies.[26]
2. Subtotal root involvement resulting in demyelination, which would not result in the characteristic changes evaluated for one needle EMG or limited axonal loss that might go undetected due to the number of axons involved

3. Circumstances in which denervation is balanced with reinnervation or old denervation where no fibrillations are seen

Some planning must be undertaken prior to performing EDX. Specifically, in lower extremity testing, a minimum of 5–6 muscles of various root and different peripheral nerve innervations should be selected for testing. Muscles in a similar region with innervation from the same peripheral nerve but different root levels should be considered. Six-muscle testing, including paraspinals, identified radiculopathy in 98–100% of patients.[27]

> In our patient, typical muscle selection would likely include lumbar paraspinals, gluteus medius, tibialis anterior, extensor hallucis longus, biceps femoris (short head), and tibialis posterior. Other muscles to consider would include tensor fascia lata, adductor longus, semitendinosus, peroneus longus, and gastrocnemius (medial/lateral head). H-wave testing may be useful specifically if S1 radiculopathy is suspected. Nerve conduction studies were performed but were normal in this patient. At 4 weeks following his injury, EDX testing demonstrated positive sharp waves and fibrillations in the extensor hallucis longus, tibialis anterior, and L5 lumbar paraspinals.

HOW IS DISC HERNIATION MANAGED?

REHABILITATION

Rehabilitation is an integral part of the comprehensive conservative management of lateral disc displacement (LDD). In addition to pharmaceutical management, physical therapy is often prescribed as an early intervention to manage symptoms and ultimately restore function in patients with LDD.[28–30] The goal of treatment is to alleviate symptoms associated with LDD, restore normal biomechanics of the spine, and guide patients to a full functional recovery. The outcome of a successful treatment is evaluated based on recovery of spine mobility, resolution of pain, restoration of function, and return to work.

LDD CLASSIFICATION

Many studies have been done to investigate effective approaches to diagnose and treat nonspecific LBP; however, successful management of LBP remains inconsistent.[31,32] Recently, there has been greater emphasis placed on investigating more specific diagnostic and treatment approaches in the rehabilitation of different types of LBP, including pain and dysfunction associated with LDD.

McKenzie is one of the early pioneers to apply the concept of response-based classification to differentially diagnose and treat LBP. McKenzie's Mechanical Diagnosis and Therapy (MDT) assesses the patient's response to treatment based on recovery of range of motion (ROM) and reduction of pain with the application of specific repetitive movement, positional modification, and spine loading techniques. With spine-related referred pain to the lower extremity, the MDT approach considers centralization of pain as an important outcome of a successful treatment.[33]

Centralization is typically defined as abolition of pain in a distal to proximal direction in response to a specific therapeutic intervention. It has been shown to be an important prognostic factor in the course of low back and related extremity pain. Patients with poor centralization in response to interventions are considered to be at greater risk of developing chronic pain.[34,35] In the presence of a multitude of treatment options (albeit limited healthcare resources), it is important that clinicians keep in mind the key prognostic factors that signpost progress and treatment outcome.

Other diagnostic and treatment classification systems can be used in managing lateral disc disease and directing rehabilitation. The work of Delitto and Erhard introduced treatment-based classification in which patients are categorized into different subgroups based on clinical signs, impairments, and types of LBP symptoms including severity and duration. Each patient subgroup is then assigned to a specific treatment based on their classification.[36] Subsequent studies refined the subgrouping of patients with LBP and examined the efficacy of specific treatments. Patients who have acute LBP and associated referred pain to the lower extremity are prescribed mobilization and exercises in the directional preference that promotes reduction of symptoms and increased spinal and functional mobility.[37,38]

Further studies are being done to fine tune the treatment-based classification algorithm and improve its clinical validity in guiding clinical decision making and the selection of effective physical therapy intervention.[39,40]

PHYSICAL THERAPY ASSESSMENT

In the case presented in this chapter, the patient suffers from L4–L5 LDD and associated pain referral to the lower extremity. A thorough physical therapy evaluation is essential and includes a subjective history and mechanism of injury, a neurological screen, assessment of motor and sensory deficits, ROM and spine mobility assessment, and, last, a postural and functional assessment that should include a standardized outcome measure.[41] The Oswestry LBP Disability Questionnaire is a valid and reliable outcome measure to assess overall patient function and progress with therapy.[42]

It is also important to assess acuteness of symptoms and tailor an appropriate treatment plan considering the patient's irritability and sensitivity in response to the intervention. With a disc displacement, the clinician should be diligent in monitoring neurological deficits and should notify the physician if significant changes are noted.[43]

Acute Phase

In the acute phase of injury, the patient may not initially tolerate aggressive exercises or manual intervention during physical therapy. As noted earlier, it is important to consider irritability and sensitivity of symptoms and monitor neurological changes when prescribing treatment for patients with LDD. To effectively manage symptoms especially in the acute phase, it is very helpful to communicate with the physician to provide adequate pharmaceutical management to control pain and inflammation so the patient can maximize benefit from physical therapy. Modalities such as electrical stimulation and ultrasound can be helpful in providing pain relief during the acute stage of injury and inflammation, although evidence is mixed with respect to their efficacy.[44,45]

Some studies advocate the use of spinal manipulation with acute LBP in a subset of patients who meet a specific clinical prediction rule.[46,47] However, in the presence of neurological deficits and radicular symptoms distal to the knee, spinal manipulation is not considered appropriate.

The clinician should initiate specific exercises indicated by the patient's directional preference and centralization of pain as soon as possible, keeping in mind the patient's tolerance to movement and general irritability of symptoms in response to treatment.[48,49] Extension-based exercises are shown to have good outcomes with patients who have LBP and referred distal lower extremity symptoms.[37] The patient is then gradually progressed to strengthening and functional training, with an emphasis on body mechanics and a gradual return to normal activities of daily living.

Subacute Phase and Return to Work

In the acute phase, rehabilitation is focused on managing pain and inflammation, restoring spine mobility, and gradual strengthening. Rehabilitation objectives differ when symptoms persist for longer durations. Maximizing function becomes the major focus in rehabilitation, whereas pain control is assigned less emphasis. Studies of subacute and chronic LBP advocate early mobilization to minimize disability and reduce sick leave resulting from work injuries.[28,50]

Also, fear avoidance behavior has been associated with a worse prognostic outlook for patients with LBP. Patients who have high fear avoidance behavior tend to have greater disability and work absenteeism.[51] It is therefore very important that the physical therapist encourages patients to stay active and engage in their normal daily activities even if they experience some increase in pain.

In the subacute phase of rehabilitation, the patient is prescribed more general strength and conditioning exercises that promote core stability and endurance. Education about positional modification, proper posture, and body mechanics will aid in preventing reinjury.[52]

In summary, rehabilitation should be tailored to the specific phase of injury and apply the appropriate therapeutic intervention to reduce pain and promote function. Communication with the physician and other members of the multidisciplinary healthcare team is important in achieving optimal and speedy patient recovery.

PHARMACOLOGICAL MANAGEMENT

Thematically, it may be important to consider the role of pharmaceutical agents in the management of pain related to lumbar disc herniation. Specifically in practice, medications are often first-line therapy with regards to early patient mobilization. Activity tolerance, particularly as it relates to physical therapy, may be significantly limited in the acute setting, and medications may allow patients to more fully participate in their treatment. Empirically speaking, NSAIDs, oral cortisone, and muscle relaxants are often considered in the acute setting, and attempts have been made to collate the role of NSAIDs and skeletal muscle relaxants on acute LBP.[53–55] Abdel Shaheed et al. concluded that there was limited evidence for efficacy of NSAIDs in the treatment of acute LBP, whereas, in 2008, Roelofs and colleagues suggested that NSAIDs were effective but their effect size was small.[53–54] In 2003, van Tulder reviewed the literature around muscle relaxants in the treatment of nonspecific acute LBP and concluded that these drugs were effective for short-term pain relief but adverse effects suggested caution in their use.[55]

Pharmacologic management with medications aimed at treating the neuropathic component of radiculopathy has achieved some albeit limited success.[56–62] These medications include gabapentinoids (pregabalin and gabapentin), the anticonvulsant topiramate, tricyclic antidepressants (such as nortriptyline), and the serotonin-norepinephrine re-uptake inhibitor antidepressant duloxetine. They are often referred to as *membrane stabilizers*.

The role of opioids in this disease state is much more controversial.[63] There is very little data to support the use of opioids beyond the acute setting in these patients. In fact, recent review articles articulate their efficacy over the short term with limited evidence for their longterm effect on or impact for improved function.

INTERVENTIONAL LIMITS OF THE MEDICAL LITERATURE

Whereas randomized clinical trials (RCTs) may represent a penultimate research standard, clinical decision making in evidence-based medical practice often relies on large well-conducted prospective and even retrospective studies. From a practical standpoint, realistic and foreseeable logistical and financial limitations will likely continually prevent the performance of RCTs on many spinal interventions.

The proper choice of comparison groups becomes a central challenge in clinical trials studying epidural injections. Because most inflammatory mediators are soluble, the selection of normal saline or local anesthetic epidural injection as control interventions may be confounded by a clinically efficacious lavage effect. As well, use of epidural lidocaine or ropivacaine alone suppresses microglial activation and cytokine production, thus possibly resulting in pain relief.[64,65]

In any study, a poorly chosen comparator group results in mathematical regression of experimental outcomes toward those seen in the control group, and, as a result, truly useful treatments may fail to demonstrate statistical efficacy with economically sized study populations. The minimal resources required to produce systematic literature reviews has led to their proliferation, which now threatens to outnumber original research trials. All derivative data analyses, including meta-analyses and systematic reviews, may be fatally poisoned by including papers lacking robust patient selection criteria. Readers are urged to read the "Methods" section in original supporting research publications before assuming that the conclusions of a published review are valid.

As will be discussed, skillfully performed ESI appear to be substantially helpful over both the short and intermediate term, and may allow patients to avoid surgery. Although large disc herniation are less successfully treated by ESI,[66] the direct mass effect of the herniated disc material compressing or impinging a nerve may be addressed, where necessary, by the using minimally invasive interventional or surgical techniques described later in this chapter to remove disc tissue.

INJECTION TECHNIQUES

When considering approaches to ESI, the anatomy and geometry of the epidural space must be taken into account. The interface between the nerve root and disc lies in the anterior epidural space; hence, medication delivered to the posterior epidural space or which otherwise fails to enter the appropriate hemiepidural space containing the anatomic target should be expectedly less effective. As in all injection techniques, absolute contraindications to epidural injection include coagulopathy, allergy to medications used, and local or systemic infection. Whereas pregnancy may contraindicate imaging with ionizing radiation, it is one of the few circumstances in which nonfluoroscopically guided ESI may be considered clinically optimal. Technical approaches to placement of an injection into the epidural space can be classified into three principal groups:

1. Posterior interlaminar approach
   a. Midline
   b. Paramedian oblique/parasagittal
2. Caudal epidural
3. Transforaminal
   a. Supraneural/subpedicular (selective nerve root)
   b. Retroneural
   c. Infraneural
   d. S1 transforaminal

The transforaminal technique is often referred to as a selective nerve root (SNR) injection, but we recommend reserving the SNR nomenclature for the anterior subpedicular technique in which the needle tip is placed just below the pedicle and posterior to the intervertebral body (Figure 12.1). Unfortunately, selectivity of the single nerve root injection is not preserved when injection volumes exceeding 0.5 mL are used,[67] but, when considering therapeutic approaches, multilevel spread may not be disadvantageous and indeed may be the basis for some efficacy.

Retroneural techniques place the needle into the upper third of the mid-posterior foramen, largely in an attempt to avoid the anterior vasculature, but ensuring injection of material into the anterior epidural space is less certain with this placement.

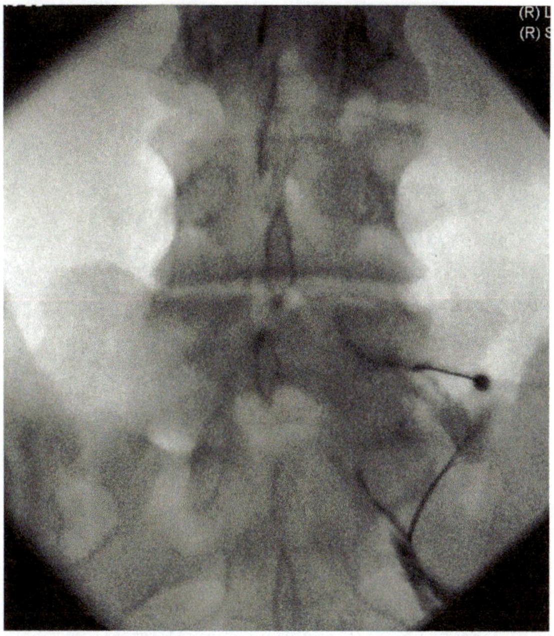

Figure 12.1 Right L5 and S1 transforaminal epidural steroid injections, subpedicular approach.

The infraneural technique uses a discography-like oblique imaging approach to place a needle or catheter just anterior of the superior articular process (which forms the posterior border of the lower lumbar foramen) and just posterior of the intervertebral disc. Jasper demonstrated that delivery of injectate to the anterolateral epidural space can be accomplished radiographically, although at the increased risk of inadvertent disc entry.[68]

Interlaminar approaches are favored by some practitioners due to the relative ease of identifying the posterior epidural space using the loss-of-resistance technique with which most anesthesiologists are familiar. Unfortunately, when performed without imaging guidance, about a third of these attempts do not access the epidural space.[69] A paramedian approach facilitates entry into a narrowed interlaminar space by avoiding the extended narrow entry trajectory imposed by adjacent dorsal spinous processes when using a midline approach (Figure 12.2). Often a pillow under the abdomen will decrease lumbar lordosis sufficiently to allow midline dorsal entry into the posterior epidural space. There remains an ongoing debate regarding the superiority of one technique versus another in the treatment of lumbar disc herniation.[70]

Injection of epidural steroid into the caudal canal to treat disc herniation at the L4–L5 and L5–S1 level has demonstrated substantial efficacy over conservative treatment,[71,72] but concerns have been raised regarding the necessity of using larger volumes of injectate with potential dilution of delivered steroid to reach the target disc/nerve level compared with interlaminar or transforaminal techniques.[73]

Although posterior interlaminar and caudal epidural approaches can be performed without imaging guidance, with historic data suggesting 50–66% rates of successful needle entry into the desired region of the lumbar epidural

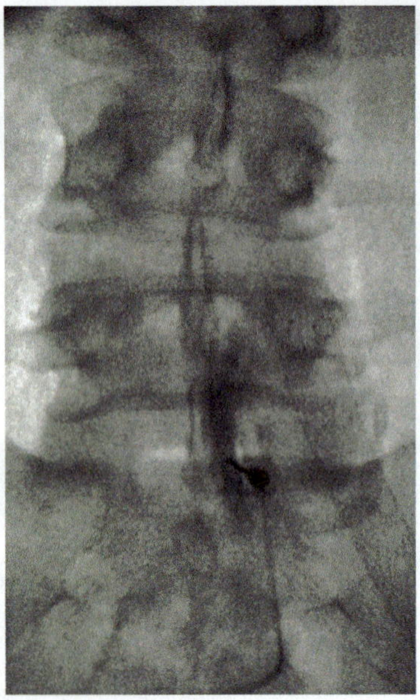

Figure 12.2 Right L5–S1 interlaminar epidural steroid injection, paramedian approach.

space, transforaminal epidural injection without image guidance has been constructively and appropriately abandoned in the United States for reasons of safety related to avoidance of needle trauma to spinal nerves.[69] Non-image-guided caudal injections have a slightly higher rate of successful entry into the caudal epidural space than do lumbar interlaminar injections but a less certain outcome. Non-image-guided injections incur lower costs, and recent changes in CPT coding have eliminated physician payment for fluoroscopic imaging, paradoxically incentivizing physicians to consider reducing efforts and expenditures by omitting fluoroscopy. Outcomes of non-image-guided lumbar epidural injections are prima facie inferior to fluoroscopically guided injections due to less frequent needle entry into a therapeutically useful anatomic space.[69] Electing to use less successful treatment strategies with lower upfront costs defers the consumption of additional healthcare resources necessary for treatment but irresponsibly imposes additional intangible costs on the patient and society resulting from reduced productivity, persisting pain, and disability. Holistic analysis shows non-imaging-guided injection to be neither clinically, economically, nor socially rational.

Risks and Complications

In discussing the interventional approach to lumbar disc herniation, issues of safety and potential complications must be considered. Principal risks of these techniques include inadvertent intravascular injection of air or drug, including gaseous or steroid particulate embolization of the arterial supply of the spinal cord, risks of direct or indirect drug toxicity, direct needle trauma to neurovascular spinal structures with resultant hematoma or neural injury, postdural puncture headaches, and infection.

The human spine has an extensive intraspinal and extraspinal vascular network, both arterial and venous. These collateral circulatory pathways involve radicular arteries, which pass through the neural foramina; lumbar spinal arteries paralleling the vertebral bodies; spinal perforating arteries; and the anterior/posterior spinal arteries, which ultimately supply the spinal cord. These arterial pathways are highly variable between individuals, and flow in these arterial systems can be easily reversed by inadvertent needle cannulation and injection during a spinal interventional procedure. Case reports of neural injury via the spinal cord arterial circulation due to embolic phenomenon have been reported with transforaminal injection, especially with upper left lumbar nerve root or S1 transforaminal approaches.[74] Remarkably, despite Furman's[75] observation of a relatively high incidence of intravascular injections following injection of radiographic contrast agent, permanent neural injury is thankfully rare.

Use of radiocontrast injection to demonstrate adequate and potentially efficacious placement provides unambiguous objective documentation of technical adequacy or, in some circumstances, of factors that prevent or limit clinical improvement with a satisfactorily placed injection, such as obstruction of epidural flow due to a large disc herniation. Smuck showed that injection of contrast agent followed by static fluoroscopic imaging is inferior to continuous fluoroscopy during contrast injection, which demonstrates inadvertent vascular injection in approximately 9% of transforaminal lumbar injections.[76] Whereas injection of contrast agent under continuous fluoroscopy often allows detection of inadvertent vascular injection, this is by no means foolproof, and this may, in part, be due to the difficulty of discerning fine detail in radiographic images where multiple overlapping structures are seen.

Jasper is first credited with suggesting the use of digital subtraction angiography (DSA) as an adjunct to spinal injection procedures in 2003.[77] Digital subtraction first obtains a digital X-ray image to form a mask that is then electronically "subtracted," pixel by pixel, from each subsequent digital image, yielding a composite image that then shows only the distribution of the injected contrast or other moving structures. The increased acquisition cost for digital subtraction capability has reduced the availability of this technology, as has concern for the increased ionizing radiation exposure incurred during DSA. The advantage of DSA is that the image of the normal osseous spinal anatomy is visually suppressed, thus allowing easier detection of the pattern of vascular or nonvascular contrast injection due to the absence of confluent radiographic shadows. As Jasper noted, the rare incidence of serious complications despite a substantial and known incidence of inadvertent intra-arterial injection during transforaminal injection would require the study of an unwieldy large population in order to prove the cost effectiveness of DSA technology in preventing neurologic injury.

McClean has shown that DSA is twice as sensitive as continuous fluoroscopy alone in detecting inadvertent vascular injection during cervical transforaminal injection (33% vs. 18%), but this incidence has not been specifically studied during lumbar transforaminal injections.[78] It is well to remember that although the risk of inadvertent injection might be dramatically reduced with DSA, a single case report has shown that, even with use of DSA, neural injury has not yet been rendered impossible.[79] The value of DSA is particularly decreased by patient movement because the pressure of injected contrast on an irritated nerve root can be exquisitely painful and lead to patient motion. Oblique views in particular may be helpful in imaging arterial flow into the lumbar or sacral radicular arteries. DSA adds an additional margin of safety, improving the sensitivity of detection of intravascular injection, but most specifically avoiding unwanted radicular artery injection although a substantial increase in X-ray exposure is incurred.

Alternative Imaging Techniques

For epidural injections, some partisans advocate imaging techniques that do not require ionizing radiation, such as ultrasound guidance. Clinical use of ultrasound, however, is limited to relatively thin patients and may be less suitable in patients with spinal deformity or prior surgery. Furthermore, ultrasound cannot routinely provide useful information to detect or prevent inadvertent vascular injection in the lumbar spine because flow in radicular arteries and epidural veins cannot be routinely visualized due to overlying echogenic osseous structures. Since Furman convincingly demonstrated that simple needle aspiration is insensitive to detect inadvertent vascular entry otherwise seen with contrast injection under fluoroscopy, ultrasound guidance combined with aspiration remains insufficient to assure safe nonvascular needle placement in the lumbar spine. At present, techniques using fluoroscopy or CT scanning must be regarded as superior to ultrasound at guiding needle placement into any desired portion of the lumbar epidural space. Ultrasound usefully demonstrates the sacral hiatus and can be used to facilitate technically adequate caudal placement. Unfortunately, ultrasound does not allow assessment of technically adequate delivery of drug to the appropriate subcompartment of the epidural space.

Where true patient allergy to the latest generation iodinated contrast agents exists, use of oral or parenteral steroid/antihistamine preoperatively may be considered to allow use of contrast agents. Consideration might be given to administration of gadodiamide, which although less radiodense than iohexol-240, may nonetheless be useful in demonstrating inadvertent vascular placement.

Particulate Versus Nonparticulate Steroids

Use of nonparticulate steroids, such as dexamethasone, has been suggested to avoid the risk of particulate emboli, which are blamed for watershed infarcts of the spinal cord and subsequent massive neurologic deficits or death. However, particulate steroid outcomes may be superior to dexamethasone, especially triamcinolone, where a 5.5/10 reduction in pain visual analog scores (VAS) was noted with ESI triamcinolone use as opposed to a 3.3/10 VAS reduction with dexamethasone.[80] Other reports on the cervical spine, however, did not find a difference between particulate and nonparticulate epidural steroids.[81] Nonetheless, powering a study to discern a difference between both types of steroids may require inclusion of hundreds of patients.[82] Betamethasone is inferred to have advantages similar to triamcinolone, but the particle size of betamethasone is smaller than that of triamcinolone, thus potentially reducing the risk of symptomatic embolic vaso-occlusion of the spinal arterial circulation.[83] The potential for gaseous emboli to create neurologic events is noted also, and practitioners are reminded to remove all air from syringes and extension tubing as a matter of good clinical practice.

Vascular Anatomy

Murthy studied thoracolumbar angiograms to quantify the course of the foraminal lumbar radicular arteries and showed that the vast majority of radicular vessels pass in the upper anterior foramen close to the usual location of the nerve, with few vessels present in the lower foramen.[84] Murthy concluded that the risk of inadvertent radicular artery injection would therefore be minimized by injection into the lower lumbar posterior foramen at nerve levels of L3 and cephalad. This finding suggested that inadvertent vascular entry might be reduced by choice of a retroneural technique.

Advantages and Disadvantages of Varied Injection Techniques

The posterior midline interlaminar epidural injection is the approach historically employed, adapted from techniques originally designed for surgical anesthesia more than a century ago. When a posterior interlaminar approach is used without fluoroscopic guidance and with a loss-of-resistance technique, approximately one-third of all injections fail to reach the desired posterior epidural space, thus increasing the likelihood of simple subcutaneous, intramuscular, or interligamentous injection of steroid.[69] Under fluoroscopic guidance, however, even adequate posterior epidural placement does not assure technically adequate delivery of medication into the anterolateral epidural space. Hogan investigated the anatomic relationship between the anterolateral and posterior epidural spaces, noting that flow into the anterolateral space depends on a pressure-driven gradient from the posterior epidural space.[85] Especially in unilateral pathology, an off-midline injection is common, and the steroid may not reach the intended anatomic target.

The interlaminar technique is typically the first, but sadly, often the only technique mastered by some practitioners. Its use may be stymied due to anterolisthesis or where reduction of disc space height narrows the interval between adjacent dorsal spinous processes. Entry into the epidural space is typically identified by loss-of-resistance technique. An alternative paramedian approach to posterior epidural space entry may be used by selecting a needle skin entry site approximately 2–3 cm inferior and 2–3 cm lateral to usual the site of midline epidural needle entry with subsequent adoption of a needle course that is more cephalad and mesiad in angulation than that usually employed for a midline entry. The needle is similarly directed through the interlaminar interval to enter the midline posterior epidural space.

Interlaminar epidural injection techniques can be modified with redirection of the needle tip to enter the dorsal epidural space in the interlaminar interval to target the lateral recess on the ipsilaterally symptomatic side. There is some speculation that this may produce superior outcomes versus approaches targeting the midline, but there is little robust data.[86] The principal risk of interlaminar injection technique in any region of the vertebral canal is dural puncture, and in patients younger than 60 years of age, a postdural puncture headache may occur.[87] This postural headache incidence should be reduced with concomitant use of fluoroscopy with loss-of-resistance technique when advancing the epidural needle, as well as with the use of smaller gauge needles and with vertical orientation of the needle bevel in line with the dural fibers.[87]

Caudal epidural injection appears to be of waning usefulness. Although not all caudal injections placed without fluoroscopy achieve entry into the caudal canal, there is less certainty of the relationship between the injected volume and the maximal cephalad level of drug delivered into the epidural space. Due to the large volume of injectate, the concentration of steroid is more dilute with caudal injection than with any other technique. Generally, if a caudal injection is contemplated, it should not be used with disc pathology at levels above L5–S1. Manchikanti reported an RCT of caudal lidocaine versus caudal steroid with roughly equal proportions of patients obtaining greater than 50% pain relief; he concluded that relief was superior after each injection in the steroid group, but each group required more than five injections on average over a 2-year period.[88] Although the control arm was clearly not a true placebo, one must question the rational clinical utility of any technique requiring more than five repetitions without demonstrated durability of response.

The S1 transforaminal injection is a special case in which the proximity and alignment of the anterior and posterior foramina allow a needle placed into the dorsal foramen to easily transit, passing misadventurously anterior to the sacrum where bowel or genitourinary entry can occur, thus opening the potential for infection as well as structural injury. As well, injected contrast often shows a predominance of contrast extravasation ventrally into the presacral space along the course of the ventral S1 nerve root and sacral plexus with little or no contrast outlining the preferred intraspinal course of the S1 nerve root. The use of lateral fluoroscopy is critical to assure that the injected contrast, and presumably any other injectate, flows cephalad along the course of the S1 nerve root.[89] Depending on the degree of sacral sagittal angulation, the AP fluoroscopic view can be misleading or confusing regarding the cephalad extent of drug or contrast spread. Achievement of cephalad contrast flow along the S1 root sometimes requires a needle tip position quite dorsal within the vertebral canal at S1. As well, often a large segmental S1 artery is present, and a live AP fluoroscopic view during contrast injection (or use of DSA) is necessary to visualize and avoid inadvertent arterial injection.

Outcomes

The transforaminal techniques are potentially the most efficacious because drug is delivered directly into the anterolateral epidural space along the course of the nerve root, an anatomically rational approach. If the disc height is normal, the typical lumbar nerve root occupies about half of the cross-sectional area at the neural foramen, except at L5–S1 where the nerve occupies about two-thirds of the area. The obvious risk of the transforaminal approach is direct needle trauma to the nerve, but inadvertent vascular entry where the radicular artery may be injected adjacent to the nerve root might be more common than expected. Unfortunately, the precise location of needle entry into the neural foramen retains a substantial bearing on clinical outcome, with Desai showing a fourfold superiority in achieving complete resolution of pain with needle placement in the superior-anterior foramen as opposed to the superior-posterior quadrant.[90]

Outcomes from transforaminal lumbar epidural techniques enjoy strong literature support as determined in contemporary reviews by Benny, Rho, Ghahreman, Manchikanti, and MacVicar with level II-1 evidence supporting their use.[91–95] Interestingly, the best outcomes from transforaminal technique involve disc herniation with only modest levels of nerve compression, with 75% of such patients having good outcomes.[96] Lee, in an unusual analysis of data, reports that superior outcomes were obtained with foraminal or extraforaminal herniation, with other MRI features being nonprognostic.[97]

Traditionally, the practitioner chooses an injection level to deliver steroid to the nerve that is anatomically compressed or impinged by the herniated disc, and this can be referred to as "postganglionic" injection. In the case of an L4–L5 disc herniation, the L4 nerve root would be considered "preganglionic" and the L5 nerve root would be considered "postganglionic." There is evidence of moderate short-term superiority of transforaminal injection made at the nerve level above the disc herniation (i.e., preganglionic). Jeong showed that at 1-month follow-up, 88% of patients treated at the preganglionic level had good to excellent results versus 71% using the postganglionic level.[98] At 6 months, however, the improvement in both groups averaged 49%, without a sustained statistically significant difference. Park's data are slightly less affirmative, but show a similar magnitude of effect.[99] These papers did not stratify foraminal from central or lateral recess herniation nor from herniated discs with extrusion.

Use of infraneural technique with injections made just caudad to the spinal nerve but immediately posterior to the disc herniation might be considered to have potential superiority by allowing both pre- and postganglionic nerve root delivery, but Park and Kim both demonstrated entirely equivalent outcomes of subpedicular and infraneural injections.[100,101] As noted earlier, infraneural techniques do substantially risk inadvertent disc entry, but Kim noted substantial reduction in the incidence of postoperative neural irritation in the infraneural injection group.[101]

Rados showed that outcomes from transforaminal ESI are superior to interlaminar approaches, with 75% versus

53% of patients having greater than 2.0 VAS improvement in pain and 66% versus 50% having greater than a 10-point gain of function on the Oswestry Disability Index (ODI). Regrettably, only 64 patients were studied in this endeavor, and statistical significance was not achieved.[102]

Of contemporary literature questioning the efficacy of ESIs, those studies based on the Spine Patient Outcomes Research Trial (SPORT) trial are the most methodologically flawed.[103] As a retrospective study of patients presenting for surgery where the stated endpoint was avoidance of surgery, 75% of patients were never considered for any type of epidural injection. The study is further confounded by failing to subdivide patients based on known prognostic factors for poor outcomes from epidural injection or by the specific technique chosen for the epidural injection. Inferior outcomes are expected from patients treated with interlaminar, caudal, or nonfluoroscopically guided injection techniques as opposed to transforaminal injections, but this analysis was not performed. The SPORT trial was uncontrolled for any other co-interventions, including physical therapy modalities. Although the authors excluded all patients who had prior ESI from analysis, nothing is known of the population denominator who underwent successful epidural injections and thus avoided surgical consultation entirely.

Necessity for Repetition of ESI

In clinical practice, many physicians repeat interlaminar or caudal epidural injections two or three times at a fixed interval of 1–3 weeks, but no published evidence specifically supports a time-contingent protocol of repeated epidural injections. The outdated but common practice of three interlaminar epidural injections performed at intervals of one to several weeks is mentioned here only to be condemned as an unsupportable and wasteful practice whose origins preceded the use of image-guided injection techniques. Best contemporary practice recommends a symptom-contingent protocol for consideration of the necessity for repeated epidural injection, although there is no literature that specifically evaluates the optimal timing of repeated injection in additional detail. There is no evidence of a cumulative or "booster" effect of repeated ESI, and any claims of this sort are unfounded. A recent review by MacVicar concludes that few patients benefit from repeated transforaminal injection.[95] This is in contrast to literature on interlaminar injections in which two, three, or more injections are often performed sometimes, but not always, based on the presence of recurrent symptoms. A yearly limit of 3 mg/kg of epidural corticosteroids has been advocated.[104]

Complications

Tarlov cysts can be present at any spinal foraminal level and personal preoperative review of the MRI is the only rational defense against this potential complication. S1 is a common level for Tarlov cysts, and interventionists are encouraged to review preoperative MRI films personally because Tarlov cysts are not reliably "read" on official radiology reports. Tarlov cysts are benign in nature, but because they are filled with CSF and in direct communication with the subarachnoid space, inadvertent injection may result in arachnoiditis with use of depot steroids and the preservatives contained within this solution or temporary spinal neuraxial blockade if local anesthetic is used.

Whereas studies have indicated minor injection site pain, worsening pain, flushing, or vasovagal symptoms, the incidence of these finding is less than 6%.[105] Incidence of postdural puncture headache is less than 1% in all series.[106] The incidence of inadvertent subarachnoid injection is not known. Epidural abscess and epidural hematoma are fortunately rare, with an incidence impossible to calculate because isolated case reports fail to provide a satisfactory denominator.

OTHER MINIMALLY INVASIVE INTERVENTIONS

No longer the exclusive domain of spinal surgeons, some pain specialists have undertaken the use of spinal endoscopy techniques with combined video and fluoroscopic guidance to remove herniated disc material under direct visualization via intradiscal or intra/transforaminal approaches. Interventionists may also use a variety of completely percutaneous systems to remove disc tissue, such as the Disc Dekompressor (Stryker), SpineJet (Hydrocision), or Coblation (Arthrocare). Limited data support the specific efficacy of use of the Disc Dekompressor and Coblation techniques in the treatment of disc herniation with radiculopathy, but Vorobeychik insightfully reviewed the Disc Dekompressor literature and concluded that the supporting studies generally lack rigor and limit the strength of recommendations that can be made.[107–109] A search for clinical series or trials on SpineJet yielded a single clinical trial (NCT0038400), begun in 2006 and completed in 2009, but the principal investigator did not publish their results. A Brazilian trial comparing SpineJet to microdiscectomy was begun in 2011. Surgical preparation of the disc space for surgical fusion using the proprietary SpineJet device is the only related publication, and no recommendations can be made for treatment of HNP with radiculopathy.[110]

The advantages of these endoscopic and percutaneous approaches as compared with open surgical approaches appear to be minimal trauma, less postoperative pain, earlier return to work, low rates of recurrent disc herniation and infection, reduced potential for epidural scarring, and reduced costs because these procedures are performed on an outpatient basis and lack any necessity for general anesthesia. With spinal endoscopic disc decompression, risk of dural puncture is greater than for microdiscectomy, but significantly fewer recurrent disc herniation events occur and less postsurgical epidural scarring results from the endoscopic technique.[111] It is notable that a lengthy physician learning curve is required to achieve competence in use of endoscopic techniques. Longer term benefits may incur to patients managed by these minimally invasive techniques resulting from avoidance of laminectomy and muscle stripping, but these are not yet proven. In addition, these techniques have largely been applied to patients with smaller sized disc protrusions.

In determining a final interventional recommendation for care of the L4–L5 central disc herniation with left L5 radiculopathy, the best evidence for an initially successful clinical outcome would suggest a left L4 or L5 transforaminal ESI via a subpedicular approach. The modestly increased likelihood of early clinical improvement with preganglionic L4 injection is offset by equivalent outcomes at 6 months. Whereas the infraneural injection technique may offer a decreased risk for vascular entry and reduced neural irritation, it is technically more difficult and increases the risk of inadvertent intradiscal injection without demonstration of superior outcomes. In some cases where the disc herniation is quite large and where contrast injection shows marked truncation of the nerve root outline by the intervertebral disc at the postganglionic injection level, some practitioners additionally perform subpedicular injection at the preganglionic nerve level, but this approach has not yet been statistically validated. Use of continuous fluoroscopy with contrast injection after needle placement is mandated. DSA is a useful but not foolproof tool, if readily available.

Alternatively, the patient may be placed on membrane stabilizers alone or concomitantly with ESI. Comparative effectiveness research studies are needed but are complex to perform and interpret. A recent three-armed study demonstrated superior efficacy of ESI combined with gabapentin/nortriptyline and physical therapy to either ESI or medications/physical therapy alone.[112] Another more recent study by the same authors examined fluoroscopically guided lumbar ESI and sham gabapentin versus sham ESI (injected intramuscular) and active gabapentin. There were only small differences in favor of ESI at 1 month in leg pain but not in overall pain and not at 3 months. However, significant limitations prevent replication of real-life scenarios in study design, such as the natural history of the condition and the potential need for multiple procedures.

If the radicular pain remains unimproved more than briefly by transforaminal ESI and the disc herniation is 5 mm or smaller on imaging studies, consideration can be given to flexion-extension lumbar MRI study or diagnostic lumbar myelography with flexion and extension views to establish whether a mass effect exists that might merit a minimally invasive or surgical disc decompressive procedure. If the disc protrusion is greater than 5 mm in size, the flexion-extension MRI result is unlikely to alter a decision to proceed with a decompressive procedure. Although endoscopic decompression of the HNP may be an appropriate option in the hands of a qualified, experienced interventionist, spinal surgical referral is an appropriate and more conventional path.

Finally, if the disc herniation is very small and no mass effect can be established, consideration can be given to the performance of provocative lumbar discography to search for annular pathology supporting a diagnosis of symptomatic internal disc disruption as the basis for radicular pain. Options for treatment of internal disc disruption include the percutaneous decompressive methods described earlier, as well as endoscopic techniques, but fuller discussion of the treatment of discogenic pain is beyond the scope of this chapter.

SURGERY

Surgery can provide significant relief in properly selected patients with a lumbar disc herniation.[113–115] The main goal of surgery is to decompress the lumbosacral nerve root causing unremitting radiculopathy and neurological deficit. In appropriately chosen patients, lumbar microdiscectomy results in an 85–90% success rate in relieving the leg pain, although the relief of back pain is less predictable.[116,117]

Outcomes Comparing Surgery to Conservative Therapy

One of the first prospective studies comparing lumbar discectomy to conservative therapy was conducted by Weber in 1983. He showed that surgery provided significant pain relief and functional improvement at 1-year follow-up; however, at 4 and 10 years, the differences between both groups were no longer significant. Of note, 26% of the conservative group eventually crossed over to receive surgery.[118]

The Maine Lumbar Spine Study Group, a prospective observational study of more than 500 patients comparing operative versus nonoperative treatment, demonstrated that surgery provided significant pain relief and improved quality of life at 1 and 5 years. At 10 years, there was no significant difference in relief of predominant symptoms between the surgical and conservative therapy group. However, patient satisfaction was markedly better in the surgically treated group.[119–121] Of note, the surgical group was significantly more symptomatic preoperatively compared to the nonoperative group. The authors noted that the most significant improvement in pain and quality of life is seen in the first 2 years postoperatively. For workers compensation patients, there was no difference in the time to return to work between either group; however, the functional status and satisfaction rate was significantly better in the operative group up to 5 years.[119–121]

The 2006 SPORT was the first multicenter, prospective RCT comparing operative versus nonoperative treatment for symptomatic lumbar disc herniations.[122] There were 501 patients with lumbar disc herniations confirmed by MRI with symptoms for at least 6 weeks. However, one of the limitations of the study was the high cross-over rate, with 50% of patients assigned to the surgical group crossing over to the nonoperative group, whereas 30% of the nonsurgical group crossed over to the operative group. Due to the lack of compliance among the assigned treatment groups, an intention-to-treat analysis did not demonstrate a significant difference between the operative and nonoperative groups. In an as-treated analysis, which accounts for the potential effects of these crossovers, patients in the surgical group reported significant improvements in ODI scores, physical function, and bodily pain compared to the nonoperative group at 4 and 8 years.[123,124]

In summary, numerous studies have shown that the majority of patients with lumbosacral radiculopathy will improve by 8 weeks without any treatment.[125–128] In the select few who continue to have unremitting radicular pain, multiple trials comparing operative versus conservative treatment have demonstrated that surgery provides improved quality of life in the first 2–5 years.[118–124] At 5–10 years, the benefits of surgery are similar to conservative therapy because both groups report a comparable overall improvement in disability and symptoms. However, those treated surgically report a higher satisfaction rate.[123,124]

Indications

An absolute indication for lumbar microdiscectomy is progressive neurological deficit or cauda equina syndrome due to a disc herniation. The American Pain Society treatment guidelines recommend lumbosacral discectomy for persistent or worsening radicular leg pain with corresponding nerve root compression confirmed by findings demonstrated by CT-myelogram/MRI in patients who have failed conservative therapy.[129]

Cauda equina syndrome is more common with a central herniation, but it can also occur due to paracentral or lateral herniations.[130–133] Diagnosis is suspected clinically with confirmation by neuroimaging. In cauda equina syndrome, the patient will complain of perineal sensory deficits, bowel or bladder incontinence, and a new or progressive neurological deficit. MRI with gadolinium contrast will demonstrate lumbosacral disc herniation compressing the cauda equina or thecal sac.[132] Urgent surgical spinal decompression is warranted because the time to decompression determines long-term neurological function.[133–135]

Duration of symptoms is one of the most significant factors in determining the decision to perform surgery. The SPORT trial required at least 6 weeks' duration of signs and symptoms for consideration of surgery.[122–124] However, multiple studies suggest that greater than 6 months of radiculopathy is associated with worse outcomes postoperatively.[136–138] Nygaard et al. showed poorer outcomes and a decreased likelihood of returning to work in patients with a symptom duration of greater than 6 months prior to surgery.[138] Hurme and Alaranta found that the best surgical results were in patients who were operated on within 2 months onset of disabling lumbosacral radiculopathy.[137]

Surgical Techniques

There are multiple surgical techniques for the excision of a herniated disc, ranging from open discectomy to newer techniques such as endoscopic microdiscectomy.[139–143] Currently, the gold standard for a lumbar disc herniation is the posterior microscopic lumbar discectomy. In 1934, Mixter and Barr published the first detailed report of an open lumbar discectomy for a herniated disc.[144] Their initial technique involved an intradural approach with an extensive laminectomy. This technique was modified over the next several decades. Current general principles include a 3- to 5-inch longitudinal incision directly over the involved lumbosacral level, dissection down to the interlaminar space, laminotomy or partial laminectomy, followed by gentle nerve retraction with direct removal of the herniated disc fragment.

The next major advancement in lumbar discectomy occurred in the late 1970s, with the introduction of microsurgical techniques. In 1977, Yasargil and Caspar independently described the use of an operating microscope to remove elements of the herniated disc through a less invasive method.[145,146] This microsurgical technique was popularized in the United States after Williams et al. published a paper outlining their experience in 532 patients in 1978.[147] The purported benefits of the microdiscectomy included a smaller incision, less trauma to the soft tissue and muscle, and less manipulation of the adjacent neural structures.[148,149] Numerous studies have demonstrated decreased morbidity, a shorter hospital stay, and faster recovery compared to the traditional open discectomy.[147–150] Microdiscectomy can be performed with magnifying loupes and a head lamp as an alternative to the operating microscope.

An alternative technique to the traditional interlaminar approach is the intertransverse approach with a paramedian incision and dissection between the multifidus and longissimus parts of the sacrospinalis muscle. It was popularized by Wiltse in the late 1970s and is used for foraminal and extraforminal lateral disc herniations.[151]

The next major advancement in lumbar discectomy occurred in 1997, when Foley and Smith described their technique for microendoscopic discectomy using a tubular retractor system.[152] Microendoscopic discectomy is becoming popular due to the advantage of an even smaller incision and less soft-tissue dissection. Multiple studies have shown that outcomes are comparable to microdisectomy,[153–156] although a recent meta-analysis revealed a higher rate of incidental durotomies with endoscopic discectomy.[153] One of the biggest disadvantages is the steep learning curve. As a result, the majority of surgeons are reluctant to adopt this technique.[157]

Postoperative Care and Rehabilitation

There are numerous studies exploring postoperative rehabilitation following lumbar microdiscectomy. Most studies have shown that early active rehabilitation versus a traditional, delayed rehabilitation program have similar overall improvements at 1 year.[158–160] Even though there is little evidence in the literature, many surgeons limit lifting and bending for 3–6 weeks after surgery. The main concern is that excessive movements in the early postoperative period may lead to reherniation or increased scarring.

Complications

Numerous complications can occur after a lumbar microdiscectomy, including incidental durotomy, reherniation, discitis, infection, and nerve root injury. This complication rate increases significantly with revision surgeries.[130,142,161–165] Depending on the study, the incidence of reherniation varies from 1% to 18%. These variations are in part due to differences in the definition of reherniation. Whereas some classify reherniation as simply recurrent sciatica, others define it as reoperation for a symptomatic reherniation at the previous discectomy level.[161,164–167] The incidence of nerve root injury is rare, with reported rates up to 1.4%.[161,163–165] Furthermore, pyogenic discitis is an infrequent complication occurring in less than 4% of patients.[163–165,168–171] Wound infections, ranging from superficial to deep, occurred in 0–4% of patients.[162–165,170,171]

The most common complication is incidental durotomy, which ranges from 1–17%, with a higher incidence occurring in revision cases.[145,161,163–165] Dural closure should be watertight to prevent a CSF leak that can lead to a postoperative headache and, rarely, the formation of a pseudomeningocele.

REFERENCES

1. Boden SC, Davis DO, Dina TS, Patronas NJ, Wiesel SW. Abnormal magnetic-resonance scans of the lumbar spine in asymptomatic subjects. *J Bone Joint Surg Am.* 1990;72(3):403–408.
2. Borenstein DG, O'Mara JW, Boden SD, et al. The value of magnetic resonance imaging of the lumbar spine to predict low-back pain in asymptomatic subjects. *J Bone Joint Surg Am.* 2001;83-A(9):1306–1311.
3. Mixter WJ, Barr, J. *Rupture of the intervertebral disc with involvement of the spinal canal. New Engl J Med.* 1934;211:210–215.
4. Kuslich, SD, Ulstrom CL, Michael CJ. The tissue origin of low back pain and sciatica: a report of pain response to tissue stimulation during operations on the lumbar spine using local anesthesia. Orthop Clin North Am. 1991;22(2):181–187.
5. Scaia, V, Baxter D, Cook C. The pain provocation-based straight leg raise test for diagnosis of lumbar disc herniation, lumbar radiculopathy, and/or sciatica: a systematic review of clinical utility. *J Back Musculoskelet Rehabil.* 2012;25(4):215–223.
6. Murata Y, et al. Local application of interleukin-6 to the dorsal root ganglion induces tumor necrosis factor-alpha in the dorsal root ganglion and results in apoptosis of the dorsal root ganglion cells. *Spine* (Phila Pa 1976). 2011;36(12): 926–932.
7. Jordan J, Konstantinou K, O'Dowd J. Herniated lumbar disc. *Clin Evid* (Online). 2011;.
8. Cohen SP, et al. Epidural steroids, etanercept, or saline in subacute sciatica: a multicenter, randomized trial. *Ann Intern Med.* 2012;156(8):551–559.
9. Golish SR, et al. Outcome of lumbar epidural steroid injection is predicted by assay of a complex of fibronectin and aggrecan from epidural lavage. *Spine* (Phila Pa 1976). 2011;36(18):1464–1469.
10. Adams MA. Biomechanics of back pain. *Acupunct Med.* 2004;22:178–188.
11. Deyo RA. Early diagnostic evaluation of low back pain. *J Gen Intern Med.* 1986;1:328–338.
12. Shahbandar L, Press J. Diagnosis and nonoperative management of lumbar disk herniation. *Oper Tech Sports Med.* 2005; 13:114–121.
13. Battie MC, Videman T, Parent E. Lumbar Disc Degeneration: epidemiology and genetic influences. *Spine.* 2004;29:2679–2690.
14. Konstantinou K, Dunn KM. Sciatica: review of epidemiological studies and prevalence estimates. *Spine.* 2008;33:2464–2472.
15. Younes M, Bejia I, Aguir Z, et al. Prevalence and risk factors of disk-related sciatica in an urban population in Tunisia. *J Bone Spine.* 2006;73:538–542.
16. Weber H. The natural course of disc herniation. *Acta Orthop Scand Suppl.* 1993;251:19–20.
17. Tarulli AW, Raynor EM. Lumbosacral radiculopathy. *Neurol Clin.* 2007;25:387–405.
18. Merskey H, Bogduk N. *Classification of Chronic Pain.* 2nd ed. Seattle, WA: IASP Press; 2012.
19. Capra F, et al. Validity of the straight-leg raise test for patients with sciatic pain with or without lumbar pain using magnetic resonance imaging results as a reference standard. *J Manipulative Physiol Ther.* 2011;34(4):231–238.
20. Walsh J, Hall. Agreement and correlation between the straight leg raise and slump tests in subjects with leg pain. *J Manipulative Physiol Ther.* 2009;32(3):184–192.
21. Alyas F, Connell D, Saifuddin A. Upright positional MRI of the lumbar spine. *Clin Radiol.* 2008;63(9):1035–1048.
22. Weishaupt D, et al. Positional MR imaging of the lumbar spine: does it demonstrate nerve root compromise not visible at conventional MR imaging? *Radiology.* 2000;215(1):247–253.
23. Zou J, et al. Missed lumbar disc herniations diagnosed with kinetic magnetic resonance imaging. *Spine* (Phila Pa 1976). 2008;33(5):E140–E144.
24. Barr K. Electrodiagnosis of lumbar radiculopathy. *Phys Med Rehabil Clin N Am.* 2013;24:79–91.
25. Kendall R, Werner RA. Interrater reliability of the needle examination in lumbosacral radiculopathy. *Muscle Nerve.* 2006;34(2):238–241.
26. Wilbourn AJ, Aminoff MJ. AAEM minimonograph 32: the electrodiagnostic examination of patients with radiculopathies. American Association of Electrodiagnostic Medicine. *Muscle Nerve.* 1998;21(12):1612–1631.
27. Dillingham TR, Lauder TD, Andary M, et al. Identifying lumbosacral radiculopathies: an optimal electromyographic screen. *Am J Phys Med Rehabil.* 2000;79(6):496–503.
28. Gellhorn AC, Chan L, Martin B, Friedly J. Management patterns in acute low back pain: the role of physical therapy. *Spine.* 2012;37(9):775–782.
29. Daffner SD, Hymanson HJ, Wang JC. Cost and use of conservative management of lumbar disc herniation before surgical discectomy. *Spine J.* 2010;10(6):463–468.
30. Hahne AJ, Ford JJ, McMeeken JM. Conservative management of lumbar disc herniation with associated radiculopathy: a systemic review. *Spine.* 2010;35(11):E488–E504.
31. Dagenais S, Tricco AC, Haldeman S. Synthesis of recommendations for the assessment and management of low back pain from recent clinical practice guidelines. *Spine J.* 2010;10(6):514–529.
32. Machado LA, Kamper SJ, Herbert RD, Maher CG, McAuley JH. Analgesic effects of treatments for non-specific low back pain: a meta-analysis of placebo-controlled randomized trials. *Rheumatology.* 2009;48(5):520–527.
33. McKenzie R, May S. *The Lumbar Spine: Mechanical Diagnosis & Therapy.* 2nd ed. Wainakae, New Zealand: Spinal Publications; 2003.
34. Long A, May S, Fung T. The comparative prognostic value of directional preference and centralization: a useful tool for front-line clinicians? *J Man Manip Ther.* 2008;16(4):248–254.
35. May S, Aina A. Centralization and directional preference: a systematic review. *Man Ther.* 2012;17(6):497–506.
36. Delitto A, Erhard RE, Bowling RW. A treatment-based classification approach to low back syndrome: identifying and staging patients for conservative treatment. *Phys Ther.* 1995;75(6):470–485.
37. Browder DA, Childs JD, Cleland JA, Fritz JM. Effectiveness of an extension-oriented treatment approach in a subgroup of subjects with low back pain: a randomized clinical trial. *Phys Ther.* 2007;87(12):1608–1618.
38. Fritz JM, George S. The use of a classification approach to identify subgroups of patients with acute low back pain. Interrater reliability and short-term treatment outcomes. *Spine.* 2000;25(1):106–114.
39. Fritz JM, Delitto A, Erhard RE. Comparison of classification-based physical therapy with therapy based on clinical practice guidelines for patients with acute low back pain: a randomized clinical trial. *Spine.* 2003;28(13):1363–1371.
40. Fritz JM, Brennan GP, Clifford SN, Hunter SJ, Thackeray A. An examination of the reliability of a classification algorithm for subgrouping patients with low back pain. *Spine.* 2006;31(1):77–82.
41. Magee DJ. *Orthopedic Physical Assessment.* 3rd ed. Philadelphia: Saunders; 1997.
42. Vainin M. Psychometric properties and clinical usefulness of the Oswestry Disability Index. *J Chiropr Med.* 2008;7(4):161–163.

43. Saunders HD, Saunders R. *Evaluation Treatment and Prevention of Musculoskeletal Disorders*. Vol. I. 3rd ed. Chaska, MN: The Saunders Group; 1995.
44. Unlu Z, Tasci S, Tarhan S, Pabuscu Y, Islak S. Comparison of 3 physical therapy modalities for acute pain in lumbar disc herniation measured by clinical evaluation and magnetic resonance imaging. *J Manipulative Physiol Ther*. 2008;31(3):191–198.
45. Buchmuller A, Navez M, Milletre-Bernardin M, Pouplin S, et al. Value of TENS for relief of chronic low back pain with or without radicular pain. *Eur J Pain*. 2012;16(5):656–665.
46. Flynn T, Fritz J, Whitman J, et al. A clinical prediction rule for classifying patients with low back pain who demonstrate short-term improvement with spinal manipulation. *Spine*. 2002;27(24):2835–2843.
47. Childs JD, Fritz JM, Flynn TW, et al. A clinical prediction rule to identify patients with low back pain most likely to benefit from spinal manipulation: a validation study. *Ann Intern Med*. 2004;141(12):920–928.
48. Long A, Donelson R, Fung T. Does it matter which exercise? A randomized control trial of exercise for low back pain. *Spine*. 2004;29(23):2593–2602.
49. Brotz D, Kuker W, Maschke E, et al. A prospective trial of mechanical physiotherapy for lumbar disk prolapse. *J Neurol*. 2003;250(6):746–749.
50. Torstensen TA, Ljunggren AE, Meen HD, et al. Efficiency and costs of medical exercise therapy, conventional physiotherapy, and self-exercise in patients with chronic low back pain. A pragmatic, randomized, single-blinded, controlled trial with 1-year follow-up. *Spine*. 1998;2616–2624.
51. Waddell G, Newton M, Henderson I, Somerville D, Main CJ. A Fear-Avoidance Beliefs Questionnaire (FABQ) and the role of fear-avoidance beliefs in chronic low back pain and disability. *Pain*. 1993;52(2):157–168.
52. Maher C, Latimer J, Refshauge K. Prescription of activity for low back pain: what works? *Aust J Physiother*. 1999;45(2):121–132.
53. Abdel Shaheed C, Maher CG, Mak W, Williams KA, McLachlan AJ. Interventions available over the counter and advice for acute low back pain: systematic review and meta-analysis. *J Pain*. 2014;15(1):2–15.
54. Roelofs PD, Deyo RA, Koes BW, Scholten RJ, van Tulder MW. Nonsteroidal anti-inflammatory drugs for low back pain: an updated Cochrane review. *Spine*. 2008;33(16):1766–1774.
55. van Tulder MW, Touray T, Furlan AD, Solway S, Bouter LM; Cochrane Back Review Group. Muscle relaxants for nonspecific low back pain: a systematic review within the framework of the Cochrane Collaboration [review]. *Spine*. 2003 1;28(17):1978–1992.
56. McCleane GJ. Does gabapentin have an analgesic effect on background, movement and referred pain? A randomized, double-blind, placebo controlled study. *Pain Clinic*. 2001;13:103–107.
57. Yildirim K, Sisecioglu M, Karatay S, et al. The effectiveness of gabapentin in patients with chronic radiculopathy. *Pain Clinic*. 2003;15:213–218.
58. Khoromi S, Cui L, Nackers L, Max MB. Morphine, nortriptyline and their combination vs. placebo in patients with chronic lumbar root pain. *Pain*. 2007; 130:66–75.
59. Baron R, Freynhagen R, Tölle TR, et al. A0081007 Investigators. The efficacy and safety of pregabalin in the treatment of neuropathic pain associated with chronic lumbosacral radiculopathy. *Pain*. 2010;150:420–427.
60. Khoromi S, Patsalides A, Parada S, Salehi V, Meegan JM, Max MB. Topiramate in chronic lumbar radicular pain. *J Pain*. 2005;6(12):829–836.
61. Muehlbacher M, Nickel MK, Kettler C, et al. Topiramate in treatment of patients with chronic low back pain a randomized, double-blind, placebo-controlled study. *Clin J Pain*. 2006;22:526–531.
62. Skljarevski V, Desaiah D, Liu-Seifert H, et al. Efficacy and safety of duloxetine in patients with chronic low back pain. *Spine* (Phila Pa 1976). 2010;35(13):E578–E585.
63. McNicol ED, Midbari A, Eisenberg E. Opioids for neuropathic pain [review]. *Cochrane Database Syst Rev*. 2013;8.
64. Toda S, et al. A local anesthetic, ropivacaine, suppresses activated microglia via a nerve growth factor-dependent mechanism and astrocytes via a nerve growth factor-independent mechanism in neuropathic pain. *Mol Pain*. 2011;;7:2.
65. Jeong HJ, et al. Delayed treatment with lidocaine reduces mouse microglial cell injury and cytokine production after stimulation with lipopolysaccharide and interferon gamma. *Anesth Analg*. 2012;114(4):856–861.
66. Sutheeranyongprasert C, Paiboonsirjit S, Kuansongtham V, Anuraklekha S, Hiranyasthiti N, Neti S. Factors predicting failure of conservative treatment in lumbar-disc herniation. *J Med Assoc Thai*. 2012;95(5):674–680.
67. Furman MB, et al. Contrast flow selectivity during transforaminal lumbosacral epidural steroid injections. *Pain Physician*. 2008;11(6):855–861.
68. Jasper JF, Lumbar retrodiscal transforaminal injection. *Pain Physician*. 2007;10(3):501–510.
69. Renfrew DL, Moore TE, Kathol MH, el-Khoury GY, Lemke JH, Walker CW. Correct placeent of epidural steroid injections: fluoroscopic guidance and contrast administration. *Am J Neurodadiol*. 1991;12(5):1003–1007.
70. Rados I, Sakic K, Fingler M, Kapural L. Efficacy of interlaminar vs transforaminal epidural steroid injection for the treatment of chronic unilateral radicular pain: prospective, randomized study. *Pain Med*. 2011;12(9):1316–1321.
71. Murakibhavi VG, Khemka AG. Caudal epidural steroid injection: a randomized controlled trial. *Evid Based Spine Care J*. 2011;2(4):19–26.
72. Bush K, Hillier S. A controlled study of caudal epidural injections of triamcinolone plus procaine for the management of intractable sciatica. *Spine* 1991;16(5):572–575.
73. Ackerman WE, Ahmad M. The efficacy of lumbar epidural steroid injections in patients with lumbar disc herniations. *Anesth Analg*. 2007;104(5):1217–1222.
74. Wybier M, et al. Paraplegia complicating selective steroid injections of the lumbar spine. *Eur Radiol*. 2010;20:181–189.
75. Furman MB, O'Brien EM, Zgleszewski TM Incidence of intravascular penetration in transforaminal lumbosacral epidural steroid injections. *Spine*. 2000;25(20):2628–2632.
76. Smuck M, et al. Accuracy of intermittent fluoroscopy to detect intravascular injection during transforaminal epidural injections. *Spine*. 2008;33(7):E205–E210.
77. Jasper JF. Role of digital subtraction fluoroscopic imaging in detecting intravascular injections. *Pain Physician*. 2003; 6(3):369–372.
78. McLean JP, et al. The rate of detection of intravascular injection in cervical transforaminal epidural steroid injections with and without digital subtraction angiography. *PM R*. 2009;1(7): 636–642.
79. Chang-Chie GC, Candido KD, Knezevic NN. Digital subtraction angiography does not reliably prevent paraplegia associated with lumbar transforaminal epidural steroid injection. *Pain Physician*. 2012;15(6):515–523.
80. Park CH, Lee SH, Kim BI. Comparison of the effectiveness of lumbar transforaminal epidural injection with particulate and nonparticulate corticosteroids in lumbar radiating pain. *Pain Med*. 2010;11(11):1654–1658.
81. Lee JW, et al. Cervical transforaminal epidural steroid injection for the management of cervical radiculopathy : a comparative study of particulate versus non-particulate steroids. *Skeletal Radiol*. 2009;38:1077–1082.
82. Dreyfuss, et al. Comparative effectiveness of cervical transforaminal injections with particulate and nonparticulate corticosteroid preparations for cervical radicular pain. *Pain Medicine*. 2006;7(3):237–242.
83. Derby R, et al. Size and aggregation of corticosteroids used for epidural injections. *Pain Med*. 2008;9(2):227–234.

84. Murthy NS, Maus TP, Behrns CL. Intraforaminal location of the great anterior radiculomedullary artery (artery of Adamkiewicz): a retrospective review. *Pain Med.* 2010;11(12):1756–1764.
85. Hogan, Q. Distribution of solution in the epidural space: examination by cryomicrotome section. Reg Anesth Pain Med. 2002;27(2):150–156.
86. Chang-Chien GC, Knezevic NN, McCormick Z, Chu SK, Trescot AM, Candido KD. Transforaminal versus interlaminar approaches to epidural steroid injections: a systematic review of comparative studies for lumbosacral radicular pain. *Pain Physician.* 2014;17(4):E509–E524.
87. Desai MJ, Dave AP, Martin MB. Delayed radicular pain following two large volume epidural blood patches for post-lumbar puncture headache: a case report. *Pain Physician.* 2010;13(3):257–262.
88. Manchikanti L, et al. Effect of fluoroscopically guided caudal epidural steroid or local anesthetic injections in the treatment of lumbar disc herniation and radiculitis: a randomized, controlled, double blind trial with a two-year follow-up. *Pain Physician.* 2012;15(4):273–286.
89. Furman MB, et al. Injectate volumes needed to reach specific landmarks in s1 transforaminal epidural injections. *Pain Med.* 2012;13(10):1265–1274.
90. Desai MJ, Shah B, Sayal PK. Epidural contrast flow patterns of transforaminal epidural steroid injections stratified by commonly used final needle-tip position. *Pain Med.* 2011;12(6):864–870.
91. Benny B, Azari P. The efficacy of lumbosacral transforaminal epidural steroid injections: a comprehensive literature review. *J Back Musculoskelet Rehabil.* 2011;24(2):67–76.
92. Rho ME, Tang CT. The efficacy of lumbar epidural steroid injections: transforaminal, interlaminar, and caudal approaches. *Phys Med Rehabil Clin N Am.* 2011;22(1):139–148.
93. Ghahreman A, Ferch R, Bogduk N. The efficacy of transforaminal injection of steroids for the treatment of lumbar radicular pain. *Pain Med.* 2010;11(8):1149–1168.
94. Manchikanti L, et al. Effectiveness of therapeutic lumbar transforaminal epidural steroid injections in managing lumbar spinal pain. *Pain Physician.* 2012;15(3):E199–E245.
95. Macvicar J, King W, Landers MH, Bogduk N. The effectiveness of lumbar transforaminal injection of steroids: a comprehensive review with systematic analysis of the published data. *Pain Med.* 2013;14(1):14–28.
96. Ghahreman A, BogdukN. Predictors of a favorable response to transforaminal injection of steroids in patients with lumbar radicular pain due to disc herniation. *Pain Med.* 2011;12(6):871–879.
97. Lee JW, et al. MR-based outcome predictors of lumbar transforaminal epidural steroid injection for lumbar radiculopathy caused by herniated intervertebral disc. *Eur Radiol.* 2013;23(1):205–211.
98. Jeong HS, et al. Effectiveness of transforaminal epidural steroid injection by using a preganglionic approach: a prospective randomized controlled study. *Radiology.* 2007;245(2):584–590.
99. Park KD, et al. Kambin triangle versus the supraneural approach for the treatment of lumbar radicular pain. *Am J Phys Med Rehabil.* 2012;91(12):1039–1050.
100. Park CH, Lee SH, Park HS. Lumbar retrodiscal versus post-ganglionic transforaminal epidural steroid injection for the treatment of lumbar intervertebral disc herniations. *Pain Physician.* 2011;14(4):353–360.
101. Kim C, et al. Retrodiscal approach of lumbar epidural block. *Ann Rehabil Med.* 2011;35(3): 418–426.
102. Rados I, et al. Efficacy of interlaminar vs transforaminal epidural steroid injection for the treatment of chronic unilateral radicular pain: prospective, randomized study. *Pain Med.* 2011;12(9):1316–1321.
103. Radcliff K, et al. The impact of epidural steroid injections on the outcomes of patients treated for lumbar disc herniation: a subgroup analysis of the SPORT trial. *J Bone Joint Surg Am.* 2012;94(15):1353–1358.
104. Manchikanti L. Role of neuraxial steroids in interventional pain management. *Pain Physician.* 2002;5(2):182–199.
105. McGrath JM, Schaefer MP, Malkamaki DM. Incidence and characteristics of complications from epidural steroid injections. *Pain Med.* 2011;12(5):726–731.
106. Manchikanti L, et al. Fluoroscopic lumbar interlaminar epidural injections in managing chronic lumbar axial or discogenic pain. *J Pain Res.* 2012;5:301–311.
107. Gerszten PC, et al. Plasma disc decompression compared with fluoroscopy-guided transforaminal epidural steroid injections for symptomatic contained lumbar disc herniation: a prospective, randomized, controlled trial. *J Neurosurg Spine.* 2010;12(4):357–371.
108. Vorobeychik Y, et al. Percutaneous mechanical disc decompression using Dekompressor device: an appraisal of the current literature. *Pain Med.* 2012;13(5):640–646.
109. Zhu H, et al. The efficacy of coblation nucleoplasty for protrusion of lumbar intervertebral disc at a two-year follow-up. *Int Orthop.* 2011;35(11):1677–1682.
110. Huh HY, et al. Comparison of SpineJet XL and conventional instrumentation for disk space preparation in unilateral transforaminal lumbar interbody fusion. *J Korean Neurosurg Soc.* 2010;47(5):370–376.
111. Kim CH, et al. Reoperation rate after surgery for lumbar herniated intervertebral disc disease: nation-wide cohort study. *Spine.* 2013 1;38(7):581–590.
112. Cohen SP, Hayek S, Semenov Y, Pasquina PF, White RL, Veizi E, et al. Epidural steroid injections, conservative treatment or combination treatment for cervical radiculopathy: a multi-center, randomized, comparative-effectiveness study. Accepted to *Anesthesiology.* In press.
113. Daneyemez M, Sali A, Kahraman S, Beduk A, Seber N. Outcome analyses in 1072 surgically treated lumbar disc herniations. *Minim Invasive Neurosurg.* 1999;42(2):63–68.
114. Davis RA. A long-term outcome analysis of 984 surgically treated herniated lumbar discs. *J Neurosurg.* 1994;80(3):415–421.
115. McCulloch JA. Focus issue on lumbar disc herniation: macro- and microdiscectomy. Spine. 1996;21(Suppl 24):45S–56S.
116. Weber H. Lumbar disc herniation. A controlled, prospective study with ten years of observation. *Spine* (Phila Pa 1976). 1983;8(2):131–140.
117. Yorimitsu E, Chiba K, Toyama Y, Hirabayashi K. Long-term outcomes of standard discectomy for lumbar disc herniation: a follow-up study of more than 10 years. *Spine.* 2001; 26(6):652–657.
118. Weber H. Lumbar disc herniation. A controlled, prospective study with ten years of observation. *Spine* (Phila Pa 1976). 1983;8(2):131–140.
119. Atlas SJ, Deyo RA, Keller RB, et al. The Maine Lumbar Spine Study, Part II: 1-year outcomes of surgical and nonsurgical management of sciatica. *Spine* (Phila Pa 1976). 1996;21:1777–1786.
120. Atlas SJ, Keller RB, Chang Y, et al. Surgical and nonsurgical management of sciatic secondary to a lumbar disc herniation: five-year outcomes from the Maine Lumbar Spine Study. *Spine* (Phila Pa 1976). 2001;26:1179–1187.
121. Atlas SJ, Keller RB, Wu YA, et al. Long-term outcomes of surgical and nonsurgical management of sciatica secondary to a lumbar disc herniation: 10 year results from the Maine Lumbar Spine Study. *Spine* (Phila Pa 1976). 2005;30:927–935.
122. Weinstein JN, Tosteson TD, Lurie JD, et al. Surgical vs nonoperative treatment for lumbar disk herniation: the Spine Patient Outcomes Research Trial (SPORT): a randomized trial. *JAMA.* 2006;296:2441–2450.
123. Weinstein JN, Lurie JD, Tosteson TD, Tosteson AN, Blood EA, Abdu WA, et al. Surgical versus nonoperative treatment for lumbar disc herniation: four-year results for the Spine Patient Outcomes Research Trial (SPORT). *Spine* (Phila Pa 1976). 2008;33(25):2789–2800.
124. Lurie JD, Tosteson TD, Tosteson AN, Zhao W, Morgan TS, Abdu WA, et al. Surgical versus nonoperative treatment for lumbar disc herniation: eight-year results for the spine patient outcomes research trial. *Spine* (Phila Pa 1976). 2014;39(1):3–16.

125. Dahm KT, Brurberg KG, Jamtvedt G, Hagen KB. Advice to rest in bed versus advice to stay active for acute low-back pain and sciatica. *Cochrane Database Syst Rev.* 2010;(6):CD007612.
126. Vroomen PC. Lack of effectiveness of bed rest for sciatica. *N Engl J Med.* 1999;340(6):418–423.
127. Hofstee DJ, Gijtenbeek JM, Hoogland PH, et al. Westeinde sciatica trial: randomized controlled study of bed rest and physiotherapy for acute sciatica. *J Neurosurg.* 2002; 96(Suppl 1):45–49.
128. Awad JN, Moskovich R. Lumbar disc herniations: surgical versus nonsurgical treatment. *Clin Orthop Relat Res.* 2006;443:183–197.
129. Ahn UM, Ahn NU, Buchowski JM, Garrett ES, Sieber AN, Kostuik JP. Cauda equina syndrome secondary to lumbar disc herniation: a meta-analysis of surgical outcomes. *Spine* (Phila Pa 1976). 2000;25(12):1515–1522.
130. Walker JL, Schulak D, Murtagh R. Midline disk herniations of the lumbar spine. *South Med J.* 1993; 86(1):13–17.
131. Tay EC, Chacha PB. Midline prolapse of a lumbar intervertebral disc withcompression of the cauda equina. *J Bone Joint Surg Br.* 1979;61(1):43–46.
132. Coscia M, Leipzig T, Cooper D. Acute cauda equina syndrome. Diagnostic advantage of MRI. *Spine* (Phila Pa 1976). 1994;19(4):475–478.
133. Nielsen B, de Nully M, Schmidt K, Hansen RI. A urodynamic study of cauda equina syndrome due to lumbar disc herniation. *Urol Int.* 1980;35(3):167–170.
134. Shapiro S. Cauda equina syndrome secondary to lumbar disc herniation. *Neurosurgery.* 1993;32(5):743–746.
135. Chou R, Loeser JD, Owens DK, Rosenquist RW, Atlas SJ, Baisden J, et al. American Pain Society Low Back Pain Guideline Panel. Interventional therapies, surgery, and interdisciplinary rehabilitation for low back pain: an evidence-based clinical practice guideline from the American Pain Society. *Spine* (Phila Pa 1976). 2009; 34(10):1066–1077.
136. Vucetic N, de Bri E, Svensson O. Clinical history in lumbar disc herniation. A prospective study in 160 patients. *Acta Orthop Scand.* 1997;68(2):116–120.
137. Hurme M, Alaranta H. Factors predicting the result of surgery for lumbar intervertebral disc herniation. *Spine* (Phila Pa 1976). 1987;12(9):933–938.
138. Nygaard OP, Romner B, Trumpy JH. Duration of symptoms as a predictor of outcome after lumbar disc surgery. *Acta Neurochir* (Wien). 1994; 128(1–4):53–56.
139. Yeung AT, Tsou PM. Posterolateral endoscopic excision for lumbar disc herniation: surgical technique, outcome, and complications in 307 consecutive cases. *Spine* (Phila Pa 1976). 2002; 27(7):722–731.
140. White AH, von Rogov P, Zucherman J, Heiden D. Lumbar laminectomy for herniated disc: a prospective controlled comparison with internal fixation fusion. *Spine* (Phila Pa 1976). 1987;12(3):305–307.
141. Tullberg T, Isacson J, Weidenhielm L. Does microscopic removal of lumbar disc herniation lead to better results than the standard procedure? Results of a one-year randomized study. *Spine* (Phila Pa 1976). 1993;18(1):24–27.
142. Soldner F, Hoelper BM, Wallenfang T, Behr R. The translaminar approach to canalicular and cranio-dorsolateral lumbar disc herniations. *Acta Neurochir* (Wien). 2002;144(4):315–320.
143. Pointillart V, Broc G, Senegas J. A novel paraspinal surgical approach for lumbar lateral extraforaminal root entrapment. *Eur Spine J.* 1997;6(2):102–105.
144. Mixter WJ, Barr JS. Rupture of intervertebral disc with involvement of the spinal canal. *N Engl J Med.* 1934;211:210–215.
145. Koebbe CJ, Maroon JC, Abla A, El-Kadi H, Bost J. Lumbar microdiscectomy: a historical perspective and current technical considerations. *Neurosurg Focus.* 2002;13(2):E3.
146. Frymoyer JW, Donaghy RM. The ruptured intervertebral disc. Follow-up report on the first case fifty years after recognition of the syndrome and its surgical significance. *J Bone Joint Surg Am.* 1985;67(7):1113–1116.
147. Williams RW. Microlumbar discectomy: a conservative surgical approach to the virgin herniated lumbar disc. *Spine* (Phila Pa 1976). 1978;3(2):175–182.
148. Kahanovitz N, Viola K, Muculloch J. Limited surgical discectomy and microdiscectomy. A clinical comparison. *Spine* (Phila Pa 1976). 1989;14(1):79–81.
149. Wilson DH, Harbaugh R. Microsurgical and standard removal of the protruded lumbar disc: a comparative study. *Neurosurgery.* 1981;8(4):422–427.
150. Vucetic N, de Bri E, Svensson O. Clinical history in lumbar disc herniation. A prospective study in 160 patients. *Acta Orthop Scand.* 1997;68(2):116–120.
151. Wiltse LL, Spencer CW. New uses and refinements of the paraspinal approach to the lumbar spine. *Spine* (Phila Pa 1976). 1988;13(6):696–706.
152. Perez-Cruet MJ, Foley KT, Isaacs RE, et al. Microendoscopic lumbar discectomy: technical note. *Neurosurgery.* 2002;51(5):S129–S136.
153. Dasenbrock HH, Juraschek SP, Schultz LR, et al. The efficacy of minimally invasive discectomy compared with open discectomy: a meta-analysis of prospective randomized controlled trials. *J Neurosurg Spine.* 2012;16(5):452–462.
154. Wu X, Zhuang S, Mao Z, Chen H. Microendoscopic discectomy for lumbar disc herniation: surgical technique and outcome in 873 consecutive cases. *Spine* (Phila Pa 1976). 2006;31(23): 2689–2694.
155. Righesso O, Falavigna A, Avanzi O. Comparison of open discectomy with microendoscopic discectomy in lumbar disc herniations: results of a randomized controlled trial. *Neurosurgery.* 2007;61(3):545–549.
156. Ruetten S, Komp M, Merk H, Godolias G. Full-endoscopic interlaminar and transforaminal lumbar discectomy versus conventional microsurgical technique: a prospective, randomized, controlled study. *Spine* (Phila Pa 1976). 2008;33(9):931–939.
157. Kaushal M, Sen R. Posterior endoscopic discectomy: results in 300 patients. *Indian J Orthop.* 2012;46(1):81–85.
158. Carragee EJ, Han MY, Yang B, Kim DH, Kraemer H, Billys J. Activity restrictions after posterior lumbar discectomy. A prospective study of outcomes in 152 cases with no postoperative restrictions. *Spine* (Phila Pa 1976). 1999;24(22):2346–2351.
159. Kjellby-Wendt G, Styf J. Early active training after lumbar discectomy. A prospective, randomized, and controlled study. *Spine* (Phila Pa 1976). 1998;23(21):2345–2351.
160. Oosterhuis T, Costa LO, Maher CG, de Vet HC, van Tulder MW, Ostelo RW. Rehabilitation after lumbar disc surgery. *Cochrane Database Syst Rev.* 2014;3:CD003007.
161. Desai A, Ball PA, Bekelis K, et al. Outcomes after incidental durotomy during first-time lumbar discectomy. *J Neurosurg Spine.* 2011;14(5):647–653.
162. Lee P, Liu JC, Fessler RG. Perioperative results following open and minimally invasive single-level lumbar discectomy. *J Clin Neurosci.* 2011;18(12):1667–1670.
163. Leung PC. Complications in the first 40 cases of microdiscectomy. *J Spinal Disord.* 1988;1(4):306–310.
164. Shamim MS, Parekh MA, Bari ME, Enam SA, Khursheed F. Microdiscectomy for lumbosacral disc herniation and frequency of failed disc surgery. *World Neurosurg.* 2010;74(6):611–616.
165. Stolke D, Sollmann WP, Seifert V. Intra- and postoperative complications in lumbar disc surgery. *Spine* (Phila Pa 1976). 1989;14(1):56–59.
166. Goffin J. Microdiscectomy for lumbar disc herniation. *Clin Neurol Neurosurg.* 1994;96(2):130–134.
167. Katayama Y, Matsuyama Y, Yoshihara H, Sakai Y, Nakamura H, Nakashima S, et al. Comparison of surgical outcomes between macro discectomy and micro discectomy for lumbar disc herniation: a prospective randomized study with surgery

performed by the same spine surgeon. *J Spinal Disord Tech.* 2006;19(5):344–347.

168. Hirabayashi S, Kumano K, Ogawa Y, Aota Y, Maehiro S. Microdiscectomy and second operation for lumbar disc herniation. *Spine* (Phila Pa 1976). 1993;18(15):2206–2211.

169. Moon MS, Kim SS, Lee BJ, Moon JL, Sihn JC, Moon SI. Pyogenic discitis following discectomy. *J Orthop Surg* (Hong Kong). 2012;20(1):11–17.

170. An HS, Simpson JM, Stein R. Outpatient laminotomy and discectomy. *J Spinal Disord.* 1999;12(3):192–196.

171. Wiese M, Krämer J, Bernsmann K, Ernst Willburger R. The related outcome and complication rate in primary lumbar microscopic disc surgery depending on the surgeon's experience: comparative studies. *Spine J.* 2004;4(5):550–556.

13.

POSTLAMINECTOMY SYNDROME

Krishna Kumar, Syed Rizvi, and Binit J. Shah

CASE PRESENTATION

A 52-year-old attorney presents with persistent low back pain (LBP) and bilateral lower extremity pain following two previous lumbar spine surgeries. Four years ago, the patient underwent emergency L5–S1 decompression secondary to acute disc herniation with foot drop. The operation was complicated by a lumbar epidural abscess noted 3 months later, and the patient had revision surgery with extension of the laminectomy to the L3–L4 level. He has been infection-free since then. The pain is described as constant in the low back and radiating to the lower extremities, more so with physical activity. The pain has burning and tingling descriptive qualities. He denies any weakness or bowel/bladder/sexual dysfunction. The patient is referred to the Interdisciplinary Back Pain clinic for further evaluation and management.

Past medical history is significant for a history of type 2 diabetes of 2 years' duration.

Review of systems is significant for obstructive sleep apnea, controlled with CPAP.

On examination, the patient weighs 89 kg and is 173 cm tall. He is afebrile with stable vital signs. His neurologic examination is significant for mild decreased sensation to pinprick in the webspace between the big toe and second toe bilaterally. He has intact motor strength, and deep tendon reflexes are within normal limits bilaterally. His lower lumbar spine is mildly tender to deep palpation.

A magnetic resonance image (MRI) of the lumbar spine is significant for grade 1 anterolisthesis of L4 on L5, moderate foraminal stenosis bilaterally at L5–S1, moderate to severe foraminal stenosis at L4–L5 on the left side, and mild on the right side.

QUESTIONS

1. What is the cause of pain in this patient?
2. What is the pathophysiology of the chronic pain state?
3. What medications may be helpful for pain control?
4. What rehabilitation techniques may be helpful in restoring function?
5. What, if any, injections or nerve blocks may be of use to control pain?
6. What is the incidence of persistent pain following lumbar spine surgery?
7. If these options are not successful at pain control, what options are left?
8. What is the long-term prognosis of persistent pain following spinal surgery?

WHAT IS THE CAUSE OF PAIN IN THIS PATIENT?

This patient has postlaminectomy syndrome, otherwise referred to as failed back surgery syndrome (FBSS). FBSS constitutes a heterogeneous group of disorders that occur post lumbosacral surgery and share pain as a common symptom.[1–3] It is an imprecise term, implying only that the outcome of lumbosacral spine surgery failed to meet the expectation of both patient and surgeon. Various case series have reported a surgical etiology in 56–90% of FBSS cases.[1–4]

Factors contributing to persistent pain in our patient are:

- Development of anterolisthesis of L4 on L5 with associated neuroforaminal stenosis (Figure 13.1)
- Bilateral foraminal stenosis at L5–S1 secondary to collapse of disc space following surgery (Figure 13.1)
- Previous surgery and subsequent complications of infection leading to epidural and perineural fibrosis
- Being overweight (body mass index [BMI] = 29.7 kg/m^2)

WHAT IS THE PATHOPHYSIOLOGY OF THE CHRONIC PAIN STATE?

Chronic pain represents aberrant somatosensory processing in the peripheral or central nervous system (CNS) that is sustained beyond the normally expected time course relative to the noxious stimulus. The pathophysiology of chronic pain arises from neuronal sensitization. Peripheral sensitization

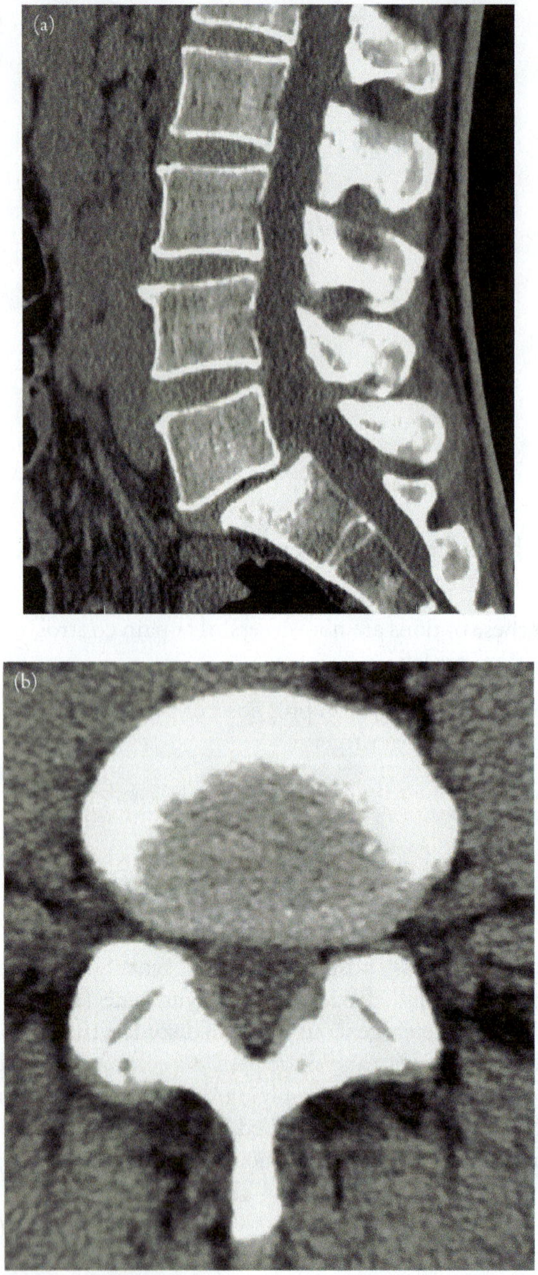

Figure 13.1 A. Sagittal computed tomography (CT) reformat indicates L5–S1 spondylolisthesis with disc bulges at L4–L5 and L5–S1. B. Axial CT image reveals foraminal stenosis at L4–L5. The spondylolisthesis resulted in back pain, whereas the foraminal stenosis produced radicular pain.

occurs through chemical products of cell destruction, whereas sensitization invokes activation of glutamate or N-methyl-D-aspartate receptor–mediated pathways in the dorsal horn of the spinal cord found in lamina II. With prolonged activation of pain pathways, augmented by sensitization, neural plasticity results in degeneration and remodeling of synapses. Changes in neuronal function may thus occur, resulting in production of pain transmitter substances by cells. These morphologic and functional changes in the nervous system cause decreased pain threshold, exaggerated activation of the pain pathway, ectopic discharges, or loss of normal inhibitory processes. Abnormal responses from the pain pathway may be described as hyperalgesia or allodynia.[5]

As its name implies, neuropathic pain originates in the nervous system and is often the consequence of traumatic damage to nervous tissue. Features of neuropathic pain include central sensitization, disinhibition (imbalance in excitatory and inhibitory inputs), and phenotypic change of mechanoreceptive fibers to begin production of substance P.[5] Neuropathic pain is usually confined to a dermatomal distribution and is characterized by a dysesthetic and burning quality. Although constant, it tends to worsen with activity. Because there is a poor concordance between radicular symptoms and standard dermatomal maps in up to 20% of patients, a transforaminal epidural injection may be used to confirm the level of pain generator. A positive response to selective nerve root block is usually associated with good surgical outcome.[2,3]

AXIAL BACK PAIN VERSUS RADICULAR LEG PAIN

Patients with FBSS are broadly divided into two groups: those with predominantly radicular leg pain and those with axial back pain as their major feature (Figures 13.2–13.5). Axial back pain may be discogenic (occurring at the index level of the prior operation or in adjacent segments), related to facet or sacroiliac (SI) joint pain, pseudo-arthrosis secondary to attempted to spinal fusion surgery, or spinal instability. Radicular leg pain is typically the consequence of nerve root

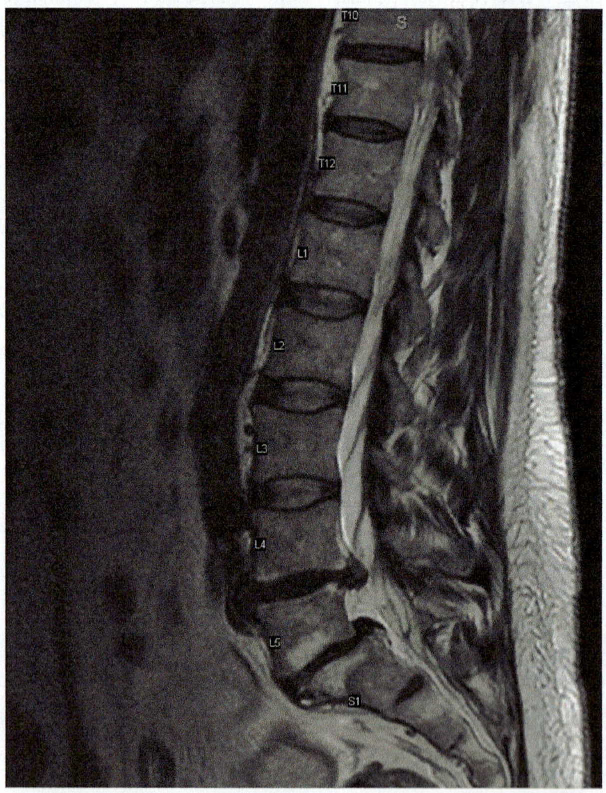

Figure 13.2 Sagittal magnetic resonance imaging (MRI) reveals a disc protrusion and retrolisthesis at L4–L5 and anterolisthesis at L5–S1. The spondylolisthesis was responsible for back pain, whereas the disc protrusion produced radicular pain.

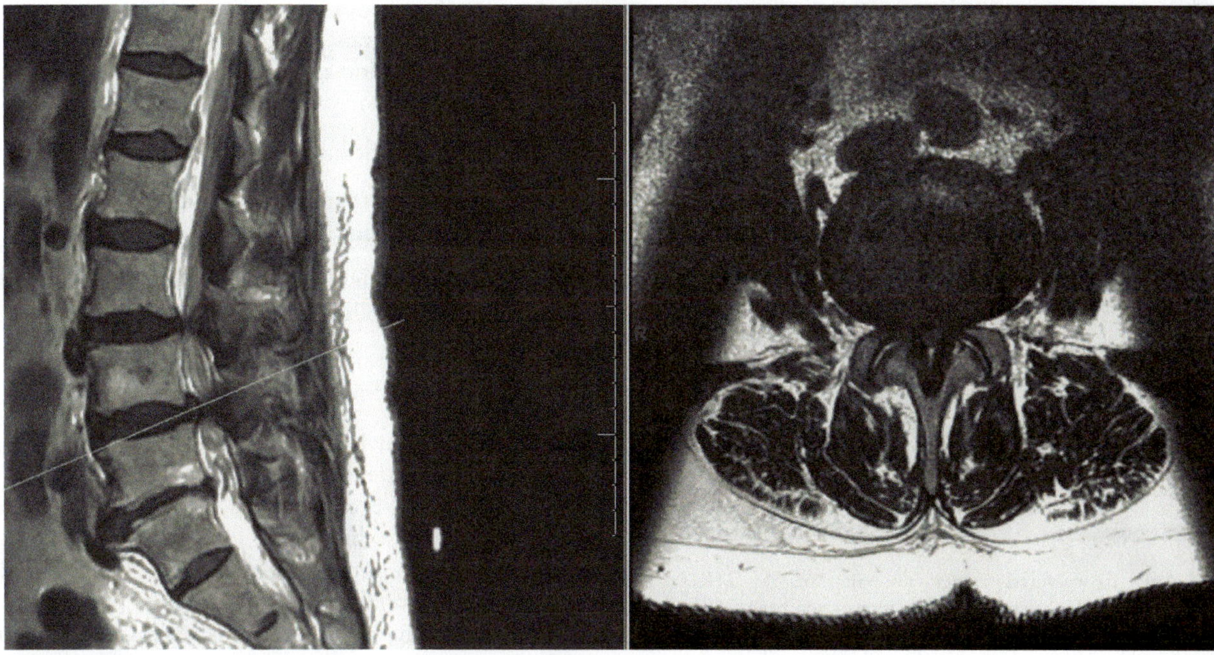

Figure 13.3 Sagittal and axial magnetic resonance imaging (MRI) reveal spinal stenosis. This can result in back and bilateral leg pain and symptoms of neurogenic claudication.

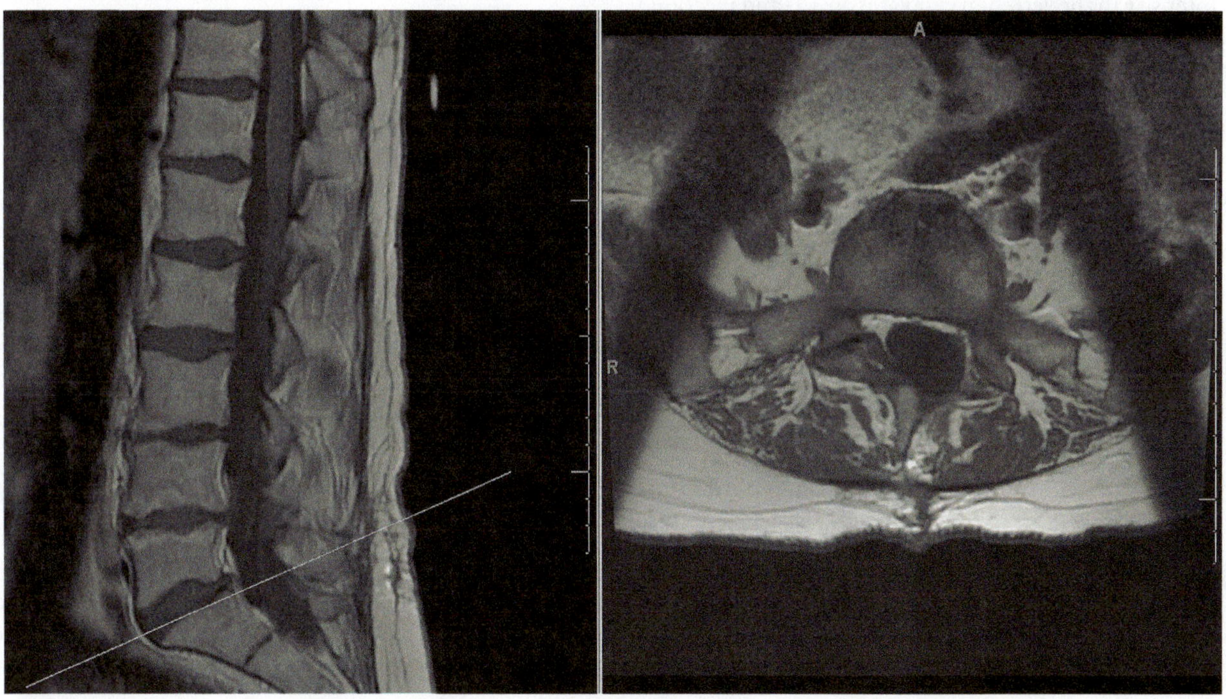

Figure 13.4 Axial postcontrast T1 (right) indicates abnormal tissue in the epidural space and around the nerve root, which enhances with contrast and is consistent with scarring. The scarring can cause nerve root irritation and displacement, resulting in radicular pain.

irritation caused by recurrent disc herniation, foraminal stenosis, epidural fibrosis, or root injury.[3]

Foraminal Stenosis

Neural foraminal stenosis produces leg pain and may occur at the level of surgery or in adjacent segments. An up-down stenosis results from loss of disc space height. A front-back stenosis is the result of facet hypertrophy and osteophyte formation. It is unclear whether neural foraminal stenosis is responsible for LBP or if the LBP results from a painful disc.[3]

Painful Disc

The diagnosis of painful disc is corroborated by MRI findings. Vertebral endplate changes are associated with degenerative

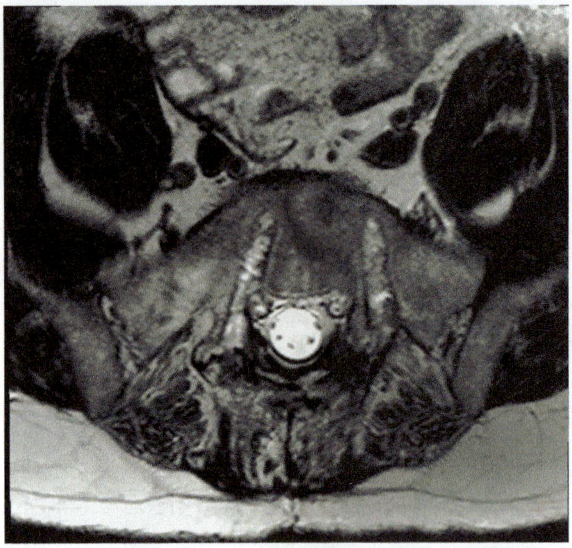

Figure 13.5 Axial T2-weighted magnetic resonance imaging (MRI) indicates failed pedicular screw fusion. The screws have been removed, but the track is visualized. Note bilateral facet degeneration. The patient continues to have back pain.

intervertebral disc disease. These changes consist of reduced signal intensity in the vertebral endplates on T1- and increased signal intensity on T2-weighted MRI sequences (Modic type I changes). They are associated with fissuring of the cartilaginous endplate. The presence of high-intensity zones in the annulus fibrosis on T2-weighted sequences correlates significantly with the presence of annular disruption and reproduction of pain. The level of painful disc can be confirmed by discography.[6] Discography, however, is known to have a high rate of false positives, and prevalence of postprocedural adverse outcomes such as disc space infections must be kept in mind.

Disc Herniation

Recurrent or residual disc herniation is best diagnosed by MRI using a combination of unenhanced and contrast-enhanced sequences. In cases where the diagnosis of recurrent disc herniation is not clear on MRI, a discogram followed by computed tomography (CT) may be helpful.[3] In certain circumstances when MRI is contraindicated (e.g., if the patient has a pacemaker, spinal cord implant, or cochlear implant), a CT myelogram is an alternative to MRI.

Patient Selection for Surgery

Appropriate patient selection and justification of surgery are the most important factors in preventing FBSS. In addition to a detail medical workup, detailed psychological workup and treatment tend to improve success rates. The indications for surgery are:

- Imaging studies (e.g., CT or MRI) indicate nerve root compression that corresponds to the clinical findings of the specific affected nerve root
- Cauda equina syndrome
- Presence of neurological abnormalities (e.g., reflex change, positive straight leg raising, sensory loss, weakness) that persist on examination and correspond to the specific affected nerve root(s)
- Progressive or significant neuromotor deficit
- Neuromotor deficit that persists after 4–6 weeks of conservative treatment
- Chronic sciatica with positive straight leg raise longer than 6 weeks or uncontrolled pain

Spinal Instability

Most cases of spondylolisthesis result either from a defect in the pars interarticubanis/interarticularis (isthmic type) or from degenerative disc and facet disease (degenerative type). Iatrogenic instability may occur after decompression of degenerative-type or isthmic spondylolisthesis. This situation is more common when parts of the facet joints have been removed during the decompression process. Pseudarthrosis may be asymptomatic or cause pain after attempted spinal fusion. Although no test is definitive, instability and pseudarthrosis are best imaged by the combination of standing X-rays with sagittal flexion and extension views and CT with three-dimensional reformatted images. After interbody fusion with a cage, nonunion may be difficult to prove. In these cases, pain failing to improve after 6 months, worsening foraminal stenosis, significant subsidence, or development of lucency around the cage is suggestive of pseudarthrosis.[3]

Facet Pain

The diagnosis of facet or SI joint pain cannot be made by history and imaging alone. The diagnosis may require the use of anesthetic injections.[2,7,8] An anesthetic block is considered positive when there is 50–80% or greater pain relief for a length of time corresponding to the local anesthetic used.[3]

Pedicular Screw Placement

New leg pain immediately after a lumbar fusion with pedicle screw placement should raise the possibility of a screw breaching the pedicle cortex. A CT scan will confirm if the screw is breaching the lateral recess and impinging the nerve root.[3]

Psychological Factors

An extensive body of literature emphasizes the role of psychological factors in surgical outcome and the development of FBSS. A recent, multivariable prospective model evaluated outcome at 12 months following decompressive surgery.[1,9]It found the most predictive factor of good outcome (global outcome of surgery using 5-point Likert scale) was lower scores of depression and somatic preoccupation. Even in less invasive/extensive surgery (e.g., lumbar discectomy) this is the case.[7,10]A systematic review of psychosocial variables affecting outcomes in lumbar surgery and spinal cord stimulation (SCS) included 25 studies, of which 92%

found a relationship between psychological factors (specifically, depression, anxiety, poor coping skills, and presurgical somatization) and poor response.[6,11] More specifically, this same finding was found in the more specific subpopulation of revision lumbar surgery patients. A retrospective cohort study followed 53 patients over 2 years to assess satisfaction following revision surgery for symptomatic same-level recurrent stenosis. Independent of improvement in pain and disability (surgical effectiveness), preoperative depression score was most associated with satisfaction.[5,12] Daubs et al. conducted a systematic review on psychological factors as a guide to fusion versus nonoperative care for chronic LBP.[2,13] Patients without a personality disorder, neuroticism, or depression had more favorable response to fusion. Their recommendations included preferential nonoperative treatment for patients with the aforementioned conditions and the use of validated screening questionnaires to identify psychopathology. In considering psychosocial factors, there is often a bias against patients from lower socioeconomic status. However, demographic factors have not shown association to pain reduction or development of subsequent lumbar postlaminectomy syndrome. Rather the most salient social issues are pending litigation, workers compensation, current sick leave, and "heavy labor job type," all of which negatively affect surgical success.[314] Most patients with chronic LBP develop symptoms of at least one psychiatric disorder, most commonly depression, substance abuse, or anxiety disorder.[15] One of the most easily assessed and directly modifiable factors is smoking cessation (see Chapter 10 on SI joint pain). Nonsmokers are more likely to have favorable outcome after fusion surgery.[4,16] Pure psychogenic pain, however, is rare in patients with FBSS. All patients exhibit some degree of pain behavior. Identification and treatment of psychiatric comorbidity is essential for enhancing treatment success and patient rehabilitation.[3,17] Given the high rates of depression and anxiety in chronic pain patients and the well-documented effects of psychological variables in spinal pain outcomes, all patients with continued pain following back surgery should be considered for psychological referral.

History provides crucial information in the evaluation of FBSS. It helps establish differential diagnoses, and it serves as an important guide for subsequent treatment decisions. Special attention must be given to descriptions of preoperative symptoms, temporal distribution of pain recurrence, current pain distribution, and type of surgical procedure initially performed. Fundamentally, it is critical to determine if the original surgery was appropriate in light of the patient's preoperative symptoms. If surgery was appropriate, consideration should be given to whether the operation was technically correct or if its outcome was marred by complications.[3]

Was the Index Operation Appropriate?

From the case history provided it appears that the index operation was justifiable. The patient had acute sciatic pain with foot drop. This patient has developed significant segmental instability due to grade 1 spondylolisthesis at L4–L5, with associated foraminal stenosis at this level that contributes to the ongoing chronic back and bilateral leg pain syndrome.

Inappropriate back surgery is an important etiologic factor for the development of FBSS. In patients who do not present with foot drop or cauda equina type syndrome, a trial of initial conservative medical management (CMM) may be in order. A randomized controlled trial (RCT) conducted in nine Dutch hospitals consisting of 283 patients with 6–12 weeks of sciatica determined that surgery was no better than CMM in the long term. The results of this RCT cannot be applied to our patient because the trial excluded patients presenting with a cauda equina syndrome or severe motor weakness (Medical Research Council score <3) and those who had identical symptoms in the previous 12 months or a history of spinal surgery, spinal stenosis, deformity, or severe comorbidity. Of the 141 patients assigned to undergo early surgery, 125 (89%) underwent microdiscectomy. Of the 142 patients assigned to conservative treatment, 62 (44%) eventually required surgery. There was no significant overall difference between treatment arms in disability scores during the first 2 years ($p = 0.25$). Improvement in leg pain was faster for patients randomized to early surgery ($p = 0.05$). This short-term benefit of early surgery was no longer significant by 6 months and continued to narrow between 6 and 24 months. At 2 years, 20% of all patients reported an unsatisfactory outcome. Early surgery achieved more rapid relief of sciatica than did conservative care, but outcomes were similar by 1 year, and these did not change during the second year.[18]

Why Does Our Patient Have Persistent LBP? What Is the Explanation for His Radicular Leg Pain?

The patient also describes radicular neuropathic pain radiating down to the lower extremities. It is dysthetic (burning) in nature and generates a tingling paresthesia. This patient does not report hyperalgesia and allodynia to suggest central sensitization. However, he has moderate foraminal stenosis bilaterally at L5–S1 and moderate to severe foraminal stenosis at L4–L5 on the left side and mild on the right side. These are responsible for root compression at the exiting neural foramen and generation of bilateral leg pain.

This patient has a neuropathic pain component that started with the underlying pathology (disc herniation) and was further complicated by discitis and abscess, resulting in a more extensive laminectomy at L3–L4. Neuropathic pain represents a reorganization of central and peripheral neuronal circuits, ephaptic transmission, recruitment of wide dynamic range neurons, and nerve ending sensitization, all of which serve to reinforce a pathologic, chronic pain state.[5]

WHAT MEDICATIONS MAY BE HELPFUL FOR PAIN CONTROL?

Combination pharmacotherapy is a cornerstone in the management of FBSS and should be utilized as part of multimodal and multidisciplinary treatment algorithm, with the aim of maximizing pain reduction and improving quality of life. Although a variety of medications with analgesic properties are available, their effect, although statistically significant, is clinically modest. On its own, conventional pharmacotherapy has a poor track record in the treatment of FBSS. Available agents include acetaminophen, nonsteroidal anti-inflammatory drugs (NSAIDs), opioids, antidepressants, anticonvulsants, and muscle relaxants.[19]

The real challenge of pharmacotherapy lies in the difficulty of balancing adequate analgesia with acceptable tolerability. Clinicians and patients are familiar with the self-perpetuating cycle of insufficient drug efficacy leading to dose escalation resulting in onset of unacceptable side effects. As a knee-jerk phenomenon, the treating physician then proceeds in dose reduction, which results in insufficient pain control. Medication side effects, inadequate analgesia, and drug tolerance drive this pattern and contribute to treatment nonadhereance.[19]

AVAILABLE AGENTS

The use of acetaminophen is ubiquitous in pain medicine. It constitutes first-line treatment for chronic LBP. However, acetaminophen has not demonstrated efficacy for neuropathic pain. NSAIDs are usually trialed after failure of or in combination with acetaminophen.[20,21] They target nociceptive pain through their effects on cyclo-oxygenase (COX)-2 and subsequently inhibit prostaglandin synthesis. These agents have not proved effective in treatment of neuropathic pain.[22] Caution is advised when prescribing an NSAID because all agents in this group appear to be associated with gastrointestinal, cardiovascular, and renal side effects.[23] NSAIDs are associated with a 42% relative increase in the incidence of serious cardiovascular events such as myocardial infarction, stroke, heart failure, and hypertension.[24] In light of the significant toxicities of treatment, the long-term use of NSAIDs in chronic pain conditions is limited, especially in the elderly and those with significant cardiac, gastrointestinal, or renal comorbidities. If used, NSAIDs should be administered for a limited period and at the lowest effective dose.[19,24]

The use of opioids in the management of chronic LBP is controversial due to concerns surrounding development of analgesic tolerance and dependence. Furlan et al. in their meta-analysis reported a dropout rate of 33% over a mean follow-up of 5 weeks. Fifteen percent left because pain relief was inadequate, and 21% withdrew because of side effects.[25] Success with opioid therapy is contingent on identification of medical and psychosocial comorbidities. Consideration should be given to choice of drug, route of administration, dosage, and monitoring. Head-to-head comparison trials of various opioids have failed to identify the superiority of one agent over another.[19]

Antidepressants are widely used because they are known to ameliorate the neuropathic component of chronic LBP. Side effects are related to their anticholinergic properties and include sedation, xerostomia, blurred vision, orthostatic hypotension, weight gain, and urinary retention. Additionally, selective serotonin reuptake inhibitors carry side effects of sexual dysfunction, and sleep disturbance. The overall benefits of antidepressants are small.[19,26] However, the serotonin-norepinephrine reuptake inhibitor (SNRI), duloxetine has shown efficacy in improving chronic LBP and is FDA approved for the treatment of chronic musculoskeletal pain.[27,28]

The use of anticonvulsant agents, notably gabapentin and pregabalin, is based on their ability to target neuropathic pain. The main side effects are somnolence, dizziness, weight gain, and peripheral edema. Gabapentin also demonstrates a complicated titration scheme requiring up to 6–8 weeks of upward titration to achieve a target dose of 1,800–3,600 mg/d as three divided doses. An adequate trial of gabapentin comprises 6–8 weeks to enable titration and a further 1–2 weeks at the maximum tolerated dose.[22] The FDA has approved pregabalin for adults in management of postherpetic neuralgia and neuropathic pain associated with spinal cord injury and diabetic peripheral neuropathy and in the treatment of fibromyalgia.[29]

COMBINATION THERAPY

FBSS is a mixed pain syndrome, encompassing both nociceptive and neuropathic mechanisms. Nonspecific nociceptive pain is the result of an inflammatory response to tissue injury. Neuropathic pain is the consequence of injury to the nervous system. For some patients, chronic LBP can be adequately managed with single-agent therapy. However, more than half of patients with CLBP have a neuropathic pain component for which combination pharmacotherapy is usually required. Several studies document improved analgesia with combination therapy and reduction of single-drug consumption (Table 13.1). Most combinations comprise an opioid/nonopioid analgesic. The drawbacks of combination therapy are adherence (especially if variable dosing schemes are employed), drug-drug interactions, and tolerability.[19] Additionally, there is a lack of evidence for long-term efficacy of opioids in chronic noncancer pain and in FBSS.

Role of Oral Pharmacotherapy

Oral pharmacotherapy by itself will likely be inadequate in alleviating our patient's symptoms, but it is helpful as part of an interdisciplinary, multimodal approach. We would propose starting this patient on combination gabapentin (300 mg, 3 times per day) titrated upward by increments of 300 mg every 3–7 days with a target dose of 1,800–2,700 mg/d for up to 3 weeks. If pain fails to respond to gabapentin, pregabalin may be substituted. The dose of pregabalin should start at 75 mg twice per day and can be increased if needed to 300–450 mg/d in divided doses over weekly increments of 75 mg as tolerated. Gabapentin or pregabalin may need to be supplemented with an opioidergic agent, initially tramadol or acetaminophen with codeine (2 tablets, 2–3 times per day). If the analgesic effect is inadequate, another long-acting opioid like morphine SR may have to be trialed. The third class of medications to add would be a tricyclic antidepressant or SNRI.

Table 13.1 INDICATIONS, MECHANISM OF ACTION, AND EVIDENCE FOR PHARMACOTHERAPY

DRUG	INDICATION	MECHANISM OF ACTION	EVIDENCE
Acetaminophen	Nociceptive pain Recommended as first-line treatment for chronic LBP	Inhibits prostaglandin synthesis by acting on the cyclo-oxygenase (COX) enzymes Reinforces descending inhibitory pain pathways	Zhang et al. (2004)[30] Meta-analysis of 10 RCTs; acetaminophen is an effective agent for pain relief due to osteoarthritis. Although safer, it is less effective than NSAIDs.
NSAIDs	Recommended for nociceptive back pain when acetaminophen fails	Traditional NSAIDs inhibit prostaglandin synthesis by acting on the COX-1 (blocks production of gastroprotective prostaglandins) and COX-2 (blocks production of pro-inflammatory prostaglandins) enzymes COX-2 agents inhibit COX-2 only	Katz et al. (2003)[31] Two 4-week, randomized, double-blind studies using rofecoxib or placebo; significant reductions in LBP intensity were observed in rofecoxib groups ($p < 0.05$); reductions were significantly greater than with placebo ($p < 0.001$)
	Caution advised when used in elderly and those with preexisting cardiovascular, renal, and gastrointestinal disease		Roelofset al. (2008)[32] Meta-analysis by Cochrane collaboration of 65 trials; NSAIDs are effective for short-term symptomatic relief in chronic LBP without sciatica; however, effect sizes are small. There is no evidence that one NSAID is more effective than another.
Opioids	Effective in nociceptive pain and moderately effective in neuropathic pain	Bind to opioid receptors in the central nervous system, modulating the pathways involved in the generation, transmission, and modulation of pain impulses and the experience of pain	Allan et al. (2005)[33] 13-month, open-label, randomized, parallel group study of transdermal fentanyl patch or sustained-release morphine 30 mg every 12 h. Transdermal fentanyl and sustained-release morphine provided similar levels of pain relief (assessed using 0–100 mm VAS), however transdermal fentanyl was associated with a lower incidence of constipation.
	Tolerability issues with opioids limit their usefulness in clinical practice		Katz et al. (2007)[34] Enriched Enrollment Randomized Withdrawal Trial (EERW) Mean pain intensity (0–100 mm VAS) decreased from 69.4 mm pre-titration to 22.7 mm post-titration ($p < 0.0001$) of oxymorphone ER. Rates of discontinuation due to lack of efficacy were significantly higher with placebo than with oxymorphone ER ($p < 0.0001$). Pain intensity increased significantly more with placebo (+26.9) than with oxymorphone ER (+10.0; $p < 0.0001$).
	Concerns surrounding development of analgesic tolerance and dependence in susceptible patients		Noble et al. (2010)[35] Meta-analysis by Cochrane collaboration; 26 studies with 27 treatment groups ($n = 4{,}893$). Discontinuation due to AEs or insufficient pain relief is common during long-term opioid therapy. Patients who continue opioid therapy long term experience clinically significant pain relief.
Antidepressants	Neuropathic pain	Noradrenaline and serotonin neurotransmission by reuptake inhibition; actions on opioid, adrenergic, serotonin, γ-aminobutyric acid and N-methyl-D-aspartate receptors; ion channel activation; and effects on inflammatory cytokines	Katz et al. (2005)[36] No significant difference between bupropion SR and placebo were observed for daily and weekly pain scores. Skljarevskiet al. (2009)[37] 13-week, multicenter, randomized, double-blind, parallel group study. Duloxetine 60 mg yielded significantly greater reductions than placebo in mean 24-h average pain (assessed using 0–10 Likert scale) during weeks 3–11, but this superiority was not maintained to week 13. Urquhart et al. (2008)[38] Meta-analysis by Cochrane collaboration. There is no clear evidence suggesting that antidepressants are more effective than placebo in the management of patients with chronic LBP.

(Continued)

Table 13.1 CONTINUED

DRUG	INDICATION	MECHANISM OF ACTION	EVIDENCE
Anticonvulsants	Neuropathic pain	Pregabalin and gabapentin exert their analgesic effects by binding to the α2-δ subunit of N-type voltage-gated calcium channels thereby modulating pathologically enhanced neurotransmission in the central terminals of primary afferent neurons	Remmerset al. (2000)[39] RCT; no significant difference was observed between pregabalin and placebo in mean pain scores. Khoromiet al. (2005)[40] No difference between topiramate and placebo in reduction of average leg pain. Percentage pain reduction scores significantly better with topiramate than with placebo for average back pain, average overall pain, and worst overall pain. Yaksiet al. (2007)[41] 4-month RCT; increase in walking distance was significantly greater with gabapentin than with placebo ($p = 0.001$). Improvements in pain scores and sensory deficit were significantly greater with gabapentin than with placebo.
Combination Therapy	Mixed Pain		Romano et al. (2009)[42] Combination therapy with pregabalin + celexocib was more effective than either monotherapy for mean pain reduction. Khoromiet al. (2007)[43] Crossover, RCT No significant reductions in mean leg pain or other leg or back pain were observed in any treatment group (morphine + nortryptyline vs. either agent alone). Pain reduction relative to placebo was 14% for nortriptyline, 7% for morphine, and 7% for combination therapy. Pelosoet al. (2004)[44] Mean final pain intensity scores (assessed using 0–100 mm VAS) were significantly lower with combination therapy with tramadol + acetaminophen (47.4) than with placebo (62.9; $p < 0.001$), as were mean final pain relief scores (assessed on 6-point Likert scale: 1.8 and 0.7, respectively, $p < 0.001$).

LBP, lower back pain; RCT, randomized controlled trial; VAS, visual analog scale

The issues of tolerability, polypharmacy, and drug-drug interactions should be kept in mind (e.g., tramadol and antidepressants). If, however, it is found that the side effects are intolerable or pain relief inadequate, serious consideration should be given to neuromodulatory techniques.

WHAT REHABILITATION TECHNIQUES MAY BE HELPFUL IN RESTORING FUNCTION?

MULTIDISCIPLINARY PAIN MANAGEMENT

Multidisciplinary management is of value in the treatment of chronic back pain in general and FBSS in particular. The typical approach includes establishment of a team consisting of a pain specialist, a physiotherapist to provide an individualized exercise and rehabilitation program, and a psychologist to help with cognitive behavioral therapy. Multidisciplinary treatment has been found to be more effective in reducing pain intensity compared with no treatment.[45] A Cochrane review concluded that there was strong evidence that an intensive multidisciplinary rehabilitation with a functional restoration approach decreased pain and improved function.[46]

Miller et al. conducted a prospective study to compare treatment responses between non-FBSS and FBSS patients with chronic LBP at a multidisciplinary clinic. They found that, overall, both FBSS and non-FBSS patients improved with regard to pain and functional level. Comparing the effects of physical therapy, the FBSS group demonstrated greater improvement versus the non-FBSS group.[47]

ACUPUNCTURE

For chronic LBP, acupuncture is modestly more effective for pain relief and functional improvement than no treatment or sham treatment in the short term. Most studies have not found acupuncture to be superior to other conventional treatments (e.g., analgesics, transcutaneous electrical stimulation [TENS], and self-care education) or alternative treatments (e.g., massage or spinal manipulation). A Cochrane review by Furlan et al. concluded that the average pain reduction in the group that received acupuncture for chronic LBP was 32% compared to 23% in those who received sham therapies and 6% in those who received no treatment.[48]

CHIROPRACTIC INTERVENTION AND SPINE MANIPULATION THERAPY (SMT)

Walker et al. reviewed 12 studies involving 2,887 participants with LBP. There was no evidence of a significant difference between chiropractic and other treatments for any outcomes for individuals with chronic or mixed duration LBP. The current evidence does not indicate that these interventions provide a clinically meaningful difference for pain or disability in people with LBP when compared to other interventions.[49] Similarly, Rubenstein et al. analyzed evidence from 26 RCTs of 6,070 patients and found no difference between SMT and other interventions for reducing pain and improving function in patients with chronic LBP.[50] The benefit of chiropractic or SMT in cases of FBSS is not documented.

EXERCISE

In a Cochrane review of 43 trials of 3,907 individuals with chronic LBP, there was strong evidence that exercise is at least as effective as other conservative treatments. Individually designed strengthening or stabilizing programs appear to be effective in healthcare settings. Although functional outcomes significantly improved, the effects were very small. Pain outcomes were also significantly improved in groups receiving exercises relative to other comparisons. Benefits were maintained over longer follow-up.[51]

MASSAGE

Furlan et al. reviewed 13 RCTs and concluded that massage might be beneficial for patients with subacute and chronic nonspecific LBP, especially when combined with exercise and education. There was insufficient evidence to verify an impact of massage on return-to-work and to determine the cost-effectiveness of massage as an intervention for LBP.[52]

TENS

In their review, van Middelkoop et al. found no difference in the effectiveness of TENS compared with sham TENS.[45] These findings were consistent with a Cochrane review of four high-quality RCTs performed by Khadilkar et al.[53] The authors concluded that evidence from placebo-controlled trials does not support the use of TENS in the routine management of chronic LBP.[53] In cases of FBSS, a positive trial of TENS tends to indicate a favorable response to SCS but not vice-versa.

Our patient was appropriately referred to a multidisciplinary back pain clinic for further evaluation and management. A trial of an interdisciplinary, multimodal treatment algorithm should continue for 4–8 weeks, with particular emphasis on pain and functional improvement (e.g., return to work, and ability to carry out activities of daily living) and downward titration of pharmacotherapy (especially opioid consumption). Objective, measurable goals should be established at the outset of therapy and continually reassessed. The evidence supports the inclusion of a pain medicine specialist, physiotherapist, and psychologist as part of a team approach. Supervised exercise is key, and therapy must be intensive (at least 100 h in duration)[46] to be of benefit. A precise structure for an "ideal" multidisciplinary treatment algorithm does not exist in the literature. An intensive treatment plan requires significant commitments by both the patient and healthcare team.

Chiropractic treatment, acupuncture, spinal manipulation, or TENS are unlikely to offer long-lasting pain relief in this case. The results of the pain clinic evaluations will be helpful in deciding if the patient requires spinal fusion and/or interventional therapy such as SCS or intrathecal drug therapy (IDT).

WHAT, IF ANY, INJECTIONS OR NERVE BLOCKS MAY BE OF USE TO CONTROL PAIN?

EPIDURAL INJECTIONS

In general, there is good evidence for epidural steroid injections (ESIs) in short-term pain relief, especially for radicular symptoms of FBSS. Long-term benefits, however, are not maintained. A recent review by Manchikanti and colleagues reported level I evidence for caudal ESI in long-term (>6 months) improvement in pain secondary to disc herniation with radiculopathy and discogenic pain without radiculopathy especially at the L5–S1 level.[54] Interlaminar ESI could be equally helpful if performed under fluoroscopy.

ESIs enable instillation of corticosteroid and/or anesthetic agents directly adjacent to suspected painful intervertebral discs with minimal systemic side effects. Corticosteroids and local anesthetics possess anti-inflammatory and neural stabilizing effects. These solutions likely exert their therapeutic benefits by bathing the posterolateral annular fibers, which are the pain triggering mechanism.[55,56]

The epidural space may be accessed via three routes, which are discussed in the following paragraphs:

- Interlaminar (ILESI)
- Transforaminal (TESI)
- Caudal (CESI)

In the interlaminar approach, the injected agent is deposited into the posterior epidural space. Although it is the most commonly employed approach, a significant limitation is that medication may not reach the site of pathology in the ventral epidural space. In their analysis, Stojanovic and colleagues performed epidurograms of 38 cervical ESIs in 31 patients. The authors found a 53% rate of false loss of resistance during the first attempt to enter the epidural space. Unilateral epidural contrast spread was found in 51%, and ventral epidural spread was found in only 28% of cases.[57] Furthermore, Fredman et al., in a study of 50 patients with FBSS, observed that even if the epidural space was successfully accessed, depot-steroid solution spread to reach the level of pathology in only 26% of cases.[58]

A fundamental shortcoming of studies evaluating the efficacy of ILESI is that injections were often performed blind, without fluoroscopic guidance. RCTs examining ILESI are listed in Table 13.2; none of these studies employed fluoroscopy. Furthermore, results of these trials do not convincingly delineate the efficacy of ILESIs for axial LBP.

The transforaminal approach has been observed to provide ventral epidural spread in virtually 100% of cases and is therefore considered superior to ILESI.[59] Fluoroscopically guided transforaminal injections may be an important tool in the nonsurgical management of lumbosacral radiculopathy secondary to a herniated nucleus pulposus. CESI is performed by inserting a spinal needle into the sacral epidural space by means of the sacral hiatus. The main advantage of this procedure is the relative ease of performance in thin individuals without requiring fluoroscopy. However, the sacral epidural space must be filled before the injected medication reaches the lumbar region, requiring large volumes that tend to dilute the steroid mixture. CESIs rarely reach the ventral epidural space or move higher than the L5–S1 segmental level.[60,61]

The heterogeneity of evidence has led to varying recommendations from several pain societies. The 2006 European guidelines for the management of CLBP reasoned that ESI be considered only for radicular pain, if a contained disc prolapse is the cause of the pain, and if the corticosteroid is injected close to the site of pathology. Moreover, injections should be fluoroscopically guided toward the ventral epidural space.[62] In its 2007 guidelines, the American Academy of Neurology reached an opposing conclusion and determined that ESI for radicular lumbosacral pain does not impact average impairment of function, need for surgery, or provide long-term pain relief beyond 3 months. They suggested that routine use was not recommended (level B evidence).[63]

The efficacy of ESI may be time-limited and route-dependent. In their review, Buenaventura et al. concluded that evidence for TESI was level II-1 for short-term relief (<6 months) and level II-2 for long-term improvement in the management of lumbar nerve root and LBP.[64] Parr and colleagues reviewed the state of the evidence for lumbar ILESI. The evidence was positive (level II-2) for short-term relief of pain of disc herniation or radiculitis utilizing blind ILESI, with lack of evidence for long-term relief for disc herniation and radiculitis. The evidence was also lacking for short- and long-term relief for spinal stenosis and discogenic pain without radiculitis or disc herniation utilizing blind epidural injections. The major limitations cited were the paucity of literature, lack of quality evidence, and lack of fluoroscopic procedures.[65]

Thomas and colleagues randomized 31 patients with discal radicular pain to receive either X-ray-guided transforaminal or blindly performed interspinous epidural corticosteroid injections. At 6 months follow-up, patients in the transforaminal injection arms showed greater improvement in pain, daily activities, work and leisure activities, anxiety, and depression.[66] Although TESI appears to afford better and longer lasting pain relief than interlaminar and caudal ESI, the added benefit must be balanced against the higher risk of the procedure. There are reports of death and paraplegia following cervical and thoracic TESI and paraplegia after lumbar TESI. By comparison, serious complications with ILESI and CESI are exceedingly rare.[67–69]

EPIDURAL ADHESIOLYSIS

Epter et al. in their systematic review of three RCTs concluded that percutaneous adhesiolysis was highly effective in the management of chronic LBP in FBSS with level I to II-1 evidence. It was superior to ESI and safe. The effectiveness of percutaneous

Table 13.2 EVIDENCE FOR EPIDURAL INJECTIONS

RCT	METHODOLOGY	RESULTS
ILESI		
Serrao et al. (1992)[70]	Epidural methylprednisolone (80 mg) compared with intrathecal midazolam (2 mg) in 28 patients with chronic LBP. Pain assessed at baseline and 2 months post-treatment using the short-form McGill Pain Questionnaire, VAS, verbal rating scales for sensory and affective components of pain experience, and pain diary.	No statistically significant difference in pain or analgesic observed between the two groups at 2 months.
Carette et al. (1997)[71]	Up to three ESIs of methylprednisolone acetate (80 mg in 8 mL of isotonic saline) or isotonic saline (1 mL) to 158 patients with sciatica due to a herniated nucleus pulposus. All patients had Oswestry disability scores higher than 20	At 3 weeks, differences in improvements between the groups were not significant, except for improvements in the finger-to-floor distance ($p = 0.006$) and sensory deficits ($p = 0.03$), which were greater in the methylprednisolone group. After 6 weeks, the only significant difference was the improvement in leg pain, which was greater in the methylprednisolone group ($p = 0.03$). After 3 months, there were no significant differences between the groups. ESI did not offer significant functional benefit nor reduce the need for surgery.
Arden at al. (2005)[72]	228 patients with unilateral sciatica of 1–18 months' duration were randomized into two groups: either (a) three lumbar ESIs of triamcinolone acetonide or (b) three lumbar ESIs of interligamentous saline injections at 3-week intervals. The main outcome measure was the Oswestry LBP disability questionnaire.	At 3 weeks, the ESI group demonstrated a transient benefit over the placebo group. No benefit was demonstrated from 6–52 weeks. ESIs did not improve physical function, hasten return to work, or reduce the need for surgery. There was no benefit of repeated ESIs over single injection. At last follow-up, patients had significant pain and disability regardless of intervention.
TESI		
Karppinen et al. (2001)[73]	160 patients with unilateral sciatica were randomized for double-blind injection with methylprednisolone bupivacaine combination or saline. Objective and self-reported outcome parameters and costs were recorded at baseline, at 2 and 4 weeks, at 3 and 6 months, and at 1 year.	Overall, no statistically significant difference was found between the methylprednisolone and saline groups at 1-year follow-up. The combination of methylprednisolone and bupivacaine seemed to have a short-term effect, but at 3 and 6 months, the steroid group experienced a "rebound" in pain. By 1 year, 18 patients in the steroid group and 15 in the saline group underwent surgery.
Vad et al. (2002)[74]	Patients received either a TESI or a saline trigger-point injection. Treatment outcome was measured using a patient satisfaction scale with choice options of 0 (poor), 1 (fair), 2 (good), 3 (very good), and 4 (excellent); Roland-Morris LBP questionnaire; a measurement of finger-to-floor distance and VAS. The final analysis included 48 patients with an average follow-up period of 16 months.	After an average follow-up period of 1.4 years, the group receiving transforaminal epidural steroid injections had a success rate of 84%, as compared with 48% for the group receiving trigger point injections ($p < 0.005$).
Ng et al. (2005)[75]	Patients with unilateral radicular pain who failed conservative management were randomized for a single injection with bupivacaine and methylprednisolone ($n = 43$) or bupivacaine only ($n = 43$). Outcome measures included the Oswestry Disability Index, VAS for back pain and leg pain, claudication walking distance, and the patient's subjective level of satisfaction of the outcome.	There was no statistically significant difference in the outcome measures between the groups at 3 months

(Continued)

Table 13.2 **CONTINUED**

RCT	METHODOLOGY	RESULTS
CESI		
Breivik et al. (1976)[76]	A parallel cohort study of 35 patients with chronic LBP and sciatic pain treated with up to three blind CESIs of either bupivicaine and methylprednisolone or bupivacaine and normal saline.	Initially, 56% of patients receiving methylprednisolone experienced significant relief compared with only 26% treated with bupivicaine/saline. In the crossover, 14% of the methylprednisolone group obtained relief from subsequent bupivicaine/saline injections, whereas 73% of the bupivicaine/saline group reported satisfactory relief after the methylprednisolone injection. Fifty percent of the methylprednisolone group and 20% of the bupivicaine group returned to work at a range of 3–17 months after treatment.
Bush et al. (1991)[77]	Assessed the efficacy of epidural injections of 80 mg triamcinolone acetonide plus 0.5% procaine hydrochloride in saline, administered via the caudal route with 1-year follow-up. Twenty-three patients were entered into the study: 12 received treatment and 11 placebo.	The active group showed significant pain relief ($p = 0.02$) and a significant increase in mobility ($p = 0.01$) at 4 weeks, which resulted in improved quality of life ($p = 0.02$). At 1 year, however, there was no statistically significant difference between both groups.
Dashfield et al. (2005)[78]	60 patients with a 6- to 18-month history of sciatica were randomized to either targeted epidural local anaesthetic or steroid placement with a spinal endoscope or caudal epidural local anaesthetic and steroid treatment. Pretreatment and 6-week, 3-month, and 6-month SF-MPQ and HAD scores were recorded.	No significant differences were found between the groups for any of the measures at any time. When analyzed individually, both techniques benefited patients.

CESI, caudal epidural space injection; ILESI, interlaminar epidural space injection; LBP, lower back pain; TESI transformainal epidural space injection adhesiolysis was demonstrated both with 1-day and 3-day procedures. The 1-day protocol involves injection of local anesthetic, hypertonic or normal saline with or without hyaluronidase, and steroid.[69] In a 3-day protocol, the first day is identical to the 1-day protocol but the remaining two days involve instillation of local anesthetic and saline into the epidural space.[80] See Table 13.3 for a summary of evidence for adhesiolysis.

FACET INTERVENTIONS

Despite their widespread use, the evidence for various facet interventions is inconclusive with little support for long-term benefit. Two of the most frequently used techniques are intra-articular corticosteroid injection and medial branch radiofrequency (RF) denervation—a neuroablative procedure that damages the afferent nerve supply to the joint(s). In their review, Cohen and Raja recognized that there was conflicting evidence for the efficacy of intra-articular steroid injections and suggested that they may provide intermediate-term relief to a small subset of patients with facet pain associated with an active inflammatory process.[84] The evidence for efficacy of this procedure is summarized in Table 13.4.

The evidence for benefit from RF neurolysis is similarly mixed. Three RCTs suggest no benefit.[89–91] Larger, prospective studies with longer follow-up are required to better delineate the risks and benefits of denervation. The evidence for efficacy of this procedure is summarized in Table 13.5.

SI JOINT INTERVENTIONS

The SI joint is accepted as a source of low back and/or buttock pain with or without lower extremity pain. The SI joint has been implicated as the primary source of pain in 10–27% of patients utilizing controlled comparative local anesthetic blocks. Rupert et al. systematically reviewed the evidence and concluded that there was level II-2 support for the diagnosis of SI joint pain utilizing comparative, controlled local anesthetic blocks. However, the authors noted the false-positive rate of single, uncontrolled SI joint injections is 20–54%. There was limited evidence (level II-3) for RF neurotomy. The limitations of the review included the paucity of literature evaluating the role of both diagnostic and therapeutic interventions and widespread methodological flaws in the studies evaluated.[92] McKenzie-Brown and colleagues in their review determined that there was moderate evidence for short-term and limited evidence for long-term relief with intraarticular SI joint injections. Evidence for RF neurotomy in managing SI joint pain was inconclusive.[93]

THERMAL ANNULAR PROCEDURES

The treatment of chronic discogenic LBP remains a challenge for patients and physicians. Intradiscal electrothermal therapy (IDET) was introduced in 2000 as a safer and less invasive alternative to treat discogenic pain. The IDET procedure involves placement of an intradiscal catheter with a

Table 13.3 EVIDENCE FOR ADHESIOLYSIS

RCT	METHODOLOGY	RESULTS
Manchikanti et al. (2005)[81]	83 patients evaluated, with 33 patients in Group I and 50 patients in Group II. Group I served as the control, with endoscopy into the sacral level without adhesiolysis, followed by injection of local anesthetic and steroid. Group II received spinal endoscopic adhesiolysis, followed by injection of local anesthetic and steroids.	Significant improvement in the spinal endoscopic adhesiolysis group occurred in 80% at 3 months, 56% at 6 months, and 48% at 12 months. The control group showed improvement in 33% of the patients at 1 month and none thereafter.
Veihelmann et al. (2006)[82]	99 patients with chronic LBP were randomly assigned either to physiotherapy ($n = 52$) or epidural neuroplasty ($n = 47$). Patients were assessed before and 3, 6, and 12 months after treatment by a blinded investigator.	After 3 months, the VAS score for back and leg pain was significantly reduced in the epidural neuroplasty group, and the need for pain medication was reduced in both groups. Furthermore, the VAS for back and leg pain as well as the Oswestry disability score were significantly reduced until 12 months for the epidural neuroplastygroup in contrast to the group that received conservative treatment.
Manchikanti et al. (2009)[83]	Patients were randomly assigned to one of two groups: Group I (60 patients) receiving caudal epidural injections with catheterization up to S3 with local anesthetic, steroids, and 0.9% sodium chloride solution serving as the control group, and Group II (60 patients) receiving percutaneous adhesiolysis with targeted delivery of lidocaine, 10% hypertonic sodium chloride solution, and non-particulate betamethasone serving as t he intervention group.	Significant pain relief (≥ 50%) and functional status improvement was recorded in 73% of patients in Group II versus 12% in Group I ($p < 0.001$). The average procedures per year were 3.5 with an average total relief of 42 out of 52 weeks in Group II and 2.2 procedures with total relief per year of 13 weeks in Group I ($p < 0.001$).

LBP, low back pain; RCT, randomized controlled trial; VAS, visual analog scale

Table 13.4 EVIDENCE FOR FACET INTERVENTIONS

RCT	METHODOLOGY	RESULTS
Lilius et al. (1989)[85]	109 patients with unilateral low back pain for more than 3 months were randomized to receive one of three types of injection treatment: cortisone and local anaesthetic injected into two facet joints ($n = 28$), the same mixture around two facet joints ($n = 39$), or physiological saline into two facet joints ($n = 42$).	A significant improvement was observed in work attendance, pain, and disability scores, in all three groups. Movements of the lumbar spine were not improved. Of the 70 patients with initial pain relief after injection, 36% reported persisting benefit at the 3-month follow-up. Remarks: In the three arms, the agent used had no bearing on outcome.
Carette et al. (1991)[86]	Patients with chronic LBP who reported immediate relief of their pain after injections of local anesthetic into the facet joints between the L4–L5 or L5–S1 vertebrae were randomly assigned to receive under fluoroscopic guidance injections of either methylprednisolone acetate (20 mg; $n = 49$) or isotonic saline ($n = 48$) in the same facet joints. Ninety-five patients were followed for 6 months, and their condition assessed with scales of pain severity, back mobility, and limitation of function.	After 1 month, none of the outcome measures evaluating pain, functional status, and back flexion differed clinically or statistically between the two study groups. The results were similar after 3 months. At the 6-month evaluation, the patients treated with methylprednisolone reported more improvement, less pain on the VAS, and less physical disability. Moreover, only 11 patients (22%) in the methylprednisolone group and five (10%) in the placebo group had sustained improvement at 6 months. Remarks: The trial failed to substantiate a long-term benefit of facet joint injections.
Marks et al. (1992)[87]	86 patients with refractory chronic LBP were randomly assigned to receive either facet joint injection or facet nerve block, using local anesthetic and steroid.	No significant difference in the immediate response. The duration of response after facet joint injection was marginally longer than after facet nerve block ($p < 0.05$ 1 month after infiltration), but for both groups the response was usually short-lived; by 3 months, only two patients continued to report complete pain relief. Remarks: The trial failed to substantiate a benefit of facet joint injections or facet nerve blocks.
Manchikanti et al. (2009)[88]	60 patients in each group with local anesthetic alone (Group I) or local anesthetic and steroids (Group II). Outcome measures included the numeric rating scale, Oswestry Disability Index, opioid intake, and work status at baseline, 3, 6, 12, 18, and 24 months.	Significant pain relief of ≥50% and functional improvement of ≥40% were observed in 85% in Group 1, and 90% in Group II at 2-year follow-up. The patients in the study experienced significant pain relief for 82–84 weeks of 104 weeks, requiring approximately 5–6 treatments with an average relief of 19 weeks per episode of treatment. Remarks: To maintain efficacy, these treatments need to repeated at regular intervals.

LBP, low back pain; RCT, randomized controlled trial; VAS, visual analog scale

Table 13.5 EVIDENCE FOR RADIOFREQUENCY DENERVATION

RCT	METHODOLOGY	RESULTS
Gallagher et al. (1994)[84]	60 patients with chronic LBP and leg pain randomized to one of three groups: Group I, RF denervation of the primary posterior ramus; Group II, RF performed using a 1.25-inch needle inserted within the area of maximum tenderness; Group III, stimulation but no coagulation (control)	In group I, 27% achieved greater than 50% pain relief at 6 months versus 53% in group II and 0% in group III Remarks: The benefits of treatment are equivalent to placebo.
Leclaire et al. (2001)[85]	70 patients with LBP and a good response after intra-articular facet injections under fluoroscopy were assigned randomly to receive percutaneous radiofrequency articular facet denervation under fluoroscopic guidance or the same procedure without effective denervation (sham therapy).	At 4 weeks, no significant treatment effect was reflected in the Oswestry or the VAS score. The only significant treatment effect was reflected in the Roland-Morris scale. At 12 weeks, neither functional disability, as assessed by the Roland-Morris scale and Oswestry scale, nor the pain level, as assessed by the VAS showed any treatment effect. Remarks: The benefits of treatment are equivalent to placebo.
Van Wijk et al. (2005)[86]	Inclusion criteria were LBP, duration more than 6 months, and ≥50% VAS reduction on diagnostic block. A total of 81 patients were randomized to undergo radiofrequency facet joint denervation or sham treatment.	The combined outcome measure (VAS, physical activities, and analgesic intake) showed no differences between radiofrequency facet joint denervation and sham. The VAS in both groups improved ($p < 0.001$). Remarks: The benefits of treatment are equivalent to placebo.

LBP, low back pain; RCT, randomized controlled trial; VAS, visual analog scale

6 cm electrothermal tip around the posterolateral border of the inner annulus, which is then heated to a peak temperature of 90°C. Mechanisms of action for IDET remain a subject of debate, but may include nociceptors denervation, collagen denaturation, and the sealing of annular tears. Several variations of IDET have emerged, including intradiscal RF intradiscal thermocoagulation, intradiscal biacuplasty, and discTRODE, in which the RF electrode is directly inserted into the posterolateral mid-annulus. The evidence supporting or refuting any of these techniques is severely limited.[94,95]

> ESIs, epidural adhesiolysis, facet and SI joint interventions do not convincingly offer sustained pain relief. There may be a role for ESI in temporary palliation of our patient's radicular pain, given its discogenic origin. The results of any of these interventions will prove unsatisfactory and fail to show durable, long-term benefit.

WHAT IS THE INCIDENCE OF PERSISTENT PAIN FOLLOWING LUMBAR SPINE SURGERY?

Despite technological advances and increasing rates of lumbosacral spinal surgery, the rates of FBSS remain unchanged. Depending on the definition of failure, the incidence of FBSS varies from 5% to 40%, with an average rate of approximately 15%.[96–99] Reoperation suffers from the law of diminishing returns. The success rate with the first operation is approximately 50%, dropping to 30% after the second surgery, 15% after the third, and 5% after the fourth.[100] It should be noted that these statistics are decades old and much has changed since these original studies were performed.

Failure rates also differ between surgical procedures and technical factors. The failure rate of lumbar fusion is quoted at between 30% and 46%. RCTs suggest that microdiscectomy is successful in 81%. Conversely, the failure rate in patients with sciatic pain due to disc herniation 2 years postsurgery is approximately 20%.[101] Ryang et al. compared the results of open microdiscectomy with minimal-access microsurgical discectomy and did not report any statistical difference between the two techniques in regard to surgical time, blood loss, complications, or pain improvement.[102]

SPINE INSTABILITY AND ADJACENT SEGMENT DISEASE FOLLOWING FUSION

Lumbar degenerative spondylolisthesis is often treated with decompression and fusion with or without instrumentation. Spinal fusion alters the biomechanics and kinematics of the lumbar spine as the mobility of adjacent segments increases after a short segment fusion. Adjacent segment disease (ASD) is recognized as an important causative factor for FBSS. This development of ASD is time-dependent. Ghiselli et al. reviewed a series of 223 patients with an average of 6.7 years of follow-up for the development of new disease requiring additional surgery because of degenerative changes adjacent to thoracolumbar, lumbar, and lumbosacral fusions. Based on a Kaplan-Meier survivorship analysis, the authors concluded that 37% of the patients in their cohort would be expected to require an additional surgical procedure for ASD of the lumbar spine within 10 years of their index procedure.[103]

The changes seen at the adjacent level following fusion include instability of the motion segment, disc space narrowing, and stenosis caused by facet degeneration and ligament flavum hypertrophy. When extensive, the movement may produce mechanical deformation of intraspinal nerve tissue and thereby induce pain or neurological deficits. Even minor instability may cause irritation of receptors related to facet joints or other components of the motion segment, resulting in local pain and/or reflexively painful muscular spasm. In a retrospective review of 39 patients with previous lumbar fusion who underwent second lumbar spine surgery for adjacent instability, clinical results were excellent or good in 76.9% of patients whereas radiographic fusion was successful in 37 (94.9%) of patients.[104]

In a study by Kim and Michelsen of revision surgery for FBSS, 81% of patients achieving successful fusion had a satisfactory outcome, compared with 23% of patients who did not achieve solid fusion.[105]

REOPERATION

The incidence of recurrent lumbar disc herniation varies between 3% and 18%, reflecting variability in follow-up, surgical technique, and management paradigms among studies.[106–109] Vik et al. reported that recurrent disc herniation at the same level was suspected before the reoperation in 18.4%, but a recurrence was found in only 8.6%. This discrepancy was due to that fact that these authors relied on CT scan findings rather than MRI to diagnosis recurrent disc herniation. Outcome score was worse among reoperated patients than among patients who only had the primary operation ($p < 0.001$).[109]

SPINAL STENOSIS

Lateral spinal canal stenosis produces lumbar radicular symptomatology and is associated with FBSS.[1–3] An 8–11% incidence of lateral root entrapment has been reported.[110–112] Burton et al. considered nonspecific lateral canal stenosis as the cause of pain in nearly 60% of patients with continued postoperative symptoms.[8] Lumbar foraminal stenosis is an important pathologic entity to identify in patients being treated for radicular symptoms.

EPIDURAL FIBROSIS

Epidural fibrosis has been implicated as an etiology of FBSS. In a prospective cohort observational study, MRI diagnosed epidural fibrosis in only 16.1% of patients, whereas on epiduroscopy 91% of all patients with persistent pain after back surgery were found to have significant (grade 2, 3, or 4) fibrosis.[113]

REVISION SURGERY

Generally, revision surgery is not recommended unless a structural lesion amenable to operative intervention is found. Patient series assessing the long-term outcome of discectomy use variable outcome criteria and report "satisfactory" or "good" results in 56–89% of patients. All studies emphasize the importance of careful preoperative patient selection and planning. All such cases should be reviewed by an expert spine surgeon.[107,108,114,115]

Despite evidence that the results of lumbar discectomy are satisfactory only in cases where the disc protrusion is well-defined and impinges on the exiting nerve root and there is radiological and clinical evidence of nerve root entrapment, lumbar discectomy rates are increasing. Some findings point to higher population-based rates of surgery being associated with inferior outcomes.[115,116] Further research on the effectiveness of discectomy is needed.

Research into reoperations after discectomy is limited. Various cohort or population-based studies cite reoperation rates after lumbar discectomy at between 5% and 19% at 4- to 10-year follow-up, but the reasons for and outcomes of reoperations are not defined.[114] Good prognostic factors for reoperation are a pain-free interval longer than 6–12 months after the index operation and a definite recurrent herniation as an intraoperative finding. Segmental fusion is only recommended if a definite recurrence occurs at the same level and can be proved clinically and radiologically again. True recurrent disc herniations (same level, same side) may associate either with a favorable or a worse outcome. Overall, good results are harder to achieve compared with the index operation. Patients undergoing lumbar discectomy with one reoperation had a 25.1% risk of further spinal surgery in the next 10 years.[114]

It is suggested that reoperations performed less than a year after the index discectomy are likely to represent an inadequate response to the initial treatment and may also represent poor patient selection.[114]

Slipman et al. in their retrospective review found an equal distribution between the incidences of nonsurgical and surgical etiologies for FBSS. The most common diagnoses identified were spinal stenosis, internal disc disruption syndrome, recurrent/retained disc, and neural fibrosis. In light of their findings, the authors suggested that the practicing spine specialist must be comfortable with diagnosing a surgical lesion in this patient population before proceeding to surgical intervention.[1]

Is surgical intervention indicated, and if so, what? Our patient was at high risk for developing FBSS due to:

1. Postsurgical complications (i.e., epidural abscess)
2. Anterolisthesis at L4–L5 level due to facet degeneration with resulting foraminal stenosis at two levels
3. Associated epidural and perineural fibrosis/scarring

Due to grade I spondylolisthesis at L4–L5 and associated foraminal stenosis at L4–L5 and L5–S1, our patient needs the following surgical interventions:

1. Spinal pedicular screw assisted fusion from L4 to S1 (Figure 13.6)
2. Bilateral foraminotomies at L4–L5 and L5–S1

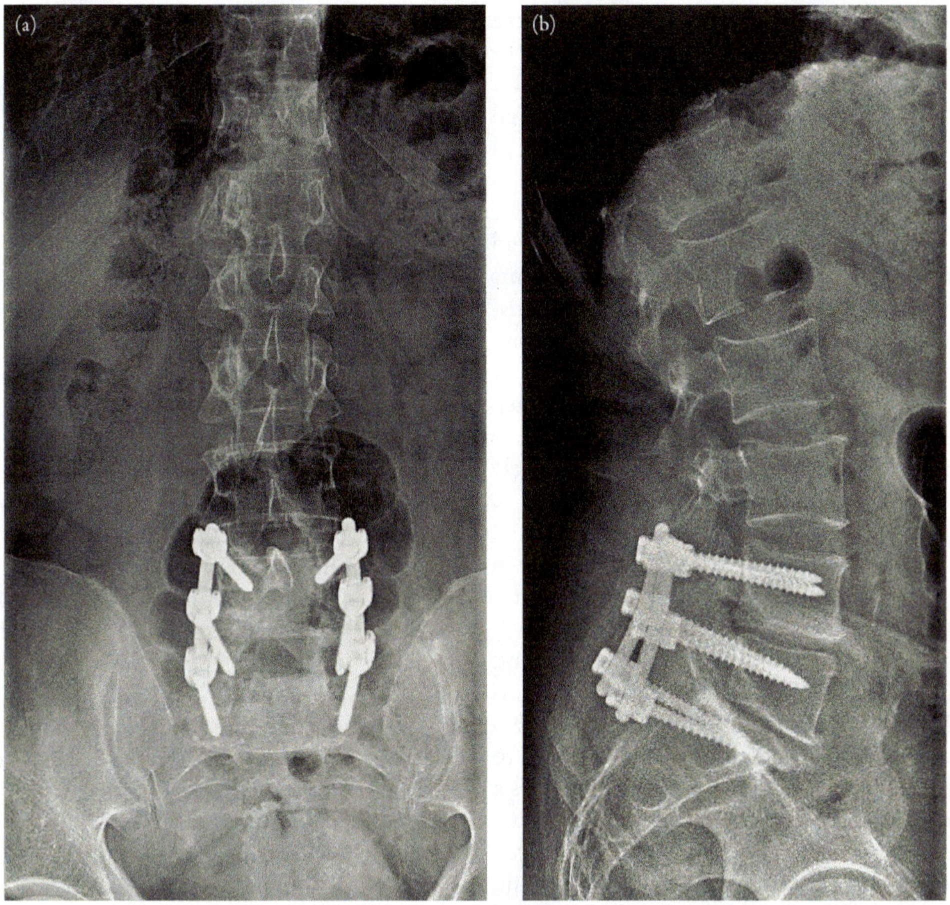

Figure 13.6 X-rays (a) anteroposterior and (b) lateral indicate pedicular screw fixation for grade I spondylolisthesis at L5–S1.

IF THESE OPTIONS ARE NOT SUCCESSFUL IN PAIN CONTROL, WHAT OPTIONS ARE LEFT?

SCS

SCS is a minimally invasive neuromodulatory technique targeted to relieve the radicular, neuropathic component of FBSS by stimulating spinal dorsal columns to generate a non-painful paresthesia that corresponds with the dermatomal distribution of pain. In the literature, FBSS cases comprise the largest group undergoing SCS treatment. SCS is approved by the U.S. FDA for treatment of chronic pain of the trunk and limbs, pain from FBSS, and intractable LBP.[117]

The efficacy of SCS in FBSS is supported by class I evidence garnered from two RCTs. North and colleagues conducted a prospective, randomized, and controlled trial to compare the outcome of SCS and repeated spine surgery in patients with FBSS. Enrolment criteria included patients with axial LBP but only if the intensity of this pain was equal to or less than that of their radicular pain. A total of 50 patients were randomized to SCS or reoperation. Outcome measures were pain relief, patient satisfaction, and rate of crossover. Patients from either group could crossover after 6 months of enrollment. Forty-five patients were available for follow-up. The authors concluded that SCS was more successful than reoperation (9 of 19 patients had a good outcome using SCS vs. 3 of 26 patients following repeat spinal surgery; $p < 0.01$). Patients initially randomized to SCS had significantly lower crossover rates than those randomized to reoperation (5 of 24 patients vs. 14 of 26 patients, $p = 0.02$). Patients assigned to reoperation required increased opioid analgesics significantly more often than those randomized to SCS ($p < 0.025$). However, other measures of activities of daily living and work status did not differ significantly between the two groups.[118]

The Prospective Randomized Controlled Multicenter Trial of the Effectiveness of Spinal Cord Stimulation (PROCESS) randomized 100 patients with FBSS who had predominant leg pain of neuropathic radicular origin to either SCS and CMM or CMM alone. CMM included oral medication (such as opioids, NSAIDs, antidepressants, antiepileptic drugs, and others), nerve blocks, epidural infiltration of steroids, physical and psychological rehabilitative therapy, and/or chiropractic care. At 6 months, results indicated that the SCS group achieved better pain relief, health-related quality of life, and functional capacity. In the intention-to-treat analysis at 6 months, 24 SCS patients (48%) and four CMM patients (9%) ($p < 0.001$) achieved the primary outcome, defined as 50% or more relief of leg pain. Five SCS patients crossed over to CMM, and 32 CMM patients crossed to SCS between 6 and 12 months after randomization. At 24 months, 46 of the 52 patients randomized to SCS and 41 of the 48 randomized to CMM were available for follow-up. The primary outcome was achieved by 17 (37%) of the SCS versus one (2%) of the CMM group (p = 0.003). Moreover, the primary endpoint was achieved by 34 (47%) of the 72 patients who received SCS as a final treatment versus one (7%) of the 15 for CMM (p = 0.02).[119,120]

Taylor et al. performed a systematic review of SCS for FBSS, which included more than 3,000 patients who had undergone implantation. Sixty-two percent of patients achieved greater than 50% pain relief, and 70% were satisfied with the treatment received.[121] In 1991, North et al. presented a case series of 50 patients with FBSS who underwent SCS. A successful outcome was defined as at least 50% sustained pain relief and patient satisfaction with the result; it was achieved in 53% of the patients 2 years postoperatively and in 47% of patients 5 years postoperatively.[122] Kumar et al. followed a cohort of 220 patients of which 184 (84%) had implantation with an SCS system. One-hundred thirty-two (60%) of the 184 patients continued to report 50% or greater pain relief over a mean follow-up of 97.6 months.[123]

The effectiveness of SCS, however, is time-dependent. An 85% long-term success rate is secured if implantation is achieved within 2 years of symptom onset; this drops to 9% if implantation delay exceeds 20 years. Most patients tend to experience wait-times of at least 4–5 years, which generates a 50% probability of long-term success.[123] The precise mechanism for declining pain control over time is unclear; however, this may relate to worsening of the pathology underlying pain, advancing age, increased mobility and activity, and patients' reframing of their original pain assessment. SCS should be considered early in the treatment continuum as part of an integrated, multidisciplinary pain management strategy.

Patient selection is critical to treatment success. In spite of appropriate screening, up to 20% may fail trial stimulation due to patient pathophysiology. During the selection process, the physician should ensure that the patient does not hold unrealistic expectations of pain relief, is able to follow directions and/or adjust programming parameters, and is without significant psychiatric comorbidity or pending litigation. Improper lead placement resulting in inadequate stimulation-paresthesia coverage to the area of pain leads to less than satisfactory pain relief. It should be kept in mind that, at present, radicular pain responds better than axial pain to SCS.[123]

SCS is a safe, reversible, and nondestructive procedure. However, the complications of SCS—largely technical and hardware-related—cause significant morbidity. Potential intraoperative risks include direct damage to the neuraxial structures (including dural puncture), bleeding, and risks inherent to surgery and anesthesia. In the early postoperative period, additional risks include infection, wound dehiscence, fluid collection (e.g., seroma, hematoma, and hygroma), pain, and poor wound healing. Over time, the patient may experience declining effective coverage, unpleasant paresthesia, and hardware failure (e.g., lead fracture/displacement, extension cable fracture, or failure of the implantable pulse generator [IPG]). A systematic review by Turner and colleagues indicated an average overall adverse occurrence rate of 34.3%. Complications cited were infection (4.5%), pain over surgical site or over IPG (5.8%), biological other than infection or local pain (2.5%), equipment failure (10.2%), stimulator revision for reasons other than battery change (23.1%), and stimulator removal (11%). Stimulator revision, the most common adverse event, was second only to lead migration/fracture.[124]

SCS is being envisioned as part of a hybrid solution to chronic pain management. Encouraging results have been reported with SCS in conjunction with IDT, peripheral field stimulation, and with combined dorsal column and dorsal root ganglion (DRG) stimulation.

The role of SCS in relieving low axial back pain is a matter of intense investigation, and early results are promising. A recent study demonstrated that tripolar leads successfully generated paresthesia in both bilateral back and leg territories in 82% of patients. Success rates of multicolumn stimulation patterns were significantly higher than for longitudinal configurations for lumbodorsal paresthesia coverage. Six months after implantation, significant pain relief was obtained compared with preoperative evaluation for global pain (visual analog scale [VAS], 2.25 vs. 8.2 preoperatively; $p < 0.05$), leg pain (VAS, 0.5 vs. 7.6 preoperatively; $p < 0.05$), and back pain (VAS, 1.5 vs. 7.8 preoperatively; $p < 0.05$). These results suggest that multicolumn leads can reliably generate back pain coverage and favor pain relief outcomes.[125] Expanding neurostimulation perspectives to intractable back pain syndromes could become realistic in the near future (Figure 13.7).

On the Horizon

Although promising, DRG stimulation and high-frequency SCS are currently not approved in the United States.

DRG Stimulation

A multicenter, prospective pilot study of 10 patients with chronic intractable pain of the trunk and/or limbs who received DRG stimulation revealed a 70% reduction in pain following stimulation (p = 0.0007). The authors concluded that DRG stimulation may offer several potential benefits over other neuromodulation techniques, including the ability to target difficult-to-reach anatomical regions such as the foot or toe.[126]

High-Frequency SCS

In a recent prospective trial, 83 patients with significant back pain were recruited for a trial of high-frequency stimulation through two percutaneous eight-contact epidural leads. In these patients with difficult-to-treat chronic back pain, high-frequency SCS provided significant and sustained LBP and leg pain relief to more than 70% of treated subjects. Notably, this was achieved without stimulation-induced paresthesia.[127]

INTRATHECAL DRUG DELIVERY SYSTEM

Where other therapies have failed, IDT is considered (Figure 13.8). Depending on the drug combination employed,

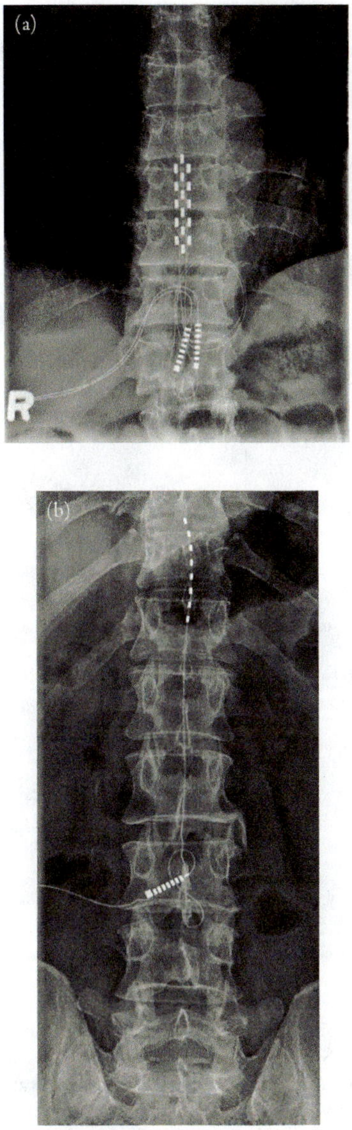

Figure 13.7 Intraoperative X-ray identifies the (a) multicolumn Specify-565™ (Medtronic Inc. Minneapolis, Minnesota) and (b) the octapolar single lead.

IDT may target both the nociceptive and neuropathic components of FBSS. A systemic review published in 2011 concluded that, based on the available evidence, the recommendation for intrathecal infusion systems is limited to moderate based on the moderate quality of evidence from nonrandomized studies for chronic nonmalignant pain. Although there is good evidence of efficacy in the short term, long-term effectiveness in persistent noncancer pain is not fully proven.[128]

A prospective study of 30 patients with FBSS treated with IDT revealed a mean VAS intensity of pain from 9.5 at baseline to 4.6 at last follow-up ($p < 0.001$). The usual mean daily dose of morphine necessary for pain control became constant after the sixth month of treatment. No difference was observed in the results between patients treated with bolus or constant infusion. Side effects were more frequent at the beginning and became less bothersome after the first month of treatment. There was improvement of the quality of life measured by the SF-36 (30.8–49.6) and in all dimensions of

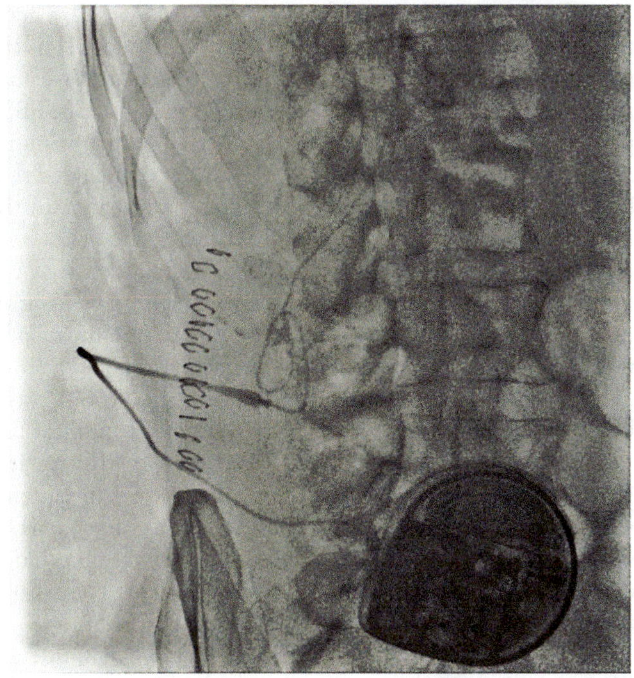

Figure 13.8 X-ray identifies the pump and catheter used in an intrathecal drug delivery system.

the Treatment of Pain Survey except for working capacity. The follow-up period ranged from 18 to 98 months (mean 46.7 months). It was concluded that intrathecal infusion of morphine is a useful and safe tool for long-term treatment of chronic nonmalignant pain.[129]

Winkelmuller followed 120 patients for 6 months to 5.7 years, 73 of whom were FBSS patients with mixed nociceptive-neuropathic pain from multiple lumbosacral operations, including spondylodesis. The best long-term benefits occurred in the management of deafferentation pain and neuropathic pain, with pain reduction (measured by a VAS) of 68% and 62%, respectively. The mean morphine dosage was 2.7 mg/d initially, which rose to 4.7 mg/d after an average of 3.4 years. Among 28 patients treated more than 4 years, 18 (64.3%) were maintained on constant doses, and 10 (35.7%) required increases to more than 6 mg/d 1 year after therapy began. Tolerance developed in seven patients, three of whom had the pump removed. During the follow-up period, 74.2% of the patients benefited from intrathecal opioid delivery. The average pain reduction was 67.4% after 6 months and 58.1% at last follow-up examination. Most patients (92%) were satisfied with therapy, and 81% reported improvement in quality of life.[130] A retrospective study with 4-year follow-up compared intrathecal treatment versus oral opioids versus pain rehabilitation program in treatment of FBSS. It found differing benefits with each treatment option. Intrathecal drug delivery provided the superior decrease in numerical pain rating scale, whereas pain rehabilitation yielded highest Quality of Well-Being score, and oral opioids were rated highest in patient satisfaction. Patients in all three groups reported overall improvement at 50–60%.[9,131]

Angel et al. studied 11 patients (nine with FBSS) referred to a neurosurgery clinic and treated with intrathecal morphine.

The patients were observed for up to 3 years. Overall, a good to excellent analgesic response was seen in 73% (8/11) of the patients. Unfortunately, the three patients judged to have poor results all had FBSS. The effective response among all the FBSS patients was 67% (6/9). Bladder dysfunction requiring pump removal occurred in two patients. The authors concluded that intrathecal morphine delivery was a viable alternative in the management of FBSS despite its limitations.[132]

In their 2007 review, Turner et al. determined that the proportion of patients with 50% or greater improvement in pain at 6 months ranged from 38% to 56%. The most commonly reported drug side effects were nausea/vomiting (33%), urinary retention (24%), and pruritus (26%). Catheter problems were most frequent. Rare but serious complications included intrathecal catheter tip granulomas. The review indicated improvement in pain and functioning in patients with chronic noncancer pain who received permanent IDT systems. However, methodological limitations precluded conclusions concerning the effectiveness of this technology long-term and as compared with other treatments.[133]

Although preservative-free morphine and ziconotide are FDA-approved for the for intrathecal administration for the treatment of chronic pain, a number of other agents including bupivacaine, clonidine, and fentanyl are used, often in combination with other agents and done so on an off-label basis. Combination therapy is likely superior to monotherapy given the complexity of pain signaling mechanisms. These assertions, although seemingly valid in animal models, have not been rigorously tested in robust clinical studies in humans. A chief concern is breakthrough pain, which can be treated with intrathecal boluses delivered through programmable pumps. Additionally, patient-controlled programming (e.g., Patient Therapy Manager, Medtronic Inc., Minneapolis, Minnesota) has provided patients with substantial potential for improved relief.[128]

Complications related to intrathecal therapy fall into one of three categories: technical, biological, or medication-related. The vast majority of complications are minor; some serious complications can occur. An increased mortality rate in patients with noncancer pain receiving intrathecal opioid therapy (mortality rate of 0.088% at 3 days after implantation, 0.39% at 1 month, and 3.89% at 1 year) was documented and likely linked to the opioids themselves.[134] Perhaps the most feared complication is granuloma formation, which may occasionally produce permanent, neurological deficits (Figure 13.9). Granuloma formation is related to the amount and concentration of opioids and is most commonly associated with morphine and hydromorphone. Surgical interventions are usually not needed because most cases resolve with drug weaning. Although granulomas may occur in as many as 3% of implanted patients, most are asymptomatic. The earliest sign of granuloma is increased pain in the setting of increasing opioid doses. Other complications include catheter kinking, catheter fracture/leakage, catheter migration, cerebrospinal fluid leak, seroma, hygroma, infection, pump erosion through the skin, and drug side effects including pruritus, nausea, vomiting, respiratory depression, and cognitive side effects.[128]

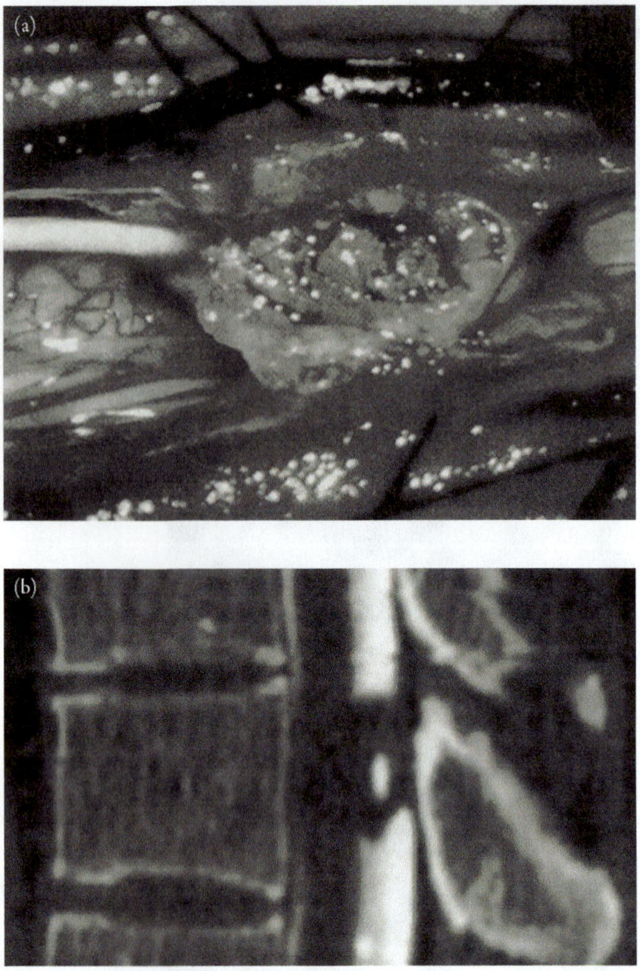

Figure 13.9 A. Intraoperative view of the intrathecal catheter and granuloma. The spinal cord to the left of the granuloma is normal in appearance. B. Sagittally reformatted postmyelographic thoracic computed tomography (CT) scan. The intrathecal catheter tip is seen within the myelographic filling defect caused by the granuloma. Reprinted from Cabell KL, Taren JA, Sagher OS. Spinal cord compression by catheter granulomas in high-dose intrathecal morphine therapy: Case report. *Neurosurgery* 1998;42:1176–1181, with permission from *Neurosurgery*.

PAIN REHABILITATION PROGRAM

Any intervention for FBSS should only be considered after an adequate trial period of intensive rehabilitation—including psychological intervention—has failed. Pain rehabilitation programs are generally effective in reducing pain levels, but there is no conclusive evidence to suggest that they improve functional status. They are employed as an adjunctive therapy to other interventional and noninterventional treatments for FBSS. A Cochrane review has found intensive interdisciplinary rehabilitation to be effective for chronic LBP. There was strong evidence that function improved with intensive interdisciplinary rehabilitation with functional restoration. There was moderate evidence that pain was improved.[45,46]

Of the interventions listed, the strongest evidence is present for neuromodulation (SCS or IDT) and a pain rehabilitation program. If CMM fails after an adequate 6- to 12-week trial, SCS should be pursued. Prior to SCS implantation, the type of pain should be determined. One should distinguish whether pain is nociceptive or neuropathic and the predominance of axial or radicular pain. This will influence lead choice, programming, level of lead placement, and whether the use of field stimulation will be needed in addition to SCS. In the absence of spinal cord compression or any other structural lesion, reoperation will yield unsatisfactory results.

WHAT IS THE LONG-TERM PROGNOSIS OF PERSISTENT PAIN FOLLOWING SPINAL SURGERY?

The long-term prognosis of persistent pain following lumbosacral spinal surgery depends on several factors and is the cumulative result of biological, morphological, and psychosocial pathology.

In light of the heterogeneity of evaluation criteria, outcome studies of lumbar disc operations indicate a success rate of 49–90%.[1] In a retrospective, long-term outcome study (mean follow-up 12.2 years) of 109 patients who underwent lumbar discectomy, 36% of patients had unsatisfactory results, 28% of patients continued to have significant back or leg pain, and 7.3% underwent reoperation, about one-third of which was due to recurrent disc herniation.[108] Similarly, Salenius and Laurent reported satisfactory early results in 70% of patients, which decreased to 56% after 6–11 years of follow-up.[135] Frymoyer et al., over a 10-year follow-up period, reported a 38% failure rate.[4] In Spangfort's study of 2,504 operations for lumbar disc herniation, more than 30% of patients complained of persistent LBP, whereas sciatic pain was found in 23% of the patients.[136]

Short-term studies with less than 2-year follow-up tend to report an optimistic success rate that exceed 90%. Studies with long-term follow-up, by contrast, have demonstrated unsatisfactory results in up to 60% of cases. It is suggested that, in order to adequately evaluate the result of surgery for herniated lumbar discs, the follow-up period should exceed 4 years.[107,108]

Comparing the outcome of operative and conservative treatment in selected patients, Weber and Nashold et al. failed to elicit any significant difference between the final results of surgical and nonsurgical treatment after 10 years and 20 years of observation.[137,138] Whether a good outcome with lumbar discectomy in the long term is due to surgery or simply a reflection of the natural history of the underlying degenerative process is a matter of debate.

PROGNOSTIC FACTORS

Loupasis et al. found on long-term follow-up that 50% of the women had an unsatisfactory result compared with 25% of the men. Jobs requiring significant strenuous physical activity had a success rate of 36% versus 81% for those with light occupational activity. Only 43% of patients involved in heavy manual labor returned to their initial occupation. Similarly, vocational education correlated positively with good outcomes—the higher the education level, the better the result. Degenerative changes at the level of surgery, presence of osteophytes, amount of disc space narrowing on postoperative radiographs, or range of motion at an operated interspace did not have any prognostic value.[108] Kohlboeck et al. determined that persistence of the Lasègue sign and depression predict poor surgical outcome.[139]

EFFECT OF WORKERS COMPENSATION CLAIMS

It is widely reported that compensation cases in general have a poorer outcome after lumbar spinal surgery. On analyzing a series of 1,000 workers compensation cases, Berger et al. discovered that after single-level disc surgery only 29% of patients had returned to work after 4 years. In contrast, if a workers compensation claimant underwent more than 1 operation, only 5% of patients returned to work. In the patients who failed to return to work neurological deficits were mild and not enough to preclude gainful employment. Therefore, the failure to return to work was attributed to chronic pain.[140]

Similarly, results of posterior spinal fusion in cases of spondylolisthesis involving workers compensation claims are poorer than in the noncompensation group. A similar trend persists in workers compensation cases of anterior fusion. It is noted that conventional lumbar discectomies showed a better outcome than anterior lumbar fusion, based on return to work rates within a year.[140,141] LBP persisting for more than half a year constitutes a watershed since little improvement can be expected even after several surgical procedures.[142] In one series, 67.7% of patients described the backache as being worse postoperation, and 55.8% stated that quality of life had suffered.[143] Anterior fusion results were poor in compensation patients, who were more often dissatisfied with the operation than were noncompensation patients.[140,143]

REFERENCES

1. Slipman CW, Shin CH, Patel RK, et al. Etiologies of failed back surgery syndrome. *Pain Med.* 2002;3:200–214.
2. Waguespack A, Schofferman J, Slosar P, et al. Etiology of long-term failures of lumbar spine surgery. *Pain Med.* 2002;3:18–22.
3. Schofferman J, Reynolds J, Herzog R, et al. Failed back surgery: etiology and diagnostic evaluation. *Spine J.* 2003;3:400–403.
4. Frymoyer JW, Cats-Baril WL. An overview of the incidences and costs of low back pain. *Orthop Clin North Am.* 1991;22: 263–271.
5. Greene SA. Chronic pain: pathophysiology and treatment implications. *Top Companion Anim Med.* 2010;25(1):5–9.
6. Thompson KJ, Dagher AP, Eckel TS, Clark M, Reinig JW. Modic changes on MR images as studied with provocative diskography: clinical relevance—a retrospective study of 2,457 disks. *Radiology.* 2009; 250:849–855.
7. Schwarzer, S. Wang, N. Bogduk, et al. Prevalence and clinical features of lumbar zygapophyseal joint pain: a study in an Australian population with chronic low back pain. *Ann Rheum Dis.* 1995;54:100–106.
8. Burton CV, Kirkaldy-Willis WH, Yong-Hing K, Heithoff KB. Causes of failure of surgery on the lumbar spine. *Clin Orthop.* 1981;157:191–199.
9. Havakeshian S, Mannion AF. Negative beliefs and psychological disturbance in spine surgery patients: a cause or consequence of

a poor treatment outcome? [published online ahead of print May 23 2013]. *Eur Spine J*. 2013.

10. Chaichana KL, Mukherjee D, Adogwa O, et al. Correlation of preoperative depression and somatic perception scales with post-operative disability and quality of life after lumbar discectomy. *J Neurosurg Spine*. 2011;14(2):261–267.
11. Celestin J, Edwards RR, Jamison RN. Pretreatment psychosocial variables as predictors of outcomes following lumbar surgery and spinal cord stimulation: a systematic review and literature synthesis. *Pain Med*. 2009;10(4):639–653.
12. Adoqwa O, Parker SL, Shau DN, et al. Preoperative Zung depression scale predicts patient satisfaction independent of the extent of improvement after revision lumbar surgery. *Spine J*. 2013;13(5):501–506.
13. Daubs MD, Norvell DC, McGuire R, et al. Fusion versus nonoperative care for chronic low back pain: do psychological factors affect outcomes? *Spine*. 2011;36(21 suppl):S96–S109.
14. Mroz TE, Norvell DC, Ecker E, et al. Fusion versus nonoperative management for chronic low back pain: do sociodemographic factors affect outcome? *Spine*. 2011;36(21 suppl):S75–S86.
15. Polatin PB, Kinney RK, Gatchel RJ, Lillo E, Mayer TG. Psychiatric illness and chronic low-back pain. The mind and the spine—which goes first? *Spine*. 1993;18:66–71.
16. Choma TJ, Schuster JM, Norvell DC, et al. Fusion versus nonoperative management for chronic low back pain: do comorbid diseases or general health factors affect outcome? *Spine*. 2011;36(21 suppl):S87–S95.
17. Carragee EJ, Alamin TF, Miller JL, Carragee JM. Discographic, MRI and psychosocial determinants of low back pain disability and remission: a prospective study in subjects with benign persistent back pain. *Spine J*. 2005;5:24–35.
18. Peul WC, van den Hout WB, Brand R, Thomeer RT, Koes BW, Leiden-The Hague Spine Intervention Prognostic Study Group. Prolonged conservative care versus early surgery in patients with sciatica caused by lumbar disc herniation: two year results of a randomised controlled trial. *Br Med J*. 2008;336:1355–1388.
19. Morlion B. Pharmacotherapy of low back pain: targeting nociceptive and neuropathic pain components. *Curr Med Res Opin*. 2011;27(1):11–33.
20. Savigny P, Kuntze S, Watson P, et al. *Low Back Pain: Early Management of Persistent Non-Specific Low Back Pain*. London: National Collaborating Centre for Primary Care and Royal College of General Practitioners; 2009.
21. Chou R, Qaseem A, Snow V, et al. Diagnosis and treatment of low back pain: a joint clinical practice guideline from the American College of Physicians and the American Pain Society. *Ann Intern Med*. 2007;147:478–491.
22. Forde G. Adjuvant analgesics for the treatment of neuropathic pain: evaluating efficacy and safety profiles. *J Fam Pract*. 2007;56:3–12.
23. Amer M, Bead VR, Bathon J, et al. Use of nonsteroidal anti-inflammatory drugs in patients with cardiovascular disease: a cautionary tale. *Cardiol Rev*. 2010;18:204–212.
24. Kearney PM, Baigent C, Godwin J, et al. Do selective cyclo-oxygenase-2 inhibitors and traditional non-steroidal anti-inflammatory drugs increase the risk of atherothrombosis? Meta-analysis of randomised trials. *Br Med J*. 2006;332: 1302–1308.
25. Furlan AD, Sandoval JA, Mailis-Gagnon A, et al. Opioids for chronic noncancer pain: a meta-analysis of effectiveness and side effects. *Can Med Assoc*. 2006;174:1589–1594.
26. Verdu B, Decosterd I, Buclin T, et al. Antidepressants for the treatment of chronic pain. *Drugs*. 2008;68:2611–2632.
27. Skljarevski V, Zhang S, Desaiah D, et al. Duloxetine versus placebo in patients with chronic low back pain: a 12-week, fixed-dose, randomized, double-blind trial. *J Pain*. 2010;11(12):1282–1290.
28. Skljarevski V, Zhang S, Chappell AS, Walker DJ, Murray I, Backonja M. Maintenance of effect of duloxetine in patients with chronic low back pain: a 41-week uncontrolled, dose-blinded study. *Pain Med*. 2010;11(5):648–657.
29. Drugs @ FDA. label approved on 08/24/2011 (PDF)11for LYRICA, NDA no. 021446. 50pp. Food & Drug Administration. Available at: www.accessdata.fda.gov/ drugsatfda_docs/label/2011/022488-s004-0211446s025lbl.pdf (accessed Feb. 15, 2013).
30. Zhang W, Jones A, Doherty M. Does paracetamol (acetaminophen) reduce the pain of osteoarthritis?: a meta-analysis of randomised controlled trials. *Ann Rheum Dis*. 2004;63:901–907.
31. Katz N, Ju WD, Krupa DA, et al. Efficacy and safety of rofecoxib in patients with chronic low back pain: results from two 4-week, randomized, placebo-controlled, parallel-group, double-blind trials. *Spine*. 2003;28:851–858.
32. Roelofs PD, Deyo RA, Koes BW, et al. Non-steroidal anti-inflammatory drugs for low back pain. *Cochrane Database Syst Rev*. 2008:CD000396.
33. Allan L, Richarz U, Simpson K, et al. Transdermal fentanyl versus sustained release oral morphine in strong-opioid naive patients with chronic low back pain. *Spine*. 2005;30:2484–2490.
34. Katz N, Rauck R, Ahdieh H, et al. A 12-week, randomized, placebo-controlled trial assessing the safety and efficacy of oxymorphone extended release for opioid-naive patients with chronic low back pain. *Curr Med Res Opin*. 2007;23:117–128.
35. Noble M, Treadwell JR, Tregear SJ, et al. Long-term opioid management for chronic noncancer pain. *Cochrane Database Syst Rev*. 2010:CD006605.
36. Katz J, Pennella-Vaughan J, Hetzel RD, et al. A randomized, placebo-controlled trial of bupropion sustained release in chronic low back pain. *J Pain*. 2005;6:656–661.
37. Skljarevski V, Zhang S, Desaiah D, et al. Duloxetine versus placebo in patients with chronic low back pain: a 12-week, randomized, double-blind trial. *J Pain*. 2010;11:1282–1290.
38. Urquhart DM, Hoving JL, Assendelft WW, et al. Antidepressants for non-specific low back pain. *Cochrane Database Syst Rev*. 2008:CD001703.
39. Remmers AE, Sharma U, Lamoreaux L, et al. Pregabalin treatment of patients with chronic low back pain [Abstract 660]. Proceedings of the 19th Annual Meeting of the American Pain Society; 2000; Atlanta, GA.
40. Khoromi S, Patsalides A, Parada S, et al. Topiramate in chronic lumbar radicular pain. *J Pain*. 2005;6:829–836.
41. Yaksi A, Ozgonenel L, Ozgonenel B.The efficiency of gabapentin therapy in patients with lumbar spinal stenosis. *Spine*. 2007;32:939–942.
42. Romano CL, Romano D, Bonora C, et al. Pregabalin, celecoxib, and their combination for treatment of chronic low-back pain. *J OrthopTraumatol*. 2009;10:185–191.
43. Khoromi S, Cui L, Nackers L, et al. Morphine, nortriptyline and their combination vs. placebo in patients with chronic lumbar root pain. *Pain*. 2007;130:66–75.
44. Peloso PM, Fortin L, Beaulieu A, et al. Analgesic efficacy and safety of tramadol/acetaminophen combination tablets (Ultracet) in treatment of chronic low back pain: a multicenter, outpatient, randomized, double blind, placebo controlled trial. *J Rheumatol*. 2004;31:2454–2463.
45. van Middelkoop M, Rubinstein SM, Kuijpers T, et al. A systematic review on the effectiveness of physical and rehabilitation interventions for chronic nonspecific low back pain. *Eur Spine J*. 2011;20:19–39.
46. Guzman J, Esmail R, Karjalainen KA, Malmivaara A, Irvin E, Bombardier C. Multidisciplinary bio-psycho-social rehabilitation for chronic low-back pain. *Cochrane Database Syst Rev*. 2006:CD000963.
47. Miller B, Gatchel RJ, Lou L, Stowell A, Robinson R, Polatin PB. Interdisciplinary treatment of Failed Back Surgery Syndrome (FBSS): a Comparison of FBSS and Non-FBSS Patients. *Pain Pract*. 2005;5:190–202.
48. Furlan AD, van Tulder MW, Cherkin D, et al. Acupuncture and dry-needling for low back pain. *Cochrane Database Syst Rev*. 2005: CD001351.

49. Walker BF, French SD, Grant W, Green S. Combined chiropractic interventions for low-back pain. *Cochrane Database Syst Rev.* 2010:CD005427.
50. Rubinstein SM, van Middelkoop M, Assendelft WJJ, de Boer MR, van Tulder MW. Spinal manipulative therapy for chronic low-back pain. *Cochrane Database Syst Rev.* 2011: D008112.
51. Hayden J, van Tulder MW, Malmivaara A, Koes BW. Exercise therapy for treatment of non-specific low back pain. *Cochrane Database Syst Rev.* 2005:CD000335.
52. Furlan AD, Imamura M, Dryden T, Irvin E. Massage for low-back pain. *Cochrane Database Syst Rev.* 2008:CD001929.
53. Khadilkar A, Odebiyi DO, Brosseau L, Wells GA. Transcutaneous electrical nerve stimulation (TENS) versus placebo for chronic low-back pain. *Cochrane Database Syst Rev.* 2008:CD003008.
54. Manchikanti L, Boswell MV, Datta S, et al. Comprehensive review of therapeutic interventions in managing chronic spinal pain. *Pain Physician.* 2009:12:E123– E198.
55. Tsantrizos A, Ito K, Aebi M, Steffen T. Internal strains in healthy and degenerated lumbar intervertebral discs. *Spine.* 2005;30:2129–2137.
56. Marchand F, Ahmed AM. Investigation of the laminate structure of lumbar disc anulusfibrosus. *Spine.* 1990;15:402–410.
57. Stojanovic MP, Vu TN, Caneris O, et al. The role of fluoroscopy in cervical epidural steroid injections: an analysis of contrast dispersal patterns. *Spine.* 2002; 27:509–514.
58. Fredman B, Nun MB, Zohar E, et al. Epidural steroids for treating "failed back surgery syndrome": is fluoroscopy really necessary? *Anesth Analg.* 1999;88:367–372.
59. Botwin KP, Natalicchio J, Hanna A. Fluoroscopic guided lumbar interlaminar epidural injections: a prospective evaluation of epidurography contrast patterns and anatomical review of the epidural space. *Pain Physician.* 2004;7:77–80.
60. Bryan BM, Lutz C, Lutz GE. Fluoroscopic assessment of epidural contrast spread after caudal injection. ISIS, 7th annual scientific meeting; August 1999; Las Vegas, NV.
61. DePalma MJ, Slipman CW. Evidence-informed management of chronic low back pain with epidural steroid injections. *Spine.* 2008;8(1):45–55.
62. Airaksinen O, Brox J, Cedraschi C, et al. European guidelines for the management of chronic nonspecific low back pain. *Eur Spine J.* 2006;15:S192–S300.
63. Armon C, Argoff C, Samuels J, Backonja M. Assessment: use of epidural steroid injections to treat radicular lumbosacral pain. *Neurology.* 2007; 68:723–729.
64. Buenaventura R, Datta S, Abdi S, Smith HS. Systematic review of therapeutic lumbar transforaminal epidural steroid injections. *Pain Physician.* 2009;12:233–251.
65. Parr AT, Diwan S, Abdi S. Lumbar interlaminar epidural injections in managing chronic low back and lower extremity pain: a systematic review. *Pain Physician.* 2009;12:163–188.
66. Thomas E, Cyteval C, Abiad L, Picot MC, Taourel P, Blotman F. Efficacy of transforaminal versus interspinous corticosteroid injection in discalradiculalgia-a prospective, randomised, double-blind study. *ClinRheumatol.* 2003;22:299–304.
67. Glaser SE, Falco F. Paraplegia following a thoracolumbar transforaminal epidural steroid injection. *Pain Physician.* 2005;8:309–314.
68. Baker R, Dreyfuss P, Mercer S, Bogduk N. Cervical transforaminal injection of corticosteroids into a radicular artery: a possible mechanism for spinal cord injury. *Pain.* 2004;103:211–215.
69. Houten JK, Errico TJ. Paraplegia after lumbosacral nerve root block: report of three cases. *Spine J.* 2002;2:70–75.
70. Serrao JM, Marks RL, Morley SJ, Goodchild CS. Intrathecal midazolam for the treatment of chronic mechanical low back pain: a controlled comparison with epidural steroid in a pilot study. *Pain.* 1992;48:5–12.
71. Carette S, Leclaire R, Marcoux S, et al. Epidural corticosteroid injections for sciatica due to herniated nucleus pulposus. *N Engl J Med.* 1997;336:1634–1640.
72. Arden NK, Price C, Reading I, et al. A multicentre randomized controlled trial of epidural corticosteroid injections for sciatica: the WEST study. *Rheumatology.* 2005; 44:1399–1406.
73. Karppinen J, Malmivaara A, Kurunlahti M, et al. Periradicular infiltration for sciatica: a randomized controlled trial. *Spine.* 2001;26(9):1059–1067.
74. Vad VB, Bhat AL, MD, Lutz GE, Cammisa F. Transforaminal epidural steroid injections in lumbosacral radiculopathy. *Spine.* 2002;27(1):11–16.
75. Ng L, Chaudhary N, Sell P. The efficacy of corticosteroids in periradicular infiltration for chronic radicular pain. *Spine.* 2005;30(8):857–862.
76. Breivik H, Helsa PE, Molnar I, Lind B. Treatment of chronic low back pain and sciatica. Comparison of caudal epidural injections of bupivacaine and methylprednisolone with bupivacaine followed by saline. In: Bonica JJ, AlbeFesard D, eds. *Advances in Pain Research and Therapy.* Vol 1. New York: Raven Press; 1976: 927–932.
77. Bush K, Hillier S. A controlled study of caudal epidural injections of triamcinolone plus procaine for the management of intractable sciatica. *Spine.* 1991;16(5):572–575.
78. Dashfield A, Taylor M, Cleaver J, Farrow D. Comparison of caudal steroid epidural with targeted steroid placement during spinal endoscopy for chronic sciatica: a prospective, randomized, double-blind trial. *Br J Anaesthesia.* 2005; 94:514–519.
79. Epter RS, Helm S, Hayek SM, Benyamin RM, Smith HS, Abdi S. Systematic review of percutaneous adhesiolysis and management of chronic low back pain in post lumbar surgery syndrome. *Pain Physician.* 2009;12:361–378.
80. Heavner J, Racz G, Raj P. Percutaneous epidural neuroplasty: prospective evaluation of 0.9% NaCl versus 10% NaCl with or without hyaluronidase. *RegAnesth Pain Med.* 1999;24:202–207.
81. Manchikanti L, Boswell MV, Rivera JJ, et al. A randomized, controlled trial of spinal endoscopic adhesiolysis in chronic refractory low back and lower extremity pain. *BMC Anesthesiol.* 2005;5:10.
82. Veihelmann A, Devens C, Trouiller H, Birkenmaier C, Gerdesmeyer L, Refior HJ. Epidural neuroplasty versus physiotherapy to relieve pain in patients with sciatica: a prospective randomized blinded clinical trial. *J Orthop Science.* 2006;11:365–369.
83. Manchikanti L, Cash KA, McManus CD, Pampati V, Singh V, Benyamin RM. The preliminary results of a comparative effectiveness evaluation of adhesiolysis and caudal epidural injections in managing chronic low back pain secondary to spinal stenosis: a randomized, equivalence controlled trial. *Pain Physician.* 2009;12:E341–E354.
84. Cohen SP, Raja SN. Pathogenesis, diagnosis, and treatment of lumbar zygapophysial (facet) joint pain. *Anesthesiology.* 2007; 106:591–614.
85. Lilius G, Laasonen EM, Harilainen A, Gronlund G. Lumbar facet joint syndrome: a randomised clinical trial. *J Bone Joint Surg.*1989;71:746–750.
86. Carette S, Marcoux S, Truchon R, et al. A controlled trial of corticosteroid injections into facet joints for chronic low back pain. *N Engl J Med.* 1991;325:1002–1007.
87. Marks RC, Houston T, Thulbourne T. Facet joint injection and facet nerve block: a randomized comparison in 86 patients with chronic low back pain. *Pain.* 1992;49:325–328.
88. Manchikanti L, Singh V, Falco FJE, Cash KA, Pampati V. Evaluation of lumbar facet joint nerve blocks in managing chronic low back pain: a randomized, double-blind, controlled trial with a 2-year follow-up. *Int J Med Sci.* 2010;7:124–35.
89. Gallagher J, Petriccione DVP, Wedley J, et al. Radiofrequency facet joint denervation in the treatment of low back pain: a prospective controlled double-blind study to assess its efficacy. *Pain Clin.*1994;7:193–198.
90. Leclaire R, Fortin L, Lambert R, Bergeron YM, Rossignol M. Radiofrequency facet joint denervation in the treatment of low back pain. *Spine.* 2001;26:1411–1417.

91. van Wijk RM, Geurts JW, Wynne HJ, et al. Radiofrequency denervation of lumbar facet joints in the treatment of chronic low back pain: a randomized, double-blind, sham lesion-controlled trial. *Clin J Pain*. 2005;21:335–344.
92. Rupert MP, Lee M, Manchikanti L, Datta S, Cohen SP. Evaluation of sacroiliac joint interventions: a systematic appraisal of the literature. *Pain Physician*. 2009;12:399–418.
93. McKenzie-Brown A, Shah RV, Sehgal N, Everett CR. A systematic review of sacroiliac joint interventions. *Pain Physician*. 2005;8:115–125.
94. Cohen SP, Larkin T, Abdi S, Chang A, Stojanovic MP. Risk factors for failure and complications of intradiscalelectrothermal therapy: a pilot study. *Spine*. 2003;28(11):1142–1147.
95. Appleby D, Andersson G, Totta M. Meta-analysis of the efficacy and safety of intradiscalelectrodthermal therapy (IDET). *Pain Med*. 2006;7(4):308–316.
96. Hirsch C, Nachemson A. The reliability of lumbar disc surgery. *Clin Orthop*. 1963;29:189–195.
97. Law JD, Lehman RA, Kirsch WM. Reoperation after lumbar intervertebral disc surgery. *J Neurosurg*. 1978;48:259–263.
98. Weir BKA, Jacobs GA. Reoperation rate following lumbar discectomy: an analysis of 662 lumbar discectomies. *Spine*. 1980;5:366–370.
99. Burton CV.Failed back surgery patients: the alarm bells are ringing. SurgNeurol. 2006;65:5–6.
100. Nachemson AL. *The natural course of low back pain. Symposium on idiopathic low back pain*. St Louis, MO: Mosby;1982:46–51.
101. Chan CW, Peng P. Failed back surgery syndrome. *Pain Med*. 2011;12:577–606.
102. Ryang YM, Oertel MF, Mayfrank L, et al. Standard open microdiscectomy versus minimal access trocar microdiscectomy: results of a prospective randomized study. *Neurosurgery*. 2008;62:174–181.
103. Ghiselli G, Wang J, Bhatia N, et al. Adjacent segment degeneration in the lumbar spine. *J Bone Joint Surg Am*. 2004;86:1497–1503.
104. Chen WJ, Lai PL, Niu CC, Chen LH, Fu TS, Wong CB. Surgical treatment of adjacent instability after lumbar spine fusion. *Spine*. 2001;26:E519–E524.
105. Kim SS, Michelsen CB. Revision surgery for failed back surgery syndrome. *Spine*. 1992;17:957–960.
106. Osterman H, Sund R, Seitsalo S, Keskimaki I. Risk of multiple reoperations after lumbar discectomy: a population-based study. *Spine*. 2003;28:621–627.
107. Davis RA. A long-term outcome analysis of 984 surgically treated herniated lumbar discs. *J Neurosurg*. 1994; 80:415–421.
108. Loupasis GA, Stamos K, Katonis PG, et al. Seven- to 20-year outcome of lumbar discectomy. *Spine*. 1999;24(22):2313–2317.
109. Vik A, Zwart JA, Hulleberg G, et al. Eight year outcome after surgery for lumbar disc herniation: a comparison of reoperated and not reoperated patients. *ActaNeurochir*. 2001;143:607–610.
110. Kunogi J, Hasue M. Diagnosis, operative treatment of intraforaminal, extraforaminal nerve root compression. *Spine*. 1991;16:1312–1330.
111. Porter R, Hibbert C, Evans C. The natural history of root entrapment syndrome. *Spine*. 1984; 9:418–421.
112. Vanderlinden R. Subarticular entrapment of the dorsal root ganglion as a cause of sciatic pain. *Spine*. 1984;9:19–22.
113. Bosscher HA, Heavner JE. Incidence and severity of epidural fibrosis after back surgery: an endoscopic study. *Pain Pract*. 2010;10:18–24.
114. Osterman H, Sund R, Seitsalo S, Keskimaki I. Risk of multiple reoperations after lumbar discectomy: a population-based study. *Spine*. 2003;28:621–627.
115. Yorimitsu E, Chiba K, Toyama Y, et al. Long-term outcomes of standard discectomy for lumbar disc herniation: a follow-up study of more than 10 years. *Spine*. 2001;26: 652–657.
116. Keller RB, Atlas SJ, Soule DN, et al. Relationship between rates and outcomes of operative treatment for lumbar disc herniation and spinal stenosis. *J Bone Joint Surg Am*. 1999;81:752–762.
117. Compton AK, Shah B, Hayek SM. Spinal cord stimulation: a review. *Curr Pain Headache Rep*. 2012;16:35–42.
118. North RB, Kidd DH, Farrokhi F, Piantadosi S. Spinal cord stimulation versus repeated lumbosacral spine surgery for chronic pain: a randomized, controlled trial. *Neurosurgery*. 2005;56:98–107.
119. Kumar K, Taylor RS, Jacques L, et al. Spinal cord stimulation versus conventional medical management for neuropathic pain: a multicenter randomised controlled trial in patients with failed back surgery syndrome. *Pain*. 2007;132:179–188.
120. Kumar K, Taylor RS, Jacques L, et al. The effects of spinal cord stimulation in neuropathic pain are sustained: a 24-month follow-up of the prospective randomized controlled multicenter trial of the effectiveness of spinal cord stimulation. *Neurosurgery*. 2008;63:762–770.
121. Taylor RS, Van Buyten JP, Buchser E. Spinal cord stimulation for chronic back and leg pain and failed back surgery syndrome: a systematic review and analysis of prognostic factors. *Spine*. 2005;30:152–160.
122. North RB, Ewend MG, Lawton MT, Kidd DH, Piantadosi S. Failed back surgery syndrome: 5-year follow-up after spinal cord stimulator implantation. *Neurosurgery*. 1991;28:692–699.
123. Kumar K, Hunter G, Demeria D. Spinal cord stimulation in treatment of chronic benign pain: challenges in treatment planning and present status, a 22-year experience. *Neurosurgery*. 2006;58:481–496.
124. Turner JA, Loeser JD, Deyo RA, Sanders SB. Spinal cord stimulation for patients with failed back surgery syndrome or complex regional pain syndrome: a systematic review of effectiveness and complications. *Pain*. 2004;108:137–147.
125. Rigoard P, Delmotte A, Dhoutaud S, et al. Back pain: a real target for spinal cord stimulation? *Neurosurgery*. 2012;70:574–585.
126. Deer TR, Grigsby E, Weiner RL, Wilcosky B, Kramer JM. A prospective study of dorsal root ganglion stimulation for the relief of chronic pain. *Neuromodulation*. 2013;16(1):67–72.
127. Van Buyten P,Al-Kaisy A, Smet I, Palmisani S, Smith T. High-frequency spinal cord stimulation for the treatment of chronic back pain patients: results of a prospective multicenter European clinical study. *Neuromodulation*. 2013;16(1):59–66.
128. Hayek SM, Deer TR, Pope JE, Panchal SJ, Patel VB. Intrathecal therapy for cancer and non-cancer pain. *Pain Physician*. 2011;14:219–248.
129. Lara NA, Jr., Teixeira MJ, Fonoff ET. Long term intrathecal infusion of opiates for treatment of failed back surgery syndrome. *ActaNeurochirSuppl*. 2011;108:41–47.
130. Winkelmüller M, Winkelmüller W. Long-term effects of continuous intrathecal opioid treatment I chronic pain of non-malignant etiology. *J Neurosurg*.1996;85:458–467.
131. Doleys DM, Brown JL, Ness T. Multidimensional outcomes analysis of intrathecal, oral opioid, and behavioral-functional restoration therapy for failed back surgery syndrome: a restrospective study with 4 years' follow-up. *Neuromodulation*. 2006;9(4):270–283.
132. Angel IF, Gould HJ III, Carey ME. Intrathecal morphine pump as treatment option in chronic pain of nonmalignant origin. *SurgNeurol*. 1998;49: 92–99.
133. Turner JA, Sears JM, Loeser JD. Programmable intrathecal opioid delivery systems for chronic noncancer pain: a systematic review of effectiveness and complications. *Clin J Pain*. 2007;23:180–195.
134. Coffey R, Owens M, Broste S, et al. Mortality associated with the implantation and management of intrathecalopoid drug infusion systems to treat noncancer pain. *Anesthesiology*. 2009;111:881–891.
135. Salenius P, Laurent LE. Results of operative treatment of lumbar disc herniation. A survey of 886 patients. *ActaOrthopScand*. 1977;48:630–634.
136. Spangfort EV. The lumbar disc herniation: a computer aided analysis of 2,504 operations. *ActaOrthopScand*. 1972;142 (Suppl):1–95.
137. Weber H. Lumbar disc herniation. A controlled, prospective study with ten years of observation. *Spine*. 1983;8:131–140.

138. Nashold BS Jr, Blaine S, Hrubec Z. *Lumbar Disc Disease. A Twenty-year Clinical Follow-up Study*. St. Louis, MO: CV Mosby Co.; 1971.
139. Kohlboeck G, Greimel KV, Piotrowski WP, et al. Prognosis of multifactorial outcome in lumbar discectomy: a prospective longitudinal study investigating patients with disc prolapse. *Clin J Pain*. 2004;20:455–461.
140. Berger E. Late postoperative results in 1000 work-related lumbar spine conditions. *SurgNeurol*. 2000;54:101–106.
141. Dowd GC, Rusich GP, Connolly ES. Herniated lumbar disc evaluation and management. *Neurosurg Quart*. 1998;8(2): 140–160.
142. Spitzer WO, LeBlanc FF, Dupuis M, et al. Scientific approach to the assessment and management of activity-related spinal disorders a monograph for clinicians. Report of the Quebec Task Force on Spinal Disorders. *Spine*.1987;12:4–55.
143. Herron L. Recurrent lumbar disc herniation results of repeat laminectomy and discectomy. *J Spinal Disord*. 1994;7:161–166.

14.

PIRIFORMIS SYNDROME

W. Evan Rivers, Honorio T. Benzon, and Binit J. Shah

CASE PRESENTATION

A 46-year-old statistician presents with a complaint of persistent right buttock pain that radiates along the posterior aspect of his thigh to the lower leg. The pain occurs mostly with prolonged sitting, making work difficult. He has been working long hours at his desk recently to meet an important project deadline, and his pain has been limiting his sitting tolerance. Physical activity also worsens his pain, and this has limited his routine jogging regimen. No weakness or changes in bowel/bladder/sexual function were noted. A course of physical therapy, nonsteroidal anti-inflammatory drugs (NSAIDs), and a muscle relaxant did not result in noticeable improvement. The patient is referred to the Interdisciplinary Back Pain Clinic for further evaluation and management.

Past medical history is significant for bipolar disorder, which the patient reports is treated with bupropion (Wellbutrin XL) 300 mg PO QAM and lamotrigine 100 mg BID.

Remainder of history and review of systems is otherwise negative.

On examination, the patient weighs 78 kg and is 174 cm tall. He is seated, leaning off to the left side. He is afebrile with stable vital signs. His neurologic examination is unremarkable. He has tenderness over the right gluteal region and the greater trochanter.

A magnetic resonance image (MRI) of the lumbar spine was obtained and was reported normal with the exception of a mild disc bulge at L2–L3.

QUESTIONS

1. What are potential pain generators in this case?
2. How is piriformis syndrome diagnosed?
3. What is the prevalence of piriformis syndrome?
4. What is the natural history of piriformis syndrome?
5. What are the clinical manifestations of piriformis syndrome?
6. How is piriformis syndrome managed?
   a. Rehabilitation
   b. Pharmacological management
   c. Interventional procedures
   d. Psychiatric interventions
   e. Surgery
7. What is the long-term prognosis of piriformis syndrome?

WHAT ARE POTENTIAL PAIN GENERATORS IN THIS CASE?

This patient has posterior pelvic pain associated with posterior thigh pain and trochanteric tenderness. Potential contributing factors to his pain syndrome include his superficial and deep gluteal muscles, sacroiliac (SI) joint, pelvic ligaments, hip joint, bursae (ischial and trochanteric), pelvic bones, and the lumbosacral plexus, as well as lumbosacral discs, zygapophyseal joints, nerve roots, and neoplasm of any of these structures.

Neoplasm of the spine has been ruled out in imaging studies. In the absence of a history of trauma or severe osteoporosis, pelvic or sacral fractures are very unlikely and are not apparent on his imaging studies. His imaging findings do not implicate a spinal cause of his pain such as focal disc pathology or stenosis, although spinal causes of pain are not always reliably imaged and the prevalence of low back pain (LBP) from discs is quite high.[1] Lumbosacral plexus involvement (postinfectious or occult neoplasm in this case because of his unremarkable history) can cause severe buttock pain and leg pain. It would also result in sensory or motor abnormalities, which are not present in this case.[2]

Zygapophyseal joint pain can refer into the buttock, but it is less likely in this case because he has no axial LBP or lumbosacral paraspinal tenderness, and pain with prolonged sitting is not consistent with this diagnosis.[3] SI joint pain could present with a syndrome similar to this, but it is uncommon in middle-aged men without other complicating inflammatory or biomechanical issues (such as seronegative spondyloarthropathies or previous lumbar fusion).[4] SI pain is usually not provoked by a prolonged sitting position, presuming his sitting posture is not remarkably abnormal. Pelvic ligaments associated with the SI joint such as the sacrotuberous, sacrospinous, and dorsal longitudinal ligaments can cause similar pain patterns, but again are uncommon for men without a history of trauma.[5]

A very similar presentation could arise with ischial bursitis,[6] with severe pain in the buttock that radiates into the posterior thigh, and trochanteric bursitis that can cause lateral thigh pain that radiates into the lateral thigh.[7] In the absence of trauma or inflammatory arthritis, bursitis typically occurs due to direct trauma, repetitive use injury, or muscle strength or flexibility imbalance, and it can coexist with enthesopathy of nearby muscle insertions. Hip joint pain should be very carefully considered in this case because hip pain can present with posterior pelvic pain and associated lateral thigh pain that radiates into the leg.[8] Furthermore, hip joint lesions can cause pain that is worse with prolonged sitting due to anterior impingement and with increased activity.

Gluteal muscle pain can present with local pain and pain radiating into the lateral and posterior thigh. For this patient with predominantly posterior pelvic pain, the gluteus maximus, gluteus minimus, gluteus medius, piriformis, obturators internus, and the deep rotators of the femur could contribute to the pain.[9] Primary gluteal muscle pain can be due to tumor; trauma; repetitive use; maladaptive motor patterns in the hip, lower extremities, or low back; weakness; or decreased flexibility. It can also be caused by imbalance of strength or flexibility between the posterior buttock muscles and anterior hip muscles such as the tensor fascia lata and iliopsoas.

The piriformis muscle is the muscle most commonly implicated in this type of syndrome. The piriformis is a muscle that originates at the anterior surface of the sacrum and nearby osseous and ligamentous structures such as the ilium, the SI joint, and the sacrotuberous ligament.[10] It extends laterally through the greater sciatic notch and has its tendinous insertion at the posteromedial aspect of the greater trochanter. Its tendon often blends with the other deep rotator muscle tendons. It is innervated by the L5 spinal nerve and the nerve to the piriformis, which is formed by the S1 and S2 spinal nerves. It functions as an external rotator of the thigh when the thigh is neutral and as an abductor when the thigh is flexed.[10]

Previous investigators have documented anatomic variations in the structure of the piriformis musculotendinous complex and its relationship to the sciatic nerve.[11–21] These abnormalities are not rare but cause sciatic nerve entrapment only infrequently; surgical case series report the prevalence of anatomic variation at the same rate as the general population.[22–24] Pelvic bone abnormalities may predispose some patients to these symptoms.[25]

This patient's presentation is most consistent with either ischial bursitis with trochanteric bursitis, hip joint pathology, or gluteal myofascial pain, which could include the gluteus maximus, medius, minimus, and piriformis. Further physical examination reveals pain exacerbation with maneuvers that place the piriformis under tension (see next section on diagnosing piriformis syndrome).

HOW IS PIRIFORMIS SYNDROME DIAGNOSED?

Unfortunately, there are no validated diagnostic criteria for piriformis syndrome. The term "piriformis syndrome" is used to describe several constellations of symptoms, including buttock tenderness without pain radiating into the leg, buttock tenderness with pain radiating into the leg, and buttock tenderness with pain and neurologic symptoms in the leg.

Freiberg defined piriformis muscle-related sciatica in 1937 as (1) tenderness at the sciatic notch, (2) positive Lasègue's sign, and (3) improvement with nonsurgical treatment.[26] Robinson described "piriformis syndrome" in 1947 as characterized by (1) history of local trauma; (2) pain localized to the SI joint, greater sciatic notch, and piriformis muscle, which extends along the course of the sciatic nerve and presents difficulty in walking; (3) acute pain brought on by stooping or lifting and relieved somewhat by traction; (4) palpable spindle- or sausage-shaped mass at the anatomic location of the piriformis muscle; and (5) positive Lasègue's sign.[27]

Criticisms of these approaches to diagnosis include the lack of specificity with Freiberg's criteria and the lack of sensitivity with Robinson's criteria, so other sets of criteria have been offered. Fishman reported a combination of three physical examination tests to support piriformis syndrome, used in conjunction with specialized nerve conduction study: pain with a flexion, adduction, and internal rotation (FAIR) test, tenderness at the intersection of the piriformis muscle and the sciatic nerve, and positive Lasègue's sign.[23] Jawish and colleagues presented six features that were present in all their cases of piriformis syndrome: absence of spinal pathology on MRI, tenderness to the sciatic spine (without pain at the SI joint or the low back), intolerance to sitting, sciatica when crossing the symptomatic leg over the other, worse sciatica with the FAIR test, and the disappearance of the common peroneal H reflex in the FAIR position.[20]

Piriformis syndrome is currently diagnosed after exclusion of concordant spine and hip pathology when there is pain in the buttock that is made worse with sitting and lower extremity activity with or without radiation of pain into the leg, with or without symptoms consistent with sciatic nerve entrapment, and confirmed with concordant physical examination findings. It can follow trauma to the buttock, but this is not a requirement.[27–29]

According to a comprehensive review, the most reliable findings for piriformis syndrome are buttock pain, aggravation of sciatica through sitting, external tenderness over the greater sciatic notch, and augmentation of the pain with maneuvers that increase piriformis muscle tension.[30] Provocation of pain with palpation of the piriformis muscle or the sciatic notch is common to every description of piriformis syndrome. Eliciting tenderness with palpation of the piriformis muscle has good interrater reliability in elderly patients with LBP, although the diagnosis of piriformis syndrome was not the goal of the study.[31] Texture changes in the piriformis muscle have been described.[27,32] The most commonly used maneuvers to increase piriformis muscle tension are:

1. *Pace sign*: pain and weakness with abduction of the hip against resistance with patient in the seated position[33]
2. *Lasègue's sign* (also known as *straight leg raise*): pain with unresisted flexion of the hip with the knee straight with patient supine.[26,27] The degree of hip flexion required to provoke symptoms may be greater than would be expected for radicular pain.[32]
3. *Freiberg's sign*: pain with internal rotation of the extended hip overcoming patient's external rotation force with patient supine.[26]
4. *FAIR test* (flexion adduction internal rotation): pain with unresisted flexion, adduction, and internal rotation of the hip with the knee bent.[20,23,34]
5. *Beatty test*: pain with holding the flexed hip in abduction against gravity lying on unaffected side[35]

Other examination findings include hip abductor weakness, leg length discrepancy, and gluteal atrophy.[27,32,36] The clinician may note an unconscious tonic external rotation position of the thigh.[34] Tenderness of the piriformis muscle by transrectal or transvaginal palpation has also been described.[37]

The diagnosis of piriformis syndrome is clinical and depends on a comprehensive history and physical. Imaging and laboratory testing should be used to rule out other conditions that can cause similar symptoms, such as radiculopathy or hip osteoarthritis.

Some authors have advocated the use of electrophysiologic studies. Fishman has described the finding of delayed H-reflex nerve conduction studies in the peroneal and tibial nerves (and reported finding more significant delay in the tibial nerve H reflex) in conjunction with the FAIR test position and has reported that using a specific combination of tests can predict patients who will reach satisfactory outcomes with physical therapy and conservative care.[23] Jawish included a similar test but believed that the peroneal H reflex in the FAIR position was a more important test.[20] These specialized electrodiagnostic tests have not been widely adopted or validated. If entrapment of the sciatic nerve is suspected, nerve conduction studies and electromyography can confirm the location of the lesion and quantify the degree and type of nerve damage, which may preferentially affect the fibular branch of the nerve.[38]

In addition to ruling out similar painful diagnoses, computed tomography (CT) and MRI have been reported in the diagnosis of piriformis syndrome. Perplexingly, both an increase and a decrease in the size of the piriformis have been described in piriformis syndrome, so it is unlikely that muscle mass changes on CT or MRI are useful in the diagnosis.[24,28,36,39,40] Another group believes that MRI neurography adds considerable value in the diagnosis of piriformis syndrome; they reported abnormalities exclusively on the symptomatic side with a very high specificity and a moderate sensitivity.[24] Bone scan does not seem to be a reliable diagnostic tool in piriformis syndrome.[41]

A test that may help confirm the diagnosis of piriformis syndrome is the image-guided injection of local anesthetic into the muscle; if this partially or completely resolves the symptoms, then the diagnosis is more likely.[24,42] The clinician must remember that diagnostic injections are not completely reliable[43] and require expert clinical judgment for appropriate interpretation.[44]

> Diagnosis of piriformis syndrome was made by confirming symptom provocation with the Pace, Freiberg, and FAIR tests. Hip joint pathology and pelvic bone lesions were ruled out using plain radiographs. Further confirmation of the diagnosis of piriformis syndrome was made using fluoroscopy or ultrasound-guided injection of 4 mL 0.25% bupivacaine with 40 mg of methylprednisolone into the right piriformis muscle, with an immediate 100% relief of his buttock and thigh pain.

WHAT IS THE PREVALENCE OF PIRIFORMIS SYNDROME?

The prevalence of piriformis syndrome has been reported to vary between 6% and 44%, depending on the population studied and the criteria for diagnosis.[45] However, piriformis syndrome may be responsible for up to 68% of patients with sciatic pain resistant to spinal intervention, based on concordant physical examination and response to either piriformis muscle local anesthetic injection or surgery.[24] There are conflicting reports of its prevalence in females and males, but it is generally considered to be more frequent in females.[42,45] In a study of elderly adults with back pain, piriformis tenderness was found in 68% of the sample, although a diagnosis of piriformis syndrome was not made, and the special tests listed earlier were not performed.[31]

> Piriformis syndrome is at least somewhat more common in women, but it is not rare in men. Our patient does not report a history of trauma to the buttock. Perhaps he has a leg-length discrepancy, a tendency to externally rotate his right leg, or one of the rare anatomic abnormalities of the piriformis muscle that leads to this syndrome.

WHAT IS THE NATURAL HISTORY OF PIRIFORMIS SYNDROME?

There have been no published studies regarding the natural history of piriformis syndrome. Furthermore, studies have only been performed that follow patients with piriformis syndrome receiving treatment (see the section "Long-Term Prognosis"). Our clinical experience indicates that most muscle-related pain resolves spontaneously within several weeks of onset and that only patients who do not improve as expected present to clinicians to then be diagnosed with piriformis syndrome. These patients are unlikely to improve spontaneously after symptoms have been present or worsening for months or years.

Our patient has had persistent pain, and a trial of medication management and physical therapy has not improved his symptoms. His pain is limiting his ability to continue vocational and avocational activity. It is unlikely that his symptoms will resolve without further intervention and certainly not before they affect his ability to meet his important deadline at work. His symptoms are also keeping him from continuing regular exercise, which is important for long-term well-being and health.

WHAT ARE THE CLINICAL MANIFESTATIONS OF PIRIFORMIS SYNDROME?

The cardinal symptoms of piriformis syndrome are buttock pain with or without radiation of pain into the posterior leg. Sometimes there are dysesthetic sensations without neurologic deficits that may be attributed to pain referral from the piriformis muscle. Rarely, there is true sensory loss and motor weakness in one or more distributions of the sciatic nerve. Patients generally complain of increased pain with prolonged sitting and prolonged activity of the affected leg. Positions and activities that result in the activation or deep stretch of the piriformis muscle, such as ambulating, stooping, or lifting, can also provoke the pain.

There is tenderness to palpation at the piriformis, which spans from the anterior surface of the sacrum to the posterior aspect of the greater trochanter. Palpation of the piriformis or the sciatic notch can often provoke leg symptoms. The physical examination maneuvers specific to piriformis syndrome previously discussed all rely on activation, deep stretch, or a combination of both to provoke symptoms from a painful piriformis muscle. A vaginal and rectal approach to palpation of the piriformis has also been described.

We recommend a full evaluation of the pelvis and low back when piriformis syndrome is suspected because piriformis muscle pain can be associated with causative or compensatory strength and flexibility deficits in the ipsilateral and contralateral hip muscles, thigh muscles, hip joints, SI joints, and lumbar spine. A brief biomechanical assessment including gait or provocative motion analysis may implicate another segment of the kinetic chain (such as abnormal motion at the knee or ankle) as a contributing factor in the patient's symptomology.[19] Some authors have linked the piriformis syndrome to coexisting SI joint pain or pathology,[9,13,26,27] whereas others have considered them exclusionary diagnoses.[20,46]

HOW IS PIRIFORMIS SYNDROME MANAGED?

A coordinated approach that uses medication and injection techniques to maximize a patient's participation in rehabilitation has the best chance of success. The goal of rehabilitation is to minimize pain-related limitations in activities that are important to the patient's work and quality of life. The approaches listed here are best combined and tailored to the needs of the patient. Conservative treatment results in satisfactory relief of symptoms for most patients.[23,36]

REHABILITATION

Physical therapy for piriformis syndrome has not been broadly standardized. There has been a published protocol for the treatment of piriformis syndrome (Box 14.1). It includes physical modalities (heat, cold, and ultrasound) to improve tolerance of treatment and compliance of the tissues, direct stretching of the piriformis perpendicular to the fibers, myofascial release of the lumbosacral paraspinal muscles, and mechanical diagnosis and treatment (also known as McKenzie) exercises targeted to "centralize" the patient's radiating pain.[23] This

---

Box 14.1 PHYSICAL THERAPY PROTOCOL FOR PATIENTS WITH PIRIFORMIS SYNDROME

Place patient in contralateral decubitus and FAIR position.[a,b]

1. Ultrasound 2.0–2.5 W/cm^2 applied in broad strokes longitudinally along the piriformis muscle from the conjoin tendon to the lateral edge of the greater sciatic foramen for 10–14 minutes.[b]
2. Wipe off ultrasound gel.[c]
3. Hot packs or cold spray at the same location for 10 minutes.
4. Stretch the piriformis muscle for 10–14 minutes by applying manual pressure to the muscle's inferior border, being careful not to press downward rather than directing pressure tangentially toward the ipsilateral shoulder.[d]
5. Myofascial release at lumbosacral paraspinal muscles.
6. McKenzie exercises.
7. Use lumbosacral corset when treating patient in the FAIR position.[e]

Duration: 2–3 times weekly for 1–3 months.

[a]Patients usually require 2–months of biweekly therapy for 60–70% improvement.

[b]Because it is painful, patients often subtly shift to prone. This must be avoided because it places the affected leg in abduction, not adduction, greatly reducing the stretch placed on the piriformis muscle.

[c]Cavitation is unreported in more than 20,000 treatments.

[d]Unless explicitly stated, therapists may tend to knead or massage the muscle, which is useless or worse. The muscle must be stretched perpendicular to its fibers, in a plane that is tangent to the buttock at the point of intersection of the piriformis muscle and the sciatic nerve, but approximately 1–1.5 inches deep to the buttock (i.e., just below the gluteus maximus).

[e]It is particularly important to avoid inducing lumbar hypermobility in patients with histories of laminectomy, fusion, or spondylolisthesis.

Reprinted from Fishman LM, Dombi GW, Michaelsen C, et al. Piriformis syndrome: diagnosis, treatment, and outcome-a 10-year study. *Archives of Physical Medicine and Rehabilitation*. 2002;83(3):295–301, with permission from Elsevier.

treatment should be followed by hip strengthening as well as lumbosacral and pelvic stabilization exercises that progress in difficulty to achieve specific functional goals.[22,47]

Treatment of the piriformis muscle may also include dry-needling, spray and stretch techniques, massage, ischemic compression, and other methods to address myofascial pain.[9,45] Nerve mobilization techniques appear to have measurable effects on the sciatic nerve and may play a role in the physical therapy regimen for piriformis syndrome.[48] Manipulation may also play a role in the treatment of piriformis syndrome even when there is a predisposing anatomical lesion.[25,49]

Physical therapists will often evaluate the entire kinetic chain to address distant joints, often in the lower extremity, that could contribute to biomechanical stresses in the piriformis muscle.[47] A heel lift can address leg length discrepancy leading to piriformis syndrome.[32] A home exercise program is often essential to maintaining the gains in strength, flexibility, and improved pain achieved with physical therapy sessions and interventional treatment.[47] A workplace ergonomic assessment and intervention could resolve his symptoms at work and could resolve his condition entirely if his positioning was responsible for his piriformis syndrome.

PHARMACOLOGICAL MANAGEMENT

No studies have investigated the effect of specific medications in the treatment of piriformis syndrome. There is modest evidence regarding medication use in muscle pain syndromes, and this is directly applicable to piriformis syndrome. The NSAIDs, specifically ibuprofen, appear to be effective only when administered in conjunction with other medications.[50] Tizanidine, but not cyclobenzaprine, was effective in the treatment of acute skeletal muscle spasms, but its use in chronic muscle pain has not been assessed. Diazepam, amitriptyline, and lidocaine patch have evidence to support their use.[50] Duloxetine has been given the broad indication for the treatment of musculoskeletal pain due to its effect in the treatment of fibromyalgia, chronic LBP, and osteoarthritis.[51] Support for anticonvulsants in the treatment of muscle pain is limited.[50] Clonazepam has been shown to relieve muscle pain, but it can cause depression, liver dysfunction, physiologic dependence, and addiction.[50] Opioid medications relieve acute and chronic musculoskeletal pain, but careful consideration is required before initiating opioids for chronic noncancer pain due to the risk of side effects, tolerance, physiologic dependence, withdrawal, misuse, abuse, and diversion.[52]

INTERVENTIONAL PROCEDURES

It is often useful to incorporate piriformis injection in the diagnosis and treatment of piriformis syndrome. Piriformis muscle injection can give temporary relief that improves tolerance of the stretching-based physical therapy treatments that are often the core of the rehabilitation program. At times, injection can give relief that lasts much longer than the duration of the anesthetic injectate, resulting in days or weeks of relief. One or two local anesthetic injections into the piriformis muscle may allow resolution of symptoms in 23% of patients, and another 37% may have recurrence of symptoms after 2–4 months.[24] A retrospective study demonstrated improvement in patients with piriformis syndrome with a combination of physical therapy and piriformis injection with local anesthetic and steroid.[23] A prospective study reported superiority sustained over 1 year for the use of local anesthetic with steroid compared to medication and physical therapy alone.[53] One study found good results using a clonidine injectate.[54] Another consideration is the perisciatic nerve injection of steroid and local anesthetic when irritation of the sciatic nerve is suspected.[55] Yet another group has recommended caudal epidural steroid injection.[56]

Piriformis injection of botulinum toxin has a high rate of success in uncontrolled studies[57–59] and in a placebo-controlled study.[60] Controlled studies using a combination of physical therapy and injection demonstrated superiority of botulinum toxin compared to local anesthetic with steroid or normal saline.[61,62]

Due to its small size compared to the glutei muscles, its proximity to neurovascular structures, and its deep location, the piriformis muscle is usually injected under radiographic (Figure 14.1) or ultrasound guidance. Piriformis injections under MRI, CT, and electromyographic guidance have also been described.[24,61,63–65] Ionizing radiation (e.g., fluoroscopy or CT) should not be used for image guidance in female patients who are pregnant.

PSYCHIATRIC INTERVENTIONS

Bipolar disorder, classically referred to as "manic-depressive" illness, has at its core the occurrence of a manic episode (for the diagnostic criteria of bipolar disorder, see the *Diagnostic and Statistical Manual of Mental Disorders*, 5th edition [DSM-5]). These are periods of elevated, expansive, or irritable

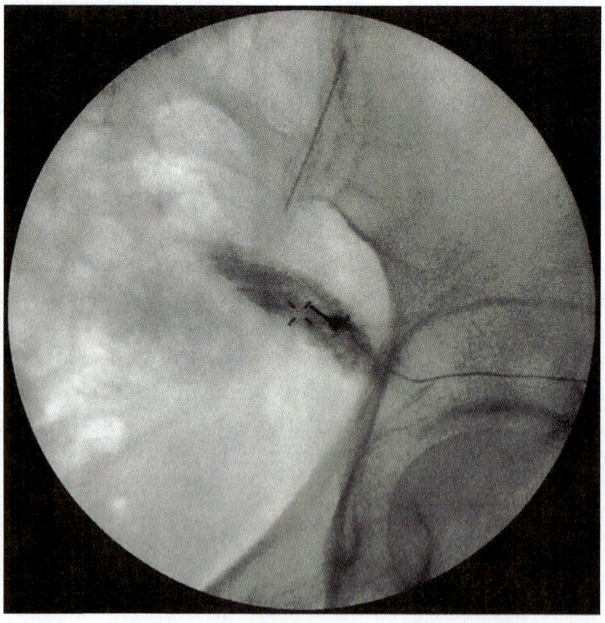

Figure 14.1 Piriformis injection under fluoroscopy guidance; note the muscle outlined by contrast.

mood that cause significant disruption in the patient's life and are generally persistent over the course of several days or weeks. During this time, a hallmark feature is the decreased need for sleep—the patient reports being well rested after only 2–3 hours of sleep or not feeling mentally/physically tired to the point that sleep seems necessary. (This is in distinction to insomnia, where the patient is unable to sleep.)

For patients who report a diagnosis of bipolar disorder, discussion with the patient's psychiatrist (or diagnosing physician) and some skepticism is warranted. The diagnosis of bipolar disorder is an oddly paradoxical one in that it is both over- and underdiagnosed. The mean age of onset is 19 years, and it shows no gender predominance.[66] The estimated 12-month prevalence is 0.6%,[67] whereas the lifetime prevalence is from 1% to 3%. This makes it slightly more common than schizophrenia but significantly less common than major depressive disorder (12-month prevalence of 10–17%, lifetime prevalence is 17–40%),[68,69] post-traumatic stress disorder (7–8% of civilians, 13–20% of military personnel),[70,71] and borderline personality disorder (prevalence of ~6%). Of DSM-5 diagnoses, these in particular have been highlighted because each has core features that involve mood lability and irritability, the grounds upon which bipolar disorder is often (mis)diagnosed. In patients initially diagnosed with major depressive disorder, 16–33% will ultimately be diagnosed as having bipolar disorder.[72,73] The literature is consistent that in patients with depression, a significant minority will develop a bipolar spectrum illness. Conversely, the majority of patients who self-report a diagnosis of bipolar disorder do not in fact have BPD. When evaluated carefully using structured clinical interviews, only 43% of patients who report a history of bipolar disorder actually have BPD.[74] Furthermore, of patients with active substance abuse who are diagnosed with BPD in the community, careful evaluation reveals that only 33% of them actually have bipolar disorder. The two clinical features commonly assumed to be suggestive of bipolar disorder—mood lability and irritability—actually have low diagnostic predictive value.[75] The Mood Disorder Questionnaire (MDQ) is often employed when patients reports these two symptoms and is the most widely used screening scale for bipolar disorder. However, positive results on it are as likely to indicate a patient has borderline personality disorder as they to have bipolar disorder.[76] At times, a diagnosis of bipolar disorder is sought out by the patient to somehow legitimize a lifetime of poor decision making and legal/criminal consequences.

Another complicating factor is the high rates of substance abuse and chronic pain among bipolar disorder patients. Among major psychiatric disorders (schizophrenia, depression, BPD) substance abuse has consistently been found to be highest among bipolar disorder patients. Three large U.S. population-based studies have found the rates of substance use disorders in this population to be 30–60%.[77–79] More recent research has explored the association of bipolar disorder and chronic pain and yielded strikingly similar results. Failde et al. found that 51% of patients with bipolar disorder and two-thirds of females with bipolar disorder complain of moderate to severe intensity chronic pain.[80] In a separate 2013 study, Subramaniam and colleagues explored comorbidity in bipolar disorder and found the most prevalent condition was chronic pain occurring in approximately 53%.[81]

The approach to treatment of manic episodes, depressive episodes, and maintenance therapy is beyond the scope of this text.[82] The literature, as highlighted here, shows the complex comorbidity involved with bipolar disorder and the confusion regarding diagnosis. The purpose, then, is to educate the reader to confirm psychiatric diagnosis and maintain vigilance when selecting appropriate pharmacotherapy, given high risk of addiction/aberrant behavior.

The patient reports that he was initially diagnosed with bipolar disorder by his PCP at the age of 27. He reports it was a rather fortuitous discovery because he had just been arrested for a DUI. He was initially started on bupropion and titrated up to his current dose to target his mental fatigue, depressive affect, and irritability. After 6 years of stable dose of medication, lamotrigine was initiated and then titrated up to his current dose of 100 mg BID. He denies ever having suicidal or homicidal ideation, auditory or visual hallucinations, or any inpatient psychiatric stays. His DUI arrest "scared [him] straight," and he has had no issues with alcohol since that time. He has never seen a psychiatrist.

The patient was referred to a psychiatrist colleague for further evaluation and management.

Diagnostic Criteria

For a diagnosis of bipolar I disorder, it is necessary to meet the DSM-5 criteria for a manic episode. The manic episode may have been preceded by and may be followed by hypomanic or major depressive episodes.

SURGERY

Surgical release of the piriformis muscle with sciatic nerve release from associated fibrous bands may be performed for cases of piriformis syndrome that do not respond to conservative treatment. Several surgical techniques have been described with relatively small groups of patients, with satisfactory outcomes and a low complication rate.[20,23,24,26–28,34,83-85] A "minimally invasive" approach has been described that may result in decreased postoperative gait disturbance.[24]

Our patient has already had a trial of physical therapy, NSAIDs, and a muscle relaxant. As part of his diagnostic evaluation, he received an injection of local anesthetic and steroid into his piriformis muscle, which resulted in complete resolution of his pain without weakness. This will likely have a longer term therapeutic effect and may give him prolonged relief. We recommend combining injection therapy with further physical therapy because his pain may have limited his participation, and long-lasting changes in the muscle fibers and motor-patterning rely on repeated and well-trained movement. If he does not have lasting relief with one or two injections and continuation of his home exercises, botulinum toxin injection could be entertained. If he continues to be limited by his symptoms, surgical evaluation would be warranted.

WHAT IS THE LONG-TERM PROGNOSIS OF PIRIFORMIS SYNDROME?

Published studies are limited by poor study methodology and reporting, inconsistent outcome selection, small sample sizes, heterogeneous patient populations, and the absence of standardized diagnostic criteria. It is generally stated that conservative care suffices for most individuals with piriformis syndrome.[36] One or two local anesthetic injections into the piriformis muscle may allow resolution of symptoms for months or years in nearly half of patients.[24] One study with a 1-year follow-up reported remarkable reduction in pain after local anesthetic with steroid injection, compared to conservative treatment alone.[53] In a large retrospective study, at least 50% improvement in pain symptoms and reported disability were achieved for most patients (67.7–83.1%) using a combination of physical therapy and piriformis injection at 10-month average follow-up.[23] Those patients with at least two of three physical examination findings (pain provoked with FAIR, Lasègue, or palpation of the piriformis) were more likely to improve and had a higher average improvement in pain rating, whereas those with at least two of three physical examination findings and a delay in the H reflex on nerve conduction velocity in the FAIR position were even more likely to benefit from this regimen.[23] Surgical outcome for carefully selected patients in recent case series was "good or excellent" for 76–100% at least 1 year after operation.[20,24,28]

> Our patient has a very good chance of significant symptom improvement at least a year from now because most individuals who have previously not responded to conservative care get relief from combined interventional and conservative management. Even among those patients who have still not improved after this management, surgical intervention has a high rate of success and a relatively low rate of significant morbidity.

REFERENCES

1. Maus T. Imaging the back pain patient. *Phys Med Rehabil Clin N Am*. 2010;21(4):725–766.
2. Ko K, Sung DH, Kang MJ, et al. Clinical, electrophysiological findings in adult patients with non-traumatic plexopathies. *Ann Rehabil Med*. 2011;35(6):807–815.
3. Van Kleef M, Vanelderen P, Cohen SP, et al. ain originating from the lumbar facet joints. *Pain Pract*. 2010;10(5):459–469.
4. Vanelderen P, Szadek K, Cohen SP, et al. 13. Sacroiliac joint pain. *Pain Pract*. 2010;10(5):470–478.
5. Hackett GS. Referred pain from low back ligament disability. *Arch Surg*. 1956;73(5):878.
6. Swartout R, Compere EL. Ischiogluteal bursitis. *JAMA*. 1974;227(5):551–552.
7. Williams BS, Cohen SP. Greater trochanteric pain syndrome: a review of anatomy, diagnosis and treatment. *Anesth Analg*. 2009;108(5):1662–1670.
8. Lesher JM, Dreyfuss P, Hager N, Kaplan M, Furman M. Hip joint pain referral patterns: a descriptive study. *Pain Med*. 2008;9(1):22–25.
9. Travell JG, Simons DG. *Myofascial Pain and Dysfunction: The Trigger Point Manual:* Vol 2. *The Lower Extremities*. Philadelphia: Lippincott, Williams, and Wilkins; 1993:132–235.
10. Salmons S. Muscle. In: Williams PL, Bannister LH, eds. *Gray's Anatomy: The Anatomical Basis of Medicine and Surgery*. New York: Churchill-Livingston; 1995:737–900.
11. Beaton LE, Anson BJ. The relation of the sciatic nerve and of its subdivisions to the piriformis muscles. *Anat Rec*. 1937;70:1–5.
12. Beaton LE, Anson BJ. The sciatic nerve and the piriformis muscle: their interrelation a possible cause of coccygodynia. *J Bone Joint Surg*. 1938;20:686–688.
13. Yeoman W. The relation of arthritis of the sacro-iliac joint to sciatica, with an analysis of 100 cases. *Lancet*. 1928;212(5492):1119–1123.
14. Pecina M. Contribution to the etiological explanation of the piriformis syndrome. *Acta Anatomica*. 1979;105(2):181–187.
15. Gotlin R. Clinical correlation of an anatomical investigation into piriformis syndrome. *Proc N Y Soc Phys Med Rehabil*. 1991; 24(6):11.
16. Benzon HT, Katz JA, Benzon HA, Iqbal MS. Piriformis syndrome: anatomic considerations, a new injection technique, and a review of the literature. *Anesthesiology*. 2003;98:1442–1448.
17. Pokorny D, Jahoda D, Veigl D, Pinskerova V, Sosna A. Topographic variations of the relationship of the sciatic nerve and the piriformis muscle and its relevance to palsy after total hip arthroplasty. *Surg Radiol Anat*. 2006;28:88–91.
18. Windisch G, Braun EM, Anderhuber F. Piriformis muscle: clinical anatomy and consideration of the piriformis syndrome. *Surg Radiol Anat*. 2007;29(1):37–45.
19. Parziale JR, Hudgins TH, Fishman LM. The piriformis syndrome. *Am J Orthop*. 1996;25:819–823.
20. Jawish RM, Assoum HA, Khamis CF, others. Anatomical, clinical and electrical observations in piriformis syndrome. *J Orthop Surg Res*. 2010;5(1):3.
21. Babinski M, Machado F, Costa W. A rare variation in the high division of the sciatic nerve surrounding the superior gemellus muscle. *Eur J Morp*. 2003;41(1):41–42.
22. Kirschner JS, Foye PM, Cole JL. Piriformis syndrome, diagnosis and treatment. *Muscle Nerve*. 2009;40(1):10–18.
23. Fishman LM, Dombi GW, Michaelsen C, et al. Piriformis syndrome: diagnosis, treatment, and outcome-a 10-year study. *Arch Phys Med Rehabil*. 2002;83(3):295–301.
24. Filler AG, Haynes J, Jordan SE, et al. Sciatica of nondisc origin and piriformis syndrome: diagnosis by magnetic resonance neurography and interventional magnetic resonance imaging with outcome study of resulting treatment. *J Neurosurg Spine*. 2005;2(2):99–115.
25. Mayrand N, Fortin J, Descarreaux M, Normand MC. Diagnosis and management of posttraumatic piriformis syndrome: a case study. *J Manipulative Physiol Ther*. 2006;29(6):486–491.
26. Freiberg AH. Sciatic pain and its relief by operations on muscle and nerve. *Arch Surg*. 1937;34:337–349.
27. Robinson D. Piriformis muscle in relation to sciatic pain. *Am J Surg*. 1947;73:355–358.
28. Benson ER, Schutzer SF. Posttraumatic piriformis syndrome: diagnosis and results of operative treatment. *J Bone Joint Surg Am*. 1999;81(7):941–949.
29. Beauchesne RP, Schutzer SF. Myositis ossificans of the piriformis muscle: an unusual cause of piriformis syndrome: a case report. *J Bone Joint Surg Am*. 1997;79(6):906–910.
30. Hopayian K, Song F, Riera R, Sambandan S. The clinical features of the piriformis syndrome: a systematic review. *Eur* Spine J. 2010;19(12):2095–2109.
31. Weiner DK, Sakamoto S, Perera S, Breuer P. Chronic low back pain in older adults: prevalence, reliability, and validity of physical examination findings. *J Am Geriatr Soc*. 2006;54(1):11–20.
32. Hallin RP. Sciatic pain and the piriformis muscle. *Postgrad Med*. 1983;74(2):69–72.
33. Pace JB, Nagle D. Piriform syndrome. *West J Med*. 1976;124:433–439.

34. Solheim LF, Siewers P, Paus B. The piriformis muscle syndrome: sciatic nerve entrapment treated with section of the piriformis muscle. *Acta Orthopaedica*. 1981;52(1):73–75.
35. Beatty RA. The piriformis muscle syndrome: a simple diagnostic maneuver. *Neurosurgery*. 1994;34(3):512–514.
36. Barton PM. Piriformis syndrome: a rational approach to management. *Pain*. 1991;47(3):345–352.
37. Durrani Z, Winnie AP. Piriformis muscle syndrome: an under diagnosed cause of sciatica. *J Pain Symptom Manage*. 1991;6(6):374–379.
38. McCrory P, Bell S. Nerve entrapment syndromes as a cause of pain in the hip, groin and buttock. *Sports Med*. 1999;27(4):261–274.
39. Rossi P, Cardinali P, Serrao M, et al. Magnetic resonance imaging findings in piriformis syndrome: a case report. *Arch Phys Med Rehabil*. 2001;82(4):519–521.
40. Jankiewicz JJ, Hennrikus WL, Houkom JA. The appearance of the piriformis muscle syndrome in computed tomography and magnetic resonance imaging. A case report and review of the literature. *Clin Orthop Relat Res*. 1991;292:205–209.
41. Fishman LM, Zybert P, et al. Electrophysiologic evidence of piriformis syndrome. *Arch Phys Med Rehabil*. 1992;73(4):359–364.
42. Kean Chen C, Nizar AJ. Prevalence of piriformis syndrome in chronic low back pain patients. A clinical diagnosis with modified FAIR test. *Pain Pract*. 2012.
43. North RB, Kidd DH, Zahurak M, Piantadosi S. Specificity of diagnostic nerve blocks: a prospective, randomized study of sciatica due to lumbosacral spine disease. *Pain*. 1996;65(1):77–85.
44. Saal JS. General principles of diagnostic testing as related to painful lumbar spine disorders: a critical appraisal of current diagnostic techniques. *Spine*. 2002;27(22):2538.
45. Cummings M. Piriformis syndrome. *AcupunctMed*. 2000; 18(2):108–121.
46. Bernard TNJ, Kirkaldy-Willis WH. Recognizing specific characteristics of nonspecific low back pain. *Clin Orthop Relat Res*. 1987;217:266–280.
47. Keskula DR, Tamburello M. Conservative management of piriformis syndrome. *J Athl Train*. 1992;27(2):102.
48. Ellis R, Hing W, Dilley A, McNair P. Reliability of measuring sciatic and tibial nerve movement with diagnostic ultrasound during a neural mobilisation technique. *Ultrasound Med Bio*. 2008;34(8):1209–1216.
49. Chapman C, Bakkum BW. Chiropractic management of a US Army veteran with low back pain and piriformis syndrome complicated by an anatomical anomaly of the piriformis muscle: a case study. *J Chiropr Med*. 2011;11(1):24–29.
50. Annaswamy TM, De Luigi AJ, O'Neill BJ, Keole N, Berbrayer D. Emerging concepts in the treatment of myofascial pain: a review of medications, modalities, and needle-based interventions. *PM R*. 2011;3(10):940–961.
51. Smith HS, Smith EJ, Smith BR. Duloxetine in the management of chronic musculoskeletal pain. *Ther Clin Risk Manag*. 2012;8:267.
52. Brennan MJ, Stanos S. Strategies to optimize pain management with opioids while minimizing risk of abuse. *PM R*. 2010;2(6):544–558.
53. Masala S, Crusco S, Meschini A, et al. Piriformis syndrome: long-term follow-up in patients treated with percutaneous injection of anesthetic and corticosteroid under CT guidance. *Cardiovasc Intervent Radiol*. 2012;35(2):375–382.
54. Naja Z, Al-Tannir M, El-Rajab M, et al. The effectiveness of clonidine-bupivacaine repeated nerve stimulator-guided injection in piriformis syndrome. *Clin J Pain*. 2009;25(3):199–205.
55. Hanania M, Kitain E. Perisciatic injection of steroid for the treatment of sciatica due to piriformis syndrome. *Reg Anesth Pain Med*. 1998;23(2):223–228.
56. Mullin V, de Rosayro M. Caudal steroid injection for treatment of piriformis syndrome. *Anesth Analg*. 1990;71(6):705–707.
57. Lang AM. Botulinum toxin type B in piriformis syndrome. *Am J Phys Med Rehabil*. 2004;83(3):198–202.
58. Fishman LM, Konnoth C, Rozner B. Botulinum neurotoxin type B and physical therapy in the treatment of piriformis syndrome: a dose-finding study. *Am J Phys Med Rehabil*. 2004;83(1):42–50.
59. Yoon SJ, Ho J, Kang HY, et al. Low-dose botulinum toxin type A for the treatment of refractory piriformis syndrome. *Pharmacotherapy*. 2007;27(5):657–665.
60. Childers MK, Wilson DJ, Gnatz SM, Conway RR, Sherman AK. Botulinum toxin type A use in piriformis muscle syndrome: a pilot study. *Am J Phys Med Rehabil*. 2002;81(10):751–759.
61. Porta M. A comparative trial of botulinum toxin type A and methylprednisolone for the treatment of myofascial pain syndrome and pain from chronic muscle spasm. *Pain*. 2000;85(1-2):101–105.
62. Fishman LM, Anderson C, Rosner B. Botox and physical therapy in the treatment of piriformis syndrome. *Am J Physical Med Rehabil*. 2002;81(12):936–942.
63. Peng P, Tumber P, et al. Ultrasound-guided interventional procedures for patients with chronic pelvic pain-a description of techniques and review of literature. *Pain Physician*. 2008;11(2):215.
64. Fishman SM, Caneris OA, Bandman TB, Audette JF, Borsook D. Injection of the piriformis muscle by fluoroscopic and electromyographic guidance. *Reg Anesth Pain Med*. 1998;23(6):554–559.
65. Finnoff JT, Hurdle MFB, Smith J. Accuracy of ultrasound-guided versus fluoroscopically guided contrast-controlled piriformis injections: a cadaveric study. *J Ultrasound Med*. 2008;27(8): 1157–1163.
66. Merikangas KR, Jin R, He JP, et al. Prevalence and correlates of bipolar spectrum disorder in the world mental health survey initiative. *Arch Gen Psychiatry*. 2011;68:241.
67. Merikangas KR, Akiskal HS, Angst J, et al. Lifetime and 12-month prevalence of bipolar spectrum disorder in the National Comorbidity Survey replication. *Arch Gen Psychiatry*. 2007;64(5):543–552.
68. Kessler RC, Berglund P, Demler O, et al. The epidemiology of major depressive disorder. *JAMA*. 2003;289:3095–3105.
69. Moffitt TE, Caspi A, Taylor A, et al. How common are common mental disorders? Evidence that lifetime prevalence rates are doubled by prospective versus retrospective ascertainment. *Psychol Med*. 2010;40:899–909.
70. Kessler RC, Berglund P, Demler O, et al. Lifetime prevalence and age-of-onset distributions of DSM-IV disorders in the national comorbidity survey replication. *Arch Gen Psychiatry*. 2005;62:593–602.
71. Tanielian T, Jaycox LH. *Invisible Wounds of War: Psychological and Cognitive Injuries, Their Consequences, and Services to Assist Recovery*. Santa Monica, CA: RAND Corporation; 2008.
72. Angst J, Azorin JM, Bowden CL, et al. Prevalence and characteristics of undiagnosed bipolar disorders in patients with a major depressive episode. *Arch Gen Psych*. 2011;68(8):791–799.
73. Dudek D, Siwek M, Zielinska D, et al. Diagnostic conversions from major depressive disorder into bipolar disorder in an outpatient setting: results of a retrospective chart review [published online ahead of print August 4 2012]. *J Affect Disord*. 2012.
74. Zimmerman M, Ruggero CJ, Chelminski I, et al. Is bipolar disorder overdiagnosed? *J Clin Psychiatry*. 2008;69:935–940.
75. Goldberg JF, Garno JL, Callahan AM. Overdiagnosis of bipolar disorder among substance use disorder inpatients with mood instability. *J Clin Psychiatry*. 2008;69(11):1751–1757.
76. Zimmerman M, Galione JN, Ruggero CJ, et al. Screening for bipolar disorder and finding borderline personality disorder. *J Clin Psychiatry*. 2010;71(9):1212–1217.
77. Regier DA, Farmer ME, Rae DS, et al. Comorbidity of mental disorders with alcohol and other drug abuse: results from the Epidemiologic Catchment Area (ECA) Study. *JAMA*. 1990;264;2511–2518.
78. Grant BF, Stinson FS, Dawson DA, et al. Prevalence and co-occurrence of substance use disorders and independent mood and anxiety disorders: results from the National Epidemiologic Survey on Alcohol and Related Conditions. *Arch Gen Psychiatry*. 2004;61:807–816.
79. Kessler RC, Nelson CB, McGonagle KA, et al. Lifetime co-occurrence of DSM-III-R alcohol abuse and dependence with other psychiatric disorders in the National Comorbidity Survey. *Arch Gen Psychiatry*. 1997;54:313–321.

80. Failde I, Duenas M, Aguera-Ortiz L, et al. Factors associated with chronic pain in patients with bipolar depression: a cross-sectional study. *BMC Psychiatry.* 2013;13:112.
81. Subramaniam M, Abdin E, Vaingankar JA, et al. Prevalence, correlates, comorbidity and severity of bipolar disorder: results from the Singapore Mental Health Study. *J Affect Disord.* 2013;146(2):189–196.
82. Hoffman BM, Papas RK, Chatkoff DK, Kerns RD. Meta-analysis of psychological interventions for chronic low back pain. *Health Psychol.* 2007;26(1):1–9.
83. Wun-Schen C. Bipartite piriformis muscle: an unusual cause of sciatic nerve entrapment. *Pain.* 1994;58(2):269–272.
84. Mizuguchi T. Division of the piriformis muscle for the treatment of sciatica: postlaminectomy syndrome and osteoarthritis of the spine. *Arch Surg.* 1976;111(6):719–722.
85. Hughes S, Goldstein M, Hicks D, Pellegrini V. Extrapelvic compression of the sciatic nerve. *J Bone Joint Surg Am.* 1992;74(10):1553–1559.

15.

WHIPLASH ASSOCIATED DISORDER AND CERVICAL FACET PAIN

Jeffrey D. Petersohn, Girish Padmanabhan, and Mehul J. Desai

CASE PRESENTATION

A 45-year-old man presents with the complaint of right-sided neck and shoulder pain for the past 6 weeks. The pain began following a motor vehicle collision whereby the patient's stopped car was rear-ended by a sports utility vehicle traveling at 20 miles per hour. There is no radiation of the pain to the upper extremities. The pain occurs mostly with ipsilateral cervical rotation, although there is complaint of pain with both extension and flexion. Pain is partly relieved by lying down. There is no weakness or changes in muscle tone. Dynamic four-view cervical spine radiographs (including flexion-extension views) reveal mild spondylotic changes. A magnetic resonance image (MRI) of the cervical spine was reported as normal with the exception of straightening of the cervical lordosis. A series of chiropractic adjustments were not helpful, and a course of physical therapy, nonsteroidal anti-inflammatory drugs (NSAIDs), and muscle relaxant did not result in noticeable improvement. The patient has not worked since the motor vehicle collision and is involved in litigation related to the accident. The patient is referred to the Interdisciplinary Pain Clinic for further evaluation and management.

Past medical history is otherwise negative.

Review of systems is otherwise negative.

Patient is self-employed.

On examination, the patient weighs 78 kg and is 180 cm tall. He is sitting comfortably. Increased muscle tone is noted over the posterior aspect of the neck with tenderness over lateral aspect of the neck on the right side. Detailed neurologic examination reveals normal sensory and motor function; reflexes are symmetric and 2+. Flexion/extension of the cervical spine produces moderate discomfort; right sided cervical pain limits right lateral rotation to 20 degrees on the right and to 50 degrees on the left.

QUESTIONS

1. What are potential pain generators in this case and the likely diagnosis?
2. How is the diagnosis confirmed?
3. What is the incidence of facet-mediated neck pain and of whiplash?
4. What is the natural history of facet-mediated neck pain and of whiplash-associated disorder (WAD)?
5. How is facet-mediated neck pain/WAD managed?
   a. Rehabilitation
   b. Pharmacological management
   c. Interventional procedures
   d. Surgery

WHAT ARE POTENTIAL PAIN GENERATORS IN THIS CASE AND THE LIKELY DIAGNOSIS?

The most common pain generators in our vignette case include the cervical facet joints, the intervertebral disc, myofascial pain, and myeloradicular mechanisms. However, a comprehensive list of potential causes is quite lengthy. Included in these potential causes are vertebral tumors, discitis, rheumatoid arthritis, and soft-tissue injuries.[1] The most likely diagnosis in the case is WAD with cervical facet syndrome. Whiplash injury typically occurs as a result of an acceleration-deceleration mechanism whereby energy is transferred to the neck in a non-linear fashion resulting in disparate rotational and translational movements of adjacent vertebrae.[2]

HOW IS THE DIAGNOSIS CONFIRMED?

A diagnostic approach to the painful cervical facet joint must begin with an appreciation of the anatomy and biomechanics of the cervical zygapophyseal joints, as well as an appreciation for the varied clinical presentations and underlying pathophysiology of cervical axial nonradicular pain.

The lateral masses are the osseous portions of the C2–C7 vertebrae interposed between the cervical pedicles anteriorly and the cervical lamina posteriorly. The cephalad and caudad surfaces of each lateral mass are covered by hyaline cartilage, and a thin fibrocartilaginous joint capsule joins the two surfaces to form the cervical zygapophyseal joint or facet joint. Redundant nomenclature commonly used in clinical practice refers to the anterior cephalad and caudad portions of the lateral mass as the superior and inferior articular processes, respectively. Seen in a true lateral radiographic projection, each lateral mass presents a trapezoidal shape with the facet joint spaces above and below, angled about 40 degrees above a transverse plane. When the fluoroscopic axis is oblique (or contralateral oblique) and the viewer is looking down the axis of a roughly ovoid neural foramen, the anteroposterior length of the lateral mass becomes markedly shortened, and the superior articular process appears as a narrow triangular shape forming the dorsal inferior portion of each cervical foramen. The corresponding inferior articular process forms the dorsal superior portion of each cervical neural foramen. Whereas Bogduk recommends use of the technically correct derivative spelling "zygopophysial," this chapter favors the American vernacular spelling, "zygapophyseal." Facet joints are also termed "z-joints" or spoken of as "zed" joints.

The surfaces of the opposed lateral masses are asymmetrical, providing a joint with a peculiarly canted primary anterior-oblique axis of rotation. Pure lateral cervical rotation or extension of the cervical spine therefore can result in impingement of the two articular facet surfaces. Injuries to the cervical facet joints are quite common in acceleration-deceleration events, commonly referred to as "whiplash."[3–5] Cervical facet injury is the most pervasive cause of persisting whiplash-associated injury, accounting for 54% of all whiplash injuries.[5] Whiplash injuries commonly occur at low to moderate velocities in which the instantaneous axis of rotation of adjacent cervical vertebrae are neither symmetrical nor parallel after impact, resulting in conjoined, but disparate angular rotational and translational moments whereby the superior articular process of the lower vertebra impinges upon and gouges the inferior articular surface of the lateral mass above.[6,7] Many high-velocity injuries have lesser relative asymmetry in adjacent vertebral axes of rotation and hence do not produce discrete facet injury. Rare exceptions are made for the "jumped facet," easily detected on X-ray and often accompanied by acute neurovascular abnormalities or the isolated fracture of a lateral mass, which may likely injure the articular surface.[8]

Approximately one patient in seven undergoing single-level cervical discectomy with fusion will develop cervical facet pain at the facet joint(s) above or below the fusion within 2 years of surgery; this is successfully treated with radiofrequency (RF) lesioning.[6,7]

Although patients with cervical facet pain often present with prominent complaints of numbness and paresthesias in the extremities, especially in the lateral hand or fingertips, this is easily differentiable from the more classical presentation of radicular pain, which is typically sharp, aching, or burning in quality and usually appears in the distribution of a specific cervical nerve root. Paresthesias and numbness are often bothersome upon awakening. Details of the patient's complaint should be documented in the history, and the result of peripheral neurological motor and deep tendon reflex examinations recorded. Sensory examination with a Wartenburg pinwheel may or may not demonstrate sensory deficits that, if present , may be nondermatomal in distribution. Positions or activities that aggravate or relieve the pain should be documented.

Although the great majority of cervical facet pain is aggravated on cervical extension or ipsilateral rotation, there are occasional exceptions. Cohen's cervical RF outcome data segregated by presenting complaint show that patient's experiencing pain on ipsilateral or contralateral cervical rotation are almost equally likely to have success with RF lesioning, but conclusions of this prescient work on RF outcomes are confounded by the use of small-gauge RF needles as well as lack of explicit exclusion of orthopedic disorders of the shoulder or coexisting lumbar facet pain.[9] A higher failure rate is anticipated when performing RF lesioning in the lumbar spine when using small-gauge as opposed to large-gauge RF needles, tined RF probes, or "cooled" RF catheter devices. This suggests that the volume of thermally lesioned tissue must be sufficient to encompass the subject nerve(s). Due to these confounders, Cohen's data on cervical RF outcomes are insufficient to refute the presumed diagnostic relevance of pain exacerbated on cervical extension and rotation.

When cervical axial pain is produced on contralateral cervical rotation, it is this author's strong recommendation to dutifully examine the ipsilateral shoulder and lumbar spine as potential sources of pain, addressing those structures by medical, interventional, or surgical means as necessary prior to further consideration of a specific cervical facet pain process. Discrete cervical pain processes often coexist with similar manifestations of pain produced by concomitant injury to the shoulder or lumbar spine. Often, a single injury event damages multiple structures, and combined injury of cervical facet and shoulder or lumbar facet structures is frequently seen clinically, thus requiring diligent sequential evaluation of each set of potentially painful structures. In this regard, however, Manchikanti's report that 94% of patients have coexisting cervical and lumbar facet pain is likely a significant overestimate due to use of nonvalidated "blocks" using 0.5 mL injection volumes containing sarapin and (variably) steroid in addition to local anesthetic.[10] In patients with apparent combined cervical and lumbar facet pain, it is my practice to address the lumbar facet process primarily because, anecdotally, cervical axial pain may resolve spontaneously after the lumbar process is treated. Although the search for a singular cause of pain is a common strategy in medical practice, it is unfortunate that patients who fail to improve after one specific interventional or surgical procedure are accounted for as "failures" instead of prompting a careful search for a coexisting injury or further consideration of a possibly flawed anatomic basis for an unsuccessful procedure.

Localization of the specific painful cervical facet joint is challenging but critical to obtaining good outcomes. Dwyer first studied pain produced on saline intra-articular facet distention in volunteers; his work yielded maps that show varying areas of pain referral for each specific cervical facet joint, with subsequent confirmation and expansion by Bogduk, Dreyfuss, Fukui, and Cooper[11–15] (Figure 15.1). Unfortunately, with significant overlap of the pain referral areas for adjacent joints, the anatomic specificity is imperfect. Pain maps have been validated in a small study ($n = 9$) by Aprill.[16]

Palpation of facets is a technique similar to traditional rheumatologic examination of peripheral joints, but the literature does not yet recognize this as diagnostically precise.[17,18] There is no literature unequivocally supporting the diagnostic utility of palpatory identification of cervical joint deformity, hypertrophy, ridging, or bogginess. The greater difficulty in examination of facet tenderness is the problem of registration; accurately identifying a specific enumerated cervical facet joint by reference to external osseous landmarks. The most useful palpable landmark for facet palpation is localization of the lateral aspect of the C2–C3 facet joint at the junction of a horizontal line drawn posterior from the retromandibular angle and a vertical line dropped from the mastoid process with the patient in anatomic position. The intersection of these lines has been radiographically proven to accurately predict the location of the underlying C2–C3 facet joint.[17] Subsequent facet joints can be palpated laterally as subcutaneous prominences, each about a thumb's breadth successively more caudad. The C6–C7 facet joint is often palpable only posteriorly. The other limiting factor on manual examination is that repetitive firm palpation of the cervical facets, often encountered when teaching residents and students, produces a patient who becomes diffusely and more expansively tender

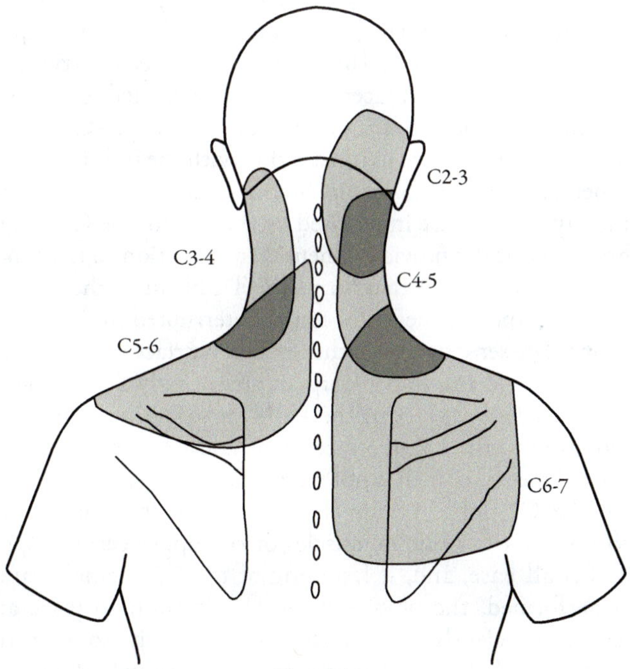

Figure 15.1 A composite map of the results in all volunteers depicting the putative characteristic distribution of pain from zygapophyseal joints at segments C2–C3 to C6–C7. From Aprill C, Dwyer A, Bogduk N. Cervical zygapophyseal joint pain patterns. I: A study in normal volunteers. *Spine* 1990;15(6):453–457, with permission from Wolters Kluwer Health.

with each additional examination, thus limiting the utility of subsequent clinical examination. Although Siegenthaler reported that measurement of pain pressure thresholds similar to that elicited on facet palpation was nondiagnostic, this conclusion is confounded and possibly invalidated in that vigorous pressure was applied over a broad area using an ultrasound transducer to first enumerate and mark the facets and only thereafter was manual force selectively applied.[19] Readers are encouraged to note how uncomfortable repetitive vigorous palpation of the facets can become and to appreciate the value of a gentle manual examination. The optimal means for precise localization of a symptomatic facet on the basis of history or physical examination remains controversial.

Whereas cervical radiculitis or radiculopathy, an irritative process in which the somatic nerve root or possibly dorsal root ganglion are mechanically or chemically irritable, can present as axial pain, most physicians assume that this process should evidence pain radiating into an extremity. Not surprisingly, because cervical nerve roots C1–C4 have little or no sensory representation in the extremity, headache, cervical axial pain, and shoulder pain are frequent clinical presentations of cervical radiculopathies and must be considered as part of any differential diagnosis. Frustratingly, mild radicular symptoms, especially due to lateral recess or foraminal stenosis in which there is only intermittent mechanical compromise of the nerve root, can produce purely axial cervical pain or headache. It is the author's experience that this frequently occurs with foraminal stenosis occuring at the C6–C7 levels and somewhat less commonly at C5–C6 levels.

Several diagnostic maneuvers are frequently used to evaluate patients for cervical foraminal stenosis including a Jackson cervical compression test, Spurling's maneuver, and modified Spurling's maneuver.

Although a Spurling's maneuver can be helpful in demonstrating clinical radiculopathy meriting clinical treatment of the compromised and symptomatic nerve root or lateral epidural space, this maneuver has only 70% clinical sensitivity and then only when considering clinical processes involving the C5 and C6 nerve roots. The C6–C7 foramen passing the seventh cervical root is minimally compromised anatomically by this maneuver, and, as noted earlier, the more cephalad nerve roots have little or no extremity representation so that the production of "radicular" extremity pain with cervical rotation and extension (classic Spurling's maneuver) or the modified Spurling's maneuver (lateral bending and extension) is limited in diagnostic sensitivity.[20] A reverse nerve tension test, the Bakody maneuver, wherein the ipsilateral shoulder is abducted to the coronal plane and the patient's palm placed on the occiput, resulting in relief of pain may be useful when considering diagnoses of axial pain where a radicular process of stenotic origin is suspected. To further complicate matters, the author has seen hundreds of examples where both a cervical facetogenic process and cervical radicular process are present simultaneously requiring specific use of relevant techniques for treatment of each type of pain process to ultimately provide successful treatment. It is the author's routine practice to first address the cervical radicular or stenotic process because this can generally be well defined on a neurologic and anatomic imaging basis whereas nomination of specific facet levels for treatment is a more artistic endeavor. For further details of diagnosis and treatment of cervical radicular pain, the reader is invited to consult Chapter 16.

Axial imaging of the cervical spine using MRI is typically considered standard of care in evaluating patients with suspected cervical facet pain. Although there are no specific or sensitive findings on MRI that can be used to diagnose or refute the diagnosis of cervical facet pain, MRI is principally appreciated for its ability to exclude other causes of severe axial cervical pain, especially the so-called red flag conditions of mass, tumor, or abscess.

Cervical foraminal stenosis is a common cause of axial pain, and MRI may be of some diagnostic utility in considering a differential diagnosis. Abnormalities of the cervical spinal cord, including myelomalacia and vascular abnormalities (e.g., vertebral artery loops), may be demonstrated. Perineural Tarlov cysts of the cervical nerve roots communicate with the cerebrospinal fluid space can be identified. Routine T1, T2, and STIR sequences with 2.5 mm thick axial sections should be obtained; there is, however, no routine diagnostic advantage to using gadolinium contrast sequences except where abscess, tumor, or vascular abnormality is suspected or the postoperative spine is encountered. MRI may also be useful in demonstrating nonsegmentation abnormalities as well as facet cysts, stenosis, herniated nucleus pulposus, and some vascular anomalies.

When ordering MRI studies of the cervical spine, routine use of closed 1.5 or 3.0 Tesla units are strongly recommended for improved spatial resolution as compared with the 0.6 Tesla open unit in which software algorithms struggle mightily—but seldom successfully—to convert low signal-to-noise ratio data into high-quality images. Sophisticated practitioners should routinely prefer use of modern MRI units with superconducting medium- and high-field magnets for cervical imaging: image voxel size and, ultimately, image spatial resolution and gray scale bit depth depends on the field strength of the magnet, and no amount of software can compensate for overly thick, poorly placed, or misaligned scan sequences. Use of older 0.3 Tesla MRI units is specifically condemned as suboptimal practice for cervical spine care. It is this author's practice to personally review all MRI images prior to performing cervical interventions. Few radiology facilities routinely and candidly report studies compromised by inadequate patient positioning, motion artifact, or where axial imaging planes were not obtained properly parallel to the anatomic planes or disc axes.

When considering the diagnosis of cervical facetogenic pain, plain cervical radiographs are of limited diagnostic value, occasionally demonstrating mild instability at the symptomatic levels. Typically, vertical lines drawn parallel to the dorsal aspect of adjacent vertebral bodies translate minimally anteroposteriorly on comparison of lateral X-ray views taken in flexed, neutral, or extended positions. Variation of more than 3 mm on these multiple lateral views is diagnostic for instability and merits spine surgery consultation. Oblique X-ray views demonstrate anatomic stenosis but at half the diagnostic sensitivity of computed tomography (CT) imaging. Often, oblique X-ray images are suboptimally aligned and do not assist in diagnosis. Dynamic lateral and oblique X-ray series incur significant ionizing radiation exposure to the patient. Where MRI study is nondiagnostic or contraindicated, the risk of ionizing radiation may be more usefully expended by obtaining a high-resolution, low-dose CT scan. If CT scan is performed, in addition to requesting 1 mm axial slice thickness, it is this author's practice to routinely request reformatted coronal and sagittal images, as well as both left and right anterior oblique reformatted images. Reformatted images may produce helpful insight into the presence of foraminal stenosis or incomplete arthrodesis, often uncertain on coronal or sagittal planar reconstructions due to beam hardening artifact produced by metallic anterior plates, cages, and screws. These anterior oblique reformatted images may be substantially more sensitive for diagnostic purposes. Reformatted images do not increase ionizing radiation exposure because they are performed on a digital workstation following image acquisition.

Sensation to the cervical facet capsule and its articular surfaces is supplied by one to four articular nerve branches that issue from the medial branch of the dorsal primary ramus as it travels along the lateral aspect of the posterior half of the lateral mass.[21] In some cases, the medial branch divides proximally into deep and superficial divisions, and the articular nerves originate from the deep division of the medial branch. A posterior Cruveilhier plexus may provide additional intersegmental sensory innervation to the posterior articular surfaces from the C1 dorsal ramus as well as the C2–C3–C4 medial branches.[22] The average cervical medial branch is approximately 1 mm or less in diameter and is typically located within 1–2 mm of the lateral surface of the osseous lateral mass. The C3 medial branch is the largest of the medial branches in the human body and issues the third occipital nerve (TON). The medial branches at the named level typically innervate the cervical facet joint, thus the medial branches of C5 and C6 innervate the C5–C6 facet. The C2–C3 facet is somewhat anomalous in innervation with the inferior surface innervated by the C3 medial branch or its deep division and the superior surface innervated by the TON. The C2 medial branch typically provides a neural contribution to the superficial division of C3 that forms the TON, and either the C2 medial branch or the TON can be interrupted to therapeutically ablate sensation from the cephalad surface of the C2–C3 facet. Govind and Bogduk argue convincingly that a series of broad RF lesions ablating the TON are sufficient to interrupt sensation to the C2–C3 facet joint and that separate RF of the C2 medial branch is not required.

The C2 dorsal ramus also provides motor innervation to the inferior oblique muscles of the upper cervical spine and skull base, and, if lesioning of the C2 medial branch is performed, the physician must be certain to place any lesion sufficiently posteriorly and inferiorly so that the more cephalad located motor branches are spared, lest the patient experience postoperative head drop. As the superficial division of C2 becomes the greater occipital nerve, postoperative anesthesia, hypesthesia, or dysesthesia in that distribution is frequently seen with C2 medial branch or TON RF lesioning. A recurrent neural arcade between C2 and C1 may carry sensory innervation from the posterior atlantoaxial joint. Tubbs, in a large cadaveric study, provides evidence for sensory innervation of the facet joint through a posterior Cruveilhier nerve plexus located posteriorly to the lateral mass in which sensory fibers anastomose with a medial branch one additional level cephalad or caudad to the expected level.[22] Thus, sensory fibers from the C1 dorsal ramus or from the C4 medial branch may provide some sensory innervation to the C2–C3 facet, perhaps accounting for a lack of satisfactory outcome following RF lesioning in some patients in whom diagnostic medial branch blocks (MBBs) have suggested that only innervation from C2 and C3/TON were responsible for nociception. In similar fashion the C3–C4 facet may include innervation from the C2 medial branch. Tubb's data distinctly conclude that the Cruveilhier plexus does not extend below C4. Unfortunately even a low-volume diagnostic MBB will likely anesthetize a large enough tissue volume to include the entire contribution from a Cruveilhier plexus, thus producing a falsely positive outcome and perhaps producing a disappointing result from an otherwise technically adequate appearing RF lesioning procedure in the upper cervical spine.

In the case of a failed RF lesioning at the C2–C3 facet joint, a C4 diagnostic MBB would be appropriate and if failed RF lesioning occurs at C3–C4, a C2 diagnostic MBB would be appropriate in consideration of a Cruveilhier plexus contribution to innervation of the painful facet and suggestion of an additional anatomic target for RF lesioning.

Regardless of the diagnostic tradition for identifying the symptomatic cervical facet joint(s) to which one may subscribe, whether relying on diligent manual palpation of the cervical facets to elicit patient complaints of pain upon palpation of a specific joint or foreswearing examination entirely and identifying symptomatic levels based on matching clinical complaints to the maps created by Dwyer and others, confirmation of the symptomatic facet joint level by interventional means is ultimately required.

Duplicate diagnostic MBB of facet joint innervation using low volumes (0.3 mL) of local anesthetic following contrast injection is the only diagnostic technique validated for confirming cervical facet joint pain. The use of injection volumes in excess of 0.5 mL is specifically condemned as compromising the anatomic specificity necessary to properly plan RF lesioning procedures. Single diagnostic blocks have 27–63% false-positive rates, but this may reflect large volumes of injectate. Although it might appear that intra-articular facet joint injection might be a useful diagnostic modality, the frequent lack of integrity of the facet articular capsule allows nonspecific spread of injectate while symptomatic subchondral injury may be unaffected by the injectate. The use of large injectate volumes all contribute to a lack of sensitivity and specificity that cannot recommend this procedure. Partisans argue that facet injection is both diagnostic and therapeutic and therefore simpler and less demanding of both physician and patient resources. Although this argument is appealing, the poor clinical outcomes from intra-articular facet injection demonstrated by Barnsley two decades prior to this writing have not been improved by time, and the argument is unsupportable by reference to the published medical literature.[23]

The necessity for duplicate diagnostic MBB has provoked the ire of many physicians. It seems quite curious that it is somehow necessary to do something poorly twice when doing it optimally once might otherwise suffice. In an informal survey of U.S. physician colleagues performing cervical RF lesioning, the experienced physicians' opinions were evenly split on the clinical necessity for the use of duplicate or comparative diagnostic blocks for diagnosis as opposed to a single diagnostic block.

It may be that customary diagnostic neural blockade at the centroid of the lateral mass is suboptimal because the articular nerves issue in the posterior half of the lateral mass, but RF lesioning is only effective when performed in the anterior half of the lateral mass, prior to emergence of the articular nerve. This anatomy may recommend use of a more anterior neural target for the purpose of diagnosis. As well, except for C5, the medial branch does not run across the centroid of the lateral mass, and perhaps use of the centroid diagnostic target is too caudad to be optimal. The medial branch is typically located in areolar tissue just off the surface of the lateral mass, and perhaps near-periosteal injection is suboptimal. Injectate may track posteriorly or may run in the course of the semispinalis muscle fibers, anesthetizing structures inappropriately or not at all. Although the technique of MBB may have been usefully optimized by various investigators in three decades of thoughtful use, demonstration of statistically superior results using modified diagnostic medial branch targets remains a tantalizing goal, as yet unconfirmed in the published literature.

In performing diagnostic MBB, patient positioning, optimal radiographic technique, and low-volume injection are crucial to technical success. Some physicians prefer prone patient position: the fluoroscopic C-arm is placed in a true AP view and the X-ray beam is then declined to identify clear, lucent facet joints above and below the lateral mass target. Needles are advanced to the centroid of each lateral mass under multiplanar fluoroscopic visualization. With initial posterior or posterolateral needle entry employing a distally curved needle and advancing into the C-shaped lateral hollow of the lateral mass, each needle is guided by sequential rotation and advancement to contact the lateral mass at the centroid as then assessed by a lateral view. Contralateral oblique fluoroscopic views are often helpful, especially when true lateral views are unabtainable. Most physicians prefer diagnostic MBB with a patient in true lateral position, which requires a shorter and more easily controllable needle path. The 2014 ISIS Practice Guidelines[23] provide comprehensive detailed instruction on technique and optimal landmarks, which are beyond the scope of this chapter.

WHAT IS THE INCIDENCE OF FACET-MEDIATED NECK PAIN AND OF WHIPLASH?

Cervical facet joints are a common source of axial neck pain (36–62%).[8, 24–28] The C2–C3 and C5–C6 joints are most commonly affected.[5,25,29] The joints have been implicated as a source of neck pain. Neck pain is quite common: systematic reviews have noted a prevalence of neck pain in the general population of 12–72%; most estimates, however, fall between 30% and 50% within 12-month prevalence.[30] In cases of trauma-related neck pain, the cervical facets are found to be involved in 50–60% of cases.[25] Specifically in patients involved in motor vehicle crashes 15–40% of patients with acute neck pain develop chronic pain.[7,31–34] Those who experience pain acutely are three times more likely to report pain 7 years later compared to those who did not have acute pain following motor vehicle collision.[34] Whiplash is a significant healthcare problem, with approximately 6.2% of Americans suffering from late whiplash syndrome.[35,36] Although most patients recover from whiplash injuries, 20–30% experience prolonged symptoms with long-term health consequences.[37,38] Poor outcomes often result from a failure to escalate treatment to incorporate inteventional modalities in a timely fashion, especially where conservative modalities have not been demonstrated to be helpful for a period of 6–12 weeks.

WHAT IS THE NATURAL HISTORY OF FACET-MEDIATED NECK PAIN AND OF WAD?

Eighty percent of patients following motor vehicle collisions begin experiencing pain the day of the collision; 60–80% of patients with acute neck pain following motor vehicle collision recover completely. Up to 40% develop mild chronic symptoms, with 5–12% developing moderate to severe pain and 5–10% experiencing permanent partial or total disability.[32–34, 39]

Multiple prospective studies have identified prognostic factors for adverse outcomes. The strongest negative predictor for poor outcome is high initial pain intensity.[39–41] Factors not necessarily implicated in poor outcomes include older age, female sex, high initial psychological response, and compensation or litigation.[41] Cote et al found that older age, female sex, radicular symptoms, multiple areas of pain, and being unprepared for impact predicted a poor prognosis.[40]

HOW IS FACET-MEDIATED NECK PAIN/WAD MANAGED?

REHABILITATION

Various structures in the neck, including those of vascular, muscular, or articular construct, may be damaged as a result of whiplash-associated injury. The results of whiplash injury may lead to both physical and psychological trauma, resulting in varying degrees of physical impairment or loss of function. The Quebec Task Force introduced a classification system that is widely utilized in delineating WADs. The classification system is as follows; WAD I neck complaints, with stiffness or tenderness in the neck region and no physical signs of injury; WAD II neck complaints, with stiffness or tenderness and some physical signs of injury, such as point tenderness or difficulty turning the head; WAD III neck complaints, with stiffness or tenderness and neurological signs of injury, such as changes to reflexes or weakness in the arms; and WAD IV neck complaints, with a fracture or dislocation of the neck.[31] The management of the patient will differ based on the severity of the injury. Physical therapy and rehabilitation have a major role in the management of WADs. There are different and varied approaches in the management of WAD-related injuries ranging from exercises, manual therapy, and education regarding the need to resume normal activities.[41,42] The main goals of physiotherapy are to improve mobility, neuromuscular function, and strength and thereby improve quality of life, participation in work activities, and function. Physical activity and therapeutic exercise are mainstays for management of musculoskeletal injury and pain of both the spine and extremity.

Patients with WADs might often present with neck movement restriction and altered muscle behavior and properties. Neck movement disorders, well documented in both acute and chronic whiplash injury, impact the ability of patients to function on a daily basis specifically due to loss of range of motion. Recent studies have documented the presence of pathological movement patterns in patients with whiplash-related neck pain. These include reduced acceleration and velocity of neck movements and reduced smoothness and irregular axis of neck movement. In patients with whiplash-related neck pain, there may be altered recruitment patterns.[43] There is reduced activation of multifidus, semispinalis cervicis, longus colli, and capitis and increased recruitment of the superficial muscles.[44–46] The deep cervical muscles have an important role in maintaining proper head control and minimizing the stress on the cervical segments during limb loading tasks. The increased activity of the superficial neck muscles may lead to pain with tasks such as typing. Also in patients with WAD, increased trapezius activation has been noted, which could lead to adverse loading of the cervical spine.[47] There is also loss of muscle endurance, which may be related to the transformation from slow-twitch to fast-twitch muscle fibers.[48]

WAD is puzzling because symptoms often persist in the absence of detectable injury or inflammation; this may be due to the presence of sensorimotor disturbances. However, there are specific features of radiculopathy that a specially trained examiner can detect and differentiate from whiplash. Patients with chronic whiplash injuries might present with neuropathic features consisting of hyperesthesia, allodynia, and hyperpathia. It is important to consider central sensitization and regional sensitization as key contributors in the perpetuation of pain in these patients as opposed to local mechanisms solely. The presence of psychological factors should not be ignored. Patients with chronic whiplash injuries often show pain-associated behavioral abnormalities including depression, anxiety disorders, and fear of movement.[49]

In addition to identifying structural injury, new evidence suggests that the clinical evaluation should attempt to identify the presence of physical and psychological impairments to provide an in-depth assessment and recognition of potential underlying mechanisms that hinder clinical improvement and full return of function.[50,51] Manual palpation and treatment lacks reliability and validity, but proper assessment of cervical mobility may be useful in guiding treatment. Assessment of motor function and useful tests like the cranial cervical flexion tests are useful. A carefully directed neurological examination is necessary. Specific sensory assessments such as measuring pain pressure threshold using pressure algometry and quantitative sensory assessment are useful in classifying patients. A few tests that are routinely used in clinical practice are listed here. It is recommended that the clinician consistently use the same assessments methods to reliably classify and treat patients.

Assessment of patients with WAD will help in their classification and treatment. In patients with mobility-based impairment, the following tests can be useful:

1. Cervical spine active range of motion (AROM)
2. Cervical and thoracic spine segmental mobility testing

In patients with suspected cervicogenic headaches and suspected movement disorders, the following tests should be utilized:

1. Cervical spine AROM
2. Cervical spine segmental mobility testing
3. Cranial cervical flexion test

In patients with suspected movement coordination problems, the following tests are useful:

1. Cranial cervical flexion test
2. Deep neck flexor endurance test

In patients with suspected cervical radiculopathy, the following tests are useful:

1. Spurling's test
2. Upper limb tension test
3. Distraction test

Clinicians should utilize easily reproducible functional restriction measures associated with their patient's neck pain to assess the changes in the patient's level of function over the episode of care. The Neck Disability Index (NDI) is commonly used in clinical practice to capture disability associated with neck pain.[52] The NDI consists of 10 items, 7 related to function, 2 related to pain, and 1 related to concentration. The NDI possesses sufficient sensitivity to measure change related to the patient reaching sufficient functional goals and work activities and patients involved in litigation.[53]

Studies comparing the treatment of WAD that compare rest, physical agents, exercise, cervical collars, neck care education, transcutaneous electrical nerve stimulation, traction, and manual therapy have not demonstrated the superiority of one intervention strategy over another.[5] There are studies that challenge the recommendation of rest and cervical collar application. Manual therapy has been shown to cause greater improvement in cervical mobility and pain reeducation compared to rest and cervical collar application.[6] Another study looking at the McKenzie approach, which utilizes repeated active submaximal movements, demonstrated similar results.[7] Active exercise programs are one of the mainstays of treating acute or chronic whiplash injuries. An exercise program should include mobility exercises with special emphasis on neuromuscular control, velocity, and proprioception. The exercise program should be individualized to the patient's needs/deficits, and emphasis should be placed on quality of movement and control. The aim of the exercise program should be to prevent a negative transition to chronicity and reduce recurrent episodes of neck pain. To do this, the exercise program should address all aspects of presenting altered muscle and behaviors and cervical movement deficits. The initial program should focus on basic recruitment of the deep cervical muscles; as the patient progresses, the therapist should introduce limb loading and more complex movement patterns. An exercise program should be multidimensional, addressing all areas of deficits including cervical mobility, neuromuscular control, endurance, and proprioception. In patients with chronic whiplash injuries, dry needling should be considered. Dry needling has been demonstrated as superior to sham in treating patients with chronic myofascial pain associated with whiplash injuries, fundamentally allowing for improvement in movement and recruitment patterns.

PHARMACOLOGICAL MANAGEMENT

Although medications often form the mainstay of front-line therapy in the treatment of acute cervical facet-mediated pain and whiplash, minimal data support this practice. Pharmacological approaches typically serve as a means to facilitate other treatment strategies, including early mobilization and physical therapy.

Acute injuries are treated with anti-inflammatory agents such as NSAIDs and skeletal muscle relaxants. Although not specifically mandated, medical treatment might follow the World Health Organization (WHO) analgesic ladder. Regarding opiate analgesics: it is important to note that opioids, if used, should only be considered for a short period, typically during the acute phase.[54] There remains a paucity of data supporting the protracted use of opioids in the setting of chronic neck pain of any etiology. Skeletal muscle relaxants such as cyclobenzaprine have been well studied and found efficacious for various musculoskeletal conditions including acute neck pain.[55,56] There is also evidence to suggest efficacy for agents such as carisoprodol, orphenadrine, and tizanidine in the acute setting.[56] Carisoprodol should be avoided due to its high potential for dependence, abuse, and withdrawal due to the properties of its metabolite meprobamate.[54]

Topical agents such as capsaicin are demonstrated to decrease neck pain.[57] Other topical agents, such as those containing local anesthetics, have not been studied in the scope of randomized trials but anecdotally appear to benefit a select group of patients.

There is even less data to guide practitioners treating patients with chronic whiplash and facetogenic pain. Typically, there is an element of trial and error that accompanies the treatment of these patients. A customized treatment plan accounting for patient response must be considered. In these patients, we favor the use of adjuvant medications such as serotonin norepinephrine reuptake inhibitors and tricyclic antidepressants along with antispasticity agents such as baclofen or tizanidine rather than traditional skeletal muscle relaxants.

INTERVENTIONAL PROCEDURES

There are three distinct paradigms commonly used for interventional treatment of cervical facet pain, the first involving injection of steroid into the facet articular joint space (facet injection) and the second recommending diagnostic neural blockade of the innervation of the joint and subsequent thermal lesioning of the innervating medial branches or deep divisions of the medial branch, typically using RF energy. The third paradigm of repeated direct application of local anesthetic with or without steroid to the medial branch is mentioned only to repudiate this technique. This technique requires an average of six procedures over 2 years to produce a greater than 50% improvement, considerably less impressive results than used to judge success in RF outcome studies. Manchikanti has published four papers on this technique using a single patient cohort, but these are methodologically flawed because no placebo or RF comparator group is used. Manchikanti's claim that the results of local anesthetic and steroid MBBs produce clinical benefit in excess of 12 weeks is profoundly inconsistent with the quotidian observations of hundreds of interventional physicians, and these results strain all credulity.[58–61] Smuck has authored an erudite critique of this technique.[62] Because there is no clinical evidence for durable clinical improvement resulting from these so-called therapeutic MBBs, and absent evidence that neurapraxic injury to the medial branch is etiologically relevant to production of cervical facet pain, a course of care using this procedure is costly, requires repetitive exposures to ionizing radiation, and represents inappropriate overutilization of physician resources.

The cervical facet capsule is frequently frankly disrupted in adults. Several excellent studies have demonstrated conclusively that the instillation of steroid by injection into the articular space is only marginally efficacious, if at all.[63] Subchondral injury may play a role in steroid nonresponsive pain. Short-term improvement following intra-articular cervical facet injection, typically 1 month or less in duration, often results. Data do not support relentless periodic repetitions of this procedure at a defined series of semi-monthly, monthly, or tri-monthly intervals based on establishment of a brief period of improvement following any one of these injections. No evidence supports an assumption of cumulative benefit accruing from multiple intra-articular or peri-articular steroid injections, although the well-known adverse systemic effects of repetitive steroid administration should serve as a sharp rebuke to this practice. In summary, despite widespread use of repetitive intra-articular cervical facet injections, no reliable evidence exists that proves cumulative intermediate or long-term efficacy.[25] In patient's enjoying only hours or several days of pain relief from facet injection, it is likely that any benefit obtained is due solely to local anesthetic effect, and repetition of this procedure is discouraged because durable benefit is unforeseeable. Due to the variable spread of the intra-articular injectate, which is seldom confined to the joint space, intra-articular injection is insufficiently target specific to function as a diagnostic standard.

The only validated paradigm for interventional treatment of cervical facet pain remains interruption of the neural pathways providing sensation to the facet joint by use of RF electrical energy at 400–550 kHz to obtain ionic heating of tissue using a so-called monopolar system with a needle electrode with an insulated shaft and a larger dispersive or return electrode applied to the skin. These produce a slender, almostcylindrical volume of thermocoagulated tissue parallel to the long axis of the RF electrode and not extending significantly distally or proximally of the uninsulated portion of the shaft. RF monopolar lesioning is the only validated technique that has demonstrated 70% or better outcomes in multiple randomized controlled trials.[25,64–65]

Whereas outcomes are generally improved in the lumbar spine with use of larger electrodes, this work is likely also applicable in the cervical spine. Lord, McDonald, and MacVicar demonstrated successful RF lesioning techniques based solely on use of anatomic radiographic landmarks to guide multiple electrode placements. Improved outcomes are thought to result from performance of multiple RF lesions that increase the likelihood that one or more of the lesion volumes will incorporate the traversing medial branch nerve. Use of cooled RF catheters or tined catheter designs may more readily accomplish the same objective by using a single lesion of larger volume that regularly encompasses the individual variability in medial branch nerve course, but robust comparative data have not yet been published.

It is common practice, prior to performance of RF lesioning, to stimulate the medial branch at 2 Hz to elicit multifidus twitch or at 50 Hz to elicit duplication of the typical pain in order to verify that the needle is appropriately proximate to the medial branch nerve for successful lesioning to occur (Figures 15.2–15.4).

Bogduk decries localization by electrical stimulation as unnecessary, relying instead on the performance of multiple anatomic lesion placements, but the majority of physicians in practice rely on it to document adequate placement as well as to ensure that the RF electrode is far enough from the somatic nerve root to avoid inadvertent thermal injury. With use of cooled RF or tined catheter designs, the electrode may be as much as 4–5 mm from the medial branch; hence, voltage stimulating thresholds may be quite high, and purely anatomic placement is required. Although these monopolar RF lesioning procedures are very safe, they are relatively contraindicated in patients with cardiac pacemakers, implantable defibrillators, spinal cord stimulators, or vagal nerve stimulators. In these circumstances, consideration may be given to the performance of bipolar RF lesions using a pair of parallel-placed RF needles that straddle the subject medial branch nerve on

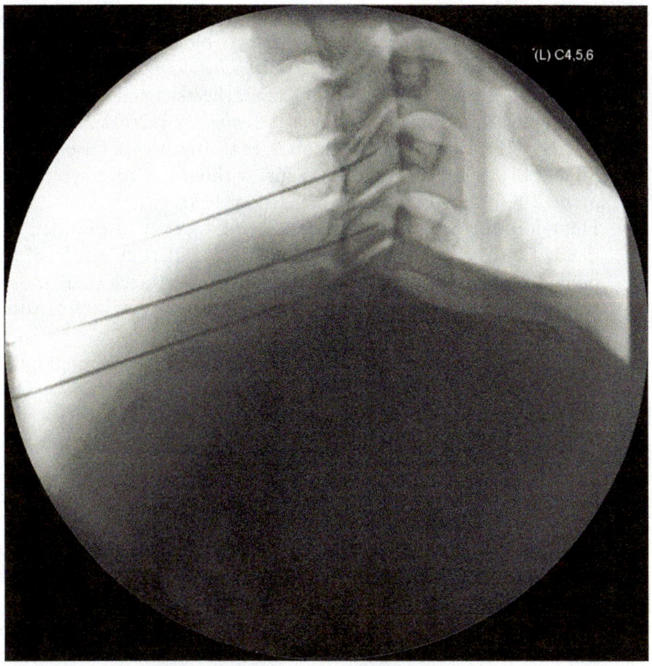

Figure 15.2 Right C4, C5, andC6 medial branch radiofrequency—lateral view.

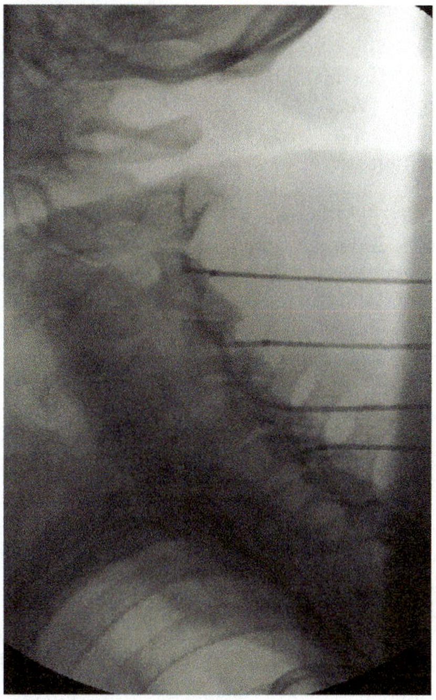

Figure 15.4 Right C3, C4, C5, and C6 medial branch radiofrequency—oblique view.

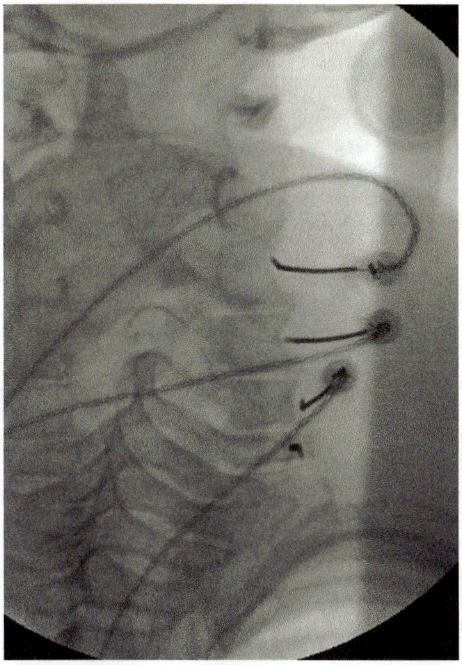

Figure 15.3 Right C3, C4, C5, and C6 medial branch radiofrequency—AP view.

the lateral aspect of the lateral mass. Caution should be exercised in use of these techniques in patient's having ventriculoperitoneal shunts or other implanted devices that cross the posterolateral cervical region.

It is this author's unpublished experience that use of a 20-gauge RF needle electrode with verification of 2 Hz multifidus stimulation at or below 0.3 volts is adequate to identify the proximity of the medial branch and electrode to assure a good clinical result. With an 18-gauge RF needle producing a larger radius of lesioned tissue, an increased 2 Hz stimulation threshold of 0.5 volts appears acceptable.

Postoperative pain and dysesthesia are common and time-limited side effects of RF lesioning. The resulting quality of pain relief is often quite dramatic, resulting in documented improved range of motion, reduced pain, and return to preinjury activities. Injury to somatic nerve roots from RF lesioning is quite rare, as are infections. Use of contralateral oblique fluoroscopic imaging is exceedingly helpful in documenting safe positioning of the RF cannula sufficiently dorsal to the neural foramen.

The durability of clinical results after cervical RF lesioning is expectedly 9–12 months, with some patients reporting greater duration of improvement. Why some patients have permanent relief of pain while others have recurrent symptoms requiring revision of the RF lesioning is not known. However, simple revision of the RF lesion is likely to be successful in reestablishing pain relief when recurrent pain is noted.

Although fine points of the interventional diagnosis and treatment of cervical facet pain remain controversial, there can be no doubt about the proven role for these techniques in clinical care of patients.

SURGERY

The treatment of axial neck pain, particularly that of facetogenic origin, with surgical fixation remains controversial in the absence of gross instability. There remains contradictory evidence regarding the efficacy of cervical discectomy and fusion or posterior fusion in the setting of WADs.[66]

REFERENCES

1. Bogduk N. The anatomy and pathophysiology of neck pain. *Phys Med Rehabil Clin N Am*. 2011;22:367–82.
2. Voyvodic F, Dolinis J, Moore VM, et al. MRO of car occupants with whiplash injury. *Neuroradiology*. 1997;39(1):35–40.
3. Bogduk N. On cervical zygapophysial joint pain after whiplash. *Spine*. 2011;36: S194–S199.
4. Jull GA, Soderlund A, Stemper BD, et al. Toward optimal early management after whiplash injury to lessen the rate of transition to chronicity [discussion paper 5]. *Spine*. 2011;36:S335–S342.
5. Barnsley L, Lord SM, Wallis BJ, Bogduk N. The prevalence of chronic cervical zygapophysial joint pain after whiplash [discussion paper 6]. *Spine* 1995;20: 20–25.
6. Pearson AM, Ivancic PC, Ito S, Panjabi MM. Facet joint kinematics and injury mechanisms during simulated whiplash. *Spine*. 2004;29:390–397.
7. Bogduk N, Yoganandan N. Biomechanics of the cervical spine Part 3: minor injuries. *Clin Biomech*. 2001;16:267–75.
8. Rabb CH, Lopez J, Beauchamp K, et al. Unilateral cervical facet fractures with subluxation: injury patterns and treatment. *J Spinal Disord Tech*. 2007;20:416–422.
9. Cohen SP, Bajwa ZH, Kraemer JJ, et al. Factors predicting success and failure for cervical facet radiofrequency denervation: a multi-center analysis. *Reg Anesth Pain Med*. 2007;32:495–503.
10. Manchikanti L, Singh V, Pampati V, et al. Is there correlation of facet joint pain in lumbar and cervical spine? An evaluation of prevalence in combined chronic low back and neck pain. *Pain physician*. 2002;5:365–371.
11. Dwyer A, Aprill C, Bogduk N. Cervical zygapophyseal joint pain patterns. I: A study in normal volunteers. *Spine*. 1990;15:453–457.
12. Bogduk N. Cervicogenic headache: anatomic basis and pathophysiologic mechanisms. *Curr Pain Headache Rep*. 2001;5:382–386.
13. Cooper G, Bailey B, Bogduk N. Cervical zygapophysial joint pain maps. *Pain Med*. 2007;8:344–353.
14. Fukui S, Ohseto K, Shiotani M, et al. Referred pain distribution of the cervical zygapophyseal joints and cervical dorsal rami. *Pain*. 1996;68:79–83.
15. Dreyfuss P, Michaelsen M, Fletcher D. Atlanto-occipital and lateral atlanto-axial joint pain patterns. *Spine*. 1994;19:1125–1131.
16. Aprill C, Dwyer A, Bogduk N. Cervical zygapophyseal joint pain patterns. II: A clinical evaluation. *Spine*. 1990;15:458–461.
17. Jull G, Bogduk N, Marsland A. The accuracy of manual diagnosis for cervical zygapophysial joint pain syndromes. *Med J Aust*. 1988;148:233–236.
18. King W, Lau P, Lees R, Bogduk N. The validity of manual examination in assessing patients with neck pain. Spine J. 2007;7:22–26.
19. Siegenthaler A, Eichenberger U, Schmidlin K, et al. What does local tenderness say about the origin of pain? An investigation of cervical zygapophysial joint pain. *Anesth Analg*. 2010;110:923–927.
20. Takasaki H, Hall T, Jull G, et al. The influence of cervical traction, compression, and Spurling test on cervical intervertebral foramen size. *Spine*. 2009;34:1658–1662.
21. Bogduk N. The clinical anatomy of the cervical dorsal rami. *Spine*. 1982;7:319–330.
22. Tubbs RS, Mortazavi MM, Loukas M, et al. Cruveilhier plexus: an anatomical study and a potential cause of failed treatments for occipital neuralgia and muscular and facet denervation procedures. *J Neurosurg*. 2011;115:929–933.
23. Barnsley L, Lord S, Wallis B, Bogduk N. False-positive rates of cervical zygapophysial joint blocks. *Clin J Pain*. 1993;9:124–130.
24. Speldewinde GC, Bashford GM, Davidson IR. Chronic cervical zygapophysial joint pain after whiplash: a placebo-controlled prevalence study. *Spine*. 1996;21:1737–1745.
25. Lord SM, Barnsley L, Wallis BJ, et al. Percutaneous radio-frequency neurotomy for chronic cervical zygapophyseal-joint pain. *N Engl J Med*. 1996;335:1721–1726.
26. Yin W, Bogduk N. The nature of neck pain in a private pain clinic in the United States. *Pain Med*. 2008;9(2):196–203.
27. Manchikanti L, Manchikanti KN, Damron KS, Pampati V. Effectiveness of cervical medial branch blocks in chronic neck pain: a prospective outcome study. *Pain Physician*. 2004;7:195–201.
28. Aprill C, Axinn MJ, Bogduk N. Occipital headaches stemming from the lateral atlanto-axial (C1-2) joint. *Cephalalgia*. 2002;22:15–22.
29. Carragee EJ, Tanner Cm, Khurana S, et al. The rates of false-positive lumbar discography in select patients without low back symptoms. *Spine*. 2000;25(11):1373–80; discussion: 1381.
30. Hogg-Johnson S, van der Velde G, Carroll LJ, et al. The burden and determinants of neck pain in the general population: results of the bone and joint decade 2000-2010 task force on neck pain and its associated disorders. *J Manipulative Physiol Ther*. 2009;32(suppl 2):S46–S60.
31. Spitzer WO, Skovron ML, Salmi LR, et al. Scientific monograph of the Quebec Task Force on Whiplash-Associated Disorders: redefining "whiplash" and its management. *Spine*. 1995;20:1S–73S.
32. Radanov BP, Sturzenegger M, Di Stefano G. Long-term outcome after whiplash injury A 2-year follow-up considering features of injury mechanism and somatic, radiologic, and pyscholosocial findings. *Medicine*. 1995;74:281–297.
33. Gozzard C, Bannister G, Langkamer G, Khan S, Gargan M, Foy C. Factors affecting employment after whiplash injury. *J Bone Joint Surg Br*. 2001;83:506–509.
34. Berglund A, Alfredsson L, Cassidy JD, Jensen I, Nygren A. The association between exposure to rear-end collision and future neck or shoulder pain: a cohort study. *J Clin Epidemiol*. 2000;53:1089–1094.
35. Karlberg M, Magnusson M, Malmstrom EM, Melander A, Moritz U. Postural and symptomatic improvement after physiotherapy in patients with dizziness of suspected cervical origin. *Arch Phys Med Rehabil*. 1996;77:874–882.
36. Freeman MD, Croft AC, Rossignol AM. "Whiplash associated disorders: redefining whiplash and its management" by the Quebec Task Force. A critical evaluation. *Spine*. 1998;23:1043–1049.
37. Bogduk N. Post whiplash syndrome. *Aust Fam Physician*. 1994;23(12):2303–2307.
38. Squires B, Gargan MF, Bannister GC. Soft-tissue injuries of the cervical spine. 15-year follow-up. *J Bone Joint Surg Br*. 1996;78(6):955–957.
39. Hendriks EJ, Scholten-Peeters GG, van der Windt DA, Neeleman-van der Steen CW, Oostendorp RA, Verhagen AP. Prognostic factors for poor recovery. *Pain*. 2005;114:408–416.
40. Cote P, Cassidy JD, Carrol L, Frank JW, Bombardier C. A systematic review of the prognosis of acute whiplash and a new conceptual framework to synthesize the literature. *Spine*. 2001;26:E445–E458.
41. Sholten-Peeters GG, Verhagen AP, Bekkering GE, et al. Prognostic factors of whiplash-associated disorders: a systematic review of prospective cohort studies. *Pain*. 2003;104:303–322.
42. Rosenfeld M, Gunnarsson R, Borenstein P. Early intervention in whiplash-associated disorders: a comparison of two treatment protocols. *Spine*. 2000;25:1782–1787.
43. Jull G, Kristjansson E, Dall'Alba P. Impairment in the cervical flexors: a comparison of whiplash and insidious onset neck pain patients. *Man Ther*. 2004;9:89–94.
44. O'Leary S, Cagnie B, Reeve A, et al. Is there altered activity of the extensor muscles in chronic mechanical neck pain? A functional magnetic resonance imaging study. *Arch Phys Med Rehabil*. 2011;92:929–934.
45. Falla DL, Jull GA, Hodges PW. Patients with neck pain demonstrate reduced electromyographic activity of the deep cervical flexor muscles during performance of the craniocervical flexion test. *Spine*. 2004;29:2108–2114
46. Jull GA. Deep cervical neck flexor dysfunction in whiplash. *J Musculoskel Pain*. 2000;8:143–154.
47. Falla D, Bilenkij G, Jull G. Patients with chronic neck pain demonstrate altered patterns of muscle activation during performance of a functional upper limb task. *Spine*. 2004;29:1436–1440.
48. Uhlig Y, Weber BR, Grob D, et al. Fiber composition and fiber transformations in neck muscles of patients with dysfunction of the cervical spine. *J Orthop Res*. 1995;13:240–249.

49. Nederhand MJ, Ijzerman MJ, Hermens HJ, Turk DC, Zilvold G. Predictive value of fear avoidance in developing chronic neck pain disability: consequences for clinical decision making. *Arch Phys Med Rehabil.* 2004; 85:496–501.
50. Sterling M. A proposed new classification system for whiplash associated disorders—implications for assessment and management. *Man Ther.* 2004;9:60–70.
51. Jull G, Kristjansson E, Dall'Alba P. Impairment in the cervical flexors: a comparison of whiplash and insidious onset neck pain patients. *Man Ther.* 2004;9:89–94.
52. Pietrobon R, Coeytux RR. Standard scales for measurement of functional outcome for cervical pain or dysfunction: a systematic review. *Spine.* 2002 1;27(5):515–522.
53. Riddle DL, Startford PW. Use of generic versus region-specific functional status measures on patients with cervical spine disorders. *Phys Ther.* 1998;78(9):951–963.
54. Pangarkar S, Lee PC. Conservative treatment for neck pain: medications, physical therapy, and exercise. *Phys Med Rehabil Clin N Am.* 2011;22:503–520.
55. Basmajian JV. Cyclobenzaprine hydrochloride effect on skeletal muscle spasm in the lumbar region and neck: two double-blind controlled clinical and laboratory studies. *Arch Phys Med Rehabil.* 1978;59(2):58–63.
56. Chou R, Peterson K, Helfand M. Comparative efficacy and safety of skeletal muscle relaxants for spasticity and musculoskeletal conditions: a systematic review. *J Symptom Manage.* 2004; 28(2):140–175.
57. Mathias BJ, Dillingham TR, Zeigler DN, et al. Topical capsaicin for chronic neck pain. A pilot study. *Am J Phys Med Rehabil.* 1995;74(1):39–44.
58. Manchikanti L, Singh V, Falco FJ, et al. Comparative outcomes of a 2-year follow-up of cervical medial branch blocks in management of chronic neck pain: a randomized, double-blind controlled trial. *Pain Physician.* 2010;13:437–450.
59. Manchikanti L, Singh V, Falco FJ, et al. Cervical medial branch blocks for chronic cervical facet joint pain: a randomized, double-blind, controlled trial with one-year follow-up. *Spine.* 2008;33:1813–1820.
60. Manchikanti L, Damron K, Cash K, et al. Therapeutic cervical medial branch blocks in managing chronic neck pain: a preliminary report of a randomized, double-blind, controlled trial: clinical trial NCT0033272. *Pain Physician.* 2006;9:333–346.
61. Manchikanti L, Manchikanti KN, Damron KS, Pampati V. Effectiveness of cervical medial branch blocks in chronic neck pain: a prospective outcome study. *Pain Physician.* 2004;7:195–201.
62. Smuck M, Levin JH. Re: Manchikanti L, Singh V, Falco FJ, et al. Cervical medial branch blocks for chronic cervical facet joint pain: a randomized, double-blind, controlled trial with one-year follow-up. *Spine.* 2008;33:1813–1820; author reply: *Spine* 2009;34:1116.
63. Barnsley L, Lord SM, Wallis BJ, Bogduk N. Lack of effect of intraarticular corticosteroids for chronic pain in the cervical zygapophyseal joints. *N Engl J Med.* 1994;330:1047–1050.
64. McDonald GJ, Lord SM, Bogduk N. Long-term follow-up of patients treated with cervical radiofrequency neurotomy for chronic neck pain. *Neurosurgery.* 1999;45:61–67; discussion 7–8.
65. MacVicar J, Borowczyk JM, MacVicar AM et al. Cervical medial branch radiofrequency neurotomy in New Zealand. *Pain Med.* 2012;13:647–654.
66. Basho R, Bhalla A, Wang JC. Neck pain from a spine surgeon's perspective. *Phys Med Rehabil Clin N Am.* 2011;22:551–555.

16.

CERVICAL RADICULAR PAIN

Jan Van Zundert, Dieter M. J. Peuskens, Peter Hallet, Koen Van Boxem, and Binit J. Shah

CASE PRESENTATION

Mr. M is a 54-year-old man referred to the pain clinic by his general practitioner with the request to perform an epidural corticosteroid infiltration at cervical level.

The patient has a history of 2 months of right-sided neck pain radiating over the shoulder into the lateral forearm and index finger. Plain X-rays of the neck indicate degenerative facet (zygapophyseal) joints, predominantly at C3.

The previous treatment consisted of paracetamol (acetaminophen) up to 4 g/d and nonsteroidal anti-inflammatory drugs (NSAIDs). Nortriptyline was used up to 50 mg 3×/day. This treatment was stopped because of intolerable side effects.

The patient received instructions for exercises (rolling neck movements and arm rotation). The patient claims having done these exercises, but pain during the exercise discourages him to continue.

QUESTIONS

1. Should patients be immediately scheduled for epidural infiltration?
2. How is the patient assessed through clinical examination?
3. Which additional examinations are useful?
4. Is a multidisciplinary evaluation recommended?
5. Which treatment should be offered?
6. How are patients followed, and how is treatment outcome registered?

SHOULD PATIENTS BE IMMEDIATELY SCHEDULED FOR EPIDURAL INFILTRATION?

Epidural corticosteroid infiltration has the objective of administering the corticosteroid close to the inflamed nerve root, thus concentrating the anti-inflammatory effects directly to the target. The efficacy of this intervention has been demonstrated in subacute cervical radicular pain. The pain specialist must confirm the diagnosis prior to planning any intervention.

HOW IS THE PATIENT ASSESSED THROUGH CLINICAL EXAMINATION?

The diagnostic process starts with an in-depth history taking. Attention is paid to the patient's history of trauma, the duration of the pain, the description of the pain, and the radiation pattern.

During history taking, indications suggestive for vascular diseases, tumor, or infection, the so-called red flags, should imperatively lead to further investigations that exclude serious pathologies.

The patient's professional situation, type of work, job satisfaction, and related issues—the so-called yellow flags—may be the cause of behavioral problems and a tendency to chronification. This type of patient may experience improvement with cognitive behavioral therapy.

When red and yellow flags are excluded, attention is directed toward the pain pattern. Patients suffering cervical radicular pain report pain in the neck that radiates over the posterior shoulder into the arm and sometimes into the hand. Radicular pain may not be confounded with radiculopathy, where an objective loss of sensory and/or motor function is noted. Radicular pain is a symptom that is caused by ectopic impulse formation, whereas radiculopathy also includes neurologic signs such as sensory or motor changes.[1] The pain radiation provides an indication of the causative level. Slipman et al.[2] performed a mechanical stimulation of the C4–C8 nerve roots and had the pain distribution noted by an independent observer. The distribution of symptom provocation resembled the classic dermatomal maps for cervical nerve roots, but symptoms were frequently provoked outside of the distribution of classic dermatomal maps, thus suggesting that the dermatomal and dynatomal maps are distinctly different. A segment-specific pattern can, however, be distinguished.

Pain originating from C4 is confined to the neck and suprascapular region. Pain originating from C5 radiates up to the upper arm, and pain from C6 and C7 radiates from the neck to the shoulder, forearm, and hand. The pain covers the posterolateral side of the upper arm, but the pain from C7 extends more dorsally.[2,3] Radicular pain can also be perceived in all structures innervated by the affected nerve roots, such as muscles, joints, ligaments, and the skin.[3]

The neurological examination includes testing sensation, strength, and tendon reflexes.[4] Table 16.1 gives a summary of the neurological characteristics of cervical radicular pain.[5]

Clinical examination of cervical radicular pain consists mainly of the use of three tests: the neck compression test (Spurling test), the shoulder abduction test, and the axial manual traction test.

For the Spurling test, the neck is extended with the head rotated to the affected shoulder while axially loaded. Reproduction of the patient's shoulder or arm pain indicates possible cervical spinal nerve root compression.

In the shoulder abduction test, the patient lifts a hand above his or her head. A positive result is the decrease or disappearance of the radicular symptom.

In the axial manual traction test, an axial traction force corresponding to 10–15 kg is applied in with the patient in the supine position. A positive finding is the decrease or disappearance of the radicular symptom.[1]

> Mr. M. does not present any red or yellow flags. The radiation pattern suggests a problem at the C6 level, and the Spurling test indicates potential nerve root compression.

Table 16.1 **CLINICAL/NEUROLOGICAL FINDINGS IN CERVICAL RADICULAR PAIN**

ROOT	ROOT PAIN DISTRIBUTION	MUSCLE WEAKNESS	SENSORY LOSS
C5	Medial scapular border, lateral upper arm to elbow	Deltoid, supraspinatus, infraspinatus	Lateral upper arm
C6	Lateral forearm, thumb and index finger	Biceps, brachioradialis, wrist extensors	Thumb and index finger
C7	Medial scapula, posterior arm, dorsum of forearm, third finger	Triceps, wrist flexors, finger extensors	Posterior forearm, third finger
C8	Shoulder, ulnar side of forearm, fifth finger	Thumb flexors, abductors, intrinsic hand muscles	Fifth finger

Adapted from Carette S, Fehlings MG. Clinical practice. Cervical radiculopathy. *N Engl J Med.*2005;353:392–399.

WHICH ADDITIONAL EXAMINATIONS ARE USEFUL?

We dispose of two additional examination means: medical imaging and electrophysiological examination. There is no direct link between medical imaging and the pain syndrome. Up to 28% of asymptomatic patients show an abnormal magnetic resonance image (MRI).[6,7] Medical imaging use has as its major objective excluding "red flags." Although computed tomography (CT) provides good images of the cortical bone structures, MRI provides better images of changes in the intervertebral discs, spinal cord, nerve roots, and surrounding tissue.[1]

Because there is no gold standard for the diagnosis of cervical radicular pain, the sensitivity and specificity of the imaging technique is not known.[8]

Electrophysiological tests, such as needle electromyography and nerve conduction tests, can be considered to differentiate between cervical radicular pain and other neurologic causes of pain in the arm and neck.[5] Electrophysiologic tests may confirm suspected nerve damage, but they do not provide any information about the pain. Quantitative sensory testing (QST) can provide more specific information about pain. This was illustrated in a QST study in which patients with cervical radicular symptoms showed an increased detection threshold for light touch and allodynia (touch-induced pain), which differed significantly from that in healthy subjects. QST confirmed the level of involvement identified by means of diagnostic selective nerve root blocks.[9]

> Mr. M's MRI showed a herniated disc at C5–C6. We found no indication for electrophysiological evaluation.

IS A MULTIDISCIPLINARY EVALUATION RECOMMENDED?

The physical therapy specialist may identify posture problems and consequently recommend a multidisciplinary rehabilitation program.[10] Psychologist and/or psychiatrist advice should be sought when the patient shows a strong dissatisfaction with the "social" situation, expresses fear of movement, or is unable to cope with the "rest pain."

The patient's attitude and posture will be indicative for the initiation of a cognitive behavioral rehabilitation program.

> Mr. M. did not require further evaluation, mainly because of the MRI-proved herniated disc at C5–C6, which corresponds with the presumed level based on the pain radiation pattern.

WHICH TREATMENT SHOULD BE OFFERED?

Every treatment strategy starts conservatively with pain medication, such as paracetamol. When the neuropathic component is prominent and pain is not satisfactory controlled with analgesic alone, antineuropathic drugs can be added. The tricyclic antidepressants and the anticonvulsants, such as carbamazepine, oxcarbazepine, gabapentin, and pregabalin, have been used with variable success in the treatment of neuropathic pain. There are, however, no studies on their effect in cervical radicular pain.[8] Exercise treatment and patient education[11] and mechanical traction were studied in Cochrane reviews that could not find evidence to support or refute those treatment options.[12]

> Mr. M. clearly suffers subacute cervical radicular pain. An epidural corticosteroid administration is indicated.

Treatment selection should be guided by the search for balance between potential beneficial effects and the risk and burden of side effects and complications. A recently published treatment guideline according to clinical diagnoses used the scoring system published by Guyatt et al.[13] "Grading strength of recommendations and quality of evidence in clinical guidelines." The method was adapted specifically for interventional pain management techniques.[14] The rating of the available evidence is summarized in Table 16.2.

Epidural corticosteroid administration can use the interlaminar or the transforaminal route. Both administration routes are illustrated in Figure 16.1.

EVIDENCE FOR INTERLAMINAR EPIDURAL CORTICOSTEROID ADMINISTRATION

Interlaminar corticosteroid administration was compared with its intramuscular administration. At 1-year follow-up, 68% of the patients in the interlaminar group had significant pain relief compared with 12% in the intramuscular group.[15] A study assessing the potential value of additional morphine administration with corticosteroid and local anesthetic revealed transient improvement in the morphine group on the first day after the injection, but in the long-term no difference between the two groups was found.[16]

A systematic review on the effectiveness of interlaminar epidural steroid injections included three randomized controlled trials (RCTs) and five observational studies of variable quality and concluded that interlaminar cervical epidural corticosteroid injections provide a significant effect on cervical radicular pain.[17]

SAFETY OF INTERLAMINAR EPIDURAL CORTICOSTEROID ADMINISTRATION

A literature review on the potential complications of interlaminar cervical corticosteroid administration showed a complication rate of less than 1% up to 16.8%, depending on the time of registration of the complications.[18]

Minor complications that spontaneously disappeared, often within 24 hours, include increasing axial neck pain, posture independent headache, facial flushing, and vasovagal episodes. Major complications mentioned included epidural hematoma and accidental subdural injection with, as a result, hypoventilation and hypotension. Accidental subdural injection-induced hypoventilation must be distinguished from the apnea and acute cardiovascular collapse that may result from an intrathecal injection. Paresthesia has been described

Table 16.2 **SUMMARY OF EVIDENCE SCORES AND IMPLICATIONS FOR RECOMMENDATION**

SCORE	DESCRIPTION	IMPLICATION
1 A +	Effectiveness demonstrated in various RCTs of good quality. The benefits clearly outweigh risk and burdens.	Positive recommendation
1 B +	One or more RCTs with methodological weaknesses demonstrate effectiveness. The benefits clearly outweigh risk and burdens.	
2 B +	One or more RCTs with methodological weaknesses demonstrate effectiveness. Benefits are closely balanced with risk and burdens.	
2B ±	Multiple RCTs with methodological weaknesses yield contradictory results better or worse than the control treatment. Benefits are closely balanced with risk and burdens, or uncertainty in the estimates of benefits, risk, and burdens.	Considered, preferably study-related
2 C +	Effectiveness only demonstrated in observational studies. Given that there is no conclusive evidence of the effect, benefits are closely balanced with risk and burdens.	
0	There is no literature or there are case reports available, but these are insufficient to suggest effectiveness and/or safety. These treatments should only be applied in relation to studies.	Only study-related
2 C –	Obational studies indicate no or too short-lived effectiveness. Given that there is no positive clinical effect, risk and burdens outweigh the benefit.	Negative recommendation
2 B–	One or more RCTs with methodological weaknesses or large observational studies that do not indicate any superiority to the control treatment. Given that there is no positive clinical effect, risk and burdens outweigh the benefit.	
2 A –	RCT of a good quality that does not exhibit any clinical effect. Given that there is no positive clinical effect, risk and burdens outweigh the benefit.	

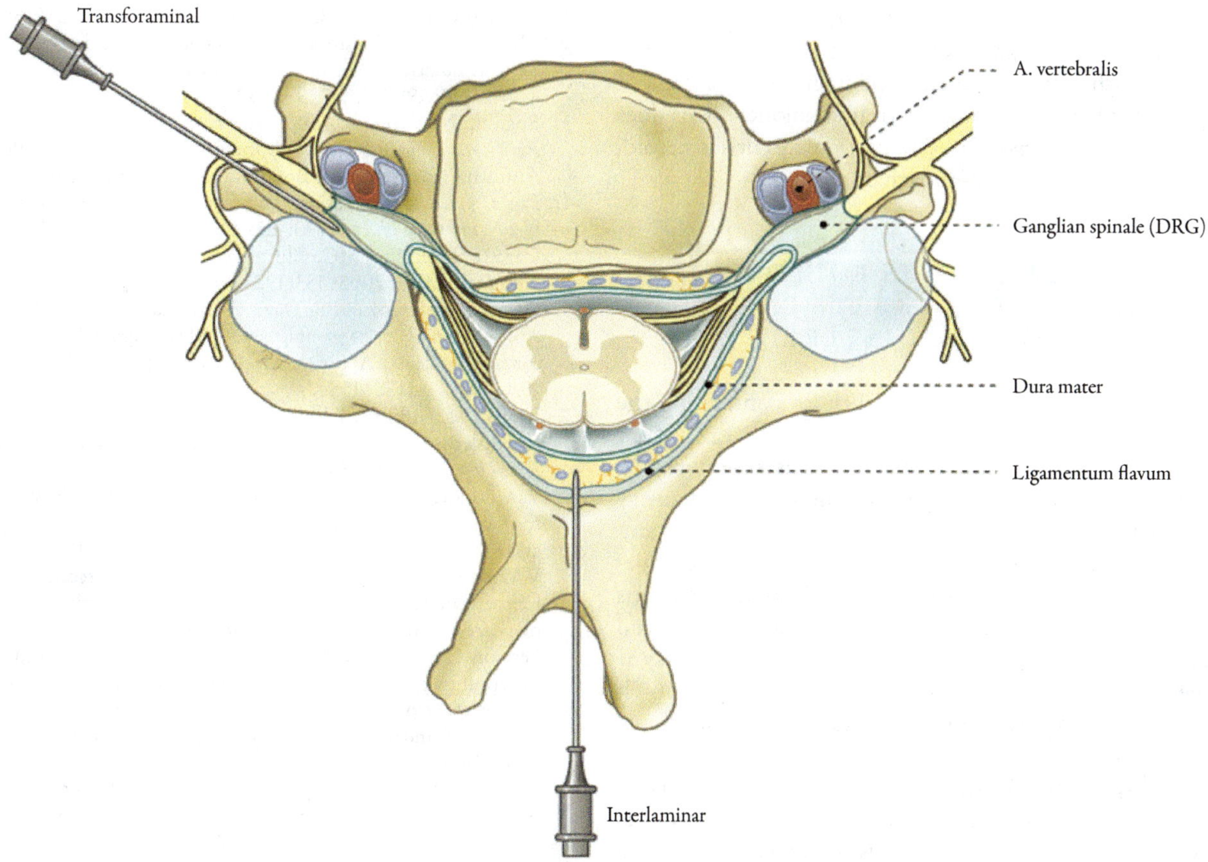

Figure 16.1 Interlaminar and transforaminal administration in the epidural space. Courtesy Rogier Trompert, Medical Art, www.medial-art.eu.

after root damage. There were two reports of permanent damage to the spinal cord in patients who were sedated and possibly unable to report warning symptoms during the procedure. Intravascular uptake of the contrast dye has also been reported, although this occurs less frequently in interlaminar administration compared to the transforaminal route.[18]

CERVICAL TRANSFORAMINAL EPIDURAL CORTICOSTEROID ADMINISTRATION: EFFICACY

An RCT compared the efficacy of transforaminal injection of corticosteroid and local anesthetic with local anesthetic and saline. At 3 weeks after the injection, no difference in the outcome was observed between the two groups.[19]

CERVICAL TRANSFORAMINAL EPIDURAL CORTICOSTEROID ADMINISTRATION: COMPLICATIONS

Alarming reports on potentially fatal neurologic complications shed an additional negative light on this treatment option. Malhotra et al.[20] summarized the published reports in a comprehensive review, but more cases have been published since.

One case report described a direct lesion of the spinal cord due to inadvertent air and contrast injection into the cervical cord,[21] and another described the consequences of a spinal cord compression due to epidural hematoma.[22] The other cases can be divided into lesions of the spinal cord caused by the anterior spinal artery syndrome[23–25] and effects on the central nervous system involving brainstem and cerebellum related to inadvertent injection of the vertebral artery.[26–33] An anatomic study on human cadavers noted several variations in the normal course of the cervical radicular arteries that may enter the intervertebral foramen near the sites recommended for transforaminal needle placement.[34]

Furthermore, upon inadvertent injection of particulate steroid into the cervical arteria radicularis, the steroid may act as an embolus and cause spinal cord infarction and permanent impairment.[1] Drawing conclusions on the role of particle size of the different corticosteroid preparation is very difficult, as illustrated in the in-depth study from Benzon et al.[35] who found that particle size depends on the concentration, the solution type, and may even be different between compounded and commercially available preparations.

An animal study confirmed the potential role of particulate steroids. Eleven pigs were instrumented and the arteriae vertebrales intentionally injected with particulate (methylprednisolone) or nonparticulate (dexamethasone) corticosteroid. The animals that received particulate corticosteroid could not be removed from life support and on histological examination there was evidence of severe tissue edema, ischemic changes, and other pathologies. In the animals injected with nonparticulate corticosteroid, no issues were noted.[36]

A small comparative trial assessing the efficacy of triamcinolone (particulate) and dexamethasone (nonparticulate) in patients with cervical radicular pain showed a slight but not significant better outcome for triamcinolone.[37] This does not justify taking the risk for using particulate corticosteroid, should the transforaminal approach be used.[1]

HOW ARE PATIENTS FOLLOWED, AND HOW IS TREATMENT OUTCOME REGISTERED?

In addition to having the responsibility for confirming the diagnosis, the pain specialist is also responsible for patient follow-up. In the short term, the patient is supervised in recovery. Special attention is paid to the patient's sensory and motor reactions. When the patient is discharged from the hospital, he or she must be accompanied by a competent person and may not drive a car. Recommendations are given to consult the emergency department if sensorial and/or neurological deficits are noted. Pain and redness at the injection site may be indicative of an infection, which equally requires immediate consultation in the emergency department.

Normally, an appointment is made to see the patient at 3 weeks and 2 months after the injection. The patient is instructed to note the evolution of his or her pain on a visual analog scale (VAS). When there has been early improvement in pain that returns to baseline value at the 3-week follow-up, a second injection can be considered.

It is also recommended to obtain the patient's Global Perceived Affect, which can be rated on a 7-point Likert scale. This global scale gives a better impression of the treatment's influence on the patient's well-being.

CONCLUSION

The pain specialist cannot perform an epidural corticosteroid administration without a careful patient assessment that should confirm or refute the diagnosis. Cervical interlaminar epidural corticosteroid administration may be considered for the management of subacute cervical radicular pain. There is evidence of its efficacy, and, when correctly performed, the technique is safe.

ACKNOWLEDGMENTS

The authors thank Nicole Van den Hecke for administrative support and coordination.

REFERENCES

1. Van Zundert J, Huntoon M, Patijn J, Lataster A, Mekhail N, van Kleef M. 4. Cervical radicular pain. *Pain Pract.* 2009;10:1–17.
2. Slipman CW, Plastaras CT, Palmitier RA, Huston CW, Sterenfeld EB. Symptom provocation of fluoroscopically guided cervical nerve root stimulation. Are dynatomal maps identical to dermatomal maps? *Spine.*1998; 23:2235–2242.
3. Bogduk N. *Medical Management of Acute Cervical Radicular Pain: An Evidence-Based Approach.* Bogduk N, ed. Newcastle, Australia: The Newcastle Bone and Joint Institute; 1999.
4. Fager CA. Identification and management of radiculopathy. *Neurosurg Clin N Am.*1993; 4:1–12.
5. Carette S, Fehlings MG. Clinical practice. Cervical radiculopathy. *New Engl J Med.* 2005; 353:392–399.
6. Boden SD, McCowin PR, Davis DO, Dina TS, Mark AS, Wiesel S. Abnormal magnetic-resonance scans of the cervical spine in asymptomatic subjects. A prospective investigation. *J Bone Joint Surg Am.*1990; 72:1178–1184.
7. Teresi LM, Lufkin RB, Reicher MA, et al. Asymptomatic degenerative disk disease and spondylosis of the cervical spine: MR imaging. *Radiology.*1987; 164:83–88.
8. Van Zundert J, Harney D, Joosten EA, et al. The role of the dorsal root ganglion in cervical radicular pain: diagnosis, pathophysiology, and rationale for treatment. *Reg Anesth Pain Med.* 2006;31:152–167.
9. Voerman VF, van Egmond J, Crul BJ. Elevated detection thresholds for mechanical stimuli in chronic pain patients: support for a central mechanism. *Arch Phys Med Rehabil.* 2000;81:430–435.
10. Persson LC, Lilja A. Pain, coping, emotional state and physical function in patients with chronic radicular neck pain. A comparison between patients treated with surgery, physiotherapy or neck collar—a blinded, prospective randomized study. *Disabil Rehabil.* 2001; 23:325–335.
11. Haines T, Gross A, Burnie SJ, Goldsmith CH, Perry L. Patient education for neck pain with or without radiculopathy. *Cochrane Database Syst Rev.* 2009:CD005106.
12. Graham N, Gross A, Goldsmith CH, et al. Mechanical traction for neck pain with or without radiculopathy. *Cochrane Database Syst Rev.* 2008:CD006408.
13. Guyatt G, Gutterman D, Baumann MH, et al. Grading strength of recommendations and quality of evidence in clinical guidelines: report from an American College of Chest Physicians task force. *Chest.* 2006; 129:174–181.
14. van Kleef M, Lataster A, Narouze S, Mekhail N, Geurts JW, van Zundert J. Evidence-based interventional pain medicine according to clinical diagnoses. 2. Cluster headache. *Pain Pract.* 2009; 9:435–442.
15. Stav A, Ovadia L, Sternberg A, Kaadan M, Weksler N. Cervical epidural steroid injection for cervicobrachialgia. *Acta Anaesthesiol Scand.*1993;37:562–566.
16. Castagnera L, Maurette P, Pointillart V, Vital JM, Erny P, Senegas J. Long-term results of cervical epidural steroid injection with and without morphine in chronic cervical radicular pain. *Pain.*1994;58:239–243.
17. Benyamin RM, Singh V, Parr AT, Conn A, Diwan S, Abdi S. Systematic review of the effectiveness of cervical epidurals in the management of chronic neck pain. *Pain Physician.* 2009; 12:137–157.
18. Abbasi A, Malhotra G, Malanga G, Elovic EP, Kahn S. Complications of interlaminar cervical epidural steroid injections: a review of the literature. *Spine.* 2007; 32:2144–2151.
19. Anderberg L, Annertz M, Persson L, Brandt L, Saveland H. Transforaminal steroid injections for the treatment of cervical radiculopathy: a prospective and randomised study. *Eur Spine J.* 2007; 16:321–328.
20. Malhotra G, Abbasi A, Rhee M. Complications of transforaminal cervical epidural steroid injections. *Spine.* 2009; 34:731–739.
21. Lee JH, Lee JK, Seo BR, Moon SJ, Kim JH, Kim SH. Spinal cord injury produced by direct damage during cervical transforaminal epidural injection. *Reg Anesth Pain Med.* 2008;33:377–379.
22. Lee JY, Nassr A, Ponnappan RK. Epidural hematoma causing paraplegia after a fluoroscopically guided cervical nerve-root injection. A case report. *J Bone Joint Surg Am.* 2007;89:2037–2039.

23. Brouwers PJ, Kottink EJ, Simon MA, Prevo RL. A cervical anterior spinal artery syndrome after diagnostic blockade of the right C6-nerve root. *Pain.* 2001; 91:397–399.
24. Rosenkranz M, Grzyska U, Niesen W, et al. Anterior spinal artery syndrome following periradicular cervical nerve root therapy. *J Neurol.* 2004; 251:229–231.
25. Ludwig MA, Burns SP. Spinal cord infarction following cervical transforaminal epidural injection: a case report. *Spine.* 2005; 30:E266–E268.
26. McMillan MR, Crumpton C. Cortical blindness and neurologic injury complicating cervical transforaminal injection for cervical radiculopathy. *Anesthesiology.* 2003;99:509–511.
27. Rozin L, Rozin R, Koehler SA, et al. Death during transforaminal epidural steroid nerve root block (C7) due to perforation of the left vertebral artery. *Am J Forensic Med Pathol.* 2003; 24: 351–355.
28. Tiso RL, Cutler T, Catania JA, Whalen K. Adverse central nervous system sequelae after selective transforaminal block: the role of corticosteroids. *Spine J.* 2004; 4:468–474.
29. Beckman WA, Mendez RJ, Paine GF, Mazzilli MA. Cerebellar herniation after cervical transforaminal epidural injection. *Reg Anesth Pain Med.* 2006;31:282–285.
30. Ziai WC, Ardelt AA, Llinas RH. Brainstem stroke following uncomplicated cervical epidural steroid injection. *Arch Neurol.* 2006;63:1643–1646.
31. Suresh S, Berman J, Connell DA. Cerebellar and brainstem infarction as a complication of CT-guided transforaminal cervical nerve root block. *Skeletal Radiol.* 2007;36:449–452.
32. Ruppen W, Hugli R, Reuss S, Aeschbach A, Urwyler A. Neurological symptoms after cervical transforaminal injection with steroids in a patient with hypoplasia of the vertebral artery. *Acta Anaesthesiol Scand.* 2008;52:165–166.
33. Muro K, O'Shaughnessy B, Ganju A. Infarction of the cervical spinal cord following multilevel transforaminal epidural steroid injection: case report and review of the literature. *J Spinal Cord Med.* 2007;30:385–388.
34. Huntoon MA. Anatomy of the cervical intervertebral foramina: vulnerable arteries and ischemic neurologic injuries after transforaminal epidural injections. *Pain.* 2005;117:104–111.
35. Benzon HT, Chew TL, McCarthy RJ, Benzon HA, Walega DR. Comparison of the particle sizes of different steroids and the effect of dilution: a review of the relative neurotoxicities of the steroids. *Anesthesiology.* 2007;106:331–338.
36. Okubadejo GO, Talcott MR, Schmidt RE, et al. Perils of intravascular methylprednisolone injection into the vertebral artery. an animal study. *J Bone Joint Surg Am.* 2008;90:1932–1938.
37. Dreyfuss P, Baker R, Bogduk N. Comparative effectiveness of cervical transforaminal injections with particulate and nonparticulate corticosteroid preparations for cervical radicular pain. *Pain Med.* 2006;7:237–242.

17.

THORACIC BACK PAIN

Shrif Costandi, Yashar Eshraghi, and Nagy Mekhail

CASE PRESENTATION

A 69-year-old woman presents with the complaint of worsening mid-back pain for the past several weeks. The pain is made worse by coughing and changing position. Staying still relieves pain. There is no reported weakness or changes in bowel or bladder function observed, and no fever is noted. Conservative treatment; including a nonsteroidal anti-inflammatory drug (NSAID) and muscle relaxant, did not result in noticeable improvement, and the patient could not tolerate physical therapy. The patient is referred to the Interdisciplinary Pain Clinic for further evaluation and management.

Past medical history is significant for osteopenia, hypertension, and hypothyroidism.

Social History: Denies smoking, reports occasional alcohol consumption.

Review of systems is significant for difficulty sleeping.

On examination, the patient weighs 62 kg and is 149 cm tall. She is sitting in mild discomfort. Musculoskeletal examination reveals tenderness over the mid-back spinous processes. Detailed neurologic examination reveals normal sensory and motor function, and reflexes are symmetric and 2+.

An X-ray of the thoracic spine reveals collapse of the superior endplate of the T6 vertebral body. Osteophytes and degenerative changes are noted diffusely. The patient has had a magnetic resonance imaging (MRI) of the thoracic spine 1 year ago, which revealed multilevel disc bulges most prominent at T7–T8 and T8–T9

QUESTIONS

1. What is the definition of thoracic back pain?
2. What are potential pain generators in this case and the likely diagnosis?
3. How is the diagnosis confirmed?
4. What is the incidence of vertebral compression fracture (VCF)?
5. What is the natural history of VCF?
6. How is VCF prevented?
7. How are thoracic back pain, VCF, thoracic disc displacement, and thoracic spondylosis managed?

WHAT IS THE DEFINITION OF THORACIC BACK PAIN?

Thoracic back pain is a term commonly used to describe mid- or upper-back pain. Thoracic back pain is much less common than neck or low back pain; therefore, the diagnosis of pain originating from thoracic region has been challenging.[1–3] Frequently, thoracic back pain has a benign musculoskeletal origin, but it may indicate a more serious underlying problem. The neural complexity of the thoracic spine, along with referred visceral pain, leads to poor pain source localization.[4,5] Many patients referred to pain specialists have seen other physicians without obtaining adequate relief. One reason is the paucity of literature regarding thoracic spine pain in comparison to the cervical and lumbar spine.

Although the incidence of spinal pain has been reported as 54–80% of the general population, the number of patients suffering from chronic upper or mid-back pain secondary to thoracic disorders is rather small, ranging from 3% to 22% of outpatient pain population.[6,7] In fact, Leboeuf-Yde et al. reported that low back pain was most common in 43% of patients, followed by neck pain in 32%, and mid-back pain in 13%.[8] Reduced physical activities and loss of function are common with thoracic pain, which can significantly affect patients' quality of life.

WHAT ARE POTENTIAL PAIN GENERATORS IN THIS CASE AND THE LIKELY DIAGNOSIS?

Before we answer this question, we need to review the functional anatomy of the thoracic vertebral segments. The thoracic area of the spine consists of 12 vertebrae (10 of which connect to ribs with costovertebral joints), intervertebral discs, supporting soft tissue, and 12 thoracic nerves. Thoracic vertebrae are considerably larger and stronger than cervical vertebrae. The spinous processes of T1 and T2 are long, laterally flattened, and directed inferiorly. On the other hand, the spinous processes of T11 and T12 are shorter, wider, and directed more posteriorly. In general, thoracic vertebrae have longer and larger transverse processes when compared to cervical vertebrae. Movements of the thoracic region are limited by the attachment of the ribs to the sternum. From a structural viewpoint, the 12 thoracic vertebrae have three separate shapes, with the smaller upper four thoracic vertebrae sharing some characteristics with the cervical vertebra and the larger lower four thoracic vertebrae sharing similar features with the lumbar vertebrae. The middle four thoracic vertebrae share characteristics with both the cervical and lumbar regions. The spinal canal has a similar diameter in the thoracic and lumbar area, but the space around the thoracic spine is narrower than lumbar spine. Thus, spinal cord compression from a herniated thoracic disk is more likely at the thoracic level. The upper thoracic vertebral interspaces from T1 to T2 and the lower thoracic vertebral interspaces from T10 to T12 are functionally equivalent to the cervical and lumbar interspaces, respectively, which facilitates placement of the epidural block in a similar fashion to the cervical and lumbar approaches. The thoracic vertebral interspaces between T3 and T9 are functionally unique because of the acute downward angle of the spinous processes. Epidural blockade of these middle thoracic interspaces requires use of the paramedian approach to the thoracic epidural space.[9]

Five facet joints, including one facet joint on either side of the vertebra, provide a minimal mobile connection between each vertebra (Figure 17.1). A distinguishing characteristic of the first 10 thoracic vertebrae is the presence of articular facets for the ribs. Thoracic vertebrae articulate with the ribs through the costovertebral joints on both sides of the vertebral body. Each of these vertebrae contains two pairs of costal demifacets on its body and one on each transverse process. Typical ribs articulate with both the inferior demifacet and transverse process of a thoracic vertebra and the superior demifacet of the vertebra below it. The 11th and 12th thoracic vertebrae lack a superior costal demifacet. The 11th and 12th ribs only articulate with the 11th and 12th thoracic vertebrae, respectively. Thoracic facet joints are more vertical than lumbar facet joints and are similarly innervated by the medial branches of the dorsal rami of the segmental nerves. Every facet joint has bisegmental innervations by the medial branch of the same vertebral level and the vertebral level above.[10–12]

Each thoracic segmental nerve divides into two main divisions: the ventral ramus and the dorsal ramus. The ventral ramus (anterior division) forms the intercostal nerve that runs in the respective intercostal space below the intercostal vessels (Figure 17.2). After its exit from the intervertebral foramen, it gives origin to both rami communicantes that synapse into the sympathetic chain. The white rami are formed by the myelinated preganglionic fibers, whereas the unmyelinated postganglionic fibers form the gray rami. As the intercostal nerve courses along the corresponding intercostal space, the lateral cutaneous branch arises and pierces the skin in the anterior axial line, where it divides into anterior and posterior branches that provide sensation to the chest wall and part of the abdominal wall. Finally, the intercostal nerve terminates as the anterior cutaneous branch that supplies the middle portion of the chest and upper abdominal wall.

The subcostal nerve is the 12th intercostal nerve and is unique in contributing to the lumbar plexus by providing a branch to the first lumbar nerve. As for the dorsal ramus (posterior division) of each thoracic nerve, it runs posteriorly and divides into medial and lateral branches. The medial branches supply mainly the facet joints, whereas the lateral branch innervates the skin and the muscles of the paraspinal area (Figure 17.3). The exact pathway of the medial branches nerves is controversial. They were not found to be crossing the junction between the superior articular process and the transverse process as do the lumbar facets medial branches. Instead,

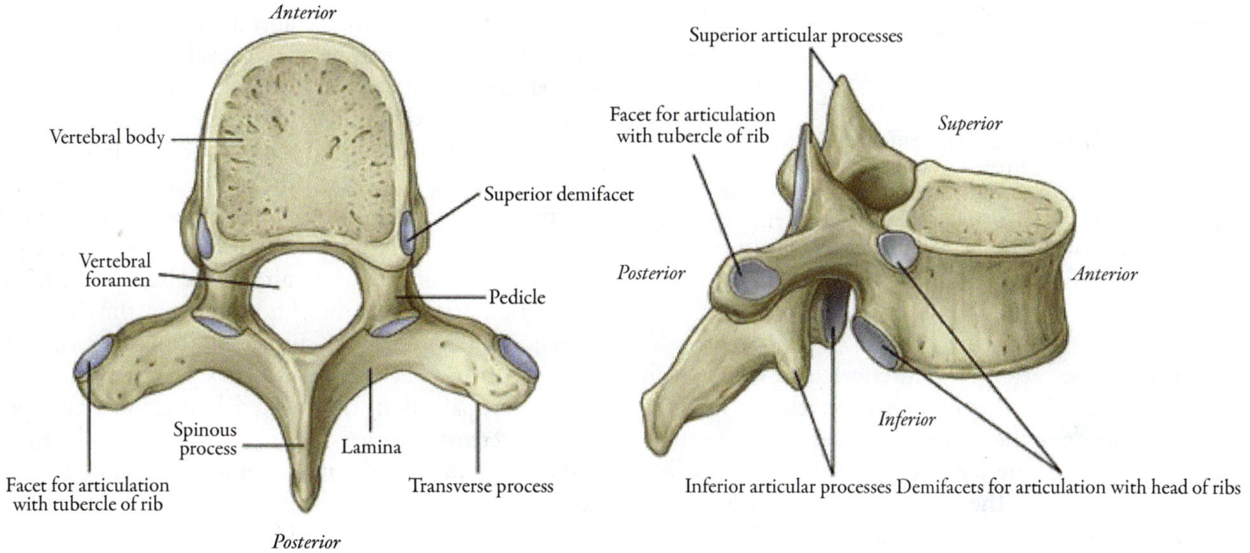

Figure 17.1 Anatomy of thoracic vertebrae. From Gray H. *Anatomy of the Human Body*. 20th ed. Lewis WH, ed. Philadelphia: Lea & Febiger, 2000.

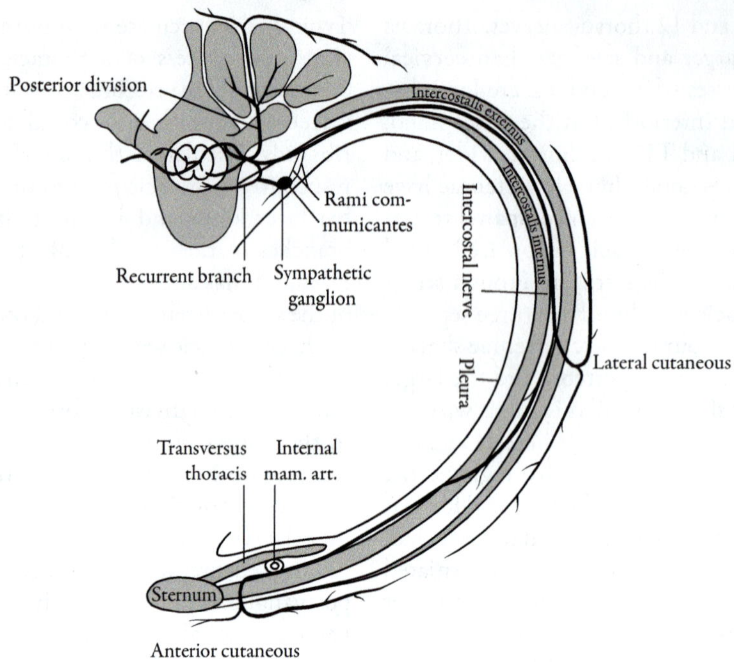

Figure 17.2 Course of a typical intercostal nerve. From Gray H. *Anatomy of the Human Body.* 20th ed. Lewis WH, ed. Philadelphia: Lea & Febiger, 2000.

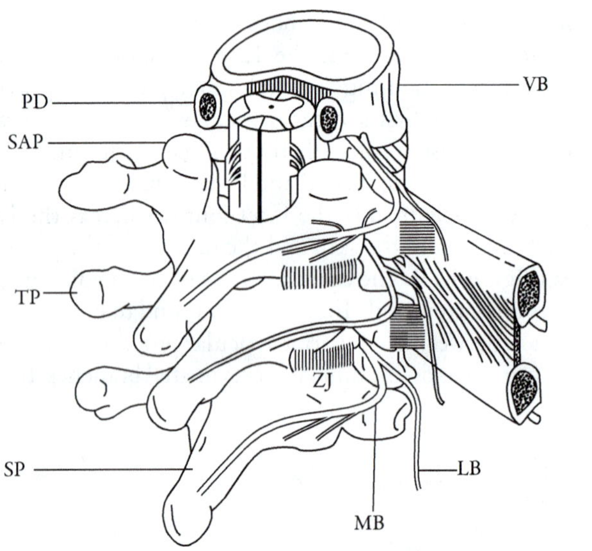

Figure 17.3 A posterior view of the course of the thoracic facet medial branches. PD, pedicle; VB, vertebral body; SAP, superior articular process; TP, transverse process; SP, spinous process; MB, medial branch; LB, lateral branch; ZJ, zygapophyseal joint; RB, rib. Reprinted from Chua WH, Bogduk N. The surgical anatomy of thoracic facet denervation. *Acta Neurochirugia* 1995;136:140–144, with permission from Springer.

they run medially, posteriorly, and inferiorly after they branch off the dorsal ramus until they come in close relation with the superolateral portion of the transverse process. They continue running medially and inferiorly across the posterior surface of the transverse process. The relation of the thoracic medial branches and the superolateral portion of the transverse process varies depending on their level. In the upper and lower thoracic levels, they come in contact with bone, whereas in mid-thoracic levels, they do not come in contact with bone but instead are suspended in the intertransverse process space.

Now back to our original question: what are the potential pain generators? Or, in other words, what is the possible etiology and pathophysiology of thoracic back pain?

Thoracic back pain can originate from different areas of thorax including surrounding soft tissues of the spine, intervertebral discs, facet joints, the spinal cord and nerve roots, or the body of the vertebra, or it can be referred pain. The pain may be the outcome of different pathological process including degenerative changes, autoimmune diseases, trauma, osteoporosis, infection, or malignancy.[2,5,13,14]

Myofascial pain is generally related to a combination of muscle and ligament sprain and inflammatory response. Poor posture and excessive sitting most usually cause thoracic back strain. Poor posture may be due to development of osteoporosis in elderly patients, which often results in excessive drooping of the neck and shoulders and decreased lumbar lordosis.

Compression of a spinal nerve root may lead to radiculopathy. Thoracic radicular pain can frequently be the result of thoracic spine degenerative changes, a neoplastic process, or trauma. The natural kyphosis of the thoracic spine places the spinal cord in close proximity to the back of the intervertebral discs, vertebral bodies, and ligaments, thus making the thoracic spinal cord more susceptible to compression from those structures. Postherpetic neuralgia may present with neuropathic pain along the affected dermatomes. Entrapment of the intercostal nerves may lead to intercostal neuralgia. Diabetes mellitus is the most common metabolic cause of radiculopathy.[10,15]

Thoracic intervertebral discs could be a potential pain generator as a result of degenerative changes or infectious processes. Pain is usually the presenting symptom in nearly 60%

Box 17.1 DIFFERENTIAL DIAGNOSIS FOR THORACIC BACK PAIN

Autoimmune diseases (e.g., ankylosing spondylitis)
Diffuse skeletal hyperostosis
Infection
Intrathoracic pathology (e.g., pleuritis, pericarditis, pneumonia, esophageal pathology)
Intraperitoneal/retroperitoneal pathology (e.g., peptic ulcer disease, pancreatitis, hepatobiliary disease)
Malignancy (lung, breast, multiple myeloma, etc.)
Myofascial pain
Spinal cord or nerve root compression
Thoracic disc degeneration
Thoracic facet arthropathy
Thoracic radiculopathy
Thoracic spondylosis
Trauma
Vascular diseases (e.g., thoracic aortic dissection and pulmonary embolism)
Vertebral fractures (pathologic fractures, osteoporotic compression fractures)

of cases. Muscle spasms or pain radiating to the front of the chest/abdomen may also be experienced.

Thoracic facet pain accounts for 42% of patients presenting with thoracic back pain.[16] Thoracic facet syndrome is commonly caused by trauma and often presents as mid-back pain with muscle spasm and loss of the normal thoracic spinal curvature.[17] Thoracic spondylosis is the result of abnormal wear and tear that causes gradual narrowing of the disc space and deformed bone growth that can lead to increased pressure on adjacent tissue and nerves, causing pain and possibly neurological symptoms. Thus, patients with thoracic facetogenic pain are generally older, whereas patients with discogenic pain are younger.

Ankylosing spondylitis often affects the entire spine with initial restriction of lumbar and chest motion and later involves the cervical spine. In those patients, pain originates from costovertebral joints, in which, prevalently, the 11th and 12th ribs and the 6th through 8th ribs are involved.[18]

The thoracic spine has the least amount of mobility in comparison to rest of the spine. Thoracic spine compression fractures commonly take place in patients with osteoporosis, but they are usually stable. Pathologic fractures can occur due to metastatic cancer from the lung, prostate, or breast. A major trauma with high energy is usually required to cause a thoracic compression fracture in a healthy vertebra. The latter is usually associated with spinal cord injury. Characteristically in osteoporotic fractures, the anterior aspects of vertebrae are affected, and compound fractures may lead to kyphosis.[14]

There are some nonspinal and possibly emergent causes of thoracic pain that should be kept in mind including vascular disease (e.g., thoracic aortic dissection, thoracic aneurysms, acute coronary syndrome, and pulmonary embolism), thoracic cavity pathology (e.g., pleuritis, pericarditis, pneumonia, lung malignancy), and abdominal pathology whether intraperitoneal or retroperitoneal (e.g., peptic ulcer disease, pancreatitis, hepatobiliary disease).[19,20] Furthermore, the differential diagnosis for thoracic pain can include major surgeries like coronary bypass, mastectomy, and thoracotomy.[21–23] Diffuse thoracic pain prevalently may result from visceral diseases like achalasia, pancreatic diseases, and esophageal cancer (Box 17.1).

In our case thoracic back pain could have been generated by any of the aforementioned conditions. The differential diagnosis list is exhaustive. How can we reach the diagnosis and the etiology of pain in our case? Are there any additional tests or imaging studies that could aid in establishing the diagnosis?

HOW IS THE DIAGNOSIS CONFIRMED?

HISTORY

Detailed physical examination and medical history play a pivotal role in detection of underlying pathology and the source of thoracic pain. Comprehensive history includes asking about pain location, radiation, intensity, quality, pattern, duration, relieving or aggravating factors, and preceding injury. Questions about recent weight loss, fever, chills, recent trauma, and chronic cough should be asked to rule out red flags.

Thoracic radicular pain is characterized by pain radiating in the area supplied by the intercostal nerve or the offended thoracic nerve root (Figure 17.4). The symptoms are usually unilateral. Unlike lumbar disc herniation, thoracic disc herniation can lead to pyramidal tract signs. Intercostal nerves overlap, thus making it difficult to identify the involved nerves. Pain in the 11th and 12th segments is often caused by irritation and compression of the subcostal nerve and is known as *12th rib syndrome*. It affects mostly middle-aged women. Intercostal neuralgia is usually described as sharp, shooting, burning pain along a certain segment supplied by certain intercostal nerves. Pain caused by rib pathology or intercostal nerve compression may vary with position; it worsens with sitting and diminishes with lying down (Box 17.2).[24]

Unilateral or bilateral thoracic paravertebral pain in a localized thoracic area may point to thoracic facet joint-mediated pain. Two studies investigated the symptoms of thoracic facet joint arthropathy and showed that they may have certain radiation patterns (Figure 17.5).[25,26] Commonly, thoracic facet-mediated pain is worsened with prolonged standing, hyperextension, or rotation of thoracic facet joints. The pain is often bilateral and involves multiple segments.

The thoracic VCF pain can vary from a dull, deep ache with minimal compression of the vertebra without nerve impingement to severe, sharp, stabbing pain that can result in major functional limitations. Deep inspiration, coughing, and any movement of the dorsal spine may trigger the pain. If an acute fracture causes pain, it is usually felt deeply at the

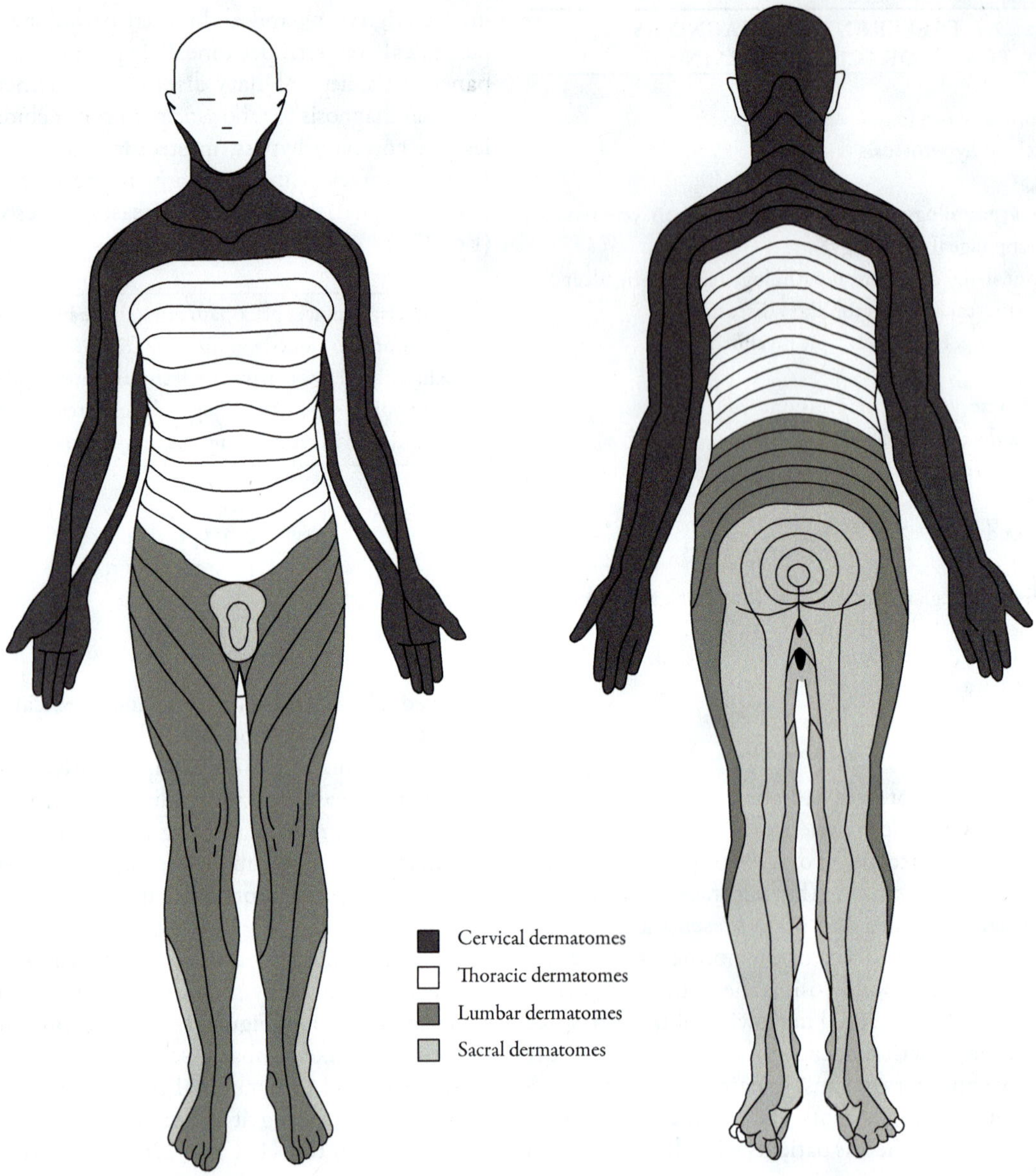

Figure 17.4 Dermatomal distribution of radicular pain.

fracture site. Cord compression, presenting with myelopathic features or with true radicular signs and symptoms, can be associated with thoracic back pain. Because any movement aggravates the acute vertebral fracture pain, the patients are most comfortable when motionless.[27–29]

PHYSICAL EXAMINATION

Complete physical examination including cardiopulmonary system and abdominal organs should be performed to rule out systemic diseases. Physical examination of the thoracic spine should start with inspection at rest and movement and palpation. The spine should be examined for any contour deformity, scars, skin changes, and tenderness in the vertebral and paravertebral areas. Eliciting pain with different spinal movements may implicate a spinal cause of the pain (e.g., vertebral metastasis). The presence of paravertebral tenderness that is usually bilateral and exacerbated with hyperextension, rotation, and/or prolonged standing is characteristic of thoracic facet pain. It is unclear whether this tenderness is related to direct stress on the facet joints or adjacent paraspinal muscles. VCF may present on examination with localized tenderness to deep palpation or percussion over the affected vertebra, and it may be associated with paraspinal muscle spasm. In trauma-related injuries, hematoma and ecchymosis overlying the fracture site may be present. In this situation, associated injury to the bony thorax and the intra-abdominal and intrathoracic organs should be considered. Neurologic signs and symptoms including range of motion (ROM), muscle strength, reflexes, and sensory signs should be evaluated. The presence of sensory disturbances may include loss of sensation, whereas hyperalgesia and allodynia are distinctive for neuropathic pain.

Box 17.2 THORACIC RADICULAR PAIN

Neuralgia:
- Intercostal neuralgia
- Postherpetic neuralgia

Pain from spinal cord:
- Thoracic intervertebral disc displacement or herniated nucleus pulposus (HNP)
- Vertebral compression fracture with retropulsion
- Vertebral metastasis

Postsurgical pain:
- Intercostobrachial neuralgia
- Postmastectomy
- Post thoracotomy

Rib pathology:
- Rib fractures
- Rib resection

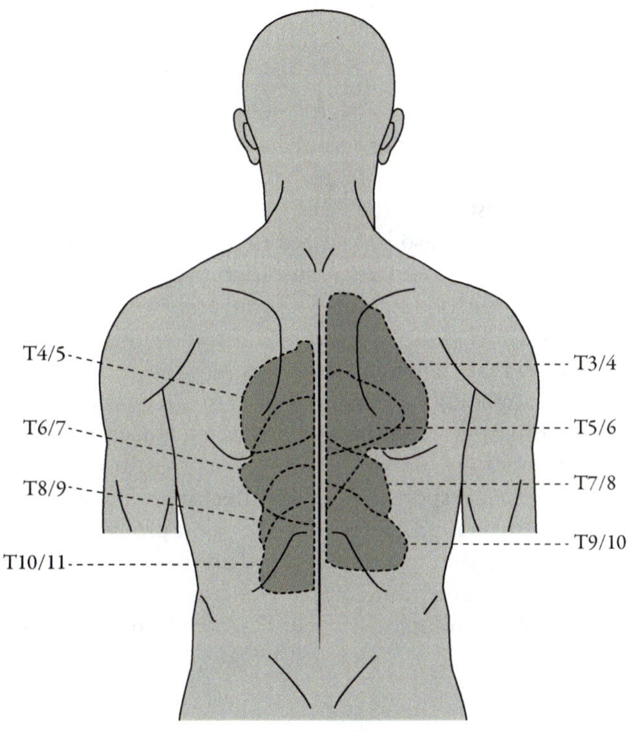

Figure 17.5 Radiation patterns of thoracic facetogenic pain.

ADDITIONAL TESTS

In addition to history and examination, diagnostic tests and imaging studies are critical in formulating a differential diagnosis. If there is suspicion of a serious condition, blood tests including a full profile of blood, urine, and electrolytes will be appropriate. Electrocardiogram is indicated to rule out cardiac contusion, particularly in patients with traumatic sternal fractures or major anterior dorsal spine trauma.

IMAGING MODALITIES

Plain radiographs, computed tomography (CT), MRI and isotope bone scan are the main imaging modalities that can help reach a precise diagnosis. Imaging studies should be ordered earlier in thoracic back pain of unknown etiology due to the lower incidence of radiculopathy and higher incidence of tumor involvement in this region. Plain radiographs are the primary diagnostic modality, and these help avoid overlooking fatal or life-threatening pathologies.[30] The occult rib fracture pain can be mistaken for cardiac or gallbladder pain and result in unnecessary cardiac and gastrointestinal workups. Plain X-ray may reveal VCF

MRI is the main imaging modality for assessment of disc degenerative disease; furthermore, one might consider short T1 inversion recovery (STIR) views when the index of suspicion for vertebral body fracture is high. This is attributed to its noninvasive nature and the superior contrast resolution. Thornbury and colleagues showed that MRI, CT myelography, and CT alone are equally accurate in evaluation of disc root compressive disease.[31] Although CT myelography is invasive, it becomes useful when MRI cannot explain the clinical findings. It is superior in differentiating bone from soft tissue. Plain CT is inexpensive and readily accessible.

MRI findings must be correlated with a physical examination because 37% of asymptomatic patients were found to have thoracic disc herniation on MRIs.[32] MRI might be needed in primary malignancies and metastatic cancers, progressive symptoms, and development of neurological deficit. The majority of the symptomatic thoracic degenerative disease occurs in the mid to lower thoracic spine. Various studies have showed that T6–T11 were the most affected levels that required interventions.[33,34] In the thoracic region, the central canal and vertebral bodies diminish in size, and thus the spatial and contrast resolution become more crucial. CT myelography has the highest spatial resolution, which facilitates demonstration of calcification within thoracic discs. Although MRI is noninvasive, it can detect signal abnormalities indicating cord edema and venous hypertension, thus elucidating the clinical significance of a visualized disc herniation.

Limited studies have addressed thoracic posterior column degeneration including the facets and costovertebral joints. Resnick and colleagues demonstrated that thoracic facet arthropathy is more common in the upper and mid-thoracic spine, with cartilage degeneration leading to joint space narrowing, sclerosis of subchondral bone, and osteophyte formation. The coronal orientation of thoracic facets renders these osteoarthritic changes not evident on plain radiographs. On the other hand, axial and sagittal images of MRI and CT are more sensitive in detecting such findings. As in the lumbar spine, morphologic degeneration does not translate to painful and symptomatic joints. Costovertebral and costotransverse joints are synovial joints that have nociceptive innervation and may become symptomatic when they undergo degeneration. Similar to the thoracic facet degeneration, these findings are difficult to detect on plain radiographs, but CT and MRI are more sensitive in detecting them. They are especially common in the T11 and T12 levels.

Our patient had an X-ray that showed collapse of the superior endplate of the T6 vertebral body. The patient had an MRI of the thoracic spine 1 year ago that revealed multilevel disc bulges most prominent at T7–T8 and T8–T9. Is a plain radiograph sufficient, or are other imaging studies necessary?

The diagnosis of thoracic VCF is usually easy in the setting of trauma, but the diagnosis might be challenging in spontaneous vertebral fracture due to osteoporosis or metastatic disease. Thoracic paraspinous muscle sprain can be confused with thoracic VCF as well. Herpes zoster pain can start 24–72 hours prior to occurrence of the rash and can potentially be mistaken for VCF. Several VCFs can occur in 5–20% of patients with a history of VCF.

The diagnostic indicators include loss of vertebral height, disruption in alignment along anterior and posterior vertebral body lines, facet dislocation, and an increase in interpedicular and interspinous distance (>7 mm). Plain radiographic films are unable to identify ligamentous injuries. Post-traumatic kyphotic angulation measurement is beneficial to assess fracture progression, particularly in the conservative management of compression fractures. Kyphotic angulation can be measured in upright radiographs as the angle between the superior endplate one level above and the inferior endplate one level below the injured portion.

Once vertebral fracture is identified with plain films, CT is primarily utilized. CT can detect anterior wedge compression fracture instability and occult bony injuries and is optimal for diagnosis of complex fractures. Other imaging modalities, such as CT myelography and MRI, are not usually needed unless there is a neurologic deficit. If the etiology of the compression fracture is an infectious or malignant process, MRI techniques can be beneficial. MRI provides better visualization of cord compression and ligamentous disruption. Cord injury can be suggested in the presence of high signal intensity. In addition, MRI with STIR views may evaluate the age of the compression fracture. Acute injuries can be detected by increased signal in T2-weighted images due to increased water content in the vertebral body as a result of bone edema (Figure 17.6).

If for any reason MRI is contraindicated, CT myelography can be helpful in assessing cord compression. Imaging modalities other than plain films should always be used in the presence of neurologic deficits because multiple compression fractures can result in severe kyphotic angulation with subsequent cord compression and progression to complete loss of neurologic function.[35,36] If a patient has a compression fracture, radiographic images of the spinal column are sufficient and will classically show a wedge-shaped defect with the anterior height being lower than the posterior. In the presence of a recent history of trauma and/or osteoporosis the final diagnosis can be made.

Bone scanning, particularly single-photon emission computed tomography (SPECT) of the spine, can be beneficial in determining the acuity of the fracture. Maynard et al. showed that increased activity on a bone scan could predict a successful clinical response to percutaneous vertebroplasty in patients with osteoporotic VCFs.[37]

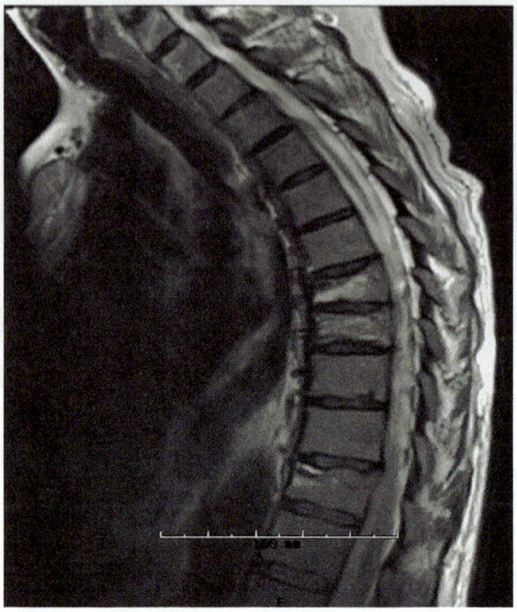

Figure 17.6 Sagittal T2-weighted magnetic resonance image of thoracic vertebral compression fracture at levels of T8 and T9.

Bone scan can also be utilized in locating tumors, infections, and occult fractures. A suspicion for intra-abdominal diseases may justify obtaining CT scan and/or ultrasound of the abdomen. In some cases, percutaneous biopsy might be necessary to make a distinct diagnosis.

Neurophysiologic procedures are required when the examination and imaging studies do not match. Electromyography, nerve conduction studies, and somatosensory evoked responses help to differentiate between spinal and peripheral problems, as well as joint problems from a radiculopathy. They can be helpful when the physical examination and imaging studies fail to match or when there is evidence of neurological deficit that needs to be further studied.

DIAGNOSTIC BLOCKS

Diagnostic blocks, such as selective nerve root blocks, paravertebral blocks, and intercostal nerve blocks, have an important role in the diagnostic algorithm. Such interventions are performed under radiological control to localize the level of pain. The level where the most pain improvement occurs is chosen for treatment. T11 and T12 intercostal nerves can be blocked via a paravertebral approach or one similar to that used in lumbar selective nerve root blocks. Intercostal nerve blocks at T10 and above are performed via the intercostal approach. This ensures peripheral spread of the injectate and avoids any epidural spread thus enhancing the selectivity of the nerve block.

Selective nerve root blocks can pinpoint the offended nerve roots responsible for thoracic radicular pain in cases of thoracic herniated discs. This could be very helpful preoperatively to ensure operating on the affected level and obtaining the best outcome. Similarly, intercostal nerve blocks and paravertebral blocks might serve as a prognostic indicator for patients who would benefit from pulsed radiofrequency (RF) to the dorsal root ganglia (DRG).

The significant reduction in pain following intra-articular injection with local anesthetic can be convincing evidence that the facet joint is the origin of pain. Medial branch blocks (MBB) can be used to diagnose facet joint pain equally.[38,39] Thoracic MBB (TMBB) is usually performed at two levels per the facet joint that correlates to the level of paravertebral pressure pain. It is essential to identify two salient points. Generally, first diagnostic injections are not accurate. However, a second injection is usually utilized as an outcome measure for treatment results.[40]

The lack of correlation between clinical and radiological findings in thoracic facet arthropathy led to the acceptance of the use of diagnostic blocks to confirm the diagnosis, whether by intra-articular thoracic facet joint injection or TMBB (see Box 17.3). IA injections are technically more challenging in the thoracic region due to the steep, frontal orientation of the facet joints. On the other hand, TMBB will temporarily block the nerves that will be eventually lesioned, which may serve as a short-lived simulation of the RF treatment. Many studies have found high rates of false diagnostic blocks whether intra-articular or TMBB. The incidence rate has been estimated to be around 58% in the thoracic area. The reasons are multifactorial and include placebo response (18–32%) to any diagnostic intervention, use of sedation, superficial use of local anesthetics, and the spread of injectate to other potential pain generators. Certain precautions have been recommended to increase the specificity of the MBBs, including avoiding the use of sedation, judicious use of superficial local anesthetics, reducing the volume injected to less than 0.5 mL, and performing either placebo-controlled blocks or comparative local anesthetic blocks.[41]

Box 17.3 **TESTS AND IMAGING STUDIES IN DIAGNOSIS OF THORACIC BACK PAIN**

- Blood tests including a full profile of blood and electrolytes
- Computed tomography (CT)
- Isotope bone scan
- Magnetic resonance imaging (MRI)
- Medial branch blocks
- Neurophysiologic procedures (electromyography, nerve conduction studies, and somatosensory evoked responses)
- Plain radiographs
- Selective nerve root blocks
- Percutaneous biopsy
- Urine analysis

Looking back to our case, the patient is presenting with pain that is worsened with coughing or any movement and is relieved by staying still. On examination, there is localized tenderness over particular thoracic spinous processes. Furthermore, plain X-ray shows a T6 VCF, which was not evident on older MRI, but could explain her mid-back pain. Based on the above findings, the diagnosis of VCF as the main etiology for her thoracic back pain is confirmed. A new thoracic MRI should be performed to determine the age and extent of the fracture and its relation to the neural elements. This will aid in determining the best treatement modality for this patient.

WHAT IS THE INCIDENCE OF VCF?

VCF is defined as more than 15% reduction in vertebral body height, which is seen on anteroposterior and lateral views of thoracolumbar spine radiographs.[27] Thoracic VCF is one of the most common etiologies of thoracic back pain. Almost 700,000 vertebral fractures take place in the United States every year.[42]

VCFs most commonly occur in the thoracolumbar region, particularly T8, T12, L1, and the lower lumbar area, mostly at the L4 level.[28,43] VCFs are categorized as wedge, biconcave, and crush fractures. The most common fractures are wedge fractures, which include more than 50% of VCFs.[44] Wedge compression fractures take place in the mid-thoracic area, and compression of the anterior segment of the vertebral body characterizes this type of fracture. Biconcave compression fractures account for around 17% of VCFs. The middle segment of the vertebral body is collapsed, whereas the anterior and posterior walls are intact. Crush compression fractures are the least frequent type of VCFs and account for 13% of the VCFs. The entire anterior column, including anterior and posterior margins, collapses in this type of fracture. The remaining 20% include complex VCFs.[44]

VCF is usually the result of osteoporosis, trauma with acceleration/deceleration, or primary tumors or metastatic disease involving the thoracic vertebra. Tussive fracture may occur with coughing. In general, patients do not recollect any memory of trauma, but they may describe physical activities like raising a window, carrying a small child or a bag of groceries, or lifting in the forward flexed posture. High-energy trauma classically occurs in younger men with normal bone density.

VCFs caused by osteoporosis are more common in the elderly, with an estimated 4 million new fractures occurring every year worldwide. Vertebral fracture risk increases in women with reaching menopause and with aging; the ratio is 2:1 for women compared to men.[42] Postmenopausal women in the United States have a 25% lifetime risk of getting a VCF; this risk increases with age, reaching up to 40% by age 80.The annual incidence of VCF is 10.7 per 1,000 women and 5.7 per 1,000 men. The risk of VCF is higher in men older than age of 65 years but is still significantly less than that for women of the same age. Asian and Caucasian women are at increased risk of VCF compared to African-American women.[45–48] Cancer-related vertebral fractures are due to skeletal metastasis. The primary sources of metastatic neoplasms to the spinal axis vary among the published series with 65% coming from carcinoma of the breast, lung, and prostate. Renal cell carcinoma and multiple myeloma may account for 10% of metastases at the spine.[49] Extradural metastases account for around 95% of secondary spinal tumors.

> The question arises: do we really need to intervene, or will the fracture eventually heal without any consequences? Intervening to fix the fracture depends on the natural history.

WHAT IS THE NATURAL HISTORY OF VCF?

Most vertebral fractures generally heal in approximately 3 months. Almost one-third of VCFs are well diagnosed, and most of them are asymptomatic or have tolerable symptoms.[45,50,51] Only about a third of VCFs are acutely symptomatic. The acute pain typically resolves after 4–12 weeks of limited activity. If the pain persists or gets worse after a period of relative improvement, this suggests additional compression or collapse. In most patients, the acute incapacitating fracture pain subsides but mechanical pain persists due to altered spinal biomechanics and myofascial fatigue. Some patients continue to experience mechanical back pain, especially with prolonged standing or walking. Chronic pain is usually more prevalent in patients with multiple fractures, loss of height, and low bone density.[27,52]

Venmans et al. assessed the natural course of osteoporotic VCFs treated conservatively, trying to identify the percentage of patients who developed chronic back pain and if there are any possible risk factors. Fifty-seven of 95 patients (60%) obtained adequate pain relief at 1-year of follow-up. Thirty-eight patients (40%) had persistent pain despite an aggressive oral analgesic regimen. No risk factors were identified. They concluded that whereas many patients with acute osteoporotic compression fractures obtained sufficient pain relief during the first 3 months with conservative measures, a considerable percentage of patients were still disabled by their pain. Therefore, vertebral augmentation procedures such as vertebroplasty should be considered for those patients.[53]

> Some would argue to manage the fracture conservatively until it heals. Are there any feared consequences while waiting for the vertebral fracture to heal? What are the clinical sequelae of inadequate pain control?

WHAT ARE THE CLINICAL CONSEQUENCES OF VCF?

The pain and functional disability associated with vertebral fractures are determined mostly by the severity of injury (e.g., the number of vertebra involved) and the nature of the injury (e.g., whether the fracture allows impingement on the spinal nerves or the spinal cord itself). Spinal nerve injury may produce abdominal ileus and severe pain with resulting splinting of the paraspinous muscles of the dorsal spine, further compromising the patient's functional capacity and pulmonary status. Inadequate pain treatment can lead to hypoventilation, atelectasis, and, ultimately, pneumonia. Undiagnosed and untreated VCFs can result in major complications such as progressive kyphosis and height loss, debilitating pain, and progressing physical, psychological, and functional morbidities. The resultant reduced ROM and prolonged inactivity can lead to collapsed lung or pneumonia, constipation due to slowing of gut motility and even possibly bowel obstruction, worsening of osteoporosis, progressive muscular weakness, loss of independence, increased risk of future VCFs, and increased mortality. Patients with compression fractures have a 15% greater risk of death compared to those who do not have a compression fracture.[35,54] Immobility predisposes patients to deep venous thrombosis and life-threatening complications such as pulmonary embolism. Pressure ulcers, pulmonary complications, urinary tract infections, and progressive deconditioning are other complications of prolonged immobility. In addition, bone mineral density (BMD) decreases 0.25% to 1.00% per week in patients who are advised bed rest.[55,56]

Development of kyphotic deformity commonly occurs in elderly female patients with osteoporosis and frequent fractures; it results from anterior vertebral collapse, creating a wedge-shaped vertebrae and severe deformed posture. Neurological complications, such as spinal stenosis, may occur due to increased pressure on the spinal cord or nerve roots. Undertreated VCFs can further be complicated with a patient's loss of independence sometimes necessitating nursing home stays or hospital admission.

Depression may occur in up to 40% of patients with VCFs because of chronic pain, body image changes, deterioration in the ability to perform self-care, and prolonged bed rest. Patients who have more than one fracture tend to be older and more socially isolated, thus, they are at a higher risk of developing depression.[57] A recent prospective cohort study showed that mortality rate is 23% higher in women age 65 or older who have five or more fractures. Interestingly, VCF was also associated with an increased risk of cancer-related death.[58] Furthermore, these fractures can result in considerable socioeconomic adverse effects. The annual costs of osteoporotic fractures are as high as $13.8 billion.[59]

HOW IS VCF PREVENTED?

Muscle mass and BMD decrease with aging and inactivity. Thus, the prevention and treatment of osteoporosis are essential considerations in the management of VCFs (Box 17.4). Women lose 3–7% of BMD around the onset of menopause followed by a 1–2% decline yearly in the postmenopausal period. Serum testosterone must be tested in men with compression fractures to rule out hypogonadism. In the presence of elevated alkaline phosphatase, osteomalacia should be suspected.[54,60] Regular weight-bearing exercise programs can improve mobility and balance with a resulting decline in risk of falls. Exercise programs need to be designed appropriately for the patient's health condition and level of function.[61–64] There are some modifiable and nonmodifiable risk factors

Box 17.4 PREVENTION OF VERTEBRAL COMPRESSION FRACTURES

Bisphosphonates
Calcium supplements
Calcitonin
Parathyroid hormone (PTH)
Selective estrogen receptor modulators (SERMs)
Vitamin D

for osteoporosis. Nonmodifiable risk factors include family history, history of fracture, race, sex, and early menopause. Modifiable risk factors include smoking, excess alcohol consumption, anticonvulsant use, long-term benzodiazepines, and steroid treatment (Box 17.5).

Adequate calcium intake during childhood can provide optimal peak bone mass in adulthood and decrease the risk of fracture. Children younger than 10 years need 700 mg of calcium intake daily, 1,300 mg of calcium daily is required for individuals between the ages of 10 and 25, and 800 mg daily is recommended for adults.[65] In addition, essential calcium intake needs to be increased to 1,500 mg/d during pregnancy and 2,000 mg/d during lactation. Alcohol, caffeine, high-fiber foods containing oxalic acid, and some medications including heparin, tetracycline, furosemide, isoniazid, corticosteroids, and drugs detoxified by P-450 hydrolase can interfere with calcium absorption and storage. Calcium supplements can decrease the speed or even prevent further bone mass loss with potentially a 3–5% improvement in femoral bone mass after 1 year of treatment. In addition to a calcium-rich diet, calcium supplements such as calcium carbonate and calcium citrate can be reliable ways to assure adequate calcium intake. Calcium citrate is a better option compared to calcium carbonate because of its easier absorption in patients with high gastric pH, and it carries less risk of renal stone formation. Vitamin D also plays an important role in the prevention of osteoporosis; the recommended dose is 400–800 IU/d. In general, vitamin D is obtained from food and sun exposure. However, supplemental vitamin D intake is recommended for people who consume a low-vitamin D diet and for those who don't receive adequate sun exposure.

Box 17.5 MODIFIABLE AND NONMODIFIABLE RISK FACTORS OF OSTEOPOROSIS

Modifiable:
- Early menopause
- Family history
- History of fracture
- Race
- Sex

Nonmodifiable:
- Anticonvulsants use
- Excessive alcohol consumption
- Long-term benzodiazepines treatment
- Long-term steroid intake
- Smoking

Newer agents such as bisphosphonates have been proved to decrease the risk of fractures.[66] They target bone mineralization and inhibit osteoclast function by binding to osteoclast resorbing cells and promoting their apoptosis.[67,68] In randomized clinical trials, alendronate was shown to reduce risk of vertebral fractures by 50% among postmenopausal women.[45] In men, alendronate was shown to decrease the risk of vertebral fractures; increase hip, spine, and total BMD; and reduce the loss of vertebral height.[69] The recommended dose of alendronate for prevention is 5 mg/d and 10 mg/d for therapeutic purposes. It must be taken by the patient while in an upright position, and the patient must avoid lying down for at least 30 minutes due to the risk of esophagitis. Etidronate has been shown to decrease the rate of vertebral fractures and increase BMD.[62,70] However, etidronate is not FDA approved, and further data are required to understand its long-term effects. Calcitonin has been used to improve spinal bone density and decrease the risk of vertebral fracture by inhibition of osteoclast activity.[71,72] Subcutaneous injection and nasal spray forms of calcitonin are available. The recommended dose of nasal spray is one spray daily containing 200 IU. If calcitonin or bisphosphonates are being used, calcium and vitamin D should be included in the regimen. This combination has been shown to decrease the incidence of fractures.[73,74]

Estrogen replacement therapy (ERT) can decrease bone loss of the hip and spine if started within 10 years of menopause and can improve BMD in patients 60 years and older.[75–77] The efficacy of ERT is enhanced if used in combination with calcium and vitamin D.[78,79] It has been shown that the benefits of ERT cease when treatment is stopped. In addition, ERT increases the risk for breast cancer, uterine cancer, and thromboembolism. Because of these adverse effects and the reported low compliance with ERT, selective estrogen receptor modulators (SERMs) have been offered to avoid ERT complications.[80–86] SERMs, including benzothiophenes, benzopyrans, tetrahydroaphthylenes, and triphenylethylene, vary in their safety and effectiveness. It has been shown that raloxifene can increase BMD and decrease the risk of vertebral fractures.[87,88] In men, testosterone replacement therapy is needed if hypogonadism is diagnosed or if there is vertebral fracture, and it is also recommended in patients taking steroids. Five percent improvement in spinal BMD has been reported in eugonadal men following testosterone treatment.[89,90] Although parathyroid hormone (PTH) is not FDA approved, it seems to have a potential role in the treatment and prevention of osteoporosis.[91,92] It has been shown that PTH treatment for 1–3 months is beneficial in postmenopausal and steroid-induced osteoporosis.[92,93] In addition, the combination of HRT and PTH treatment can result in a 5.5% increase in vertebral area density compared with a 2% increase with HRT treatment alone.[94]

It is believed that sodium fluoride increases bone remodeling by stimulating osteoblast proliferation, but its benefit in increasing BMD and decreasing the rate of fracture is controversial. Daily treatment with 30 mg of sodium fluoride has been reported to improve spinal bone mass.[95] The adverse effects of sodium fluoride treatment include painful lower extremity syndrome, gastrointestinal discomfort, frank hematemesis and melena.

HOW ARE THORACIC BACK PAIN, VCF, THORACIC DISC DISPLACEMENT, AND THORACIC SPONDYLOSIS MANAGED?

A multidisciplinary approach is necessary for the management of thoracic back pain, including physical or occupational therapy, drug therapy, bed rest, and interventional management. The importance of intensive interdisciplinary approaches in the management of thoracic back pain disability is undeniable. The treatment team should include cognitive-behavioral therapists, psychologists, psychiatrists, biofeedback therapists, massage therapists, kinesiologists, occupational therapists, physiotherapists, and physicians. Usually, a specialized physician experienced and trained in this area of chronic pain leads the team (Box 17.6).

PHYSICAL REHABILITATION

The physiotherapist employs manual and manipulative therapy appropriate to each patient's specific presentation.[96–99] The physiotherapist also prescribes and monitors compliance and outcomes of the exercise program.[100,101] Education on the patient's condition, hurt versus harm, posture, core stability and motor control retraining, scapular stabilization, stretches, and strengthening are important parts of the program.[99,102–110] Transcutaneous electrical nerve stimulation (TENS) is an alternative option that can be used by physical therapists for the treatment of thoracic back pain.

A kinesiologist working under the direction of the physiotherapist supervises the exercise program. The kinesiologist encourages patients to use their pain management strategies during functional activities while at the clinic and incorporates regular relaxation practice as a standard part of the treatment schedule. Eventually, the physiotherapist and the medical consultant make recommendations for permanent restrictions and temporary limitations of function for each patient, if necessary.

In a trial to try to normalize the soft tissues affected by injury and stress, massage therapy is used selectively with conditions such as myofascial trigger points, hypertonicity, muscle spasm, fibrosis, and contracture. The appropriate therapeutic massage techniques, such as effleurage, pétrissage, friction, tapotement, vibration, myofascial trigger points, and fascial release, are used based on the unique clinical presentation of each of these conditions.[111–116] Recently, botulinum toxin (Botox) injections also have been demonstrated to be beneficial in localized myofascial pain syndrome.[117,118]

The occupational therapist's goal is to improve the skills acquired by the patient through in-home visits, job site analyses, and return-to-work program design and implementation. The education component of the occupational therapy services includes graded activity, energy conservation, work simplification techniques, joint sparing techniques, pacing, training in body mechanics, and proper posture and positioning.[119–121] In addition, the occupational therapist makes recommendations for the provision of assistive devices and ergonomic equipment, as well as for environmental modifications. A gradual return-to-work plan is developed jointly with the patient and the employer and is carried out under the close supervision of the occupational therapist.[121]

As for our patient with VCF, should any certain measures be considered? Treatment of VCF is based on the severity of symptoms.[122,123] Conservative management includes a short period of bed rest followed by gradual mobilization with external orthoses.[124] Prolonged bed rest in the elderly patient may result in deconditioning, accelerated bone loss, deep venous thrombosis, pneumonia, pressure ulcers, disorientation, and depression. Many VCFs respond appropriately to nonsurgical care while the fracture heals. Avoiding strenuous activity or exercise like heavy lifting or anything else that puts stress on the spine is recommended. In some patients, bed rest may be required. Since VCFs are flexion-compression injuries, a hyperextension brace may be used to keep the patient from bending forward, support the spine, and take pressure off the fractured vertebra. These braces are usually beneficial for the first few months, until the pain resolves. Although younger patients tolerate bracing well, elderly patients generally do not[123] because of increased pain with bracing. Thus, elderly patients tend to require more bed rest. The appropriate duration of bracing is not well studied. For the majority of patients, 2–3 months is recommended. Prolonged bracing can result in muscular atrophy, skin breakdown, increased segmental motion at the upper and lower ends of the orthosis, and declined pulmonary capacity.[125,126] The local application of heat and cold can be helpful for symptomatic relief of the pain of VCF as well.

Physical therapy and rehabilitation are important factors that expedite healing and aim at improved ROM along with

Box 17.6 TREATMENT OPTIONS FOR THORACIC BACK PAIN

- Acupuncture
- Botulinum toxin injections
- Cognitive-behavioral therapy
- Medical treatment (NSAIDS, muscle relaxants, steroids, opioids, topical medication, nerve membrane stabilizers)
- Physical/occupational therapy
- Intercostal nerve blocks
- Spinal cord stimulation (SCS)
- Surgery
- Transcutaneous electrical nerve stimulation (TENS)
- Thoracic epidural steroid injections
- Thoracic facet medial branch blocks
- Thoracic facet medial branch radiofrequency
- Vertebral augmentation procedure (kyphoplasty and vertebroplasty)

muscular strengthening. While the acute fracture pain subsides, a walking program can be started, with gentle strengthening exercises focusing on spinal extensor muscles. A home physical therapist may aid with early ambulation and mobilization in some patients. More aggressive physical therapy should be started after 3–4 months to strengthen the spinal extensor and abdominal muscles.[127]

PSYCHOLOGICAL INTERVENTIONS

The psychologist directs the treatment team to optimally manage the emotional, cognitive, and personality issues that might influence the patient's clinical presentation and treatment progress. In addition, the psychologist provides individual therapy, focusing on the patient's identified psychological and emotional problems related to the pain disorder. This management addresses social, occupational, and emotional adjustment issues impeding the patient's best possible functioning, including the use of pain management strategies.[128,129]

The cognitive-behavioral therapist works with the patient to identify how his thought process and behaviors influence his mood and pain levels. Treatment plans include the detection and correction of distorted cognitive patterns, such as confusion over hurt versus harm and managing fear avoidance. Patients are educated to utilize a diversity of strategies to overcome the difficulties related to their condition. Psychoeducational components may include the pain system, the hurt-harm distinction, sleep hygiene, medication scheduling or reduction, emotional reaction to pain, anger management, mind-body connection, self-talk, assertiveness, stress management, goal setting, and relaxation therapy. In addition, core family members are invited to the clinic, informed about the program's objectives, and educated in cognitive-behavioral therapy principles and goals.[130]

A biofeedback therapist reports to the rest of the team on stress triggers and successful strategies specific to the individual patient. The goal of this therapy is to identify and correct dysfunctional muscular activation patterns and stress responses that might be contributing to the patient's pain.[131–133]

These components are planned to augment the patient's perspective of chronic pain and to promote effective use of pain management skills. Patients are taught effective physical and mental pain coping techniques within a supportive, goal-oriented atmosphere to increase self-efficacy in pain management. Individualized goals are negotiated with the patient and often include improving the patient's functional abilities and work status. In support of these goals, treatment is also directed at lifestyle changes that allow patients to use their pain management strategies throughout the day, to improve sleeping patterns, to rationalize and reduce unnecessary pain medications, and to improve their emotional state and their ability to handle future pain exacerbations. The team members communicate on a regular basis to discuss problems and improve programming. When appropriate, team members meet with the patient to discuss obstacles and solutions.[129]

As in treating other causes of thoracic back pain, in VCF, the physiotherapist employs manual and manipulative therapy appropriate to patient's specific presentation.[96–99] In addition, the physiotherapist prescribes and monitors compliance with and outcomes of the exercise program.[100,101]

PHARMACOLOGIC MANAGEMENT

Medical treatment with analgesic drugs may provide good short-term relief of thoracic back pain. In addition to pain control, these drugs may permit earlier ambulation and thus avoid the adverse effects of prolonged bed rest.[27] NSAIDs and muscle relaxants may be helpful to control thoracic pain. The adverse effects of NSAIDs include gastrointestinal discomfort, renal insufficiency, and congestive heart failure.[134–136] Opioids should be reserved for patients who receive inadequate relief in spite of regular analgesic consumption. Adverse effects of opioids include physical dependence, development of addiction, gastrointestinal dysmotility, and cognitive deficits. Prophylactic laxative treatment may need to be started at the same time the opioid is prescribed. Given that opioid analgesics have the potential to suppress respiratory drive, careful patient monitoring and adequate pulmonary toilet techniques instruction are required. Topical pain treatment medications such as transdermal lidocaine patches may be beneficial as well. Systemic steroids can be prescribed in certain situations such as nerve root impingement by disk protrusion. The local application of heat and cold may also be useful to provide symptomatic relief of the pain. Antidepressants like amitriptyline and anticonvulsants like gabapentin and pregabalin are used to manage thoracic radicular pain with neuropathic features.

The treatment of VCF may include pain medications that help to control pain but do not actually help to heal the fracture. To achieve adequate pain reduction and thus promote early mobilization with conservative management, analgesics need to be prescribed carefully. Primary treatment of pain due to VCF should include a combination of simple analgesics and NSAIDs or cyclo-oxygenase-2 (COX-2) inhibitors. If these medications do not adequately relieve the patient's symptoms, short-acting potent opioid analgesics can be considered as a next treatment step. The adverse effects of NSAIDs are remarkably higher in the elderly patients.[134–136] Hence, pure analgesics, whether opioid or nonopioid, might be preferred to NSAIDs, especially in older patients with VCF.

Calcitonin, which is available in subcutaneous, intranasal, or rectal forms, can have analgesic properties in compression fractures caused by osteoporosis and in patients with metastatic bone pain that might be due to elevated plasma endorphin levels.[137] Patients who develop VCF secondary to osteoporosis are at greater risk of developing additional fractures in the future; thus, these patients should be placed on preventive medications to halt the progression of the disease (see the section "How Is VCF Prevented?")

INTERVENTIONAL PROCEDURES

Thoracic Radicular Pain

Interventional management of thoracic radicular pain includes intercostal nerve block and pulsed RF treatment of the dorsal root ganglion (DRG) or intercostal nerves. Successful results have been reported in utilizing pulsed RF treatment in thoracic radicular back pain management. Stolker et al. showed significant pain relief after pulsed RF treatment in more than 70% of patients for 13–46 months.[138] Furthermore, van Kleef and Spaans reported similar results, with remarkable pain improvement in 52% of the patients for 9–39 months following the procedure.[139] The efficacy of the treatment was reduced when multiple segments were involved as a cause of pain. There is only one retrospective report of a comparison between pulsed RF treatment of the intercostal nerves and DRGs. In this study, pulsed RF of the DRG showed a higher rate of success and longer duration of pain relief. The efficacy of standard RF therapy is superior but causes DRG injury.[140] Localized pain may occur for several days following the majority of these procedures. Pain after RF treatment was reported in 20% of patients and lasted up to a few weeks. The most important adverse event in thoracic blocks is pneumothorax. If the physician is suspicious, a chest X-ray will rule out the presence of pneumothorax.

Patients with displaced thoracic intervertebral discs or herniated nucleus pulposus (HNP) impinging on the intrathecal space may attempt initially a trial of conservative treatment with oral medications. For those who do not respond to noninvasive treatment modalities, thoracic epidural steroid injections (ESI) are usually the most reasonable next step, provided there are no signs of progressive neurological deficits that necessitate surgical decompression (Figure 17.7). Other indications of thoracic ESI include postherpetic neuralgia (PHN).

Due to the fact that thoracic back pain is less prevalent compared to lumbar and cervical pain, thoracic ESIs are less commonly performed compared to lumbar or cervical ESI, which explains the paucity of literature. Cohen et al. indicated in their review of ESIs that there is strong evidence (level I) in favor of the use of intrathecal steroids for PHN and moderate evidence to support the early use of ESI in acute herpes zoster to prevent the development of PHN.[141,142] In a randomized controlled study, the incidence of PHN among those who received ESI was less compared to the control group who received parenteral acyclovir and steroids.

Similarly, in another trial, there was lower incidence of PHN at 1 month, but not at 3 or 6 months after ESI.[143,144] Benyamin et al. conducted a systematic review of the role of thoracic epidural ESI in the treatment of chronic mid and upper back pain due to various conditions including disc herniation and radiculitis, axial or discogenic pain, spinal stenosis, post thoracic surgery syndrome, and post thoracotomy pain syndrome. They concluded that there is fair evidence in favor of ESI in the management of thoracic back pain secondary to thoracic disk herniation and disk degeneration, based on one double-blinded randomized trial.[145,146]

Spinal cord stimulation (SCS) might be considered in controlling pain on a long-term basis in selected groups of patients, especially in those who have undergone spine surgery with residual pain.

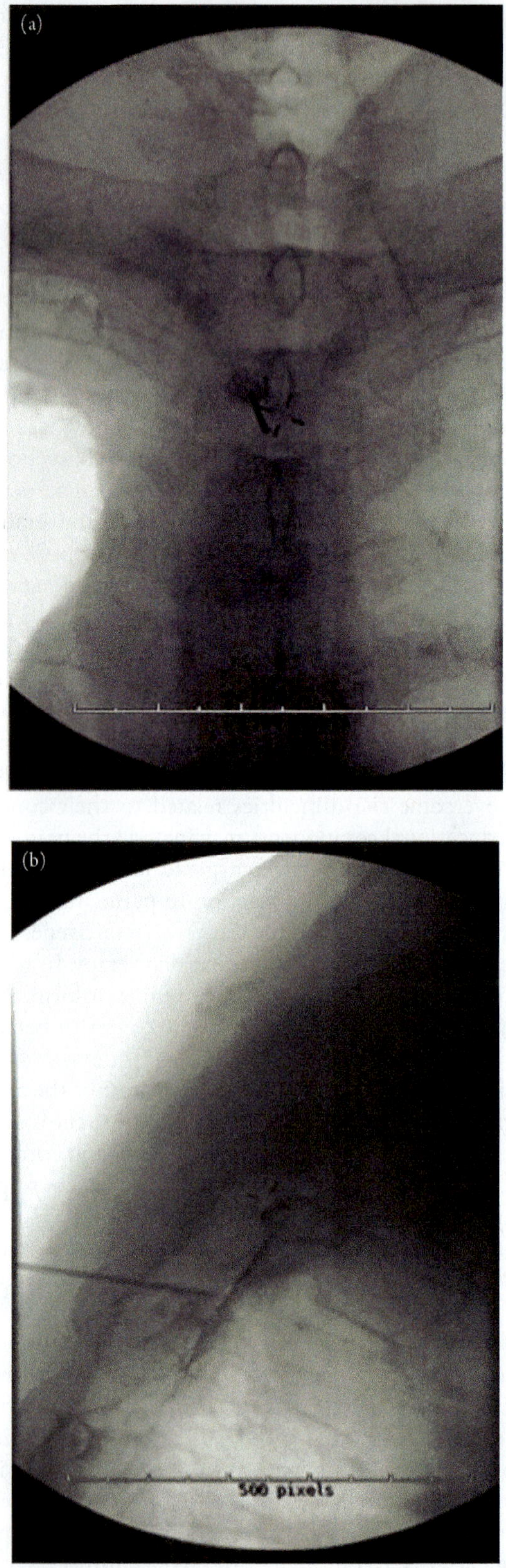

Figure 17.7 Anteroposterior (A) and lateral (B) views of thoracic epidural steroid injection for thoracic radicular pain.

Thoracic Spondylosis

The benefit of intra-articular local anesthetic and steroid injections for the diagnosis and treatment of facet joint pain is controversial. Whereas most of the studies have been performed on lumbar facet joints, the results could still be extrapolated cautiously and applied to thoracic facet joints. Long-term pain relief following intra-articular steroid injection has been reported from 18% to 63%.[147–150] Other studies have showed intermediate pain improvement with intra-articular local anesthetic alone and hyaluronic acid.[151,152] Review articles have shown that studies are equally divided regarding the efficacy of the intra-articular steroids.[153–155] Based on basic science studies, intra-articular steroid injections may provide intermediate pain relief in a subset of patients with actively inflamed zygapophyseal joints.[156,157]

TMBBs are diagnostic to confirm the diagnosis of thoracic facet arthropathy. However, they can still be potentially therapeutic and provide longer term relief lasting for a few months. Manchikanti et al. reported significant pain reduction with TMBB up to 1 year.[158] Other studies have failed to reproduce such results. Nevertheless, there is a small subset of patients who will obtain sustained pain relief following TMBB. Therefore, percutaneous denervation of the thoracic facet medial branches should follow diagnostic blocks as a definitive method of treatment.

Limited numbers of studies are available regarding the effectiveness of RF treatment of thoracic facet-mediated pain. In a prospective uncontrolled study involving 40 patients with thoracic pain that failed conservative measures, Stokler et al. obtained substantial results with thoracic facet rhizotomy. The diagnosis was established based on clinical criteria and positive response to TMBB. At 2 months follow-up, 47.5% patients had complete resolution of their pain, 35% of patients obtained more than 50% reduction of their pain, and 17.5% reported no relief. At 31 months following the procedure, 44% remained pain free, 39% continued to have more than 50% reduction of their pain, and 17% still experienced fair relief.[159] In another study, Tzaan and Tasker studied 17 patients with acquiring substantial pain relief.[160] In an attempt to identify the factors associated with successful treatments, Cohen and coworkers studied 192 patients in three teaching hospitals after these patients had received a single positive MBB. Among other variables, paraspinal tenderness was found to be the highest factor associated with successful RF treatment. Upon return of pain 6–12 months after the treatment, repeat of neurotomy was similarly effective as the initial procedure. Although sensory stimulation (<0.5) has been used to confirm the proximity of the probe to the medial branches, many patients may falsely report stimulation if the probe is placed in the muscle far away from the nerves.[161,162]

A major limitation to the success of rhizotomy treatment is the anatomic variability of the thoracic facets' medial branches, especially those of the middle thoracic levels. An evolving and promising technique is the use of cooled RF technology to produce a larger lesion and thus ensure denervation of the nerves despite anatomic variability of medial branches (Figure 17.8). Postprocedure complications include increased pain following treatment and pneumothorax. Appropriate technique and monitoring is essential to decrease the incidence of complications.

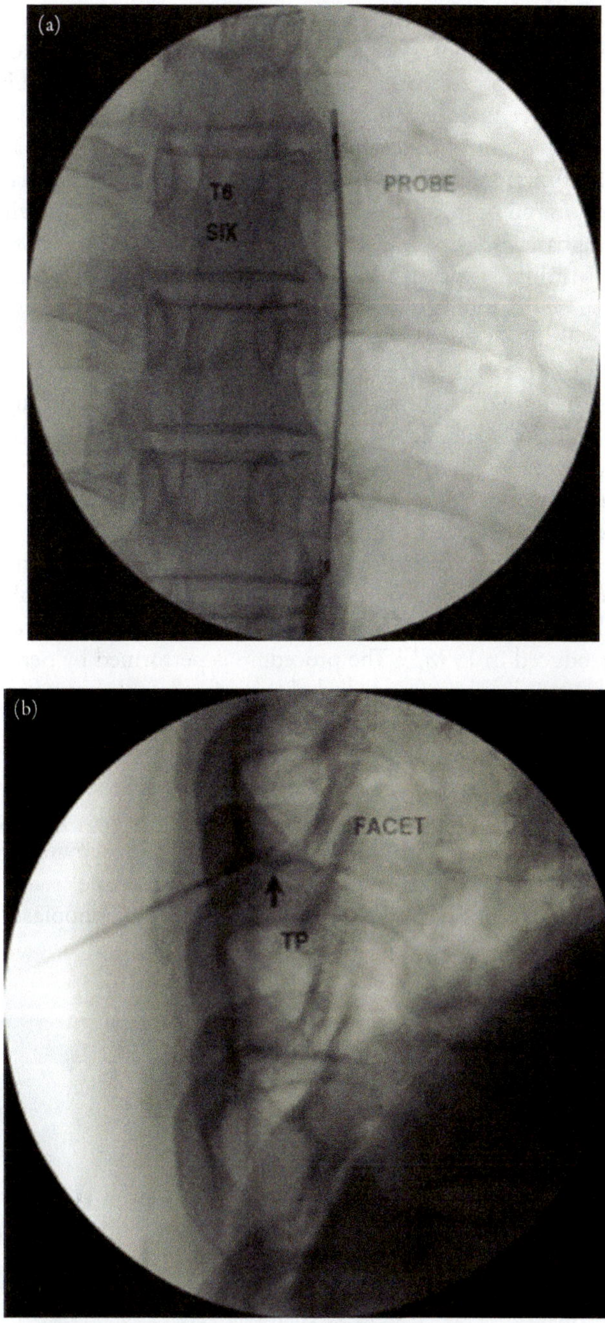

Figure 17.8 Anteroposterior (A) and lateral (B) views of cooled radiofrequency ablation of the thoracic medial branches for thoracic facet-mediated pain.

> If our patient mentioned in the case fails to respond to conservative measures, what are her other options?

Thoracic VCFs

Management of VCF needs to address acute fracture pain control, chronic mechanical sequelae, and the prevention of additional compression fractures with treatment of underlying osteoporosis. As for patients with pathologic compression fractures due to tumor involvement, a course of radiotherapy may be indicated if the tumor is radiosensitive. Radiotherapy provided pain relief in approximately 50% of patients with VCFs due to myeloma or prostate or breast cancer.[163]

Patients with recent fracture who continue to have pain regardless of conservative management may benefit from percutaneous vertebral augmentation procedures (VAP). These procedures have gained in popularity because they produce rapid, significant, and sustained improvements in back pain, function, and quality of life.[164] Additionally, they have been found to provide spinal stabilization in patients with malignancies.[165]

Minimally invasive VAPs, like kyphoplasty and percutaneous vertebroplasty, are among the most popular procedures (Figure 17.9).[166,167]

Percutaneous vertebroplasty is a common method for treatment of VCFs by augmenting the vertebral body through injection of polymethylmethacrylate (PMMA).[166] A bone marrow biopsy needle is placed into the compressed vertebra via a posterior approach under fluoroscopy or CT guidance. Methylmethacrylate cement is then injected.[48,168–170]

Another treatment option for vertebral body augmentation is kyphoplasty, which includes placement of an inflatable balloon in the fractured vertebral body. This procedure was introduced in 1998.[171] The procedure is performed by percutaneous insertion of a needle holding an inflatable bone tamp into the fractured vertebra. The balloon is inflated to create a cavity that can later be filled with PMMA or other types of bone cement. The risks associated with this procedure are similar to percutaneous vertebroplasty; however, lower rates of cement leakage into the spinal canal have been shown.[164]

Vertebroplasty is most effective when done within 6 months of compression fractures.[172–174] Kyphoplasty's success rate is highest when it is performed within 3 months of the fracture or pain onset.[112,164,175] Although selection criteria for kyphoplasty versus vertebroplasty in patients with acute fracture are yet to be determined, both techniques provide significant pain relief in patients with VCF.[173]

The primary goal of vertebroplasty is pain relief by stabilizing the fracture, with subsequent improvement in pulmonary function and quality of life. Studies showed 75–100% pain relief after vertebroplasty, which also increases functional capacity by stabilizing the fracture and preventing further vertebral collapse.[48,168–170] Although Rousing et al. showed no greater improvement in back pain in patients treated with vertebroplasty when compared to medical therapy, they found a significant improvement in function 12 months after the procedure. In spite of primary encouraging results of vertebroplasty for VCFs, some studies found no beneficial effect of vertebroplasty when compared to a sham procedure. Buchbinder et al. showed that vertebroplasty offered no benefit to patients with fresh and painful VCFs. A similar study also found that vertebroplasty and a sham procedure had equivalent results.[176,177] Based on these results, some practitioners abandoned the use of vertebroplasty, whereas others challenge the quality of those trials.[172,176–178]

Following kyphoplasty, 85–100% of patients may experience good to moderate pain relief.[114,173] A multicenter randomized controlled trial showed better functional recovery after kyphoplasty, with a lower incidence of adverse events compared to nonsurgical management.[174,179,180] Kyphoplasty may reverse spinal kyphosis and potentially prevent the

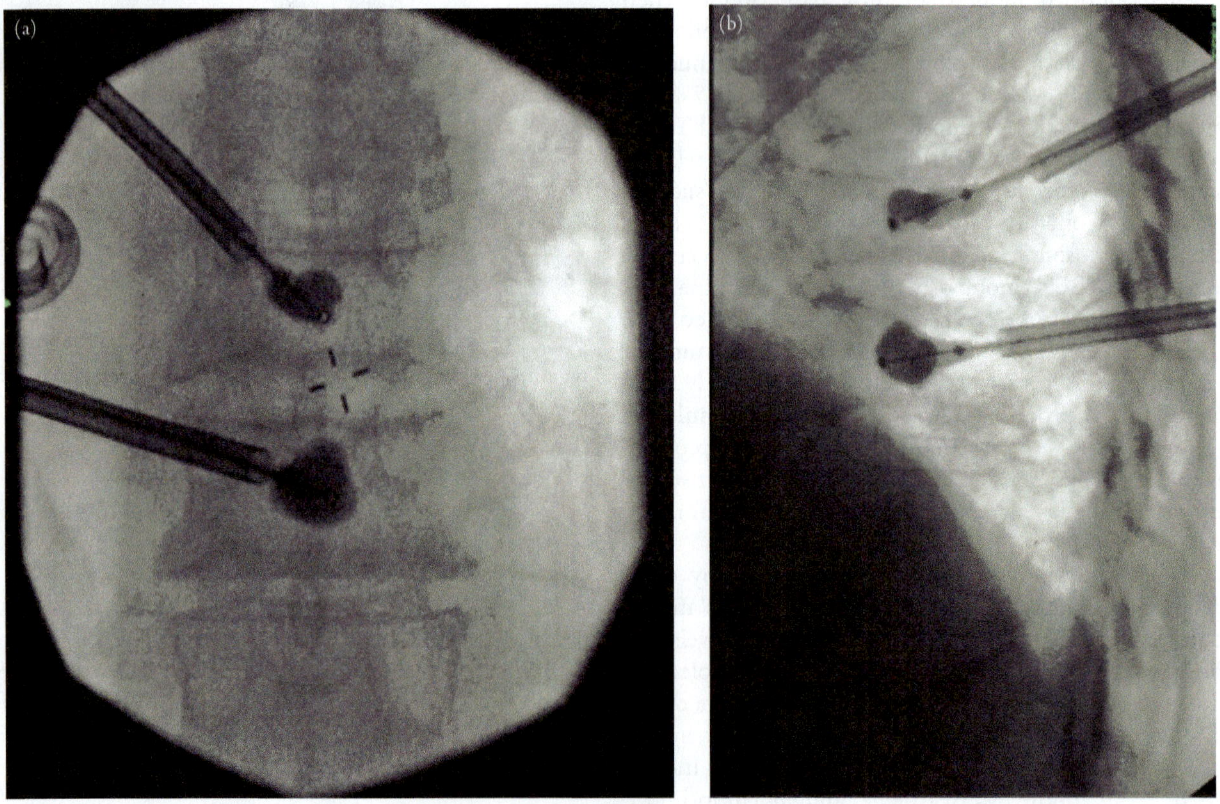

Figure 17.9 Anteroposterior (A) and lateral (B) views of kyphoplasty procedure for T8 and T9 osteoporotic compression fracture.

pulmonary and gastrointestinal complications associated with severe kyphosis.[30,173] Osteoporotic kyphotic compression fractures may result in an anterior shift of the sagittal plumb line and augmented load on the anterior vertebral column, which can be complicated with further compression fractures. These sequential compression fractures can ultimately cause the typical hump of the elderly, with considerable thoracic kyphosis and low pelvic incidence, forcing the patient to bend hips and knees to maintain sagittal balance. The fundamental rationale for kyphoplasty is to increase anterior column load with progressing kyphosis. Kyphoplasty may also restore vertebral body height and prevent progressive kyphosis in osteoporotic compression fractures. In a recent retrospective review of 67 consecutive patients who underwent single or multilevel kyphoplasty to quantify the restoration of lost vertebral height, the authors noted restoration of 45% of the lost vertebral height. The incidence of restoration of vertebral height was observed in 98% of treated vertebral bodies (N = 118). The significant diminution in pain is objectively translated into daily morphine consumption reduction, along with improvement in functional outcome measures.[181] The incidence of height restoration varied from 58% to 92%.[181,182] In a similar study (N = 49), a mean of 47% of lost vertebral height was restored using the adjacent vertebral body as a reference measure.[30] Earlier intervention with kyphoplasty in VCF patients may lead to more successful results.[183]

Long-term outcomes were evaluated in a prospective controlled study (N = 40). In addition to maintenance of pain reduction (p = .0008) and mobility improvement (p = .308) up to 3 years, the incidence of new vertebral fractures was less compared to the control group (p = .0341).[184] Similarly, when long-term outcomes of vertebroplasty were prospectively assessed, it was found to provide significant and clinically meaningful reduction in pain, oral analgesic intake, and disability when compared with conservative therapy. There was no clear increased risk of new vertebral fractures.[185] This disproves earlier fears of an increased risk of new VCFs in the adjacent segments after vertebral body augmentation procedures, which was believed to be induced by the increased stiffness of treated vertebra compared to adjacent vertebral bodies.[175]

A number of potentially serious complications of intraosseous injection of bone cement have been reported in the literature. One such complication is cement leakage, which ranged from 3% to 75%. Leakage into the spinal canal may result in neurologic deficit, such as radiculopathy or spinal cord compression. Other complications include cement leakage from a vertebra to the paravertebral muscles, such as the psoas, which can result in severe pain due to a localized thermal reaction. Leakage of cement into the venous circulation may cause a systemic toxic reaction. Garfin et al. found that short-term complications from kyphoplasty were related to cement extravasation and damage from heat and pressure on the spinal cord and nerve roots.[164] Pulmonary embolism can occur if the cement enters the inferior vena cava. The risk of complications can be reduced by utilizing venography prior to the injection of cement and by injecting an appropriate dose of cement.[186–188] Long-term consequences of cement in a vertebral body are still not well investigated.[183]

Contraindications of VAP include infection of the vertebral body, coagulopathy, bone fragment retropulsion, and allergy to any of the substances used during the procedure, including PMMA cement and contrast agent.[164,183,189]

New techniques have been developed to minimize the risks of complications from kyphoplasty. Vesselplasty was developed to decrease the rate of cement leakage: the inflatable balloon is left in the patient and filled with cement, thus reducing the risk of cement leakage. Alternatives to PMMA were also explored; however, these substances produced a greater physiologic load transfer thus increasing the risk for development of new VCFs.[190–192]

> The MRI performed to our patient showed an acute T6 vertebral compression fracture with resultant loss of 40% of the vertebral height and no retropulsion. Since our patient failed to respond to conservative management and tolerate physical therapy, the patient is likely to benefit from kyphoplasty to be followed by physical therapy.

SURGERY

Thoracic Herniated Discs or Thoracic Radicular Pain

Various surgical options aim at spinal decompression, correction of deformity, and instrumented stabilization/fusion. Deciding on the best approach depends on the extent and location of the pathology and the degree of instability. The posterior laminectomy approach is commonly performed for spinal canal decompression. The anterior approach is implemented in the presence of anterior vertebral collapse or spinal cord compression. In cases of tumors impinging on the spinal cord, timely intervention is crucial to ensure resolution of neurological dysfunction. Pain and neurological deficits may improve substantially with the use of high-dose steroid in the process of planning for surgical or oncological treatment.[193]

Radical surgical excision is usually sufficient for benign spinal tumors. On the other hand, the majority of malignant spinal tumors are managed with palliative radiotherapy and/or chemotherapy unless there is neurological compression and deformity and instability. Surgical intervention in these patients has not been shown to have any survival benefit over oncological treatment. Patients presenting with early signs of neurological deficits due to compression often respond to urgent radiotherapy. For severe and rapidly progressive cases, surgical decompression may provide a more immediate response.

Thoracic Spondylosis

Patients with nonradicular, localized back pain tend to respond poorly to thoracic discectomy and fusion. Surgery is indicated if any of the patients shows any signs of neurological deficits or if pain is refractory to conservative measures including oral medications, physical therapy, and ESIs. Deciding on the appropriate surgical approach depends on many factors.

Anterior approaches are used for centrally located disc prolapses, intradurally eroded discs, and heavily calcified discs requiring significant manipulation. A posterior approach excision can pose significant risks of spinal cord injury in such cases. However, posterior approaches are indicated for lateral and soft anterolateral prolapses, which require minimal manipulation of the spinal cord. To improve surgical access, the facet joint or pedicle can be partially excised. However, this may eventually lead to spinal instability and thus the performance of a simultaneous fusion procedure should be considered.[194]

Thoracic VCF

Surgical intervention for thoracic VCF is indicated for patients when there is evidence of impending or existing neurologic deficit, long-standing myelopathy, progressive symptoms, or severe spinal deformity.[195] However, surgical management of elderly patients does carry increased risk of morbidities.[60,123,166] A major surgical procedure to treat a VCF is infrequently necessary and is performed only if there is severe spinal instability. There are several surgical options for the management of painful osteoporotic fractures. Spinal fusion surgery can be used to eliminate vertebral movement through the fusion of two or more spinal vertebrae to create a solid bone bridge between the vertebrae. Open surgery is indicated in the presence of neurological deficit, long-standing myelopathy, and progressive symptoms (Box 17.7). Some patients fail to improve neurological deficits brought about by neural compression.[195] This compression is due to retropulsed bony fragments from the delayed collapsed vertebral body restricting the spinal canal. In patients with multiple VCFs that are complicated with kyphosis associated with fixed sagittal imbalance, a cement augmentation procedure may improve fracture pain but not the overall imbalance. Significant spinal imbalance can lead to a significant functional disability and subsequent worsening quality of life. In addition, excess kyphosis can later result in a VCF due to increased anterior load. The anterior location of the sagittal plumb line in fixed sagittal imbalance may be the cause of falls, with possible further fractures and morbidity. Thus, the correction of global sagittal imbalance may be indicated in severe cases. Because both open and closed wedge procedures are associated with adverse outcomes leading to disabling morbidity, surgeons are often hesitant to proceed with these operations in patients with multiple comorbidities. Long instrumentation times are required for these patients due to poor bone quality, and these patients are at an increased risk of adjacent VCF and pedicle fractures.[196–198]

Box 17.7 **INDICATIONS FOR SURGICAL INTERVENTION**

Progressive spinal deformity
Radio-resistant tumors
Spinal Instability
Solitary lesions not responding to adjuvant treatment
Static or progressive neurological dysfunction

Anterior instrumentation surgery is one surgical treatment options. The benefits of anterior instrumentation surgery with a vertebral spacer include the direct resection of the retropulsed bony fragment and the reconstruction of the stable anterior spinal column. Additional posterior reinforcement might be required in some patients because of multiple-level vertebral collapse, steroid-induced osteoporosis, or low BMD.[199,200] With regard to open sagittal corrections, there is growing evidence that the posterior-only pedicle subtraction osteotomy is preferred to multiple Smith-Petersen osteotomies due to better correction with shorter operation time.[201]

Other methods include the use of the OsseoFix Spinal Fracture Reduction System and internal bracing. More invasive techniques, such as anterior and posterior decompression and stabilization with placement of screws, plates, cages, and rods, are also available. These procedures, however, are challenging because it is difficult to achieve adequate fixation in osteoporotic bone.[55]

Combined cement augmentation and posterior instrumentation has been discussed as an alternative therapy. In some cases, further splintering of the fractured vertebra with posterior dislocation of an instable fragment is a potentially severe complication. Therefore, several surgeons perform posterior instrumentation of the adjacent vertebrae to protect the posterior wall and to improve the sagittal profile. This can be done via a percutaneous approach or with a conventional open technique. Possible disadvantages of this technique include increased load on the adjacent segments with degeneration due to segmental fusion and possible implant loosening with loss of correction due to low bone quality. Cement augmentation of the implanted pedicle screws can reduce the complication rate regarding low bone quality.[202–206]

CONCLUSION

Thoracic back pain has been historically problematic with extensive differential diagnoses. Detailed history and thorough physical examination along with diagnostic tests play a pivotal role in detecting the underlying pathology. An appropriate multidisciplinary approach should be implemented for the management of thoracic back pain patients. Physical therapy is imperative in the long-term management of these patients. In addition to pharmacological and interventional treatments, psychological aspects of chronic pain and functional loss should be addressed as well. Timely interventions may be warranted to prevent further clinical sequelae and functional disability resulting from inadequate pain control.

REFERENCES

1. Benhamou CL, Roux C, Tourliere D, Gervais T, Viala JF, Amor B. Pseudovisceral pain referred from costovertebral arthropathies. twenty-eight cases. *Spine* (Phila Pa 1976). 1993;18(6):790–795.
2. Fruth SJ. Differential diagnosis and treatment in a patient with posterior upper thoracic pain. *Phys Ther*. 2006;86(2):254–268.

3. Yelland MJ. Back, chest and abdominal pain. How good are spinal signs at identifying musculoskeletal causes of back, chest or abdominal pain? *Aust Fam Physician*. 2001;30(9):908–912.
4. Stolker RJ, Groen GJ. Medical and invasive management of thoracic spinal pain. In: Gile LGF, Singer KP, eds. *The Clinical Anatomy and Management of Thoracic Spine Pain*. Oxford: Butterworth-Heinemann; 2000:206.
5. Groen GJ, Stolker RJ. Thoracic neural anatomy. In: Giles LGF, Singer KP. *The Clinical Anatomy and Management of Thoracic Spine Pain*. Oxford: Butterworth-Heinemann; 2000:114.
6. Manchikanti L, Singh V, Datta S, et al. Comprehensive review of epidemiology, scope, and impact of spinal pain. *Pain Physician*. 2009;12(4):E35–E70.
7. Manchikanti L, Boswell MV, Singh V, et al. Comprehensive evidence-based guidelines for interventional techniques in the management of chronic spinal pain. *Pain Physician*. 2009;12(4):699–802.
8. Leboeuf-Yde C, Nielsen J, Kyvik KO, Fejer R, Hartvigsen J. Pain in the lumbar, thoracic or cervical regions: do age and gender matter? A population-based study of 34,902 Danish twins 20-71 years of age. *BMC Musculoskelet Disord*. 2009;10:39.
9. Waldman SD. Functional anatomy of the thoracic vertebrae. *Pain review*. 2009:71.
10. Maarten va Kleef RJS, Lataster A, Geurts JW, Benzon HT, Mekhail N. Evidence-based interventional pain management according to clinical diagnosis. *Pain Practice*. 2010;(10):327–338.
11. Tortora GJ, Derrickso BH. *The Skeleton System: The Axial Skeleton, Principles of Physiology and Anatomy*. 12th ed.Wiley & Sons Inc.; 2009:222.
12. Chua WH, Bogduk N. The surgical anatomy of thoracic facet denervation. *Acta Neurochir* (Wien). 1995;136(3-4):140–144.
13. Berger A, Henry L, Goldberg M. Surgical palliation of thoracic malignancies. *Surg Oncol Clin N Am*. 2004;13(3):429–453.
14. Chowdary MU. Intradural thoracic disc protrusion. *Spine*. 1987;(12):718–719.
15. Nguyen TH, Randolph DC. Non-specific low back pain and return to work. *Am Fam Pract*. 2007;76:1497.
16. Manchikanti L, Boswell, M V, Singh V, Pampati V, Damron K S, Beyer, CD. Prevalence of facet joint pain in chronic spinal pain of cervical, thoracic, and lumbar regions. *BMC Musculoskelet Disord*. 2004;5:15.
17. Manchikanti L, Pampati V, Fellows B, Baha AG. The inability of the clinical picture to characterize pain from facet joints. *Pain Physician*. 2000;3(2):158–166.
18. Sidiropoulos PI, Hatemi G, Song, IH, et al. Evidence-based recommendations for the management of ankylosing spondylitis: systematic literature search of the 3E Initiative in Rheumatology involving a broad panel of experts and practising rheumatologists. *Rheumatology* (Oxford). 2008;47(3):355–361.
19. Gerwin RD. Myofascial and visceral pain syndromes: visceral-somatic pain representations. *J Musculoskeletal Pain*. 2002;10:165–175.
20. Lillegard WA. Medical causes of pain in the thoracic region. In: Flynn TW, ed. *The Thoracic Spine and Rib Cage: Musculoskeletal Evaluation and Treatment*. Boston: Butterworth-Heinemann; 1996:107–120.
21. Karlson KA. Thoracic region pain in athletes. *Curr Sports Med Rep*. 2004; 3(1):53–57.
22. Kost RG,Straus SE. Postherpetic neuralgia—pathogenesis, treatment, and prevention. *N Engl J Med*. 1996;335(1):32–42.
23. Wanek S, Mayberry JC. Blunt thoracic trauma: flail chest, pulmonary contusion, and blast injury. *Crit Care Clin*. 2004;20(1):71–81.
24. McBeath AA,Keene JS. The rib-tip syndrome. *J Bone Joint Surg Am*. 1975;57(6):795–797.
25. Dreyfuss P, Tibiletti C, Dreyer SJ. Thoracic zygapophyseal joint pain patterns. A study in normal volunteers. *Spine* (Phila Pa 1976). 1994;19(7):807–811.
26. Fukui, S., K. Ohseto, and M. Shiotani, Patterns of pain induced by distending the thoracic zygapophyseal joints. *Reg Anesth*. 1997;22(4):332–336.
27. Silverman SL. The clinical consequences of vertebral compression fracture. *Bone*. 1992;13(suppl 2):S27–S31.
28. Patel U, Skingle S, Campbell GA, Crisp AJ, Boyle IT, et al. Clinical profile of acute vertebral compression fractures in osteoporosis. *Br J Rheumatol*. 1991;30(6):418–421.
29. Nevitt MC, Ettinger B, Black DM, et al. The association of radiographically detected vertebral fractures with back pain and function: a prospective study. *Ann Intern Med*. 1998;128(10):793–800.
30. Lieberman IH, Dudeney S, Reinhardt MK, Bell G. Initial outcome and efficacy of "kyphoplasty" in the treatment of painful osteoporotic vertebral compression fractures. *Spine* (Phila Pa 1976). 2001;26(14):1631–1638.
31. Thornbury JR, Fryback DG,mTurski PA, et al. Disk-caused nerve compression in patients with acute low-back pain: diagnosis with MR, CT myelography, and plain CT. *Radiology*. 1993;186(3):731–738.
32. Wood KB, Garvey TA, Gundry C, Heithoff KB. Magnetic resonance imaging of the thoracic spine. Evaluation of asymptomatic individuals. *J Bone Joint Surg Am*. 1995;77(11):1631–1638.
33. Stillerman CB, Chen TC, Couldwell WT, Zhang W, Weiss MH. Experience in the surgical management of 82 symptomatic herniated thoracic discs and review of the literature. *J Neurosurg*. 1998;88(4):623–633.
34. Lyu RK, Chang HS, Tang LM, Chen ST. Thoracic disc herniation mimicking acute lumbar disc disease. *Spine* (Phila Pa 1976). 1999;24(4):416–418.
35. Alexandru D, So W. Evaluation and management of vertebral compression fractures. *Perm J*. 2012;16(4):46–51.
36. Epstein O, Ludwig S, Gelb D, Poelstra K, O'Brien J. Comparison of computed tomography and plain radiography in assessing traumatic spinal deformity. *J Spinal Disord Tech*. 2009;22(3):197–201.
37. Maynard AS, Jensen ME, Schweickert PA, Marx WF, Short JG, Kallmes DF. Value of bone scan imaging in predicting pain relief from percutaneous vertebroplasty in osteoporotic vertebral fractures. *Am J Neuroradiol*. 2000;21(10):1807–1812.
38. Bogduk N. International Spinal Injection Society guidelines for the performance of spinal injection procedures. Part 1: zygapophysial joint blocks. *Clin J Pain*. 1997;13(4):285–302.
39. Dreyfuss PH, Dreyer SJ, NASS. Lumbar zygapophysial (facet) joint injections. *Spine J*. 2003;3(3 suppl):50S–59S.
40. North RB, Kidd DH, Zahurak M, Piantadosi S. Specificity of diagnostic nerve blocks: a prospective, randomized study of sciatica due to lumbosacral spine disease. *Pain*. 1996; 65(1):77–85.
41. Cohen SP, Larkin TM, Chang AS, Stojanovic MP. The causes of false-positive medial branch (facet joint) blocks in soldiers and retirees. *Mil Med*. 2004;169(10):781–786.
42. Cooper C, Atkinson EJ, O'Fallon WM, Melton LJ 3rd. Incidence of clinically diagnosed vertebral fractures: a population-based study in Rochester, Minnesota, 1985-1989. *J Bone Miner Res*. 1992;7(2):221–227.
43. Riggs BL, Melton LJ 3rd. The worldwide problem of osteoporosis: insights afforded by epidemiology. *Bone*. 1995;17(5 suppl):505S–511S.
44. Black DM, Arden NK, Palermo L, Pearson J, Cummings SR. Prevalent vertebral deformities predict hip fractures and new vertebral deformities but not wrist fractures. Study of Osteoporotic Fractures Research Group. *J Bone Miner Res*. 1999;14(5):821–828.
45. Black DM, Cummings SR, Karpf DB, et al. Randomised trial of effect of alendronate on risk of fracture in women with existing vertebral fractures. Fracture Intervention Trial Research Group. *Lancet*. 1996;348(9041):1535–1541.
46. Felsenberg D, Silman AJ, Lunt M, et al. Incidence of vertebral fracture in Europe: results from the European Prospective Osteoporosis Study (EPOS). *J Bone Miner Res*. 2002;17(4):716–724.
47. Kanis JA. Diagnosis of osteoporosis and assessment of fracture risk. *Lancet*. 2002;359(9321):1929–1936.
48. Fourney DR, Schomer DF, Nader R, et al. Percutaneous vertebroplasty and kyphoplasty for painful vertebral body fractures in cancer patients. *J Neurosurg*. 2003;98(1 suppl):21–30.

49. Dahan A, Yassen A, Bijl H, Romberg R,Sarton E, Teppema L, Olofsen E, Danhof, M. Comparison of the respiratory effects of intravenous buprenorphine and fentanyl in humans and rats. *Br J Anaesth.* 2005;94(6):825–834.
50. Klazen CA, Lohle PN, de Vries J, et al. Vertebroplasty versus conservative treatment in acute osteoporotic vertebral compression fractures (Vertos II): an open-label randomised trial. *Lancet.* 2010;376(9746):1085–1092.
51. Johnell O, Kanis JA. An estimate of the worldwide prevalence and disability associated with osteoporotic fractures. *Osteoporos Int.* 2006;17(12):1726–1733.
52. Lukert BP. Vertebral compression fractures: how to manage pain, avoid disability. *Geriatrics.* 1994;49(2):22–26.
53. Venmans A, Klazen CA, Lohle PN, Mali WP, van Rooij WJ. Natural history of pain in patients with conservatively treated osteoporotic vertebral compression fractures: results from VERTOS II. *Am J Neuroradiol.* 2012;33(3):519–521.
54. Meunier PJ, Delmas PD, Eastell R, et al. Diagnosis and management of osteoporosis in postmenopausal women: clinical guidelines. International Committee for Osteoporosis Clinical Guidelines. *Clin Ther.* 1999;21(6):1025–1044.
55. Leblanc AD, Schneider VS, Evans HJ, Engelbretson DA, Krebs JM. Bone mineral loss and recovery after 17 weeks of bed rest. *J Bone Miner Res.* 1990;5(8):843–850.
56. Krolner B, Toft B. Vertebral bone loss: an unheeded side effect of therapeutic bed rest. *Clin Sci* (Lond). 1983;64(5):537–540.
57. Yoon SP, Lee SH, Ki CH, Lee YT, Hong SH, Lee HM, Moon SH. Quality of life in patients with osteoporotic vertebral fractures. Asian Spine J. 2014;8(5): 653–8.
58. Kado DM, Browner WS, Palermo L, Nevitt MC,Genant HK,Cummings SR.Vertebral fractures and mortality in older women: a prospective study. Study of Osteoporotic Fractures Research Group. *Arch Intern Med.* 1999;159(11):1215–1220.
59. Truumees E. Osteoporosis. *Spine* (Phila Pa 1976). 2001;26(8):930–932.
60. Kim DH, Vaccaro AR. Osteoporotic compression fractures of the spine; current options and considerations for treatment. *Spine J.* 2006;6(5):479–487.
61. Cohn SH, Vartsky D, Yasumura S, Sawitsky A, Zanzi I, Vaswani A, Ellis KJ. Compartmental body composition based on total-body nitrogen, potassium, and calcium. *Am J Physiol.* 1980;239(6):E524–E530.
62. Evans WJ, Campbell WW. Sarcopenia and age-related changes in body composition and functional capacity. *J Nutr.* 1993;123(2 suppl):465–468.
63. Lord SR, Ward JA, Williams P, Strudwick M. The effect of a 12-month exercise trial on balance, strength, and falls in older women: a randomized controlled trial. *J Am Geriatr Soc.* 1995;43(11):1198–1206.
64. Shumway-Cook A, Gruber W, Baldwin M, Liao S. The effect of multidimensional exercises on balance, mobility, and fall risk in community-dwelling older adults. *Phys Ther.* 1997; 77(1):46–57.
65. No F. *Osteoporosis: Physician's Guide to Prevention and Treatment of Osteoporosis.* Belle Mead, NJ: Excerpta Medica; 1998.
66. Resch A, Schneider B, Bernecker P, Battmann A, Wergedal J, Willvonseder R, Resch H. Risk of vertebral fractures in men: relationship to mineral density of the vertebral body. *Am J Roentgenol.* 1995;164(6):1447–1450.
67. Rogers MJ, Gordon S, Benford HL, Coxon FP, Luckman SP, Monkkonen J, Frith, JC. Cellular and molecular mechanisms of action of bisphosphonates. *Cancer.* 2000;88(12 suppl):2961–2978.
68. Coxon FP, Benford HL, Russell RG, Rogers MJ. Protein synthesis is required for caspase activation and induction of apoptosis by bisphosphonate drugs. *Mol Pharmacol.* 1998;54(4):631–638.
69. Orwoll E, Ettinger M, Weiss S, et al. Alendronate for the treatment of osteoporosis in men. *N Engl J Med.* 2000;343(9):604–610.
70. Watts NB, Harris ST,Genant HK, et al. Intermittent cyclical etidronate treatment of postmenopausal osteoporosis. *N Engl J Med.* 1990;323(2):73–79.
71. Overgaard K, Hansen MA, Nielsen VA, Riis, BJ, Christiansen C. Discontinuous calcitonin treatment of established osteoporosis—effects of withdrawal of treatment. *Am J Med.* 1990; 89(1):1–6.
72. Silverman SL, Calcitonin. *Am J Med Sci.* 1997;313(1):13–16.
73. Chapuy MC, Arlot ME, Duboeuf F, et al. Vitamin D3 and calcium to prevent hip fractures in the elderly women. *N Engl J Med.* 1992;327(23):1637–1642.
74. Dawson-Hughes B, Harris SS, Krall EA, Dallal GE. Effect of calcium and vitamin D supplementation on bone density in men and women 65 years of age or older. *N Engl J Med.* 1997;337(10):670–676.
75. Cauley JA, Seeley DG, Ensrud K, Ettinger B, Black D, Cummings SR. Estrogen replacement therapy and fractures in older women. Study of Osteoporotic Fractures Research Group. *Ann Intern Med.* 1995;122(1):9–16.
76. Lindsay R, Bush TL, Grady D, Speroff L, Lobo RA. Therapeutic controversy: estrogen replacement in menopause. *J Clin Endocrinol Metab.* 1996;81(11):3829–3838.
77. Schneider DL, Barrett-Connor EL, Morton DJ. Timing of postmenopausal estrogen for optimal bone mineral density. The Rancho Bernardo Study. *JAMA.* 1997;277(7):543–547.
78. Naessen T, Berglund L, Ulmsten U. Bone loss in elderly women prevented by ultralow doses of parenteral 17beta-estradiol. *Am J Obstet Gynecol.* 1997;177(1):115–119.
79. Prestwood KM, Pannullo AM, Kenny AM, Pilbeam CC, Raisz LG. The effect of a short course of calcium and vitamin D on bone turnover in older women. Osteoporos Int. 1996;6(4): 314–9.
80. Felson DT, Zhang Y, Hannan MT, Kiel DP, Wilson PW, Anderson JJ. The effect of postmenopausal estrogen therapy on bone density in elderly women. *N Engl J Med.* 1993;329(16):1141–1146.
81. Colditz G, Hankinson SE, Hunter DJ, et al. The use of estrogen and progestins and the risk of breast cancer in postmenopausal women. *N Engl J Med.* 1995;332:1589–1593.
82. Beresford SA, Weiss NS, Voigt LF, McKnight B. Risk of endometrial cancer in relation to use of oestrogen combined with cyclic progestagen therapy in postmenopausal women. *Lancet.* 1997;349(9050):458–461.
83. Grady D, Rubin SM, Petitti DB, et al. Hormone therapy to prevent disease and prolong life in postmenopausal women. *Ann Intern Med.* 1992;117(12):1016–1037.
84. Daly E, Vessey MP, Hawkins MM, Carson JL, Gough P, Marsh S. Risk of venous thromboembolism in users of hormone replacement therapy. *Lancet.* 1996;348(9033):977–980.
85. Jick H, Derby LE, Myers MW, Vasilakis C, Newton KM. Risk of hospital admission for idiopathic venous thromboembolism among users of postmenopausal oestrogens. *Lancet.* 1996;348(9033):981–983.
86. Ravnikar VA. Compliance with hormone replacement therapy: are women receiving the full impact of hormone replacement therapy preventive health benefits? *Womens Health Issues.* 1992;2(2):75–80; discussion 80–82.
87. Delmas PD, Bjarnason NH, Mitlak BH, et al. Effects of raloxifene on bone mineral density, serum cholesterol concentrations, and uterine endometrium in postmenopausal women. *N Engl J Med.* 1997;337(23):1641–1647.
88. Lufkin EG, Whitaker MD, Nickelsen T, et al. Treatment of established postmenopausal osteoporosis with raloxifene: a randomized trial. *J Bone Miner Res.* 1998;13(11):1747–1754.
89. Katznelson L, Finkelstein JS, Schoenfeld DA, Rosenthal DI, Anderson EJ, Klibanski A. Increase in bone density and lean body mass during testosterone administration in men with acquired hypogonadism. *J Clin Endocrinol Metab.* 1996;81(12) :4358–4365.
90. Anderson FH, Francis RM, Peaston RT, Wastell HJ. Androgen supplementation in eugonadal men with osteoporosis: effects of six months' treatment on markers of bone formation and resorption. *J Bone Miner Res.* 1997;12(3):472–478.
91. Finkelstein JS, Arnold AL. Increases in bone mineral density after discontinuation of daily human parathyroid hormone and gonadotropin-releasing hormone analog administration in women with endometriosis. *J Clin Endocrinol Metab.* 1999;84(4):1214–1219.

92. Lane NE, Sanchez S, Modin GW, Genant HK, Pierini E, Arnaud, CD. Parathyroid hormone treatment can reverse corticosteroid-induced osteoporosis. Results of a randomized controlled clinical trial. *J Clin Invest.* 1998;102(8):1627–1633.
93. Hodsman AB, Fraher LJ, Watson PH, et al. A randomized controlled trial to compare the efficacy of cyclical parathyroid hormone versus cyclical parathyroid hormone and sequential calcitonin to improve bone mass in postmenopausal women with osteoporosis. *J Clin Endocrinol Metab.* 1997;82(2):620–628.
94. Lindsay R, Cosman C, Nieves J, Woelfert L. Does treatment with parathyroid hormone increase vertebral size? [abstract]. *Osteoporosis Int* (Suppl). 2000;2:S206.
95. Riggs BL, Hodgson SF, O'Fallon WM, et al. Effect of fluoride treatment on the fracture rate in postmenopausal women with osteoporosis. *N Engl J Med.* 1990;322(12):802–809.
96. Bronfort G, Evans R, Nelson B, et al. A randomized clinical trial of exercise and spinal manipulation for patients with chronic neck pain. *Spine* (Phila Pa 1976). 2001;26(7):788–797; discussion 798–799.
97. Gross AR, Hoving JL, Haines TA, et al. A Cochrane review of manipulation and mobilization for mechanical neck disorders. *Spine* (Phila Pa 1976). 2004;29(14):1541–1548.
98. Machado LA, de Souza Mv, Ferreira PH, Ferreira ML. The McKenzie method for low back pain: a systematic review of the literature with a meta-analysis approach. *Spine* (Phila Pa 1976). 2006;31(9):E254–E262.
99. O'Sullivan PB, Beales DJ, Beetham JA, Cripps J, Graf F, Lin IB, et al. Altered motor control strategies in subjects with sacroiliac joint pain during the active straight-leg-raise test. *Spine.* 2002;27:E1–E8.
100. Kay TM, Gross A, Goldsmith C, et al. Exercises for mechanical neck disorders. *Cochrane Database Syst Rev.* 2005(3):CD004250.
101. Hayden JA, van Tulder MW, Malmivaara A, Koes BW. Exercise therapy for treatment of non-specific low back pain. *Cochrane Db Syst Rev.* 2005;4. doi:10.1002/14651858.CD000335.pub2
102. Hodges PW, Richardson CA. Contraction of the abdominal muscles associated with movement of the lower limb. *Phys Ther.* 1997;77(2):132–142; discussion 142–144.
103. Hodges PW, Butler JE, McKenzie DK, Gandevia, SC. Contraction of the human diaphragm during rapid postural adjustments. *J Physiol.* 1997;505(Pt 2):539–548.
104. Hodges PW, Gandevia SC, Richardson CA. Contractions of specific abdominal muscles in postural tasks are affected by respiratory maneuvers. *J Appl Physiol.* 1997;83:753–760.
105. Hodges P, Cresswell A, Thorstensson A. Preparatory trunk motion accompanies rapid upper limb movement. *Exp Brain Res.* 1999;124(1):69–79.
106. O'Sullivan PB, Phyty GD, Twomey LT, Allison GT. Evaluation of specific stabilizing exercise in the treatment of chronic low back pain with radiologic diagnosis of spondylolysis or spondylolisthesis. *Spine* (Phila Pa 1976). 1997;22(24):2959–2967.
107. Hides JA, Jull GA, Richardson CA. Long-term effects of specific stabilizing exercises for first-episode low back pain. *Spine.* 2001;26:E243–E248.
108. Sapsford RR, Hodges PW. Contraction of the pelvic floor muscles during abdominal maneuvers. *Arch Phys Med Rehabil.* 2001;82(8):1081–1088.
109. Hagins M, Adler K, Cash M, Daugherty J, Mitrani G. Effects of practice on the ability to perform lumbar stabilization exercises. *J Orthop Sports Phys Ther.* 1999;29(9):546–555.
110. Jull G, Trott P, Potter H, et al. A randomized controlled trial of exercise and manipulative therapy for cervicogenic headache. *Spine* (Phila Pa 1976)., 2002;27(17):1835–1843; discussion 1843.
111. Wright A, Sluka KA. Nonpharmacological treatments for musculoskeletal pain. *Clin J Pain.* 2001;17(1):33–46.
112. Hanten W, Olson SL, Hodson J, Imler V, Knab V, Magee J. The effectiveness of CV-4 and resting position techniques on subjects with tension-type headaches. *J Man Manip Ther.* 1999;7:64–70.
113. Wylie KR, Jackson C, Crawford PM. Does psychological testing help to predict the response to acupuncture or massage/relaxation therapy in patients presenting to a general neurology clinic with headache? *J Tradit Chin Med.* 1997;17:130–139.
114. Preyde, M. Effectiveness of massage therapy for subacute low-back pain: a randomized controlled trial. *Can Med Assoc J.* 2000;162(13):1815–1820.
115. Walach H, Guthlin C, Konig M. Efficacy of massage therapy in chronic pain: a pragmatic randomized trial. *J Altern Complement Med.* 2003;9:837–846. doi:10.1089/107555303771952181.
116. Furlan AD, Imamura M, Dryden T, Irvin E. Massage for low-back pain. *Cochrane Database Syst Rev.* 2008(4):CD001929.
117. Burchiel KJ, Anderson VC, Brown FD, et al. Prospective, multicenter study of spinal cord stimulation for relief of chronic back and extremity pain. *Spine* (Phila Pa 1976). 1996;21(23):2786–2794.
118. Graboski CL, Gray DS, Burnham RS. Botulinum toxin A versus bupivacaine trigger point injections for the treatment of myofascial pain syndrome: a randomised double blind crossover study. *Pain.* 2005;118(1-2):170–175.
119. Strong J, Incorporating cognitive-behavioral therapy with occupational therapy: a comparative study with patients with low back pain. *J Occup Rehabil.* 1988;8(1):61–71.
120. Birkholtz M, Aylwin L, Harman RM. Activity pacing in chronic pain management: one aim, but which methods? Part 2: National Activity Pacing Survey. *Brit J Occup Ther.* 2004;67:481–487.
121. Harden RN, Swan M, King A, Costa B, Barthel J. Treatment of complex regional pain syndrome: functional restoration. *Clin J Pain.* 2006;22(5):420–424.
122. Lindsay R, Silverman SL, Cooper C, et al. Risk of new vertebral fracture in the year following a fracture. *JAMA.* 2001; 285(3):320–323.
123. Truumees E, Hilibrand A, Vaccaro AR. Percutaneous vertebral augmentation. *Spine J.* 2004;4(2):218–229.
124. Gardner MJ, Demetrakopoulos D, Shindle MK, Griffith MH, Lane JM. Osteoporosis and skeletal fractures. *HSS J.* 2006; 2(1):62–69.
125. Bonner FJ, Chesnut CH, Fitzsimmons A, et al. Osteoporosis. In: Delisa JA, Gans BM, Bockenek WL, et al, eds. *Rehabilitation Medicine: Principles and Practice.* 3rd ed. Philadelphia: Lippincott-Raven; 1998:1453–1476.
126. Fisher SV, Winter RB, Spinal orthoses in rehabilitation. In: Braddom RL, ed. *Physical Medicine and Rehabilitation.* Philadelphia: W.B. Saunders Company; 1996:359–368.
127. Rapado, A. General management of vertebral fractures. *Bone.* 1996;18(3 Suppl):191S–196S.
128. Brown KS, Folen RA. Psychologists as leaders of multidisciplinary chronic pain management teams: a model for health care delivery. *Prof Psychol Res Pr.* 2005;36:587–594. doi:10.1037/0735-7028.36.6.587
129. Bosy D, Etlin D, Corey D, Lee JW. An interdisciplinary pain rehabilitation programme: description and evaluation of outcomes. *Physiother Can.* 2010;62(4):316–326.
130. Novy DM. Invited special review: psychological approaches for managing chronic pain. *J Psychopathol Behav Assess.* 2004;26:279–288. doi:10.1023/B:JOBA.0000045343.08494.34
131. Geisser ME, Ranavaya M, Haig AJ, et al. A meta-analytic review of surface electromyography among persons with low back pain and normal, healthy controls. *J Pain.* 2005;6(11):711–726.
132. Donaldson S, Donaldson M, Snelling L. SEMG evaluations: an overview. *Appl Psychophysiol Biofeedback.* 2003;28(2):121–127.
133. Drost G, Stegeman DF, van Engelen BG, Zwarts MJ. Clinical applications of high-density surface EMG: a systematic review. *J Electromyogr Kinesiol.* 2006;16(6):586–602.
134. Lyles KW, Gold DT, Shipp KM, et al. Association of osteoporotic vertebral compression fractures with impaired functional status. *Am J Med.* 1993;94(6):595–601.
135. Wolfe MM, Lichtenstein DR, Singh G. Medical progress: gastrointestinal toxicity of nonsteroidal anti-inflammatory drugs. *N Engl J Med.* 1999;340:1888–1899.
136. Heerdink ER, Leufkens HG, Herings RM, et al. NSAIDs associated with increased risk of congestive heart failure in elderly patients taking diuretics. *Arch Intern Med.* 1998;158(10):1108–1112.

137. Laurian L, Oberman Z, Graf E, Gilad S, Hoerer E, Simantov R. Calcitonin induced increased ACTH, β-endorphin andcortical secretion. *Horm Metab Res*. 1981;18:268–271.
138. Stolker RJ, Vervest AC, Groen GJ., The treatment of chronic thoracic segmental pain by radiofrequency percutaneous partial rhizotomy. *J Neurosurg*. 1994;80(6):986–992.
139. van Kleef M, Barendse GA, Dingemans WA, et al. Effects of producing a radiofrequency lesion adjacent to the dorsal root ganglion in patients with thoracic segmental pain. *Clin J Pain*. 1995; 11(4):325–332.
140. Cohen SP, Sireci A, Wu CL, et al. Pulsed radiofrequency of the dorsal root ganglia is superior to pharmacotherapy or pulsed radiofrequency of the intercostal nerves in the treatment of chronic postsurgical thoracic pain. *Pain Physician*. 2006; 9(3):227–235.
141. Cohen SP, Bicket MC, Jamison D, Wilkinson I, Rathmell JP. Epidural steroids: a comprehensive, evidence-based review. *Reg Anesth Pain Med*. 2013;38(3):175–200.
142. Benzon HT, Chekka K, Darnule A, et al. Evidence-based case report: the prevention and management of postherpetic neuralgia with emphasis on interventional procedures. *Reg Anesth Pain Med*. 2009;34(5):514–521.
143. Pasqualucci A, Pasqualucci V, Galla F, et al. Prevention of post-herpetic neuralgia: acyclovir and prednisolone versus epidural local anesthetic and methylprednisolone. *Acta Anaesthesiol Scand*. 2000;44(8):910–918.
144. van Wijck AJ, Opstelten W, Moons KG, et al. The PINE study of epidural steroids and local anaesthetics to prevent postherpetic neuralgia: a randomised controlled trial. *Lancet*. 2006;367(9506):219–224.
145. Manchikanti L, Cash KA, McManus CD, Pampati V, Benyamin RM. A preliminary report of a randomized double-blind, active controlled trial of fluoroscopic thoracic interlaminar epidural injections in managing chronic thoracic pain. *Pain Physician*. 2010;13(6):E357–E369.
146. Benyamin RM, Wang VC, Vallejo R, Singh V, Helm Ii S. A systematic evaluation of thoracic interlaminar epidural injections. *Pain Physician*. 2012;15(4):E497–E514.
147. Destouet JM, Gilula LA, Murphy WA, Monsees B. Lumbar facet joint injection: indication, technique, clinical correlation, and preliminary results. *Radiology*. 1982;145(2):321–325.
148. Long DM, BenDebba M, Torgerson WS, et al. Persistent back pain and sciatica in the United States: patient characteristics. *J Spinal Disord*. 1996;9(1):40–58.
149. Murtagh FR. Computed tomography and fluoroscopy guided anesthesia and steroid injection in facet syndrome. *Spine* (Phila Pa 1976). 1988;13(6):686–689.
150. Lippitt AB. The facet joint and its role in spine pain. Management with facet joint injections. *Spine* (Phila Pa 1976). 1984;9(7):746–750.
151. Fairbank JC, Park WM, McCall IW, O'Brien JP. Apophyseal injection of local anesthetic as a diagnostic aid in primary low-back pain syndromes. *Spine* (Phila Pa 1976). 1981;6(6):598–605.
152. Fuchs S, Erbe T, Fischer HL, Tibesku CO. Intraarticular hyaluronic acid versus glucocorticoid injections for nonradicular pain in the lumbar spine. *J Vasc Interv Radiol*. 2005; 16(11):1493–1498.
153. Cohen SP, Raja SN. Pathogenesis, diagnosis, and treatment of lumbar zygapophysial (facet) joint pain. *Anesthesiology*. 2007;106(3):591–614.
154. Bogduk N. A narrative review of intra-articular corticosteroid injections for low back pain. *Pain Med*. 2005;6(4):287–296.
155. Slipman CW, Bhat AL, Gilchrist RV, et al. A critical review of the evidence for the use of zygapophysial injections and radiofrequency denervation in the treatment of low back pain. *Spine J*. 2003;3(4):310–316.
156. Willburger RE, Wittenberg RH. Prostaglandin release from lumbar disc and facet joint tissue. *Spine* (Phila Pa 1976). 1994;19(18):2068–2070.
157. Igarashi A, Kikuchi S, Konno S, Olmarker K. Inflammatory cytokines released from the facet joint tissue in degenerative lumbar spinal disorders. *Spine* (Phila Pa 1976). 2004;29(19):2091–2095.
158. Manchikanti L, Manchikanti KN, Manchukonda R, Pampati V, Cash KA. Evaluation of therapeutic thoracic medial branch block effectiveness in chronic thoracic pain: a prospective outcome study with minimum 1-year follow up. *Pain Physician*. 2006;9(2):97–105.
159. Stolker RJ, Vervest AC, Groen GJ. Percutaneous facet denervation in chronic thoracic spinal pain. *Acta Neurochir* (Wien). 1993;122(1-2):82–90.
160. Tzaan WC, Tasker RR. Percutaeous radiofrequency facet rhizotomy—experience with 118 procdedures and reappraisal of its value. *Can J Neurol Sci*. 2000;27(2):125–130.
161. Dreyfuss P, Halbrook B, Pauza K, et al. Efficacy and validity of radiofrequency neurotomy for chronic lumbar zygapophysial joint pain. *Spine* (Phila Pa 1976). 2000;25(10):1270–1277.
162. van Kleef M, Barendse GA, Kessels A, et al. Randomized trial of radiofrequency lumbar facet denervation for chronic low back pain. *Spine* (Phila Pa 1976). 1999;24(18):1937–1942.
163. Sundaresan N, Krol G, Steinberger AA, Moore F. Management of tumors of the thoracolumbar spine. *Neurosurg Clin N Am*. 1997;8(4):541–553.
164. Garfin SR, Buckley RA, Ledlie J. Balloon kyphoplasty for symptomatic vertebral body compression fractures results in rapid, significant, and sustained improvements in back pain, function, and quality of life for elderly patients. *Spine* (Phila Pa 1976. 2006;31(19):2213–2220.
165. Triano JJ, , Erwin M, Hansen DT. Costovertebral and costotransverse joint pain: a commonly overlooked pain generator. *Top Clin Chiropractic*. 1999;6(3):79–92.
166. Bostrom MP, Lane JM. Future directions. Augmentation of osteoporotic vertebral bodies. *Spine* (Phila Pa 1976). 1997;22(24 Suppl):38S–42S.
167. Vaccaro AR, Kim DH, Brodke DS, et al. Diagnosis and management of thoracolumbar spine fractures. *Instr Course Lect*. 2004;53:359–373.
168. Barr JD, Barr MS, Lemley TJ, McCann RM. Percutaneous vertebroplasty for pain relief and spinal stabilization. *Spine* (Phila Pa 1976). 2000;25(8):923–928.
169. McKiernan F, Faciszewski T, Jensen R. Quality of life following vertebroplasty. *J Bone Joint Surg Am*. 2004;86-A(12):2600–2606.
170. Lo YP, Chen WJ, Chen LH, Lai PL. New vertebral fracture after vertebroplasty. *J Trauma*. 2008;65(6):1439–1445.
171. Wu SS, Lachmann E, Nagler W. Current medical, rehabilitation, and surgical management of vertebral compression fractures. *J Womens Health* (Larchmt). 2003;12(1):17–26.
172. Miller FG, Kallmes DF. The case of vertebroplasty trials: promoting a culture of evidence-based procedural medicine. *Spine* (Phila Pa 1976). 2010;35(23):2023–2026.
173. Gaitanis IN, Hadjipavlou AG, Katonis PG, et al. Balloon kyphoplasty for the treatment of pathological vertebral compressive fractures. *Eur Spine J*. 2005;14(3):250–260.
174. Rohlmann A, Klockner C, Bergmann G. [The biomechanics of kyphosis]. *Orthopade*. 2001;30(12):915–918.
175. Shen MS, Kim YH. Vertebroplasty and kyphoplasty: treatment techniques for managing osteoporotic vertebral compression fractures. *Bull NYU Hosp Jt Dis*. 2006;64(3-4):106–113.
176. Buchbinder R, Osborne RH, Ebeling PR, et al. A randomized trial of vertebroplasty for painful osteoporotic vertebral fractures. *N Engl J Med*. 2009;361(6):557–568.
177. Kallmes DF, Comstock BA, Heagerty PJ, et al. A randomized trial of vertebroplasty for osteoporotic spinal fractures. *N Engl J Med*. 2009;361(6):569–579.
178. Rousing R, Andersen MO, Jespersen SM, Thomsen K, Lauritsen J. Percutaneous vertebroplasty compared to conservative treatment in patients with painful acute or subacute osteoporotic vertebral fractures: three-months follow-up in a clinical randomized study. *Spine* (Phila Pa 1976). 2009;34(13):1349–1354.

179. Lee JS, Kim KW, Ha KY. The effect of vertebroplasty on pulmonary function in patients with osteoporotic compression fractures of the thoracic spine. *J Spinal Disord Tech*. 2011;24(2):E11–E15.
180. Wardlaw D, Cummings SR,Van Meirhaeghe J, et al. Efficacy and safety of balloon kyphoplasty compared with non-surgical care for vertebral compression fracture (FREE): a randomised controlled trial. *Lancet*. 2009;373(9668):1016–1024.
181. Tolba R, Bolash RB,Shroll J, Costandi S, Dalton JE, Sanghvi C, Mekhail N. Kyphoplasty increases vertebral height, decreases both pain score and opiate requirements while improving functional status. Pain Pract. 2014 Mar;14(3):E91–97.
182. Resnick DK, Garfin SR. *Vertebroplasty and Kyphoplasty*. New York: Thieme;2005:10–13.
183. Garfin SR, Reilley MA. Minimally invasive treatment of osteoporotic vertebral body compression fractures. *Spine J*. 2002;2(1):76–80.
184. Kasperk C, Grafe IA, Schmitt S, et al. Three-year outcomes after kyphoplasty in patients with osteoporosis with painful vertebral fractures. *J Vasc Interv Radiol*. 2010;21(5):701–709.
185. Thillainadesan J, Schlaphoff G, Gibson KA, Hassett GM, McNeil HP. Long-term outcomes of vertebroplasty for osteoporotic compression fractures. *J Med Imaging Radiat Oncol*. 2010;54(4):307–314.
186. Mathis JM, Barr JD, Belkoff SM, et al. Percutaneous vertebroplasty: a developing standard of care for vertebral compression fractures. *Am J Neuroradiol*. 2001;22(2):373–381.
187. Jensen ME, Evans AJ, Mathis JM, et al. Percutaneous polymethylmethacrylate vertebroplasty in the treatment of osteoporotic vertebral body compression fractures: technical aspects. *Am J Neuroradiol*. 1997;18(10):1897–1904.
188. Cotten A, Boutry N, Cortet B, et al. Percutaneous vertebroplasty: state of the art. *Radiographics*. 1998;18(2):311–320; discussion 320–323.
189. Kumar K, Nguyen R, Bishop S. A comparative analysis of the results of vertebroplasty and kyphoplasty in osteoporotic vertebral compression fractures. *Neurosurgery*. 2010;67(3 Suppl Operative):171–188; discussion 188.
190. Flors L, Lonjedo E, Leiva-Salinas C, et al. Vesselplasty: a new technical approach to treat symptomatic vertebral compression fractures. *Am J Roentgenol*. 2009;193(1):218–226.
191. Xiong J, Dang Y, Jiang BG, Fu ZG, Zhang, DY. Treatment of osteoporotic compression fracture of thoracic/lumbar vertebrae by kyphoplasty with SKY bone expander system. *Chin J Traumatol*. 2010;13(5):270–274.
192. Gilula L, Persenaire M. Subsequent fractures post-vertebral augmentation: analysis of a prospective randomized trial in osteoporotic vertebral compression fractures. *Am J Neuroradiol*. 2013;34(1):221–227.
193. Palumbo MA, Hilibrand AS, Hart RA, Bohlman HH. Surgical treatment of thoracic spinal stenosis: a 2- to 9-year follow-up. *Spine* (Phila Pa 1976). 2001;26(5):558–566.
194. Epstein NE, Schwall G. Thoracic spinal stenosis: diagnostic and treatment challenges. *J Spinal Disord*. 1994;7(3):259–269.
195. Sudo H, Ito M, Abumi K, et al. One-stage posterior instrumentation surgery for the treatment of osteoporotic vertebral collapse with neurological deficits. *Eur Spine J*. 2010;19(6):907–915.
196. Hato T, Kawahara N, Tomita K, et al. Finite-element analysis on closing-opening correction osteotomy for angular kyphosis of osteoporotic vertebral fractures. *J Orthop Sci*. 2007; 12(4):354–360.
197. Daubs MD, Lenke LG, Cheh G, Stobbs G, Bridwell KH. Adult spinal deformity surgery: complications and outcomes in patients over age 60. *Spine* (Phila Pa 1976). 2007;32(20):2238–2244.
198. DeWald CJ, Stanley T. Instrumentation-related complications of multilevel fusions for adult spinal deformity patients over age 65: surgical considerations and treatment options in patients with poor bone quality. *Spine* (Phila Pa 1976). 2006;31(19 suppl):S144–S151.
199. Kaneda K, Taneichi H, Abumi K, et al. Anterior decompression and stabilization with the Kaneda device for thoracolumbar burst fractures associated with neurological deficits. *J Bone Joint Surg Am*. 1997;79(1):69–83.
200. Uchida K, Kobayashi S, Nakajima H, et al. Anterior expandable strut cage replacement for osteoporotic thoracolumbar vertebral collapse. *J Neurosurg Spine*. 2006;4(6):454–462.
201. Kim YJ, Bridwell KH, Lenke LG, Cheh G, Baldus C. Results of lumbar pedicle subtraction osteotomies for fixed sagittal imbalance: a minimum 5-year follow-up study. *Spine* (Phila Pa 1976). 2007;32(20):2189–2197.
202. Robinson Y, Tschoke SK, Stahel PF, Kayser R, Heyde CE. Complications and safety aspects of kyphoplasty for osteoporotic vertebral fractures: a prospective follow-up study in 102 consecutive patients. *Patient Saf Surg*. 2008;2:2.
203. Patel AA, Vaccaro AR, Martyak GG, et al. Neurologic deficit following percutaneous vertebral stabilization. *Spine* (Phila Pa 1976). 2007;32(16):1728–1734.
204. Noldge G, DaFonseca K, Grafe I et al. Balloon kyphoplasty in the treatment of back pain. *Radiologe*. 2006;46(6):506–512.
205. Verlaan JJ, Dhert WJ, Verbout AJ, Oner FC. Balloon vertebroplasty in combination with pedicle screw instrumentation: a novel technique to treat thoracic and lumbar burst fractures. *Spine* (Phila Pa 1976). 2005;30(3):E73–E79.
206. Aydogan M, Ozturk C, Karatoprak O, Tezer M, Aksu N, Hamzaoglu A. The pedicle screw fixation with vertebroplasty augmentation in the surgical treatment of the severe osteoporotic spines. *J Spinal Disord Tech*. 2009;22(6):444–447.

SECTION IV

VISCERAL PAIN

18.

PAIN FROM CHRONIC PANCREATITIS

Leonardo Kapural, Martine Puylaert, R. Matthew Walsh, and Giries W. Sweis

CASE PRESENTATION

A 42-year-old woman continues to have abdominal pain 4 years after her last hospitalization for exacerbation of chronic pancreatitis (CP) due to unknown cause. She has constant pain and intermittent exacerbations that can be severe. She is treated with short-acting opioid analgesics by her primary care physician, but the same physician will no longer prescribe more opiates because she has been asking for a dose increase. She is treated with hydrocodone/APAP 10/325 mg PO q6h PRN; her primary care physician suggested an antidepressant, but she is hesitant to use it.

Past medical history is significant for migraine and hypertension.

Past surgical history: tonsillectomy.

On examination, the patient's abdomen is soft and tender in the epigastrium, as well as in the right upper quadrant. No allodynia is noted, but some hyperalgesia is observed. Carnett sign is negative.

QUESTIONS

1. How is pain generated in CP?
2. What is the etiology of CP?
3. How is CP clinically presented?
4. How is a diagnosis of CP established?
5. How is the pain from CP managed?
   a. Conservative treatment
   b. Psychological interventions
   c. Nerve blocks and ablative and neuromodulation procedures
   d. Surgical interventions

HOW IS PAIN GENERATED IN CP?

Chronic pancreatitis is a frequently painful disease state, and its pain can be caused by several mechanisms. Localized inflammatory infiltration of sensory nerves can produce a nociceptive type of pain. In human and animal models, the degree of inflammation correlates with the severity of the pain.[1] Pressure changes in the pancreatic duct secondary to obstruction may also cause such nociceptive pain, thus suggesting that decompression procedures may relieve it.[2] A neuropathic pain component can occur in CP and may be relayed through direct changes in the dorsal root ganglia of neurons innervating the pancreas.[3] Patients with CP may develop visceral hyperalgesia that may perpetuate neuropathic pain.[4] Central and peripheral sensitization does develop in animals with CP.[5]

WHAT IS THE ETIOLOGY OF CP?

Various causes of CP have been identified including autoimmune, hereditary (e.g., cystic fibrosis gene mutation), metabolic, and idiopathic, but the most predominant cause is still alcoholism, in about 51% of patients. Although a hereditary form of CP is clinically seen relatively early in life, alcoholic pancreatitis is mainly present after 40 years of age.[6] Autoimmune pancreatitis may be an IgG4-related disease with onset after the age of 50; it occurs mainly in men. Obstruction of the main pancreatic ducts may be caused by scarring, tumors, intraductal stones, or stenosis of the papilla of Vater. Obstructive CP can be caused by narrowing or stricture of the main pancreatic duct. A large subset of patients requiring surgery have no discernible cause and are considered to have idiopathic pancreatitis.

HOW IS CP CLINICALLY PRESENTED?

Abdominal pain is the most predominant symptom, one that can influence quality of life, reduce food intake, and result in an excessive use and misuse of narcotic analgesics. Many patients complain of epigastric pain that may radiate to the back, may increase after fatty food ingestion, and is described as boring, deep, sharp, and penetrating. It is often associated with nausea and vomiting.

When pancreatic lipase secretion is significantly reduced, steatorrhea will occur. This is a symptom of advanced CP in which most of the acinar cells have been destroyed, but significant weight loss due to maldigestion is uncommon. Endocrine insufficiency may result in diabetes mellitus in up to 80% of the patients with CP. Other symptoms include jaundice, painful joints, abdominal distension, shortness of breath and pleural effusions, and pancreatic ascites.

HOW IS A DIAGNOSIS OF CP ESTABLISHED?

Physical examination does not give much additional information except for abdominal tenderness and possibly jaundice from distal biliary obstruction. In contrast to acute pancreatitis, serum lipases and amylase are normal in CP. Complete blood count, electrolytes, and liver function tests are often normal. Elevated serum bilirubin and alkaline phosphates can be indicative of intrapancreatic bile duct compromise.

It seems that functional pancreatic activity assessment (secretin and cholecystokinin [CCK]) is unnecessary in advanced chronic disease because imaging tests typically reveal morphologic changes, and these images can also be used as a guide to enzyme therapy. Quantifying enzymes (tryptase, amylase, lipase) and bicarbonate levels helps in assessing the residual functional mass of pancreas. A low level of trypsinogen has a high specificity for CP.

Five pancreatitis susceptibility genes are established: cystic fibrosis transmembrane conductance regular gene (CFTR), pancreas secretory trypsin inhibitor gene (SPINK-1), chymotrypsinogen Cgene (CTRC), calcium sensing receptor gene (CASR), and cationic trypsinogen gene (PRSS); these are linked to hereditary pancreatitis. However, routine full genetic analysis is not recommended in CP; these tests are expensive and do not contribute to establishing a diagnosis.

Diffuse calcifications on plain X-ray or computed tomography (CT) are pathognomonic for CP, but they frequently occur late in the disease course. Better specificity can be obtained by endoscopic ultrasound, which can show parenchymal changes (atrophic and fibrosis) and ductal features suggestive of CP. A reproducible set of endoscopic ultrasound criteria, the Rosemont criteria, help categorize the often subtle morphologic changes in the gland. CT with contrast provides more details about pancreatic inflammatory mass, calcifications, and duct dilation and can additionally identify pseudocysts, splenic artery pseudoaneurysms, and biliary duct involvement.[7] Unlike CT, magnetic resonance imaging (MRI) presents no radiation risk, and it can detail calcifications, atrophy, ductal abnormalities, fluid-filled cysts, and neoplastic masses. MRI better defines the biliary and pancreatic ductal anatomy and is currently preferred for surgical planning in lieu of endoscopic retrograde cholangiopancreatography (ERCP).

ERCP is used in complicated acute and chronic pancreatitis, principally for therapeutic interventions. A differential retrograde epidural block is a diagnostic test used for initial evaluation of the neural mechanisms in chronic abdominal pain. In patients with visceral pain, a differential retrograde epidural block is used as a diagnostic modality to identify which patients should receive celiac, splanchnic, or hypogastric blocks. The specificity, sensitivity, and predictive value of this test still need to be established.[8,9]

HOW IS THE PAIN FROM CP MANAGED?

CONSERVATIVE TREATMENT

The management of CP is mainly directed at the treatment of persistent pain. Some lifestyle changes are necessary, such as abstinence from alcohol even in those forms of pancreatitis that are not linked to alcohol consumption. Smoking cessation is essential. These lifestyle adjustments may reduce pain and improve life expectancy.[10,11]

Pharmacological management of chronic pain from CP may be complicated by liver and renal insufficiency, and the medication schedule needs to be adjusted accordingly.

Acetaminophen can be used for mild pain, and the use of nonsteroidal anti-inflammatory drugs (NSAIDs) can be justified despite their potential side effects that may include dyspepsia, gastric ulcerations, and even renal toxicity. Short-acting opioid preparations are suitable for more severe breakthrough pain, whereas long-acting preparations are used for more severe constant pain with or without breakthroughs. It may be necessary to combine both in some patients with persistent severe pain with breakthroughs. Their common side effects, such as nausea and vomiting, can be managed with low doses of a centrally acting antiemetic, whereas constipation can be managed with laxatives. Opioids bind to opioid receptors (μ, κ, and δ) that are invariably found in the sphincter of Oddi. Opioids may result in an increase in the contraction frequency, amplitude, and tonic rest pressure of the sphincter of Oddi muscular valve. Because this effect can only partly be counteracted by naloxone (an opioid antagonist), it is likely that the effect of morphine, or possibly other opioids, on the sphincter of Oddi is mediated by several opioid receptors. It is not clear if such increased sphincter pressure may indirectly cause development or deterioration of acute or CP.[12–14]

Membrane stabilizers and antidepressants for chronic pain are used predominantly for neuropathic pain but can be used for the treatment of CP. Tricyclic antidepressants, selective serotonin reuptake inhibitors (SSRIs), and serotonin norepinephrine reuptake inhibitors (SNRIs) are frequently prescribed. Calcium channel blockers like pregabalin or gabapentin are effective in treatment of chronic pain from CP and may provide an opioid-sparing effect.[15,16]

Ketamine in various doses has been used for treatment of chronic pain. An S-ketamine infusion for chronic pain from CP reduces hyperalgesia immediately after such infusion.[17]

Pancreatic enzyme supplementation may help in controlling chronic pain by, in optimal dosing, degrading CCK-releasing factor and thus lowering the CCK levels. The best results of therapeutic pancreatic enzyme supplementation were achieved in small duct disease or minimal-change

CP.[18] Octreotide, an inhibitor of the exocrine secretion of the pancreas, may provide analgesia by anti-inflammatory action, reduction of sphincter of Oddi pressure, and inhibition of neural stimulation.[18]

Various endoscopic and percutaneous interventions may provide pain relief in patients with CP. If the pancreatitis is caused by intraductal stones, extracorporal shock wave lithotripsy combined with endoscopic extraction of the stones has a relatively high success rate.[19] If the pancreatitis is caused by strictures of the main duct, stenting with endoscopic drainage seems to be the therapy of choice.[20] Pancreatic sphincterotomy should be performed prior to any stricture treatment.[21,22] Pancreatic pseudocysts can be also drained endoscopically; this approach has lower costs but may provide a therapeutic effect similar to that achieved by surgery.

PSYCHOLOGICAL INTERVENTIONS

Psychological treatments can improve chronic abdominal pain, and such treatment should be considered in most patients with persistent pain from CP. Those who have moderate or severe symptoms or whose pain is potentiated by stress or emotional symptoms should be provided with such a comprehensive approach.[23,24] It is the opinion of this group of physicians that such therapy should be initiated in parallel with other listed therapeutic approaches presented here and, if appropriate, continued throughout the course of treatment.

Biofeedback is one of the therapeutic approaches used to allow a patient to regain control of his or her physiological systems' functioning through the use of various mechanisms that demonstrate changes in the activity of those same systems brought about by the patient's activity. Studies on biofeedback have been promising, but current clinical evidence is rather insufficient to support its use in some painful abdominal states.[25] Previously, at least one study using thermal biofeedback suggested benefits for treatment of recurrent abdominal pain,[26] and electromyelographic (EMG) biofeedback may be beneficial in reducing constipation.[27,28] Relaxation training involving progressive muscle relaxation, thermal biofeedback, cognitive therapy, and education implemented through biofeedback training may provide some relief from chronic abdominal pain, particularly in irritable bowel syndrome (IBS).[29,30]

Hypnosis has been utilized in the treatment of various chronic pains, despite a lack of knowledge on how analgesic hypnosis actually works. In general, induction of relaxed states of focused attention and inner absorption, with a relative suspension of peripheral awareness, is combined with suggestions for pain control.[31] The primary focus of hypnotherapy research, when it comes to abdominal pain, is on IBS, with three randomized studies providing evidence for a reduction of IBS symptoms and improvement in quality of life.[32] Hypnotherapy also improved visceral pain thresholds, which could suggest similar effects in other chronic abdominal pain states.[33]

Cognitive-behavioral therapy (CBT) is psychotherapeutic approach focusing on those thoughts and feelings that influence a patient's behaviors. CBT implements various behavioral (e.g., relaxation, coping skills training) and cognitive approaches to reduce pain and pain-related disability.[34] CBT was mainly studied for pain control in IBS, with mixed results.[35,36]

A multidisciplinary chronic pain rehabilitation program that includes patient education, physical therapy, occupational therapy, medication management, individual psychotherapy, group therapy, cognitive therapy, thermal biofeedback, weaning of opioids and habituating substances, substance use education, and progressive muscle relaxation may provide both short- and long-term benefits in improving chronic pain.[37,38]

NERVE BLOCKS AND ABLATIVE AND NEUROMODULATION PROCEDURES

Nerve blocks, ablative procedures, and neuromodulating techniques aim at interrupting or modulating neural/pain conduction; when used for abdominal pain relief, multiple mechanisms of action have been speculated.

Historically, splanchnic nerves, mainly greater and lesser, and the celiac plexus were considered likely targets for pain control. In general, sympathetic innervation of the abdominal organs consists of preganglionic fibers of T5–T12 that merge with the ventral rami. Together with communicating rami, they course in the direction of the sympathetic chain. They synapse at the level of the celiac, aortorenal, and superior mesenteric ganglion.

Splanchnic nerves confluence with the vagal preganglionic parasympathetic fibers, sensory fibers of the phrenic nerve, and postganglionic sympathetic fibers to form the celiac plexus, which is widely spread around the abdominal aorta, especially anteriorly. The location of the splanchnic nerves is in a narrow space between the lateral border of the vertebra and medial pleura.[39]

Although commonly used nerve blocks using long-acting local anesthetic may significantly reduce the pain caused by pancreatic cancer and pancreatitis, neurolysis of the celiac plexus using alcohol or phenol provides prolonged pain relief in those patients with end-stage pancreatic cancer.[40] Limited use of such neurolytic agents in cancer patients is advised due to the unpredictable flow of the agent and therefore uncontrolled lesion size; this can result in rare catastrophic consequences like paraplegia and retroperitoneal fibrosis.

Splanchnic and celiac plexus blocks are performed percutaneously under fluoroscopic guidance. Several approaches, such as transaortic, retrocrural, and transdiscal, are used without a clear advantage accruing to the use one over another[41] (Figure 18.1).

Although computed tomography (CT) guidance provides better visualization of the anatomic structures during more demanding neurolytic celiac plexus block, in patients with nonmalignant pain, repeated exposure to radiation and the expense of CT guidance does not justify its use.[42]

Endoscopic ultrasound guidance for celiac plexus block or celiac plexus neurolysis provides good pain relief in only 55% of patients at 4 and 8 weeks follow-up. Complications from the endoscopic approach are at about 1.8%, and these include the possibility of major complications such as paraplegia.[44]

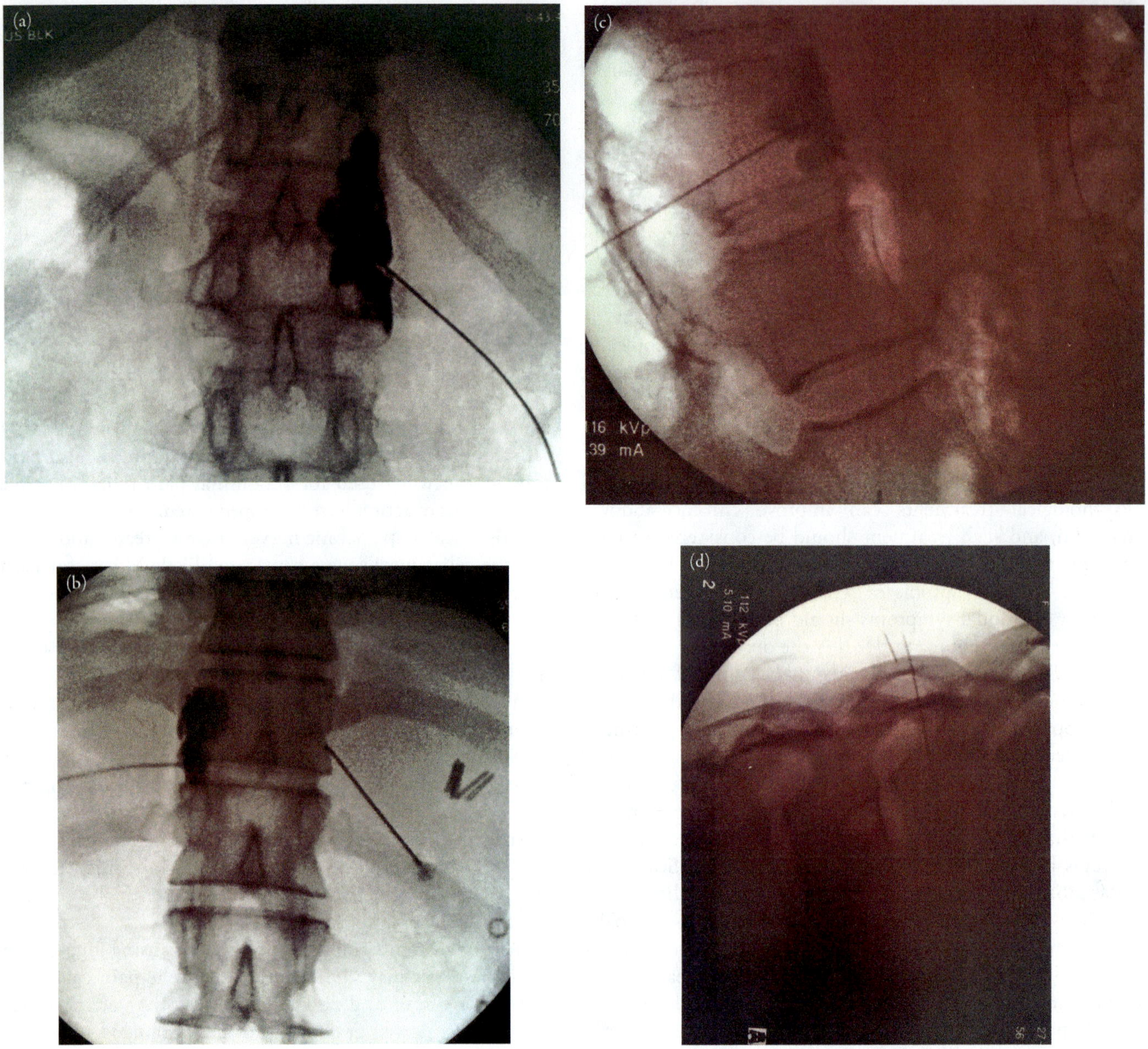

Figure 18.1 Celiac plexus (A) and splanchnic nerve block (B) needle and contrast position in AP intraprocedural fluoroscopic view. Approximately 20 cc of 0.375% bupivacaine was injected bilaterally during celiac plexus block (A) and 10 cc bilaterally during splanchnic nerve block (B) following contrast dye verification of proper needle placement. Notice that the needle at the T11 level (B) when used for the splanchnic block is kept in contact with the concavity of the T11 vertebral body and in the posterior third of the body width. Needle passage to the vertebral body is always maintained at the top of the corresponding foramina in order to minimize the frequency of possible paresthesias.

Splanchnic nerve blocks are frequently followed by radiofrequency (RF) denervation for prolonged pain relief (Figure 18.2). Predictable nerve position and a low frequency of serious complications compared to neurolytics are advantages of splanchnic RF.

Contrast should be used before lesioning to ensure extravascular and extrapleural position of the RF needles. The RF generator is adjusted to 70°C, and lesioning time is 90 seconds.

Two larger case series on the use of RF ablative procedures suggested a significant improvements in pain scores for patients who suffer from CP[45,46]; 73 out of 107 patients who positively responded to a diagnostic block were followed prospectively. Whereas 38 of them received another block, 31 received RF treatment. In both groups, pain relief of greater than 50% was found in 40% of patients. Another study[46] described the long-term effects of splanchnic RF in 10 patients with a follow-up of about 18 months. A significant reduction of pain scores, use of opiates, and frequency of acute hospitalization was reported.

Better pain control was also reported over a mean period of 45 weeks in 11 out of 18 patients, and opioid use was significantly reduced.[47] Patients with previous positive responses had repeated denervation with repetitive comparable therapeutic effect. Return of abdominal pain was speculated to be caused by nerve regeneration. Complications may include postprocedural neuritis and, more frequently, hypotension and diarrhea.

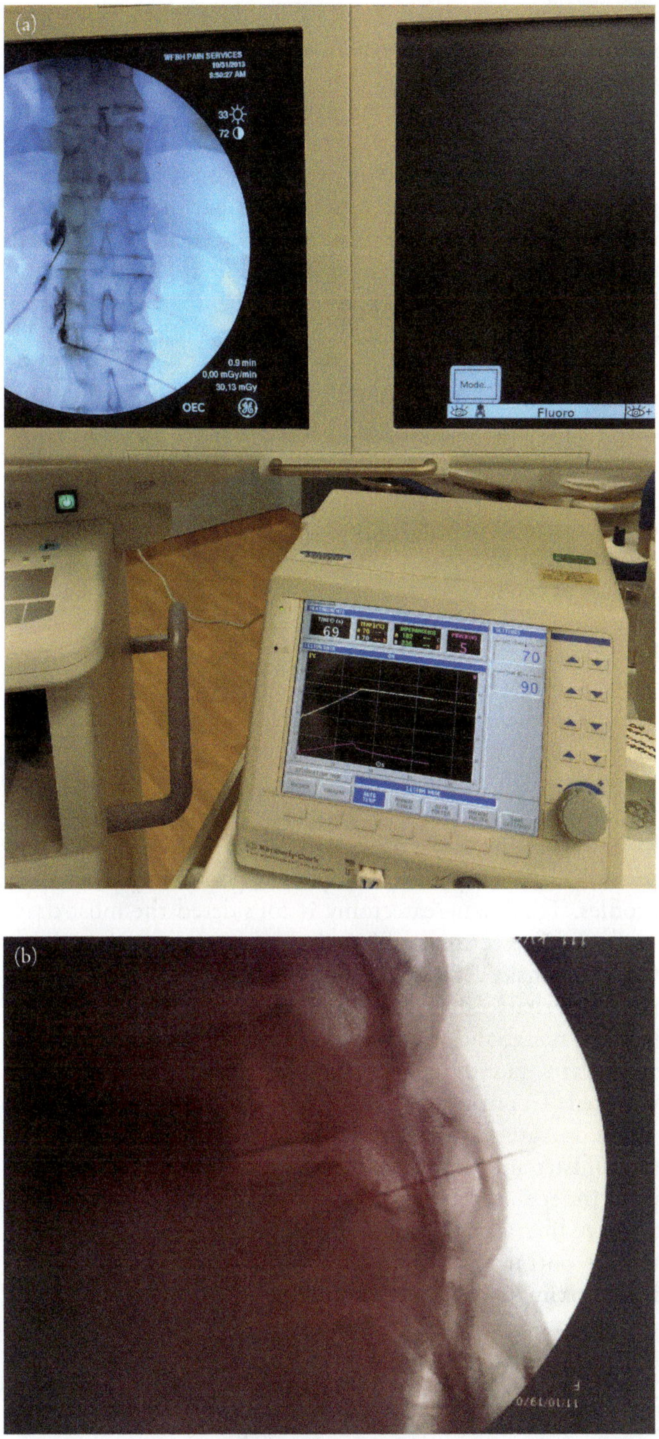

Figure 18.2 Radiofrequency (RF) denervation of splanchnic nerves. A. The RF setup during splanchnic denervation showing in the upper left corner a proper AP fluoroscopic view of the electrodes. In this case 20-gauge, 100 mm, 10 mm active tip curved RF needles were positioned on the left side of vertebral body of T11 and T12.

Despite the fact that thoracoscopic splanchnicectomy for pancreatic pain is, at least initially, a highly successful procedure in alleviating pain from CP, patients' chronic pain returns at 6 months in about 25% of those treated and in more than 50% of patients in the long-term. Splanchnicectomy is an extensive procedure involving dissection of the parietal pleura and transection of the splanchnic nerve fibers at the thoracic level, and the risks of anesthesia with an endotracheal double-lumen tube in the prone position cannot be discounted. Interestingly, it appears that additional vagotomy does not provide additional pain relief.[48,49]

The use of spinal cord stimulation (SCS) to treat visceral pain and pain from CP was initially presented via several case reports.[50,51] More recently, several larger retrospective publications provided further evidence that SCS may be an effective long-term solution for those patients with severe CP. Two of these studies included patients with clearly identified but various causes of chronic abdominal pain and visceral hyperalgesia,[52,53] whereas a third study included 54 patients with only CP (Figure 18.3). The first study involved 30 out of 35 patients who reported 50% or greater relief of pain at the end of the SCS trial.[52] They were followed for more than 1 year, and they maintained similar pain relief.

A comprehensive national survey on SCS for chronic abdominal pain that followed this retrospective study included 76 case reports, and its results were consistent in the technical aspects of SCS implantation, as well as in the opioid use and pain score improvements.[53] Both studies suggested that the "sweet spot" for SCS when it comes to various causes of chronic abdominal pain is a standard octrapolar lead tip placed near the top of the fifth thoracic vertebral body in the posterior epidural space. Pain relief exceeded 50% in most of the patients, and their long-term opioid use decreased by more than two-thirds.[52–53] In both studies, the largest numbers of participants were patients with severe CP:[52,53] 26 out of 35 patients in the retrospective study and 26 out of 70 patients in

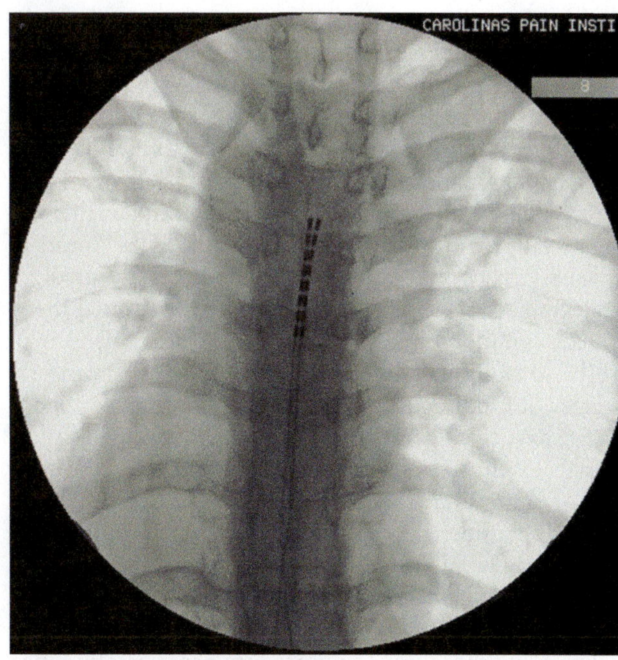

Figure 18.3 Anteroposterior view of the epidural leads using intraoperative fluoroscopy during positioning of two octrode leads. The most common "sweet spot" to achieve proper stimulation within the abdominal area is the midline positioned lead near the top of the T5 vertebral body. Such posterior epidural position was also confirmed in the lateral view.

the survey study carried a diagnosis of CP. Data from the subgroup of the patients with CP showed similar improvements in pain and opiate use to those in patients with other sources of chronic abdominal pain.

Subsequent retrospective analysis examined 30 consecutive patients with severe pain due to CP who underwent a trial with SCS for 7–14 days. Twenty-four patients reported 80% pain relief at the end of the trial period. After definite implantation, one patient was lost to follow-up, and in three patients the system had to be removed because of infection. At 1-year follow-up, visual analog (VAS) pain scores and opioid consumption were both profoundly reduced, reflecting the results of previous studies.[54] The main complications of SCS are wound infection and lead migration.

An attempt was also made to directly stimulate splanchnic nerves, and this resulted in long-term pain reduction and decreased opioid consumption in one case report of a patient with CP. Octapolar leads were placed along the mid-vertebral body of T11–T12 and connected to an implantable pulse generator using a relatively simple approach with stable lead placement. This therapy should be investigated further.[55]

SURGICAL INTERVENTIONS

Surgery for pain relief in CP should be considered if medical or endoscopic treatments do not provide satisfactory pain relief. Chronic pain from CP can be improved by using a variety of surgical procedures tailored to the specific morphology of the disease. The two general surgical procedures are duct decompression with or without resection. The goal of surgical treatment is to alleviate all manifestations of the disease while minimizing parenchymal loss.[56,57]

A lateral pancreaticojejunostomy, the Partington-Rochelle modification of the Puestow procedure, is a proven procedure that purely achieves ductal drainage. This spleen-preserving longitudinal drainage procedure can be accomplished with low morbidity and mortality rates. This procedure has been one of the dominant pancreatic procedures; short-term pain relief is achieved in more than 75% of patients, but this success rate falls off over time to roughly 50% at 5–7 years of follow-up. Other procedures that are principally used for ductal drainage include any of the sphincter-directed therapies, such as minor sphincteroplasty for pancreatic divisum or dual (biliary and main pancreatic duct) sphincteroplasty for sphincter of Oddi dysfunction. These procedures for ductal drainage have the highest degree of parenchymal sparing.

Some extent of resection is a component of all other forms of surgical treatment for CP. The procedures most commonly considered to be extensions of ductal drainage are the Frey and DuVal procedures. The Frey procedure includes incomplete resection of the pancreatic head in conjunction with the later longitudinal drainage of the duct, as is done in a Puestow procedure. The procedure has generally superseded the Puestow procedure in most patients requiring ductal drainage, especially if there is an inflammatory head mass. The Frey procedure has been shown to have superior results compared to other pancreatic head resections in randomized trials. The DuVal procedure includes a short distal pancreatectomy with drainage of the duct into a Roux jejunal limb for ductal decompression. More extensive resections occur in distal or subtotal pancreatectomy, Whipple, Beger, and Berne procedures. Distal pancreatectomy of any amount that does not include ductal drainage should be reserved for patients with clearly focal disease in the body and tail of the pancreas.[57] The Whipple procedure is performed similarly to the operation done for pancreatic cancer, and, in fact, the concern for pancreatic cancer in a patient with CP would be a reason to select this procedure. The operation includes cholecystectomy and excision of the distal bile duct, duodenum, and head of the pancreas. It is particularly useful in patients with multiple complications of CP, including biliary or duodenal obstruction, particularly with a head mass. In the United States, it is the most common resection done for CP involving the pancreatic head. The Berger procedure is a duodenum-preserving resection of the pancreatic head that includes subtotal resection of the pancreatic head, transection of the neck of the pancreas, and drainage by pancreaticojejunostomy. The Berne procedure includes an isolated head resection, similar to the Beger, but without division of the pancreatic neck. Both Beger and Berne procedures have the advantage of not including resection of the duodenum, which may contribute to the favorable results shown in clinical trials when compared to the Whipple procedure. All of these head resections are more complex procedures with higher morbidity than other pancreatic procedures, but, for properly selected patients, they show good early pain relief profiles. Total pancreatectomy is considered the most drastic form of resection and is indicated in some patients with CP. It is considered for patients with disabling quality of life from CP that is due to genetic abnormalities or idiopathic CP. The metabolic consequences of total pancreatectomy are significant, but the procedure treats completely the organ involved. To mitigate the metabolic endocrine consequences of the operation, specialized centers have included the addition of islet autotransplantation. This allows partial or complete independence from exogenous insulin by native islets that are liberated from the gland and infused into the liver via the portal vein. Complete insulin independence occurs in approximately in 25–35% of patients, but the remainder of patients are usually pleased with the small amounts of insulin they require for glucose control. The operation is effective in pain control and improvement in quality of life in properly selected patients.[57]

Recent studies suggest that preoperative opioid use is a negative predictor of long-term pain relief after either surgical or endoscopic interventions. It could be that central sensitization or opioid dependency may be causes.[58,59] Earlier surgical interventions likely provide better pain relief compared to endoscopic interventions, and they carry similar complication rates.[60,61]

CONCLUSION

When establishing a pharmacological treatment plan for chronic abdominal pain, nonanalgesic drugs should also be considered. Membrane stabilizers and antidepressants for pain, such as calcium channel blocking agents or norepinephrine reuptake inhibitors, seem to be effective. Other potential targets in the treatment of chronic abdominal pain are nerve growth factor inhibitors and the TRPV1 antagonist. Concerning central sensitization, indirect N-methyl-D-aspartate (NMDA) receptor antagonists may be found useful in the future despite their very narrow therapeutic window.

Chronic abdominal pain is a complex physical and psychological problem that requires an understanding of its clinical, physical, and psychosocial features and providing treatment options tailored to the needs of patients. An integrated biopsychosocial treatment plan combined with comprehensive treatment for chronic abdominal pain may offer better clinical outcomes.

Despite the fact that celiac and splanchnic nerve blocks were long a part of the armamentarium of pain physicians, RF denervation of the greater and lesser splanchnic nerves to provide prolonged treatment effects needs to be studied in a formal, randomized, prospective study. SCS appears to be a robust yet minimally invasive therapy that has a promising future when it comes to pain control from CP. Comparative studies between surgery and endoscopic treatment show evidence in favor of early surgery.

REFERENCES

1. Anaparthy R, Pasricha PJ. Pain and chronic pancreatitis: is it the plumbing or the wiring? Current gastroenterology reports. *Curr Gastroenterol Rep.* 2008;10:101–106.
2. Lieb JG, 2nd, Forsmark CE. Review article: pain and chronic pancreatitis. *Aliment Pharmacol Ther.* 2009;29:706–719.
3. DiMagno MJ, DiMagno EP. Chronic pancreatitis. *Curr Opin Gastroenterol.* 2012;28:523–531.
4. Pasricha PJ. Unraveling the mystery of pain in chronic pancreatitis. *Nat Rev Gastroenterol Hepatol.* 2012;9:140–151.
5. Pasca di Magliano M, Forsmark C, Freedman S, et al. Advances in acute and chronic pancreatitis: from development to inflammation and repair. *Gastroenterology.* 2013;144:e1–e4.
6. Yadav D, Lowenfels AB. The epidemiology of pancreatitis and pancreatic cancer. *Gastroenterology.* 2013;144:1252–1261.
7. Kim HC, Yang DM, Kim HJ, Lee DH, Ko YT, Lim JW. Computed tomography appearances of various complications associated with pancreatic pseudocysts. *Acta Radiol.* 2008;49:727–734.
8. Rizk MK, Tolba R, Kapural L, et al. Differential epidural block predicts the success of visceral block in patients with chronic visceral abdominal pain. *Pain Pract.* 2012;12:595–601.
9. Bielefeldt K, Gebhart G. Visceral pain. In: Benzon HT, Rathmell J, Wu C, Turk D, Argoff C, eds. *Raj's Practical Management of Pain.* 4th ed. Philadelphia: Mosby Elsevier; 2008:529–540.
10. Lankisch PG, Lohr-Happe A, Otto J, Creutzfeldt W. Natural course in chronic pancreatitis. Pain, exocrine and endocrine pancreatic insufficiency and prognosis of the disease. *Digestion.* 1993;54:148–155.
11. Layer P, Yamamoto H, Kalthoff L, Clain JE, Bakken LJ, DiMagno EP. The different courses of early- and late-onset idiopathic and alcoholic chronic pancreatitis. *Gastroenterology.* 1994;107:1481–1487.
12. Radnay PA, Brodman E, Mankikar D, Duncalf D. The effect of equi-analgesic doses of fentanyl, morphine, meperidine and pentazocine on common bile duct pressure. *Anaesthesist.* 1980;29:26–29.
13. Helm JF, Venu RP, Geenen JE, et al. Effects of morphine on the human sphincter of Oddi. *Gut.* 1988;29:1402–1407.
14. Gachago C, Draganov PV. Pain management in chronic pancreatitis. *World J Gastroenterol.* 2008;14:3137–3148.
15. Olesen SS, Bouwense SA, Wilder-Smith OH, van Goor H, Drewes AM. Pregabalin reduces pain in patients with chronic pancreatitis in a randomized, controlled trial. *Gastroenterology.* 2011;141:536–543.
16. Olesen SS, Graversen C, Olesen AE, et al. Randomised clinical trial: pregabalin attenuates experimental visceral pain through sub-cortical mechanisms in patients with painful chronic pancreatitis. *Aliment Pharmacol Ther.* 2011;34:878–887.
17. Bouwense SA, Buscher HC, van Goor H, Wilder-Smith OH. S-ketamine modulates hyperalgesia in patients with chronic pancreatitis pain. *Reg Anesth Pain Med.* 2011;36:303–307.
18. Lieb JG, 2nd, Forsmark CE. Review article: pain and chronic pancreatitis. *Aliment Pharmacol Ther.* 2009;29:706–719.
19. Nguyen-Tang T, Dumonceau JM. Endoscopic treatment in chronic pancreatitis, timing, duration and type of intervention. Best practice & research. *Clin Gastroenterol.* 2010;24:281–298.
20. Dumonceau JM, Delhaye M, Tringali A, et al. Endoscopic treatment of chronic pancreatitis: European Society of Gastrointestinal Endoscopy (ESGE) Clinical Guideline. *Endoscopy.* 2012;44:784–800.
21. Ponchon T, Bory RM, Hedelius F, et al. Endoscopic stenting for pain relief in chronic pancreatitis: results of a standardized protocol. *Gastrointest Endosc.*1995;42:452–456.
22. Smits ME, Badiga SM, Rauws EA, Tytgat GN, Huibregtse K. Long-term results of pancreatic stents in chronic pancreatitis. *Gastrointest Endosc.*1995;42:461–467.
23. Drossman DA, Camilleri M, Mayer EA, Whitehead WE. AGA technical review on irritable bowel syndrome. *Gastroenterology.* 2002;123:2108–2131.
24. Palsson OS, Whitehead WE. Psychological treatments in functional gastrointestinal disorders: a primer for the gastroenterologist. *Clin Gastroenterol Hepatol.* 2013:11(3):208–216.
25. Coulter ID, Favreau JT, Hardy ML, Morton SC, Roth EA, Shekelle P. Biofeedback interventions for gastrointestinal conditions: a systematic review. *Altern Ther Health Med.* 2002;8(3):76–83.
26. Humphreys P, Gevirtz R. Treatment of recurrent abdominal pain: components analysis of four treatment protocols. *J Pediatr Gastroenterol Nutr.* 2000;31:47–51.
27. Bassotti G, Chistolini F, Sietchiping-Nzepa F, De Roberto G, Morelli A, Chiarioni G. Biofeedback for pelvic floor dysfunction in constipation. *Br Med J.* 2004;328(7436):393–396.
28. Chiarioni G, Salandini L, Whitehead WE. Biofeedback benefits only patients with outlet dysfunction, not patients with isolated slow transit constipation. *Gastroenterology.* 2005;129(1):86–97.
29. Blanchard EB, Schwarz SP, Suls JM, Gerardi MA, Scharff L, Greene B, et al. Two controlled evaluations of multicomponent psychological treatment of irritable bowel syndrome. *Behav Res Ther.* 1992;30(2):175–189.
30. Schwarz SP, Blanchard EB, Neff DF. Behavioral treatment of irritable bowel syndrome: a 1 year follow-up study. *Biofeedback Self Regul.* 1986;11(3):189–198.
31. Kupers R, Faymonville ME, Laureys S. The cognitive modulation of pain: hypnosis and placebo induced analgesia. *Rog Brain Res.* 2005;150:251–269.
32. Blanchard EB, Scharff L. Psychosocial aspects of assessment and treatment of irritable bowel syndrome in adults and recurrent abdominal pain in children. *J Consult Clin Psychol.* 2002; 70:725–738.
33. Lea R, Houghton LA, Calvert EL, Larder S, Gonsalkorale WM, Whelan V, et al. Gut-focused hypnotherapy normalizes disordered rectal sensitivity in patients with irritable bowel syndrome. *Aliment Pharmacol Ther.* 2003;17:635–642.
34. Sullivan MJ, Thorn B, Haythornthwaite JA, Theoretical perspectives on the relation between catastrophizing and pain. *Clin J Pain.* 2001;17:52–64.
35. Blanchard EB, Keefer L, Galovski TE, Taylor AE, Turner SM. Gender differences in psychological distress among patients with irritable bowel syndrome. *J Psychosom Res.* 2001;50:271–275.

36. Drossman DA, Toner BB, Whitehead WE. Cognitive-behavioral therapy versus education and desipramine versus placebo for moderate to severe functional disorders. *Gastroenterology.* 2003;125:19–31.
37. Schwarz SP, Taylor AE, Scharff L, Blanchard EB. Behaviorally treated irritable bowel syndrome patients: a four-year follow-up. *Behav Res Ther.* 1990;28:331–335.
38. Blanchard EB, Schwarz SP, Neff DF. Two-year follow-up of behavioral treatment of irritable bowel syndrome. *Behav Ther.* 1988;19(1):67–73.
39. Puylaert M, Kapural L, Van Zundert J, et al. 26. Pain in chronic pancreatitis. Pain Pract. 2011; Sep-Oct;11(5):492–505.
40. Vissers KC, Besse K, Wagemans M, et al. 23. Pain in patients with cancer. Pain Pract. 2011; Sep-Oct;11(5):453–75.
41. Eisenberg E, Carr DB, Chalmers TC. Neurolytic celiac plexus block for treatment of cancer pain: a meta-analysis. *Anesth Analg.*1995;80:290–295.
42. Rathmell JP, Gallant JM, Brown DL. Computed tomography and the anatomy of celiac plexus block. *Reg Anesth Pain Med.* 2000;25:411–416.
43. Gress F, Schmitt C, Sherman S, Ciaccia D, Ikenberry S, Lehman G. Endoscopic ultrasound-guided celiac plexus block for managing abdominal pain associated with chronic pancreatitis: a prospective single center experience. *Am J Gastroenterol.* 2001; 96:409–416.
44. Mittal MK, Rabinstein AA, Wijdicks EF. Pearls & oysters: acute spinal cord infarction following endoscopic ultrasound-guided celiac plexus neurolysis. *Neurology.* 2012;78:e57–e59.
45. Prithvi Raj P, Sahinder B, Lowe M. Radiofrequency lesioning of splanchnic nerves. *Pain Practice.* 2002;2:241–247.
46. Garcea G, Thomasset S, Berry DP, Tordoff S. Percutaneous splanchnic nerve radiofrequency ablation for chronic abdominal pain. *ANZ J Surg.* 2005;75:640–644.
47. Verhaegh BP, van Kleef M, Geurts JW, et al. Percutaneous radiofrequency ablation of the splanchnic nerves in patients with chronic pancreatitis: results of single and repeated procedures in 11 patients. *Pain Pract.* 2013; Nov;13(8):621–626.
48. Buscher HC, Jansen JB, van Dongen R, Bleichrodt RP, van Goor H. Long-term results of bilateral thoracoscopic splanchnicectomy in patients with chronic pancreatitis. *Br J Surg.* 2002;89:158–162.
49. Howard TJ, Swofford JB, Wagner DL, Sherman S, Lehman GA. Quality of life after bilateral thoracoscopic splanchnicectomy: long-term evaluation in patients with chronic pancreatitis. *J Gastrointest Surg.* 2002;6:845–852; discussion 853–844.
50. Khan I, Raza S, Khan E. Application of spinal cord stimulation for the treatment of abdominal visceral pain syndromes: case reports. *Neuromodulation.* 2005;8:14–27.
51. Kapural L, Rakic M. Spinal cord stimulation for chronic visceral pain secondary to chronic non-alcoholic pancreatitis. *J Clin Gastroenterol.* 2008;42:750–751.
52. Kapural L, Nagem H, Tlucek H, Sessler DI. Spinal cord stimulation for chronic visceral abdominal pain. *Pain Med.* 2010;11:347–355.
53. Kapural L, Deer T, Yakovlev A, et al. Technical aspects of spinal cord stimulation for managing chronic visceral abdominal pain: the results from the national survey. *Pain Med.* 2010;11:685–691.
54. Kapural L, Cywinski JB, Sparks DA. Spinal cord stimulation for visceral pain from chronic pancreatitis. *Neuromodulation.* 2011;14:423–426; discussion 426–427.
55. Goroszeniuk T, Khan R. Permanent percutaneous splanchnic nerve neuromodulation for management of pain due to chronic pancreatitis: a case report. *Neuromodulation.* 2011;14:253–257; discussion 257.
56. Strate T. Resection vs drainage in treatment of chronic pancreatitis: long-term results of a randomized trial. *Gastroenterology.* 2008;134:1406–1411.
57. Mullhaupt B, Ammann RW. Total pancreatectomy for intractable pain in chronic pancreatitis? *Pancreas.* 2010;39:111–112.
58. Ahmed AU, Nieuwenhuijs VB, van Eijck CH, et al. Clinical outcome in relation to timing of surgery in chronic pancreatitis: a nomogram to predict pain relief. *Arch Surg.* 2012;147:925–932.
59. Negi S, Singh A, Chaudhary A. Pain relief after Frey's procedure for chronic pancreatitis. *Br J Surg.* 2010;97:1087–1095.
60. Dite P, Ruzicka M, Zboril V, Novotny I. A prospective, randomized trial comparing endoscopic and surgical therapy for chronic pancreatitis. *Endoscopy.* 2003;35:553–558.
61. Cahen DL, Gouma DJ, Nio Y, et al. Endoscopic versus surgical drainage of the pancreatic duct in chronic pancreatitis. *New Engl J Med.* 2007;356:676–684.

19.

CHRONIC PELVIC PAIN

Thomas C. Chelimsky, Jeffrey Janata, Susie As-Sanie, Frank F. Tu, and Denniz Zolnoun

CASE PRESENTATION

Lori is a 19-year-old young woman in her second year of college. After the semester break, over the past 2 months, she has developed severe, aching pelvic pain. She was previously sexually active, but her dyspareunia has been so severe that she had to stop all sexual activity. The pain is not affected by body position, such as sitting or lying flat. She has experienced some urgency and frequency, 14 times per day, and nocturia about 4 times per night. The pain is slightly worse with a full bladder and improves temporarily after she voids, from 7 to 6/10. The pain ranges from 4 to 9/10. There are no associated bowel complaints. The pain worsens slightly with her menstrual periods, which have become heavier but are still regular.

Her evaluation, performed at an outside hospital, included normal pelvic ultrasound, normal Pap smear, and normal pelvic exam (except for severe tenderness on insertion of both the examining finger and the speculum). She saw several physicians near her college, and she was ultimately placed on hydromorphone 4 mg BID because the pain was so severe. This relieved her pain for 3 hours or so. Because of night pain, she was prescribed lorazepam 2 mg at bedtime, which helped her get to sleep and stay asleep, although her sleep did not provide her with any energy in the morning.

QUESTIONS

1. What is the differential diagnosis of chronic pelvic pain (CPP)?
2. What are the methods of assessing CPP?
3. What is the pathophysiology of CPP ?
4. How are the psychological aspects of pelvic pain managed?

WHAT IS THE DIFFERENTIAL DIAGNOSIS OF CPP?

This history is very typical for one of the CPP disorders, particularly myofascial pelvic pain (MPP) or interstitial cystitis/bladder pain syndrome (IC/BPS). Typical features include onset in a young adult, without clear cause, severe pain localized to the pelvis, and severe dyspareunia. Features that distinguish IC include pain more localized to the bladder, significantly worse when the bladder is full and often greatly diminished once the bladder is empty, and the constant feeling of having a urinary tract infection despite negative studies. Examination of MPP is visually and anatomically normal but demonstrates exquisite tenderness of the pelvic floor muscles, usually not present in isolated IC, although the two conditions often coexist. Isolated IC will usually demonstrate tenderness on palpation of the bladder and may show petechial hemorrhages (glomerulations) or Hunner's ulcers on cystoscopy.[1]

Examination shows severely tender abdominal musculature and adductor muscles in all three segments, distal at the knee, at the mid thigh, and at the proximal thigh. Pelvic examination is visually normal. The pelvic and abdominal muscles are exquisitely tender to palpation, including both levator ani complexes, both internal obliques, and the perineal body. Palpation of the bladder, uterus, and fornices, as well as a bimanual and rectovaginal examination, show no specific abnormalities (e.g., nodules, fixed masses) or tenderness. In addition, examination for fibromyalgia reveals 14 of 18 possible tender points. There are no other findings.

Based on this examination, we suspect that pelvic structural pathology is less likely causing our patient's pain. In addition, the tenderness of all muscles speaks of a generalized pelvic pain process, such as MPP, with IC being less likely given the absence of any bladder tenderness. Furthermore, the tenderness of the adductors and of the body muscles reflected in the 14 of 18 tender points on fibromyalgia examination suggests a diffuse process that extends beyond the pelvis. It will be important to determine what other support is found for such a diffuse process, in particular by assessing comorbidities.

Further history reveals that she has had other pain syndromes in her life. She had menstrual migraines since age 14, occurring 4–5 times per year, which have become almost daily since the onset of her pelvic pain. In the past 6 months, she has experienced abdominal pain prior to some bowel movements, and those tend to be loose although not watery or bloody. At age 16, she was diagnosed with a panic disorder and generalized anxiety, both of which were well managed with a combination of selective serotonin reuptake inhibitors (SSRIs) and behavior therapy until the past few months. Finally, her sleep has been disrupted, and she seldom wakes up feeling refreshed, even when she sleeps late into the morning. Social history is remarkable for a major change in her school life. She is in her second year of college, having received mostly A's in her freshman year. However, she is currently on leave and living at home, because she was unable to attend classes due to pain.

Beyond fibromyalgia, we now have evidence of several other comorbid disorders, including migraine headaches since age 14, panic and generalized anxiety since age 16, and, more recently, probable irritable bowel syndrome (IBS) and a major disruption in sleep effectiveness. In addition, it is important to attend to the changes that have occurred in her life functions. She has become debilitated to the point of putting a hold on a promising college trajectory. More than likely, her comorbidities play a major role in this decision, although, from the patient's perspective, the entire focus of her complaint is on her pelvic pain. The next major questions will emphasize her family—both family history and exposure to early trauma.

WHAT ARE THE METHODS OF ASSESSING CPP?

FAMILY HISTORY

Family history reveals that her mother, one of three sisters, and three maternal aunts have migraine headaches; her mother has IBS and fibromyalgia; she also has a sister, maternal aunt, and three cousins with postural tachycardia syndrome (POTS). Another sister has biopsy-proven endometriosis and a generalized anxiety disorder. Her mother remarried when our patient was 8 years old, and, when she was diagnosed with generalized anxiety, a history of sexual abuse of our patient over a 4-year period by her stepfather (who is now in jail) was uncovered.

Extensive family history of these same comorbidities is the rule. Specific disorders that should be sought in the family include migraine headache, IBS, pelvic pain, Raynaud syndrome, functional dyspepsia, functional abdominal pain, cyclic vomiting syndrome, idiopathic chronic nausea, POTS, syncope, panic and anxiety disorders, temporomandibular joint disorder, complex regional pain syndrome, and fibromyalgia. It is unclear at this point whether this familiality represents common environmental and behavioral factors, epigenetic factors, genetic factors, or some combination. Unfortunately, the history of sexual abuse is common and will require specific therapy if it has not already been addressed.[2] This issue should be inquired about in a delicate manner and can be left to the psychologist in an interdisciplinary team.

BEDSIDE SENSORY TESTING

In this chapter's case study, local sensory testing was not particularly revealing. However, in other cases involving a postsurgical pain syndrome or in any setting associated with a specific traumatic event, a detailed bedside sensory examination may provide highly clinically significant diagnostic information. A few clinical caveats need to be stated to provide a context for the final diagnosis of neuropathic pain and the location of sensory abnormalities. First and foremost, the pelvic region has poor point discrimination, making it difficult for patients to identify the exact location of their pain. Second, the standard dermatome maps detailed in any textbook, with their cleanly delineated dermatomes, is for demonstrative purposes only, and there is a significant overlap in innervation distribution, as with all dermatomes in the body. Third, the anatomical landmarks and corresponding sensory innervation in the genital region (particularly in women) are not characterized and hence are the focus of ongoing investigation.

The following steps may help to provide an accurate evaluation.

Step 1: Orientation and Situating the Patient

- The patient is directed to point to the area of maximal pain to the best of her ability. The objective is to examine the least sensitive region first in order to avoid triggering a diffuse pain response.
- In general, the abdomen will be examined first, followed by the pelvis.
- Patients are oriented to verbal cues and sensation. For example, using unaffected skin, patients are oriented to cottons swab, pinprick, and gentle stroke sensation using a wooden cotton swab. Gentle stroke is the experience of moving the cotton swab across skin. Pinprick is the sensation of touching the skin with a sharp wooden stick, approximately the caliber of a toothpick. The cotton swab stimulus requires the cotton swab to be applied perpendicular to the skin with enough force to indent the skin.

Step 2: Assessment of Symmetry for Perception of Gentle Stroking

- The examination proceeds from the unaffected side to the affected side. The examiner strokes the cotton swab laterally to medially along the dermatome starting at the bellybutton (approximately T10) and alternating from side to side across dermatomes and moving downward toward the mons (approximate level of L1). Skin regions reported as having abnormal sensation (dysesthesia; abnormal sensation) are demarcated (e.g., numbness, rawness, etc.) with a marker.
- This process clarifies the abnormal region or regions in the abdomen and pelvis (or lack thereof) and their (a) symmetry.

Step 3: Assessment of Allodynia

- Examination for abnormal sensation by perpendicular application of the cotton swab is primarily done in the vulvar region. The objective is to identify abnormal sensation of the vulvar mucosa whereby perpendicular application of cotton swab is misperceived as pinprick (allodynia).

Step 4. Assessment of Pinprick Hyperalgesia

- The last part of the sensory assessment involves examining the affected area with a wooden stick (toothpick) for sensitivity. The objective of this test is to localize the primary region of pain to determine if a diagnostic nerve block might be useful. Normally, the repetitive application of the wooden stick leads to temporal summation whereby repetitive stimulation becomes progressively more painful. For example, a pinprick that is perceived as 1 (on a scale of 0 being no pain and 10 being the most intense pain imaginable) becomes a 6 or 7 after repetitive stimulation of the same area after upward of 12 stimulations are administered less than 2 seconds apart. In a person with nerve irritation/injury, pain levels as high as 10 can be reached with as few as 3–4 repetitive stimulations, thus flagging the possibility of neuropathic pain.

Following the examination and using a mirror to help the patient understand the discussion, the examination findings are discussed with the patient. The therapeutic approach is primarily guided by the elements of the history and examination findings, specifically the extent to which the pain can be localized to a specific region.[3]

Structural examination should focus on the palpation of the soft and bony tissues of the back, abdomen, and pelvis and include assessment for emergent and systemic disease, such as appendicitis or inflammatory bowel disease. We prefer to evaluate the musculoskeletal elements and lumbosacral peripheral nerve function as described in detail earlier prior to the gynecologic examination because these are often ignored by general women's health practitioners. The assessment should be concerned with both the somatic and visceral tissues of the abdomen, back, hips, and pelvis. The single-digit exam consists of superficial and deep palpation and can differentiate between superficial allodynia and myofascial pain of the abdominal wall versus deeper visceral pain. Screening for evidence of neuropathy or neuralgia in the ilioinguinal, iliohypogastric, genitofemoral, pudendal, and posterior femoral cutaneous nerve distributions (as described earlier) with evidence of both electrical or burning pain in the appropriate dermatome upon tapping the nerve (a Tinel's sign) can then be followed up with selective nerve blocks to determine if there is a significant nerve component contributing to symptoms. This is particularly important if the history identifies prior surgical or external trauma in the appropriate areas, or, in the case of perineal pain syndromes, if patients report difficulty with sitting or wearing tight pants.[4] If focal areas of taut bands and muscle spasm are present in pelvic or abdominal muscles, trigger point injections may help assess whether pain is predominantly of somatic origin, although the evidence base is still sparse at this writing.[5] Likewise, transvaginal evaluation can distinguish forniceal pain, uterine pain, and bladder pain (visceral elements) from obturator or levator ani pain (somatic sources). An expert pelvic surgeon notably may be able to identify restrictions in the normal mobility of pelvic organs when assessing the cul de sac on pelvic exam, thus allowing identification of those patients who will likely benefit from excisional therapy of endometriotic lesions involving broad areas of the peritoneum, which can severely scar the uterosacral ligaments to the ovaries, rectum, and posterior aspect of the uterus. When stage IV endometriosis is suspected in these rare cases, it is important not to limit therapy to conventional neurological or hormonal therapy (see later discussion).

LABORATORY TESTS

In our experience, there is an excessive use of repeated tests for infection and imaging studies in CPP management. Simple laboratory studies should be obtained in order to exclude other processes, such as a routine pregnancy test in reproductive-age women, a complete blood count, and pelvic cultures to rule out pelvic inflammatory disease. However, careful attention to the key elements of the historical features of the onset, location, and quality of pain, paired with a deliberate physical examination, are more valuable in identifying the source of pain than any laparoscopy or magnetic resonance imaging (MRI) study. For example, a diagnosis of "endometriosis" (a sometimes painful visceral disorder in the pelvic cavity) is not compatible with an isolated complaint of external vulvar pain (a somatic pain condition). Indeed, in determining a diagnostic strategy, it is most helpful to group testing in visceral symptom versus somatic symptom categories.

IMAGING STUDIES

Appropriate diagnostic imaging should be conducted on all patients with a pelvic examination suggestive of acute infection or a pelvic mass. Ultrasonography can assist in identifying the origin of the mass as uterine, adnexal, gastrointestinal, or from the bladder. Although MRI and ultrasound are good tests for characterizing suspected uterine disorders (leiomyoma, adenomyosis) and pelvic masses such as endometriomas, they do not provide good, nonspecific screening tools to identify a potentially painful end organ. Pelvic computed tomography (CT) is most advantageous in identifying intra-abdominal infection or bowel issues, and therefore it is most useful for confirmation of diagnoses suggested by the examination. MRI and electromyography and nerve conduction studies (EMG/NCS) may be helpful in evaluating a nerve or muscle entrapment such as piriformis syndrome or a pudendal neuralgia. In certain patients, transfundal retrograde venography or MR venograms can image the pelvic venous system to determine if pelvic varicosities or pelvic congestion syndrome is present. According to recent reviews, however, we and others find no high-quality evidence to suggest which clinical characteristics (location of findings, pain features, demographic factors) predict response to treatments for venous congestion. Indeed, the whole concept of this pathophysiology is being called into question by the absence of test-retest reliability for abnormal pelvic venograms.[6]

FURTHER EVALUATION WHEN VISCERAL DYSFUNCTION IS SUSPECTED

Symptoms suggestive of bowel or bladder pathology will warrant selective colonoscopy or cystoscopy, particularly in the presence of occult bleeding. Urgency and frequency with bladder pain (suggesting a diagnosis of IC/BPS) do not in themselves require cystoscopy. Bladder evaluation during hydrodistension (typically 80 cm of H_2O pressure, held under general anesthesia for 8 minutes) is no longer endorsed by the American Urologic Association in part due to the risk of bladder rupture.[7] Simple documentation of whether the patient reports pain with bladder palpation vaginally may be more effective in determining if bladder-specific therapy is appropriate.[8] Similarly, in the absence of significant weight loss or other signs of potential malignancy or of other bowel symptoms suggesting mucosal dysfunction, colonoscopy is generally unnecessary in defining IBS. Diagnostic pelvic laparoscopic evaluation ideally should focus on those patients with prominent visceral pain with specific features, such as painful periods or pain readily reproducible on internal examination of the uterus, adnexa, or fornices (pointing to potential peritoneal inflammation). In such a setting, endometriosis or adhesions will be found 90% of the time.[9] A major advantage of this approach is the ability to treat identified problems at the time of diagnosis. The surgeon must be careful not to overlook atypical or subtle areas of disease, ideally performing a biopsy on all suspicious lesions to rule out endometriosis.

Conscious laparoscopic pain mapping, performed under local anesthesia and rapidly reversible sedation (dexmetomedine or propofol) using instruments inserted transabdominally through 5 mm or smaller incisions, has been suggested as a way to allow patients to identify focal intra-abdominal pain generators. However, a modern view of pain processing that encompasses top-down, experientially driven cortical modulation and interpretation of peripheral nociceptive signals renders the findings of blunt palpation of pelvic organs perhaps less relevant in defining "true pain sources" (if such a concept is still viable) and thus remains unproved in its generalizability or efficacy. In addition, it is not something most gynecologists are trained to perform.

In Lori's case, the presentation does not appear to require significant imaging. The practitioner should carefully explain to her why initial laparoscopy and cystoscopy will not contribute much. If initial therapy fails, the clinical team should not wait too long to consider either or both to ensure that this is not an odd presentation of intravesical or peritoneal disease. Referring the patient to a specialized physical therapist to do connective tissue release and biomechanical strengthening/training of the abdominal/pelvic complex has been shown to be effective for many pelvic pain patients and likely should include internal pelvic floor targeted therapy.[10]

WHAT IS THE PATHOPHYSIOLOGY OF CPP?

The pathophysiology of CPP has been discussed extensively elsewhere.[11,12] Much of the literature focuses on various forms of pelvic pathology, such as IC/BPS, endometriosis, MPP, and venous engorgement. Although the pathophysiology and mechanism of afferent input are not fully understood and likely vary among these conditions, a common underlying theme in pelvic pain and nearly all other chronic pain conditions is the notion that persistent pain is a central nervous system problem. Chronic pain has been consistently shown to be related to central amplification of pain processing, which likely occurs at various levels of the nervous system.[13] Many potential mechanisms are thought to contribute to augmented central pain processing and are generally related to amplification of pain signals (e.g., central sensitization) and/or a loss of descending analgesia.[14,15] In line with this evidence, structural and functional alterations in brain regions associated with pain perception and modulation have also been identified. The most reproducible findings are alterations in excitatory and inhibitory neurotransmitters levels, changes in the cerebral connectivity, and associated decreases in gray matter volume in the thalamus, cingulate cortex, and insular cortex.[13,16,17] It is postulated that such changes in regional brain morphology and function may be responsible not only for the evolution and maintenance of the chronic pain state, but might also contribute to other common comorbid clinical traits, such as mood disorders and cognitive impairment.

Although central changes associated with pelvic pain are not as well studied as in other pain syndromes, there is increasing evidence that CPP correlates more closely with central changes rather than with pelvic pathology. Using voxel-based morphometry to evaluate differences in regional gray matter volume, women with CPP display decreased gray matter volume in key regions of the brain involved in pain perception, including the thalamus, cingulate gyrus, putamen, and insula.[18] Decreases in gray matter volume were seen in women with CPP, regardless of an underlying diagnosis of endometriosis and were not identified in women with pain-free endometriosis. Interestingly, women with pain-free endometriosis demonstrated an increase in gray matter volume in the periaqueductal gray, a key structure in the antinociceptive system. Given these findings and the absence of other gray matter changes seen in endometriosis patients with CPP, it is tempting to hypothesize that pain-free endometriosis patients (probably the majority) experience little if any pain due to adaptive changes in the brain that down-regulate peripheral nociceptive input. Like most other studies to date, the cross-sectional design of this study does not allow inferences about whether these central changes are the cause or consequence of the chronic pain experience. Despite this, it remains quite clear that chronic pain represents a multidimensional experience that is dependent less on nociceptive input from the periphery and more on the extensive modulation of that input by affective and cognitive mechanisms.

Such novel concepts highlight the critical importance of assessing these high-level changes in affect and cognition in planning management for two reasons: first, the variety of disorders associated with pelvic pain at the end-organ level is large, with presumably different afferent input mechanisms including, but not limited to IC/BPS, MPP, endometriosis, adhesions, chronic pelvic inflammatory disorder, and venous engorgement. Second, where investigation at the end-organ level has been extensive, as in IC/BPS, it has not been particularly fruitful in leading to helpful treatments. In contrast, treatment that focuses on higher level processing utilizing, for example, the biopsychosocial model of pain, carries the strongest evidence base of benefit. This discussion therefore focuses on these aspects.

> If we revisit the case presentation that began this chapter, several critical points emerge. Her history included sexual abuse as well as post-traumatic stress disorder (PTSD), unfortunately a common finding. The pathophysiologic role of sexual abuse in CPP is unclear, although others have explored obvious logical connections. A second major point revolves around the presence of so many painful comorbidities, such as fibromyalgia, migraine headaches, and the like, and of autonomic comorbidities such as POTS.

Emerging information suggests that, at very high cortical levels, the anterior cingulate cortex influences the balance of lateral and medial prefrontal cortex input to the periaqueductal gray region. When the lateral prefrontal cortex dominates, ascending pain signals are inhibited, whereas medial prefrontal cortex permits their access to higher order structures. Because prefrontal cortex is generally considered to represent a major site for executive control, engaging these areas may be one mechanism for the critical role of cognitive-behavioral therapy. Involvement of this network could also eventually help to explain the role of early life stress such as sexual abuse and the widespread pain and autonomic comorbid disorders.[19]

HOW ARE THE PSYCHOLOGICAL ASPECTS OF PELVIC PAIN MANAGED?

> It is likely that Lori does not make an attributional connection between her pain and her history of trauma. Both she and her sister have been diagnosed with generalized anxiety disorder, which may, on more careful evaluation, prove to be better understood as PTSD. Her sleep is disrupted and nonrestorative despite (likely *because* of) the use of lorazepam, and she reports dyspareunia, which loads more heavily on psychological than physical contributions. Finally, she has interrupted a promising college career, thus giving evidence that her overall level of function is deteriorating.

Most women with pelvic pain interpret their pain as a purely sensory phenomenon, and they seek relief by attending to the apparent peripheral source. The challenge for clinicians is to help the patient reconceptualize her pain as having sensory, affective, and cognitive dimensions, each of which demands attention before pain relief and return to normal function can be achieved.[20] Unfortunately, this can be difficult. Our patient wants relief, but effective treatment is elusive, and Lori is experiencing a gradual sense of loss of control. As she loses a sense of self-efficacy at coping with pain, she also gradually relies more on external measures to relieve pain. The psychological construct called *locus of control* refers to the extent to which individuals believe that they can control events that affect them, and it ranges along a scale from internal to external, from belief in one's own control to the sense that pain is controlled by factors that the patient cannot influence and whose amelioration must come from external sources.[21] Our task is to help Lori regain a sense of control, to recognize aspects of her situation that she can address, and to collaborate with us in pursuit of reduced pain and improved function.

We begin by addressing her insomnia, which is a common accompaniment to pelvic pain but that also can be symptomatic of depression. Although sleep onset insomnia is often correlated with pain and anxiety, sleep maintenance insomnia is often a characteristic of clinical depression.[22] Lorazepam, a benzodiazepine that has been termed "alcohol in a pill" by one of our colleagues, creates a risk for dependence and tolerance but also is very likely to degrade sleep architecture.[23] A tricyclic antidepressant with serotonergic and noradrenergic properties, such as amitriptyline, is useful for its analgesic properties as well as for treating insomnia. Research additionally supports the efficacy of behavioral sleep hygiene strategies that emphasize homeostatic, adaptive, and circadian aspects of sleep control; how to avoid sleep deprivation; and how to respond to unwanted middle-of-the-night awakenings.[24]

The discussion about insomnia leads rather naturally to a review of depressive symptoms. Pain is corrosive of mood, and patients typically are open to an examination of this normal depressive response. Vegetative signs, like insomnia, appetite, and cognition, are reviewed, along with psychological symptoms of demoralization, anergia, amotivation, and anhedonia (an inability to experience pleasure from activities usually found enjoyable). We assess mood stability to rule out bipolar symptoms. Because there is a high incidence of suicide in chronic pain conditions, we conduct a careful examination of suicidal ideation, intent, and plan.

There is also a high risk of substance misuse or dependence that a series of studies have suggested includes as many as 35% of patients with chronic pain.[25, 26] Therefore, we take a careful history of substance use, employ questionnaires like the CAGE, and utilize pharmacy confirmation to help determine the risk of a comorbid addictive process.

Finally, we address anxiety, beginning with symptoms consistent with her previously diagnosed generalized anxiety disorder, which is characterized by excessive, irrational worry that is disproportionate to the actual content of the worry. Patients are understandably agitated by pain, and their cognitive process is characterized by pain catastrophizing, with excessive rumination, symptom magnification, and helplessness. Studies have shown a strong correlation between intensity of pain catastrophizing and physical and psychological disability associated with pain.[27] As evaluation of anxiety proceeds, symptoms of PTSD can be addressed. The therapist should be forewarned that Lori may transiently worsen as she re-experiences flashbacks or nightmares of the original sexual trauma. She may strive to avoid stimuli associated with the trauma, experience periods of increased arousal (e.g., insomnia), and have unpredictable episodes of anger and nociceptive hypervigilance.

A behavioral approach to pelvic pain broadly addresses these biopsychosocial aspects of pain and can help patients regain a sense of control. Function is emphasized more than relief of pain as Lori is encouraged to take an active role in managing her pelvic pain. A truly interdisciplinary approach to pelvic pain requires the active participation of a psychologist, psychiatrist, or both to enhance Lori's return to function and amelioration of pain.

CONCLUSION

Although CPP is highly complex from pathophysiologic, neural network, and psychological perspectives, a simple approach emphasizing careful neurophysiologic examination of the pelvis and a history and examination that conceptually extend well beyond the pelvic region to capture comorbid disorders in both the patient and the family (e.g., such as migraine, fibromyalgia, IBS, and orthostatic intolerance) will provide the needed information to treat the patient's entire problem. This may be best accomplished in an interdisciplinary clinic setting. Successful treatment will emphasize the principles of the biopsychosocial over the purely biologic model of chronic pain.

REFERENCES

1. Nordling J, et al. eds. *Bladder Pain Syndrome: A Guide for Clinicians*. New York: Springer Science+Business Media; 2013.
2. Curtis Nickel J, Tripp DA, Pontari M, et al. Childhood sexual trauma in women with interstitial cystitis/bladder pain syndrome: a case control study. *Can Urol Assoc J*. 2011;5(6):410–415.
3. Haanpaa MR, Rowbotham M. Diagnosing neuropathic pain: clinical examination, neurophysiology, and neuroimaging. Paper presented at: 14th World Congress on Pain; 2012.
4. Robert R, Prat-Pradal D, Labat JJ, et al. Anatomic basis of chronic perineal pain: role of the pudendal nerve. *Surg Radiol Anat*. 1998;20(2):93–98.
5. Shah JP, Phillips TM, Danoff JV, Gerber LH. An in vivo microanalytical technique for measuring the local biochemical milieu of human skeletal muscle. *J Appl Physiol (1985)*. 2005;99(5):1977–1984.
6. Tu FF, Hahn D, Steege JF. Pelvic congestion syndrome-associated pelvic pain: a systematic review of diagnosis and management. *Obstet Gynecol Surv*. 2010;65(5):332–340.
7. Hanno PM, Burks DA, Clemens JQ, et al. AUA guideline for the diagnosis and treatment of interstitial cystitis/bladder pain syndrome. *J Urol*. 2010; 185(6):2162–2170.
8. Peters KM, Carrico DJ, Diokno AC. Characterization of a clinical cohort of 87 women with interstitial cystitis/painful bladder syndrome. *Urology*. 2008;71(4):634–640.
9. Howard FM. The role of laparoscopy in chronic pelvic pain: promise and pitfalls. *Obstet Gynecol Surv*. 1993;48(6):357–387.
10. FitzGerald MP, Payne CK, Lukacz ES, et al. Randomized multicenter clinical trial of myofascial physical therapy in women with interstitial cystitis/painful bladder syndrome and pelvic floor tenderness. *J Urol*. 2013;187(6):2113–2118.
11. Nazif O, Teichman JM, Gebhart GF. Neural upregulation in interstitial cystitis. *Urology*. 2007;69(4 suppl):24–33.
12. Potts JM, Payne CK. Urologic chronic pelvic pain. *Pain*. 2012;153(4):755–758.
13. Lee MC, Tracey I. Imaging pain: a potent means for investigating pain mechanisms in patients. *Br J Anaesth*. 2013;111(1):64–72.
14. Cruz-Almeida Y, Fillingim RB. Can quantitative sensory testing move us closer to mechanism-based pain management? *Pain Med*. 2014;15:61–72.
15. Phillips K, Clauw DJ. Central pain mechanisms in chronic pain states—maybe it is all in their head. *Best Pract Res Clin Rheumatol*. 2011;25(2):141–154.
16. Harris RE, Clauw DJ. Imaging central neurochemical alterations in chronic pain with proton magnetic resonance spectroscopy. *Neurosci Lett*. 29 2012;520(2):192–196.
17. Smallwood RF, Laird AR, Ramage AE, et al. Structural brain anomalies and chronic pain: a quantitative meta-analysis of gray matter volume. *J Pain*. 2013;14(7):663–675.
18. As-Sanie S, Harris RE, Napadow V, et al. Changes in regional gray matter volume in women with chronic pelvic pain: a voxel-based morphometry study. *Pain*. 2012;153(5):1006–1014.
19. Schweinhardt P, Bushnell MC. Pain imaging in health and disease—how far have we come? *J Clin Invest*. 2010;120(11):3788–3797.
20. Keane TM, Taylor KL, Penk WE. Differentiating post-traumatic stress disorder (PTSD) from major depression (MDD) and generalized anxiety disorder (GAD). *J Anxiety Disord*. 1997;11(3):317–328.
21. Lefcourt H. *Locus of Control: Current Trends in Research and Theory*. Hillsdale, NJ: Lawrence Erlbaum Associates; 1982.
22. Singh A, Ghazvini P, Robertson N, Massey A, Kirksey O, Honeywell M. Sleep disturbances in patients with psychiatric illnesses. *J Pharm Practice*. 2006;19(6):369–378.
23. Roth T, Hartse KM, Saab PG, Piccione PM, Kramer M. The effects of flurazepam, lorazepam, and triazolam on sleep and memory. *Psychopharmacology (Berl)*. 1980;70(3):231–237.
24. Murtagh DR, Greenwood KM. Identifying effective psychological treatments for insomnia: a meta-analysis. *J Consult Clin Psychol*. 1995;63(1):79–89.
25. Boscarino JA, Rukstalis M, Hoffman SN, et al. Risk factors for drug dependence among out-patients on opioid therapy in a large US health-care system. *Addiction*. 2010;105(10):1776–1782.
26. Ewing JA. Detecting alcoholism. The CAGE questionnaire. *JAMA*. 1984;252(14):1905–1907.
27. Tripp DA, Nickel JC, Wang Y, et al. Catastrophsizing and pain-contingent rest predict patient adjustment in men with chronic prostatitis/chronic pelvic pain syndrome. *J Pain*. 2006;7(10):697–708.

20.

CHRONIC REFRACTORY ANGINA

Philippe Mavrocordatos, Dag Söderström, and Mike J. L. DeJongste

CASE PRESENTATION

A 62-year-old cook sells ice cream and pancakes in his shop during the summer season and oysters, foie gras, and champagne in winter. He lives like a "bon vivant," working with his only son. The son got married 2 years ago and now intends to leave and open a similar shop in another town. The patient's past medical history recalls no psychiatric symptoms, but his mother has an anxious personality. He suffers from diabetes, hypercholesterolemia, and mild hypertension for the past 12 years. He has never smoked, and there is no significant family history of cardiovascular disease.

He is obese (body mass index [BMI] 37.8). In the past 10 years, he has suffered from recurrent episodes of angina. At first, the angina was mild and responsive to medication. However, this has progressed in intensity and frequency despite optimal antianginal medication, multiple coronary percutaneous procedures with stenting, and two open coronary artery bypass grafting (CABG) procedures.

Four years ago, 3 months after his last CABG, severe angina recurred. At that time, his quality of life was described as poor. He was unable to work and needed help with most daily activities. Despite optimal medication management, he was again suffering from recurrent chest discomfort radiating to the left arm with a Numeric Rating Scale (NRS) of between 4 and 6 (on an 11-point scale). He cannot walk more than 500 meters or carry weight due to his angina and shortness of breath. He wakes up at least four times per night with extremely anxious feelings, which causes a deficient sleeping pattern. When he finally falls asleep due to exhaustion, he often wakes up imagining he is going to die during his sleep. Because no cardiac medication or cardiac interventional options seem appropriate, he is referred to the Interdisciplinary Pain Clinic for evaluation.

Relevant on examination: The patient is 61 years old, 172 cm, 112 kg. Massive abdominal obesity, deconditioned. No shortness of breath at rest, no pain during examination.

Cardiovascular examination: No jugular distension. Pulse rate: 62 bpm. Blood pressure 135/85 mm Hg. Cardiac sounds are difficult to hear. No S3 or S4, murmurs, or rubs. No chest pain elicited through palpation of the chest.

Pulmonary examination reveals symmetrical auscultation without wheezes, crackles, or rales.

Extremities: No edema; pulse is palpable in all extremities.

Medication when evaluated at the pain clinic: Acetylsalicylate 100 mg/daily; metoprolol 200 mg BID; long-acting nitrates 120 mg/d; amlodipine 10 mg BID; rosuvastatin 10 mg/d; enalapril 10 mg/d; esomeprazole 40 mg BID; metformin 3 g/d; insulin sc BID.

Past surgical history:

1995 knee arthroscopy

2006 CABG (left internal mammary artery [LIMA] on anterior wall [LAD] and vein-graft on posterior wall [RDP-LPL])

2010 CABG (right internal mammary artery [RIMA] on lateral wall [D1] and vein-graft on inferolateral wall [MO1-2])

Active medical problems: Long-standing controlled hypertension, type 2 diabetes, hypercholesterolemia, central sleep apnea (on CPAP at night). Former smoker of 28 pack/year; stopped 13 years ago.

Coronarography: Diffuse atherosclerosis with multiple significant stenoses in the periphery of the large coronary arteries. LIMA and RIMA are patent. Vein-graft on MO1-2 is patent. Vein-graft on RPL-RDP is occluded.

Echocardiography (difficult to visualize): Left ventricular (LV) ejection fraction 48% (Simpson's formula). Inferior wall shows hypokinetic movement. No severe valve dysfunction was observed.

Radionuclide myocardium perfusion scan with sestamibi and adenosine stress showed inferoseptal, inferior, and posterior mismatch in perfusion.

The diagnosis of chronic angina resistant to standard therapies was established, a condition also known as *chronic refractory angina* (CRA).

QUESTIONS

1. What is the definition of CRA?
2. What is physiopathology of CRA?
3. Does a patient with stable angina differ from a patient with CRA?
4. What is the prevalence and incidence of refractory angina?
5. What is the cost and burden of refractory angina?

6. What is the natural history of CRA and life expectancy?
7. How do you evaluate patients with refractory angina?
8. What parameters are essential in following CRA patients?
9. What are the psychosocial aspects of CRA?
10. Is patient-centered or disease-centered care preferable?
11. What are emerging therapeutic alternative options for CRA?

WHAT IS THE DEFINITION OF CRA?

Since the classical description of angina pectoris by William Heberden in 1768, the clinical syndrome has attracted the interest of generations of clinicians.[1] More recently, basic scientists provided mechanistic evidence for relating physical or mental stress with symptoms. To date, significant atherosclerotic coronary artery disease is considered a characteristic result of stress with subsequent induced symptoms of angina. To quote Heberden, angina pectoris was "brought on by the motion of a horse," "increased by disturbance of the mind," and "relieved by wine, spirituous liquors and opium."

Over the centuries, superior therapies for angina were developed. Glycerin trinitrate in 1879 was an important launch.[2] From then on, a better understanding of the underlying mechanisms of the disease provided a platform for the progress made in its pharmacological and surgical treatment. This development led to the current effective spectrum of therapies. Accordingly, quality of life and life expectancy have increased dramatically. However, a subgroup of patients surviving their atherosclerotic disease do not experience sufficient pain relief from the conventional armamentarium of anti-ischemic treatments. These patients are suffering from chronic angina symptoms.[3] Angina, usually felt in the chest, often radiating to arm, neck, jaw, and sometimes back, is visceral in origin and is therefore commonly associated with anxiety, stress, or fear of death. Severe complaints of angina most often result in a poor quality of life.[4] As such, a patient suffering from lasting symptoms, who at first was a "cardiac patient," becomes progressively a chronic pain patient. The support, evaluation, follow-up, and treatment of angina therefore become more complex as psychosocial aspects add to the already severe biological problem. Different terms, including end-stage coronary artery disease, no-option coronary vascular disease, and intractable chronic angina have been used to describe this clinical syndrome. Although debatable whether CRA can be considered a separate stable angina entity, the ESC (Joint Study Group of the European Society of Cardiology on the treatment of Refractory Angina) defined the condition in 2002:[5] "Refractory angina pectoris is a chronic condition characterized by the presence of angina caused by coronary insufficiency in the presence of coronary artery disease which cannot be controlled by a combination of medical therapy, angioplasty and coronary bypass surgery. The presence of reversible myocardial ischaemia should be clinically established to be the cause of the symptoms. Chronic is defined as a duration of more than 3 months."

Defining CRA was important for building up an appropriate framework for basic science and clinical research, increasing awareness among clinicians, and establishing an adequate clinical pathway to evaluate and treat this specific group of patients.

> Our patient displays most of the conditions described in the definition: a long-lasting history of therapeutic failures linked to a lack of understanding of the particular patient is a very common feature of this clinical syndrome.

WHAT IS THE PATHOPHYSIOLOGY OF CRA?

Angina pectoris is considered a specific kind of pain experience because angina as a visceral provoked discomfort has emotional components. Furthermore, due to its visceral component, the symptoms of angina are quite often vaguely projected onto the trunk, which makes the diagnosis of a cardiac origin sometimes difficult. Before describing the complexity of chronic angina refractory to conventional therapies and its related symptoms, we therefore discuss pain in general.

First, in concert with many pain syndromes, symptoms resulting from specific underlying mechanisms are usually related to their etiology. Moreover, the symptoms may or may not be present all the time because the mechanisms participate either simultaneously or sequentially in the disease process.[6] Second, comorbidities and psychosocial factors must be taken into account. Specifically, affective influences may have an impact on the course of disease.[7]

Until recently and due to our lack of knowledge, the *Cartesian model* of pain was popular. In this model, pain was considered as a symptom only. The pain generator was located in the periphery, activated through a wound, a broken limb, or a failing organ. A model for the complexity of pain pathways, proposed by Patrick Wall and Ron Melzack[8] in the mid-1960s still stands, although their theory is no longer entirely justifiable. Studies of pain pathways and chronic pain mechanisms have demonstrated that pain and nociception are not only expressions of symptoms generated by a failing structure but may also be generated through modifications of the pain pathways or pain mechanisms. As a consequence, pain does not always reflect an "excess" of nociception but may also reflect abnormal modulation.[9] All chronic pain conditions, including refractory angina, must be judged with respect to this latter concept. Although in refractory angina we likely do face an excess of nociception, modulation of the symptoms, given the persistence of the disease, may also affect the condition.

Taking the complexity of chronic pain conditions into account, we further focus on the present understanding of the pathophysiology of refractory angina starting from peripheral mechanisms and moving up to central pathways.

THE PAIN GENERATOR

In general, angina pectoris is a perceived symptom resulting from a mismatch of oxygen supply and demand in the myocardium. Oxygen delivery to the myocytes (mDO_2) depends on cardiac output, patency of coronary arteries, hemoglobin binding capacity, cellular environment, myocyte function, and oxygen concentration in the blood. Myocardial O_2 consumption (mVO_2) is linearly related to the product of heart rate and systolic blood pressure (double product or rate pressure product) and varies in concert with local tissue metabolism. So, mVO_2 adapts to the instant requirements of the body, up to the point at which mDO_2 becomes insufficient. In general, if mDO_2 diminishes critically, the impending reduction in mVO_2 reduces the function of the heart to adjust to body needs.[10] When compromised blood flow caused by obstructive coronary artery disease limits regional myocardial perfusion, the metabolic demands of the myocardial tissue will not be met. The resulting myocardial ischemia initiates a sequence of events as a consequence of regional metabolic changes and acidosis (Figure 20.1). This condition generates nociceptive stimuli.[11]

MYOCARDIAL ISCHEMIA AS A NOCICEPTIVE TRIGGER

By definition, ischemia induces anaerobic metabolism and triggers inflammation.[12] The production of an array of chemical mediators further activates and sensitizes nociceptors. Among them, bradykinin, lactate, and proton production (H+) have been recognized as important factors,[13] as have adenosine and substance P.[14] More recently, a study by Pan and Chen[15] confirmed earlier observations by Albutahi et al.[16] and Foreman et al.[17] that ischemia might directly sensitize afferent nociceptors via a subcategory of capsaicin receptors, the transient receptor potential vanilloid 1 (TRPV1). TRPV1 receptors, being involved in cardiac nociception, are highly expressed on sensory nerve ending at the surface of the heart located at the peripheral extremities of the nociceptor.[16]

These fibers convey from the heart to the spine stimuli resulting from input of chemical and mechanical receptors. However, the potential role of mechanoreceptors in angina has been discussed for many years even as a variety of evidence challenges the concept.[12] Following activation of cardiac afferent nociceptive fibers, the first afferent neurons synapse in the dorsal horn and second-order neurons forward the signal to the brain.

$$\text{Myocardial ischemia} = \text{decreased ratio } \frac{\text{Oxygen supply}}{\text{Oxygen demand}}$$

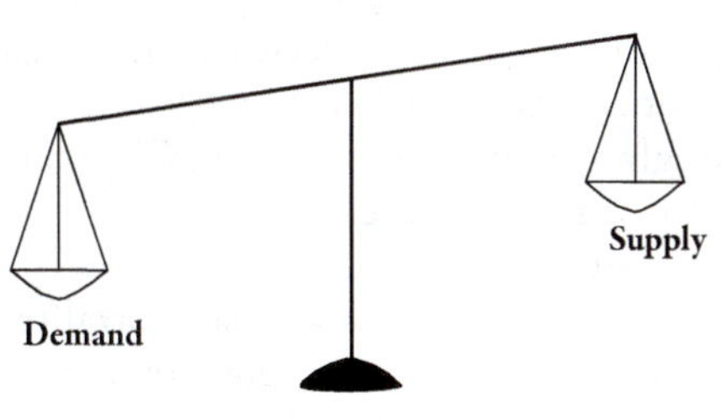

Demand ischemia:
–Ischemia during stress

Determinants of demand
- Heart rate
- Systolic blood pressure
- Myocardial wall stress
- Myocardial contractility

Supply ischemia:
–Ischemia at rest

Determinants of supply
- Coronary artery diameter and tone
- Collateral blood flow
- Perfusion pressure
- Heart rate (duration of diastole)

Figure 20.1 mVO_2 balance. Reprinted with permission from DeJongste MJL, Foreman RD. Spinal cord stimulation for refractory angina. *Neuromodulation* 2009;2:831–843.

REFERRED PAIN AND THE SPINAL INTERNEURON NETWORK

Initially, the model explaining referred pain was based on the idea that multiple peripheral branches innervating both visceral and somatic structures produced viscerosomatic convergence in primary afferent fibers. A number of studies showed that the number of these fibers was insufficient to support this hypothesis.[18] Based on extensive documentation, it is demonstrated that both somatic and visceral afferents synapse onto the same second-order sensory neurons located in the outer layers of the dorsal horn.[19,20] At this point, a complex inhibitory (GABAergic) and excitatory (glutamatergic) interneuron network allows modulation of ascending and descending signals. This network has complex multilevel connections.[21] The second-order neurons ascend to deep brain structures via multiple pathways, including the spinothalamic tracts, the spinoamygdaloid tract, and the spinohypothalamic pathway.[22]

CENTRAL PATHWAY AND MECHANISMS

Most second-order neurons synapse in the thalamus (ventroposterior lateral nucleus). The thalamus is considered a second gating system[22] that enables the modulation of signals. In conjunction with third-order neurons, the information is further transferred to the frontal cortex. Other inputs activate the reticular formation and hypothalamus, initiating arousal, fear, and autonomic system.

Different cortical areas participate in pain sensation, perception, and identification and in pain-related behavior. The cortical areas are activated at different intervals. The S1 and S2 areas of the somatosensory cortex are activated early, within milliseconds, and participate in early identification and sensory discrimination. Affective reactions are mediated later through the prefrontal cortex and the limbic system, and evaluation and sustained behavior are processed by the orbitofrontal cortex, hippocampus, and, later, by the entorhinal cortex.[23]

Descending inhibitory and excitatory pathways have also been identified. These project from the brain to the spinal cord. Serotonin axons descend from the medullary raphe nuclei and noradrenergic axons from the lateral pons. In the search for new therapeutic targets and following their suggested involvement in stimulation-produced analgesia, the serotonergic axons have been the focus of extensive research.[24]

BRAIN IMAGING AND ANGINA

Rosen and coworkers measured cerebral blood flow in patients experiencing dobutamine-induced angina symptoms.[25] The results of this positron emission tomography (PET) study showed involvement of the hypothalamus, periaqueductal gray, thalamus, lateral prefrontal cortex, and anterocrural cingulate cortex. Their findings were confirmed by a PET study making use of an implantable neurostimulator for refractory angina. During neurostimulation, activation of overlapping brain centers was identified, as during the induction of angina in the earlier study.[26]

When dobutamine was withheld during the study on angina and symptoms resolved, thalamic but not cortical activation was still present. The authors hypothesized that the thalamus could act as a gate to afferent pain signals.[25] Based on this hypothesis, the same authors studied silent ischemia.[27] Because thalamic but not cortical activity was similar with or without angina symptoms, they postulated that abnormal central processing could be involved in the pathophysiology of silent ischemia. In electrophysiologic studies, Droste and Roskamm showed that patients suffering from silent ischemia had a higher pain perception threshold compared to patients experiencing symptoms of angina.[28] Do patients with refractory angina have a lower pain perception threshold? Although unknown, it is tempting to hypothesize that patients suffering from refractory angina have a sensitized threshold for cardiac nociception (i.e., the high-thresholds receptors have become low-threshold receptors).

DOES A PATIENT WITH STABLE ANGINA DIFFER FROM A PATIENT WITH CRA?

Two centuries ago, the British physician Heberden was the first to describe *angina pectoris*.[1] In addition to his description, he noted "but it is not to be expected, that much could have been done towards establishing the method of cure for a distemper hitherto so unnoticed, that it has not yet, as far as I know, found a place or a name in the history of diseases." Many studies have since demonstrated that during either mentally or physically induced stress, oxygen supply is no longer capable meeting the oxygen demand of the heart muscle in significantly narrowed coronary arteries. The subsequent shift in oxygen balance induces so-called (reversible) myocardial ischemia. So, in the absence of myocardial hypertrophy, "demand" ischemia usually results from an increased heart rate, most often exercise induced, in conjunction with one or more atherosclerotic stenoses in coronary arteries. Exercise-induced myocardial ischemia most often provokes angina pectoris of a chronic and stable kind.[12] It is characterized by a localized discomfort in the chest provoked during stress and relieved with short-acting nitrates or rest. Following (temporary) occlusion of a coronary artery through atherosclerotic plaque rupture or coronary spasm, supply ischemia induces an acute coronary syndrome (ACS). In the presence of an ACS, complaints of angina are felt at rest and are most often associated with vaguely distributed anxious feelings.

CHRONIC ANGINA REFRACTORY TO CONVENTIONAL THERAPIES

The main objectives of therapies for chronic stable angina are to relieve symptoms and to prevent progression of the atherosclerotic coronary artery disease. In addition, therapeutic strategies are developed to decrease oxygen demand and increase oxygen supply. The latter is attained by providing sufficient blood supply to the myocardium and is performed by means of a revascularization procedure. Revascularization can be executed by either dilating the supplying coronary artery with percutaneous coronary intervention (PCI) or by creating a bypass vessel with CABG. The supply-demand balance is also influenced by anti-ischemic drugs such as calcium channel blockers, β-blocking agents, and sinus node (*If* channel) inhibitors. Furthermore, reduction of preload is achieved with nitrates and, with regard to endothelial function, statins and angiotensin-converting enzyme inhibitors are given in conjunction with inhibitors of thrombocyte aggregation.

Patients with long-lasting severe angina—Canadian Cardiovascular Society Class III–IV despite optimal pharmacological therapy—who are not suitable candidates for revascularization (either PCI or CABG) are defined as suffering from CRA by the Joint Study Group of the ESC [5] (Box 20.1). Most often, patients with refractory angina can be considered disabled by their severely restricted exercise capacity. Moreover, this limited life exposure frequently results in a significantly decreased quality of life. The fear of a menacing cardiac event and subsequent hospitalization decreases the remaining quality of life of patients even further.

Interestingly, patients suffering from CRA can be considered survivors of their disease. In the presence of end-stage coronary artery disease in conjunction with reversible myocardial ischemia, the relatively low annual mortality is thought to be the consequence of lack of severe arrhythmias and a frequently maintained LV function. So, on the one hand, these patients are facing a relatively good prognosis whereas, on the other hand, quality of life is severely reduced. In this respect, any therapy that improves the quality of life of these patients without aggravating their prognosis is worth being taken into consideration.

> The evolution of our patient toward chronicity is paved with typical landmarks: progressive onset of angina, first responding to anti-angina medication, recurrence of symptoms, interventional revascularization procedures, ultimately failing to reduce complaints of angina, and, finally, resistance to all conventional therapies focused on the heart.

Box 20.1 **THE MOST COMMON REASONS THAT FURTHER REVASCULARIZATION PROCEDURE IS NOT POSSIBLE**

- Unsuitable anatomy, such as diffuse coronary sclerosis, often with well-preserved left ventricular function; sometimes called *end-stage angina*
- One or several previous CABGs and/or PTCAs that exclude further benefit or possibility of further revascularization
- Lack of graft material
- Impaired LV function in patients with previous CABG and/or PTCA
- Extracardiac diseases that increase perioperative/postoperative morbidity or mortality, such as general arteriosclerotic disease, renal insufficiency, carotid stenosis, and pulmonary disease
- Age, often in combination with the above-mentioned factors

Reprinted with permission from C Mannheimer, P Camici, MR Chester, et al. The problem of CRA. Report from the ESC Joint Study Group on the Treatment of Refractory Angina. *Eur Heart J* 2002;23:355–370.

WHAT IS THE PREVALENCE AND INCIDENCE OF REFRACTORY ANGINA?

GENERAL CONSIDERATIONS

In the wake of improved survival from ischemic heart diseases in the Western world, the number of patients suffering from CRA is increasing.[5] In this perspective, refractory angina draws attention to a growing social, emotional, and medical problem.

Indicators of morbidity and mortality are basic tools of epidemiology. They help healthcare providers to understand community issues and define priorities in public health. Assessing these indices affects the perspective one has, broadens the view on a disease, and may provide solutions to manage the disease. In addition, epidemiology studies provide information about pathological states and help in formulating hypotheses of causality, testing them, and evaluating their efficacy. These studies usually do not offer a qualitative assessment of morbidity, survival, or quality of life.

There are two types of indicators, direct and indirect. The indirect category often evaluates but does not diagnose the health state of a population. Indirect indicators focus mainly on changes that may have an impact on a defined situation. An example of an indirect index is the number of hospitalizations due to recurrent episodes in patients suffering from severe coronary disease. This parameter only indirectly reflects chronic angina morbidity. When direct morbidity indicators, prevalence, and incidence of the disease are not available, indirect indicators are used to draw the best possible picture. In this regard, as a consequence of improved strategies, the prevalence of stable angina is increasing.[29]

INCIDENCE

The incidence of angina is the number of new patients suffering from this condition within a given period of time. Duration of the disease does not have an impact on incidence, so incidence directly quantifies the progression of the disease. As more patients survive coronary events, it is estimated that the incidence of angina is increasing. However, exact numbers on patients suffering from refractory angina are difficult to obtain because no large epidemiological study has focused on refractory angina only.[30] Moreover, the condition of refractory angina may represent at least four different phenotypes.[29]

PREVALENCE

Prevalence of refractory angina is the total number of subjects suffering from the disease at a given period of time, be it week, month, or year. Subjects already suffering from the condition, deceased or not, and new cases are counted. This means that duration of the disease will impact on prevalence. In refractory angina, this effect will become even more important as therapies for stable angina therapy improve.[31] The population of survivors will increase and so will the number of patients becoming progressively refractory to conventional anti-angina treatments.[5]

CURRENT SITUATION IN REFRACTORY ANGINA

Although we have a definition of refractory angina,[5] it remains difficult to differentiate stable angina from refractory angina because patients may move from one category to the other. Moreover, objective morbidity is not accessible because it would require a study of the whole population. Therefore, epidemiologic studies have been performed.[32]

An estimation of the incidence can be executed through dividing the numbers of performed coronary angiography (per country) by the number of patients with nonrevascularizable significant coronary arteries and multiplying the outcome by the population. This computation provides an estimated incidence of 6.8% of patients suffering from angina, which equals 150,000 patients in the United States.[33] By the same token, through estimating the number of patients per cardiologist with refractory angina,[32–34] the prevalence of patients with refractory angina in a population can be calculated. It is estimated that a cardiologist usually has two or three patients with CRA. In the United States, there are about 60,000 practicing cardiologists. So, the prevalence of refractory angina can be extrapolated to at least 150,000 subjects in the United States, a figure that fits nicely with the calculation made by Mukherjee et al.[35] Furthermore, mortality from CRA seems to be relatively modest.[33]

By integrating available data, direct and indirect indicators are the most appropriate way to obtain the best possible picture of the incidence and prevalence of refractory angina.

One of these indicators is provided by cardiac catheterization registries in the United States and Europe. Registries suggest that between 5% and 10% of patients investigated for symptomatic angina are unsuitable for revascularization and therefore fulfil the definition of refractory angina.[33,36] A second indicator derives from stable angina prevalence and the guessed estimated proportion of refractory angina cases.[30] From this approximation, it is estimated that 3–7 per 1,000 patients aged 45–74 years suffer from refractory angina.[37] Based on multiple variables, Mukherjee et al. evaluated the incidence of patients who are not candidates for revascularization therapy to be around 100,000–200,000 per year in the United States and a comparable number of patients in Europe.

The different indirect parameters suggest the approximate prevalence and incidence of the disease. To clarify the burden of the pathology, epidemiology studies specifically focused on refractory angina are clearly needed.

WHAT IS THE COST AND BURDEN OF REFRACTORY ANGINA?

A cost-of-illness analysis consists of the identification, measurement, and valuation of all resources related to an illness. It should include costs falling inside and outside the healthcare sector, including, for example, loss of productivity associated with morbidity or premature death. Such extensive work has been done for cardiovascular diseases in general, but refractory angina as clinical entity has not been the specific focus of such cost-of-illness studies. All the information gathered here is derived from chronic stable angina economic burden studies or from cost-utility studies comparing refractory angina treatments.

Cardiovascular disease is the leading cause of death in United States. It is responsible for 17% of national health expenditures.[38] In the past decade, the medical costs of cardiovascular diseases have grown at an average rate of 6% per year.[39] Looking forward, the American Heart Association developed a methodology to project future costs of care for hypertension, coronary heart disease, heart failure, and other cardiovascular pathologies. Using this model, it has been forecast that between 2010 and 2030, real direct medical costs would triple, jumping from $273 billion to $818 billion in the United States.[40] Previous reports about the increasing incidence of cardiovascular pathologies including refractory angina are unfortunately confirmed by this worrying forecast.[5]

Looking at the situation in the United Kingdom, Stewart and coworkers studied the cost of angina pectoris during 2000. Including the cost of hospital admissions, revascularization procedures, hospital outpatient consultations, general practice consultations, and prescribed drugs, the total expenditure was £60.5 million. During this period, 1.1% of the population consulted for angina.[41]

Reynolds et al. studied the economic burden of chronic angina in a 2004 systematic review.[42] Among the 47 selected studies, 10 directly addressed the cost. The annual direct costs ranged from $1,937 for medically managed patients to almost 10 times that amount for patients with advanced illness and refractory angina ($18,467 in 1997). Severity of illness, then, clearly matters. Two other studies by Schofield in 1999 and Kandzari in 2001 focused on "severe angina" patients. These two studies also found that costs were much higher than for "medically managed" chronic angina.[43,44]

However, looking at refractory angina simply as a subgroup of cardiovascular disease is probably too reductive. As a chronic condition, it may induce other expenses not accounted for in cost-of-illness studies addressing only cardiac diseases. Such a chronic handicap is usually linked to an increased requirement of psychosocial resources. Refractory angina should be differentiated from its origin (i.e., ischemic heart diseases in general) in regard to the burden it represents. This has been recognized only recently, and, consequently, its management has significantly changed.[45]

Cost-utility studies may also provide information on specific costs. Although they focus mainly on therapy, the cost of illness has also been evaluated. Most studies evaluated the use of spinal cord stimulation or percutaneous laser revascularization. In these studies, the cost-of-illness before and after treatment was evaluated [46–48] and/or the costs of the two arms of the study were calculated.[49–51] Overall, the numbers are similar to those found in previously mentioned articles. In summary, the economic burden is huge, and, not surprisingly, the severity of the disease seems to have a clear impact on the expenses. Moreover, we believe that the situation of patients suffering from refractory angina requires even more healthcare and social resources due to the chronic aspect of the handicap. These aspects have not been considered yet.

> The total cost of our patient's entire treatment is, of course, very high—particularly CABG surgery. The only positive aspect is that this independent worker continued to run his shop despite his physical limitations and fatigue. Usually, the cost of disability must be added to the expenses directly linked to therapy.

WHAT IS THE NATURAL HISTORY OF CRA AND LIFE EXPECTANCY?

Coronary artery disease is a progressive, low-grade inflammatory disease, resulting in thickening of the vascular wall through formation of atherosclerotic obstructive plaques. When stenosis of the artery limits oxygen supply, a point may be reached at which myocytic oxygen needs are not met and local ischemia occurs. In general, symptoms related to the ischemic event are felt when oxygen needs are increased by exercise, meals, cold, or mental stress,[52,53] but, as the disease progresses, angina pectoris "translating" myocardial ischemia may even occur with minimal exercise.

Angina pectoris is not a very sensitive marker of myocardial ischemia; however, it is a key symptom of coronary artery disease. In this regard, in the presence of myocardial ischemia, complaints of angina are often expressed late, inconsistently, or may be even completely absent in 30% of patients.[54] Myocardial ischemia occurs when coronary artery diameter is already narrowed at least by 70% but may also appear later, when the stenosis exceeds 90%. Angina is not a proportional indicator of the severity of occlusive coronary disease. So angina should not be considered as a reliable maker of the underlying pathological process of atherosclerosis. However, angina remains the key symptom of the clinical presentation of myocardial ischemia and an important clinical guide of the therapeutic effect of the treatment. The Canadian Cardiovascular Society (CCS) proposed a modification of the New York Heart Association's (NYHA) classification to improve the classification of angina.[55]

The desired effects of therapy for stable angina are to relieve symptoms, prevent progression to future cardiac events, and improve survival. Pharmacological treatment as well as revascularization procedures are meant to restore the oxygen demand-supply balance and reverse myocardial ischemia episodes. When pharmacological and conservative treatment fails, patients undergo coronary angiography to determine their eligibility for revascularization.

At this point in the evolution of coronary artery disease, some patients will benefit from revascularization procedures and some will not. Mukherjee et al. reviewed 500 patients with documented and symptomatic ischemia. Decision for revascularization was taken after coronary angiography and according to strict criteria established by consensus among reviewers and interventional cardiologists.[56] Patients were unsuitable for PCI if one or more of the following existed: chronic total occlusion with unfavorable morphologic features, degenerated vein graft, and multiple restenoses. For CABG ineligibility criteria were poor target, no conduit, and no severe comorbidities. Even though a vast majority of patients were appropriate candidates for PCI or CABG, between 7% and 12% were excluded following these criteria.[5] This group of nonrevascularizable patients suffering from symptoms refractory to conventional therapies find themselves in a critical situation.

At this point, it is important to further categorize these patients in order to determine their best possible options. Assessment of patients should focus on both exclusion criteria for revascularization and inclusion in the definition of refractory angina. In 2002, the ESC joint study group on the treatment of refractory angina agreed on the definition provided earlier, in the section "What Is the Definition of CRA?"[5] This definition takes into account the exclusion parameters for revascularization but also states that other causes of chronic chest pain should have been excluded.

Because patients with refractory angina are considered survivors of their coronary artery disease, they have been studied as such and present common features including a long history of coronary artery disease (8 years on average), a relatively young age (mean age 63 years), a predominantly male gender, a moderate reduced LV ejection fraction, and an elevated fibrinogen level.[57]

The situation of these patients is difficult because many aspects of their life are severely impaired. Chronicity of symptoms becomes as invalidating as the symptoms themselves, and morbidity goes beyond the border of most cardiac pathologies. In addition to the biological aspects, the patient may suffer from psychological distress, and social issues may arise including loss of productivity, limited social life, and isolation. All these aspects must be addressed, and thus the "only cardiac" management becomes multidisciplinary pain (angina) management.

This group suffers a rather high morbidity considering the occurrence of ACS, hospital admissions, and concomitant diseases, especially given that mortality is relatively low (5–7% per year) in these no-option patients.[58] In a study by TenVaarwerk et al., 66% of the patients had experienced myocardial infarctions and 17% underwent percutaneous transluminal coronary angioplasties. In addition, bypass surgery was performed in 58% of the participants. During a median follow-up of 23 months (range 0–128), 103 patients died (52 from a cardiac cause, 25 from a noncardiac cause, and 26 from an unknown cause).[58]

These patients are survivors of their disease also in terms of psychological and social issues. The quality of life of these patients is severely impaired and depression, anxiety, and stress must be evaluated and treated to the same extent as the coronary disease.

> To the classical cardiovascular-associated risk factors, our patient adds ongoing unhealthy behaviors, obesity, stress, and fatigue. The only positive aspect is that he stopped smoking years ago. When the diagnosis of CRA was established, a review of his medication was performed and the interdisciplinary cardiovascular team, including (interventional) cardiologists and thoracic surgeons, agreed not to proceed with any further cardiac interventions.

HOW DO YOU EVALUATE PATIENTS WITH REFRACTORY ANGINA?

Patient evaluation should include a set of defined criteria to render the best possible picture of the patient at a given time. Because it is advisable to reuse these same criteria to qualify and quantify the biological, psychological, and social evolution of the patient, the importance of the baseline evaluation become clear.

In addition to the patient history and physical examination, reliable objective and semi-objective parameters must be recorded. They should be collected and easily retrievable.

The adjective "chronic refractory" makes a world of difference in the assessment and management approach because it introduces the concept of intractability with conventional strategies. It is essential that the reader understand this change of paradigm because treatment then evolves from that of a "cardiac" symptom translating the underlying disease to that of a chronic pain condition. CRA in all its bio-psychosocial issues then becomes the predominant aspect of the problem and the primary target of the patient's management and treatment.

The first step of the evaluation is to establish the diagnosis of refractory angina pectoris.[59] The aim of this procedure is to establish whether a patient on optimal anti-ischemic pharmacological therapy is inaccessible to further revascularization.[5] An algorithm for assessment was proposed by the Joint Study group on the treatment of refractory angina in 2002 and is presented in Box 20.1. This algorithm addresses the following issues: ineligibility for revascularization, on optimal medication regimen and adherence to medication regimen, exclusion of nonischemic etiology of angina symptoms, and evaluation of aggravating psychological factors.[5]

INELIGIBILITY FOR REVASCULARIZATION

A team of interventional cardiologists and cardiac surgeons should consult together on the possibility of revascularization based on a recent angiogram. The most common reasons that further revascularization procedures are not possible are listed in Table 20.1.

OPTIMAL MEDICATION AND COMPLIANCE

Before establishing the diagnosis of refractory angina, one must assure the failure of all prior interventions. A critical review of medication and therapeutic strategies must therefore be applied. Treatment and patient compliance should be assessed and optimized as much as possible. In 2005, Osterberg et al. reviewed overall adherence to medication. From the patient point of view, reasons for noncompliance with medications included forgetfulness (30%), other priorities (16%), decision to omit (11%), lack of information (9%), emotional factors (7%), and no reason provided (27%). Physician's contribution to poor adherence was linked to complex regimens, failing to explain benefits and side effects, not considering the patient's lifestyle or cost of medication, and a poor therapeutic relationship.[60]

Table 20.1 **CHARACTERISTICS OF PATIENTS (N = 517) SUFFERING FROM CHRONIC REFRACTORY ANGINA PECTORIS**

Sex	71% male
Age (years)	63.9 (10.1)
Clinical presentation	
Duration of angina pectoris (years)	8.1 (6.3)
NYHA class (mean)	3.5 (0.7)
LVEF <40%	24%
Previous myocardial infarction	66%
Three vessel disease	68%
PTCA	17%
CABG	58%
Risk factors	
Family CAD	61%
Hypertension	39%
Hypercholesterolemia	28%
Smoking	21%
IDDM	14%

Patient characteristics modified from Ten Vaarwerk.

CAD, coronary artery disease; CABG, coronary artery bypass graft surgery; IDDM, insulin dependent diabetes mellitus; LVEF, left ventricular ejection fraction; NYHA, New York Heart Association functional class; PTCA, percutaneous transluminal coronary angioplasty.

Reprinted with permission from MJL DeJongste, RA Tio, RD Foreman. Chronic therapeutically refractory angina pectoris. *Heart* 2004;90:225–230.

EXCLUSION OF NONISCHEMIC ETIOLOGY OF ANGINA SYMPTOMS

Questioning the origin of chest pain is essential at this point. It is crucial to exclude other causes for chest discomfort, such as those from psychological stress (hyperventilation, panic disorders), pulmonary, abdominal (gastrointestinal), or musculoskeletal origin even in the presence of myocardial ischemia.[61]

AGGRAVATING PSYCHOLOGICAL FACTORS

Ongoing pain is a major burden in life and, in the majority of patients with chronic pain, psychosocial issues emerge. It is not easy to evaluate these aspects in relation to baseline characteristics such as comorbidities and personality.

Multiple questionnaires are available and helpful, but most of them have been validated in a specific population (e.g., back pain patients or neuropathic syndromes). Although some disease-specific questionnaires are available, such as the Seattle Angina Questionnaire (SAQ),[64] most often disease-generic questionnaires are used, such as the Hospital Anxiety and Depression Score (HADS)[65] and Short Form-36 (SF-36). No questionnaire has been specifically developed for CRA patients. All these questionnaires are indicative of significant psychosocial factors and can be used to re-evaluate the situation later to determine the efficacy of the applied therapy or progression of the disease. The questions and answers may also provide an interesting medium and a very practical tool through which to discuss the current situation with the patient. However, the best option—if available—is to organize a formal psychological assessment with the assistance of a psychologist or psychiatrist.

In addition to these aspects, the patient's socioeconomic situation should be considered in further management and treatment planning.

Multidisciplinary assessment is at this point important to establish a clear baseline. It will help build a clear management and treatment plan aimed at optimizing the evaluated parameters. Finally, given the frequent concomitant presence of comorbidities and the psychosocial effects of chronic refractory ischemic heart disease on these patients, a multidisciplinary team approach is required for optimal overall treatment.

When the patient was diagnosed with CRA and referred to us for pain management, we first reviewed the situation, making sure nothing was omitted. Medication had to be optimized, so patient compliance and reinforcement of already given instructions were checked. We further ascertained that the patient had been evaluated by a team of cardiologists, rehabilitation specialists, and cardiothoracic surgeons and that no revascularization procedure was feasible. Baseline bio-psychosocial questionnaires were filled out by the patient. Our pain management center uses a standard selection of questionnaires for all chronic pain patients: a numeric rating scale of pain at rest and exercise scored from 0 to 5. The Oswestry Disability Questionnaire score was 42% (moderate disability) and the Depression/Anxiety/Stress Scale (DASS) scores were 12/27/34 showing moderate to severe psychological impact. A review of all these aspects was performed.

The first consultations focused on the chronic aspect of the disease and on pain management. Instead of the cardiac-related problems, we focused on habits, social life, and daily activities. We looked at psychological issues, including anxiety, stress, and depression. Anxiety and stress indicators were extremely high, but depression was not present. Quality of life was very poor, and sleep deprivation was the most important complaint. Rehabilitation addressing behavioral changes was planned, and possible therapeutic options were reconsidered.

WHAT PARAMETERS ARE ESSENTIAL IN FOLLOWING CRA PATIENTS?

Because of their chronic condition, patients suffering from refractory angina require long-term management and follow-up. Aiming for best quality of life without adversely affecting their disease course, multidisciplinary care should be focused on pain management, psychological support, and (potential) cardiac concerns.[66] Subsequently, to further improve adherence to medical strategies, patient-centered care is preferable in comparison with disease-centered care.[67] In this regard, a more holistic assessment of patients suffering from chronic diseases is needed to understand how the condition affects both patients and relatives.[68]

To guarantee adequate follow-up, objective and semi-objective tests are required for the interdisciplinary baseline evaluation. Because healthcare providers are facing a chronic pain syndrome in conjunction with a progressive cardiac disease, parameters should be categorized into biological, psychological, and social aspects.

BIOLOGICAL PARAMETERS

Follow-up biological parameters should ideally be indicative of outcomes. Furthermore, optimal management of convalescence, quality of life, and physical function measures are preferred. Because these kinds of indicators have not been specifically defined or studied within any one study, outcome studies most often report a series of characteristics, differentiating survivors and nonsurvivors[58] (Table 20.1). These measurable, discriminative variables are indicators of disease processes and include CCS classification, LV function, medication use, hospital admissions, number of myocardial infarcts, and chronic comorbidities, such as diabetes, chronic obstructive pulmonary disease (COPD), end-stage renal insufficiency, rheumatoid arthritis, and more. Current smoking history and obesity have a direct effect on oxygen supply and demand. Finally, patients with CRA are frequently also suffering from multiple comorbidities.[62,63]

PSYCHOLOGICAL PARAMETERS

Most chronic pain syndromes may induce anxiety, stress, and severe depressive states. Asking patients to fill in questionnaires on a regular basis provides a general idea of the psychological impact of their disease. As a potential outcome of the obtained scores, it may be of relevance to advise the patient to seek professional psychological support. Among numerous questionnaires, the web site www.angina.org recommends the HADS and the 5-point Liverpool Angina Questionnaire.[64,65]

SOCIAL PARAMETERS

Refractory angina patients are severely restricted in daily activities. Their physical disability has an important impact on their social life because it may lead to isolation and increased dependence on families and healthcare providers. Again, questionnaires on perceived quality of life are useful tools with which to evaluate these issues as they pertain to patients with CRA.[5]

WHAT ARE THE PSYCHOSOCIAL ASPECTS OF CRA?

CRA AND PANIC DISORDER: EVIDENCE FOR COMORBIDITY?

Psychiatric disorders are very common in patients referred for pain as a first symptom. However, anxiety disorders often precede the onset of pain, whereas depressive disorders follow the appearance of chronic pain syndrome. In addition, there is abundant evidence that depression, irrespective whether preceding or following a myocardial infarction, adversely affects the prognosis of these patients.[69] From a psychosocial point of view, refractory angina is a chronic pain condition that requires the consideration of psychiatric diagnoses as causes, as well as their consequences for pain conditions. Moreover, we should also look more closely at their interactions because these complex relationships may be a type of comorbidity in that they share the autonomic activation of the sympathetic system and may induce a vicious cycle.[69]

Anxiety can lead to panic attacks and mimic an ACS. This syndrome includes fear of dying, which may further trigger a myocardial infarction. CRA is a threat that can easily trigger anxiety and related symptoms. Understanding and treating underlying psychiatric disorders, such as panic disorder and depression, is imperative.

WHAT PSYCHIATRIC DIAGNOSES SHOULD BE CONSIDERED?

In the emergency room, panic attack is the most common psychiatric disorder to consider in the presence of chest pain and dyspnea. Panic attack is a severe and unpredictable anxiety reaction with a sudden onset of apprehension, fear, or terror, often associated with feelings of impending doom. The ICD-10 (a classification of mental and behavioral disorders developed by the World Health Organization in 1992) classifies panic disorder as recurrent, unpredictable panic attacks with palpitations, chest pain, shocking sensations, dizziness, and feelings of unreality, often with associated fear of dying, losing control, or going mad.[70] For a definite diagnosis, several severe attacks of autonomic anxiety should have occurred within a period of 1 month: (a) in circumstances where there is no objective danger; (b) without being confined to known or predictable situations; and (c) with comparative freedom from anxiety symptoms between attacks (although anticipatory anxiety is common).

HOW OFTEN DOES THIS DIAGNOSIS APPEAR IN ANGINA PATIENTS IN THE EMERGENCY ROOM?

During a 24-month period, 301 patients presenting with chest pain and dyspnea were randomly selected: 27% were diagnosed with musculoskeletal chest pain, 19% with ACS, and 12% with panic attack. The other cardiac diagnoses were myocardial infarction, unstable angina pectoris, cardiac arrhythmia, and heart failure.

When excluding patients with previous heart disease, the prevalence of psychiatric disorders in patients with chest pain reported in a Norwegian study was 39%: 14% panic disorder, 14% somatoform disorders, and 5% major depression.[71] Furthermore, in patients with atypical/nonanginal chest pain and normal angiograms, the prevalence of panic disorder ranged between 34% (32 out of 94) and 57% (59 out of 103).[72]

These observations imply that one-third of patients presenting with an ACS are actually experiencing a panic attack. The panic attack may mimic the clinical presentation of an ACS to the point of being clinically indistinguishable without appropriate investigations. This ability to mimic symptoms of acute coronary insufficiency has led to costly and unnecessary medical evaluations and prolonged mismanagement of underlying panic disorder. However, establishing the diagnosis of panic disorder is difficult. Often, physicians are either not aware of the differential diagnosis of panic disorder or coarsely underestimate its severity.[73,74] With respect to symptoms, the two conditions usually can be differentiated (Table 20.2).

However, the literature actually demonstrates that the two conditions are more related than simply as differential diagnosis alternates. Panic disorder, a psychiatric condition with recurrent panic attacks, has been found to be an independent risk factor for subsequent coronary events. Mental stress, such as that produced by panic disorders, may induce (spasm-generated) vasoconstriction and subsequently provoke ischemic pain. As a consequence of vasoconstriction (e.g., an increase in both blood pressure and resistance of coronary vessels), heart rate increases.[75] Furthermore, a panic disorder is also capable of directly inducing myocardial ischemia.[76] In a review of the literature, Soh and Lee show that through activation of the sympathetic system by differing upstream mechanisms, the two conditions have similar presentations.[77]

Table 20.2 **SYMPTOMS OF A PANIC ATTACK COMPARED WITH ACUTE CORONARY SYNDROME**

PANIC ATTACK	ACUTE CORONARY SYNDROME
1. Palpitations, pounding heart, or accelerated heart rate	1. Palpitations
2. Sweating	2. Diaphoresis
3. Trembling or shaking	3. Pain (usually described as pressure, squeezing/burning sensation across the precordium and may radiate to the neck, shoulder, jaw, back, upper abdomen, or either arm)
4. Sensations of shortness of breath or smothering	4. Exertional dyspnea
5. Feeling of choking	5. Nausea
6. Chest pain or discomfort	6. Decreased exercise tolerance
7. Nausea or abdominal distress	7. Atypical presentations in elderly and/or diabetic: • Fatigue • Syncope • Weakness • Lightheadedness • Altered mental status • Asymptomatic
8. Feeling dizzy, unsteady, lightheaded or faint	
9. Feelings of unreality (derealization) or of being detached from oneself (depersonalization)	
10. Feeling of losing control or going crazy	
11. Fear of dying	
12. Numbness and tingling sensations	
13. Chills and hot flushes	
>4 of the above symptoms, as defined by the DSM-IV-TR1	

Reprinted from Keng Chuan Soh, Cheng Lee, Panic Attack and its Correlation with Acute Coronary Syndrome—More Than Just a Diagnosis of Exclusion. *Ann Acad Med Singapore.* 2010;39:197–202.

Panic disorder is strongly related to depression. Sometimes panic attack is the only symptom of an underlying depression, particularly in men, and it should be considered as secondary to the depressive disorder.

In the workup of patients with CRA, the presence of panic symptoms should be routinely assessed. Chest pain and psychiatric illness represent a very complex relationship. Katon et al. in their first study evaluating psychiatric diagnoses showed that more than 70% of patients with chest pain and a coronary arteriography without significant stenosis had either panic disorder, major depression, or both illnesses compared with about 9% of patients with chest pain and coronary arteriography with significant stenosis.[78] Moreover, the importance of accurate diagnosis and treatment of psychiatric disease is emphasized by follow-up studies of patients with chest pain who have apparently normal coronary angiograms. Normal coronary angiographies do not seem to reassure patients sufficiently.

DIFFERENTIAL DIAGNOSIS AND CLINICAL CASE

A differential diagnosis should be made following a panic attack (Table 20.2). Panic attack can be diagnosed by negative findings of cardiovascular disease but also by looking for positive signs. The positive signs for panic attack are feelings of fear and a patient history of anxiety and/or depression. Nausea, dizziness, paresthesia, dissociative feelings, and autonomic symptoms, as well as feelings of losing reality are also positive signs for panic attack. Because panic attacks often co-occur with depression, other signs of depression, such as negative thoughts, pervasive guilt or worthlessness, low self-esteem, and sleep disturbance, will help in establishing the diagnosis.

Our clinic psychiatrist took a careful history to examine childhood markers of anxiety such as repeated nightmares, enuresis, repeated somatic symptoms, and history of separation anxiety disorder. A careful examination of current symptomatology revealed the diagnoses of both panic disorder and major depressive disorder. Practice guidelines for the American Psychiatric Association and the National Institute for Health and Clinical Excellence (NICE) both recommend first-line treatment with selective serotonin reuptake inhibitor (SSRI)/serotonin norepinephrine reuptake inhibitor (SNRI) medications, not benzodiazepines.[79,80] Among these, sertraline specifically has the most evidence supporting cardiovascular stability and should be considered a first-line agent.[81]

IS PATIENT-CENTERED OR DISEASE-CENTERED CARE PREFERABLE?

Until recently, medical care was focused mainly on pathophysiology and (directly) related therapeutical strategies. Physicians appraised the underlying mechanisms of the disease process and, in doing so, most often neglected other relevant issues in a patient's life.[82]Following this paradigm, in general, physicians do not differentiate the approach between chronic and acute pathological conditions and thus act in a similar manner in both conditions. Subsequently, the patient and relatives sometimes have to deal with challenging psychosocial problems that are not recognized or addressed by the medical world.

Recently, the management focus on chronic diseases—particularly of chronic pain—has shifted from the interdependence of organs to the importance of an interdisciplinary approach to the entire patient. Both psychosocial and quality of life determinants of a patient are now recognized as essential to encompassing a holistic approach. The latter are addressed as such and have become one of the goals of medical therapy that moves beyond treating the biological components of disease.[68]

With patients suffering from CRA, we are facing the limits of curative therapy. Thus, the interdisciplinary therapeutic concept used in the management of noncancer chronic pain patients also applies to CRA patients. This concept was introduced and applied to CRA by M. Chester and colleagues in 1998.[67] In opposition to the traditional medical approach centered on the disease process only, the emphasis was placed instead on the patient and on improving his or her quality of life. This innovative idea was rewarded many times. Patient-centered care is a complex, time-consuming process and involves a drastic change in the education, understanding, and behavior of practicing physicians. It involves a clear understanding of the chronic disease process and also requires an ability to collaborate with the patient. The endpoint of this collaboration is to establish goals and therapeutic options, putting the emphasis on patient's expectations.[67]

During the first few months, it was very difficult for the patient to accept that no further revascularization options existed. His anxiety and stress were difficult to control, and he even asked for a second opinion. When he realized that there were no alternatives to holistic approaches and pain management, he began to accept and was able to cope with his situation. Subsequently, he followed most suggestions, including physical activities, an adequate nutritional program, and work-related stress control.

WHAT ARE EMERGING THERAPEUTIC ALTERNATIVES FOR CRA?

In CRA, healthcare providers face a situation defined as a chronic condition that cannot be controlled by a combination of medical therapy, angioplasty, and coronary bypass surgery. We are thus looking either at palliative approaches or evolving therapies, many of which are still under investigation.

Rehabilitation programs have already been discussed. In addition, it is important to stress that noninvasive and safe, reversible options should be considered first; a "traditional" approach focused on the disease will frequently promote the use of high-risk, invasive techniques. The available therapeutic options are discussed in the following sections.

PHARMACOTHERAPEUTICS

One option is the addition of analgesic medication to the anti-angina treatment. Opioids are often used and may be appropriate. However, most patients suffer from intermittent episodes of chest pain, and the effect of oral or even transmucosal medication is generally slightly delayed and therefore not fast enough to cover breakthrough pain. It is therefore difficult to obtain immediate pain relief. In addition, the omnipresent opioid concerns of tolerance, dependence, and addiction limit the usefulness of these analgesics. The use of opioids should only be initiated with the support of expert opinion.[83]

NERVOUS SYSTEM: NEUROMODULATION AND ABLATIVE TECHNIQUES

Transcutaneous Electrical Nerve Stimulation (TENS)

TENS is a simple technique that applies low-voltage electrical current via pads placed on the skin in the area of pain. It has been used in a variety of pain syndromes, and different mechanisms of action have been proposed. One of the first was the gate control theory of pain that postulates that, via the stimulation of large nerve fibers, an inhibition of the activity of small-diameter fibers is achieved and results in reduced pain. A second proposed mechanism is the activation of endogenous opioid pathways because it has been shown that the effect of TENS is reversed by naloxone.[84]

Clinical studies demonstrate the benefits of TENS in refractory angina patients. Mannheimer et al. showed that in pacing induced angina, patients treated with TENS had an increased tolerance to pacing, less ST-segment depression, and improved lactate metabolism.[85] The advantages of TENS are that it is a safe, noninvasive, and user-friendly method. It can be applied at home by the patient after adequate training. It may induce skin irritation (orthoergic reaction), which makes it difficult for long-term use. Although it seems to be safe and adequate, this cheap, noninvasive option for refractory angina is no longer advocated in the NICE guidelines. In addition, TENS is not approved by the FDA for application over the chest wall.

Spinal Cord Stimulation

Spinal cord stimulation (SCS) is a reversible procedure in which electrodes are implanted in the epidural space to stimulate the dorsal columns of the spinal cord. For many years, SCS has been used to relieve chronic pain in neuropathic syndromes, peripheral ischemia, and CRA. The electrode is positioned in the epidural space to produce paresthesia in the painful area. In the case of refractory angina, the induced paresthesia should cover the region of anginal pain radiation. This technique has been the focus of numerous studies.[86] SCS is listed in the joint guidelines for the treatment of angina of the American College of Cardiology 2002[87] and the American Heart Association (evidence class IIb) and in the recent guidelines of the ESC.[88] Despite the abundant evidence and symptomatic relief provided to CRA patients (equivalent to CABG), it has not yet been adopted by the cardiology community. One meta-analysis of seven randomized control trials (including 270 patients) performed on SCS and refractory angina patients was published in 2009 and reviews most aspects of the therapy.[89] A recent meta-analysis from observational studies confirms the safety and effectiveness of SCS in refractory angina.[90] Because the underlying mechanisms of pain are multifactorial, pain relief can be addressed at many levels. Although not completely understood, increase in and redistribution of regional cardiac blood flow and normalization of the intrinsic cardiac nervous system and spinal mechanisms in SCS are likely to be responsible for symptom reduction.[91–93]

Indications for SCS in refractory angina are NYHA class III and IV patients experiencing angina despite optimal medical therapy with no foreseen benefits from CABG or percutaneous myocardial revascularization procedures.[89]

Complications of the technique are rare and include mainly infections and lead migration, but these are correctable and usually minor.[94] No cardiac-based increased morbidity has been observed when compared to other treatments. Of note, many reports indicate that angina symptoms are not concealed during acute ischemic syndromes.[58] In this regard, electrical neuromodulation is deferring (i.e., normalizing) the sensitized angina threshold rather than abolishing complaints of angina. Outcome studies showed improvement in exercise capacity, significant reduction in nitrate drug consumption, and significant improvement in quality of life (both generic and disease-specific). In one of the controlled randomized trials performed on SCS, the Epidural Spinal Cord Stimulation vs Bypass Surgery (ESBY) study, morbidity was similar in the SCS group compared to the high operation risk CABG group; however, cardiac mortality was higher in the CABG group than in the SCS group.[95]

Left Stellate Ganglion Blockade

This rather old technique was used before CABG became available in the 1950s and has regained some interest recently because it is technically simple to execute, inexpensive, and easily available. The technique has not been adequately studied, however, has serious potential complications and side effects, and has not gained enough evidence to be listed as an option in the strategy of refractory angina therapy.[96]

THORACIC EPIDURAL ANESTHESIA

In thoracic epidural anesthesia, a catheter is placed in the epidural space to achieve pain relief during and after thoracic and high abdominal surgery. It provides efficient analgesia via the infusion of local anesthetics into the epidural space, corresponding spinal roots are anesthetized, and the innervated pain and sensibility of the targeted areas are reduced or abolished according to the drug used. The technique has been shown to be extremely effective in acute and subacute ischemic animal models, as well as in humans.[97] For technical reasons, it is not very attractive for chronic use and therefore it has not been well documented.

TRANSMYOCARDIAL PERFUSION AND VESSEL FORMATION

Transmyocardial (TMR) and percutaneous myocardial laser revascularization (PMR) techniques aim to improve flow through the myocardium by creating channels with laser beams.[98] The first technique, used to channel the myocardium via the epicardium, has been associated with high complication rates. It has been outstripped by PMR, which is safer, nonsurgical, and percutaneously performed via the femoral artery approach. In PMR, a catheter is retrogradely passed through the aortic valve into the left ventricle under fluoroscopy and echographic control. The hypothesis for both techniques was to improve transmyocardial flow; however, it was shown that the channels were closed in less than 24 hours after the procedure. The second hypothesis was that angiogenesis and vessel neoformation was induced by TMR or PMR, although this could not be demonstrated either.

Even though a few studies showed reduction in angina episodes and an increased exercise tolerance, clinical studies were not able to show evidence to support the use of these techniques.[99]

ANGIOGENESIS, CELL AND GENE THERAPY

These new approaches are innovative attempts to improve myocardial perfusion. The idea of in vivo repair of the ischemic myocardium is losing favor to research focused on the role of circulating cells differentiating from bone marrow, termed *endothelial progenitor cells* (EPC). These EPCs have the capacity to proliferate, migrate, and differentiate into endothelial lineage cells.[100,101] Stem cells are also currently under investigation, but, as of yet, only a few clinical studies have been published.

Another promising option is gene therapy, applied by direct intramyocardium injection of naked DNA encoding for vascular endothelial growth factor (VEGF), a heparin-binding glycoprotein.[102] Angiogenesis seems to be highly dependent on the presence of VEGF and significant improvement in flow to ischemic areas in peripheral arteries as well as to the heart.

ENHANCED EXTERNAL COUNTERPULSATION (EECP)

The aim of this treatment is to improve diastolic coronary blood flow using external compression cuffs wrapped around the legs. Myocardial perfusion has been shown to improve using this system.[103] The outcomes of EECP seem comparable to those of SCS.[104]

HEART TRANSPLANTATION

This therapy is not considered feasible for these patients in general[5] because safe, reversible therapies are available. However, when patients also have a severe reduction in LV performance without being candidates for resynchronization therapy, heart transplantation may be considered.

CONCLUSION

Although promising techniques are under investigation, current therapeutic options are still limited for patients with refractory angina. Until more evidence or clinical applications are available for cell and gene therapy, better acceptance of available techniques like electrical neuromodulation, usually executed through SCS, would probably benefit a majority of patients.[55]

> Our patient underwent most therapeutic options, including opiates, which he did not tolerate well. At first, he used weak analgesics, over-the-counter medications, and acupuncture. TENS was also used, but there was difficulty maintaining adhesion to the patient's chest due to abundant chest hair. He began a trial of sertraline, which was up-titrated to effect, and he continued to follow-up regularly with the psychiatrist. The best results in reduction of complaints and improvement in quality of life were obtained with SCS. Like many patients, he was initially hesitant because he worried that when we covered the area where angina was felt with paresthesias he would be unable to feel a significant ischemic event. Finally, he was so disabled by complaints of angina that he agreed to undergo an SCS trial period with an external generator. The result was excellent, and a device was implanted 2 weeks after. Since that moment and for the first time in the past 7 years, he was able to walk and return to work without angina. He started exercising on his home bicycle and finally was able to cycle 20 km at a tailored pace. Unfortunately, one day he burned himself on the oven at work at the site of the SCS implant (left abdomen). Not conscious of the severity of the wound, he covered it with a simple dressing for several days. The pocket became infected and when he finally consulted us, we had no other option but to remove the device, culture bacteria, and start antibiotics. The patient was released after 1 week. After recovering and normalization of infection parameters, a new SCS system was implanted.
>
> So, SCS was successful in improving symptoms, but did it affect his prognosis? That question remains unanswered.

REFERENCES

1. Heberden W. Some account of a disorder of the breast. *Medical Transactions of the College of Physicians*. 1786;II:59–67.
2. Murrel W. Nitro-glycerine as a remedy for angina pectoris. *Lancet*. 1879;1:80.
3. Mulcahy D, Knight C, Stables R. Lasers, burns, cuts, tingles and pumps: a consideration of alternative treatments for intractable angina [editorial]. *Br Heart J*. 1994;71:406–407.
4. Vulink NC, Overgaauw DM, Jessurun GA, et al. The effects of spinal cord stimulation on quality of life in patients with therapeutically chronic refractory angina pectoris. *Neuromodulation: Technology at the Neural Interface*. 1999;2(1):33–40.
5. Mannheimer C, Camici P, Chester MR, et al. The problem of chronic refractory angina. Report from the ESC Joint Study Group

on the Treatment of Refractory Angina. *European Heart Journal.* 2002;23:355–370.
6. Attal N, Fermanian NC, Fermanian J, Lanteri-Minet M, Alchaar H, Bouhassira D. Neuropathic pain: Are there distinct subtypes depending on the aetiology or anatomical lesion? *Pain.* 2008:138(2): 343–353.
7. Stewart S. Refractory to medical treatment but not to nursing care: can we do more for patients with chronic angina pectoris? *Eur J Cardiovasc Nurs.* 2003;2:169–170.
8. Melzack R, Wall PD. Pain mechanisms: a new theory. *Science.* 1965;150(3699):971–979.
9. Latremoliere A, Woolf CJ. Central sensitization: a generator of pain hypersensitivity by central neural plasticity. *J Pain.* 2009;10(9):895–926.
10. Nathan AT, Singer M. The oxygen trail: tissue oxygenation. *Br Med Bull.* 1999; 55(1):96–108.
11. Wang H, Ehnert C, Brenner GJ, Woolf CJ. Bradykinin and peripheral sensitization. *Biol Chem.* 2006;387(1):11–14.
12. Foreman RD. Mechanisms of cardiac pain. *Annu Rev Physiol.* 1999;61:143–167.
13. Mazzone A, Cusa C, Mazzucchelli I, et al. Increased production of inflammatory cytokines in patients with silent myocardial ischemia. *J Am Coll Cardiol.* 2001;38:1895–1901.
14. Crea F, Pupita G, Galassi A, et al. Role of adenosine in pathogenesis of angina pain. *Circulation.* 1990;81:164–172.
15. Pan HL, Chen SR. Sensing tissue ischemia: another new function for capsaicin receptors? *Circulation.* 2004;110:1826–1831.
16. Albutaihi IA, Hautvast RW, DeJongste MJ, Ter Horst GJ, Staal MJ. Cardiac nociception in rats: neuronal pathways and the influence of dermal neurostimulation on conveyance to the central nervous system. *J Mol Neurosci.* 2003;20(1):43–52.
17. Qin C, Farber JP, Miller KE, Foreman RD. Responses of thoracic spinal neurons to activation and desensitization of cardiac TRPV1-containing afferents in rats. *Am J Physiol Regul Integr Comp Physiol.* 2006;291(6):R1700–R1707.
18. Habler HJ, Koltzenburg M, Jänig W. Dichotomizing unmyelinated afferents supplying pelvic viscera and peritoneum are rare in the sacral segments of the cat. *Neurosc Lett.*1988 94:119–124.
19. Cervero F. Visceral pain: mechanisms of peripheral and central sensitization. *Ann Med.* 1995;27:235–239.
20. Cervero F, Laird JM. Understanding the signaling and transmission of visceral nociceptive events. *J Neurobiol.* 2004;61:45–54.
21. Zeilhofer H U. The glycinergic control of spinal pain processing. *Cell Mol Life Sci.* 2005. 62(18):2027–2035.
22. Brooks J, Tracey I. From nociception to pain perception: imaging the spinal and supraspinal pathways. *J Anat.* 2005;207:19–33.
23. Casey K, Tran T. Cortical mechanisms mediating acute and chronic pain in humans. In Cervero F, Jensen TS, eds. *Handbook of Neurology.* 2006; 81. 3rd series. *Pain.* Elsevier B.V.
24. Miletic V, Hoffert MJ, Ruda MA, Dubner R, Shigenaga Y. Serotoninergic axonal contacts on identified cat spinal dorsal horn neurons and their correlation with nucleus raphe magnus stimulation. *J Comp Neurol.* 1984;228:129–141.
25. Rosen S, Paulesu E, Frith C, Frackowiak R, Jones T, Camici P. Central nervous pathways mediating angina pectoris. *Lancet.* 1994;344: 147–150.
26. Hautvast RW, Ter Horst GJ, DeJong BM, et al. Relative changes in regional cerebral blood flow during spinal cord stimulation in patients with refractory angina pectoris. *Eur J Neurosci.* 1997;9(6):1178–1183.
27. Rosen S, Paulesu E, Nihoyannopoulos P, et al. Silent ischaemia as a central problem: regional brain activation compared in silent and painful myocardial ischemia. *Ann Int Med.* 1996; 124:939–949.
28. Droste C, Roskamm H. Experimental pain measurement in patients with asymptomatic myocardial ischemia. *J Am Coll Cardiol.* 1983;81: 164–172.
29. Jolicoeur EM, Cartier R, Henry TD, et al. Patients with coronary artery disease unsuitable for revascularization: definition, general principles, and a classification. *Can J Cardiol.* 2012;28(2 suppl):S50–S59.
30. Khan SN, Dutka P. A systematic approach to refractory angina. *Curr Opin Support Palliat Care.* 2008;2:247–251.
31. DeJongste MJL. Neurostimulation as an adjuvant therapy for patients with intractable angina pectoris. In: *Kader Presentation Service.* Annen, NL. 1994:16.
32. TenVaarwerk IA, Jessurun GA, DeJongste MJ, et al. Clinical outcome of patients treated with spinal cord stimulation for therapeutically refractory angina pectoris. The Working Group on Neurocardiology. *Heart.* 1999;82(1):82–88.
33. Williams B, et al. Patients with coronary artery disease not amenable to traditional revascularization: prevalence and 3-year mortality. *Catheter Cardiovasc Interv.* 2010;75:886–891.
34. Gibbons RJ, Abrams J, Chatterjee K, et al. ACC/AHA 2002 guideline update for the management of patients with chronic stable angina—summary article: a report of the American College of Cardiology/American Heart Association Task Force on practice guidelines (Committee on the Management of Patients With Chronic Stable Angina). *J Am Coll Cardiol.* 2003;41:159–168.
35. Mannheimer C, Eliasson T, Augustinsson LE, et al. Electrical stimulation versus coronary artery bypass surgery in severe angina pectoris: the ESBY study. *Circulation.* 1998;97:1157–1163.
36. Cosın J, Ası'n E, Marrugat J, et al. Prevalence of angina pectoris in Spain. PANES Study group. *Eur J Epidemiol.* 1999;4:323–330.
37. Mukherjee D, Bhatt DL, Matthew TR, Patel V, Ellis VG. Direct myocardial revascularization and angiogenesis—how many patients might be eligible? *Am J Cardiol.* 1999;84:157–161.
38. Lloyd-Jones D, Adams RJ, Brown TM, et al. Heart disease and stroke statistics—2010 update: a report from the American Heart Association. *Circulation.* 2010;121:e46–e215 [published correction appears in *Circulation.* 2010;121:e260].
39. Roehrig C, Miller G, Lake C, Bryant J. National health spending by medical condition, 1996-2005. *Health Aff (Millwood).* 2009;28:w358–w367.
40. Heidenreich PA, Trogdon JG, Khavjou OA, et al. Forecasting the future of cardiovascular disease in the united states: a policy statement from the American Heart Association. *Circulation.* 2011;123:933–944.
41. Stewart S, Murphy N, Walker A, McGuire A, McMurry JJ. The current cost of angina pectoris to the National Health Service in the UK. *Heart.* 2003;89:848–853.
42. Reynolds MW, Frame D, Scheye R, et al. A systematic review of the economic burden of chronic angina. *Am J Manag Care.* 2004;10:S347–S357.
43. Schofield PM, Sharples LD, Caine N, et al. Transmyocardial laser revascularisation in patients with refractory angina: a randomised controlled trial. *Lancet.* 1999;353:519–524.
44. Kandzari DE, Lam LC, Eisenstein EL, et al. Advanced coronary artery disease: appropriate end points for trials of novel therapies. *Am Heart J.* 2001;142:843–851.
45. National Institute for Health and Clinical Excellence. Guidelines for diagnosis and treatment of panic disorder. 2011.
46. Murray S, Carson KGS, Ewings PD, Collins PD, James MA. Spinal cord stimulation significantly decreases the need for acute hospital admission for chest pain in patients with refractory angina pectoris. *Heart.* 1999;82:89–92.
47. Rasmussen MB, Hole P, Andersen C. Electric Spinal Cord Stimulation (SCS) in the treatment of angina pectoris: a cost-utility analysis. *Neuromodulation.* 2004;7(2):89–96.
48. Simpson EL, Duenas A, Holmes MW, Papaioannou D, Chilcott J. Spinal cord stimulation for chronic pain of neuropathic or ischaemic origin: systematic review and economic evaluation [review]. *Health Technol Assess.* 2009;13(17):iii, ix–x, 1–154.
49. Dyer MT, Goldsmith KA, Khan SN, et al. Clinical and cost-effectiveness analysis of an open label, single-centre, randomised trial of spinal cord stimulation (SCS) versus percutaneous myocardial laser revascularisation (PMR) in patients with refractory angina pectoris: The SPiRiT trial. *Trials.* 2008;9:40.

50. Taylor RS, De Vries J, Buchser E, Dejongste MJ. Spinal cord stimulation in the treatment of refractory angina: systematic review and meta-analysis of randomised controlled trials. *BMC Cardiovasc Disord.* 2009;9:13.
51. Andréll P, Ekre O, Eliasson T, Blomstrand C, et al. Cost-effectiveness of spinal cord stimulation versus coronary artery bypass grafting in patients with severe angina pectoris—long-term results from the ESBY study. *Cardiology.* 2003;99(1):20–24.
52. Deanfiel JE, Shea M, Kensett M, Horlock P. Silent myocardial ischemia due to mental stress. *Lancet.* 1984;2:1001–1005.
53. Kim CK, Bartholomew BA, Mastin ST, Taavan VC, Carson KM, Sheps DS. Detection and reproducibility of mental stress-induced myocardial ischemia with Tc- 99m sestamibi SPECT in normal and coronary artery diseased populations. *J Nucl Cardiol.* 2003;10:56–62.
54. Deedwania PC, Carbajal EV. Silent ischemia during daily life is an independent predictor of mortality in stable angina. *Circulation.* 1990;81:748–756
55. Goldman L, Hashimoto B, Cook EF, Loscalzo A. Comparative reproducibility and validity of systems for assessing cardiovascular functional class: advantages of a new specific activity scale. *Circulation.* 1981;64(6):1227–1234.
56. Mukherjee D, Bhatt DL, Roe MT, Patel V, Ellis SG. Direct myocardial revascularization and angiogenesis—how many patients might be eligible? *Am J of Cardiol.* 1999;598–600.
57. Schoebel FC, Frazier OH, Jessurun GA, et al. Refractory angina pectoris in end- stage coronary artery disease: evolving therapeutic concepts. *Am Heart J.* 1997;134(4):587–602.
58. TenVaarwerk IAM, Jessurun GAJ, DeJongste MJL, et al. Clinical outcome of patients treated with spinal cord stimulation for therapeutically refractory angina pectoris. *Heart.* 1999;82:82–88.
59. Schoebel F, Frazier H, Jessurun G, et al. Refractory angina pectoris in end-stage coronary artery disease: Evolving therapeutic concepts. *Am Heart J.* 1997;134:587–602.
60. Osterberg L, Blaschke T. Adherence to medication. *N Engl J Med.* 2005;353:487–497.
61. Hurst J, Morris DC. *Chest Pain.* Armonk, NY: Futura; 2001.
62. Jitta DJ, DeJongste MJ, Kliphuis CM, Staal MJ. Multimorbidity, the predominant predictor of quality-of-life, following successful spinal cord stimulation for angina pectoris. *Neuromodulation.* 2011;14(1):13–18.
63. Vulink NC, Overgaauw DM, Jessurun GA. The effects of spinal cord stimulation on quality of life in patients with therapeutically chronic refractory angina pectoris. *Neuromodulation.* 1999; 2(1):33–40.
64. Spertus JA, Winder JA, Dewhurst TA, et al. Development and evaluation of the Seattle Angina Questionnaire: a new functional status measure for coronary artery disease. *J Am Coll Cardiol.* 1995;25(2):333–341.
65. Zigmond AS, Snaith RP. The hospital anxiety and depression scale. *Acta Psych Scan.* 1983;67(1):361–370.
66. Herta F, Fydrich T, Turk DC. Efficacy of multidisciplinary pain treatment centers: a meta-analytic review. *Pain.* 1992;49:221–230.
67. Moore RK, Groves D, Bateson S, et al. Health related quality of life of patients with refractory angina before and one year after enrolment onto a refractory angina program. *Eur J Pain.* 2005;9(3):305–310.
68. www.angina.org.
69. Monteleone P. The association between depression and heart disease: the role of biological mechanisms. In: Glassman A, Maj M, Sartorius N, eds. *Depression and Heart Disease.* Oxford, UK: Wiley-Blackwell; pp.39–56. 2011.
70. *The ICD-10 Classification of Mental and Behavioural Disorders.* Geneva: World Health Organization; 1992.
71. Rohacek M, Bertolotti A, Grützmüller N, et al. The challenge of triaging chest pain patients: the Bernese University Hospital experience. *Emergency Medicine International* 2012. doi:10.1155/2012/975614.
72. Jonsbu E, Dammen T, Morken G, Lied A, Vik-mo H, Martinsen E. Cardiac and psychiatric diagnoses among patients referred for chest pain and palpitations. *Scan Cardiovasc J.* 2009;43:256–259.
73. Beitman BD, Basha I, Flaker G, DeRosear L, Mukerji V, Trombka L, et al. Atypical or nonanginal chest pain. Panic disorder or coronary artery disease? *Arch Intern Med.* 1987;147:1548–1552.
74. Beitman BD, Mukerji V, Lamberti JW, Schmid L, DeRosear L, Kushner M, et al. Panic disorder in patients with chest pain and angiographically normal coronary arteries. *Am J Cardiol.* 1989;63:1399–1403.
75. Katon WJ. Chest pain, cardiac disease, and panic disorder. *J Clin Psychiatry.* 1990; 51(suppl):27–30; discussion 50–53.
76. Soares-Filho GL, Mesquita CT, Mesquita ET, et al. Panic attack triggering myocardial ischemia documented by myocardial perfusion imaging study. A case report. *Int Arch Med.* 2012;5(1):24.
77. Keng CS, Lee C. Panic attack and its correlation with acute coronary syndrome –more than just a diagnosis of exclusion. *Ann Acad Med Singapore.* 2010;39:197–202.
78. Katon, et al. Chest pain and psychiatric illness. *Am J Med.*1988;84(1):1–9.
79. J Read, R Bentall. Negative chilhood experiences and mental health, theoretical, clinical and primary prevention implications. *Br J Psychiatry.* 2012;200:89–91.
80. Rutter M. Resilience as a dynamic concept. *Dev Psychopathology.* 2012;24(2):335–344.
81. Shapiro PA, Lesperance F, Frasure-Smith N, et al. An open-label preliminary trial of sertraline for treatment of major depression after acute myocardial infarction (the SADHAT trial). Sertraline anti-depressant heart attack trial. *Am Heart.* 1999;137(6):1100–1106.
82. Bensing J. Bridging the gap. The separate worlds of evidence-based medicine and patient-centered medicine. *Patient Education and Counseling.* 2000;39: 17–25.
83. Collett B. Chronic opioid therapy for non-cancer pain. *Br J Anaesth.* 2001;87:133–143.
84. Mannheimer C, Emanuelsson H, Waagstein F. The effect of transcutaneous electrical nerve stimulation (TENS) on catecholamine metabolism during pacing-induced angina pectoris and the influence of naloxone. *Pain.* 1990;41(1):27–34.
85. Mannheimer C, Carlsson C-A, Emanuelsson H, Vedin A, Waagstein F, Wilhelmsson C. The effects of transcutaneous electrical nerve stimulation in patients with severe angina pectoris. *Circulation.* 1985;71:308–316.
86. Hegarty D. Spinal cord stimulation: the clinical application of new technology. *Anesthesiology Research and Practice.* 2012. doi:10.1155/2012/375691.
87. Braunwald E, Antman E, Beasley J, et al. ACC/AHA 2002 guideline update for the management of patients with unstable angina and non–ST-segment elevation myocardial infarction—summary article. *J Am Coll Cardiol.* 2002;40(7):1366–1374.
88. Fox K, et al. Guidelines on the management of stable angina pectoris: executive summary The Task Force on the Management of Stable Angina Pectoris of the European Society of Cardiology. *Eur Heart J.* 2006;27(11):1341–1381.
89. Taylor RS, De Vries J, Buchser E, Dejongste MJ. Spinal cord stimulation in the treatment of refractory angina: systematic review and meta-analysis of randomised controlled trials. *BMC Cardiovasc Disord.* 2009;9:13.
90. Lanza GA, Barone L, Di Monaco A. Effect of spinal cord stimulation in patients with refractory angina: evidence from observational studies. *Neuromodulation.* 2012;15:542–549.
91. De Landsheere CH, Mannheimer C, Habets A, et al. Effect of spinal cord stimulation on regional myocardial perfusion assessed by positron emission tomography. *Am J Cardiol.* 1992;69:1143–1149.
92. De Vries J, Foreman RD, DeJongste MJ. The anti-ischemic effects of electrical neurostimulation in the heart. *Cleve Clin J Med.* 2007;74(suppl 1):S42–S47.
93. Hautvast RWM, DeJongste MJL, Blanksma PK, et al. Spinal cord stimulation causes redistribution in myocardial perfusion during dipyridamole stress testing in patients with refractory angina pectoris as assessed by 13 NH3-positron emission tomography. *Am J Cardiol.* 1996;77:462–467.

94. Turner JA, Loeser JD, Deyo RA, Sanders SB. Spinal cord stimulation for patients with failed back surgery syndrome or complex regional pain syndrome: a systematic review of effectiveness and complications. *Pain*. 2004;108(1-2):137–147.
95. Mannheimer C, Eliasson T, Augustinsson LE, et al. Electrical stimulation versus coronary artery bypass surgery in severe angina pectoris: the ESBY study. *Circulation*. 1998;97: 1157–1163.
96. Chester M, Hammond C, Leach A. Long-term benefits of stellate ganglion block in severe chronic refractory angina. *Pain*. 2000;87:103–105.
97. Olausson K, Magnusdottir H, Lurje L, Wennerblom B, Emanuelsson H, Ricksten S. Anti-ischemic and anti-anginal effects of thoracic epidural anesthesia versus those of conventional medical therapy in the treatment of severe refractory unstable angina pectoris. *Circulation*. 1997;96:2178–2182.
98. Lauer B, Junghans U, Stahl F, Kluge R, Oesterle SN, Schuler G. Catheter-based percutaneous myocardial laser revascularization in patients with end-stage coronary artery disease. *J Am Coll Cardiol*. 1999;34(6):1663–1670.
99. McNab D, Khan SN, Sharples LD, et al. An open label, single-centre, randomized trial of spinal cord stimulation vs. percutaneous myocardial laser revascularization in patients with refractory angina pectoris: the SPiRiT trial. *Eur Heart J*. 2006;27:1048–1053.
100. Losordo DW, Henry TD, Davidson C. Intramyocardial, autologous CD34^{+} cell therapy for refractory angina. *Circ Res*. 2011;109:428–436.
101. van Ramshorst J, Bax JJ, Beeres SL, et al.Intramyocardial bone marrow cell injection for chronic myocardial ischemia: a randomized controlled trial. *JAMA*. 2009;301:1997–2004.
102. Madlav L, Gundewar S, Lefe DJ. Gene therapy for ischemic heart disease *J Mol Cell Cardiol*. 2011;50(5):742–750.
103. Stys TP, Lawson WE, Hui JC, et al. Effects of enhanced external counterpulsation on stress radionuclide coronary perfusion and exercise capacity in chronic stable angina pectoris. *Am J Cardiol*. 2002;89:822–824.
104. Bondesson S, Pettersson T, Erdling A, Hallberg IR, Wackenfors A, Edvinsson L. Comparison of patients undergoing enhanced external counterpulsation and spinal cord stimulation for refractory angina pectoris. *Coron Artery Dis*. 2008;19(8):627–634.

SECTION V

PERSISTENT POSTSURGICAL PAIN

21.

POSTSURGICAL THORACIC PAIN

Dalia H. Elmofty, Asokumar Buvanendran, and Jennifer Moore Brandstetter

CASE PRESENTATION

A 35-year-old woman with intraductal carcinoma of the right breast underwent a modified radical mastectomy and a right video-assisted thoracic surgery (VATS) for excision of a lung nodule 7 months ago. She has unrelenting, severe, right chest wall pain over the breast scar that occasionally radiates to the back in a band-like distribution; it is unresponsive to medical treatment since surgery. Her case has been complicated by issues of noncompliance. While hospitalized, the patient would accept prescribed pain medications (both opioid and nonopioid); however, she failed to refill her pregabalin prescription after discharge. Furthermore, she has missed some follow-up appointments and even routine scans have had to be rescheduled.

Chief complaint: Severe burning pain over the right chest wall unresponsive to medications

Allergies: no known drug allergies

Family: mother deceased from breast cancer

Social history: married, no tobacco use, no alcohol use, no illicit drug use

Review of systems: severe burning pain over the right scar on chest wall associated with numbness and tingling, radiating to back, along T4 dermatome

Physical examination: Vital signs: BP 137/73 mm Hg, heart rate 61 bpm, respiratory rate 16 breaths per minute, oxygen saturation 97% at room air, body mass index (BMI) 36

The chest wall has a clean, healed right breast scar that is hypersensitive to light touch and associated with an area of numbness on the right upper inner arm. Sensation to coldness and wetness has decreased over the right T4 dermatome distribution.

The patient is able to move all four extremities, 2+ reflexes, normal sensory response on all four extremities except for the right upper inner arm. Her ability to lift the right arm above her head is limited. A right winged scapula is noted.

The patient is given a diagnosis of postsurgical neuropathic pain.

QUESTIONS

1. What is the definition of postsurgical neuropathic pain syndrome?
2. What is the prevalence of postsurgical neuropathic pain syndrome?
3. What are the risk factors for developing postsurgical neuropathic pain syndrome?
4. What is the innervation of the breast?
5. What are the different types of breast cancer surgery?
6. What is the innervation of the chest?
7. What are the different types of thoracic surgery?
8. What is the underlying etiology/pathophysiology of postsurgical neuropathic pain syndrome)?
9. What are the clinical characteristics of postsurgical neuropathic pain syndrome?
10. How is postsurgical neuropathic pain syndrome diagnosed?
11. How can postsurgical neuropathic pain syndrome be prevented?
12. What are the treatment options for postsurgical neuropathic pain syndrome?
13. What behavioral and psychological factors need to be considered?

WHAT IS THE DEFINITION OF POSTSURGICAL NEUROPATHIC PAIN SYNDROME?

Chronic pain, as defined by the International Association for the Study of Pain (IASP), is pain without biological value that has persisted beyond the normal tissue healing time, usually 3 months.[1] Neuropathic pain is defined by the IASP as pain "caused by a lesion of the somatosensory nervous system." [1] Post-mastectomy, post-thoracotomy, and post-sternotomy pain are types of chronic neuropathic pain syndromes that can develop after surgery, otherwise known as postsurgical neuropathic pain syndromes.

POST-MASTECTOMY PAIN SYNDROME

Based on current incidence rates, breast cancer will affect 12.4% of women born in the United States.[2] Most women with breast cancer will eventually have some type of surgery. Surgery can range from modified radical mastectomy to breast-conserving surgery with sentinel lymph node biopsy or axillary lymph node dissection. Persistent pain after breast surgery is defined as post-mastectomy pain syndrome.[3] This chronic pain syndrome can burden patients in multiple domains: socioeconomic, psychological, and qualitative. Patients with post-mastectomy pain syndrome report a poor health-related quality of life (HRQoL).[4]

POST-THORACOTOMY PAIN SYNDROME

Post-thoracotomy pain syndrome produces persistent pain in the area of a thoracotomy incision or dermatomal distribution of the intercostal nerves for at least 2 months following surgery.[5] It was first described in 1944 by army surgeons[6] who noticed persistent chest wall pain in soldiers after thoracotomies for war wounds to the chest. The data are inconsistent on the effect that post-thoracotomy pain has on a patient's HRQoL. In a nationwide questionnaire given to patients with post-thoracotomy pain syndrome after lung cancer surgery, pain-related reduction in the activities of daily living affected more than 50% of the patients.[7]

POST-STERNOTOMY PAIN SYNDROME

Post-sternotomy pain syndrome is defined as pain along the sternum arising after surgeries requiring a sternotomy and persisting for longer than 3 months. It can affect daily activities and sleep.[8]

> By definition, our patient appears to have chronic pain after surgery. She had a right modified radical mastectomy and right video-assisted thoracic surgery 7 months ago and continues to have pain at the surgical site.

WHAT IS THE PREVALENCE OF POSTSURGICAL NEUROPATHIC PAIN SYNDROME?

It has been estimated that 10-50% of patients suffer from neuropathic pain after common surgical procedures.[9] The prevalence of post-mastectomy pain syndrome is reported at 25–50%.[10] In a prospective cohort study of women who had breast cancer surgery in Brazil, 52% of the patients reported persistent postsurgical pain at the 6-month follow-up visit.[11] In a population-based study in Denmark, the prevalence rate was 24% as determined from questionnaires mailed to patients 1.5 years after breast cancer surgery.[12] The incidence of post-thoracotomy pain at 6 months has been reported at 25–60%.[13] In a prospective study to evaluate the incidence of chronic post-sternotomy pain in 318 patients who had cardiac surgery, 28% reported chest discomfort 1 year after surgery. The prevalence of post-sternotomy pain has been reported at approximately 30%.[14] The variability in incidence rates may be attributed to a lack of standard criteria to classify postsurgical neuropathic pain.

WHAT ARE THE RISK FACTORS FOR DEVELOPING POSTSURGICAL NEUROPATHIC PAIN SYNDROME?

Risk factors for the development of postsurgical neuropathic pain syndrome may be identified as pre-, intra-, or postoperative (Figure 21.1). Knowledge of the risks identifies patients most vulnerable to developing postsurgical neuropathic pain syndrome so that preventative strategies can be implemented.

POST-MASTECTOMY PAIN SYNDROME

Several risk factors have been identified for post-mastectomy pain syndrome, and these appear in Table 21.1. Preoperative risk factors identified include psychological factors, age, and weight. A positive correlation exists between the presence of anxiety and depression and the development of post-mastectomy pain syndrome.[15] The presence of preoperative pain in the breast, younger age, and high BMI are also predictive factors.[16] Intraoperative risk factors depend on the surgical procedure performed. Patients undergoing axillary lymph node dissection have an increased risk for post-mastectomy pain syndrome compared to patients without axillary dissection or sentinel lymph node biopsy.[17] Data regarding injury to the intercostobrachial nerve have been inconsistent. In a prospective, randomized, controlled study, no difference was found at 3 months between patients with preserved or sacrificed intercostobrachial nerve during axillary dissection.[18] Postoperative risk factors may include the administration of adjuvant therapy. Radiation therapy is one risk factor for post-mastectomy pain.[19] Although

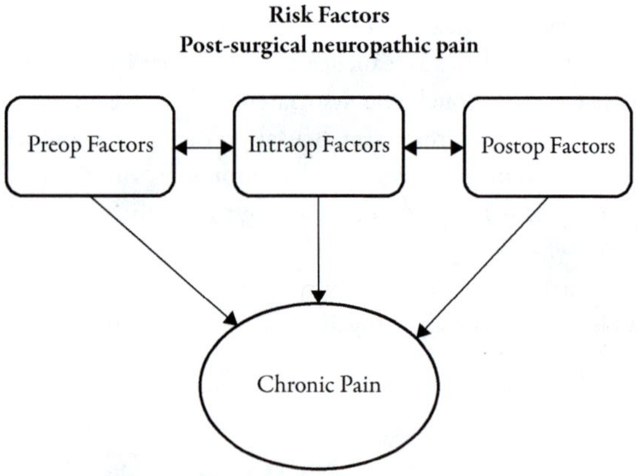

Figure 21.1 Preoperative, intraoperative, and postoperative factors can play a significant role in the development of postsurgical neuropathic pain. Proper identification of these risk factors is important in the implementation of preventative strategies.

Table 21.1 **RISK FACTORS FOR DEVELOPING POST-MASTECTOMY PAIN SYNDROME**

Preoperative	Anxiety, depression, young age, high BMI, pain in breast
Intraoperative	Axillary lymph node dissection
Postoperative	Radiation therapy, uncontrolled postoperative pain

BMI, body mass index

chemotherapy has been identified as a risk factor, its effect, along with endocrine therapy, is uncertain at this time. Uncontrolled acute postoperative pain predisposes to post-mastectomy pain syndrome.[20] In one prospective study aimed at developing a screening tool to identify risk factors of developing persistent pain after breast cancer surgery, patients completed questionnaires the day before surgery and 6 months after surgery. Six factors were identified: previous chronic pain, high number of previous operations, preoperative pain in the area to be operated on, high BMI, history of smoking, and older age.[21]

POST-THORACOTOMY PAIN SYNDROME

Data on the role of psychosocial factors and preoperative pain in the development of post-thoracotomy pain are limited. In a prospective study of patients who had elective thoracic surgery, no relationship was found between the presence of preoperative anxiety or depression and the post-thoracotomy pain syndrome. The Hospital Anxiety and Depression Score was used for measurement.[22] No difference in the incidence of post-thoracotomy pain syndrome was found when different surgical approaches were compared, such as muscle-sparing posterolateral versus posterolateral thoracotomy[23] or muscle-sparing posterolateral thoracotomy versus video-assisted thoracic surgery.[24] Video-assisted thoracic surgery reduced the incidence of post-thoracotomy pain syndrome compared to muscle-sparing posterolateral thoracotomy in another retrospective study.[25] Patients who had video-assisted thoracic surgery experienced less acute postoperative pain,[26] yet a significant number still suffered from post-thoracotomy pain syndrome.[27] No clear relationship was found between the intensity of acute postoperative pain and the development of post-thoracotomy pain syndrome.[28]

POST-STERNOTOMY PAIN SYNDROME

There is limited data on the risk factors for post-sternotomy pain syndrome (Figure 21.1).

> The patient has identifiable pre-, intra-, and postoperative risk factors that predispose her to post-mastectomy pain and post-thoracotomy pain syndrome. She is young and has a high BMI. She has had a modified radical mastectomy, which involves axillary node dissection. The patient also underwent a right video-assisted thoracic surgery, which can injure intercostal nerves. Uncontrolled postoperative pain predisposes her to postsurgical neuropathic pain syndrome.

WHAT IS THE INNERVATION OF THE BREAST?

The breast tissue overlies the pectoralis major and minor muscle, and the intercostal and anterior serratus muscle. The pectoralis muscles are innervated by the lateral (C5–C7) and medial cords (C8, T1) of the brachial plexus. The serratus anterior muscle is innervated by the long thoracic nerve that arises from C5–C7 nerve roots. The thoracodorsal nerve, arising from C6, innervates the latissimus dorsi muscle and runs through the axilla. The breast tissue is innervated by the anterior and lateral cutaneous branches of the third, fourth, fifth, and sixth intercostal nerves (Figure 21.2). The nipple-areola complex is innervated by the fourth thoracic spinal nerve. The supraclavicular nerve from the lower branches of the superficial cervical plexus innervates the upper and lateral portion of the breast. The lateral cutaneous branch of the second intercostal nerve (T2) innervates the axilla and upper medial portion of the arm and is known as the intercostobrachial nerve (Figure 21.2).

WHAT ARE THE TYPES OF BREAST CANCER SURGERY?

Breast cancer surgery can range from radical or modified radical mastectomy to breast-conserving surgery with sentinel lymph node biopsy or axillary lymph node dissection. Radical mastectomy involves removal of skin, fat, breast, underlying muscles (pectoralis major and minor),

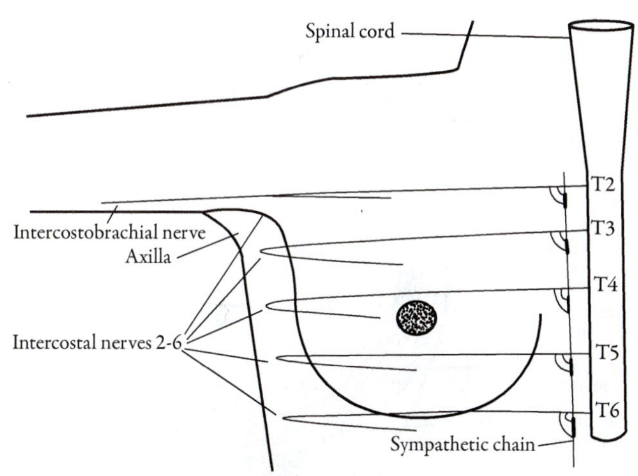

Figure 21.2 Innervation of the breast and axilla. Intercostal nerves 3–6 innervate the breast. The second intercostal nerve (known as the intercostobrachial nerve [ICBN]) innervates the axilla and upper medial portion of the arm. Reprinted from Wallace AM, Wallace MS. Post-mastectomy and post-thoracotomy pain. Anesthesiol Clin N Am. 1997;15(2):353–370, with permission from Elsevier.

and axillary lymph nodes. It is extremely disfiguring and rarely performed today. Modified radical mastectomy involves removal of the skin, fat, breast, and lymph nodes. In breast-conserving surgery, a lumpectomy is performed to remove tumor and a margin of normal tissue in patients who have breast cancer in situ. Some patients undergo sentinel lymph node biopsy; only those who have a positive sentinel node have axillary lymph node dissection. Patients who have breast-conserving surgery may undergo postoperative radiation.

WHAT IS THE INNERVATION OF THE CHEST?

The skin, muscle, ribs, and parietal pleura are innervated by the corresponding intercostal nerves.[29] The vagus nerve conducts noxious stimuli from the visceral pleura and lung parenchyma. The phrenic nerve carries noxious stimuli from the mediastinum and diaphragm.[30] The muscle and nerve innervation of the chest wall is demonstrated in Figure 21.3.

WHAT ARE THE TYPES OF THORACIC SURGERY?

Among the many types of thoracic procedures are posterolateral or modified muscle-sparing posterolateral thoracotomy and video-assisted thoracic surgery.[31] In the posterolateral approach, the latissimus dorsi and the serratus anterior muscles are cut. In the modified muscle-sparing posterolateral method, these muscles are preserved by retracting the latissimus dorsi and serratus anterior muscle. In video-assisted thoracic surgery, several minute incisions are made at multiple intercostal levels for placement of the scopes. After resection, the lung tissue is extracted through the ports.

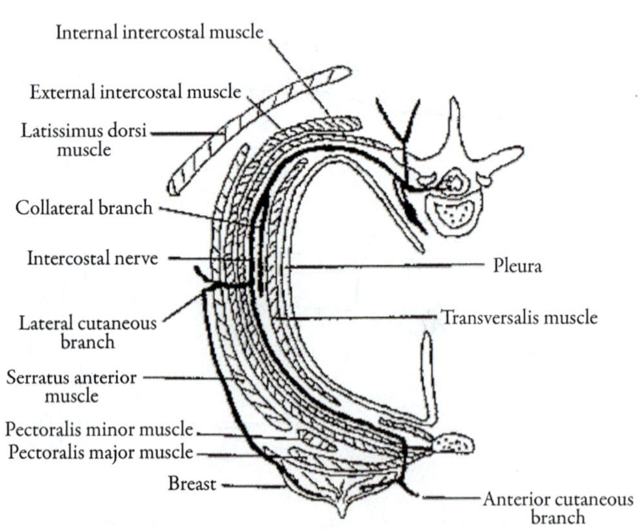

Figure 21.3 Muscles and nerves of the chest wall. Reprinted from Wallace AM, Wallace MS. Post-mastectomy and post-thoracotomy pain. Anesthesiol Clin N Am. 1997;15(2):353–370, with permission from Elsevier.

WHAT IS THE UNDERLYING ETIOLOGY/PATHOPHYSIOLOGY OF POSTSURGICAL NEUROPATHIC PAIN?

The mechanism of postsurgical neuropathic pain is complex, and the cascade of events in the peripheral and central nervous system (CNS) is not fully understood. With initial surgical insult, high-threshold peripheral nociceptors are activated. As the stimulus subsides, the nociceptors should deactivate, but a lesion in the afferent pathway predisposes to neuropathic pain. Injury of neural tissue results in peripheral sensitization, an inflammatory response, and a state of hyperexcitability in the primary afferent nociceptors with spontaneous neuronal discharge. Primary afferent neurons and sympathetic nerves sprout in the dorsal root ganglion. Spinal reorganization and a decrease in descending inhibitory pathways can develop.[32] Prolonged afferent nociceptor input increases CNS hyperexcitability, known as *central sensitization*. If there is inadequate analgesia perioperatively, the nociceptive drive continues and increases excitability in central nociceptive pathways and results in central sensitization.[33]

POST-MASTECTOMY PAIN SYNDROME

Post-mastectomy pain, a complex pain syndrome, can arise from a number of contributing factors. Breast cancer therapy often involves surgical and nonsurgical treatment modalities. Surgical treatment options have been described earlier. Nonsurgical treatment includes chemotherapy, radiation, or endocrine therapy, all of which can predispose to post-mastectomy pain syndrome.

Wallace et al. described the origination of post-mastectomy pain from tissue or nerve trauma (Table 21.2).[34] Tissue trauma, being nociceptive in nature, results from muscle injury. Nerve trauma, from surgical or nonsurgical insult, results in neuropathic pain. Neuropathic pain after breast cancer surgery can be neuroma pain, phantom breast, intercostobrachial neuralgia, or pain from injury to motor nerves.[35] Injury to small cutaneous sensory nerves produces cutaneous scar neuroma.[36] Tasmuth et al. found that patients who had lumpectomy were more likely to have neuroma pain than were patients who had a modified radical mastectomy.[37] The prevalence of neuroma pain following breast cancer surgery has been reported at 23–49%.[35] Phantom breast pain is a sensation that the removed breast is present and painful after modified radical mastectomy. The prevalence of phantom breast pain has been reported at 13–44%.[35] Intercostobrachial neuralgia is likely if the intercostobrachial nerve is damaged during axillary node dissection and is the most common cause of post-mastectomy pain syndrome. The prevalence of intercostobrachial neuralgia is reported at 13–68%.[35] Forceful traction during surgery may injure the medial and lateral pectoral nerve or long thoracic and thoracodorsal nerve. Although motor nerves are less

Table 21.2 ETIOLOGY AND CLINICAL CHARACTERISTICS OF POST-MASTECTOMY PAIN SYNDROME

TISSUE TRAUMA NOCICEPTIVE	CLINICAL CHARACTERISTICS	NERVE TRAUMA NEUROPATHIC	CLINICAL CHARACTERISTICS
Muscle Injury Myofascial pain	Aching muscle pain associated with stiffness and limited range of motion with palpable trigger points	Neuroma	Hyperalgesia or allodynia over breast scar
		Phantom breast	Knife-like, shooting or pricking in area of surgically removed breast
		Intercostobrachial neuralgia	Aching, burning or stabbing pain, numbness, and other sensory changes in the upper, medial aspect of the arm
		Injury to motor nerves	
		Medial and lateral pectoral nerve	Paralysis and atrophy of pectoral muscle
		Long thoracic nerve (*notalgia paresthetica*)	Burning pain between the medial border of the scapula and spine on the affected side with winging of the scapula.
		Thoracodorsal nerve	Paralysis of the latissimus dorsi muscle and weakness with adduction and internal rotation of the shoulder

likely to be a source of neuropathic pain, they have sensory nervi nevorum and may be susceptible.[35]

POST-THORACOTOMY PAIN SYNDROME

The pathogenesis of post-thoracotomy pain syndrome remains unclear and complex. Both peripheral and central sensitization may give rise to postsurgical neuropathic pain. Similar to post-mastectomy pain syndrome, post-thoracotomy pain syndrome can originate from tissue or nerve trauma (Table 21.3).[34] Tissue trauma can result from muscle injury to the intercostal, serratus anterior, pectoralis major and minor, latissimus dorsi, levator scapulae, and teres major and minor. This can result in myofascial pain. Tumor recurrence in surrounding structures also causes pain. Because intercostal nerves transverse the intercostal space, they are prone to surgical trauma from rib retraction, rib resection, or a compressing suture.[38] The incidence of post-thoracotomy pain resulting from rib retraction has been reported as 1–8%; from rib resection, 10–15%.[34] Video-assisted thoracic surgery can also damage the intercostal nerves by trocar insertion or excessive torque on the instruments. If microneuroma forms within a scar, pain may be persistent.

POST-STERNOTOMY PAIN SYNDROME

Several factors are responsible for the development of post-sternotomy pain syndrome. Osteomyelitis, incomplete healing of the sternum, and sternocostal chondritis have been implicated.[39] Post-sternotomy pain can originate from tissue or nerve trauma (Table 21.4). Tissue injury creates myofascial pain. Nerve injury results from damage of the intercostal nerves or the brachial plexus. Anterior chest wall pain, also known as *internal mammary artery syndrome*, has been described as burning chest wall pain after damage to intercostal nerves during dissection and harvesting of the internal mammary artery.[40] Nerves can be entrapped during sternal wire closure. Injury to the brachial plexus from first rib fractured fragments and from positioning of the patient during surgery and during dissection of the internal mammary artery can cause post-sternotomy pain.[41]

Table 21.3 ETIOLOGY AND CLINICAL CHARACTERISTICS OF POST-THORACOTOMY PAIN SYNDROME

TISSUE TRAUMA NOCICEPTIVE	CLINICAL CHARACTERISTICS	NERVE TRAUMA NEUROPATHIC	CLINICAL CHARACTERISTICS
Muscle Injury Myofascial pain	Aching muscle pain associated with stiffness and limited range of motion with palpable trigger points	Microneuroma	Hyperalgesia or allodynia over thoracic scar, reproduced by palpating
		Intercostal neuralgia	Severe, paroxysmal sharp pain along dermatome, wrap around trunk in band-like distribution

Table 21.4 ETIOLOGY AND CLINICAL CHARACTERISTICS OF POST-STERNOTOMY PAIN SYNDROME

TISSUE TRAUMA NOCICEPTIVE	CLINICAL CHARACTERISTICS	NERVE TRAUMA NEUROPATHIC	CLINICAL CHARACTERISTICS
Muscle injury, myofascial pain	Aching muscle pain associated with head, neck, shoulder, and between scapula	Anterior chest wall pain Internal mammary artery syndrome	Anterior chest wall pain on left side described as sharp, aching, burning, cutting or heavy character with altered sensation; hypoesthesia, hyperalgesia, or allodynia
		Brachial plexopathy	Upper extremity pain and chest pain along the T1 dermatome

The patient's symptoms are a result of surgical trauma leading to tissue and nerve injury. The patient underwent a modified radical mastectomy and a right video-assisted thoracic surgery, both of which can cause peripheral nerve injury, peripheral and central sensitization, and postsurgical neuropathic pain syndrome.

WHAT ARE THE CLINICAL CHARACTERISTICS OF POSTSURGICAL NEUROPATHIC PAIN SYNDROME?

Postsurgical neuropathic pain is often associated with hyperalgesia (increased sensitivity to painful stimuli), allodynia (pain from a stimulus not usually painful), paresthesia (abnormal nonpainful sensations, such as tingling), or dysesthesia (unpleasant but not necessarily painful sensations).

POST-MASTECTOMY PAIN SYNDROME

Post-mastectomy pain syndrome appears as a sensory disturbance in the area of the breast tissue, chest wall, axilla, or the medial upper arm.[42] Its characteristics are summarized in Table 21.2.

Neuroma pain can be nonspecific, ranging from aching to burning or electrical sensation in a distinct area of the scar. Hyperalgesia or allodynia may be present. The patient may report a decreased sensation to coldness (ice) or wetness (alcohol swab) over the area. The pain is reproduced by percussion of the scar.

Phantom breast pain is the perception of pain in a breast that has been surgically removed. It can range from nonpainful to painful. It has been described as severe knife-like, shooting, or pricking pain.[43]

Intercostobrachial neuralgia pain results from damage to the intercostobrachial nerve during breast surgery with axillary node dissection.[44] It presents as aching, burning or stabbing pain, numbness, and other sensory changes in the upper medial aspect of the arm.

Injury to the motor nerves can occur during surgery for breast cancer. Damage to the medial and lateral pectoral nerves may lead to paralysis or atrophy the pectoral muscle. From injury to the long thoracic nerve, also known as *notalgia paresthetica*,[45] burning pain may be felt between the medial border of the scapula and spine on the affected side. On examination, a winging of the scapula may be observed. Injury to the thoracodorsal nerve paralyzes the latissimus dorsi muscle, and there is weakness with adduction and internal rotation of the shoulder.

POST-THORACOTOMY PAIN SYNDROME

Patients with microneuromas at an incisional scar site may describe the pain as aching or burning. Numbness or tingling can be reproduced by palpation. Patients with intercostal neuralgia from rib resection or rib retraction report sharp, severe paroxysmal pain along the affected nerve(s) and dermatome(s). The pain can wrap around the trunk in a band-like distribution. Myofascial pain syndrome from muscle trauma is aching muscle pain associated with stiffness and limited range of motion with palpable trigger points. The characteristics of post-thoracotomy pain are summarized in Table 21.3.

POST-STERNOTOMY PAIN SYNDROME

Patients with post-sternotomy pain complain of pain in the chest, head, neck, shoulder, or between the scapulae. Pain may worsen with movement. Nerve injury produces anterior chest wall pain (internal mammary artery syndrome) that is usually left sided. The chest pain is described as sharp, aching, burning, cutting, or heavy. It can be associated with hypoesthesia, hyperalgesia, or allodynia and can be spontaneous or evoked pain. It is thought to be the result of intercostal nerve damage. Brachial plexopathy manifests as upper extremity pain and chest pain along the T1 dermatome.[14] The characteristics of post-sternotomy pain are summarized in Table 21.4.

The patient appears to have the symptoms of neuropathic pain. Based on her clinical presentation, she has breast scar neuroma pain, intercostobrachial neuralgia, long thoracic nerve injury, and intercostal neuralgia. She reports burning pain and hyperalgesia at the site of the breast scar, most likely because of neuroma pain. She reports decreased sensation over the right upper arm indicating intercostobrachial neuralgia. On examination, she has winging of the scapula most likely from long thoracic nerve injury. She also reports severe, sharp pain in a band-like distribution across her right upper chest wall, which indicates intercostal neuralgia from intercostal nerve injury during the right video-assisted thoracic surgery.

HOW IS POSTSURGICAL NEUROPATHIC PAIN SYNDROME DIAGNOSED?

Assessing subjective pain is a challenge. The accuracy of measuring the experience of pain is undetermined. A thorough history and physical examination are fundamental in the investigation. A detailed medical history is taken regarding the onset of the pain and its proximity to surgical trauma. Standardized neuropathic pain screening tools (Leeds Assessment of Neuropathic Symptoms and Signs [LANSS], Neuropathic Pain Questionnaire [NPQ], DN4, Pain-Detect, and ID Pain) aid clinicians in the assessment of neuropathic pain.[46] A careful examination includes assessing sensory signs (the response to pinprick, touch, pressure, cold and heat), motor signs (atrophy and paresis), and autonomic signs (skin color and temperature changes). Electrophysiological and quantitative sensory testing can be useful for diagnostic evaluation.

> Based on history and physical examination, the patient has neuropathic pain. She complains of a burning pain in her chest wall associated with numbness and tingling. She has allodynia. Quantitative sensory testing may be helpful in the diagnosis of postsurgical neuropathic pain to measure sensory thresholds to pain, touch, and temperature.

HOW CAN POSTSURGICAL NEUROPATHIC PAIN SYNDROME BE PREVENTED?

Neuropathic pain is difficult to treat. Prevention is as important as treatment. The first step in prevention is identifying patients at risk. There is growing evidence that psychophysical measures can identify patients who are susceptible to developing chronic postsurgical pain. Quantitative sensory testing utilizes psychophysical measures to assess pain perception and modulation. Diffuse noxious inhibitory control and temporal summation are dynamic psychophysical measures of pain modulation, both sensitization and inhibition. Pain modulation testing can identify patients with abnormal pain processing who are predisposed to suffering from chronic pain after surgery.[47]

Postsurgical neuropathic pain can be influenced by interventions (medications and procedures) perioperatively. Preemptive analgesia, "stopping pain before it starts," is essential in the prevention of postsurgical neuropathic pain by inhibiting surgically induced central sensitization. No single analgesic technique has been proved to prevent postsurgical neuropathic pain, but a multimodal approach, with medications and interventions, may be beneficial. In a systematic review of the efficacy and safety of perioperative gabapentin and pregabalin for patients undergoing surgical procedures, gabapentinoids effectively reduced postoperative pain scores, opioid consumption, and opioid-related side effects.[48] In a randomized, double-blinded clinical trial, perioperative administration of venlafaxine extended-release reduced the incidence of postsurgical mastectomy pain at 6 months.[49] The role of thoracic epidural analgesia has been controversial in the prevention of postsurgical neuropathic pain. In a prospective, randomized, single-blinded trial, the use of thoracic epidural analgesia perioperatively reduced the risk of post-thoracotomy pain syndrome at 6 month.[50] In another prospective, randomized, double-blinded study that compared initiation of thoracic epidural analgesia 20 minutes before incision with initiation after completion of thoracotomy, patients with epidural analgesia before incision had lower pain scores postoperatively and at 6 months.[51] Paravertebral blocks and paravertebral catheters have recently emerged as alternatives to thoracic epidural analgesia. Paravertebral blocks have fewer adverse effects on hemodynamics than does thoracic epidural analgesia. They are associated with less serious neurological complications and may be useful in patients with preexisting coagulopathy. Data are limited regarding its role in the prevention of postsurgical neuropathic pain. In a prospective, randomized trial, patients who received preincisional paravertebral blocks for radical breast cancer surgery had less chronic postoperative pain than those who did not.[52] In another study, interpleural and intercostal nerve blocks did not reduce post-thoracotomy pain syndrome.[38] Minimizing surgical trauma and nerve injury, however, is as important as controlling pain perioperatively.

> A perioperative, multimodal analgesic plan could have been implemented to prevent postsurgical neuropathic pain. Our patient had several identifiable risk factors. After certain surgical procedures, such as mastectomies, thoracotomies, and amputations, postsurgical neuropathic pain syndrome should be anticipated. Quantitative sensory testing may be helpful in identifying patients who may succumb to postsurgical neuropathic pain syndrome. Such patients exhibit changes in diffuse noxious inhibitory control and temporal summation preoperatively. Preoperative initiation of gabapentin, venlafaxine, and/or regional techniques, such as thoracic epidural analgesia, could have been considered as preemptive measures for this patient.

WHAT ARE THE TREATMENT OPTIONS FOR POSTSURGICAL NEUROPATHIC PAIN SYNDROME?

The broadness of this chronic pain syndrome and its coexistence with other types of pain makes the underlying mechanism of postsurgical neuropathic pain relatively complex. Animal models of neuropathic pain have provided valuable information. Human pain research has flourished in the past decade, but very few randomized, double-blinded, placebo-controlled trials exist for the treatment of post-mastectomy pain syndrome, post-thoracotomy pain, or post-sternotomy pain syndrome. The use of evidence-based medicine in combination with individualizing treatment options is recommended. A patient's comorbidities should be considered when determining the plan of management. A multidisciplinary plan with preventative, pharmacological, nonpharmacological, and interventional treatment options is preferred. Figure 21.4 shows a diagram of multidisciplinary approaches for the treatment of postsurgical neuropathic pain syndromes.

NONPHARMACOLOGIC TREATMENT

Among psychotherapeutic treatments for chronic pain are cognitive-behavioral therapy, biofeedback, hypnosis, operant-behavioral therapy, and meditation. The goal of these therapies is to help the patient function in spite of pain.[53] Physical therapy also plays an important role and helps to improve of range of motion.

PHARMACOLOGIC TREATMENT

The mainstay of treatment for postsurgical neuropathic pain, as for other neuropathic pain syndromes, is medication. Cross-sectional studies of chronic neuropathic pain have shown that even with pharmacological treatment, patients continue to experience moderate or severe pain.[54] The evidence-based literature shows that combination therapy has been more beneficial in the treatment of neuropathic pain than single-agent therapy.[55–57] Common agents used in the treatment of neuropathic pain include anticonvulsants, antidepressants, and opioids.

The Neuropathic Pain Special Interest Group of the International Association for the Study of Pain, the Canadian Pain Society, and the European Federation of Neurological Societies have published evidence-based clinical guidelines for the pharmacological treatment of neuropathic pain (Table 21.5).[58–60] The choice of the pharmacological agent for treatment depends on the potential benefit. Medications are introduced at separate time frames to determine efficacy and to observe side effects. With a multimodal approach, different receptors can be targeted to maximize analgesia and minimize drug doses to reduce adverse effects.

Antiepileptic Drugs

Gabapentin and pregabalin are second-generation antiepileptic drugs used to treat neuropathic pain. Both bind to the $\alpha 2\delta$ subunit of the voltage-gated calcium channel that is overexpressed in sensory neurons after nerve injury and reduce the release of excitatory neurotransmitters.[61] They have minimal drug interactions, and adverse effects may include dizziness, drowsiness, nausea, lower extremity edema, and weight gain. Their efficacy in the treatment of neuropathic pain has been demonstrated in randomized

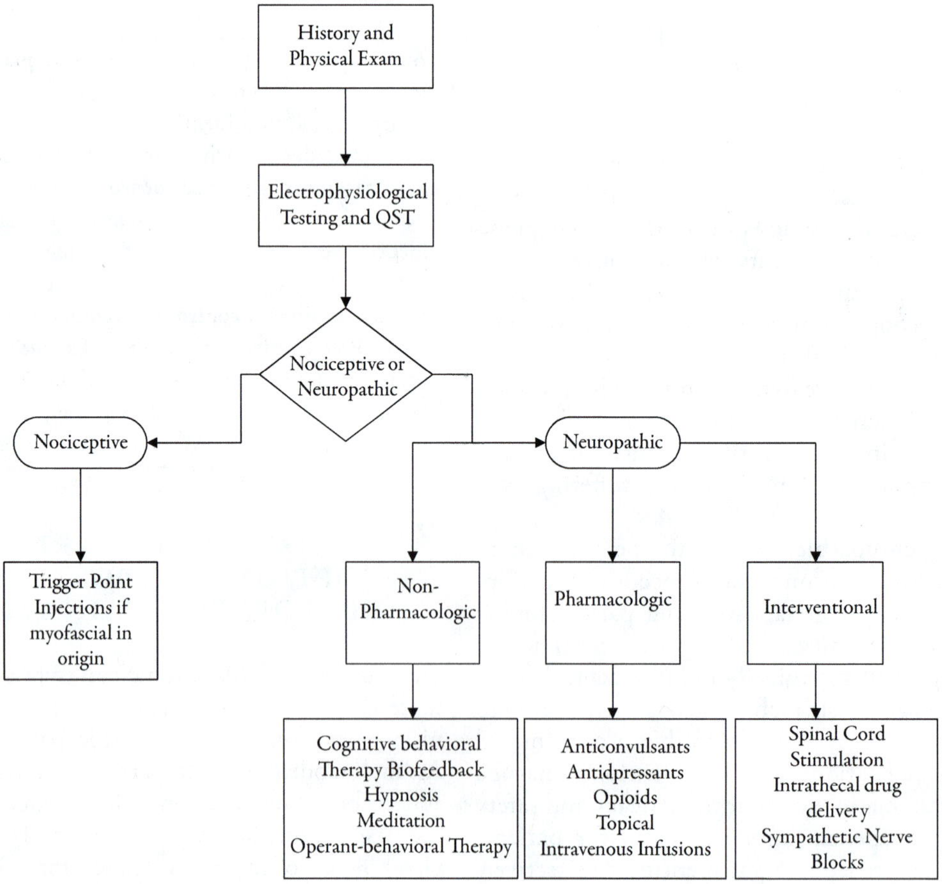

Figure 21.4 Multidisiplinary approach in the treatment of postsurgical neuropathic pain.

Table 21.5 **PHARMACOLOGICAL TREATMENT OF NEUROPATHIC PAIN: RECOMMENDATIONS OF THE NEUROPATHIC PAIN SPECIALISTS INTEREST GROUP AND THE CANADIAN PAIN SOCIETY**

RECOMMENDATIONS	NEUROPATHIC PAIN SPECIAL INTEREST GROUP	CANADIAN PAIN SOCIETY
First Line Treatment	Antidepressants (secondary amine TCAs, SNRIs) Anticonvulsants (gabapentin, pregabalin) Topical Lidocaine	Antidepressants (TCAs) Anticonvulsants (gabapentin, pregabalin)
Second Line Treatment	Tramadol Opioids (oxycodone, methadone, morphine)	SNRIs (duloxetine, venlafaxine) Topical lidocaine
Third Line Treatment	NMDA antagonists Topical capsaicin Mexiletine Other anticonvulsants (exp. carbamazepine, lamotrigine, topiramate, valproic acid, oxcarbazepine) Other antidepressant (exp. bupropion, citalopram, paroxetine)	Tramadol Extended-release opioids
Fourth Line Treatment	Nonapplicable	Cannabinoids Methadone Other anticonvulsants (topiramate, lamotrigine, valproic)

TCAs, tricyclic antidepressants; SNRIs, selective norepinephrine reuptake inhibitors; NMDA, N-methyl-D-aspartate

controlled trials. Gabapentin was found to reduce the incidence of chronic pain after breast cancer surgery.[62,63]

Antidepressants

Tricyclic antidepressants (TCAs) were introduced in the 1950s. TCAs were effective in numerous, randomized, blinded, and placebo-controlled studies. In a Cochrane review, TCAs were found to have a number needed to treat (NNT) of approximately 3.[64] The exact mechanism of action for the analgesic effect is still unclear. TCAs act primarily by inhibiting reuptake of norepinephrine and serotonin. They are also antagonistic at the N-methyl-D-aspartate (NMDA) receptor and act as sodium-channel antagonists. They have effects on several systems: anticholinergic (altered mental status, dry mouth, mydriasis), CNS (myoclonus, syncope), cardiac (tachycardia, orthostatic hypotension), and gastrointestinal (deceased bowel motility). Caution is necessary when TCAs are prescribed for the elderly or patients with cardiovascular comorbidities. An electrocardiogram is recommended before initiating therapy. There are two classes of TCAs, tertiary and secondary amines. The tertiary amines (amitriptyline) inhibit serotonin reuptake more than the secondary amines do. Tertiary amines have a tendency to cause sedation, anticholinergic-like side effects, and orthostatic hypotension. Secondary amines (nortriptyline and desipramine) enhance inhibition of norepinephrine reuptake and have a more favorable side-effect profile than the tertiary amines but can cause irritability and disturbed sleep. Tertiary amines may be beneficial in a patient who has insomnia; secondary amines, for patients with chronic fatigue. In a randomized, double-blind, placebo-controlled crossover study, amitriptyline was found to be effective in relieving neuropathic pain following treatment for breast cancer.[65]

Serotonin and Norepinephrine Reuptake Inhibitors (SNRIs) and Others

SNRIs (venlafaxine, milnacipran, duloxetine) exert balanced inhibition of reuptake of serotonin and norepinephrine that can be dose-dependent. Venlafaxine was as effective in the treatment of neuropathic pain as were TCAs.[64] Perioperative administration of venlafaxine reduced the incidence of post-mastectomy pain syndrome.[48,66] Selective serotonin reuptake inhibitors (SSRIs) do not appear to be as efficacious as TCAs for treatment of neuropathic pain.[67,68] Data on the use of norepinephrine and dopaminergic reuptake inhibitors are limited. Bupropion, a norepinephrine and dopamine reuptake inhibitor, was effective in the treatment of neuropathic pain.[69]

Capsaicin

Capsaicin, an extract from chili peppers, is available as a topical ointment or dermal patch. When capsaicin binds to the transient receptor potential cation channel subfamily V member 1 (TRPV1), otherwise known as the capsaicin receptor, substance P, an excitatory neurotransmitter for pain, is depleted. Topical capsaicin has been beneficial in the treatment of post-mastectomy pain.[70,71]

Lidocaine

Lidocaine, a local anesthetic, is also available as a topical ointment or a dermal patch. It causes temporary loss of sensation in the area of application. The dermal patch has been used in the treatment of neuropathic pain and can reduce allodynia.[72]

Opioids

The use of opioids for the treatment of neuropathic pain remains controversial. Opioids can be administered to patients severely incapacitated from pain until antidepressant and anticonvulsant therapies are titrated to efficacy. Opioid agonists are also initiated if patients cannot tolerate antidepressant and/or anticonvulsant therapy. In a systematic review of randomized controlled trials of opioid agonists for the treatment of neuropathic nonmalignant pain, short-term trials (opioid administered <24 h) and intermediate-term trials (opioid administered 8–56 days) were identified. Results of short-term studies were equivocal; intermediate-term trials were efficacious for the treatment of neuropathic pain.[73]

Intravenous Infusion Therapy

Intravenous lidocaine and ketamine infusions have been used to treat neuropathic pain.[74,75] Lidocaine is a sodium channel blocker that is postulated to act centrally.[76] Ketamine is an NMDA receptor antagonist. NMDA receptor activation is associated with neuropathic pain.[77] Ketamine also has been used to treat cancer pain, postherpetic neuralgia, and diabetic neuropathy,[78] but it has not been beneficial in preventing post-thoracotomy pain syndrome. In a double-blinded, placebo-controlled trial, patients undergoing thoracic surgery were randomized into treatment group (ketamine 1 mg/kg at induction followed by 1 mg/kg/h infusion during surgery) or placebo group. Although ketamine lessened acute postsurgical pain, it did not prevent chronic pain.[79]

INTERVENTIONAL OPTIONS

Complex pain syndromes require treatment strategies that include interventional options. Evidence-based data support the use of spinal cord stimulation (SCS),[80] intrathecal drug delivery,[81] and sympathetic nerve blocks for the treatment of neuropathic pain.

SCS

SCS can be an alternative treatment for certain types of neuropathic pain. It was first used in 1967 to treat neuropathic cancer pain.[82] In 2007, the European Federation of Neurological Societies proposed guidelines for the use of neurostimulation for neuropathic pain.[80] The mechanism of action of SCS still remains unclear. The gate control theory of pain proposed by Melzack and Wall provides some of the basic concepts behind neurostimulation.[83]

Cost-effectiveness studies also have favored SCS. In a randomized, controlled crossover trial, cost-effectiveness of SCS or reoperation was compared in 42 patients with neuropathic pain from failed back surgery syndrome. SCS was more cost-effective than reoperation but was less effective after reoperation.[84] In the PR Prospective, Randomized, Controlled Multicenter Trial of the Effectiveness of Spinal Cord Stimulation (PROCESS) study, SCS was associated with higher health costs at 6 months but improved HRQoL at 3 and 6 months compared to conventional medical management in patients with neuropathic pain from failed back surgery syndrome.[85] The 24-month follow-up study reported sustained improvement of HRQoL.[86]

SCS has been described for post-mastectomy and post-thoracotomy pain syndrome with lead placement between T1 and T4 (Figure 21.5).[87] One lead is placed midline to capture stimulation for anterior chest wall pain, whereas the other lead is placed laterally for coverage of lateral and posterior chest wall pain. To date, there are no reported studies on the use of SCS for the treatment of post-mastectomy pain syndrome or post-sternotomy pain syndrome. Successful use of SCS with complete resolution of symptoms was described for persistent post-thoracotomy pain syndrome resistant to other modalities.[88]

Intrathecal Drug Delivery

The first administration of an intrathecal medication is credited to Leonard Corning in 1885.[89] The identification of opioid receptors in the substantia gelatinosa of the dorsal horn of the spinal cord led to the use of intrathecal opioid analgesia. Intrathecal treatment for neuropathic pain should be considered when conservative measures have failed because it has been shown to be beneficial.[81] Opioids suitable for intrathecal administration include morphine, hydromorphone, and fentanyl. The main advantage of intrathecal opioids is that the dose needed is lower than that for opioids taken orally,

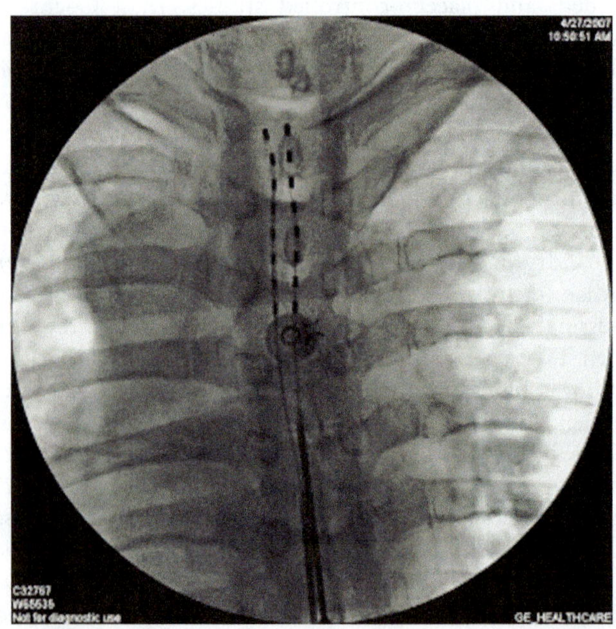

Figure 21.5 Thoracic epidural spinal cord stimulation lead placement between T1 and T4. Reprinted from de Leon OA. Casasola, spinal cord and peripheral nerve stimulation techniques for neuropathic pain. *J Pain Sympt Manage.* 2009;38(2):S28–S38, with permission from Elsevier.

resulting in fewer adverse effects. One disadvantage is the formation of granulomas at the catheter tip, which can lead to spinal cord compression.

Granuloma formation has been associated with escalating doses and concentrations of intrathecal morphine or hydromorphone.[90] Intrathecal local anesthetics, such as bupivacaine, are also effective in the treatment of neuropathic pain.[91] Dosage is adjusted to prevent numbness and weakness. Ziconotide, an intrathecally administered calcium channel blocker, has been beneficial in the treatment of refractory neuropathic pain.[92] Other agents that can be administered intrathecally include α_2 agonists (clonidine) and γ-aminobutyric acid agonists (baclofen). Dosing recommendations for intrathecal infusions were made at the polyanalgesic consensus conference held in 2012.[93]

Sympathetic Nerve Blocks

A dysfunction in the sympathetic nervous system can cause neuropathic pain. Sympathetic nerve fibers sprout into the dorsal root ganglia resulting in sympathetically maintained pain. Sympathetic nerve blocks have been studied for the treatment of neuropathic pain[94] and can be incorporated as part of the diagnostic and treatment algorithm in selected cases. The stellate ganglion is formed by the union of the inferior cervical ganglion and the first thoracic ganglion. It is found in the anterolateral aspect of the seventh cervical vertebral body. Stellate ganglion blocks have been described in the literature as a possible therapeutic intervention for post-mastectomy pain syndrome.[95]

WHAT BEHAVIORAL AND PSYCHOLOGICAL METHODS FOR ARE USED AS TREATMENT?

Patients with chronic pain from breast cancer surgery have been found to have greater psychological stress and psychiatric comorbidities than the general population.[96] Pain is no longer thought to be caused only by pathophysiological changes in the pain pathways; it also involves psychosocial changes. Pain is the result of biological and psychosocial variables; this is otherwise known as the *biopsychosocial model*.[97] Psychotherapeutic treatments such as cognitive-behavioral therapy, biofeedback, hypnosis, operant-behavioral therapy, and meditation may be helpful in the treatment of postsurgical neuropathic pain.

The physician-patient relationship is important in the management of chronic pain. Realistic goals, from both the physician's and patient's prospective, should be discussed. Measures to achieve the goals must be defined clearly. Treatment options—nonpharmacologic, pharmacologic, and interventional—were discussed with the patient. Because the literature supports the use of antiepileptic drugs and antidepressant therapy for neuropathic pain, gabapentin was initiated. Additional considerations included antidepressant therapy, topical capsaicin, opioids (tramadol), and, if pain was still refractory, a trial of intravenous infusion therapies with ketamine or lidocaine. More advanced interventional options can be initiated if conservative medical management fails to improve quality of life. The safety, tolerability, cost, and adherence to the regimen are factors. Unfortunately, our patient was poorly compliant with medical care.

PSYCHOLOGICAL AND BEHAVIORAL FACTORS IN THIS CASE

As clinicians, we have all experienced cases where behavioral or psychological factors negatively impact treatment and/or increase risk to the patients. The *Diagnostic and Statistical Manual of Mental Disorder 5* (DSM-5)[98] conceptualizes this aspect of illness and provides criteria for diagnosis when it becomes clinically significant (see Box 21.1).The criteria account for common etiologies and negative impacts, both in terms of direct effect of the behavior and on increased risk to a patient. The criteria specify that the factor must be present prior to the medical diagnosis and is not a result thereof, which would be better described as an adjustment disorder. The factor must cause significant adverse effect to a present medical condition, further described through severity modifiers. Finally, the factor cannot be better explained by another mental disorder. Although prevalence data are not available, it has been noted that this diagnosis is more common than somatic symptom disorders when reviewing insurance claims. This may be due to the stigma surrounding somatic disorders and psychiatric diagnosis.

One particular factor that is common across specialties is nonadherence and noncompliance. Compliance, as defined in *Stedman's Medical Dictionary*,[99] is the consistency and accuracy with which a patient follows the prescribed regimen by a physician or other healthcare professional. Adherence is defined as the extent to which a patient continues treatment under limited supervision. These terms are often used interchangeably and frequently coexist. They do encompass different aspects of the same concept, however; namely, that compliance is following the doctor's orders overall and adherence is doing so without direct supervision. The difference can be understood in the following example: a patient who refuses to take the prescribed medication while in the hospital is noncompliant, whereas a patient who will take the medication when given but does not take it on his or her own is nonadherent. Clinically, this distinction may not be as significant, particularly in the outpatient setting. It does highlight how there could be an assortment of reasons and motives leading to the behavior. Although many explanations could fit either scenario, the patient refusing the offered treatment may disagree with the treatment plan or have had an adverse effect, whereas the patient who will cooperate in the hospital but not continue at home may have a limited understanding of the treatment or disease, may be forgetful and unintentionally is nonadherent, or may have adverse effects but is willing to tolerate these in order to not be oppositional to hospital staff.

Box 21.1 **PSYCHOLOGICAL FACTORS AFFECTING OTHER MEDICAL CONDITIONS**

Diagnostic Criteria

A. A medical symptom or condition (other than a mental disorder) is present.
B. Psychological or behavioral factors adversely affect the medical condition in one of the following ways:
   1. The factors have influenced the course of the medical condition as shown by a close temporal association between the psychological factors and the development or exacerbation of, or delayed recovery from, the medical condition.
   2. The factors interfere with the treatment of the medical condition (e.g., poor adherence).
   3. The factors constitute additional well-established health risks for the individual.
   4. The factors influence the underlying pathophysiology, precipitating or exacerbating symptoms or necessitating medical attention.
C. The psychological and behavioral factors in Criterion B are not better explained by another mental disorder (e.g., panic disorder, major depressive disorder, posttraumatic stress disorder).

Specify current severity:

Mild: Increases medical risk (e.g., inconsistent adherence with antihypertension treatment)
Moderate: Aggravates underlying medical condition (e.g., anxiety aggravating asthma)
Severe: Results in medical hospitalization or emergency room visit
Extreme: Results in severe, life-threatening risk (e.g., ignoring heart attack symptoms)

This patient shows evidence of both noncompliance and nonadherence. In certain cases, she fails to follow through on beginning or initiating recommendations (missing scheduled radiologic follow-up). In addition, she has initially taken other medications while in a supervised setting (pregabalin while hospitalized) but fails to continue this when left to her own devices, despite the fact that she reports benefit from it.

Epidemiology

Statistics vary across the literature, although most studies report around 50% of patients are nonadherent with medical treatment. This results in increased costs of healthcare as well as poor outcomes for patients. When nonadherence does not meet the criteria for psychological factors affecting other medical conditions, it has in fact been given its own specification with a V-code in DSM-5 stating that nonadherence is severe enough to warrant independent clinical attention. In this case, nonadherence does not meet criteria for psychological factors affecting medical condition. The fact that there is a V-code illustrates how universal and significant nonadherence is in patient care and highlights the importance of monitoring for nonadherence in clinical practice.

This patient meets criteria for psychological factors affecting other medical conditions. Her underlying medical condition (breast cancer and postsurgical neuropathic pain) has been affected due to her noncompliance/nonadherence. The fact that she has missed a scheduled imaging examination may lead to undetected progression/recurrence of her cancer. In addition, she has visited the emergency room for pain control, therefore the specifier would be "severe."

Reasons for Nonadherence

Whether the issue is nonadherence, noncompliance, or both, it is essential to understand the reasons for the behavior in order to intervene and improve treatment outcomes. There is no single method of improving compliance in patients, and each case must be taken individually. For this reason, it is important to have an open conversation with patients about their treatment compliance. As mentioned earlier, noncompliance is ubiquitous, and so it is important to ask patients whether they are taking their medication. To be effective, this must be done without judgment or scolding. An effective method of asking about compliance is to say, "It must be difficult keeping up with all your medications. Often, patients will forget or miss a dose here and there. Does this ever happen to you?" The exchange normalizes the behavior and allows patient to admit nonadherence without feeling chastised. This also will open the door for a conversation about the patient's compliance and adherence, one in which the clinician should seek to understand the contributing factors, thus bridging the way for an appropriate, and likely more effective, intervention.

There are many reasons that patients are noncompliant. Some of the main reasons identified include adverse effects, cost, regimen complexity, scheduling conflicts, poor understanding of illness/treatment, and different belief systems between patient and provider. From this list, there are several different aspects that would each require specific interventions. For example, if cost was the concern, an alternative medication could be substituted. Medi-sets or simplified dosing schedules help with complicated regimens, and alarms can be used to help remind forgetful patients. Clinicians should provide education about the disease and treatment and screen for understanding when applicable. It is important to be cognizant of patient education levels because providing a handout will not be effective to a patient who is illiterate or has poor literacy. It is estimated that 25% of American adults fall into this category and is often underrecognized.

Other times, the noncompliance is more complicated than the fairly straightforward reasons just discussed. Certain psychological factors can have a negative impact and are often more difficult to identify and treat. Some of these factors include humiliation, feelings of helplessness, anger toward physician or self, and a lack of trust/paranoia. An astute clinician will be able to recognize these and intervene early, before the patient and the team are at odds.

Feelings of humiliation and helplessness are common in patients who have otherwise been healthy and are now ill and require increased assistance. Patients often do not want to burden family and friends to the detriment of their own health. Another common scenario is a patient who was previously independent and is now in the hospital, where the schedule is out of his control: the only way he can exert control is by refusing treatment. Brief supportive therapy can be quite helpful, allowing the patient to be heard with an empathic ear. Also, it can be helpful to allow the patient to make choices about less regimented aspects of his care, if at all possible.

Anger at the physician can be due to a variety of reasons, some warranted and some not. It is essential that the clinician not take such feelings personally and to admit missteps or unintentional offense when it occurs. The patient with anger at self often blames himself for his health or sees it as a deserved punishment; this anger is often subconscious and difficult to treat, particularly if unrecognized. If a patient is paranoid, it is important to be open and honest in the treatment and consider referral for treatment if it is part of a psychotic illness.

Strategies for Noncompliance

Having reviewed many of the common reasons that patients are nonadherent, it is easy to see why intervention can be so complicated. Most clinicians underestimate how many of their patients are nonadherent, so a good start is to simply ask patients about compliance. As discussed previously, this can be effective when done in a neutral, nonjudgmental fashion without scolding or shaming the patient. The question not only opens discussion of why the patient is nonadherent, but the question itself can be therapeutic in that it conveys concern and compassion to the patient. During this discussion, emphasizing that you, the clinician, are invested in the patient's care and improvement will increase the likelihood that he or she will adhere to treatment.

A generally helpful strategy is to request that each patient bring in pill bottles for counts. although this is not foolproof and patients could simply throw out their medications, it can be effective for some patients by increasing their accountability. Monitoring refills is another method, although many pharmacies now have automatic refill systems that may mask nonadherence.

Another helpful method is to involve family or ancillary staff, including case managers and nursing, in monitoring adherence. Many patients may have family members in charge of administering medication to improve adherence. Home health nurses can visit weekly to fill medi-sets or, more often, to help administer medications. Certain pharmacies will fill all prescriptions weekly in a medi-set for patients with complicated regimens. These interventions are particularly helpful for patients with cognitive impairment.

Drug levels and urine drug screens are helpful in applicable situations, although this is clearly not available for all medications. In particular, urine drug screens for opiate use can be monitored to ensure patients are taking their medication, if diversion is a concern, and to screen for recreational use that may interfere with treatment. State prescription monitoring registries are another helpful way to monitor drugs with abuse potential to ensure that patients do not have multiple providers and are not receiving multiple prescriptions. With the rising number of deaths from accidental overdoses, it is imperative that physicians prescribing controlled substances monitor their patients.

Nonadherence and Pain

Nonadherence and pain often go hand in hand, but the literature is limited. There are several limitations to such studies including the logistics of measuring adherence. Self-report is the most straightforward method, although patients over-report compliance. Pill counts are also subject to patient misrepresentation, and pharmacy records do not necessarily correlate to compliance. Direct observation is difficult both logistically and can be cost prohibitive.

The available literature confirms that many patients are noncompliant, and, for pain treatment, underuse is often more common than overuse.[100,101] Characteristics of underuse include younger age, higher number of analgesics in the regimen, nonopioid medications, lower pain intensity, and less anxiety. Overuse is associated with current smoker, more frequent dosing, more complicated regimens, and higher comorbid depression and anxiety.[100,101] It is important to note that depression does not have a higher rate of nonadherence,[102]but some symptoms of depression, including decreased energy and motivation, can impact an otherwise adherent patient. It is not a given that a patient with psychiatric comorbidity is nonadherent; however, treating the comorbidity may improve nonadherence if it is present.

Adherence in pain management does have an extra layer of complication given its potential lethality. Close monitoring and open dialogue are paramount to address concerns early. Regimens should be simplified as much as possible, and contracts and drug screens are pertinent as well as prudent. Open discussion and honesty provide improved outcomes and improved adherence. Having family input will again reinforce adherence. Rating scales are another useful clinical tool for addressing adherence, especially the Drug Abuse Screening Test (DAST) and Screener and Opioid Assessment for Patients with Pain-Revised (SOAPP-R). The DAST is a 28-question yes-no self-questionnaire that has a sensitivity of 81–96% and a specificity of 71–94% and is modifiable to different clinical settings. The SOAPP-R is a 14-question self-report measure with a sensitivity of 0.82 and specificity of 0.52. These assessment tools are particularly helpful in cases of previous substance abuse.[103–105]

When the patient presented for her next scheduled follow-up visit, the team discussed with her their concern with her progress. She was reminded that she reported good relief of pain with pregabalin, but did not continue to use the medication. The patient was asked if there was something the team could do differently to help her continue with medication. Furthermore, she was provided with education regarding the benefit of routine scanning in disease surveillance.

After this honest, nonjudgmental discussion, the patient hesitantly revealed her shame and guilt in not being able to comply with recommendations. She had previously been working full-time and had anticipated going back to work full-time when her active breast cancer treatment was completed. The severity of her pain prevented this, however, and she felt this to be a personal failing. Due to her reduced income, she was not able to afford the pregabalin. Her husband continued to work full-time and had taken considerable work leave during the more active phase of her treatment. This had caused some increased work and marital stress, so the patient was hesitant to ask him to drive her to appointments.

Several changes were made to accommodate the patient's situation. First, the patient was transitioned to gabapentin, which she could obtain at a reasonable cost. Second, she was connected to the hospital social worker who established transportation vouchers. Third, multiple appointments were scheduled on one day to prevent disruption in her schedule and save her time and money because she lived 1.5 hours from the medical center.

In summary, psychological and behavioral factors impact healthcare costs and outcomes. In particular, nonadherence is ubiquitous and underrecognized in clinical practice. The first step is vigilance to adherence, followed by an open, honest approach to understand the reasons for nonadherence and to address each case individually. It is essential to work with the patient, and often family, to develop strategies for improving adherence. Pain management brings another layer of complexity to patient adherence and often requires further monitoring and testing, including urine drug screens and assessment measures for screening for abuse. As always, good rapport improves all areas of patient care and is important to patient adherence.[106–108]

CONCLUSION

Postsurgical neuropathic pain syndrome is multifactorial. Identifying predisposing risk factors, preventative or timely detection, and pain management referral are imperative to treating postsurgical neuropathic pain syndromes. Surgeons and anesthesiologists can prevent postsurgical neuropathic pain by identifying high-risk patients and high-risk surgery types. Collaborative efforts are needed to implement a multimodal perioperative analgesic plan.

REFERENCES

1. IASP Task Force on Taxonomy. Part III: Pain terms, a current list with definitions and notes on usage. In: Merskey H, Bogduk N, eds. *Classification of Chronic Pain*. 2nd ed. Seattle, WA: IASP Press; 1994:209–214.
2. Howlader N, Noone AM, Krapcho M, et al., eds. *SEER Cancer Statistic Review, 1975–2009*. Bethesda, MD: National Cancer Institute; 2012.
3. Granek I, Ashikari R, Foley K. The post-mastectomy pain syndrome: clinical and anatomical correlates. *Proc Am Soc Clin Oncol.* 1984;3:122.
4. Peuckmann V, Ekholm O, Rasmussen NK, et al. Chronic pain and other sequelae in long-term breast cancer survivors: nationwide survey in Denmark. *Eur J Pain*. 2009;13:478–485.
5. Merskey H. Classification of chronic pain: description of chronic pain syndromes and definitions of pain terms. *Pain*. 1986;3:S138–S139.
6. Blade B, Dugan DJ. War wounds of the chest. *J Thorac Surg.* 1944;13:294–306.
7. Wildgaard K, Ravn J, Nikolajsen L, et al. Consequences of persistent pain after lung cancer surgery: a nationwide questionnaire study. *Acta Anaesthesiol Scand*. 2011;53:60–68.
8. Eisenberg E, Pultorak Y, Pud D, Bar-EL Y. Prevalence and characteristics of post coronary artery bypass graft surgery pain (PCP). *Pain*. 2001;92(1-2):11–17.
9. Kehlet H, Jensen TS, Woolf CJ. Persistent postsurgical pain: risk factors and prevention. *Lancet*. 2006;367(9522):1618–1625.
10. Gartner R, Jensen MB, Nielsen J, Ewertz M, Kroman N, Kehlet H. Prevalence of and factors associated with persistent pain following breast cancer surgery. *JAMA*. 2009;302(18):1985–1992.
11. Alves Nogueira Fabro E, Bergmann A, do Amaral E, Silva B, et al. Post-mastectomy pain syndrome: incidence and risk. *Breast*. 2012;12(3):321–325.
12. Vilholm OJ, Cold S, Rasmussen L, Sindrup SH. The post-mastectomy pain syndrome: epidemiology study on the prevalence of chronic pain after surgery for breast cancer. *Br J Cancer*2008;99:604–610.
13. Gottschalk A, Cohen SP, Yang S, Ochroch EA. Preventing and treating pain after thoracic surgery. *Anesthesiology*. 2006;104(3):594–600.
14. Van Leersum NJ, van Leersum RL, Verwey HF, Klautz RJM. Pain symptoms accompanying chronic poststernotomy pain: a pilot study. *Pain Med*. 2010;11:1628–1634.
15. Kudel I, Edwards RR, Kozachik S, et al. Predictors and consequences of multiple persistent postmastectomy pains. *J Pain Symptom Manage*. 2007;34:619–627.
16. Andersen KG, Kehlet H. Persistent pain after breast cancer treatment: A critical review of risk factors and strategies for prevention. *J Pain*. 2011;12(7):725–746.
17. Peintinger F, Reitsamer R, Stranzl H, Ralph G. Comparison of quality of life and arm complaints after axillary lymph node dissection vs sentinel lymph node biopsy in breast cancer patients. *Br J Cancer*. 2003;89:648–652.
18. Abdullah TI, Iddon J, Barr L, Baildam AD, Bundred NJ. Prospective randomized controlled trial of preservation of the intercostobrachial nerve during axillary node clearance for breast cancer. *Br J Surg*. 1998;85:1443–1445.
19. Ishiyama H, Niino K, Hosoya T, Hayakawa K. Results of a questionnaire survey for symptom of late complications caused by radiotherapy in breast conserving therapy. *Breast Cancer*. 2006;13:197–201.
20. Poleshuck EL, Katz J, Andrus CH, et al. Risk factors for chronic pain following breast cancer surgery: A prospective study. *J Pain*. 2006;7:626–634.
21. Sipila R, Estlander AM, Tasmuth T, Kataja M, Kalso E. Development of a screening instrument for risk factors of persistent pain after breast cancer surgery. *Br J Cancer*. 2012;(107): 1459–1466.
22. Maguire MF, Latter JA, Mahajan R, Beggs FD, Duffy JP. A study exploring the role of intercostal nerve damage in chronic pain after thoracic surgery. *Eur J Cardiothorac Surg*. 2006;29:873–879.
23. Landrenaeu RJ, Pigula F, Luketich JD, et al. Acute and chronic morbidity differences between muscle-sparing and standard lateral thoracotomies. *J Thorac Cardiovasc Surg*. 1996;112(5):1346–1350.
24. Kirb TJ, Mack MJ, Landreneau RC, Rice TW. Lobectomy-video-assisted thoracic surgery versus muscle-sparing thoracotomy. A randomized trial, *J Thorac Cardiovasc Surg*. 1995;109(5):997–1001.
25. Landreneau RJ, Mack MJ, Hazelrigg SR, et al. Prevalence of chronic pain after pulmonary resection by thoracotomy or video-assisted thoracic surgery. *J Thorac Cardiovasc Surg*. 1994;107(4):1079–1085.

26. Landreneau RJ, Hazelrigg SR, Mack MJ, et al. Postoperative pain-related morbidity: video-assisted thoracic surgery versus thoracotomy. *Ann Thorac Sur.* 1993;56(6):1285–1289.
27. Passlick B, Born C, Sienel W, Thetter O. Incidence of chronic pain after minimal-invasive surgery for spontaneous pneumothorax. *Eur J Cardiothorac Surg.* 2001;19(3):355–358.
28. Tippana E, Nilsson E, Kalso E. Post-thoracotomy pain after thoracic epidural analgesia: a prospective follow-up study. *Acta Anaesthesiol Scand.* 2003;47:433–438.
29. Hazelrigg SR, Cetindag IB, Fullerton J. Acute and chronic pain syndromes after thoracic surgery. *Surg Clin North Am.* 2002;82:849–865.
30. Slater B, Frost E. Pain management after thoracic surgery. *Top Pain Manage.* 2012;28(3):1–8.
31. Koehler RP, Keenan RJ. Management of post-thoracotomy pain: acute and chronic. *Thorac Surg Clin.* 2006;16:287–297.
32. Bridges D, Thompson SW, Rice AS. Mechanisms of neuropathic pain. *Br J Anaesth.* 2001;87(1):12–26.
33. Woolf CJ. Central sensitization: implications for the diagnosis and treatment of pain. *Pain.* 2011;152:S2–S15.
34. Wallace A, Wallace M. Post-mastectomy and post-thoracotomy pain. *Anesthesiol Clin N Amer.* 1997;15(2):353–370.
35. Jung BF, Ahrnedit GM, Oaklander AL, Dworkin RH. Neuropathic pain following breast cancer surgery: proposed classification and research update. *Pain.* 2003;104:1–13.
36. Barelka P, Carroll IR. Chronic pain after surgery for breast cancer. In: Dirbas F, Scott-Conner C, eds. *Breast Surgical Techniques and Interdisciplinary Management.* New York: Springer; 2011:1029–1037.
37. Tasmuth T, von Smitten K, Hietanen P, Kataja M, Kalso E. Pain and other symptoms after different treatment modalities of breast cancer. *Ann Oncol.* 1995;6:453–459.
38. Wildgaard K, Ravn J, Kehlet H. Chronic post-thoracotomy pain: a critical review of pathogenic mechanisms and strategies for prevention. *Eur J Cardiothorac Surg.* 2009;36:170–180.
39. Kalso E, Mennander T, Tasmuth T, Nilsson E. Chronic post-sternotomy pain. *Acta Anaesthesiol Scand.* 2001;45:935–939.
40. Mailis A, Chan J, Basinski A, et al. Chest wall pain after aortocoronary bypass surgery using internal mammary artery graft: a new pain syndrome? *Heart Lung.* 1989;18:553–558.
41. Sharma AD, Parmley CL, Sreeram G, Grocott HP. Peripheral nerve injuries during cardiac surgery: risk factors, diagnosis, prognosis, and prevention. *Anesth Analg.* 2000;91:1358–1369.
42. Gartner R, Jensen MB, Nielsen J, Ewertz M, Kroman N, Kehlet H. Prevalence of and factors associated with persistent pain following breast cancer surgery. *JAMA.* 2009;302(18):1985–1992.
43. Jackson MA, Simpson KH. Pain after amputation. *Contin Educ Anaesth Crit Care Pain.* 2004;4(1):20–23.
44. Vecht CJ. Arm pain in the patient with breast cancer. *J Pain Symptom Manage.* 1990;5:109–117.
45. Tacconi P, Manca D, Tamburini G, Cannas A, Giagheddu M. Notalgia paresthetica following neuralgic amyotrophy: a case report. *Neurol Sci.* 2004;25:27–29.
46. Bennet MI, Attal N, Backonja MM, et al. Using screening tools to identify neuropathic pain. *Pain.* 2007;127:199–203.
47. Granot M. Can we predict postoperative pain by testing preoperative experimental pain? *Curr Opin Anaesthesiol.* 2009;22:425–430.
48. Tiippana EM, Hamunen K, Kontinen VK, Kalso E. Do surgical patients benefit from perioperative gabapentin/pregabalin? A systematic review of efficacy and safety. *Anesth Analg.* 2007;104:1545–1556.
49. Amr Y, Yousef A. Evaluation of the efficacy of the perioperative administration of venlafaxin or gabapentin on acute or chronic post-mastectomy pain. *Clin J Pain.* 2012;26(5):381–385.
50. Senturk M, Ozcan PE, Talu GK, et al. The effects of three different analgesia techniques on long-term post-thoracotomy pain. *Anesth Analg.* 2002;94:11–15.
51. Obata H, Saito S, Fujita N, Fuse Y, Ishizaki K, Goto F. Epidural block with mepivacaine before surgery reduces long-term post-thoracotomy pain. *Can J Anaesth.* 1999;46(12):1127–1132.
52. Ibarra MM, S-Carralero GC, Vincente GU, et al. Chronic postoperative pain after general anesthesia with or without a single-dose pre-incisional paravertebral nerve block in radical breast cancer surgery. *Rev Esp Anestesiol Reanim.* 2011;58:290–294.
53. Songer D. Psychotherapeutic approaches in treatment of pain. *Psychiatry.* 2005;2(5):19–24.
54. O'Connor A. Neuropathic pain. Quality-of-life impact, costs, and cost effectiveness of therapy. *Pharmacoeconomics.* 2009;27(2): 95–112.
55. Gilron I, Bailey JM, Tu D, Holden RR, Weaver DF, Houlden RL. Morphine, gabapentin, or their combination for neuropathic pain. *N Engl J Med.* 2005;352:1324–1334.
56. Hanna M, O'Brien C, Wilson MC. Prolonged-release oxycodone enhances the effects of existing gabapentin therapy in painful diabetic neuropathy patients. *Eur J Pain.* 2008;12:804–813.
57. Chaparro LE, Wiffen PJ, Moore RA, Gilron I. Combination pharmacotherapy for the treatment of neuropathic pain in adults. *Cochrane Database Syst Rev.* 2012;7CD008943.
58. Dworkin RH, O'Connor AB, Backonja M, et al. Pharmacologic management of neuropathic pain: Evidence-based recommendations. *Pain.* 2007;132:237–251.
59. Moulin DE, Clark AJ, Gilron I, et al. Pharmacological management of chronic neuropathic pain. Consensus statement and guidelines from the Canadian Pain Society. *Pain Res Manage.* 2007;12(1):13–21.
60. Attal N, Cruccu G, Baron R, et al. EFNS guidelines on the pharmacological treatment of neuropathic pain: 2010 revision. *Eur J Neurol.* 2010;17:1113–1123.
61. Dooley DJ, Taylor CP, Donevan S, et al. Ca2+ channel alpha2-delta ligands: novel modulators of neurotransmission. *Trends Pharmacol Sci.* 2007;28:75–82.
62. Fassoulaki A, Triga A, Melemeni A, Sarantopoulos C. Multimodal analgesia with gabapentin and local anesthetic prevents acute and chronic pain after breast surgery for cancer. *Anesth Analg.* 2005;101:1427–1432.
63. Fassoulaki A, Patris K, Sarantopoulos C, Hogan Q. The analgesic effect of gabapentin and mexiletine after breast surgery for cancer. *Anesth Analg.* 2002;95:985–991.
64. Saarto T, Wiffen PJ. Antidepressants for neuropathic pain. *Cochrane Database Syst Rev.* 2007;4CD005454.
65. Kalso E, Tasmuth T, Neuvonen PJ. Amitriptyline effectively relieves neuropathic pain following treatment of breast cancer. *Pain.* 1995;64:293–302.
66. Reuben SS, Makari-Judson G, Lurie SD. Evaluation of efficacy of the perioperative administration of venlafaxine XR in the prevention of postmastectomy pain syndrome. *J Pain Symptom Manage.* 2004;27:133–139.
67. Finnerup NB, Otto M, Jensen TS, Sindrup SH. Algorithm for neuropathic pain treatment: an evidence based proposal. *Pain.* 2005;118:289–305.
68. Max MB, Lynch SA, Muir J, Shoaf S, Smoller B, Dubner R. Effects of desipramine, amitriptyline, and fluoxetine on pain in diabetic neuropathy. *N Engl J Med.* 1992;326:1250–1256.
69. Semenchuk MR, Sherman S, Davis B. Double-blind, randomized trial of bupropion SR for the treatment of neuropathic pain. *Neurology.* 2001;57:1583–1588.
70. Watson C, Evans R. The post-mastectomy pain syndrome and topical capsaicin: a randomized trial. *Pain.* 1992;51:375–379.
71. Dini D, Bertelli G, Gozza A, Forno GG. Treatment of the post-mastectomy pain syndrome with topical capsaicin. *Pain.* 1993;54:223–226.
72. Galer BS, Jensen MP, Ma T, et al. The lidocaine patch 5% effectively treats all neuropathic pain qualities: results of a randomized, double-blind, vehicle-controlled, 3-week efficacy study with use of the neuropathic pain scale. *Clin J Pain.* 2002;18:297–301.
73. Eisenberg E, McNicol ED, Carr DB. Efficacy and safety of opioid agonists in the treatment of neuropathic pain of nonmalignant origin. Systematic review and meta-analysis of randomized controlled trials. *JAMA.* 2005;293(24):3043–3052.

74. Park CH, Jung SH, Han CG. Effects of intravenous lidocaine on the neuropathic pain of failed back surgery syndrome. *Korean J Pain*. 2012;25(2):94–98.
75. Kvarnstrom A, Karsten R, Quiding H, Emanuelsson BM, Gordh T. The effectiveness of intravenous ketamine and lidocaine on peripheral neuropathic pain. *Acta Anaesthesiol Scand*. 2003;47:868–878.
76. Finnerup N, Biering-Sorensen F, Johannesen IL, et al. Intravenous lidocaine relieves spinal cord injury pain: a randomized controlled trial. *Anesthesiology*. 2005;102:1023–1030.
77. Petrenko AB, Yamakura T, Baba H, et al. The role of N-methyl-D-aspartate (NMDA) receptor in pain: a review. *Anesth Analg*. 2003;97:25–28.
78. Patil SK, Anitescu M. Efficacy of outpatient ketamine infusions in refractory chronic pain syndromes: a 5 year retrospective analysis. *Pain Med*. 2012;13:263–269.
79. Duale C, Sibaud F, Guastella V, et al. Perioperative ketamine does not prevent chronic pain after thoracotomy. *Eur J Pain*. 2009;13:497–505.
80. Cruccu G, Aziz TZ, Garcia-Larrea L, et al. EFNS guidelines on neurostimulation therapy for neuropathic pain. *Eur J Neurol*. 2007;14(9):952–970.
81. Jamison DE, Wilkinson IM, Cohen SP. Intrathecal drug delivery for neuropathic pain. *US Neurology*. 2011;7(2): 154–162.
82. Shealy CN, Mortimer JT, Reswick JB. Electrical inhibition of pain by simulation of the dorsal columns: preliminary clinical report. *Anesth Analg*. 1967;46 (4):489–491.
83. Melzack R, Wall PD. Pain mechanisms: a theory. *Science*. 1965; 150(699):971–979.
84. North R, Kidd D, Shipley J, Taylor R. Spinal cord stimulation versus reoperation for failed back surgery syndrome: A cost effectiveness and cost utility analyses based on randomized control trial. *Neurosurgery*. 2007;61(2):361–369.
85. Manca A, Kumar K, Taylor R, et al. Quality of life, resource consumption and cost of spinal cord stimulation versus conventional medical management in neuropathic pain patients with failed back surgery syndrome (PROCESS trial). *Eur J Pain*. 2008;12(8):1047–1058.
86. Kumar K, Taylor R, Jacques L, et al. The effects of spinal cord stimulation in neuropathic pain are sustained: A 24-month follow-up of the prospective randomized controlled multicenter trial of the effectiveness of spinal cord stimulation. *Neurosurgery*. 2008; 63:762–770.
87. de Leon-Casasol OA. Spinal cord and peripheral nerve stimulation techniques for neuropathic pain. *J Pain Symptom Manage*. 2009;38(25):S28–S38.
88. Graybill J, Conermann MD, Kabazie ME, Chandy S. Spinal cord stimulation for treatment of pain in a patient with post-thoracotomy pain syndrome. *Pain Physician*. 2011;14:441–445.
89. Corning JL. Spinal anesthesia and local medication of the cord. *NY Med J*. 1885;42:483–485.
90. Gradert TL, Baze WB, Satterfield WC, Hildebrand KR, Johansen MJ, Hassenbusch SJ. Safety of chronic intrathecal morphine infusion in a sheep model. *Anesthesiology*. 2003;99:188–198.
91. Osenbach R. Intrathecal drug delivery in the management of pain. In: Fishman SM, Ballantyne JC, Rathmell JP, eds. *Bonica's Management of Pain*. 4th ed. Philadelphia: Lippincott Williams and Wilkins; 2010:1437–1458.
92. Rauck RL, Wallace MS, Burton AW, Kapural L, North JM. Intrathecal ziconotide for neuropathic pain: a review. *Pain*. 2009;9(5):327–337.
93. Deer TR, Prager J, Levy R, et al. Polyanalgesic consensus conference 2012: recommendations for the management of pain by intrathecal (intraspinal) drug delivery: report of an interdisciplinary expert panel. *Neuromodulation*. 2012;15(5):436–466.
94. Straube S, Derry S, Moore RA, McQuay HJ. Cervico-thoracic or lumbar sympathectomy for neuropathic pain and complex regional pain syndrome. *Cochrane Database Syst Rev*. 2010;7 CD002918.
95. Abbas DN, Abd el Ghafar EM, Ibrahim WA, Omran AF. Fluoroscopic stellate ganglion block for post-mastectomy pain: a comparison of the classic anterior approach and the oblique approach. *Clin J Pain*. 2011;27:207–213.
96. Tasmuth, T, Estlanderb A, Kalso E. Effect of present pain and mood on the memory of past postoperative pain in women treated surgically for breast cancer. *Pain*. 1996;68:343–347.
97. Turk DC, Flor H. Chronic pain: a biobehavioral perspective. In: Gatchel RJ, Turk DC, eds. *Psychosocial Factors in Pain: Critical Perspectives*. New York: Guilford Press; 1999:18–34.
98. American Psychiatric Association. *Diagnostic and Statistical Manual of Mental Disorders*. 5th ed. Arlington, VA: APA; 2013.
99. Stegman JK. *Stedman's Medical Dictionary for the Health Professional and Nursing*. 5th ed. Baltimore, MD: Lippincott Williams & Wilkins; 2005.
100. Broekmans S, Dobbels F, Milisen K, Morlion B, Vanderschueren S. Pharmacologic pain treatment in a multidisciplinary pain center: do patients adhere to the prescription of the physician? *Clin J Pain*. 2010;26:81–86.
101. Broekmans S, Dobbels F, Milisen K, Morlion B, Vanderschueren S. Determinants of medication underuse and overuse in patients with chronic nonmalignant pain: a multicenter study. *Int J Nurs Stud*. 2010;47:1408–1417.
102. Cramer JA, Rosenheck R. Compliance with medication regimens for mental and physical disorders. *Psychiatric Services*. 1998;49(2). Retrieved from http://ps.psychiatryonline.org/article.aspx?articleID=81035
103. Ballantyne JC, Cousins MJ, Giamberardino MA, et al. Screening for opioid use potential. *Pain Clinical Update*. 2008;XVI(7). Available at: www.iasp-pain.org/AM/Template.cfm?Section=Home&CONTENTID=15335&SECTION=Home,HOME&TEMPLATE=/CM/ContentDisplay.cfm
104. Calcaterra S, Glanz J, Binswanger IA. National trends in pharmaceutical opioid related overdose deaths compared to other substances related overdose deaths: 1999-2009. *Drug Alcohol Depend*. 2013;131(1):263–270.
105. Annemans L. Pharmacoeconomic impact of adverse events of long-term opioid treatment for the management of persistent pain. *Clin Drug Investig*. 2011;31(2):73–86.
106. Levenson JL. *The Textbook of Psychosomatic Medicine: Psychiatric Care of the Medically Ill*. 2nd ed. Arlington, VA: American Psychiatric Association Publishing; 2011.
107. Davis TC, Wolf MS. Health literacy: implications for family medicine. *Family Med*. 2004;36(8): 595–598.
108. Philbrick KL, Rundell J, Netzel PJ, Levenson JL. *Clinical Manual of Psychosomatic Medicine: A Guide to Consultation-liaison Psychiatry*. 2nd ed. Arlington, VA: American Psychiatric Publishing; 2011.

22.

POST-HERNIORRHAPHY PAIN

David A. Edwards, James P. Rathmell, and Binit J. Shah

CASE PRESENTATION

A 34-year-old man presents with a 10-month history of right groin pain. The pain started following lifting a heavy object and was initially intermittent. Evaluation revealed a right inguinal hernia, and the patient underwent an open herniorrhaphy 6 months earlier; the pain has been persistent since surgery. He describes the pain as a constant burning sensation in the area of the inguinal incision with occasional radiation to the scrotum. It is worsened by physical activity. A trial of nonsteroidal anti-inflammatory drugs (NSAIDs) was not helpful. He was referred for a second opinion to one of your colleagues—a general surgeon—who in turn refers him to the Interdisciplinary Pain Clinic.

Past medical history is otherwise negative.

Social history: The patient previously worked at a factory job that involved moderate lifting. Since his pain began, he has been put on "light duty."

Review of systems is otherwise positive only for "social" alcohol use.

On examination, the patient weighs 72 kg and is 178 cm tall. There is a well-healed surgical incision and moderate right groin tenderness to palpation. Neurologic examination is significant for decreased sensation to light touch and cold in the area below the scar but above the inguinal ligament.

QUESTIONS

1. What is the differential diagnosis for the etiology of the pain in this case?
2. What further history may be useful in establishing the diagnosis?
3. What other examination findings may be pertinent?
4. What diagnostic studies may be helpful?
5. What is the pathophysiology of persistent postoperative pain?
6. How would you manage the patient's medications?
7. What other approaches would you consider for managing this patient?

WHAT IS THE DIFFERENTIAL DIAGNOSIS FOR THE ETIOLOGY OF THE PAIN IN THIS CASE?

When evaluating a patient with pain after hernia repair, it is reasonable to first consider those factors related to the surgery. Chronic postoperative pain is the most frequently recognized complication of herniorrhaphy since the advancement of surgical technique and the reduction in the incidence of recurrent hernia.[1–4] Still, in the case of pain in the inguinal region, there are many possibilities, and the differential is broad (Box 22.1). Proper consideration of the entire differential is prudent before moving on to more likely perioperative causes.

WHAT FURTHER HISTORY MAY BE USEFUL IN ESTABLISHING THE DIAGNOSIS?

Consider that, in the United States, more than 800,000 hernia repair operations are performed every year, making it the most common general surgical procedure (Scott et al. 2002).[5] The overall incidence of chronic pain after herniorrhaphy is estimated at approximately 12%.[6] This suggests that every year nearly 80,000 people in the United States acquire this chronic pain syndrome and underscores the fact that our patient scenario is a common one in the surgical clinic. When taking a patient's history, it is useful to try to determine if they are having pain from chronic inflammation or nerve injury or if there is a continuous noxious stimulus that can be alleviated, such as with irritation from mesh or staples or recurrent hernia. It is also important to consider the patient's risk factors in the preoperative, operative, and postoperative settings (Table 22.1).

Pain following herniorrhaphy falls into two general categories: neuropathic pain due to nerve injury and non-neuropathic pain. Patients often describe neuropathic pain as sharp, shooting, burning, pricking, and radiating, but these descriptors are nonspecific.[7,8] Herniorrhaphy is considered a high-risk surgery for nerve injury given the close association of several sensory nerves along the

Box 22.1 **DIFFERENTIAL DIAGNOSES FOR CHRONIC INGUINAL PAIN**

- Postsurgical
  - Inflammation
  - Infection
  - Nerve injury
  - Adhesions/scar tissue
  - Staple/mesh irritation
- Gastrointestinal
  - Recurrent/persistent hernia
  - Appendicitis
  - Diverticulitis
  - Meckel diverticulitis
  - Colitis
  - Adhesions
- Neurologic
  - Neurofibromatosis
  - Lumbosacral radiculopathy
  - Spinal tumors
- Urological
  - Epididymitis
  - Cystitis
  - Nephrolithiasis
  - Prostatitis
  - Testicular torsion
  - Urinary tract infection
  - Urethral extravasation
  - Vas granuloma/fibrosis
  - Aneurysm/pseudoaneurysm
  - Thrombosis
  - Hematoma
  - Vascular graft
- Musculoskeletal
  - Sacroiliitis
  - Avascular necrosis
  - Hip osteoarthritis
  - Hip chondritis
  - Trochanteric bursitis
  - Pelvic insufficiency fracture
  - Spondylolisthesis
  - Spondylolysis
  - Lumbar disc disease
  - Adductor strain, "sports hernia"
- Gynecological
  - Endometriosis
  - Ovarian cystitis
  - Cervical disorders
- Infectious
  - Abscess
  - Tuberculosis
  - HIV
  - Lyme disease
  - Herpes zoster
  - Lymphadenitis

Table 22.1 **RISK FACTORS FOR CHRONIC POST-HERNIORRHAPHY PAIN**

PREOPERATIVE	OPERATIVE	POSTOPERATIVE
Younger age	Surgical technique	Pain level
Sex		Infection
Recurrent hernia		Hematoma
Degree of pain		Psychological: low perceived control over pain
Obesity		
Psychological: low optimism		
Employment		

inguinal canal: the ilioinguinal, iliohypogastric, genital branch of the genitofemoral, lateral femoral cutaneous, and the femoral nerves (Figure 22.1). Careful dissection along proper tissue planes and identification of these five major nerves can help reduce the complication of chronic groin pain after surgery.[9]

The anterior rami of T12 and L1 nerve roots bifurcate into the superior iliohypogastric nerve and the inferior ilioinguinal nerve (Table 22.2). The iliohypogastric nerve runs lateral with the 12th thoracic nerve and then anteriorly between the transversalis muscle and the internal oblique muscle. It provides sensation to the hypogastric and suprapubic regions. The ilioinguinal nerve initially runs parallel to the iliohypogastric and enters the inguinal canal anteriorly. The ilioinguinal nerve provides sensation to the pubic region, upper medial thigh, mons pubis, labium majus, root of the penis, and upper scrotum. The genitofemoral nerve originates from the L1 and L2 lumbar nerve roots, pierces and then runs along the psoas anteriorly where it divides into a genital branch and femoral branch. The genital branch pierces the transversalis fascia and enters the inguinal canal, then exits to innervate the labium majus and the mons pubis or scrotum and cremaster muscle. The femoral branch runs along the psoas major under the inguinal ligament to innervate the femoral triangle and anterolateral thigh. Injury through transection or entrapment of these nerves may lead to neuroma formation and persistent pain.

Non-neuropathic pain following herniorrhaphy is the result of nociceptive signaling, either somatic or visceral, typically from the presence of excessive scar tissue, pressure from bulky or heavy mesh used in repair, or mechanical distortion of viscera due to recurrent hernia and adhesions. The quality of this type of pain may be described as aching, throbbing, constricting, tender, shooting, drilling, and gnawing.[7,10]

PREOPERATIVE RISK FACTORS

Several preoperative factors that correlate with the development of chronic pain after hernia surgery have been identified, including age, the severity of acute hernia-related pain, the presence of chronic pain of any type prior to herniorrhaphy, employment status, and psychological factors such as anxiety, depression, and catastrophizing behavior.[11,12]

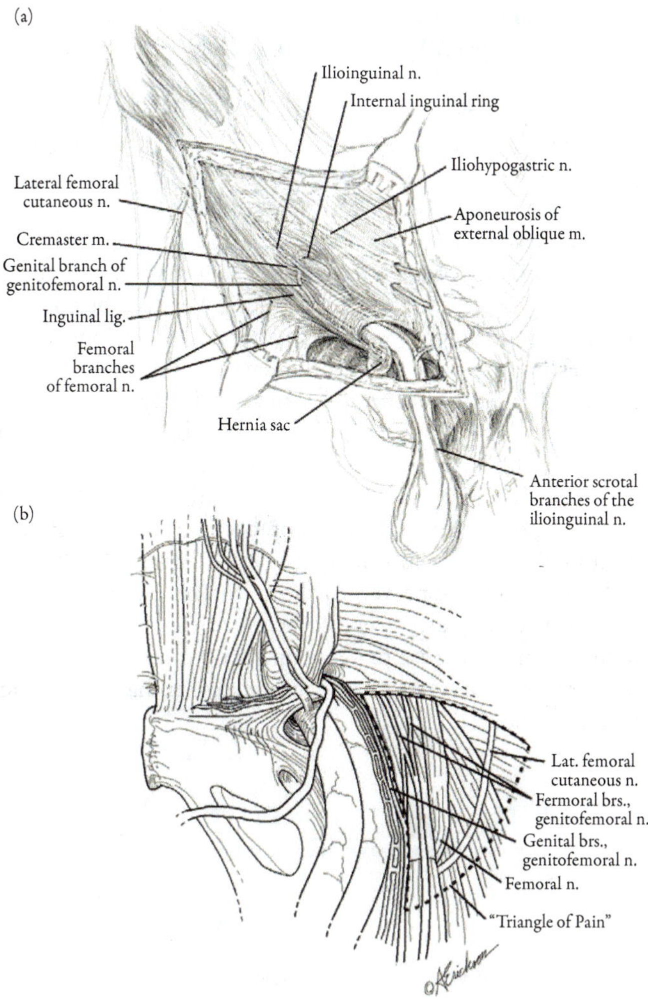

Figure 22.1 A. Open inguinal neural anatomy. B Laparoscopic view of inguinal anatomy. Reprinted with permission from Ferzli GS, et al. Postherniorrhaphy groin pain and how to avoid it. *Surg Clin N Am.* 2008;88(1):203–16, x–xi.

Age

The age of the patient may determine his or her likelihood to develop chronic pain after hernia repair. The risk of chronic pain in children is significantly lower than that in adults. In one follow-up study, children who underwent herniorrhaphy at an average age of 4.6 years were asked about their pain 3 years afterward; the prevalence of chronic pain was found to be 5.1%[13] compared to an overall incidence in adult patients of approximately 12%.[3] In older patients, the outcomes are less clear. Aasvang et al. found no difference in the rate of chronic pain among age groups between 26 and 93 years,[7] whereas Massaron et al. found nearly twice the risk in patients less than 66 years old.[10]

Preexisting Preoperative Pain

Patients who report severe pain before hernia surgery are more likely to report chronic pain at follow-up after surgery.[14–16] The hernia itself may be complicated with entrapment of bowel, stretching of nerves, and inflammation. Susceptible patients

Table 22.2 **NERVES IN THE INGUINAL REGION**

NERVE	ROOT	INNERVATION
Iliohypogastric	T11, T12, L1	Lower abdomen, suprapubic region
Ilioinguinal	T12, L1	Lower abdomen, mons pubis, labium majus, root of penis, upper scrotum, proximal medial thigh
Genitofemoral	L1, L2	Mons pubis, labium majus, scrotum, motor to cremaster muscle, inguinal region, upper medial thigh, anterolateral thigh
Lateral femoral cutaneous	L2, L3	Anterolateral thigh
Femoral	L2, L3	Anterior thigh, motor to quadriceps

may already be sensitized to pain by the presence of preexisting chronic pain elsewhere, unrelated to the hernia.[17]

Psychological Factors

Psychological risk factors for chronic pain after surgery include depression and anxiety.[18] In a prospective study of 135 patients who underwent hernia repair, among the psychological factors assessed (anxiety, depression, fear-avoidance, activity avoidance, catastrophizing, worry about the operation, activity expectations, perceived pain control and optimism), only low preoperative optimism was found to be an independent predictive factor of chronic postoperative pain.[19] In a recent prospective cohort study, postoperative lower perceived control over pain was an independent risk factor for development of chronic pain at 4 months after inguinal surgery.[19]

Employment Status

Several studies suggest there may be a positive association between being gainfully employed or having private health insurance and chronic pain after herniorrhaphy, but the significance or clinical utility of these findings is unclear.[16] A matched case control study from Seattle, Washington, compared 22 consecutive workers compensation recipients to 22 consecutive patients with commercial insurance who underwent inguinal herniorrhaphies. The duration of postoperative pain following herniorrhaphy correlated strongly with the type of employment/insurance coverage. Compared to commercial insurance carriers, the duration of postoperative pain was six times longer for workers compensation patients, and the number of days of work was three times longer.[20]

SURGICAL RISK FACTORS

Surgical Technique

Over the years, the pain outcomes associated with new surgical approaches for hernia repair have been compared with older techniques. In the traditional Shouldice repair, the hernia operation is done through an open incision, and sutures are used to close the defect. This technique is criticized because the sutures can create tension and contribute to post-operative pain. Newer techniques include open repair using mesh and staples or mesh and glue instead of sutures.

Among open techniques, the Lichtenstein repair is the American College of Surgeons' gold standard for inguinal hernia repair.[21] Here, a polypropylene mesh is placed over the front of the defect in the anterior abdominal wall, in front of the transversalis fascia, thus providing a "tension-free" patch.[22] Alternatively, in a posterior approach, mesh can be placed behind the transversalis fascia in the preperitoneal space. The posterior approach requires greater surgical skill and carries an increased risk of hematoma and injury to pelvic structures.[23] The advantage of the posterior approach for the skilled surgeon is that the mesh overlays the hernia defect directly and results in lower rate of hernia recurrence.

The Lichtenstein repair, although tension-free, still results in unacceptable levels of chronic pain. Comparing Lichtenstein to the preperitoneal approach, two trials suggest less chronic pain after preperitoneal approach, whereas a third trial suggests the opposite.[24] In a retrospective review comparing Lichtenstein to preperitoneal approaches, there was no difference in the incidence of chronic pain.[25] The same authors proceeded with a randomized trial and showed an incidence of chronic pain at 1 year of 3.5% in the preperitoneal repair group compared to 12.9% in the Lichtenstein group.[26]

Laparoscopic approaches require greater skill and are gaining in popularity. There are two main laparoscopic approaches: the transabdominal preperitoneal (TAPP) approach and the totally extraperitoneal (TEP) repair. Fewer patients report chronic pain after laparoscopic hernia repair compared to open surgery.[4,27–29] In a prospective randomized controlled trial of 314 patients comparing TAPP versus TEP repair, chronic pain assessed at 3, 6, and 12 months was similar between groups.[30]

Mesh and Fixatives

Lichtenstein and laparoscopic approaches use mesh to fortify the abdominal wall defect. Since mesh repair has become common, the incidence of recurrent hernia has fallen,[5] but the incidence of chronic pain remains high. Mesh may be a source of chronic irritation and inflammation. With a mesh implant, there is an initial foreign body reaction that may persist beyond 3 months. So, recent studies involving a mesh have begun to look at pain at 6 months to 1 year in order to avoid this confounder. If staples are used to secure the mesh, they may entrap nerves causing continuous noxious pain. In a meta-analyses comparing open suture repair to mesh repair it is unclear if mesh repair has decreased the incidence of chronic pain.[5,31] In a retrospective questionnaire of 2,612 Danish patients, there was no difference in incidence of chronic pain among open mesh (Lichtenstein) and open suture repairs (Shouldice or Marcy).[32] Use of a fibrin sealant to anchor the mesh instead of staples or sutures may[33–36] or may not[37,38] reduce chronic pain.

WHAT OTHER EXAM FINDINGS MAY BE PERTINENT?

A careful history with a thorough physical exam will likely be all that is needed to diagnose the most likely etiology of post-herniorrhaphy pain. Recurrent hernia may be visible, and hernia and excessive scar tissue may be palpable.[39] Diagnosis of primary hernia by physical exam has a sensitivity of 74.5–92% and a specificity of 93%.[40] Sensory exam may show hypoesthesia, hyperalgesia, or allodynia along the distribution of a named nerve. Among published reports, descriptions of sensory testing methods are poorly defined.[6] For example, in a study of 276 patients, chronic pain at 1 year significantly correlated with the presence of numbness,[41] but the method of evaluation is undefined. On the other hand, numbness or pain along the distribution of a named nerve (ilioinguinal, iliohypogastric, genitofemoral) has not been shown to correlate with improved pain following surgical intervention aimed at that corresponding nerve.[6] In those who have previously had surgery, the diagnosis may also be more difficult to establish with certainty because patients may have excess scarring and wider areas of numbness. In such cases, other diagnostic studies may be needed.

WHAT DIAGNOSTIC STUDIES MAY BE HELPFUL?

ULTRASOUND

Ultrasound is a versatile and inexpensive technique with the advantage of not exposing patients to radiation. Ultrasound for diagnosis of occult hernia was found to be 86% sensitive and 77% specific.[39] It is also useful for differentiating whether a growing mass is due to recurrent hernia or fluid collections such as seromas, hematomas, or abscesses. If due to a fluid collection, real-time treatment by aspiration can be performed. The disadvantage of ultrasound is that it is user dependent, and variables such as patient obesity, fibrous scar tissue, and pain may result in a poor examination and decreased sensitivity.[42]

MAGNETIC RESONANCE IMAGING (MRI)

MRI with Valsalva is recommended if ultrasound diagnosis of recurrent hernia is negative. MRI has specificity of 94.5% and sensitivity of 96.3% for detection of primary inguinal hernias. Furthermore, it more clearly shows musculoskeletal pathology that may be within the differential diagnosis for inguinal pain. MRI is more sensitive than ultrasound for diagnosis of adhesions.[43] In addition, the status of the primary hernia repair, including mesh and tack position, can be evaluated.

COMPUTED TOMOGRAPHY (CT)

CT is 80% sensitive and 65% specific for occult hernia detection.[39] It is also more sensitive than ultrasound when differentiating seromas from infection or hematoma[44] and depends less on operator skill and the patient's body habitus. It is also more useful than ultrasound for visualizing mesh migration or contraction. If infection or inflammation were a concern, CT would be the study of choice to differentiate these. CT exam following herniography added no increased sensitivity.[45]

HERNIOGRAPHY

Herniography employs plain radiographs after ingestion of radiographic contrast media to outline the contours of the gastrointestinal tract. Herniography is more sensitive than physical examination for the diagnosis of recurrent hernia.[46] The sensitivity for occult hernia detection using herniography is 91% and specificity is 83%[39] but is decreased to 60% specificity in recurrent hernia.[45] The use of herniography is historical at this point, given its invasiveness and that comparable outcomes have been attained with ultrasound and MRI. Plain X-ray gastrointestinal contrast studies may be useful for diagnosing bowel obstruction due to recurrent hernia, adhesions, or constipation.

FLUOROSCOPY

Fluoroscopy with contrast can also be useful for finding bowel obstruction or recurrent hernia if the contrast extends beyond the boundary of the abdominal wall, but it is not as sensitive as herniography or CT.[39]

ELECTROMYOGRAPHY (EMG) AND QUANTITATIVE SENSORY TESTING (QST)

Significant nerve injury can occur during herniorrhaphy.[47,48] EMG and QST may be helpful in this situation[49,50] in clearly defining the extent of neurologic injury when major sensory or motor deficits are apparent in the history or physical examination.

SELECTIVE NERVE BLOCKS

Selectively blocking the ilioinguinal, iliohypogastric, genitofemoral, or lateral femoral cutaneous nerves has been suggested as a means to diagnose the source of post-herniorrhaphy pain prior to surgical neurectomy.[51–53] However, studies in which patients had a decrease in pain with nerve block failed to show a correlation with improved pain outcome following surgical neurectomy or re-exploration and mesh removal.[6] Nerve blocks have not been shown to provide long-term pain relief for patients with post-herniorrhaphy pain.

Our patient is a seemingly uncomplicated young man with a typical history leading to hernia repair who goes on to suffer from persistent post-herniorrhaphy pain. By history, the only preoperative risk factor he has is young age. His pain has already persisted 6 months after the operation. If mesh was used, the inflammatory process can prolong the expected duration of postoperative pain. However, after 6 months, persistent pain due to normal postoperative inflammation is an unlikely explanation, and spontaneous resolution would not be expected. There is numbness above the inguinal ligament in the lower abdomen suggesting injury to the iliohypogastric or ilioinguinal nerves. Physical examination and ultrasound can be used to rule out recurrent hernia. CT can be useful in assessing the position of the mesh, and MRI can help identify the etiology in those where musculoskeletal pathology is suspected (e.g., radiculopathy associated with spinal stenosis producing pain referred to the inguinal region). Selectively blocking nerves may provide short-term pain relief, but does not provide reliable prognostic information prior to surgical re-exploration or neurectomy.

WHAT IS THE PATHOPHYSIOLOGY OF PERSISTENT POSTOPERATIVE PAIN?

It is thought that chronic pain occurs as the final step along a pathway that began as acute pain. Surgical incision and subsequent dissection causes tissue damage that, were the patient not anesthetized, would be perceived as acutely painful. Despite lack of awareness by the patient under anesthesia, peripheral nervous tissue responds protectively to noxious stimuli. In the acute postoperative phase, a region of increased sensitivity to both light touch (allodynia) and lightly painful stimuli (hyperalgesia) develops and can persist for months while the healing process proceeds. This increase in sensitivity in the injured area serves as a protective response, warning the individual to protect the injured area from recurrent injury while healing ensues. When these normal painful responses, including increase in sensitivity in the injured area, persist after the injured region appears to have completely healed, chronic neuropathic pain is present.[18] The transition from normal, acute, protective pain to abnormal, persistent, neuropathic pain is not well understood and remains an area of active research.

MECHANISM OF ACUTE PAIN

Nociception is the detection of noxious stimuli and begins at the primary afferent terminals of first-order neurons that have their cell bodies within the dorsal root ganglia.[54,55] These neurons include medium-sized myelinated Aδ and small unmyelinated C fibers, both of which detect stimuli through free nerve endings. Aδ fibers transmit fast well-localized pain, whereas C fibers transmit delayed and poorly localized pain. The Aδ fibers are subdivided into two types: type I are high-threshold fibers that detect mechanical and chemical stimuli as well as heat at a higher threshold (>50°C). Type II fibers detect mechanical stimuli and heat at a lower threshold (43°C). C fibers are also divided into subtypes that respond to heat, mechanical, and chemical signals. One subclass of C fiber, the "silent" nociceptor, signals only in the presence of tissue injury.[56] Peptidergic C fibers release neuropeptide neurotransmitters (substance P, calcitonin-gene related peptide [CGRP], neuropeptide Y) and glutamate, whereas nonpeptidergic C fibers release glutamate only.

Painful sensation is initiated at the site of tissue injury when ion channels are activated along the free ends of afferent sensory nerve terminals. Heat is detected by activation of nonselective cation channels called *transient receptor potential* (TRP) channels.[57] Activation of TRPV-1 by capsaicin, a receptor ligand and pungent compound found in chili peppers, causes a burning sensation. The receptor molecules that respond to mechanical stimuli (pressure) have not yet been clearly identified, but candidate channels under investigation include acid-sensitive ion channels (ASICs) that detect tissue acidosis in musculoskeletal and ischemic pain,[58] other TRP channels (TRPV2, TRPV4, TRAPA1), and KCNK potassium channels.[54] Chemical irritants, as found in the endogenously produced inflammatory milieu after tissue injury, result in nociception via activation of several TRP channel subtypes (TRPV1, TRPM8, TRPA1).[54]

Peripheral nociceptive signals are transduced to electrical signals and conducted centrally along an axon by sodium channel-mediated action potentials. Nociceptor axons contain the voltage-gated sodium channel subtypes Nav1.7 (tetrodotoxin sensitive) and Nav1.8 and 1.9 (tetrodotoxin resistant).[54] Aδ and C fibers terminate in laminae I–II of the dorsal horn onto second-order neurons that are specific to Aδ or C fibers or are nonspecific (wide-dynamic range neurons).[55] With the arrival of the action potential at the central synapse within the dorsal horn, voltage-gated calcium channels (N-, P/Q-, and T-type) are activated and neurotransmitters are released into the synaptic cleft. Neuropeptide neurotransmitters (substance P, CGRP, and neuropeptide Y) activate postsynaptic G-protein coupled receptors and cause slow postsynaptic potentials. Fast pain is transmitted by the neurotransmitter glutamate, which activates AMPA/kainate receptors postsynaptically. Prolonged repetitive stimulation results in activation of N-methyl-D-aspartate (NMDA) channels by removing its magnesium blockade and is followed by influx of sodium and by calcium that signals downstream cascades and results in modification of the synaptic terminal.

Second-order neurons carry the signal to the brain through ascending pathways from laminae I and V along the anterolateral tract to the thalamus and along the spinobulbar tracts to the periaqueductal gray (PAG) and parabrachial region of the pons. From the thalamus, third-order neurons transmit discriminatory pain sense to the somatosensory cortex. Projections to the limbic and frontal brain regions mediate the affective component of pain; projections from the parabrachial pons to the amygdala mediate the aversive response to pain.

Higher brain centers can enhance or suppress nociceptive signal intensity by way of descending pathways. The cortex, hypothalamus, and amygdala modulate nociceptive input via pathways through the PAG and rostral ventromedial medulla. These regions project to lamina I and V of the dorsal horn where C-fiber signals are inhibited.[55] Descending inhibition is primarily mediated by the neurotransmitter norepinephrine but also by serotonin and endogenous opioids (enkephalins, dynorphins, endorphins).[59,60]

MECHANISM OF PERSISTENT PAIN

Acute nociceptive pain is detected, conducted, and transmitted only while the painful stimulus is present; once the stimulus is removed, nociception ends. If the painful stimulus persists or the intensity is severe, tissue damage, including nerve injury, can occur. When tissue is damaged, proalgesic and proinflammatory mediators are released from the destroyed tissue and from basal cells, mast cells, and macrophages. This "inflammatory soup" consists of cytokines, chemokines, neurotrophins, peptides (substance P, CGRP, bradykinin), and eicosanoids (cannabinoids, leukotrienes, thromboxanes, prostaglandins) that have profound modulatory effects on pain pathways. Peripheral and central nociceptive pathways are enhanced as neurons become more excitable, synaptic signaling more efficacious, and the threshold for painful stimuli is decreased.[61]

Peripheral sensitization occurs when proalgesic and proinflammatory molecules modulate receptors and the transduction and conduction of peripheral neurons.[62] The thermal threshold for activation of TRPV1 is decreased through direct interaction of extracellular protons and lipids and indirectly through activation of second-messenger systems by bradykinin, adenosine triphosphate (ATP), and nerve growth factor (NGF). TRPA1 is modulated directly by prostaglandins and indirectly by bradykinin. ASIC channels are activated in the presence of protons, such as occurs with pH decline in tissue ischemic acidosis. This state of increased sensitivity, where responses to noxious stimuli are exaggerated and prolonged, is called *primary hyperalgesia*.

Secondary hyperalgesia, pain that spreads beyond the site of injury, is the result of neuroplastic changes within the central nervous system (CNS), called *central sensitization*.[63] Central sensitization is pain hypersensitivity that results from activity-dependent synaptic plasticity and requires intense, repetitive, and sustained noxious stimuli with or without tissue damage. The early phase of central sensitization is phosphorylation-dependent and results in glutamate receptor and ion channel sensitivity.[61] The heightened level of sensitivity is a protective mechanism to allow for prolonged time to heal. Even though it may last for months, hyperalgesia is not necessarily irreversible; in the absence of further noxious stimuli, the changes may revert to the prior level of sensitivity.[62]

MECHANISM OF CHRONIC PAIN

During late-phase central sensitization, changes in transcription and translation underlie longer lasting change seen in pathological states.[62] Pain is pathological when it persists despite the absence of a noxious stimulus and when it outlives the normal period of hyperalgesia with wound healing. Both neuropathic pain and inflammatory pain can outlive the initial injury and persist as pathological pain.

Neuropathic Pain

Neuropathic pain can be caused during surgery if nerves are transected or damaged. When C fibers are injured, they may continue to fire spontaneously. Activity-dependent central sensitization in the dorsal horn is maintained by this continuous ectopic firing.[64] Transcriptional changes occur in the C-fiber cell bodies of dorsal root ganglia altering expression of ion channels, receptors, neurotransmitters, and cell scaffolding molecules.[65] Damage to A-fibers results in a change in transcription and new neurotransmitter release. Typically non-nociceptive A-fibers now release substance P and brain-derived neurotrophic factor (BDNF) at central synapses in the dorsal horn and sustain central sensitization.[65–67]

Continual and prolonged activation of NMDA receptors postsynaptically causes excitotoxicity and apoptosis of interneurons.[68] The resultant loss of GABAergic and glycinergic transmission further decreases inhibition, thus leading to more excitation.[69] C-fiber terminals degenerate in lamina II[70,71] allowing Aβ fibers to sprout in. Low-threshold stimuli that would normally transmit light touch sensation via Aβ fibers now cause painful sensation by transmission to nociceptive-specific second-order neurons.[72,73]

Dorsal horn astrocytes and microglia are also activated following neuron injury. Activated microglia release BDNF that changes chloride channel (KCC2) expression and abolishes normal inhibition of neurons dependent on chloride gradients.[74] Activated astrocytes release ATP, nitric oxide (NO), cytokines, and chemokines enhancing and maintaining neuronal hypersensitivity.[62,75]

Inflammatory Pain

Even in the absence of nerve injury, postsurgical inflammation causes a phenotypic switch in primary sensory neurons that induces central sensitization.[62] Aβ fibers begin to express substance P and BDNF at central synapses and transmit low-threshold innocuous sensation onto nociceptive second-order neurons in the superficial dorsal horn.[76,77] Activation here drives cyclo-oxygenase-2 (COX-2) production of prostaglandin E2 and enhances glutamate receptor sensitivity. Activation of microglia results in release of pro-inflammatory cytokines that enhance excitatory and reduce inhibitory currents and further promote central sensitization.[78]

> Herniorrhaphy is a surgery that carries a high risk for nerve injury. The duration and characteristics of our patient's persistent postsurgical pain make it likely that he is experiencing chronic neuropathic pain. If mesh were used in the original hernia repair, then the postsurgical inflammatory phase would be prolonged. However, he is now 6 months postoperative, so we suspect that there is peripheral enhancement of neuronal signaling and development of central sensitization.

HOW WOULD YOU MANAGE THE PATIENT'S MEDICATIONS?

The International Association for the Study of Pain (IASP)'s Neuropathic Pain Interest Group formulated guidelines for the medical management of neuropathic pain.[79] As first-line agents, they recommend calcium channel ligands (gabapentin and pregabalin), topical lidocaine, tricyclic antidepressants (TCAs), and serotonin and norepinephrine reuptake inhibitors (SNRIs) (Table 22.3). The IASP, Latin American experts, and the Canadian Pain Society group neuropathic pain as a single entity, whereas the European Federation of Neurological Societies (EFNS) splits neuropathic pain into different conditions. None of these expert groups divides out or provides treatment recommendations specifically aimed at postsurgical neuropathic pain. As a result, medical treatment for chronic postsurgical neuropathic pain follows the guidelines of neuropathic pain treatment in general.[80]

FIRST-LINE MEDICATION THERAPY

Calcium Channel Ligands (Gabapentin, Pregabalin)

Gabapentin and pregabalin target the $\alpha_2\delta$ subunit of a voltage-gated calcium channel known to be involved in maintenance of central sensitization and chronic pain.[81] Their action results in decreased neuronal excitability, thus their advantage as antiepileptics at higher doses.[81] The recommended dose of gabapentin for neuropathic pain is 600 mg three times daily and can be increased up to 1,200 mg three times daily. This must be adjusted in renal insufficiency. Slow titration up to the recommended dose over 3–8 weeks may help obtain pain relief with minimal side effects such as somnolence and dizziness. The effective dose for pregabalin is 150–600 mg/d in divided doses two or three times daily. A recommended starting dose is 75 mg twice daily or 50 mg three times daily for the first 3–5 days, then followed by an increase to 300 mg/d in divided doses. Titration is also recommended to avoid early side effects similar to those of gabapentin (dizziness, somnolence, headache, peripheral edema). Renal adjustment for pregabalin is also necessary.

Topical Lidocaine

Topical lidocaine is recommended for patients with localized peripheral neuropathic pain, particularly those with localized

Table 22.3 **MEDICATION TREATMENT RECOMMENDATIONS FOR POSTSURGICAL CHRONIC PAIN**

FIRST-LINE	SECOND-LINE	THIRD-LINE
Calcium channel ligands	*Opioids*	*Other antiepileptics*
Gabapentin		Lamotrigine
Pregabalin	Tramadol	Carbamazepine
TCAs		Oxcarbazepine
Nortriptyline		Topiramate
Amitriptyline		Levetiracetam
Desipramine		Zonisamide
Imipramine		*Other antidepressants*
SNRIs		Bupropion
Duloxetine		Paroxetine
Venlafaxine		Citalopram
Lidocaine 5% topical		Mexiletine
		Capsaicin cream

sensitivity to light touch (allodynia), and is available commercially as a 5% patch for topical application. Up to 3 patches can be applied for 12 hours with minimal blood levels.[82] Side effects are limited to rash or erythema from the patch adhesive.

TCAs: Nortriptyline, Desipramine, Amitriptyline, Imipramine

TCAs inhibit the reuptake of the biogenic amines serotonin and norepinephrine. Placebo-controlled trials consistently support the use of TCAs for neuropathic pain.[79,83] Secondary amines (nortriptyline and desipramine) are preferred over tertiary amines (amitriptyline and imipramine) given the lower incidence of side effects and better safety profile.[84–86] Nortriptyline and gabapentin have been shown to provide better pain control in combination, thus allowing for reduced dose and limiting side effects.[87] The most common side effects of TCAs include sedation, tachycardia, dry mouth, constipation, urinary retention, and orthostatic hypotension. At doses of greater than 100 mg/d there may be an increased risk of sudden cardiac death.[88] Caution should be used when prescribing TCAs in patients with cardiac risk factors,[89] in the elderly with cognitive impairment or at risk for falls, and in those at risk for suicide. Titrate TCAs up until pain control is reached or the dose becomes limited by side effects. It is recommended to start at a low dose of 10–25 mg at bedtime and gradually increase to 150 mg or until limited by side effects.[90]

SNRIs: Duloxetine, Venlafaxine

Duloxetine inhibits the reuptake of both serotonin and norepinephrine. It is useful for treating neuropathic pain at doses between 30 and 120 mg/d. A recommended titration is to start at 30 mg/d and then after 5–7 days increase to 60 mg/d to avoid the main side effect of nausea.[91]

SECOND-LINE MEDICATION THERAPY

Opioid Analgesics

Opioid analgesics may be first-line agents in the treatment of certain chronic pain conditions such as in cancer-related care. In chronic noncancer pain, opioids are considered second-line agents and are used when first-line drugs fail to provide significant relief. Although opioids are effective in treating neuropathic pain,[92–94] the benefit is a tradeoff with the increased risk for side effects,[95] tolerance, and dependence. The most common side effects of opioids are nausea and somnolence, which may be transient, and constipation. Long-term use has been associated with immunosuppression,[96,97] hypogonadism, adrenal suppression,[98,99] and hyperalgesia in experimental models. Treatment of neuropathic pain with opioids should be reserved for those patients who have failed first-line therapy or as part of a strategy to control breakthrough pain and infrequent acute exacerbations, or while titrating other medications to effective doses.[100]

Tramadol

Tramadol is a weak μ-opioid agonist as well as an SNRI. It has been shown to reduce pain in several neuropathic pain syndromes.[79] Side effects include somnolence, dizziness, nausea, orthostatic hypotension, and constipation. As with other opioids, there is a risk for abuse. In combination with other serotonin reuptake inhibitors, there is an increased risk for serotonin syndrome. The starting dose is 50 mg once or twice daily, preferably on an as-needed basis. The maximum daily dose is 100 mg q6h (400 mg/d).

Third-Line Medication Therapy

Third-line agents for the treatment of neuropathic pain include antiepileptics (lamotrigine, carbamazepine, oxcarbazepine, topiramate, valproic acid), other antidepressants (bupropion, citalopram, paroxetine), mexiletine, and capsaicin cream. The effectiveness for pain management of these agents is less supported.[101–103]

Pre-emptive and Preventative Analgesia

Since the discovery of pre- and perioperative pain as a strong risk factor for the development of chronic postsurgical pain, several preventative therapies have been studied. A meta-analysis using preoperative gabapentin or pregabalin showed at least a moderate reduction in chronic postsurgical pain with either drug[104]; however, the exclusion of several large trials on pregabalin has called the methodology and results into question.[105] Etanercept is a tumor necrosis factor (TNF)-α inhibitor that may prevent initiation of the inflammatory cascade that leads to development of chronic pain. A randomized-controlled trial of a single 50 mg preoperative dose of etanercept showed no reduction in postoperative pain at 24 hours (the primary outcome measure), or at 3, 6, and 12 months (secondary outcomes) after surgery.[106] Perioperative pregabalin showed improved pain control at 3 months following major spinal surgery, but there was no difference at 1 year.[107] It is unclear if the administration of any of these agents immediately prior to the surgical intervention will reduce the probability of persistent postsurgical pain. Although some agents show promise, none is universally effective, and this remains an area of active research.

A young person who was previously trialed on an NSAID is not likely to have renal impairment, so he could reasonably be started on any of the first-line agents such as gabapentin. Beginning with gabapentin 300 mg at night for 3 days and, if side effects are tolerable, increasing to 300 mg twice daily for 3 days and further increasing to 600 mg three times daily would be a reasonable approach. He should be on an effective dose of 600–1,200 mg three times daily for 2 weeks to properly assess benefit. If, after a trial period, he is not obtaining benefit, then titrate back down while initiating a trial of another first-line agent. Alternatively, if he experiences partial benefit or is limited by side effects at higher doses, then the addition of another agent such as nortriptyline or duloxetine in combination with gabapentin would be reasonable.[95] If his pain is localized and accompanied by sensitivity to light touch (allodynia), then addition of a topical lidocaine patch is warranted. Risks of heart disease and depression should be assessed prior to starting a TCA.

WHAT OTHER APPROACHES WOULD YOU CONSIDER FOR MANAGING THIS PATIENT?

BEHAVIORAL

The presence of constant and unrelenting pain is a psychological burden that affects patients in multiple ways, often resulting in anxiety, depression, poor sleep, stress in social relationships, and overuse of medications.[108] Among psychological treatments, the most frequently used are behavioral (biofeedback, relaxation, exposure) and cognitive behavioral (learning coping strategies while recognizing the effect their thoughts may have on their pain). Comprehensive reviews of these behavior treatments suggest that cognitive behavior therapy (CBT) can be moderately effective in reducing chronic pain and disability and in improving mood in patients with medical[109] or surgical[110] reasons for chronic pain. Behavioral therapies may be ineffective.[109] The efficacy of behavioral treatments for chronic pain has not been studied specifically in postherniorrhaphy patients.

Alcohol Use

Alcohol is the most commonly used and abused substance in the United States—80% have used alcohol at some point in their lives and 65% have drank alcohol in the last year.[111] Of these, more than 23% have engaged in binge drinking in the past 30 days.[112] Correspondingly, the 12-month prevalence of alcohol use disorders (AUD) is 4.6% in those 12–17 and 8.5% in those 18 and older.[113]

There is a significant association with ethnicity, showing that AUD is most common among Native Americans, then Caucasians, Hispanics, African Americans, and, last, Asians. Geographically, the highest rates of AUD are found in Eastern Europe.[114] AUD is more common among those who are male, have a history of military experience, younger age, single, and of lower socioeconomic status.[113,115]

Among patients who develop an AUD, first use often occurs during the teenage years, with 90% developing problem drinking by the age of 40.[116,117] There is a strong genetic predisposition to alcoholism, with a three to four times increased risk among children of an alcoholic parent. This risk is greatest in the son of an alcoholic father.[118,119]

Alcohol use is significantly associated with mortality to self and others. Alcohol use is involved in 40% of all traffic fatalities.[120] In addition, 7% of patients with AUDs will attempt suicide versus 1% of the general population.[121–123]

Previously, separate diagnoses were given for the lesser alcohol abuse and the more severe alcohol dependence. Largely, the boundary between the two was artificial and not representative of severity of alcohol use. Therefore, the new term *alcohol use disorder* has been adopted for the *Diagnostic and Statistical Manual of Mental Disorders Fifth Edition* (DSM-5). This term represents problem use of alcohol with associated psychological and behavioral complications and is analogous to the term "alcoholism." Although there are physical findings and lab work that are associated with alcohol abuse, the diagnosis is based on clinical interview. The National Institute on Alcohol Abuse and Alcoholism (NIAAA) also states that, based on epidemiological evidence, passing certain thresholds of drinking is suggestive of problem use: more than 14 drinks/week for men and more than 7 drinks/week for women.[124]

The United States Preventive Services Task Force (USPSTF) recommends that all adults are screened for AUDs.[125] Patients with chronic pain have very high rates of substance abuse: 46% have a history of substance abuse and 8–23% are current abusers.[126,127] Trauma is a primary source of the development of chronic pain, and up to 50% of patients are intoxicated at the time of injury.[128] Therefore, it is even more essential to screen for alcoholism in these patients.

There are several validated methods for screening, from single questions to multiple-item tools (see Table 22.4). A positive screen should result in further discussion with the patient regarding concern of use and referral to an addiction specialist. In patients unwilling to consider further evaluation and treatment, the management of chronic pain will be difficult if not impossible. It is against the standard of care to prescribe opioids to patients with ongoing substance abuse issues. In addition, use of membrane stabilizers carries significantly greater risk due to the additive CNS depressant effects when combined with alcohol. The exceptions may be gabapentin and topiramate. Both medications have largely been found to be safe when combined with alcohol, have efficacy in treating neuropathic pain, and have been shown to effectively treat AUDs.[129–139] Strong consideration should be given to using these medications as "first-line" agents in patients with a combination of AUDs and chronic pain.

Another issue is that alcoholics, when sober, have been found to have a lower pain threshold than controls.[140] For most patients with an AUD, then, a multimodal approach will be necessary to optimize pain control.

The treatment for AUDs is based around the goal of abstinence. There is no "safe level" of alcohol intake. Toward this end, a combination of motivational enhancement therapy (MET) along with pharmacologic intervention may be appropriate. There are currently three FDA-approved medications for alcoholism: disulfiram, naltrexone, and acamprosate. In addition, there is evidence in the literature for nalmefene, varenicline, gabapentin, and topiramate, among others. A full review of treatment for alcohol dependence is beyond the scope of this chapter.

On initial evaluation in the multidisciplinary pain clinic, a single-item screening question was given, and the patient reports drinking more than five drinks in one sitting at least

20 times in the past year. Based on this finding, a more thorough discussion was engaged regarding psychiatric symptoms and other substance abuse. The patient reports he started drinking at the age of 15 with friends and would primarily engage in binge drinking on the weekends. He reports "blacking out" on several occasions. He notes no difficulties with drinking until he graduated high school and began work. His drinking began to expand to Thursday, Friday, and Saturday nights. By the age of 25, he was drinking at least 5 nights/week and had one DUI. He reports stopping drinking completely at this point for 2 months before going back to "social" drinking. This quickly escalated to his current drinking level of six beers/night within 1 year. He reports he has to have a drink in the morning to calm himself enough to get to work and has missed work because of being hung over. Most of his nights are spent are home, drinking, to the point that he socializes very little and no longer plays in his basketball league. The patient is ambivalent regarding whether alcohol use is a problem for him. He firmly denies any depressive symptoms, anxiety symptoms, or psychotic symptoms and any suicidal/homicidal ideation. He feels he can stop if he chooses to.

The patient is diagnosed with an AUD. Subsequently, he is given several options. If he is unwilling to change his level of alcohol consumption, then there are few treatments that will be available, and his long-term prognosis is very poor. If, in fact, alcohol use is not a problem and he can stop any time, he will stop immediately. If that is difficult for him to do, then a referral will be made to see addiction psychiatry. On reflection, the patient accepts the referral.

SURGERY

Surgical re-exploration may be necessary, especially if there is concern for recurrent hernia, mesh migration, nerve compression, or nerve irritation from staples or scar tissue. Attempts to identify the affected nerve (ilioinguinal, iliohypogastric, or genitofemoral) beforehand through ultrasound-guided blocks have not shown a correlation with pain reduction following neurectomy of the corresponding nerve.[6] In one report, 16 of 19 patients obtained complete pain relief following ilioinguinal neurectomy, and 8 out of 12 patients obtained relief after genitofemoral neurectomy.[52] Amid describes a triple neurectomy procedure for postherniorrhaphy chronic pain that involves ligation of the ilioinguinal, iliohypogastric, and genitofemoral nerves.[1] In three studies involving 49,[141] 225,[21] and 16 patients,[1] respectively, nearly 80% had complete pain relief after neurectomy 1 month later; however, long-term assessment was not done. Case reports show reduction in pain after mesh or tack removal.[142–145] Numbness, loss of cremaster reflex, and testicular atrophy are among reported adverse outcomes of neurectomy.[52,143]

More recently, Aasvang and Kehlet performed a prospective cohort study of 21 patients.[146] They looked at pain-related impairment of everyday activities as a primary outcome after reoperation that included mesh removal and neurectomy in patients with pain after open hernia repair. Eighteen patients underwent one or two neurectomies, and all had the mesh removed. Interestingly, in 11 of 18 patients, the mesh was twisted and some were strangulating the vas deferens. The ilioinguinal, iliohypogastric, and genitalis nerves were identified, and many were found to be sutured or embedded in a

Table 22.4 ALCOHOL USE SCREENING TOOLS

METHOD	DETAILS	SCORING
Single-item	How many times in the past year have you had five (four for women) or more drinks in a day?	Any score >0 has an 82% sensitivity and 79% specificity for unhealthy alcohol use.[155]
AUDIT-C (Alcohol Use Disorders Identification Test)	3 questions: • How often do you have a drink containing alcohol? • How many drinks containing alcohol do you have on a typical day when you are drinking? • How often do you have 6 or more drinks on one occasion?	Each item has 5 choices, and is scored 0-4 (total 0-12). 80-90% sensitivity and specificity (both are higher with higher scores).[156,157] Available for free from SAMHSA.[158]
CAGE	4-item screen: • Have you ever felt you should Cut down on your drinking? • Have people Annoyed you by criticizing your drinking? • Have you ever felt bad or Guilty about your drinking? • Have you ever taken a drink first thing in the morning (Eye-opener) to steady your nerves or get rid of a hangover?	2 positive responses have 77% sensitivity and 79% specificity for AUD.[159]
MAST (Michigan Alcohol Screening Test)	22-item self-administered; well validated Focuses more on lifetime use rather than current use Compared to other screens, more accurate in women and elderly	Each item scores one point (total 0–22) ≥6 indicates unhealthy alcohol use and further in-depth evaluation.[160–164]
ASSIST (Alcohol, Smoking and Substance Involvement Screening Test)	80+ items Specifically inquires about alcohol, cannabis, cocaine, amphetamine, inhalant, sedative/hypnotic, hallucinogen and opioid abuse Not practical for daily clinical use	Gives specific levels of risk (low, moderate, high) for each substance[165] More involved scoring

conglomerate of mesh and scar tissue. If the nerves were macroscopically intact, they were not ligated; otherwise, neurectomy was performed. Patient's outcome was measured at 3 and 6 months using a validated activities assessment scale (AAS) and compared to their function preoperatively. There was significant improvement in AAS from 13 patients at 6 months, but three patients worsened.

Vuilleumier et al. performed surgical revision, mesh removal, and neurectomy on 43 patients with neuropathic pain after prior herniorrhaphy.[147] All operations were done by the same surgeon, and both the ilioinguinal nerve and iliohypogastric nerves were removed in a standardized procedure. In 35 patients, the ilioinguinal nerve was found to be entrapped, damaged, or transected, and, in 10 patients, the iliohypogastric nerve was damaged. The genitofemoral nerve was not found to be affected. Median VAS scores decreased, with 41 of 43 patients experiencing complete pain relief (VAS score of 0), and all 43 patients returned to work within 6 weeks.

INTERVENTIONAL PAIN TREATMENTS

Interventional treatments, considered within the realm of conservative management with the potential to preclude the need for reoperation, include procedures such as directed nerve blocks, radiofrequency nerve ablation, cryoablation, and neuromodulation. Most of these have not been studied in systematic clinical trials.

Nerve Blocks

Ultrasound-guided or nerve stimulator-guided nerve blocks using local anesthetic and/or steroid are in regular use for treatment of postherniorrhaphy pain although with little consistent evidence for efficacy. In a randomized double-blind, placebo-controlled crossover trial of ultrasound-guided ilioinguinal and iliohypogastric nerve blocks using lidocaine in patients with persistent post-herniorrhaphy pain, no relief of pain was obtained as measured by quantitative sensory testing and patient reporting.[148] In a questionnaire study of 38 patients who had received a block for chronic post-herniorrhaphy pain, 55.3% no longer described neuropathic pain at a median of 16 months; however, no improvement in VAS scores was found between the patients who were blocked using ultrasound versus a nerve stimulator.[149]

Radiofrequency (RF) Ablation

There is limited evidence for use of RF techniques. A recent review of the literature found a total of four case reports and one letter in which pulsed RF (PRF: an insulated needle with an active tip delivers voltage in the RF range of 300–500 kHz at ≤42°C) was used on a total of eight patients.[150] There were no reports using conventional RF (CRF: the treatment cannula reaches temperatures between 45°C and 80°C). Five patients had at least 90% pain relief with follow-up assessment between 3 and 9 months.

Cryoablation

An advantage of cryoablation is its reduced incidence of neuroma formation and exacerbation of deafferentation pain. There is a single case report of this technique being used successfully for postherniorrhaphy pain.[151] The genitofemoral nerve was identified under ultrasound guidance, and, after the pain was reproduced with low-intensity stimuli, the nerve was treated with cryoablation. The patient reported significant reduction in pain at 3 months.

Neuromodulation

Spinal cord stimulation (SCS) for pain of the low back and groin, representing the distribution of the low thoracic and high lumbar nerve roots, can be difficult to target given the deeper relative location of these nerve fibers in the posterior columns. In a single case report, two patients were successfully treated with SCS for intractable inguinal pain.[152] In another case series, SCS was combined with peripheral nerve field stimulation with some success.[153] In a larger series, 23 patients underwent laparoscopic implantation of a neuroprosthesis, the so-called LION procedure, for intractable post-herniorrhaphy pain. Nineteen obtained greater than 50% pain relief at a minimum of 6 months follow-up.[154]

Rehabilitation

There is no available literature to guide the use of rehabilitation approaches for treating patients with post-herniorrhaphy pain. Although the pain can often be severe and markedly limit some activities, it is unusual for post-herniorrhaphy pain to limit mobility. In those with limited mobility where specific goals can be ascertained in advance, a course of physical therapy aimed at optimizing function would be reasonable.

There is little evidence to support interventional pain treatment techniques for our patient. In many pain clinics, he would likely undergo a peripheral nerve block, and this may help to confirm the neuropathic origin of the pain if it is relieved by the injection of local anesthetic. It is unclear if this will provide any long-term benefit. The risks of any intervention must be weighed against the severity of the symptoms and the likelihood of benefit. His level of disability, anxiety, and depression should be gauged. If this is having a significant impact on his life, he should be referred for behavioral treatments. Surgical exploration and neurectomy may be the treatment method, with the most evidence of benefit for relief of pain, but there is also the risk of worsened pain. The risks of repeat surgical intervention must be weighed, and only after taking into account that he may have failed all other conservative measures. Whereas use of rehabilitation approaches is not typically needed, in those with significant limitations in physical function, targeted physical therapy may help improve functional status.

REFERENCES

1. Amid PK, Chen DC. Surgical treatment of chronic groin and testicular pain after laparoscopic and open preperitoneal inguinal hernia repair. *J Am Coll Surg.* 2011;213(4):531–536.
2. Wake BL, McCormack K, Fraser C, et al. Transabdominal pre-peritoneal (TAPP) vs totally extraperitoneal (TEP) laparoscopic techniques for inguinal hernia repair. *Cochrane Database Syst Rev.* 2005(1):CD004703.
3. Aasvang E, Kehlet H. Chronic postoperative pain: the case of inguinal herniorrhaphy. *Br J Anesth.* 2005a;95(1):69–76.
4. Anon. Laparoscopic versus open repair of groin hernia: a randomised comparison. The MRC Laparoscopic Groin Hernia Trial Group. *Lancet.* 1999;354(9174):185–190.
5. Scott NW, Go PM. Graham P, et al. Open mesh versus non-mesh for repair of femoral and inguinal hernia. *Cochrane Database Syst Rev.* 2001(4):CD002197.
6. Aasvang E, Kehlet H. Surgical management of chronic pain after inguinal hernia repair. *Br J Surg.* 2005b;92(7):795–801.
7. Aasvang EK, Bay-Nielsen M, Kehlet, H. Pain and functional impairment 6 years after inguinal herniorrhaphy. *Hernia.*2006;10(4):316–321.
8. Kalliomäki M-L, Meyerson J, Gunnarsson U, et al. Persistent pain after groin hernia surgery: a qualitative analysis of pain and its consequences for quality of life. *Acta Anaesthesiol Scand.* 2009;53(2):236–246.
9. Ferzli GS, Edwards E, Al-Khoury G, et al. Postherniorrhaphy groin pain and how to avoid it. *Surg Clin North Am.* 2008;88(1):203–216.
10. Massaron S, Bona S, Fumagalli U, et al. Analysis of post-surgical pain after inguinal hernia repair: a prospective study of 1,440 operations. *Hernia.* 2007;11(6):517–525.
11. Macrae WA. Chronic pain after surgery. *Br J Anesth.* 2001;87(1):88–98.
12. Perkins FM, Kehlet H. Chronic pain as an outcome of surgery. A review of predictive factors. *Anesthesiology.* 2000;93(4):1123–1133.
13. Kristensen AD, Ahlburg P, Lauridsen M, et al. Chronic pain after inguinal hernia repair in children. *Br J Anesth.* 2012;109(4):603–608.
14. Poobalan AS, Bruce J, King PM, et al. Chronic pain and quality of life following open inguinal hernia repair. *Br J Surg.* 2001;88(8):1122–1126.
15. Courtney CA, Duffy K, Serpell MG, et al. Outcome of patients with severe chronic pain following repair of groin hernia. *Br J Surg.* 2002;89(10):1310–1314.
16. Fränneby U, Sandblom G, Nordin P, et al. Risk factors for long-term pain after hernia surgery. *Ann Surg.* 2006;244(2):212–219.
17. Callesen T, Bech K, Kehlet H. Prospective study of chronic pain after groin hernia repair. *Br J Surg.* 1999;86(12):1528–1531.
18. Kehlet H, Jensen TS, Woolf CJ. Persistent postsurgical pain: risk factors and prevention. *Lancet.* 2006;367(9522):1618–1625.
19. Powell R, Johnston M, Smith WC, et al. Psychological risk factors for chronic post-surgical pain after inguinal hernia repair surgery: a prospective cohort study. *Eur J Pain* (London). 2012;16(4): 600–610.
20. Salcedo-Wasicek MC, Thirlby RC. Postoperative course after inguinal herniorrhaphy. A case-controlled comparison of patients receiving workers' compensation vs patients with commercial insurance. Arch Surg. 1995;130(1):29–32.
21. Amid PK. Causes, prevention, and surgical treatment of postherniorrhaphy neuropathic inguinodynia: triple neurectomy with proximal end implantation. *Hernia.* 2004a;8(4):343–349.
22. Lichtenstein IL, Shulman AG. Ambulatory outpatient hernia surgery. Including a new concept, introducing tension-free repair. *Int Surg.* 1986;71(1):1–4.
23. Amid PK. Groin hernia repair: open techniques. *World J Surg.* 2005;29(8):1046–1051.
24. Willaert W, De Bacquer D, Rogiers X, et al. Open preperitoneal techniques versus Lichtenstein repair for elective inguinal hernias. *Cochrane Database Syst Rev.* 2012;7:CD008034.
25. Koning GG, Koole D, de Jongh MAC, et al. The transinguinal preperitoneal hernia correction vs Lichtenstein's technique: is TIPP top? *Hernia.* 2011;15(1);19–22.
26. Koning GG, Keus F, Koeslag L, et al. Randomized clinical trial of chronic pain after the transinguinal preperitoneal technique compared with Lichtenstein's method for inguinal hernia repair. *Br J Surg.* 2012;99(10):1365–1373.
27. McCormack K, Scott NW, Go PM, et al. Laparoscopic techniques versus open techniques for inguinal hernia repair. *Cochrane Database Syst Rev.* 2003;(1):CD001785.
28. Bozuk M, Schuster R, Stewart D, et al. Disability and chronic pain after open mesh and laparoscopic inguinal hernia repair. *Am Surg.* 2003;69(10):839–841.
29. Bignell M, Partridge G, Mahon D, et al. Prospective randomized trial of laparoscopic (transabdominal preperitoneal-TAPP) versus open (mesh) repair for bilateral and recurrent inguinal hernia: incidence of chronic groin pain and impact on quality of life: results of 10 year follow-up. *Hernia.* 2012;16(6):635–640.
30. Bansal VK, Misra MC, Babu D, et al. A prospective, randomized comparison of long-term outcomes: chronic groin pain and quality of life following totally extraperitoneal (TEP) and transabdominal preperitoneal (TAPP) laparoscopic inguinal hernia repair. *Surg. Endosc.* 2013;27(7):2373–2382.
31. Grant, AM, EU Hernia Trialists Collaboration. Open mesh versus non-mesh repair of groin hernia: meta-analysis of randomised trials based on individual patient data [corrected]. *Hernia* 2002;6(3):130–136.
32. Bay-Nielsen M, Nilsson E, Nordin P, et al. Chronic pain after open mesh and sutured repair of indirect inguinal hernia in young males. *Br J Surg.* 2004;91(10):1372–1376.
33. Benizri EI, Rahili A, Avallone S, et al. Open inguinal hernia repair by plug and patch: the value of fibrin sealant fixation. *Hernia.* 2006;10(5):389–394.
34. Schwab R, Willms A, Kröger A, et al. Less chronic pain following mesh fixation using a fibrin sealant in TEP inguinal hernia repair. *Hernia.* 2006;10(3):272–277.
35. Canonico S, Benevento R, Perna G, et al. Sutureless fixation with fibrin glue of lightweight mesh in open inguinal hernia repair: effect on postoperative pain: a double-blind, randomized trial versus standard heavyweight mesh. *Surgery.* 2013;153(1):126–130.
36. Campanelli G, et al. Reducing postoperative pain: the use of Tisseel for mesh fixation in inguinal hernia repair. *Surg Tech Int.* 2012;22(Dec):134–139.
37. Lau H. Fibrin sealant versus mechanical stapling for mesh fixation during endoscopic extraperitoneal inguinal hernioplasty: a randomized prospective trial. *Ann Surg.* 2005;242(5):670–675.
38. Wong J-U, Leung T, Huang C, et al. Comparing chronic pain between fibrin sealant and suture fixation for bilayer polypropylene mesh inguinal hernioplasty: a randomized clinical trial. *Am J Surg.* 2011;202(1):34–38.
39. Robinson A, Light D, Kasim A, et al. A systematic review and meta-analysis of the role of radiology in the diagnosis of occult inguinal hernia. *Surg Endoscop.* 2013;27(1):11–18.
40. Kraft BM, Kolb H, Kuckuk B, et al. Diagnosis and classification of inguinal hernias. *Surg Endoscop.* 2003;17(12):2021–2024.
41. Cunningham J, Temple WJ, Mitchell P, et al. Cooperative hernia study. Pain in the postrepair patient. *Ann Surg.* 1996;224(5):598–602.
42. Simons MP, Aufenacker T, Bay-Nielsen M, et al. European Hernia Society guidelines on the treatment of inguinal hernia in adult patients. *Hernia.* 2009;13(4):343–403.
43. Mussack T, Fischer T, Ladurner R, et al. Cine magnetic resonance imaging vs high-resolution ultrasonography for detection of adhesions after laparoscopic and open incisional hernia repair: a matched pair pilot analysis. *Surg Endoscop.* 2005;19(12):1538–1543.
44. Baker ME, Blinder RA, Rice RP. Diagnostic imaging of abdominal fluid collections and abscesses. *Crit Rev Diagn Imaging.* 1986;25(3):233–278.

45. Markos V, Brown EF. CT herniography in the diagnosis of occult groin hernias. *Clin Radiol.* 2005;60(2):251–256.
46. Hamlin JA, Kahn AM. Herniography: a review of 333 herniograms. *Am Surg.* 1998;64(10):965–969.
47. Karakayali F, Karatas M, Ozcelik U, et al. Influence of synthetic mesh on ilioinguinal nerve motor conduction and chronic groin pain after inguinal herniorrhaphy: a prospective randomized clinical study. *Int Surg.* 2007;92(6):344–350.
48. Kocijan R, Sandberg S, Chan Y, et al. Anatomical changes after inguinal hernia treatment: a reason for chronic pain and recurrent hernia? *Surg Endoscop.* 2010;24(2):395–399.
49. Linderoth G, Kehlet H, Aasvang EK, et al. Neurophysiological characterization of persistent pain after laparoscopic inguinal hernia repair. *Hernia.* 2011;15(5):521–529.
50. Aasvang EK, Brandsborg B, Christensen B, et al. Neurophysiological characterization of postherniotomy pain. *Pain.* 2008;137(1):173–181.
51. Deysine M, Deysine GR, Reed WP. Groin pain in the absence of hernia: a new syndrome. *Hernia* 2002;6(2):64–67.
52. Starling JR, Harms BA. Diagnosis and treatment of genitofemoral and ilioinguinal neuralgia. *World J Surg.* 1989;13(5):586–591.
53. Bower S, Moore BB, Weiss SM. Neuralgia after inguinal hernia repair. *Am Surg.* 1996;62(8):664–667.
54. Basbaum AI, Bautista DM, Scherrer G, et al. Cellular and molecular mechanisms of pain. *Cell.* 2009;139(2):267–284.
55. Voscopoulos C, Lema M. When does acute pain become chronic? *Br J Anesth.* 2010;105(suppl 1):i69–i85.
56. Schmidt R, Schmelz M, Forster C, et al. Novel classes of responsive and unresponsive C nociceptors in human skin. *J Neurosci.* 1995;15(1 Pt 1):333–341.
57. Cesare P, McNaughton P. A novel heat-activated current in nociceptive neurons and its sensitization by bradykinin. *Proc Natl Acad Sci USA.* 1996;93(26):15435–15439.
58. Immke DC, McCleskey EW. Protons open acid-sensing ion channels by catalyzing relief of Ca2+ blockade. *Neuron.* 2003;37(1):75–84.
59. Millan MJ. Descending control of pain. *Prog Neurobiol.* 2002;66(6):355–474.
60. D'Mello R, Dickenson AH. Spinal cord mechanisms of pain. *Br J Anesth.* 2008;101(1):8–16.
61. Woolf CJ, Salter MW. Neuronal plasticity: increasing the gain in pain. *Science.* 2000;288(5472):1765–1769.
62. Latremoliere A, Woolf CJ. Central sensitization: a generator of pain hypersensitivity by central neural plasticity. *J Pain.* 2009;10(9):895–926.
63. Woolf CJ. Evidence for a central component of post-injury pain hypersensitivity. *Nature.* 1983;306(5944):686–688.
64. Koltzenburg M, Wahren LK, Torebjörk HE. Dynamic changes of mechanical hyperalgesia in neuropathic pain states and healthy subjects depend on the ongoing activity of unmyelinated nociceptive. *Pflügers Archive* 1992;R52.
65. Costigan M, Befort K, Karchewski L, et al. Replicate high-density rat genome oligonucleotide microarrays reveal hundreds of regulated genes in the dorsal root ganglion after peripheral nerve injury. *BMC Neurosci.* 2002;3:16.
66. Fukuoka T, Kondo E, Dai Y, et al. Brain-derived neurotrophic factor increases in the uninjured dorsal root ganglion neurons in selective spinal nerve ligation model. *J Neurosci.* 2001; 21(13):4891–4900.
67. Noguchi K, Kawai Y, Fukuoka T, et al. Substance P induced by peripheral nerve injury in primary afferent sensory neurons and its effect on dorsal column nucleus neurons. *J Neurosci.* 1995;15(11):7633–7643.
68. Scholz J, Broom D, Youn D, et al. Blocking caspase activity prevents transsynaptic neuronal apoptosis and the loss of inhibition in lamina II of the dorsal horn after peripheral nerve injury. *J Neurosci.* 2005;25(32):7317–7323.
69. Moore KA, Kohno T, Karchewski LA, et al. Partial peripheral nerve injury promotes a selective loss of GABAergic inhibition in the superficial dorsal horn of the spinal cord. *J Neurosci.* 2002;22(15):6724–6731.
70. Arvidsson J, Ygge J, Grant G. Cell loss in lumbar dorsal root ganglia and transganglionic degeneration after sciatic nerve resection in the rat. *Brain Res.* 1986;373(1-2):15–21.
71. Kapadia SE, LaMotte CC. Deafferentation-induced alterations in the rat dorsal horn: I. Comparison of peripheral nerve injury vs. rhizotomy effects on presynaptic, postsynaptic, and glial processes. *J Comp Neurol.* 1987;266(2):183–197.
72. Lekan HA, Carlton SM, Coggeshall RE. Sprouting of Aβ fibers into lamina II of the rat dorsal horn in peripheral neuropathy. *Neurosci Lett.* 1996;208(3):147–150.
73. Mannion RJ, Doubell TP, Coggeshall RE, et al. Collateral sprouting of uninjured primary afferent A-fibers into the superficial dorsal horn of the adult rat spinal cord after topical capsaicin treatment to the sciatic nerve. *J Neurosci.* 1996;16(16):5189–5195.
74. Coull JAM, Beggs S, Boudreau D, et al. BDNF from microglia causes the shift in neuronal anion gradient underlying neuropathic pain. *Nature.* 2005;438(7070):1017–1021.
75. Svensson CI, Tran TK, Fitzsimmons B, et al. Descending serotonergic facilitation of spinal ERK activation and pain behavior. *FEBS Lett.* 2006;580(28-29):6629–6634.
76. Ma QP, Woolf CJ. Progressive tactile hypersensitivity: an inflammation-induced incremental increase in the excitability of the spinal cord. *Pain.* 1996;67(1):97–106.
77. Mannion RJ, Costigan M, Decosterd I, et al. Neurotrophins: peripherally and centrally acting modulators of tactile stimulus-induced inflammatory pain hypersensitivity. *Proc Natl Acad Sci USA.* 1999;96(16):9385–9390.
78. Raghavendra V, Tanga FY, DeLeo JA. Complete Freunds adjuvant-induced peripheral inflammation evokes glial activation and proinflammatory cytokine expression in the CNS. *Eur J Neurosci.* 2004;20(2):467–473.
79. Dworkin RH, O'Connor AB, Backonja M, et al. Pharmacologic management of neuropathic pain: evidence-based recommendations. *Pain.* 2007;132(3):237–251.
80. de Leon-Casasola O. New developments in the treatment algorithm for peripheral neuropathic pain. *Pain Med.* 2011;12(suppl 3):S100–S108.
81. Taylor CP. The biology and pharmacology of calcium channel alpha2-delta proteins. Pfizer Satellite Symposium to the 2003 Society for Neuroscience Meeting; 2003 November 10; New Orleans, LA. *CNS Drug Rev.* 2004:183–188.
82. Gammaitoni AR, Davis MW. Pharmacokinetics and tolerability of lidocaine patch 5% with extended dosing. *Ann Pharmacother.* 2002;36(2):236–240.
83. Vadalouca A, Siafaka I, Argyra E, et al. Therapeutic management of chronic neuropathic pain: an examination of pharmacologic treatment. *Ann NY Acad Sci.* 2006;1088:164–186.
84. Max MB, Lynch SA, Muir J, et al. Effects of desipramine, amitriptyline, and fluoxetine on pain in diabetic neuropathy. *N Engl J Med.* 1992;326(19):1250–1256.
85. Rowbotham MC, Reisner RA, Davies PS, et al. Treatment response in antidepressant-naïve postherpetic neuralgia patients: double-blind, randomized trial. *J Pain.* 2005;6(11):741–746.
86. Watson CP, Vernich L, Chipman M, et al. Nortriptyline versus amitriptyline in postherpetic neuralgia: a randomized trial. *Neurology.* 1998;51(4):1166–1171.
87. Gilron I, Bailey JM, Tu D, et al. Nortriptyline and gabapentin, alone and in combination for neuropathic pain: a double-blind, randomised controlled crossover trial. *Lancet.* 2009;374(9697):1252–1261.
88. Ray WA, Meredith S, Thapa PB, et al. Cyclic antidepressants and the risk of sudden cardiac death. *Clin Pharmacol Ther.* 2004;75(3):234–241.
89. Dworkin RH, Backonja M, Rowbotham MC, et al. Advances in neuropathic pain: diagnosis, mechanisms, and treatment recommendations. *Arch Neurol.* 2003;60(11):1524–1534.

90. Beniczky S, Tajti J, Timea Varge E, Vecsei L. Evidence-based pharmacological treatment of neuropathic pain syndromes. *J Neur Trans* (Vienna, 1996). 2005;112(6):735–749.
91. Dunner DL, Wohlreich MM, Mallinckrodt CH. Clinical consequences of initial duloxetine dosing strategies: comparison of 30 and 60 mg QD starting doses. *Curr Ther Res.* 2005;66:522–540.
92. Gimbel JS, Richards P, Portenoy RK. Controlled-release oxycodone for pain in diabetic neuropathy: a randomized controlled trial. *Neurology*, 2003;60(6):927–934.
93. Morley JS, Bridson J, Nash TP, et al. Low-dose methadone has an analgesic effect in neuropathic pain: a double-blind randomized controlled crossover trial. *Palliat Med.* 2003;17(7):576–587.
94. Rowbotham MC, et al. Oral opioid therapy for chronic peripheral and central neuropathic pain. *N Engl J Med.* 2003;348(13):1223–1232.
95. Gilron I, Bailey JM, Tu D, et al. Morphine, gabapentin, or their combination for neuropathic pain. *N Engl J Med.* 2005;352(13):1324–1334.
96. Vallejo R, de Leon-Casasola O, Benyamin R. Opioid therapy and immunosuppression: a review. *Am J Ther.* 2004;11(5):354–365.
97. Sacerdote P. Opioid-induced immunosuppression. *Curr Op Supp Palliat Care.* 2008;2(1):14–18.
98. Daniell HW. Hypogonadism in men consuming sustained-action oral opioids. *J Pain.* 2002;3(5):377–384.
99. Daniell HW. Opioid endocrinopathy in women consuming prescribed sustained-action opioids for control of nonmalignant pain. *J Pain.* 2008;9(1):28–36.
100. Højsted J, Sjøgren P. Addiction to opioids in chronic pain patients: a literature review. *Eur J Pain* (London). 2007;11(5):490–518.
101. Finnerup NB, Otto M, McQuay HJ, et al. Algorithm for neuropathic pain treatment: an evidence based proposal. *Pain.* 2005;118(3):289–305.
102. Silver M, Blum D, Grainger J, et al. Double-blind, placebo-controlled trial of lamotrigine in combination with other medications for neuropathic pain. *J Pain Symptom Manage.* 2007;34(4):446–454.
103. Mason L, Moore RA, Derry S, et al. Systematic review of topical capsaicin for the treatment of chronic pain. *Br Med J* (Clinical research ed.). 2004;328(7446):991.
104. Clarke H, Bonin RP, Orser BA, et al. The prevention of chronic postsurgical pain using gabapentin and pregabalin: a combined systematic review and meta-analysis. *Anesth Analges.* 2012;115(2):428–442.
105. Chelly JE. Pregabalin effective for the prevention of chronic postsurgical pain: really? *Anesth Analges.* 2013;116(2):507–508.
106. Cohen SP, Galvagno SM, Plunkett A, et al. A multicenter, randomized, controlled study evaluating preventive etanercept on postoperative pain after inguinal hernia repair. *Anesth Analges.* 2013;116(2):455–462.
107. Gianesello L, Pavoni V, Barboni E, et al. Perioperative pregabalin for postoperative pain control and quality of life after major spinal surgery. *J Neurosurg Anesthesiol.* 2012;24(2):121–126.
108. Siddall PJ, Cousins MJ. Persistent pain as a disease entity: implications for clinical management. *Anesth Analges.* 2004;99(2):510–520.
109. Eccleston C, Morley SJ. Williams AC de C. Psychological approaches to chronic pain management: evidence and challenges. *Br J Anesth.* 2013;111(1):59–63.
110. Henschke N, Ostelo RW, van Tulder MW, et al. Behavioural treatment for chronic low-back pain. *Cochrane Database Syst Rev.* 2010;(7):CD002014.
111. Pleis JR, Ward BW, Lucas JW. *Summary Health Statistics for U.S. Adults: National Health Interview Survey, 2009.* National Center for Health Statistics. Vital Health Stat 10. 2010;249:1–207; tables 26 and 27.
112. Substance Abuse and Mental Health Services Administration. *Results from the 2008 National Survey on Drug Use and Health: National Findings.* (Office of Applied Studies, Substance NSDUH Series H-36, HHS Publication No. SMA 09-4434). Rockville, MD; 2009.
113. Hasin DS, Stinson FS, Ogburn E, Grant BF. Prevalence, correlates, disability, and comorbidity of DSM-IV alcohol abuse and dependence in the United States: results from the National Epidemiologic Survey on Alcohol and Related Conditions. *Arch Gen Psychiatry.* 2007;64:830.
114. Rehm J, Mathers C, Popova S, et al. Global burden of disease and injury and economic cost attributable to alcohol use and alcohol-use disorders. *Lancet.* 2009;373(9682):2223–2233.
115. Jacobson IG, Ryan MA, Hooper TI, et al. Alcohol use and alcohol-related problems before and after military combat deployment. *JAMA.* 2008;300:663.
116. Gossop M, Moos R. Substance misuse among older adults: a neglected but treatable problem. *Addiction.* 2008;103(3):347–348.
117. Schuckit MA, Smith TL. Onset and course of alcoholism over 25 years in middle class men. *Drug Alcohol Depend.* 2011;113(1):21–28, 2011.
118. Nurnberger JI Jr, Bierut LJ. Seeking the connections: alcoholism and our genes. *Sci Am.* 2007;296(4):46–53.
119. Schuckit MA. An overview of genetic influences in alcoholism. *J Subst Abuse Treat.* 2009:36(1):S5–S14.
120. National Highway Traffic Safety Administration (NHTSA). *Traffic safety facts 2000: alcohol.* Available from: www.nhtsa.dot.gov
121. Yaldizli O, Kuhl HC, Graf M, et al. Risk factors for suicide attempts in patients with alcohol dependence or abuse and a history of depressive symptoms: a subgroup analysis from the WHO/ISBRA study. *Drug Alcohol Rev.* 2010;29:64.
122. Ohberg A, Vuori E, Ojanperä I, Lonngvist J. Alcohol and drugs in suicides. *Br J Psychiatry.* 1996;169:75.
123. Hingson R, Heeren T, Winter M, Wechsler H. Magnitude of alcohol-related mortality and morbidity among U.S. college students ages 18–24: changes from 1998 to 2001. *Annu Rev Public Health.* 2005;26:259.
124. National Institute on Alcohol Abuse and, Alcoholism. *Helping Patients Who Drink Too Much: A Clinician's Guide: Updated 2005 Edition.* Bethesda, MD: National Institutes of Health; 2007.
125. U.S. Preventive Services Task Force. Screening and behavioral counseling interventions in primary care to reduce alcohol misuse: recommendation statement. *Ann Intern Med.* 2004; 140:554.
126. Manchikanti L, Cash KA, Malla Y, et al. A prospective evaluation of psychotherapeutic and illicit drug use in patients presenting with chronic pain at the time of initial evaluation. *Pain Phys.* 2013;16:E1–E13.
127. Manchikanti L, Damron KS, McManus CD, et al. Patterns of illicit drug use and opioid abuse in patients with chronic pain at initial evaluation: a prospective, observational study. *Pain Phys.* 2004;7:431–437.
128. Gentilello LM, Donovan DM, Dunn CW, Rivara FP. Alcohol interventions in trauma centers. Current practice and future directions. *JAMA.* 1995;274(13):1043–1048.
129. Codd EE, Martinez RP, Molino L, et al. Tramadol and several anticonvulsants synergize in attenuating nerve injury-induced allodynia. *Pain.* 2008;134:254–262.
130. Muehlbacher M, Nickel MK, Kettler C, et al. Topiramate in treatment of patients with chronic low back pain. *Clin J Pain.* 2006;22(6):526–531.
131. Shinn AK, Greenfield SF. Topiramate in the treatment of substance-related disorders: a critical review of the literature. *J Clin Psychiatry.* 2010;71(5):634–648.
132. Mariani JJ, Rosenthal RN, Tross S, et al. A randomized, open-label, controlled trial of gabapentin and Phenobarbital in the treatment of alcohol withdrawal. *Am J Addict.* 2006;15:76–84.
133. Myrick H, Malcolm R, Randall PK, et al. A double blind trial of gabapentin versus lorazepam in the treatment of alcohol withdrawal. *Alcohol Clin Exp Res.* 2009;33:1582–1588.
134. Furieri FA, Nakamura-Palacios EM. Gabapentin reduces alcohol consumption and craving: a randomized, double-blind, placebo-controlled trial. *J Clin Psychiatry.* 2007;68:1691–1700.

135. Anton RF, Myrick H, Baros AM, et al. Efficacy of a combination of flumazenil and gabapentin in the treatment of alcohol dependence: relationship to alcohol withdrawal symptoms. *J Clin Psychopharmacol.* 2009;29:334–342.
136. Bisaga A, Evans SM. The acute effects of gabapentin in combination with alcohol in heavy drinkers. *Drug Alcohol Depend.* 2006;83:25–32.
137. Anton RF, Myrick H, Wright TM, et al. Gabapentin combined with naltrexone for the treatment of alcohol dependence. *Am J Psychiatry.* 2011;168:709–17.
138. Hyrick H, Malcolm R, Randall PK, et al. A double blind trial of gabapentin vs lorazepam in the treatment of alcohol withdrawal. *Alcohol Clin Exp Res.* 2009;3(9):1582–1588.
139. Brower KJ, Kim HM, Strobbe S, et al. A randomized double-blind pilot trial of gabapentin vs placebo to treat alcohol dependence and comorbid insomnia. *Alcohol Clin Exp Res.* 2008;32(8):1429–1438.
140. Brown RA, Cutter HS. Alcohol, customary drinking behavior, and pain. *J Abnorm Psychol.* 1977;86(2):179–188.
141. Amid PK. A 1-stage surgical treatment for postherniorrhaphy neuropathic pain: triple neurectomy and proximal end implantation without mobilization of the cord. *Arch Surg* (Chicago, 1960). 2002;137(1):100–104.
142. Wong J, Anvari M. Treatment of inguinodynia after laparoscopic herniorrhaphy: a combined laparoscopic and fluoroscopic approach to the removal of helical tackers. *Surg Laparos Endosc Percutan Tech.* 2001;11(2):148–151.
143. Heise C, Starling JR. Mesh inguinodynia: a new clinical syndrome after inguinal herniorrhaphy? *J Am Coll Surg.* 1998;187(5):514–518.
144. Seid AS, Amos E. Entrapment neuropathy in laparoscopic herniorrhaphy. *Surg Endoscop.* 1994;8(9):1050–1053.
145. Sampath P, Yeo CJ, Campbell JN. Nerve injury associated with laparoscopic inguinal herniorrhaphy. *Surgery.* 1995;118(5):829–833.
146. Aasvang EK, Kehlet H. The effect of mesh removal and selective neurectomy on persistent postherniotomy pain. *Ann Surg.* 2009;249(2):327–334.
147. Vuilleumier H, Hübner M, Demartines N. Neuropathy after herniorrhaphy: indication for surgical treatment and outcome. *World J Surg.* 2009;33(4):841–845.
148. Bischoff JM, Koscielniak-Nielsen ZJ, Kehlet H, et al. Ultrasound-guided ilioinguinal/iliohypogastric nerve blocks for persistent inguinal postherniorrhaphy pain: a randomized, double-blind, placebo-controlled, crossover trial. *Anesth Analges.* 2012;114(6):1323–1329.
149. Thomassen I, van Suijlekom JA, van de Gaag A, et al. Ultrasound-guided ilioinguinal/iliohypogastric nerve blocks for chronic pain after inguinal hernia repair. *Hernia.* 2013;17(3):329–332.
150. Werner MU, Bischoff JM, Rathmell JP, et al. Pulsed radiofrequency in the treatment of persistent pain after inguinal herniotomy: a systematic review. *Reg Anesth Pain Med.* 2012;37(3):340–343.
151. Campos NA, Chiles JH, Plunkett AR. Ultrasound-guided cryoablation of genitofemoral nerve for chronic inguinal pain. *Pain Phys.* 2009;12(6):997–1000.
152. Elias M. Spinal cord stimulation for post-herniorrhaphy pain. *Neuromodulation.* 2000;3(3):155–157.
153. Lepski G, Vahedi P, Tatagiba MS, et al. Combined spinal cord and peripheral nerve field stimulation for persistent post-herniorrhaphy pain. *Neuromodulation.* 2013;16(1):84–88; discussion 88–89.
154. Possover M. Use of the LION procedure on the sensitive branches of the lumbar plexus for the treatment of intractable postherniorrhaphy neuropathic inguinodynia. *Hernia.* 2013;17(3):333–337.
155. Dawson DA, Compton WM, Grant BF. Frequency of 5+/4+ drinks as a screener for drug use and drug-use disorders. *J Stud Alcohol Drugs.* 2010;71:751.
156. Bush K, Kivlahan DR, McDonell MB, et al. The AUDIT alcohol consumption questions (AUDIT-C): an effective brief screening test for problem drinking. *Arch Intern Med.* 1998;3:1789–1795.
157. Bradley KA, Bush KR, Epler AJ, et al. Two brief alcohol-screening tests from the Alcohol Use Disorders Identification Test (AUDIT): validation in a female Veterans Affairs patient population. *Arch Internal Med.* 2003;163:821–829.
158. http://www.integration.samhsa.gov/images/res/tool_auditc.pdf
159. Maisto SA, Saitz R. Alcohol use disorders: screening and diagnosis. *Am J Addict.* 2003;12(suppl 1):S12.
160. Selzer ML. The Michigan Alcoholism Screening Test (MAST): the quest for a new diagnostic instrument. *Am J Psychiatry.* 1971;127:1653–1658.
161. Maisto SA, Connors GJ, Allen JP. Contrasting self-report screens for alcohol problems: a review. *Alcohol Clin Exp Res.* 1995;19(6):1510–1516.
162. Bradley KA, Boyd-Wickizer J, Powell SH, Burman ML. Alcohol screening questionnaires in women: a critical review. *JAMA.* 1998;280(2):166–171.
163. Teitelbaum L, Mullen, B. Validity of the MAST in psychiatric settings: a META-analytic integration. *J Stud Alcohol.* 2000;61(2):254–261.
164. Hirata ES, Almeida OP, Funari RR, Klein EL. Validity of the Michigan Alcoholism Screening Test (MAST) for the detection of alcohol-related problems among male geriatric outpatients. *Am J Geriatr. Psych.* 2001;9:30–34.
165. Humeniuk R, Ali R, Babor TF, et al. Validation of the Alcohol, Smoking and Substance Involvement Screening Test (ASSIST). *Addiction.* 2008;103:1039.

SECTION VI

CANCER-RELATED PAIN

23.

PALLIATIVE CANCER PAIN

Mellar P. Davis, Harold Goforth, and Pam Gamier

CASE PRESENTATION

A 47-year-old man developed shoulder pain that subsequently radiated to his little finger over 4 months and increased in severity. He initially took nonsteroidal anti-inflammatory drugs (NSAIDs). His primary care physician ordered a chest X-ray (read as normal) and believed that this patient had a rotator cuff tear. He completed 1 month of rehabilitation without improvement.

Due to persistent pain and smoking history, a computed tomography (CT) scan of the chest was obtained that demonstrated a right apical mass. A transthoracic needle biopsy demonstrated squamous carcinoma. He also developed a right-sided ptosis for which he sought medical treatment. With the diagnosis of a Pancoast-type tumor involving the apex of the right lung, he underwent a positron emission tomography (PET) CT scan that demonstrated disease limited to the apex.

He received combination cisplatin and etoposide chemotherapy for three cycles plus simultaneous radiation therapy. He was placed on sustained-release morphine 60 mg twice a day with 15 mg every 4 hours as needed and was started on gabapentin 300 mg three times daily.

During the day, he noted increasing fatigue and avolition, which worsened significantly during chemotherapy. In addition to weakness, he reports significant nausea and vomiting, particularly during the week of chemotherapy. Chemotherapy and radiation were completed, and a surgical opinion was obtained for consideration of resection of residual disease.

The patient became demoralized over the course of his treatment. He had significant financial concerns because his resulting disability prevented him from working in construction. He noted that his sleep has worsened since diagnosis as well, and he attributes these both to the anxiety surrounding his condition and to uncontrolled pain at night. He also noted the onset of numbness and paresthesias in his bilateral lower extremities, which he fears may be related to his cancer.

He underwent resection but developed post-thoracotomy pain, and, 3 months following resection, he developed recurrent right shoulder and hand pain, as well as swelling of the right arm and hand. The pain was a burning type in his right hand coupled with mechanical allodynia and motor weakness in the same region. The pain was unremitting, and averaged 7/10 in severity despite morphine and gabapentin. A PET/CT scan demonstrated a recurrent mass surrounding the brachial plexus, mediastinal adenopathy, and a left adrenal metastasis.

He worried excessively regarding his declining medical condition and was especially concerned with what may happen following his death with regards to his wife and two young children. He also has great concern over the increasing loss of his mobility because he is a laborer and has few other job-related resources.

Past medical history is significant only for hypertension and tobacco abuse.

Past surgical history is significant for tonsillectomy and adenoidectomy as a child.

Current medications at time of presentation included only hydrochlorothiazide.

On examination: The right hand demonstrates allodynia and appears hyperemic. There is thenar wasting, as well as atrophy of the biceps and triceps muscles. Strength testing is impaired, and it is difficult for the patient to maintain strength against gravity (3/5) in the biceps and triceps muscle groups. His bilateral lower extremities show diminished light touch discrimination. His affect appears anxious and distraught.

QUESTIONS

1. What is the presentation of a Pancoast tumor?
2. How does one manage superior sulcus cancers?
3. What interventional approaches can be done for a brachial plexopathy?
4. What is the pathophysiology of cancer-related neuropathy? How is cancer-related neuropathy managed?
5. How is chemotherapy-induced neuropathy managed?
6. How is depression and anxiety diagnosed in the context of a cancer pain diagnosis?
7. What is the role of insomnia in mood and pain perception?
8. How are depression, anxiety, and insomnia most effectively managed in a cancer pain population?

WHAT IS THE PRESENTATION OF A PANCOAST TUMOR?

A cancer presenting in the superior sulcus of the lung poses a significant challenge both diagnostically and therapeutically. Superior sulcus tumors are in proximity to the brachial plexus, major vasculature, and cervical and upper thoracic spine. These structures determine presentation and therapeutic options.[1–5] The superior sulcus is not an anatomic site but a groove formed by vessels crossing the lung apex.[6] A subset of superior sulcus cancers that involve the brachial plexus are called Pancoast tumors.[7] Most cancers that involve the brachial plexus arise from the breast or lung or occasionally from the head and neck region; these tumors grow caudally, invading the superior portion of the plexus.[8] Pancoast cancers make up 5% of lung cancers; 90% are squamous or adenocarcinomas, rarely, small-cell carcinomas.[6] Pain is the most common presenting symptom of Pancoast tumors (75%), usually located over the shoulder and into the axilla. Pain often radiates down the medial forearm to the fourth and fifth finger.[9–10] Motor weakness and abnormal upper extremity reflexes occur in 75%, usually from involvement of the lower plexus divisions (C8–T1), the remaining involve more widespread brachial plexus involvement.[9–10] Vertebral extension frequently occurs through the intervertebral foramen. Involvement may also comprise sympathetic ganglia in 23%, resulting in an ipsilateral Horner syndrome. The presentation of a Horner syndrome implies proximity to the spinal cord and warrants a magnetic resonance imaging (MRI) of cervical and thoracic spine to exclude epidural extension of cancer.[9] Lymphedema is an uncommon presentation (15%) for tumor-related brachial plexopathy but is more commonly seen after radiation therapy. The ipsilateral phrenic nerve may become involved, leading to an elevated diaphragm. Recurrent laryngeal nerve involvement leads to hoarseness. Ipsilateral reflex sympathetic dystrophy, superior vena cava syndrome, and supraclavicular adenopathy may occasionally accompany a Pancoast cancer.[6]

Misdiagnosis or delay in diagnosis is not uncommon with superior sulcus tumors and Pancoast cancers. Patients are often mistaken for having periarthritis, bursitis, rotator cuff tears, humeroscapularis, cervical neck osteoarthritis, and even pulmonary tuberculosis.[11–16] The fact that superior sulcus lung cancers present in the periphery of the lung means that the usual symptoms associated with lung cancer (cough, dyspnea, and hemoptysis) are unusual.[6] The average delay in diagnosis is 13 months, with a range of 2–24 months.[17]

Symptoms of a Pancoast cancer briefly outlined here can be understood by a basic understanding of the brachial plexus anatomy (Figure 23.1). The brachial plexus arises from the roots of ventral rami of the C5–T1 spinal nerves. The C5–C7 roots exit above the vertebral bodies; the C8 and T1 below. The roots unite in the neck between the anterior and middle scalene muscle.[18] Segmental nerve innervation to paravertebral and scalene muscles, the dorsal scapular nerve from C5, the long thoracic nerve from C5–C7, and the first intercostal nerve from T1 arise from the plexus before forming trunks. The phrenic nerve arises from the C4 nerve root but often receives contribution from the C5 nerve root as it descends. The brachial plexus trunks are located in the lower part of the posterior cervical triangle. The upper trunk is formed from

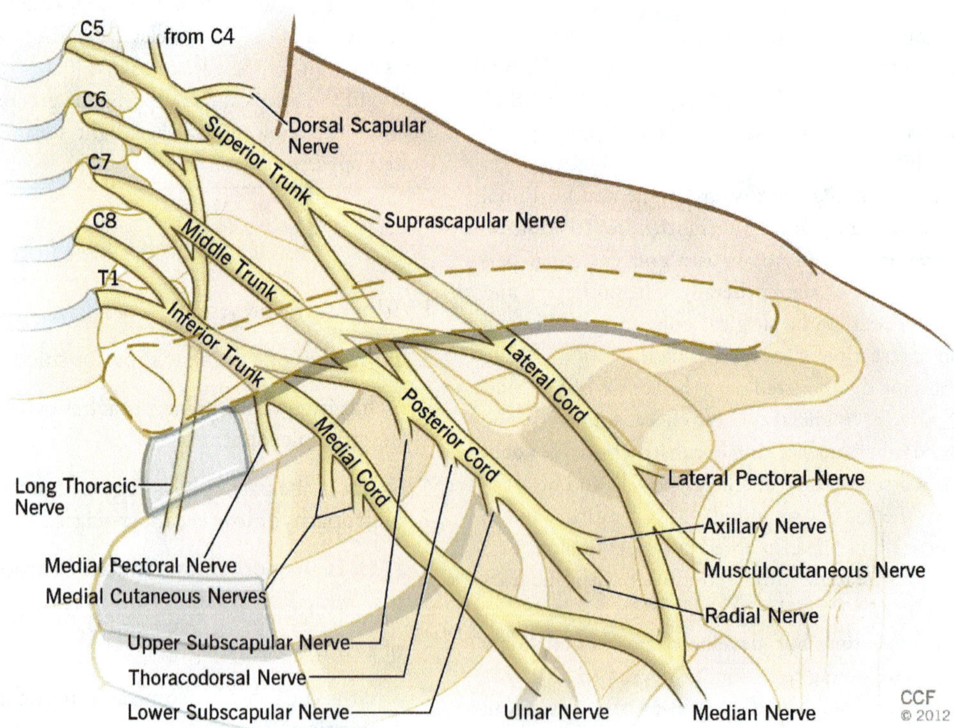

Figure 23.1 Anatomy of the brachial plexus. Reprinted with permission from the Cleveland Clinic Center for Medical Art & Photography ©2012. All Rights Reserved.

C5 and C6, the middle from C7, and the lower trunk from C8 and T1. Each divides anteriorly and posteriorly under the clavicle. The divisions converge on the axilla and form cords beneath the pectoralis minor muscle. The cords are named based on their location relative to the axillary artery. The posterior cord is formed from the posterior divisions of C5–T1. The posterior cord eventually becomes the radial nerve. The lateral cord is made up of divisions from C5–C7 and gives off the lateral pectoralis nerve and terminates as the musculocutaneous and lateral root of the median nerve. The medial cord is most often invaded by superior sulcus tumors and is made up of divisions from a C8 and T1. The medial cord gives off the medial pectoralis nerve, the medial brachial cutaneous nerve, and the medial anterior brachiocutaneous nerve and finally contributes to the median nerve and terminates as the ulnar nerve. The shoulder muscles are supplied by the C5 and C6 nerve roots. The C7 root contributes to elbow, wrist, and finger extensors. The C8 and T1 contribute to the long finger flexors and intrinsic hand muscles. Because superior sulcus tumors often invade the medial cord, pain occurs in an ulnar distribution and medial forearm. There is often loss of finger flexion and intrinsic hand muscle function.

Surgical approaches to superior sulcus tumors divide the sulcus into anterior, middle, and posterior compartments. The anterior compartment is anterior to the anterior scalene and contains the subclavian vein, internal jugular vein, and sternocleidomastoid muscle. The middle compartment between anterior and middle scalene muscle contains the subclavian artery, trunks of the brachial plexus, and phrenic nerve. The posterior compartment, which is most often involved with Pancoast cancer contains the nerve roots of the brachial plexus, stellate ganglia, vertebral column. A Horner syndrome is a result of posterior compartment invasion and consists of miosis, ptosis, and anhydrosis.[19–22] Radiation-induced brachial plexopathy most frequently involves the upper trunks of the brachial plexus. Upper trunk palsies produce an internally rotated and abducted shoulder, extended elbow, and pronated forearm with a flexed wrist and digits.[18] Brachial plexopathy involving the lower trunk present with extended fingers and pain and numbness in the fifth and fourth finger on the involved side.

Radiation therapy has been used to treat Pancoast cancers for decades.[23–26] Historically, radiation dose constraints of the brachial plexus were 60–66 Gy.[27] In recent studies, radiation-induced brachial plexopathy has been reported in 12% from 3–6.5 years after radiation.[28] Time from radiation therapy to onset of plexopathy can be as short as 6 months and peaks at 10–20 months.[29–30] Independent risk factors for radiation plexopathy are brachial plexus doses of greater than 69 Gy, maximum doses greater than 75 Gy to 2 cm^3 of the brachial plexus, and previous brachial plexus injury.[31] There is also evidence that combining chemotherapy with radiation therapy will increase plexus injury.[29–30] Radiation-induced brachial plexopathy often produces a causalgic dysesthesia, numbness, and lymphedema, with greater sensory deficits than seen with tumor-related brachial plexopathy; late-onset pain and motor weakness are common. The latter occurs in approximately 60% of cases, whereas 50% may experience numbness and paresthesias. Radiation damage occurs more often to the C5–C7 roots (77%), whereas tumor usually involves the lower plexus. Ribs, clavicle, and upper chest wall soft tissues may partially protect the lower brachial plexus from radiation therapy. The overlying skin may have telangiectasias, soft tissues may feel "woody" and firm, and the upper lobe will be fibrotic and retracted on X-ray. Radiation plexus injury is due to direct adverse effects on the vaso nervorum resulting in microinfarcts of the nerve.[9] Modern radiation techniques limit skin damage, and so these findings will be less evident. Radiation-induced brachial plexopathy can overlap with cancer-related plexopathy if tumor recurs locally or if the cancer is poorly responsive to radiation or radiation plus chemotherapy and it cannot be resected. Progression of brachial plexopathy, therefore, may be related to therapy, or cancer, or both. Clinicians can be misled into thinking that cancer has locally recurred if additional deficits are experienced over time.[32] Stereotactic body radiation is now more frequently used to treat localized peripheral lung cancers. Radiation doses of greater than 26 Gy to the upper lobe will produce a brachial plexopathy in 46% of individuals, whereas doses of less than 26 Gy cause plexopathy in 8% of cases. If stereotactic radiation surgery is considered, doses should be less than 26 Gy given in 3–4 fractions.[33]

HOW ARE SUPERIOR SULCUS CANCERS MANAGED?

CT scans and ultrasound-guided transthoracic needle biopsies will have a diagnostic yield in 90% of cases.[34] Bronchoscopy has a diagnostic yield of only 30–40% because of the peripheral location of superior sulcus cancers. However, bronchoscopy will assess proximal airways for metachronous cancers, and the addition of endoscopic ultrasound is used to stage mediastinal nodes, which influences treatment and prognosis.[35–37] MRI of the brachial plexus allows visualization of branches of the brachial plexus including trunk and cords. MRI should be multiplanar for full evaluation of the brachial plexus.[38] T1- and T2-weighted images demonstrate tumor infiltrating the plexus. Radiation-induced brachial plexopathy will have diffuse thickening of the cords or trunk without a T2-weighted soft-tissue component. T2-weighted signals are low with radiation-induced brachial plexopathy and enhanced with tumor.[38]

Treatment of Pancoast tumor has evolved over time. From 1956 to the 1990s, bimodality therapy consisting of preoperative radiation followed by resection was the standard of care.[39–40] Survival was 30% at 5 years.[41] Treatment began to change in the 1980s. The surgery changed such that an anterior approach was taken for anterior compartment involvement. Aggressive surgical resections included vertebrectomy and reconstruction for individuals with contiguous vertebral body involvement.[19,42] The subclavian artery was resected for middle compartment cancers.[19] Resection of the T1 nerve root could be accomplished without producing much disability, whereas resection of the C8 nerve root led to loss of hand and arm function. At the same time, trimodal therapy was being investigated for locally advanced non-small cell lung cancer. Preoperative chemoradiation therapy led to pathologic complete responses in one-third of individuals. CT scans prior to surgery overstaged patients. Fifty-five percent of those with a "stable" CT scan after chemoradiation therapy had either a pathologic complete response or only microscopic residual disease upon pathologic review of resected specimens. Five-year survival was 53% for those with a complete pathologic response, 41% for all patients. Relapse with trimodal therapy switched to predominant distant relapse, with only 12% relapsing locally.[19,43–45] Postoperative complications were not greater in those who underwent chemoradiation therapy compared to those who received radiation only prior to surgery. Poor prognostic findings were mediastinal nodal involvement, incomplete resections and spinal cord compression, and subclavian vessel involvement.[20,22,46–47]

WHAT INTERVENTIONAL APPROACHES CAN BE DONE FOR A BRACHIAL PLEXOPATHY?

Regional interventional techniques have been used to control brachial plexus-related pain. Brachial plexus pain is relatively resistant to opioids and adjuvant analgesics.[48–49] Almost all individuals with cancer pain from superior sulcus tumors have neuropathic pain, whereas only 25% of patients with lung cancer in general will have neuropathic pain.[50] Regional interventional techniques can be used as ancillaries to systemic analgesics and rarely as primary therapy. Most evidence for benefit is based on case reports, case series, and, in a few circumstances, large prospective studies. There are no randomized control trials comparing different interventional techniques or systemic analgesics. In addition, the clinical experience with regional analgesia varies widely and is operator dependent. Although there is a significant amount of evidence for regional analgesia in managing postoperative pain, there is less evidence for brachial plexus injury and largely anecdotal experience when managing cancer-related brachial plexopathy. Because chest wall invasion is not uncommon, the neuropathic pain may be mixed with nociceptive somatic pain. As a result, opioids are frequently used as first-line analgesics in contradistinction to noncancer neuropathic pain.

Nondestructive regional approaches to pain management include peripheral repetitive magnetic stimulation over the superior trapezius muscle and regional blocks. Repetitive magnetic stimulation has been done for dramatic brachial injuries but not for neoplastic brachial plexopathy. This has been done during conventional physical therapy in a randomized study compared with sham magnetic stimulation. Motor recovery and pain improved with magnetic stimulation.[51] Continuous brachial plexus blocks have been performed using axillary catheters and local anesthetics, usually in the postoperative setting, for shoulder surgery. Pain improved as measured by a visual analog scale (VAS) over and above pain relief provided by analgesics and adjuvants in a group of patients with brachial plexopathy.[52] Regional blocks have been performed using different approaches to the brachial plexus. Interscalene, infraclavicular, perivascular axillary, and suprascapular approaches have been described with or without stimulating catheters.[53–60] Almost all these approaches have been used for postoperative analgesia but could be adopted to manage brachial plexus pain associated with cancer. The choice would depend on the location of the cancer, which compartment the cancer invades, and its proximity to the vertebral column.

Other noninvasive unique approaches to pain management include motor cortex stimulation either by direct current or by transcranial magnetic stimulation. Stimulation of motor cortex in the motor cortex (M1) region can improve pain.[61] There are limitations to noninvasive motor cortex stimulation for pain control. Motor cortex stimulation is ineffective in managing paroxysmal pain from brachial plexus injury but is moderately effective for continuous pain from the same cause.[62]

Neuromodulation by way of a spinal cord stimulator has been reported to improve deafferentiated pain from a brachial plexus injury.[63] Tumors proximate to the vertebral body and radiation field overlaps may render this option less attractive. However, there would be little neurologic disability produced by this procedure.

In a subset of individuals who experience sympathetically mediated pain, a stellate ganglion block or radiofrequency neurolysis under CT scan guidance has been shown to reduce pain in half of individuals.[64] There is some disability caused by these two procedures. Ultrasound-guided percutaneous ablation of the dorsal cervical nerve roots and dorsal root entry zone have reduced the difficult of managing neuropathic pain. Both paroxysmal and continuous pain responds to these approaches.[65–71]

WHAT IS THE PATHOPHYSIOLOGY OF CANCER-RELATED NEUROPATHY? HOW IS CANCER-RELATED NEUROPATHY MANAGED?

Neuropathic pain is initiated by a primary lesion in the somatosensory nervous system.[72] It arises as a direct consequence of the lesion or disease adversely affecting the somatosensory system.[73] Neuropathic pain is, in fact, not the result of a single mechanism, but rather arises through the action of several different mechanisms. In time, the pain generator may become maladaptive (i.e., without biologic purpose to the sufferer).[74] Mechanisms are protean, extending from peripheral nociceptors to the highest brain center. The pain generator may change and move centrally in time. Even within a single disease entity, such as diabetes, there are several pain mechanisms resulting in different clinical phenotypes; analgesic responses will vary between phenotypes. It is unlikely that a single analgesic will be effective in managing all neuropathic pain. Insult to the nervous system can cause a neuroplastic cascade of events, and, as a result, pain becomes chronic after the initiating event resolves and healing takes place.

Two basic mechanisms lead to chronic neuropathic pain: loss of normal inhibitory mechanisms and gain in nociception. Neuropathic pain is paradoxically associated with hypersensitivity, allodynia, hyperalgesia, and/or hyperpyrexia in an area of sensory deficit and/or motor deficit. Regeneration and/or disinhibition in response to loss of normal afferent input causes these "positive" symptoms in an area of sensory loss.[75–76] Neuropathic pain is generally less responsive to analgesics such as opioids; higher doses and the use of adjuvant analgesics are frequently needed for pain control.[49,77–78] Only one-third of individuals respond with current single-agent analgesics, as determined by numbers needed to treat.[79–80]

Knowledge of the neuroanatomy of the spinal cord is important for an understanding of neuropathic pain (Figure 23.2). Understanding neuropathic pain mechanisms provides insight into why opioids are less effective and provides a rationale for treatment with adjuvant analgesics. Low threshold Aβ fibers synapse in the innermost lamina II of the dorsal horn and ascend in the dorsal column, whereas nociceptive specific C fibers and Aδ fibers synapse in the superficial dorsal horn (lamina I), cross, and ascend in the contralateral spinothalamic tract. Wide dynamic range neurons (WDR) in the deep dorsal horn (lamina V) are responsible for wind-up and are subject to long-term potentiation. Both second-order nociceptive specific neurons and WDRs ascend together in the dorsal horn.[81] There is a "silent" circuit between Aβ fibers and nociceptive-specific neurons within lamina II that is governed by excitatory and γ-aminobutyric acid (GABAergic)/glycinergic inhibitory interneurons. Loss of inhibitory interneuron function or gain of excitatory interneuron activity causes disinhibition. This disinhibition leads to "gating" of Aβ activity through nociceptive specific C-fiber neurons, causing allodynia and mechanical hypersensitivity. The Aβ fibers do not contain μ receptors; therefore, pain generated by this mechanism will be relatively morphine resistant.[82] Neuropathic injury also leads to a neuron phenotypic switch from nociceptive-specific to WDR neurons within the spinal cord. This increases the activation of the neuron as measured by c-fos expression and lowers thresholds of mechanical stimulation.[83] Damage to primary afferents can lead to development of ectopic pacemaker activity as membrane potentials fall below thresholds to generate action potentials.[84] This leads to paroxysmal pain. Opioid receptor expression on C fibers is reduced with neuropathic injury, thus rendering pain less responsive to opioids.[85] Ion channels, which regulate action potentials, are altered favoring depolarization of neurons.[86–87] Up-regulation of voltage-gated calcium channels occurs with neuropathic injury and increases neuron activation.[88] Gabapentin and pregabalin target certain calcium channel subunits and down-regulate calcium channel expression, which improves pain.[89] Large-size Aβ neurons normally do not express neuroexcitatory transmitters but change phenotype and begin to express substance P and calcitonin gene-related peptide as well as brain-derived neurotrophic factor.[90–91] Structural plasticity also occurs when afferent neurons develop collateral sproutingat multiple locations, The result will extend the receptive area of pain from the site of primary injury and generate sympathetically mediated pain.[92–94]

Inhibitory pathways to spinal nociception and presumably pain processing in humans involve interneurons found in laminae II, which are GABAergic. Nonsegmental inhibitory pathways include monoaminergic descending pathways from brainstem rostral ventromedial medulla and subnucleus reticularis dorsalis. The latter pathway involves diffuse noxious inhibitory control tested by conditioning pain modulation. All three inhibitory pathways may be impaired by neuropathic injury.[81,95–98] In certain clinical circumstances, it may be important to know the mechanism of disinhibition. For instance, duloxetine improves diffuse noxious inhibitory

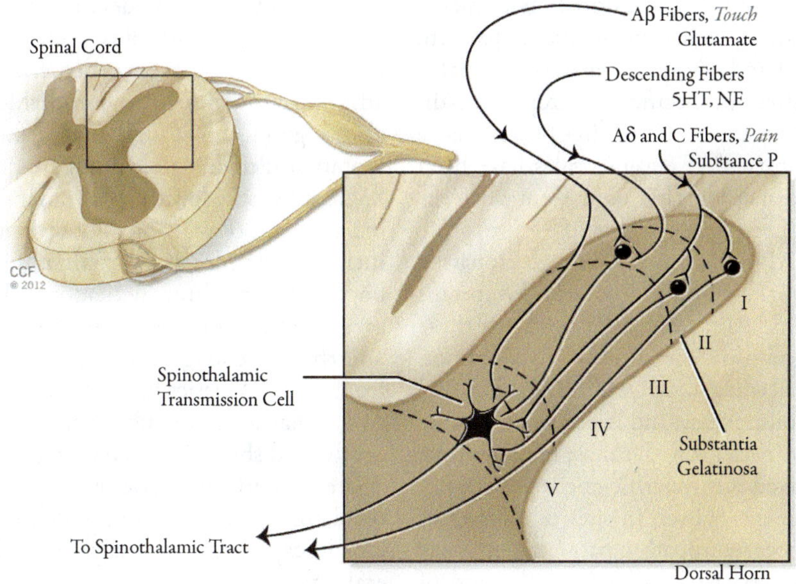

Figure 23.2 Neuroanatomy of nociception. Reprinted with permission from the Cleveland Clinic Center for Medical Art & Photography ©2012. All Rights Reserved.

control and neuropathic pain in the subset of patients with diabetic neuropathy with impaired conditioning pain modulation.[98]

Non-neural glia cells are involved in sensory neurotransmission. Glia enhance excitatory interneuron signaling in pathologic states.[99–100] Astroglia consists of astrocytes and microglia and are intimately involved in synapse function. Glia contain glutamate transporters that remove neuroexcitatory glutamate from synapses. Glutamate transporters are down-regulated when microglia are activated.[101] Microglia and astrocytes produce cytokines in response to neuropathic injury, leading to activation of nociceptive sensitive neurons. Interleukin-1β and tumor necrosis factor derived from glia increase WDR neuron firing. Cytokines and chemokines derived from microglia trigger spontaneous postsynaptic potentials.[102–103] Prostaglandins released as a result of neural injury contribute to pain hypersensitivity.[104] Prostaglandin E2 (PGE2) contributes to signaling between microglia and neurons. PGE2-dependent, ERK1/2-regulated microglia-neuron signaling pathways mediate the microglial component of pain maintenance.[104] Clinically, although NSAIDs are not extensively used for neuropathic pain, responses have been reported anecdotally.[105–107]

Causes for neuropathic pain include chemotherapy, nutritional deficiencies, metabolic disturbances, opportunistic infections, and paraneoplastic neurologic disorders.[108] Hence, depending on the clinical presentation and history and physical examination, laboratory tests such as thyroid function tests, B_{12} and folate, glucose, and hemoglobin A1c may need to be performed.

Pain assessment is often the rate-limiting step to good pain control. Quantifying pain is essential to choosing initial therapy and monitoring the impact of the intervention on patients. Intensity can be "quantified" using a numerical rating scale (NRS), VAS, and/or categorical scale. A numerical rating of greater than 4 (0 no pain, 10 most severe pain) requires further assessment, including the impact of pain severity on daily function.[109–110] Additional assessments should include pain location, radiation, temporal pattern, quality, associated physical and emotional distress, and palliating factors. Questionnaires not specific to neuropathic pain but helpful in this regard are the McGill Pain Questionnaire and the Brief Pain Inventory.[111–112] Several scales have been developed to differentiate neuropathic pain from nociceptive pain, including the Leeds Assessment of Neuropathic Signs and Symptoms (LANSS), Pain ID, the Neuropathic Pain Symptom Inventory, the Neuropathic Trial Symptoms Scale, and the Neuropathic Pain Scale.[113–117] Some of these scales require a physical examination to complete. Common descriptors are pins and needles, heat or burning, impaired temperature sensation, numbness, and electric shock-like spontaneous pain.[118] Many patients with cancer have multiple pain syndromes and mixed neuropathic-nociceptive pain, which complicates assessment.[119] Even in sites of metastases where one would not expect neuropathic pain, patients may describe neuropathic features. For instance, a subgroup of patients with bone metastases (17%) has neuropathic pain by the LANSS. This subgroup has higher pain scores on the Brief Pain Inventory.[120] A corollary to this can be found in animal models of bone metastases where a neuropathic "signature" can be seen in the spinal cord manifested by microglia activation.[121] The clinical relevance of this can be seen in a subset of individuals with bone metastases who respond to adjuvant analgesics commonly used for neuropathic pain.[122] In addition, neuropathic pain features from bone metastases may respond better to multiple fractions of radiation rather than a single fraction (although randomized trials will be necessary to confirm this).[123] Bone pain with neuropathic features may require a different therapeutic approach.

In general, questionnaires fail to identify 10–20% of patients with neuropathic pain. Hence, clinical judgment cannot be replaced by routine use of questionnaires. Quantitative sensory testing (QST) is particularly appropriate for positive symptoms such as mechanical and thermal allodynia and/or hyperalgesia.[124] QST is rarely done in palliative care settings due to limited survival of patients. Electromyography/nerve conduction studies are the best methods for verifying lesions of large peripheral nerve fibers.[125] Such tests should be done only if it would make a difference in managing pain. If a central lesion is suspected based on physical examination and/or history, an MRI should be obtained. Pain-evoked potentials and functional neuroimaging may have some clinical utility, as would skin biopsies in certain settings.[124,125] This would largely depend upon the goals of care and is more often done in the research setting. Those with a short expected survival should not be put through extensive testing but should be treated empirically. In those whose cause for pain is quite evident, there is less of a role for extensive diagnostic procedures.

Cancer neuropathic pain is often managed by the World Health Organization analgesic stepladder guidelines. Analgesic choices are based on pain severity rather than pain mechanism (nociceptive vs. neuropathic), which may be a drawback. In addition, adjuvant analgesics are suggested to be used with each of the three steps, but when to start them and which adjuvant to use are not explicitly outlined.[126] The starting opioid for moderate pain can be tramadol, tapentadol, or oxycodone plus acetaminophen or hydrocodone plus acetaminophen or codeine.[127–128] Tramadol may be an advantage in treating neuropathic pain.[129] Oxycodone is also a good choice in light of published experience.[130–135] Compounded analgesic doses are limited by acetaminophen. Some substitute low doses of potent opioids for a "weak" opioid as a step II analgesic. Potent opioids used for severe pain include oxycodone, morphine, fentanyl, hydromorphone, buprenorphine, and methadone. There is no advantage of one potent opioid over another when comparing efficacy, and there is enough evidence for any of these opioids to be front-line analgesics.[127,136–137] Although methadone is effective, it has a unique pharmacokinetic and drug interaction profile and should be used only by experienced prescribers.[138] There is insufficient evidence to support any particular protocol for opioid titration.[139] Published dosing strategies are largely experience- rather than evidence-based.[140] As a general strategy, an opioid is titrated to pain control then continued around-the-clock at dosing intervals based on drug half-life.[128,140] Laxatives are started with the first opioid dose to prevent constipation. Around-the-clock dosing is normally every 4 hours for immediate-release opioids and every 12–24 hours for sustained-release opioids. The usual starting immediate release dose for the opioid naive is 5 mg of morphine, 5 mg of oxycodone, 1 mg of hydromorphone, and fentanyl 12 mcg an hour.[140] Transdermal fentanyl should be used only after titration when pain is under control; parenteral fentanyl titration is done before switching to transdermal patch. Transdermal fentanyl patches are changed at 72 hours and, rarely, at 48 hours. Doses need to be adjusted due to individual variability in fentanyl cutaneous absorption.[141–143] Absorption can be altered at the end of life, particularly for those who are elderly and those who are cachectic.[143] Individuals with chronic cancer pain often experience transient flares of pain requiring rescue opioids. It is reasonable to use one-sixth of the total daily opioid as the starting rescue dose.[144] Several transmucosal and intranasal fentanyl preparations have been developed to manage breakthrough pain. However, the effective dose for breakthrough pain does not correlate with the around-the-clock opioid dose, and so transmucosal and intranasal fentanyl need to be titrated independently to response.[145]

Errors in prescribing opioids include starting opioid doses too high for the elderly.[128] Severity of pain in the opioid naive does not predict the final effective opioid dose. Opioids may mistakenly be given at greater than drug half-life intervals, thus resulting in resurgence of pain or withdrawal between doses.[128] Clinicians may fail to give around-the-clock doses for continuous pain or fail to provide a rescue dose for flares of pain.[146] Titration may be too slow. Opioid doses should be increased by at least 25% to have an appreciable analgesic effect.[128] On the other hand, continuous opioid dosing may be increased too rapidly before reaching steady state, leading to delayed opioid toxicity. Around-the-clock immediate-release opioid doses should be adjusted not more frequently than every 24 hours, sustained-release opioids every 48 hours, and transdermal fentanyl at 48–72 hours. If pain is still moderate to severe before reaching steady state, the rescue dose should be titrated and rescue doses added to the around-the-clock dose once reaching steady state. Clinicians may use multiple opioids at low doses rather than titrating a single opioid to response.[146] Not more than one change at a time should be done, and the patient is assessed for response after each change. Either an increase in the rescue dose, an increase in the around-the-clock dose, or adding an adjuvant should be done for poorly controlled pain. Alternatively, opioid rotation or route conversion may be a choice, particularly if opioid toxicity is occurring with inadequately controlled pain. Switching opioids in the face of inadequate pain control will improve pain control and reduce side effects in at least half of individuals.[147] Common conversion ratios are morphine to oxycodone (equivalents 1.5–1), oxycodone and to hydromorphone (equivalents 4–1), morphine to hydromorphone (equivalents 5–1), morphine to fentanyl (equivalents 100–1), and morphine to buprenorphine (equivalents 75–1).[127] Doses should be reduced by 25–50% when rotating because of analgesic non-cross-tolerance. Subcutaneous infusions of potent opioids (except for methadone) are simpler, better tolerated, and have fewer adverse effects than intravenous infusions.[127] Psychosocial and spiritual distress can be somatized as "physical pain" and will not respond to an opioid.[148]

Opioids should be used with caution in organ failure. Fentanyl, buprenorphine, or methadone may be preferred when the glomerular filtration rate (GFR) is less than 30 mL per minute.[149–151] In those with moderate to severe hepatic failure, morphine or hydromorphone should be considered.[152–153]

Adjuvant analgesics are second-line therapy for cancer-related neuropathic pain.[128,154] Most guidelines for cancer neuropathic pain rely on evidence derived from noncancer neuropathic pain trials. Gabapentin is the only adjuvant that has randomized controlled trial evidence of benefit for cancer neuropathic pain.[155–156] Most comparisons between analgesics for noncancer neuropathic pain are indirect; only 27% of trials are head-to-head comparisons.[157] The mean trial size is 45, so most are underpowered; power calculations were performed in only 31% of studies. Less than one-third are of high quality; only 35 of 129 studies have an explicit intent to treat analysis. Outcome measures were explicitly stated in only half of studies.[157] If one extrapolates treatment to cancer neuropathic pain based on studies for noncancer neuropathic pain, there is no difference between the gabapentinoids, lamotrigine, and tricyclic antidepressants (TCAs) when comparing response rates defined as the number of individuals with a 50% reduction in pain intensity.[158] Serotonin norepinephrine reuptake inhibitors (SNRIs; duloxetine and venlafaxine) are just as effective. Either gabapentin or pregabalin are preferred due to reduced side effects and drug interactions. Based on efficacy, gabapentinoids, TCAs, or SNRIs would be reasonable first choices to add to an opioid. Lacosamide, by indirect comparison, appears to be inferior to gabapentin, pregabalin, and SNRIs. For cancer neuropathic pain, a combination of low-dose gabapentin (400–800 mg/d) plus an opioid is equivalent to low-dose imipramine plus an opioid.[158] A triple drug combination of low-dose gabapentin plus low-dose imipramine plus an opioid is superior to the double drug combination of an opioid plus gabapentin or an opioid plus imipramine.[159–160] A small trial that combined venlafaxine with gabapentinoids in diabetic neuropathy found the combination superior to gabapentin alone in diabetic neuropathy.[161] A combination of gabapentin plus an SNRI would be a reasonable option in those who failed to respond to a single adjuvant analgesic. Additional evidence in noncancer neuropathic pain trials suggests that gabapentin plus nortriptyline, gabapentin plus venlafaxine, gabapentin plus morphine, pregabalin plus oxycodone, and pregabalin plus celecoxib are superior to monotherapy.[133,162–167] Not all trials of combination therapy are positive.[168] The same is true for cancer neuropathic pain. In a small placebo-controlled crossover study, the addition of amitriptyline to morphine was not better than morphine alone.[169] This study was underpowered because only 16 patients participated. To date, the number of clinical studies addressing the value of combination analgesics for cancer neuropathic pain is very limited. Many are small and underpowered and so have the same limitations as studies for noncancer neuropathic pain. Individuals often had mixed pain syndromes, and outcomes were not uniform, thus making it difficult to offer a firm recommendation in regards to the value of combination analgesics. Which combinations are best and at what dose still needs to be explored in randomized studies.[170–171]

Despite the lack of quality trials, a treatment algorithm has been piloted in a group of cancer patients with neuropathic pain. In this study, neuropathic pain was predominantly due to chemotherapy. A numerical rating scale (Neuropathic Pain-NRS) was used as primary outcome. Most individuals were on opioids. Step 1 of the algorithm was assessment. Step 2 included the topical Lidoderm patch 5% for localized pain. Step 2b was gabapentin titrated to 2,700–3,600 mg. Step 2c involved short-acting opioids (oxycodone plus acetaminophen, tramadol, or morphine) for those not on an opioid. Step 3 was nonpharmacologic therapy such as physical and occupational therapy, exercises, adaptive therapy, and energy conservation. Step 4 involved drug rotations to pregabalin, nortriptyline, duloxetine, or a different opioid if pain was poorly controlled.[172] One patient dropped out of study. Pain, sleep, and life enjoyment significantly improved using this algorithm. This study, however, involved only 20 patients and was not randomized, so the true benefits to this approach are not established. Gabapentin dose titration in this study was relatively slow. Gabapentin can usually be titrated quickly to 900 mg within 3 days without significant toxicity.[173] Within step 2c and 4, TCAs or SNRIs should not be combined with tramadol because there is an increased risk for a serotonin syndrome.[174]

It would be rational to take the approach of adding a complementary analgesic when neuropathic pain is poorly controlled. One would start with an opioid for those with cancer neuropathic pain and add either a gabapentinoid or an antidepressant as a second step. The third step would be to add the alternative psychotropic (a gabapentinoid for those on an antidepressant or an antidepressant for those on a gabapentinoid).[76] Alternatively, rotating the opioid within the combination would be a fourth step. Switching from gabapentin to pregabalin has also been reported to improve pain control.[175] A fifth step would be interventional approaches.

HOW IS CHEMOTHERAPY-INDUCED NEUROPATHY MANAGED?

Chemotherapy-induced peripheral neuropathy (CIPN) produces a "stocking-and-glove" distribution of numbness, paresthesias, and burning pain. Motor weakness may be seen clinically with foot drop. Patellar reflexes may be lost. Autonomic neuropathy is manifested as orthostatic hypotension and cardiovascular, erectile, or gastrointestinal dysfunction.[176] Autonomic neuropathy can be seen without peripheral neuropathy.[177] Symptoms usually start to improve once chemotherapy is stopped (the exception to this is cisplatin).[178–179] The differential diagnosis includes diabetic- or alcohol-related neuropathy, thyroid dysfunction, nutritional deficiencies (in particular B_{12} and folate), monoclonal gammopathy, infectious etiology, paraneoplastic, leptomeningeal carcinomatosis, intramedullary metastases, or epidural metastases.[177] Chemotherapy agents commonly associated with neuropathic pain are taxanes, platinum compounds, vinca alkaloids, bortezomib, thalidomide and its derivatives, etoposide, and procarbazine.[180–182] If the peripheral neuropathy does not follow the course of treatment or fails to improve off therapy (with the exception of cisplatin), or if the history and physical examination suggests another cause, then laboratory studies similar to those obtained for cancer neuropathic pain, including hemoglobin A1c, thyroid function tests, B_{12} and folate, venereal disease screening, monoclonal antibody screen, anti-HU antibody studies, serum ANA, and Westergren sedimentation rate, should be obtained.[177] Nerve conduction studies and electromyography, as well as QST, may help differentiate CIPN from other causes. These are rarely needed with initial detection.[183] These ancillary studies may be important in clinical trials that involve both objective and subjective outcomes.[184]

There are multiple potential causes for CIPN. Microtubular structures may be damaged, which influences axonal transport. DNA damage leads to neuron death. Mitochondria are damaged by taxanes and platinum compounds causing deficits in adenosine triphosphate (ATP) production.[185–190] Individuals differ in the clinical expression of CIPN, which may be genetically determined.[190–191] Chemotherapy neuron damage leads to neuroplastic changes, which may ultimately lead to pain. Voltage-gated sodium and calcium channels are upregulated.[181,192] Central sensitization may occur due to dropout of inhibitory neurons within the dorsal horn. Increased pain facilitation results from plastic changes within the periaqueductal gray and rostral ventromedial medulla. Diffuse noxious inhibitory control becomes impaired.[193] Glia are activated within the dorsal root ganglia.[194] Acute paclitaxel pain, which is unique, peaks 3 days after administration and is associated with up-regulation of transcription factor-3 within the dorsal root ganglia.[195]

Several trials have been published that explore the use of agents to prevent chemotherapy-related neuropathy. Present evidence does not support the use of amifostine, calcium, or magnesium in the prevention of cisplatin neuropathy.[196] N-acetyl cysteine, a precursor of glutathione, was reported to reduce oxaliplatin neuropathy in a small, randomized study.[197] Glutamine was effective in reducing or preventing neuropathy from paclitaxel and oxaliplatin.[198–199] Oxcarbazepine reduced the incidence of oxaliplatin neuropathy.[200] Allopregnanolone, which interacts on $GABA_a$ receptor and calcium channels, reduced vincristine-induced nerve conduction abnormalities in an animal model.[201] Clinical benefits are unknown, and confirmation is needed. In animal models, acetyl L-carnitine prevents mitochondrial damage by paclitaxel and oxaliplatin. The incidence and severity of neuropathy is significantly reduced in animal models.[186,202–205] This has been confirmed in small clinical trials.[206–207] Venlafaxine prevents oxaliplatin acute neurosensory symptoms and cold intolerance. Venlafaxine 50 mg is given prior to oxaliplatin, and 37.5 mg is given on days 2 through 11.[208]

To date, no therapy has been licensed or approved to treat CIPN.[108] Both nortriptyline and amitriptyline are ineffective in managing CIPN, as demonstrated by prospective studies.[209–210] In a double-blind randomized crossover study, gabapentin was no better than placebo.[211] Pregabalin was reported to be effective in a small single-arm study to treat oxaliplatin neuropathy.[212] This needs to be confirmed in a randomized trial, particularly since the gabapentin study was negative. Lamotrigine was found to be no better than placebo in a randomized trial.[213] Mexiletine has been used in animal models with some benefit, but there are no clinical studies.[193] In the same manner, cannabinoids have been used in animal models of vinca and paclitaxel neuropathy.[214–216] However, there are no clinical trials available to confirm the benefits seen with animal models. Opioids have been tested in animal models using paclitaxel. Both morphine and methadone were reported to be effective.[217] No randomized controlled trials of opioids for CIPN have been published. Duloxetine has been reported to improve oxaliplatin-related peripheral neuropathy in a single-arm study.[218] Anecdotal reports suggest that duloxetine plus pregabalin improve paclitaxel related pain.[219] There are no randomized trials of duloxetine alone or in combination with other adjuvant analgesics. α-Lipoic acid with doses up to 600 mg three times a day in a small single-arm study reduced platinum related neuropathy.[220–221] In a single-arm study acetyl L-carnitine 1 g three times a day reduced paclitaxel- and cis-platinum-related neuropathy.[222] However, there are no randomized prospective studies to confirm these benefits.

Topical analgesics have been used for pain management. Topical doxepin has been used for mucositis as an oral rinse and topically for complex regional pain syndromes.[223–224] There are no reports of topical doxepin use for CIPN. Capsaicin at low doses (0.075%) and high doses (8%) has been used for peripheral neuropathy and combined with doxepin.[225–228] However, there are no trials of capsaicin or a combination capsaicin plus doxepin for CIPN. Topical combination therapy consisting of amitriptyline (40 mg), ketamine (20 mg), and baclofen (10 mg) in pluronic lecithin organogel (BAK-Plo) in a randomized 4-week trial improved CIPN compared to placebo. None of the three drugs was absorbed, as determined by blood levels.[229]

Current recommendations for the treatment of CIPN consist of choosing an agent based on experience, efficacy, and safety.[108] Based on randomized controlled trials, single-agent gabapentin, amitriptyline, and nortriptyline should be avoided. This does not exclude their potential benefits in combination. Based on single-arm studies, pregabalin and duloxetine have some activity. The evidence for opioids is in animal models only, but many patients with advanced cancer require opioids because of moderate to severe pain from concurrent somatic and/or visceral metastases. For those survivors who are cancer free but suffer from CIPN, start with pregabalin or duloxetine and switch or add the alternative drug if the initial drug is not effective. A trial of topical amitriptyline, ketamine, and baclofen may also be considered if there is access to a compounding pharmacy.

Nonpharmacologic approaches to managing CIPN include acupuncture and neurostimulation (neuromodulation with MC5-A Calmare, Scrambler Therapy, Competitive Technologies Inc., Fairfield, Connecticut).[230–233] Scrambler therapy is U.S. Food and Drug Administration (FDA) approved. Both are operator dependent. Evidence of benefit with acupuncture or scrambler therapy has been in small single-arm studies. Repetitive transcranial magnetic stimulation (rTMS) over the motor cortex at high frequencies (5–10 Hz) reduces pain refractory to other modalities.[234–236] rTMS has successfully managed neuropathic pain syndromes.[237–241] Repetitive noninvasive stimulation of the motor cortex works by improving GABAergic inhibitory activity.[242] However, there are no studies of rTMS in CIPN. Transcutaneous electrical nerve stimulation (TENS) appears to alter CNS pain processing through the CNS pain matrix.[243] There is little evidence that TENS benefits those suffering from cancer pain and no reports of its use in CIPN.[244] Anecdotally, spinal cord stimulation may be helpful in refractory cases of chemotherapy-induced neuropathy.[245]

Acupuncture, scrambler therapy, and rTMS are low-risk, noninvasive, nondestructive procedures that do not have the side effects of analgesics. The addition of scrambler therapy to guideline-based management of neuropathic pain has been reported to improve pain control compared to drug management alone in a small randomized study.[231] At present, a comprehensive evidence-based approach to CIPN prevention and treatment is lacking. Randomized trials of single agents, drug combinations, drug plus nonpharmacologic management, and comprehensive assessment of multimodality approaches are needed.

HOW IS DEPRESSION AND ANXIETY DIAGNOSED IN THE CONTEXT OF A CANCER PAIN DIAGNOSIS?

Diagnostic classification systems for depression have been criticized when dealing with medically ill patients because many symptoms of systemic illness can lead to similar symptoms of depression and lead to an overdiagnosis of mood disorders in this population. One potential solution to this diagnostic quandary would be to remove the neurovegetative symptoms from this diagnostic scheme, which may be overrepresented in medically ill populations, but this may lead to the population being underdiagnosed for these conditions that are both disabling and treatable. The controversy over this topic continues, and a consensus opinion has not been possible to date.[245]

A review of the literature on depression in palliative cancer care by Wasteson et al. (2009) systematically identified the assessment methods and classification systems used in studies of depression in this population. In the 202 identified papers, 106 different assessment methods were used, and 65 were used only once. The most commonly used scale was the Hospital Anxiety and Depression Scale (HADS), which dominated the European literatures but was less used in the United States and Canada. Notably, most prevalence and intervention studies did not make an explicit reference to a diagnostic system, utilizing instead cutoff scores on various rating scales. Less than one-third of the assessments in the review accounted for the duration of the symptoms, and less than one-fifth assessed consequences and impact on functioning. This review points to a need for some degree of consensus on the assessment and conceptualization of depression and mood disorders in palliative care populations.[246]

While acknowledging shortcomings in the available classification schemes of mental disorders in a medically ill population, it is clear that anxiety and depressive symptoms are common and disabling. A descriptive study of 266 consecutive palliative patients in Western Australia and New South Wales utilizing the HADS demonstrated significant levels of both anxiety and depression. These patients represented a real-world sample recruited from a combination of palliative settings including home care, hospices, and private and tertiary hospitals. Utilizing recommended cutoff scores on the HADS, it was determined that 46% of patients were possibly depressed and 23% probably depressed. Similarly, 37% were possibly anxious, whereas 20% were probably anxious. One-quarter of the population showed comorbid symptoms of both anxiety and depression. Although systematic diagnostic interviews were not conducted with this population to determine syndromal diagnoses, the data are clear that a majority of patients do experience clinically significant anxiety and depressive symptoms.[247]

Other studies have also demonstrated high levels of mood disturbances among individuals with advanced cancer or medical illness. A retrospective survey of 216 patient records of prior study participants demonstrated that 37% showed clinically significant symptoms of depression and 44% anxiety. Importantly, those with clinically significant levels of depression or anxiety expressed both higher frequencies and higher intensities of physical symptoms including drowsiness, nausea, pain, dyspnea, diminished appetite, and overall well-being.[248]

Another study demonstrated that the presence of depression in palliative care patients hospitalized for cancer, heart failure, and chronic obstructive pulmonary disease (COPD) predicted additional symptom burden at follow-up in 2 weeks.[249] These studies support that those palliative patients who report a high frequency and intensity of physical symptoms or persistent physical symptoms that remain even after attempts at treatment should be more carefully screened for mood and anxiety disturbances.

Finally, a meta-analysis of depression, anxiety, and adjustment disorder in oncological, hematological, and palliative care settings identified 94 interview-based studies. Twenty-four of these took place in palliative care settings. Depression defined by the DSM or ICD criteria was 16.5% for major depression. Anxiety disorders had a prevalence of 9.8% in this meta-analysis. There were no significant differences between palliative care settings and oncological settings in this study.[250] Importantly, when looking at impact on disease state and quality of life, even mild depressive episodes show significant impact on perception of wellness and life satisfaction.

When examining anxiety in particular, relatively less attention has been given to it in palliative care settings in contrast to depression, in spite of its being linked to lower quality of life, increased insomnia, decreased trust in physicians, and nonadherence to prescribed treatment. Estimates of anxiety disorder prevalence range from 2% to 14%, with generalized anxiety disorder and panic disorder being the most common diagnoses. The prevalence rates of both generalized anxiety (4.8–5.8%) and panic disorder (5.5%) have been noted to be greater than in the general adult population. In addition to those with definable anxiety disorder, 25–48% of the advanced cancer population has been estimated to experience clinically significant anxiety. Rates appear increased among females, unmarried patients, and those with poor physical functioning. Conflicting evidence exists whether or not progression of illness is associated with worsening anxiety.[251]

Kolva et al. also sought to identify predictors of anxiety, focusing on treatment-related variables, and prospectively collected data from patients in two New York City area hospitals, all of whom had a diagnosis of Stage IV cancer and life expectancy of less than 1 year. Approximately half were recruited from a 200-bed palliative care hospital, with the remainder from a tertiary-care cancer center where they were receiving aggressive life-prolonging interventions. Anxiety and depression were measured using the HADS to exclude the somatic symptoms that confound assessment of anxiety and depression in medically ill patients. Anxiolytics and antidepressants were commonly prescribed, with approximately 24% taking one or the other, and 10% taking both. Sleep aids were prescribed to 10% of the population.[251]

Approximately 19% of the same patients scored in a range suggesting moderate clinically significant anxiety, and an additional 12% reported high levels of anxiety. The presence of worrying thoughts was the most common item endorsed by participants. Anxiety was positively correlated with other psychological distress including depression, hopelessness, and desire for hastened death, with women reporting significantly higher levels of anxiety than men. Mixed anxiety and depressive symptoms were most common in this group, and this group in particular reported more hopelessness and a desire for a hastened death. The severity of anxiety across the two groups (palliative vs. life-sustaining treatment) did not differ, which suggests that patients do not become more anxious as they approach death when cancer is already advanced. Other studies suggest worsening anxiety across disease progression, but all participants in this study had advanced cancer already. Other elements of psychological distress did appear to increase as participants approached death, including depression and a desire for a hastened death.[251]

The detection and treatment of depressive and anxiety disorders in cancer populations can be challenging, but these syndromes are treatable. In a well-designed study utilizing the HADS as a screening tool, 32 patients were found to have significant mental distress. The screening was followed by other standardized assessments by a psychiatrist to improve diagnostic validity. It was found that adjustment disorders were most common, followed by depressive disorders and anxiety disorders. Most subjects in this trial were prescribed psychotropics: mirtazapine to 15, citalopram to 13, and escitalopram to 4. Improvements in symptoms of depression and anxiety were observed on all measures, suggesting that this population does respond well to pharmacological intervention.[252]

WHAT IS THE ROLE OF INSOMNIA ON MOOD AND PAIN PERCEPTION?

Insomnia is one of the more common disorders among adults, and some studies have suggested that up to one-third of adults have experienced insomnia within the preceding 12 months. A smaller percentage of adults (10–15%) have more severe current insomnia. Insomnia has been strongly linked to major depression and anxiety disorders in adults, and insomnia is a strong predictor of future major depressive episodes. Ford and Kamerow found those with chronic insomnia were up to 40 times more likely to have major depression and six times more likely to have an anxiety disorder compared to those without insomnia.[253] Other studies have also linked insomnia to the development of major depressive disorder, anxiety, and suicide, with odds for suicidality increased from 2–5 times compared to those without insomnia.[254–256]

Comparatively little data have examined the role of mental disorders on creating insomnia; typically, more attention has been given to the impact of insomnia on creating other disorders.[257] Johnson notes that prevalence rates of insomnia occurred prior to a first episode of anxiety less than 20% of the time, occurred at the same time in 39%, and insomnia occurred after the anxiety disorder in 44%.[257] In contrast, insomnia predated the diagnosis of major depressive disorder 41% of the time, simultaneously in 29%, and following the occurrence of the mood disorder in 29%. Johnson speculates that, based on these limited data, insomnia may have a different relationship with anxiety disorders than with depression or other mood disorders.

Johnson notes that although it is clear that there is a relationship between insomnia, anxiety, and depression, it remains unclear whether the relationship is bidirectional. It also raises the issue of whether insomnia is a prodromal condition or simply a risk factor for the development of anxiety and depression.[257,258]

As with insomnia and mood disorders, insomnia and pain share a complex relationship. Recent population data from Australia demonstrated a prevalence of insomnia of approximately 5%, and insomnia was associated with increasing age, pain, and psychological distress. Controlling for these variables, insomnia remains associated with increased disability dates, difficulty of daily activities, life dissatisfaction, and greater visits to general practitioners.[259] In addition to these items, insomnia has been noted to play a role in both pain perception as well as fatigue in patients with advanced cancer.[260]

Insomnia has been noted to be common among cancer patients and occurs in approximately 30–50% of the cancer population. Theobald notes that pain is one of the more common symptoms experienced by cancer patients, with prevalence rates of up to 80% in some cancer types; it is also one of the most important identifiable and treatable causes of insomnia in this population. Conversely, whereas pain contributes to fatigue directly, it also appears to have an indirect influence on fatigue via its disruption of sleep patterns and insomnia. Other notable causes for insomnia in cancer patients include depression, anxiety, and post-traumatic stress disorder that may be precipitated by a cancer diagnosis or cancer treatment. Insomnia may have another important role in cancer patients in that it has been recognized that insomnia can be associated with aberrant patterns of cortisol secretion, which may additively depress immune function. Whether there is a difference with respect to cancer outcome remains speculative.[261]

In addition to insomnia being a marker for mood disorders and diminished quality of life, it has also been shown to have an association with other symptoms in patients with advanced cancer. Sleep disturbances can lead to declines in cognitive function, inability to engage in work and recreational activities, and anhedonia. Sela et al. demonstrated that, in a multidisciplinary pain and symptom control clinic, there were high correlations among sleep disturbances, fatigue, and anxiety. In particular, post-traumatic experiences were the strongest predictors of sleep quality, along with urinary frequency and dyspnea.[262] Another study by Gibbins et al. showed that among patients with advanced cancer, sleep disturbance was associated with higher anxiety and increased body pain.[263] These associations were confirmed in a prospective study by Delgado-Guay et al. who found that the presence of sleep disturbance was significantly associated with pain, depression, anxiety, and reduced sense of well-being. This strengthens the argument that in individuals with elevated pain scores, a sleep assessment should be performed along with an evaluation of underlying anxiety or depressive symptoms.[264]

Treatment of insomnia with associated improvements in function have been shown to improve overall health perceptions and perceived quality of life. It is recognized that insomnia within cancer populations is likely undertreated, and treatment should be incorporated into a global plan designed to ameliorate the sleep disturbance by either addressing it directly or identifying and addressing the factors leading to the sleep disturbance.[261]

Other mental health conditions have also been noted to have an impact on the perception of depression and pain, among these coping styles. Coping styles have received increased attention in recent years because they appear to not only predispose to affective disorder, but also appear to play a major influence in longitudinal models of chronic disease and disease outcome.[265] Coping styles have been shown also to be related to pain and adjustment in chronic illness. In a secondary analysis of a group of lung cancer patients, those utilizing coping mechanisms demonstrated lower scores for pain quality, pain catastrophizing, and depression.[266] These data suggest that early psychological intervention in patients displaying significant anxiety may be helpful as an overall pain management strategy.

HOW ARE DEPRESSION, ANXIETY, AND INSOMNIA MOST EFFECTIVELY MANAGED IN A CANCER PAIN POPULATION?

Available treatments for depression, anxiety, and insomnia can all be divided into psychotherapeutic versus pharmacological and somatic modalities. Somatic modalities including electroconvulsive therapy, deep brain stimulation, and vagal nerve stimulation will not be discussed because they are rarely utilized in populations with advanced malignancies. Psychotherapy and pharmacotherapy are the mainstays of treatment and have the bulk of available evidence for treatment.

Selective serotonin reuptake inhibitors (SSRIs) and SNRIs have emerged as first-line medications for both depressive and anxiety disorders. They share many advantages over older classes of medications, such as TCAs and monoamine oxidase inhibitors, in that they have fewer drug-drug interactions, have a wider margin of safety in use and dosing, produce fewer side effects, and are better tolerated (Table 23.1). Available SSRIs include fluoxetine, paroxetine, sertraline, citalopram, escitalopram, and fluvoxamine. All these medications have data supporting their use in depression and anxiety, and there is no convincing superiority data available to suggest one is more effective than another. Fluoxetine, fluvoxamine, and paroxetine are highly protein bound and are potent inhibitors of CYP 2D6 and/or the 3A4 enzyme systems, making their use more complicated in patients on multidrug regimens.[267]

Citalopram has recently received a black-box warning from the FDA regarding the dose-dependent QTc prolongation if dosed above 40 mg/d for adults or 2 0mg/d for geriatric patients. To date, this black-box warning has not been extended to escitalopram, which appears to be a potentially safer alternative.[268]

Dosing SSRIs for anxiety or depressive disorder does require some degree of patience on the part of clinicians and patients because effects are delayed typically 4–6 weeks after initiating dosing. Treating patients who are highly anxious with SSRIs can also be challenging in that most SSRIs may exacerbate anxiety initially prior to its effective treatment; thus, beginning with smaller and potentially subtherapeutic doses until tolerance is achieved is sometimes necessary, which may delay effective treatment in a population with limited life-expectancy. The advantage of these medications is that they are well tolerated and quite effective, with a low deliriogenic potential—especially in patients with generalized anxiety disorder, panic disorder, or social phobias.

SNRIs are largely limited to three agents at this point: duloxetine, venlafaxine, and desvenlafaxine. Duloxetine enjoys FDA approval for major depressive disorder, generalized anxiety disorder, fibromyalgia, chronic low back pain, and diabetic sensory neuropathy. Duloxetine is also the one antidepressant outside the TCAs that has accumulated the most data supporting its role in treating pain. Thus, it may enjoy significant advantages in a population where pain complaints commonly coexist with symptoms of depression and anxiety.[269]

Table 23.1 ANTIDEPRESSANTS, COMMON INTERACTIONS, AND POTENTIAL ADVANTAGES

ANTIDEPRESSANT	METABOLISM	COMMON INTERACTIONS	POTENTIAL USES AND ADVANTAGES
Escitalopram	3A4, 2C19	Few drug-drug interactions	SSRI with most evidence in painful conditions Starting dose of 10 mg is also therapeutic dose
Citalopram	3A4, 2C19	Dose-dependent QTc prolongation; max dose is 20 mg/d in patients 65 or older; 40 mg/d otherwise	Well-studied during pregnancy/ breast-feeding Generic form available
Sertraline	3A4 inhibition in high doses (150 mg/d or greater) only	Tamoxifen if at high doses; otherwise, few drug-drug interactions	Best cardiac safety data of antidepressants
Fluoxetine/ Paroxetine	2D6 and 3A4 inhibition	Tamoxifen, beta-blockers, calcium channel blockers, multiple others including antiarrhythmics	Available in once-weekly formulation Associated with increased energy; enhances concentration
Mirtazapine	2D6, 1A2, 3A4	Few drug-drug interactions	Treats insomnia, anorexia, few sexual side effects
Bupropion	2B6	Sorafenib	Causes weight loss, increased energy; treatment for ADHD; antismoking approval
Duloxetine	1A2, 2D6	Few relevant drug-drug interactions; rare cases of hepatotoxicity; avoid with underlying hepatic disease (HCV, alcoholic cirrhosis)	Treats painful diabetic neuropathy, low back and chronic musculoskeletal pain, other painful neuropathies
Venlafaxine	2D6	Can result in diastolic blood pressure increases that are dose related Generally felt to be safe with tamoxifen use	Treats painful neuropathies (although less data than with duloxetine), treats hot flashes and perimenopausal symptoms

Mirtazapine is an interesting agent that is often used in palliative medicine because it has also been shown to have antidepressant, antianxiolytic, and sleep properties that can ameliorate these problems that are common in advanced cancer populations. Mirtazapine acts on multiple receptor types including 5-HT_2, 5-HT_3, α_2, and H_1. This multiplicity of action yields a wide array of effects, but, notably, the agent has been shown to be effective in addressing anxiety, depression, and insomnialargely through its antagonism of 5-HT_2, a trait it shares with trazodone.[267] It has also been shown to have positive effects on nausea as well.[270–271] Data to support its use in treating anxiety and depression in cancer populations do exist, and it has been shown to be effective in these conditions as well as effective for improving quality of life in patients with advanced cancer.[272]

A Turkish study comparing mirtazapine to imipramine (TCA with antianxiolytic properties) to placebo (three-arm trial) found mirtazapine to be superior for initial, middle, and late insomnia. HADS scores were also significantly better for the group taking mirtazapine as compared to imipramine. Differences between the groups for measures of pain, nausea, vomiting, or appetite loss were nonsignificant.[273] Another 4-week, prospective, open-label trial in cancer patients found mirtazapine to be effective in the management of nausea as well as the total night sleep time from day 1 of the treatment phase. Depression and anxiety scores also improved significantly after the first week on the medication, reinforcing it as a potential antidepressant with a more rapid onset of action as compared to traditional SSRI/SNRI alternatives. Mirtazapine was well tolerated in the latter study, but daytime drowsiness developed in approximately one-third of subjects, although it dissipated gradually over several days.[274]

Available long-term data regarding mirtazapine used for depression in cancer patients also reinforce its role in this population, although the total quantity of any long-term antidepressant treatment data in cancer populations is scarce. An open-label naturalistic study of 21 consecutive depressed oncology patients showed that mirtazapine was helpful in managing depression by the end of month 1, and the improvement was maintained for the remaining 23 weeks of the study. Importantly, the magnitude of improvement in this population as defined by the Hamilton Rating Scale for Depression-17 (HAM-D-17) was impressive. Prior to treatment, the HAM-D-17 average score was 21.4 + 4.9, indicative of moderate depression severity; following treatment at 1 month, HAD-D-17 scores has dropped to 6.5 + 3.2, indicative of remission of depressive symptoms. Side effects were self-limiting and described as mild-moderate.[275]

In addition, mirtazapine's antihistamine effects aid in sleep maintenance, and it appears to increase appetite, which may give it a role in cancer-related cachexia. A small prospective study of 17 subjects found that approximately 25% gained 1kg or more at a 4-week endpoint using an intention to treat analysis. Although absolute effect size is small, there may be a role for this agent in such populations.[276] It has the added advantage of having virtually no drug-drug interactions, which makes it a safer agent in such complex populations. Of note, there are also reports of intolerance to this agent in advanced cancer with resultant hypersomnia.[277]

Trazodone is one of the older antidepressant agents and is virtually free of anticholinergic effects, making it one of the safer agents in terms of deliriogenic potential. Its mechanism of action blocks postsynaptic serotonin 5-HT_{2a} and 5-HT_{2c} receptors, which gives it a preferential effect in improving sleep continuity. It is metabolized by cytochromes CYP1A2, CYP2D6, and CYP3A4, so drug interactions are a risk when using trazodone in this population.[278,279] Inhibition of CYP3A4 especially inhibits the clearance of trazodone neuroactive metabolite mCPP, which can lead to anxiety, nightmares, and potentially increased pain sensation. Its use in a palliative care population has not been substantiated with large-scale trials, but, nevertheless, it is commonly prescribed with available data supporting its role in managing sleep disturbances.[280] Older data have compared its effectiveness to chlorazepate in the treatment of adjustment disorders (anxious type) in cancer and HIV populations and found the agent to be superior to chlorazepate in both populations, although numbers treated were not adequate to power the study for true statistical differences. Nevertheless, given that trazodone is largely devoid of abuse risk, it seems to be a viable alternative to benzodiazepine-based treatments of anxiety.[281,282] It was also as effective as amitriptyline on measures of pain intensity and sleep in another randomized double-blind study examining deafferentation pain.[283]

Whereas, in the past, conventional wisdom held that all the newer antidepressants produced roughly equivalent results, more recent data based on meta-analyses do show some trends toward relative superiority. A meta-analysis examining 117 randomized controlled trials (25,928 participants) from 1991 to 2007 in patients with unipolar depression found that mirtazapine, escitalopram, venlafaxine, and sertraline were significantly more efficacious than other antidepressants. Additionally, escitalopram and sertraline demonstrated the best acceptability profile, which led to fewer discontinuations in this group when compared to all other antidepressants. Importantly, escitalopram and sertraline also have fewer drug-drug interactions than do alternate SSRI antidepressants, so it may emerge as the preferred agents in this category. Both are available generically in the United States.[284]

Psychostimulants also have a long history of use within palliative medicine, both as antidepressant agents as well as agents that can counteract some of the side effects of opioid-based analgesia. Methylphenidate (MPH) is the CNS stimulant with the most data for use in cancer patients, but it is approved for use only in attention deficit hyperactivity disorder and narcolepsy. Its mode of action is not fully understood, but it appears to block the reuptake of dopamine by binding to the dopamine transporter in the presynaptic cell member, thus increasing extracellular dopamine levels. It also appears to block the reuptake of serotonin and norepinephrine as well, although its effect on the latter two is weaker compared to dopamine. It has a brief half-life of approximately 3–5 hours. It is also a relatively safe drug with few adverse events seen in clinical practice and trial settings—insomnia and nervousness are the two most common. Other adverse events (AEs) seen in less than 10% of patients included cardiovascular effects (tachycardia), CNS effects (headache, dizziness, hypomania, psychosis), GI effects (anorexia at higher doses, nausea), and skin-related effects (rash, urticaria). However, minimal cardiovascular changes are seen with doses of less than 30 mg/d. The most important drug-drug interactions occur with warfarin, anticonvulsants, TCAs, monoamine oxidase inhibitors, and alcohol. All MPH preparations are Schedule II under the Drug Enforcement Administration.[285]

Cancer-related fatigue is defined as an unusual, persistent, and subjective sense of tiredness that is related to cancer or cancer treatment and interferes with usual functioning. Its current construct is that of a multidimensional syndrome that includes cachexia, depression, pain, opioid and medication side effects, anemia, antineoplastic treatments, and deconditioning. Few of these have definitive pharmacological treatments, making cancer-related fatigue a challenge to treat. MPH is a psychostimulant that has been used successfully to manage opioid-induced sedation, cognitive failure associated with brain tumors, and depression.[286] It has also been shown to provide early benefit in HIV-related fatigue, which is a construct not dissimilar to cancer-related fatigue.[287] It has also been presented as being effective in biological models of fatigue, such as interferon-induced fatigue in melanoma patients.[288]

Fatigue has long been an issue almost universally present in advanced cancer patients, and it is also a symptom that is often misdiagnosed as depression. However, comorbid depression can also exacerbate fatigue, making its recognition important when treating this population. Fatigue has been noted to be multidimensional and impairs sense of well-being, activities of daily living, relationships with others, and adherence to therapy. The use of MPH in treating both fatigue and depression has been evaluated in double-blind, placebo-controlled trials and was found to be rapidly efficacious. Kerr at al. demonstrated that, among hospice patients, fatigue was the most distressing symptom identified by the study participants. Study participants taking MPH were found to have significantly and clinically meaningful responses in fatigue scores by day 14 following initiation with MPH, with a mean average effective dose of 20 mg on day 14. All subjects receiving MPH were started at 5 mg/d and then titrated to effect and tolerability. Placebo-treated individuals showed no improvement in fatigue during the study. Similarly, for patients with clinically significant depression as measured by the ESAS or Beck Depression Inventory, treatment with MPH was associated with significant improvements in depressive symptom burden by day 14. The effects of MPH appeared to be dose dependent and sustained over the duration of the study.[289] Although the magnitude of response is impressive, perhaps more important is the rapidity of response, which is important in those patients with limited life expectancy who may not see the benefit of starting an antidepressant.

In addition to MPH's role in treating cancer-related fatigue, it has also been investigated to reverse opioid-induced somnolence and potentially augment an opioid-mediated analgesic response. Three randomized double-blind, placebo-controlled trials involving just 95 patients have examined the efficacy of MPH for reducing opioid-induced somnolence and potentiation analgesia. All showed significant improvements in pain, activity, cognitive function, and drowsiness, but additional studies are required to further assess the true role of MPH on the treatment of cancer-related pain and opioid toxicity.[285]

Studies examining the characteristics of patients responding to MPH clinically have showed a response rate of greater than 50% but also found that the severity of baseline fatigue correlated positively to the degree of MPH response. Interestingly, the response to treatment on day 1 following MPH dosing predicted response at day 8 as well. Response to MPH was not associated with depression or degree of opioid-associated sedation.[290]

Dosing of MPH has generally been twice daily, and most have advocated dosing times of early morning followed by a second dose at 12–2 p.m. Dosing later than this risks nocturnal insomnia. However, Bruera and colleagues have noted that given MPH's short half-life and rapid onset of action, it may be feasible to allow patients to self-administer treatment based on the time of day during which they are most bothered by fatigue. A preliminary investigation designed to assess this approach found that MPH use improved fatigue rapidly and significantly over a 1-week time frame. Other positively affected variables included measures of well-being, anxiety, appetite, pain, nausea, depression, and drowsiness. Importantly, more than 90% of the study group took three or more doses daily, and all patients took afternoon or evening doses. No serious side effects were reported.[286]

A longer term study looking at the effects of MPH on cancer fatigue also supported the increased dosing protocol. Subjects with a fatigue score of 4/10 or greater and a hemoglobin level of 10 g/dL were included and assigned to MPH 5 mg PO q2h as needed (maximum 20 mg/d) or placebo for 7 days. Symptoms were then assessed periodically through 36 days. Fatigue intensity was shown to improve significantly on day 8 for both placebo and MPH; however, both groups tolerated the intervention well, and no significant toxicities were observed even with this more aggressive dosing regimen.[291]

ANXIETY

With regards to treating anxiety in cancer population, much depends on the stage of cancer and expected longevity of the patient. SSRIs remain first-line agents for the majority of anxiety disorders, and strong data exist for their use in generalized anxiety, social phobia, post-traumatic stress disorder, and panic disorder. In addition, they are also effective in atypical depression, which can appear clinically as an anxiety disorder. Just as when being used for depression, the SSRIs and SNRIs typically take between 4–6 weeks prior to produce onset of symptomatic improvement, and they may take as long as 8–12 weeks for peak improvement. In general, as when being used for antidepressant effects, most SSRIs are equivalent in terms of overall efficacy so are dosed based on desired pharmacokinetics and side-effect profiles. However, there are emerging data suggestive that escitalopram may have superior efficacy and tolerability compared to other choices in this group.[292]

If anxiety is acute or severe, a benzodiazepine can be helpful for control of anxiety-based symptoms, but these agents can also be quite deliriogenic in medically complex and failing patients. A careful risk-benefit consideration is required prior to their addition in advanced cancer patients due to this reason. Additionally, benzodiazepines vary widely in terms of their half-lives and pharmacokinetic properties. Lorazepam, oxazepam, and temazepam undergo only hepatic conjugation, so they are potentially better tolerated and more easily cleared than other potential alternatives. All have half-lives that range from 6 to 10 hours. Conversely, diazepam and chlordiazepoxide have half-lives that can be more than 100 hours, have multiple active metabolites, and require complex oxidative reactions prior to elimination.[293] Caution should be utilized when using compounds with long half-lives and complicated metabolism in medically ill individuals.

There is also a growing body of literature incorporating atypical antipsychotics into pharmacy regimens for depression and anxiety as adjunctive or augmentation agents. Prior utilization studies show that the most common off-label uses of these agents include as treatments for depression, obsessive-compulsive disorder, post-traumatic stress disorder, personality disorder, Tourette syndrome, autism, and agitation in dementia.[294] There appears to be some advantage to this strategy in that antidepressant and antianxiety responses appear more complete and occur more rapidly than when using an antidepressant agent alone.[295–297] Quetiapine, olanzapine, and aripiprazole have received FDA approval for depression augmentation when used in conjunction with an antidepressant agent, but available data also support the use of atypical antipsychotics in managing refractory or severe anxiety. Current data indicate that quetiapine, risperidone, and olanzapine are all effective when used as either monotherapy or adjunctive therapy for generalized anxiety disorder.[298,299] Typical augmentation doses are lower than comparable antipsychotic doses of these agents (e.g., risperidone 0.25–0.5 mg PO qhs; olanzapine 2.5–5 mg PO qhs).

SLEEP DISTURBANCES

Sleep disorders remain prevalent in the U.S. population and can best be understood and treated within a logical framework if one divides them into disorders of insomnia and disorders of excessive sleepiness. *Primary insomnia* refers to persistent difficulty in initiating or maintaining sleep that is not secondary to another mental disorder or the result of a medical condition.

In advanced cancer patients, making a diagnosis of primary insomnia is very challenging because their medical burden and associated stressors often impact sleep continuity. However, in large part, treatments for insomnia have been validated in cancer populations and have been shown to be effective in improving sleep parameters. It is important, however, to understand the type of sleep disruption experienced by the patient because treatment selection will depend heavily on whether it is a disorder of impaired sleep initiation or sleep maintenance. For disorders of sleep initiation, preference should be given to an agent with a rapid onset of action and rapid peak effect. On the other hand, if the patient suffers from disorders of sleep maintenance with frequent nocturnal awakenings, then more careful consideration should be given to an agent with a longer half-life that will remain at therapeutic levels across the night.

Of the benzodiazepines available and FDA-approved for insomnia as hypnotics, none is optimal. Flurazepam, quazepam, estazolam, and temazepam are the four traditional benzodiazepines approved for use as hypnotics. The initial three have long half-lives, and both flurazepam and quazepam have active metabolites that extend their half-lives to more than 100 hours. Estazolam has a half-life of approximately 24 hours. Thus, whereas all may be effective in isolated doses, there is an increased risk of daytime sedation and drowsiness associated with these agents. Temazepam has a short half-life and a more rapid peak onset than the other classic hypnotic agents (with a half-life that ranges from 4 to 15 hours), so it can be a reasonable alternative for both sleep onset as well as sleep maintenance insomnia.[293]

The newest category of sleep aids are the "benzodiazepine-like" agents, which includes zolpidem, zolpidem extended release, zaleplon, and eszopiclone. Chemically, these agents are not true benzodiazepines but act at the site of the benzodiazepine receptor; they appear to also increase cellular Cl– influx into neurons, as do typical benzodiazepines and barbiturates. Zaleplon is an agent that has an exquisitely short half-life of 1 hour and a time to peak effect of 1 hour, making it very suitable for those individuals who have only sleep-onset insomnia. Alternatively, it can also be taken in the middle of the night for those with intermittent sleep maintenance issues, with only a minimal likelihood of daytime sedation effects.[300] Zolpidem has the cost advantage of being generically available and has a rapid onset of action (approximately 1 hour) with a relatively short half-life of 4–5 hours, similar to triazolam. Eszopiclone enjoys the most data for use in concurrently painful conditions, and it appears to not only improve sleep, but also may improve pain perception as well, independent of its sleep effect.[301,302] Additionally, it has data supporting chronic use up to 6 months with continued efficacy.[303] It is rapidly absorbed (1–1.5 hours) and has a somewhat longer half-life, thus making it appropriate for sleep-maintenance insomnia as well. For those patients with sleep-onset insomnia alone, then reducing the dose is recommended (e.g., 2 mg for adults and 1 mg for geriatric patients).

Other agents have long histories of being used off-label for sleep effects, and these include trazodone, mirtazapine, hydroxyzine, TCAs, and even atypical antipsychotics for refractory cases. Trazodone is a 5-HT_2 serotonin antagonist with prominent sedative effects, and it is a widely prescribed sleep aid in the United States. Although its efficacy in models of primary insomnia are somewhat lacking, it has robust data for treating the insomnia that co-occurs with major depressive disorder and has been shown to improve slow wave sleep and improve overall sleep architecture as compared to the benzodiazepines. Trazodone also has a wide margin of safety and wide range of dosing for insomnia, ranging from 25 to 300 mg. It is generically available and is effective for both sleep initiation as well as sleep maintenance subtypes of insomnia.[304,305]

Histamine is a naturally occurring activating neurotransmitter that naturally declines in late afternoon through the night and begins to peak in the morning hours during times of natural awakenings. Blocking the effect of this agent through the night to promote sleep is the mechanism of action behind antihistaminic agents for sleep, including the actions of TCAs and mirtazapine.[304] Mirtazapine has a host of other effects as well, including its antidepressant effects; it may stimulate hunger in a substantial portion of the population and has been shown to be effective for nausea in phase II trials.[270]

One can also use TCAs in low dosages for sleep effects, and they have been shown to be effective for insomnia in doses far lower than those required for antidepressant effects. Doxepin has been shown to be effective for both sleep initiation and sleep maintenance over long periods of time at doses as low as 6 mg orally at bedtime, and a generic formulation of a 10 mg capsule is commercially available.[306] Given their widely reported efficacy in controlling neuropathic pain, a member of this class may be the preferred agent when dealing with patients with concurrent neuropathic pain complaints.

For those patients with refractory insomnia or contraindications to other therapies, atypical antipsychotics have been used for their sleep inducing and maintaining properties. These agents are especially useful when used in patients with underlying psychotic disorders or delirium, or for those with contraindications to benzodiazepine-like agents.[307] A comprehensive review of the action of these agents on sleep in schizophrenia was completed in 2008 and notes that, of the available agents, quetiapine and risperidone have the most rapid peak effect, with quetiapine having the greatest impact on total sleep time and shortening the sleep onset latency while reducing awakening after sleep onset. Olanzapine is another agent that shares these effects on sleep architecture while also promoting slow wave sleep, although its peak onset is up to 5 hours following administration, and its half life is substantially longer at 30 hours. Chlorpromazine is another viable alternative in this patient group as well.[308]

THE INFLUENCE OF DEPRESSION AND ANXIETY ON CANCER PAIN SEVERITY

There is a conventional wisdom that untreated depression and anxiety increase the perceived severity of cancer pain; however, there are limited good data to support this assertion. A systematic review in 2009 examining the relationship between cancer pain and depression found the mean prevalence of both depression and pain to be 36.5%: 892 articles were identified by a computer search, with 41 articles being independently reviewed. Fourteen articles were included in the systematic review. In 9 of 14 studies, a statistically significant association was demonstrated between pain and depression, with pain intensity correlating with depression. Interestingly, items on the Brief Pain Inventory such as "worst pain" and "enjoyment of life" also correlated significantly with depression. Similarly, the longer the duration of pain, the higher the risk of depression. At this point, there still have been no appropriately designed studies to show a causal relationship between pain and depression, but associations between the two have been shown to be present across many studies.[309]

The adverse impact of a high somatic burden in patients with pain and depression is well established for primary care, and cancer populations have appeared to mirror those findings. Among a population of cancer patients experiencing pain and depression, there appears to be perhaps an overreporting of somatic symptoms, with 15 of 22 symptoms being reported by more than 50% of the population. Pain and depression were also associated with increased scores on the Sheehan Disability Scale, with a mean number of 16.9 disabled days in the past month. This supports available data encouraging routine screening and management of depression in this population, given the impact that depression appears to have not only on pain itself, but also on overall disability.[310,311]

Similarly, a study examining physical symptom profiles of depressed and nondepressed patients with cancer demonstrated that those with depression displayed a higher symptom burden that those without depression. Insomnia, pain, anorexia, fatigue, and wounds and pressure sores occurred more frequently in depressed patients. The most prevalent symptom in the study was insomnia, illustrating the value in screening for this symptom among at-risk populations.[312]

A secondary analysis of the telephone care Indiana Cancer Pain and Depression trial was completed and showed that greater improvement in depression also contributed to both continuous and categorical pain improvement over time.[313] Conversely, one can infer that depression appeared to be an independent item that worsened pain in those patients. It does support treating depression in a rigorous manner in an effort to improve both quality of life and pain scores.

The role of depression on pain has also been assessed in women with breast cancer, and the presence of breast cancer (among other types) has been linked to a greater risk for depression. In 191 couples coping with metastatic breast cancer (patient and caregiver), multilevel models showed that depression mediated associations between the patient's and partner's report of pain and pain behaviors and accounted for up to 71% of the variance. This is suggestive that pain management programs in metastatic cancer models should incorporate both the patient's as well as the caregiver's depression levels when systematically assessing for pain.[314]

DEMORALIZATION AND ITS ROLE IN CANCER PAIN MANAGEMENT

Levels of hope appear to be negatively correlated with average pain intensity, worst pain intensity, pain interference with function, and anxiety and depression in a convenience sample of 78 patients enrolled in a comprehensive cancer center who were concurrently receiving both oncology and supportive care. However, after controlling for depression and spiritual well-being with regression analysis, the relationship between pain intensity and hope was no longer significant, indicating a role of depression on pain perception in this group of individuals.[315] Other studies have also noted a relationship between levels of hopelessness and depression.[316]

Desire for a hastened death has been reported as common among cancer patients with pain, and little evidence has shown that by treating the pain this desire lessens. One study looking at desire for a hastened death among those with cancer pain and depression did find that depression was likely underdiagnosed and undertreated in this population, and only 40% of patients with moderate to severe depression were prescribed antidepressants. Even though depression scores remained stable over the course of the study, rates of desire for a hastened death increased and appeared to be partly correlated with depression, low social support, poor spiritual well-being, lower physical functioning, and pain interference. Improvement in pain was not predictive of improvement in a desire for a hastened death. However, a change in depression severity was predictive of hastened death desire, thus illustrating that depression needs to be both better recognized as well as better treated in this population.[317]

REFERENCES

1. Kamman GR, Ikeda K. Superior pulmonary sulcus tumor (Pancoast tumor). *Minn Med.* 1946;29(11):1134–1138.
2. Walker JE. Superior sulcus pulmonary tumor (Pancoast syndrome). *J Med Assoc Ga.* 1946;35(12):364.
3. Mowrey FH. Thoracic inlet tumor (Pancoast syndrome) a case report and review. *Bull U S Army Med Dep.* 1949;9(9):755–759.
4. Huehnergarth KV, Lipsky BA. Superior pulmonary sulcus tumor with Pancoast syndrome. *Mayo Clin Proc.* 2004;79(10):1268.
5. Narayan S, Thomas CR, Jr. Multimodality therapy for Pancoast tumor. *Nat Clin Pract Oncol.* 2006;3(9):484–491.
6. Peedell C, Dunning J, Bapusamy A. Is there a standard of care for the radical management of non-small cell lung cancer involving the apical chest wall (Pancoast tumours)? *Clin Oncol* (R Coll Radiol). 2010; 22(5):334–346.
7. Herbut PA, Watson JS. Tumor of the thoracic inlet producing the Pancoast syndrome: a report of 17 cases and a review of the literature. *Arch Pathol* (Chic). 1946;42:88–103.
8. Kori SH, Foley KM, Posner JB. Brachial plexus lesions in patients with cancer: 100 cases. *Neurology.* 1981;31(1):45–50.
9. Jaeckle KA. Neurological manifestations of neoplastic and radiation-induced plexopathies. *Semin Neurol.* 2004;24(4):385–393.
10. Arcasoy SM, Jett JR. Superior pulmonary sulcus tumors and Pancoast's syndrome. *N Engl J Med.* 1997;337(19):1370–1376.
11. Deng PB, Luo YY, Hu CP, Zhou LH. Misdiagnosis of Pancoast cancer: analysis of 26 cases. *Zhonghua Jie He He Hu Xi Za Zhi.* 2011;34(9):663–665.
12. Becker J. Clinical significance of Pancoast syndrome: a reference to the early diagnosis of the bronchial cancer. *Med Klin* (Munich). 1953;48(46):1689–1691.
13. Gal J, Sai-Halasz A. Lung cancer causing dorsal radicular syndrome: dorsal Pancoast syndrome. *Nervenarzt.* 1957;28(10):474–476.
14. Simon H, Moon AC. Pitfalls in the diagnosis of Pancoast tumor. *Radiology.* 1964;82:235–239.
15. Yacoub M, Hupert C. Shoulder pain as an early symptom of Pancoast tumor. *J Med Soc N J.* 1980;77(9):583–586.
16. Kovach SG, Huslig EL. Shoulder pain and Pancoast tumor: a diagnostic dilemma. *J Manipulative Physiol Ther.* 1984;7(1):25–31.
17. Villas C, Collia A, Aquerreta JD, et al. Cervicobrachialgia and Pancoast tumor: value of standard anteroposterior cervical radiographs in early diagnosis. *Orthopedics.* 2004;27(10):1092–1095.
18. Kattan AE, Borschel GH. Anatomy of the brachial plexus. *J Pediatr Rehabil Med.* 2011;4(2):107–111.
19. Rusch VW. Management of Pancoast tumours. *Lancet Oncol.* 2006;7(12):997–1005.
20. Bilsky MH, Vitaz TW, Boland PJ, Bains MS, Rajaraman V, Rusch VW. Surgical treatment of superior sulcus tumors with spinal and brachial plexus involvement. *J Neurosurg.* 2002;97(3 suppl):301–309.
21. Rusch VW, Giroux DJ, Kraut MJ, et al. Induction chemoradiation and surgical resection for non-small cell lung carcinomas of the superior sulcus: initial results of Southwest Oncology Group Trial 9416 (Intergroup Trial 0160). *J Thorac Cardiovasc Surg.* 2001;121(3):472–483.
22. Rusch VW, Parekh KR, Leon L, et al. Factors determining outcome after surgical resection of T3 and T4 lung cancers of the superior sulcus. *J Thorac Cardiovasc Surg.* 2000;119(6):1147–1153.
23. Bradley JD, Moughan J, Graham MV, et al. A phase I/II radiation dose escalation study with concurrent chemotherapy for patients with inoperable stages I to III non-small-cell lung cancer: phase I results of RTOG 0117. *Int J Radiat Oncol Biol Phys.* 2010;77(2):367–372.
24. Okubo K, Wada H, Fukuse T, et al. Treatment of Pancoast tumors. Combined irradiation and radical resection. *Thorac Cardiovasc Surg.* 1995;43(5):284–286.
25. Detterbeck FC. Changes in the treatment of Pancoast tumors. *Ann Thorac Surg.* 2003;75(6):1990–1997.
26. Millward M. Treatment of superior sulcus non-small cell lung cancer. *Asia Pac J Clin Oncol.* 2010;6(1):1–2.
27. Emami B, Lyman J, Brown A, et al. Tolerance of normal tissue to therapeutic irradiation. *Int J Radiat Oncol Biol Phys.* 1991;21(1):109–122.
28. Eblan MJ, Corradetti MN, Lukens JN, et al. Brachial plexopathy in apical non-small cell lung cancer treated with definitive radiation: dosimetric analysis and clinical implications. *Int J Radiat Oncol Biol Phys.* 2012;85(1):175–181.
29. Olsen NK, Pfeiffer P, Johannsen L, Schroder H, Rose C. Radiation-induced brachial plexopathy: neurological follow-up in 161 recurrence-free breast cancer patients. *Int J Radiat Oncol Biol Phys.* 1993;26(1):43–49.
30. Olsen NK, Pfeiffer P, Mondrup K, Rose C. Radiation-induced brachial plexus neuropathy in breast cancer patients. *Acta Oncol.* 1990;29(7):885–890.
31. Amini A, Yang J, Williamson R, et al. Dose constraints to prevent radiation-induced brachial plexopathy in patients treated for lung cancer. *Int J Radiat Oncol Biol Phys.* 2012;82(3):e391–E398.
32. Boyaciyan A, Oge AE, Yazici J, Aslay I, Baslo A. Electrophysiological findings in patients who received radiation therapy over the brachial plexus: a magnetic stimulation study. *Electroencephalogr Clin Neurophysiol.* 1996;101(6):483–490.
33. Forquer JA, Fakiris AJ, Timmerman RD, et al. Brachial plexopathy from stereotactic body radiotherapy in early-stage NSCLC: dose-limiting toxicity in apical tumor sites. *Radiother Oncol.* 2009;93(3):408–413.
34. Paulson DL, Weed TE, Rian RL. Cervical approach for percutaneous needle biopsy of Pancoast tumors. *Ann Thorac Surg.* 1985;39(6):586–587.
35. Maxfield RA, Aranda CP. The role of fiberoptic bronchoscopy and transbronchial biopsy in the diagnosis of Pancoast's tumor. *N Y State J Med.* 1987;87(6):326–329.
36. Davis GA, Knight SR. Pancoast tumors. *Neurosurg Clin N Am.* 2008;19(4):545–557, v–vi.
37. Detterbeck FC. Pancoast (superior sulcus) tumors. *Ann Thorac Surg.* 1997;63(6):1810–1818.
38. Wittenberg KH, Adkins MC. MR imaging of nontraumatic brachial plexopathies: frequency and spectrum of findings. *Radiographics.* 2000;20(4):1023–1032.
39. Chardack WM, Maccallum JD. Pancoast tumor: five-year survival without recurrence or metastases following radical resection and postoperative irradiation. *J Thorac Surg.* 1956;31(5):535–542.

40. Shaw RR, Paulson DL, Kee JL. Treatment of superior sulcus tumor by irradiation followed by resection. *Ann Surg.* 1961;154(1):29–40.
41. Paulson DL. Carcinomas in the superior pulmonary sulcus. *J Thorac Cardiovasc Surg.* 1975;70(6):1095–1104.
42. York JE, Walsh GL, Lang FF, et al. Combined chest wall resection with vertebrectomy and spinal reconstruction for the treatment of Pancoast tumors. *J Neurosurg.* 1999;91(1 suppl):74–80.
43. Kwong KF, Edelman MJ, Suntharalingam M, et al. High-dose radiotherapy in trimodality treatment of Pancoast tumors results in high pathologic complete response rates and excellent long-term survival. *J Thorac Cardiovasc Surg.* 2005;129(6):1250–1257.
44. De Leyn P, Vansteenkiste J, Lievens Y, et al. Survival after trimodality treatment for superior sulcus and central T4 non-small cell lung cancer. *J Thorac Oncol.* 2009;4(1):62–68.
45. Kappers I, Belderbos JS, Burgers JA, van Zandwijk N, Groen HJ, Klomp HM. Non-small cell lung carcinoma of the superior sulcus: favourable outcomes of combined modality treatment in carefully selected patients. *Lung Cancer.* 2008;59(3):385–390.
46. Alifano M, D'Aiuto M, Magdeleinat P, et al. Surgical treatment of superior sulcus tumors: results and prognostic factors. *Chest.* 2003;124(3):996–1003.
47. Komaki R, Mountain CF, Holbert JM, et al. Superior sulcus tumors: treatment selection and results for 85 patients without metastasis (Mo) at presentation. *Int J Radiat Oncol Biol Phys.* 1990;19(1):31–36.
48. Geertzen JH, Groothoff JW, Nicolai JP, Rietman JS. Brachial plexus neuropathy. A long-term outcome study. *J Hand Surg Br.* 2000;25(5):461–464.
49. Smith HS. Opioids and neuropathic pain. *Pain Physician.* 2012;15(3 suppl):ES93–ES110.
50. Wilkie DJ, Huang HY, Reilly N, Cain KC. Nociceptive and neuropathic pain in patients with lung cancer: a comparison of pain quality descriptors. *J Pain Symptom Manage.* 2001;22(5):899–910.
51. Khedr EM, Ahmed MA, Alkady EA, Mostafa MG, Said HG. Therapeutic effects of peripheral magnetic stimulation on traumatic brachial plexopathy: clinical and neurophysiological study. *Neurophysiol Clin.* 2012;42(3):111–118.
52. Vranken JH, Zuurmond WW, de Lange JJ. Continuous brachial plexus block as treatment for the Pancoast syndrome. *Clin J Pain.* 2000;16(4):327–333.
53. De Tran QH, Clemente A, Doan J, Finlayson RJ. Brachial plexus blocks: a review of approaches and techniques. *Can J Anaesth.* 2007;54(8):662–674.
54. Buttner J, Meier G. Regional anesthesia—approaches to the brachial plexus. *Anasthesiol Intensivmed Notfallmed Schmerzther.* 2006;41(7-8):491–497.
55. Stevens MF, Werdehausen R, Golla E, et al. Does interscalene catheter placement with stimulating catheters improve postoperative pain or functional outcome after shoulder surgery? A prospective, randomized and double-blinded trial. *Anesth Analg.* 2007;104(2):442–447.
56. van de Putte P, van der Vorst M. Continuous interscalene block using a stimulating catheter: a review of the technique. *Acta Anaesthesiol Belg.* 2005;56(1):25–30.
57. Li PY, Che XH, Gu HH, Liang WM. Influence of stimulating different cords on the efficacy of infraclavicular brachial plexus block. *Zhonghua Yi Xue Za Zhi.* 2007;87(29):2058–2061.
58. Fernandes MR, Barbosa MA, Sousa AL, Ramos GC. Suprascapular nerve block: important procedure in clinical practice. Part II. *Rev Bras Reumatol.* 2012;52(4):616–622.
59. Fernandes MR, Barbosa MA, Sousa AL, Ramos GC. Suprascapular nerve block: important procedure in clinical practice. *Rev Bras Anestesiol.* 2012;62(1):96–104.
60. Capdevila X, Ponrouch M, Choquet O. Continuous peripheral nerve blocks in clinical practice. *Curr Opin Anaesthesiol.* 2008;21(5):619–623.
61. Zaghi S, Thiele B, Pimentel D, Pimentel T, Fregni F. Assessment and treatment of pain with non-invasive cortical stimulation. *Restor Neurol Neurosci.* 2011;29(6):439–451.
62. Ali M, Saitoh Y, Oshino S, et al. Differential efficacy of electric motor cortex stimulation and lesioning of the dorsal root entry zone for continuous vs paroxysmal pain after brachial plexus avulsion. *Neurosurgery.* 2011;68(5):1252–1257.
63. Brill S, Aryeh IG. Neuromodulation in the management of pain from brachial plexus injury. *Pain Physician.* 2008;11(1):81–85.
64. Kastler B, Michalakis D, Clair CH, et al. Stellate ganglion radiofrequency neurolysis under CT guidance. Preliminary study. *JBR-BTR.* 2001;84(5):191–194.
65. Aichaoui F, Mertens P, Sindou M. Dorsal root entry zone lesioning for pain after brachial plexus avulsion: results with special emphasis on differential effects on the paroxysmal versus the continuous components. A prospective study in a 29-patient consecutive series. *Pain.* 2011;152(8):1923–1930.
66. Gofeld M, Bhatia A. Alleviation of Pancoast's tumor pain by ultrasound-guided percutaneous ablation of cervical nerve roots. *Pain Pract.* 2008;8(4):314–319.
67. Teixeira MJ, Fonoff ET, Montenegro MC. Dorsal root entry zone lesions for treatment of pain-related to radiation-induced plexopathy. *Spine* (Phila Pa 1976). 2007;32(10):E316–E319.
68. Zheng Z, Hu Y, Tao W, Zhang X, Li Y. Dorsal root entry zone lesions for phantom limb pain with brachial plexus avulsion: a study of pain and phantom limb sensation. *Stereotact Funct Neurosurg.* 2009;87(4):249–255.
69. Tomycz ND, Moossy JJ. Follow-up 26 years after dorsal root entry zone thermocoagulation for brachial plexus avulsion and phantom limb pain. *J Neurosurg.* 2011;114(1):196–199.
70. Forouzanfar T, van Kleef M, Weber WE. Radiofrequency lesions of the stellate ganglion in chronic pain syndromes: retrospective analysis of clinical efficacy in 86 patients. *Clin J Pain.* 2000;16(2):164–168.
71. Arai YC, Nishihara M, Aono S, et al. Pulsed radiofrequency treatment within brachial plexus for the management of intractable neoplastic plexopathic pain. *J Anesth.* 2012;27(2):298–301.
72. Merskey H. Clarifying definition of neuropathic pain. *Pain.* 2002;96(3):408–409.
73. Treede RD, Jensen TS, Campbell JN, et al. Neuropathic pain: redefinition and a grading system for clinical and research purposes. *Neurology.* 2008;70(18):1630–1635.
74. Costigan M, Scholz J, Woolf CJ. Neuropathic pain: a maladaptive response of the nervous system to damage. *Annu Rev Neurosci.* 2009;32:1–32.
75. Jensen TS, Gottrup H, Sindrup SH, Bach FW. The clinical picture of neuropathic pain. *Eur J Pharmacol.* 2001;429(1-3):1–11.
76. Jensen TS, Madsen CS, Finnerup NB. Pharmacology and treatment of neuropathic pains. *Curr Opin Neurol.* 2009;22(5):467–474.
77. Przewlocki R, Przewlocka B. Opioids in neuropathic pain. *Curr Pharm Des.* 2005;11(23):3013–3025.
78. Katz N, Benoit C. Opioids for neuropathic pain. *Curr Pain Headache Rep.* 2005;9(3):153–160.
79. Finnerup NB, Otto M, McQuay HJ, Jensen TS, Sindrup SH. Algorithm for neuropathic pain treatment: an evidence based proposal. *Pain.* 2005;118(3):289–305.
80. Attal N, Cruccu G, Haanpaa M, et al. EFNS guidelines on pharmacological treatment of neuropathic pain. *Eur J Neurol.* 2006;13(11):1153–1169.
81. Berger JV, Knaepen L, Janssen SP, et al. Cellular and molecular insights into neuropathy-induced pain hypersensitivity for mechanism-based treatment approaches. *Brain Res Rev.* 2011;67(1-2):282–310.
82. Miraucourt LS, Moisset X, Dallel R, Voisin DL. Glycine inhibitory dysfunction induces a selectively dynamic, morphine-resistant, and neurokinin 1 receptor-independent mechanical allodynia. *J Neurosci.* 2009;29(8):2519–2527.
83. Zhang ET, Ossipov MH, Zhang DQ, Lai J, Porreca F. Nerve injury-induced tactile allodynia is present in the absence of FOS labeling in retrogradely labeled post-synaptic dorsal column neurons. *Pain.* 2007;129(1-2):143–154.

84. Amir R, Michaelis M, Devor M. Membrane potential oscillations in dorsal root ganglion neurons: role in normal electrogenesis and neuropathic pain. *J Neurosci.* 1999;19(19):8589–8596.
85. Hervera A, Negrete R, Leanez S, Martin-Campos JM, Pol O. Peripheral effects of morphine and expression of mu-opioid receptors in the dorsal root ganglia during neuropathic pain: nitric oxide signaling. *Mol Pain.* 2011;7:25.
86. Cummins TR, Waxman SG. Downregulation of tetrodotoxin-resistant sodium currents and upregulation of a rapidly repriming tetrodotoxin-sensitive sodium current in small spinal sensory neurons after nerve injury. *J Neurosci.* 1997;17(10):3503–3514.
87. Cregg R, Momin A, Rugiero F, Wood JN, Zhao J. Pain channelopathies. *J Physiol.* 2010;588(Pt 11):1897–1904.
88. Li L, Cao XH, Chen SR, Han HD, et al. Up-regulation of Cavbeta3 subunit in primary sensory neurons increases voltage-activated Ca2+ channel activity and nociceptive input in neuropathic pain. *J Biol Chem.* 2012;287(8):6002–6013.
89. Heblich F, Tran Van Minh A, Hendrich J, Watschinger K, Dolphin AC. Time course and specificity of the pharmacological disruption of the trafficking of voltage-gated calcium channels by gabapentin. *Channels* (Austin). 2008;2(1):4–9.
90. Berman RM, Anand A, Cappiello A, et al. The use of pindolol with fluoxetine in the treatment of major depression: final results from a double-blind, placebo-controlled trial. *Biol Psychiatry.* 1999;45(9):1170–1177.
91. Michael GJ, Averill S, Shortland PJ, Yan Q, Priestley JV. Axotomy results in major changes in BDNF expression by dorsal root ganglion cells: BDNF expression in large trkB and trkC cells, in pericellular baskets, and in projections to deep dorsal horn and dorsal column nuclei. *Eur J Neurosci.* 1999;11(10):3539–3551.
92. Diamond J, Foerster A. Recovery of sensory function in skin deprived of its innervation by lesion of the peripheral nerve. *Exp Neurol.* 1992;115(1):100–103.
93. Doubell TP, Mannion RJ, Woolf CJ. Intact sciatic myelinated primary afferent terminals collaterally sprout in the adult rat dorsal horn following section of a neighbouring peripheral nerve. *J Comp Neurol.* 1997;380(1):95–104.
94. Deng YS, Zhong JH, Zhou XF. Effects of endogenous neurotrophins on sympathetic sprouting in the dorsal root ganglia and allodynia following spinal nerve injury. *Exp Neurol.* 2000; 164(2):344–350.
95. Leong ML, Gu M, Speltz-Paiz R, et al. Neuronal loss in the rostral ventromedial medulla in a rat model of neuropathic pain. *J Neurosci.* 2011;31(47):17028–17039.
96. Jaggi AS, Singh N. Role of different brain areas in peripheral nerve injury-induced neuropathic pain. *Brain Res.* 2011;1381:187–201.
97. Nahman-Averbuch H, Yarnitsky D, Granovsky Y, et al. Pronociceptive pain modulation in patients with painful chemotherapy-induced polyneuropathy. *J Pain Symptom Manage.* 2011;42(2):229–238.
98. Yarnitsky D. Conditioned pain modulation (the diffuse noxious inhibitory control-like effect): its relevance for acute and chronic pain states. *Curr Opin Anaesthesiol.* 2010;23(5):611–615.
99. Austin PJ, Moalem-Taylor G. The neuro-immune balance in neuropathic pain: involvement of inflammatory immune cells, immune-like glial cells and cytokines. *J Neuroimmunol.* 2010;229(1-2):26–50.
100. De Leo JA, Tawfik VL, LaCroix-Fralish ML. The tetrapartite synapse: path to CNS sensitization and chronic pain. *Pain.* 2006;122(1-2):17–21.
101. Sung B, Lim G, Mao J. Altered expression and uptake activity of spinal glutamate transporters after nerve injury contribute to the pathogenesis of neuropathic pain in rats. *J Neurosci.* 2003;23(7):2899–2910.
102. Berger JV, Deumens R, Goursaud S, et al. Enhanced neuroinflammation and pain hypersensitivity after peripheral nerve injury in rats expressing mutated superoxide dismutase 1. *J Neuroinflammation.* 2011;8:33.
103. Kawasaki Y, Zhang L, Cheng JK, Ji RR. Cytokine mechanisms of central sensitization: distinct and overlapping role of interleukin-1beta, interleukin-6, and tumor necrosis factor-alpha in regulating synaptic and neuronal activity in the superficial spinal cord. *J Neurosci.* 2008;28(20):5189–194.
104. Zhao P, Waxman SG, Hains BC. Extracellular signal-regulated kinase-regulated microglia-neuron signaling by prostaglandin E2 contributes to pain after spinal cord injury. *J Neurosci.* 2007;27(9):2357–2368.
105. Kausar F, Davis MP. Ketorolac in neuropathic pain. *J Pain Symptom Manage.* 2006;32(3):202–204.
106. Ma W, Eisenach JC. Morphological and pharmacological evidence for the role of peripheral prostaglandins in the pathogenesis of neuropathic pain. *Eur J Neurosci.* 2002;15(6):1037–1047.
107. Ripamonti C, Ticozzi C, Zecca E, Rodriguez CH, De Conno F. Continuous subcutaneous infusion of ketorolac in cancer neuropathic pain unresponsive to opioid and adjuvant drugs. A case report. *Tumori.* 1996;82(4):413–415.
108. Stubblefield MD, Burstein HJ, Burton AW, et al. NCCN task force report: management of neuropathy in cancer. *J Natl Compr Canc Netw.* 2009;7(suppl 5):S1–S26; quiz S7–S8.
109. Oldenmenger WH, de Raaf PJ, de Klerk C, van der Rijt CC. Cut Points on 0-10 Numeric Rating Scales for symptoms included in the Edmonton symptom assessment scale in cancer patients: a systematic review. *J Pain Symptom Manage.* 2012;45(6): 1083–1093.
110. Given B, Given CW, Sikorskii A, et al. Establishing mild, moderate, and severe scores for cancer-related symptoms: how consistent and clinically meaningful are interference-based severity cut-points? *J Pain Symptom Manage.* 2008;35(2):126–135.
111. Melzack R. The McGill Pain Questionnaire: major properties and scoring methods. *Pain.* 1975;1(3):277–299.
112. Cleeland CS, Ryan KM. Pain assessment: global use of the Brief Pain Inventory. *Ann Acad Med Singapore.* 1994;23(2):129–138.
113. Bennett M. The LANSS Pain Scale: the Leeds assessment of neuropathic symptoms and signs. *Pain.* 2001;92(1-2):147–157.
114. Portenoy R. Development and testing of a neuropathic pain screening questionnaire: ID pain. *Curr Med Res Opin.* 2006;22(8):1555–1565.
115. Bouhassira D, Attal N, Fermanian J, et al. Development and validation of the Neuropathic Pain Symptom Inventory. *Pain.* 2004;108(3):248–257.
116. Bastyr EJ, 3rd, Price KL, Bril V. Development and validity testing of the neuropathy total symptom score-6: questionnaire for the study of sensory symptoms of diabetic peripheral neuropathy. *Clin Ther.* 2005;27(8):1278–1294.
117. Galer BS, Jensen MP. Development and preliminary validation of a pain measure specific to neuropathic pain: the Neuropathic Pain Scale. *Neurology.* 1997;48(2):332–338.
118. Cleeland CS, Farrar JT, Hausheer FH. Assessment of cancer-related neuropathy and neuropathic pain. *Oncologist.* 2010;15(suppl 2):13–18.
119. Goudas LC, Bloch R, Gialeli-Goudas M, Lau J, Carr DB. The epidemiology of cancer pain. *Cancer Invest.* 2005;23(2):182–190.
120. Kerba M, Wu JS, Duan Q, Hagen NA, Bennett MI. Neuropathic pain features in patients with bone metastases referred for palliative radiotherapy. *J Clin Oncol.* 2010;28(33):4892–4897.
121. Jimenez-Andrade JM, Mantyh WG, Bloom AP, Ferng AS, Geffre CP, Mantyh PW. Bone cancer pain. *Ann N Y Acad Sci.* 2010;1198:173–181.
122. Caraceni A, Zecca E, Martini C, Pigni A, Bracchi P. Gabapentin for breakthrough pain due to bone metastases. *Palliat Med.* 2008;22(4):392–393.
123. Dennis K, Chow E, Roos D, et al. Should bone metastases causing neuropathic pain be treated with single-dose radiotherapy? *Clin Oncol* (R Coll Radiol). 2011;23(7):482–484.
124. Cruccu G, Sommer C, Anand P, et al. EFNS guidelines on neuropathic pain assessment: revised 2009. *Eur J Neurol.* 2010;17(8):1010–1018.

125. Haanpaa M. Are neuropathic pain screening tools useful for patients with spinal cord injury? *Pain.* 2011;152(4):715–716.
126. Marinangeli F, Ciccozzi A, Leonardis M, et al. Use of strong opioids in advanced cancer pain: a randomized trial. *J Pain Symptom Manage.* 2004;27(5):409–416.
127. Caraceni A, Hanks G, Kaasa S, et al. Use of opioid analgesics in the treatment of cancer pain: evidence-based recommendations from the EAPC. *Lancet Oncol.* 2012;13(2):e58–e68.
128. Dy SM. Evidence-based approaches to pain in advanced cancer. *Cancer J.* 2010;16(5):500–506.
129. Duhmke RM, Cornblath DD, Hollingshead JR. Tramadol for neuropathic pain. *Cochrane Database Syst Rev.* 2004(2): CD003726.
130. Cartoni C, Brunetti GA, Federico V, et al. Controlled-release oxycodone for the treatment of bortezomib-induced neuropathic pain in patients with multiple myeloma. *Support Care Cancer.* 2012;20(10):2621–2626.
131. Hermanns K, Junker U, Nolte T. Prolonged-release oxycodone/naloxone in the treatment of neuropathic pain—results from a large observational study. *Expert Opin Pharmacother.* 2012;13(3):299–311.
132. Barrera-Chacon JM, Mendez-Suarez JL, Jauregui-Abrisqueta ML, Palazon R, Barbara-Bataller E, Garcia-Obrero I. Oxycodone improves pain control and quality of life in anticonvulsant-pretreated spinal cord-injured patients with neuropathic pain. *Spinal Cord.* 2011;49(1):36–42.
133. Gatti A, Sabato AF, Occhioni R, Colini Baldeschi G, Reale C. Controlled-release oxycodone and pregabalin in the treatment of neuropathic pain: results of a multicenter Italian study. *Eur Neurol.* 2009;61(3):129–137.
134. Nunez Olarte JM. Oxycodone and the challenge of neuropathic cancer pain: a review. *Oncology.* 2008;74(suppl 1):83–90.
135. Watson CP, Babul N. Efficacy of oxycodone in neuropathic pain: a randomized trial in postherpetic neuralgia. *Neurology.* 1998;50(6):1837–1841.
136. Caraceni A, Pigni A, Brunelli C. Is oral morphine still the first choice opioid for moderate to severe cancer pain? A systematic review within the European Palliative Care Research Collaborative guidelines project. *Palliat Med.* 2011;25(5):402–409.
137. Mercadante S, Porzio G, Ferrera P, et al. Sustained-release oral morphine versus transdermal fentanyl and oral methadone in cancer pain management. *Eur J Pain.* 2008;12(8):1040–1046.
138. Nicholson AB. Methadone for cancer pain. *Cochrane Database Syst Rev.* 2007(4):CD003971.
139. Davis MP, Weissman DE, Arnold RM. Opioid dose titration for severe cancer pain: a systematic evidence-based review. *J Palliat Med.* 2004;7(3):462–468.
140. Walsh D, Rivera NI, Davis MP, Lagman R, Legrand SB. Strategies for pain management: Cleveland Clinic Foundation guidelines for opioid dosing for cancer pain. *Support Cancer Ther.* 2004;1(3):157–164.
141. Solassol I, Caumette L, Bressolle F, et al. Inter- and intra-individual variability in transdermal fentanyl absorption in cancer pain patients. *Oncol Rep.* 2005;14(4):1029–1036.
142. Solassol I, Bressolle F, Caumette L, et al. Inter- and intraindividual variabilities in pharmacokinetics of fentanyl after repeated 72-hour transdermal applications in cancer pain patients. *Ther Drug Monit.* 2005;27(4):491–498.
143. Van Nimmen NF, Poels KL, Menten JJ, Godderis L, Veulemans HA. Fentanyl transdermal absorption linked to pharmacokinetic characteristics in patients undergoing palliative care. *J Clin Pharmacol.* 2010;50(6):667–678.
144. Mercadante S. Pharmacotherapy for breakthrough cancer pain. *Drugs.* 2012;72(2):181–190.
145. Caraceni A, Bertetto O, Labianca R, et al. Episodic (breakthrough) pain prevalence in a population of cancer pain patients. Comparison of clinical diagnoses with the QUDEI—Italian questionnaire for intense episodic pain. *J Pain Symptom Manage.* 2012;43(5):833–841.
146. Shaheen PE, Legrand SB, Walsh D, et al. Errors in opioid prescribing: a prospective survey in cancer pain. *J Pain Symptom Manage.* 2010;39(4):702–711.
147. Nalamachu SR. Opioid rotation in clinical practice. *Adv Ther.* 2012;29(10):849–863.
148. Hanks GW, Forbes K. Opioid responsiveness. *Acta Anaesthesiol Scand.* 1997;41(1 Pt 2):154–158.
149. Droney J, Levy J, Quigley C. Prescribing opioids in renal failure. *J Opioid Manag.* 2007;3(6):309–316.
150. Dean M. Opioids in renal failure and dialysis patients. *J Pain Symptom Manage.* 2004;28(5):497–504.
151. Tegeder I, Geisslinger G, Lotsch J. Therapy with opioids in liver or renal failure. *Schmerz.* 1999;13(3):183–195.
152. Davis M. Cholestasis and endogenous opioids: liver disease and exogenous opioid pharmacokinetics. *Clin Pharmacokinet.* 2007;46(10):825–850.
153. Murphy EJ. Acute pain management pharmacology for the patient with concurrent renal or hepatic disease. *Anaesth Intensive Care.* 2005;33(3):311–322.
154. Ross JR, Goller K, Hardy J, et al. Gabapentin is effective in the treatment of cancer-related neuropathic pain: a prospective, open-label study. *J Palliat Med.* 2005;8(6):1118–1126.
155. Caraceni A, Zecca E, Bonezzi C, et al. Gabapentin for neuropathic cancer pain: a randomized controlled trial from the Gabapentin Cancer Pain Study Group. *J Clin Oncol.* 2004;22(14):2909–2917.
156. Gilron I, Bailey JM, Tu D, Holden RR, Weaver DF, Houlden RL. Morphine, gabapentin, or their combination for neuropathic pain. *N Engl J Med.* 2005;352(13):1324–1334.
157. Sauzet O, Williams JE, Ross J, et al. The characteristics and quality of randomized controlled trials in neuropathic pain: a descriptive study based on a systematic review. *Clin J Pain.* 2012;29(7):591–599.
158. Selph S, Carson S, Fu R, et al. Neuropathic Pain: Final Update 1 Report, Drug Class Reviews. Portland (OR): Oregon Health & Science University; 2011.
159. Arai YC, Matsubara T, Shimo K, et al. Low-dose gabapentin as useful adjuvant to opioids for neuropathic cancer pain when combined with low-dose imipramine. *J Anesth.* 2010;24(3):407–410.
160. Keskinbora K, Pekel AF, Aydinli I. Gabapentin and an opioid combination versus opioid alone for the management of neuropathic cancer pain: a randomized open trial. *J Pain Symptom Manage.* 2007;34(2):183–189.
161. Simpson DA. Gabapentin and venlafaxine for the treatment of painful diabetic neuropathy. *J Clin Neuromuscul Dis.* 2001;3(2):53–62.
162. Gilron I, Bailey JM, Tu D, Holden RR, Jackson AC, Houlden RL. Nortriptyline and gabapentin, alone and in combination for neuropathic pain: a double-blind, randomised controlled crossover trial. *Lancet.* 2009;374(9697):1252–1261.
163. Hanna M, O'Brien C, Wilson MC. Prolonged-release oxycodone enhances the effects of existing gabapentin therapy in painful diabetic neuropathy patients. *Eur J Pain.* 2008;12(6):804–813.
164. Rowbotham M, Harden N, Stacey B, Bernstein P, Magnus-Miller L. Gabapentin for the treatment of postherpetic neuralgia: a randomized controlled trial. *JAMA.* 1998;280(21):1837–1842.
165. Romano CL, Romano D, Bonora C, Mineo G. Pregabalin, celecoxib, and their combination for treatment of chronic low-back pain. *J Orthop Traumatol.* 2009;10(4):185–191.
166. Dworkin RH, Corbin AE, Young JP, Jr., et al. Pregabalin for the treatment of postherpetic neuralgia: a randomized, placebo-controlled trial. *Neurology.* 2003;60(8):1274–1283.
167. Sabatowski R, Galvez R, Cherry DA, et al. Pregabalin reduces pain and improves sleep and mood disturbances in patients with post-herpetic neuralgia: results of a randomised, placebo-controlled clinical trial. *Pain.* 2004;109(1-2):26–35.
168. Zin CS, Nissen LM, O'Callaghan JP, Duffull SB, Smith MT, Moore BJ. A randomized, controlled trial of oxycodone versus placebo in patients with postherpetic neuralgia and painful diabetic neuropathy treated with pregabalin. *J Pain.* 2010;11(5):462–471.

169. Mercadante S, Arcuri E, Tirelli W, Villari P, Casuccio A. Amitriptyline in neuropathic cancer pain in patients on morphine therapy: a randomized placebo-controlled, double-blind crossover study. *Tumori.* 2002;88(3):239–242.
170. Chaparro LE, Wiffen PJ, Moore RA, Gilron I. Combination pharmacotherapy for the treatment of neuropathic pain in adults. *Cochrane Database Syst Rev.* 2012;7:CD008943.
171. Vorobeychik Y, Gordin V, Mao J, Chen L. Combination therapy for neuropathic pain: a review of current evidence. *CNS Drugs.* 2011;25(12):1023–34.
172. Smith EM, Bakitas MA, Homel P, et al. Preliminary assessment of a neuropathic pain treatment and referral algorithm for patients with cancer. *J Pain Symptom Manage.* 2011;42(6):822–838.
173. Fisher RS, Sachdeo RC, Pellock J, Penovich PE, Magnus L, Bernstein P. Rapid initiation of gabapentin: a randomized, controlled trial. *Neurology.* 2001 27;56(6):743–748.
174. Sansone RA, Sansone LA. Tramadol: seizures, serotonin syndrome, and coadministered antidepressants. *Psychiatry* (Edgmont). 2009;6(4):17–21.
175. Saldana MT, Perez C, Navarro A, Masramon X, Rejas J. Pain alleviation and patient-reported health outcomes following switching to pregabalin in individuals with gabapentin-refractory neuropathic pain in routine medical practice. *Clin Drug Investig.* 2012;32(6):401–412.
176. Visovsky C, Daly BJ. Clinical evaluation and patterns of chemotherapy-induced peripheral neuropathy. *J Am Acad Nurse Pract.* 2004;16(8):353–359.
177. Kaley TJ, Deangelis LM. Therapy of chemotherapy-induced peripheral neuropathy. *Br J Haematol.* 2009;145(1):3–14.
178. Kannarkat G, Lasher EE, Schiff D. Neurologic complications of chemotherapy agents. *Curr Opin Neurol.* 2007;20(6):719–725.
179. Windebank AJ. Chemotherapeutic neuropathy. Curr Opin Neurol. 1999;12(5):565–571.
180. Wickham R. Chemotherapy-induced peripheral neuropathy: a review and implications for oncology nursing practice. *Clin J Oncol Nurs.* 2007;11(3):361–376.
181. Windebank AJ, Grisold W. Chemotherapy-induced neuropathy. *J Peripher Nerv Syst.* 2008;13(1):27–46.
182. Visovsky C. Chemotherapy-induced peripheral neuropathy. *Cancer Invest.* 2003;21(3):439–451.
183. Ocean AJ, Vahdat LT. Chemotherapy-induced peripheral neuropathy: pathogenesis and emerging therapies. *Support Care Cancer.* 2004;12(9):619–625.
184. Postma TJ, Heimans JJ. Grading of chemotherapy-induced peripheral neuropathy. *Ann Oncol.* 2000;11(5):509–513.
185. Zheng H, Xiao WH, Bennett GJ. Mitotoxicity and bortezomib-induced chronic painful peripheral neuropathy. *Exp Neurol.* 2012;238(2):225–234.
186. Zheng H, Xiao WH, Bennett GJ. Functional deficits in peripheral nerve mitochondria in rats with paclitaxel- and oxaliplatin-evoked painful peripheral neuropathy. *Exp Neurol.* 2011;232(2):154–161.
187. Xiao WH, Zheng H, Zheng FY, Nuydens R, Meert TF, Bennett GJ. Mitochondrial abnormality in sensory, but not motor, axons in paclitaxel-evoked painful peripheral neuropathy in the rat. *Neuroscience.* 2011;199:461–469.
188. Xiao WH, Zheng H, Bennett GJ. Characterization of oxaliplatin-induced chronic painful peripheral neuropathy in the rat and comparison with the neuropathy induced by paclitaxel. *Neuroscience.* 2012;203:194–206.
189. Goswami C. TRPV1-tubulin complex: involvement of membrane tubulin in the regulation of chemotherapy-induced peripheral neuropathy. *J Neurochem.* 2012;123(1):1–13.
190. Podratz JL, Knight AM, Ta LE, et al. Cisplatin induced mitochondrial DNA damage in dorsal root ganglion neurons. *Neurobiol Dis.* 2011;41(3):661–668.
191. Inada M, Sato M, Morita S, et al. Associations between oxaliplatin-induced peripheral neuropathy and polymorphisms of the ERCC1 and GSTP1 genes. *Int J Clin Pharmacol Ther.* 2010;48(11):729–734.
192. Baron R, Binder A, Wasner G. Neuropathic pain: diagnosis, pathophysiological mechanisms, and treatment. *Lancet Neurol.* 2010;9(8):807–819.
193. Pachman DR, Barton DL, Watson JC, Loprinzi CL. Chemotherapy-induced peripheral neuropathy: prevention and treatment. *Clin Pharmacol Ther.* 2011;90(3):377–387.
194. Warwick RA, Hanani M. The contribution of satellite glial cells to chemotherapy-induced neuropathic pain. *Eur J Pain.* 2012;17(4):571–80.
195. Peters CM, Jimenez-Andrade JM, Kuskowski MA, Ghilardi JR, Mantyh PW. An evolving cellular pathology occurs in dorsal root ganglia, peripheral nerve and spinal cord following intravenous administration of paclitaxel in the rat. *Brain Res.* 2007;1168:46–59.
196. Albers J, Chaudhry V, Cavaletti G, Donehower R. Interventions for preventing neuropathy caused by cisplatin and related compounds. *Cochrane Database Syst Rev.* 2007(1):CD005228.
197. Lin PC, Lee MY, Wang WS, et al. N-acetylcysteine has neuroprotective effects against oxaliplatin-based adjuvant chemotherapy in colon cancer patients: preliminary data. *Support Care Cancer.* 2006;14(5):484–487.
198. Stubblefield MD, Vahdat LT, Balmaceda CM, Troxel AB, Hesdorffer CS, Gooch CL. Glutamine as a neuroprotective agent in high-dose paclitaxel-induced peripheral neuropathy: a clinical and electrophysiologic study. *Clin Oncol* (R Coll Radiol). 2005;17(4):271–276.
199. Wang WS, Lin JK, Lin TC, et al. Oral glutamine is effective for preventing oxaliplatin-induced neuropathy in colorectal cancer patients. *Oncologist.* 2007;12(3):312–319.
200. Argyriou AA, Chroni E, Polychronopoulos P, et al. Efficacy of oxcarbazepine for prophylaxis against cumulative oxaliplatin-induced neuropathy. *Neurology.* 2006;67(12):2253–2255.
201. Meyer L, Patte-Mensah C, Taleb O, Mensah-Nyagan AG. Allopregnanolone prevents and suppresses oxaliplatin-evoked painful neuropathy: multi-parametric assessment and direct evidence. *Pain.* 2011;152(1):170–181.
202. Jin HW, Flatters SJ, Xiao WH, Mulhern HL, Bennett GJ. Prevention of paclitaxel-evoked painful peripheral neuropathy by acetyl-L-carnitine: effects on axonal mitochondria, sensory nerve fiber terminal arbors, and cutaneous Langerhans cells. *Exp Neurol.* 2008;210(1):229–237.
203. Flatters SJ, Xiao WH, Bennett GJ. Acetyl-L-carnitine prevents and reduces paclitaxel-induced painful peripheral neuropathy. *Neurosci Lett.* 2006;397(3):219–223.
204. Ghirardi O, Lo Giudice P, Pisano C, et al. Acetyl-L-Carnitine prevents and reverts experimental chronic neurotoxicity induced by oxaliplatin, without altering its antitumor properties. *Anticancer Res.* 2005;25(4):2681–2687.
205. Ghirardi O, Vertechy M, Vesci L, et al. Chemotherapy-induced allodinia: neuroprotective effect of acetyl-L-carnitine. *In Vivo.* 2005;19(3):631–637.
206. De Grandis D. Acetyl-L-carnitine for the treatment of chemotherapy-induced peripheral neuropathy: a short review. *CNS Drugs.* 2007;21(suppl 1):39–43; discussion 5–6.
207. Maestri A, De Pasquale Ceratti A, Cundari S, Zanna C, Cortesi E, Crino L. A pilot study on the effect of acetyl-L-carnitine in paclitaxel- and cisplatin-induced peripheral neuropathy. *Tumori.* 2005;91(2):135–138.
208. Durand JP, Deplanque G, Montheil V, et al. Efficacy of venlafaxine for the prevention and relief of oxaliplatin-induced acute neurotoxicity: results of EFFOX, a randomized, double-blind, placebo-controlled phase III trial. *Ann Oncol.* 2012;23(1):200–205.
209. Kautio AL, Haanpaa M, Saarto T, Kalso E. Amitriptyline in the treatment of chemotherapy-induced neuropathic symptoms. *J Pain Symptom Manage.* 2008;35(1):31–39.
210. Hammack JE, Michalak JC, Loprinzi CL, et al. Phase III evaluation of nortriptyline for alleviation of symptoms of cis-platinum-induced peripheral neuropathy. *Pain.* 2002;98(1-2):195–203.
211. Rao RD, Michalak JC, Sloan JA, et al. Efficacy of gabapentin in the management of chemotherapy-induced peripheral neuropathy: a

phase 3 randomized, double-blind, placebo-controlled, crossover trial (N00C3). *Cancer.* 2007;110(9):2110–2118.
212. Saif MW, Syrigos K, Kaley K, Isufi I. Role of pregabalin in treatment of oxaliplatin-induced sensory neuropathy. *Anticancer Res.* 2010;30(7):2927–2933.
213. Rao RD, Flynn PJ, Sloan JA, et al. Efficacy of lamotrigine in the management of chemotherapy-induced peripheral neuropathy: a phase 3 randomized, double-blind, placebo-controlled trial, N01C3. *Cancer.* 2008;112(12):2802–2808.
214. Rahn EJ, Zvonok AM, Thakur GA, Khanolkar AD, Makriyannis A, Hohmann AG. Selective activation of cannabinoid CB2 receptors suppresses neuropathic nociception induced by treatment with the chemotherapeutic agent paclitaxel in rats. *J Pharmacol Exp Ther.* 2008;327(2):584–591.
215. Rahn EJ, Makriyannis A, Hohmann AG. Activation of cannabinoid CB1 and CB2 receptors suppresses neuropathic nociception evoked by the chemotherapeutic agent vincristine in rats. *Br J Pharmacol.* 2007;152(5):765–777.
216. Hohmann AG. A cannabinoid pharmacotherapy for chemotherapy-evoked painful peripheral neuropathy. *Pain.* 2005;118(1-2):3–5.
217. Pascual D, Goicoechea C, Burgos E, Martin MI. Antinociceptive effect of three common analgesic drugs on peripheral neuropathy induced by paclitaxel in rats. *Pharmacol Biochem Behav.* 2010;95(3):331–337.
218. Yang YH, Lin JK, Chen WS, et al. Duloxetine improves oxaliplatin-induced neuropathy in patients with colorectal cancer: an open-label pilot study. *Support Care Cancer.* 2012;20(7): 1491–1497.
219. Takenaka M, Iida H, Matsumoto S, Yamaguchi S, Yoshimura N, Miyamoto M. Successful treatment by adding duloxetine to pregabalin for peripheral neuropathy induced by paclitaxel. *Am J Hosp Palliat Care.* 2012;30(7):734–736.
220. Gedlicka C, Scheithauer W, Schull B, Kornek GV. Effective treatment of oxaliplatin-induced cumulative polyneuropathy with alpha-lipoic acid. *J Clin Oncol.* 2002;20(15):3359–3361.
221. Gedlicka C, Kornek GV, Schmid K, Scheithauer W. Amelioration of docetaxel/cisplatin induced polyneuropathy by alpha-lipoic acid. *Ann Oncol.* 2003 ;14(2):339–340.
222. Bianchi G, Vitali G, Caraceni A, et al. Symptomatic and neurophysiological responses of paclitaxel- or cisplatin-induced neuropathy to oral acetyl-L-carnitine. *Eur J Cancer.* 2005;41(12): 1746–1750.
223. McCleane G. Topical application of doxepin hydrochloride can reduce the symptoms of complex regional pain syndrome: a case report. Injury. 2002 Jan;33(1):88–89.
224. Epstein JB, Truelove EL, Oien H, Allison C, Le ND, Epstein MS. Oral topical doxepin rinse: analgesic effect in patients with oral mucosal pain due to cancer or cancer therapy. *Oral Oncol.* 2001;37(8):632–637.
225. Backonja M, Wallace MS, Blonsky ER, et al. NGX-4010, a high-concentration capsaicin patch, for the treatment of postherpetic neuralgia: a randomised, double-blind study. *Lancet Neurol.* 2008;7(12):1106–1112.
226. Simpson DM, Estanislao L, Brown SJ, Sampson J. An open-label pilot study of high-concentration capsaicin patch in painful HIV neuropathy. *J Pain Symptom Manage.* 2008;35(3): 299–306.
227. Simpson DM, Brown S, Tobias J. Controlled trial of high-concentration capsaicin patch for treatment of painful HIV neuropathy. *Neurology.* 2008;70(24):2305–2313.
228. McCleane G. Topical application of doxepin hydrochloride, capsaicin and a combination of both produces analgesia in chronic human neuropathic pain: a randomized, double-blind, placebo-controlled study. *Br J Clin Pharmacol.* 2000;49(6):574–579.
229. Barton DL, Wos EJ, Qin R, et al. A double-blind, placebo-controlled trial of a topical treatment for chemotherapy-induced peripheral neuropathy: NCCTG trial N06CA. *Support Care Cancer.* 2011;19(6):833–841.
230. Wong R, Sagar S. Acupuncture treatment for chemotherapy-induced peripheral neuropathy—a case series. *Acupunct Med.* 2006;24(2):87–91.
231. Marineo G, Iorno V, Gandini C, Moschini V, Smith TJ. Scrambler therapy may relieve chronic neuropathic pain more effectively than guideline-based drug management: results of a pilot, randomized, controlled trial. *J Pain Symptom Manage.* 2012;43(1):87–95.
232. Sabato AF, Marineo G, Gatti A. Scrambler therapy. *Minerva Anestesiol.* 2005;71(7-8):479–482.
233. Smith TJ, Coyne PJ, Parker GL, Dodson P, Ramakrishnan V. Pilot trial of a patient-specific cutaneous electrostimulation device (MC5-A Calmare(R)) for chemotherapy-induced peripheral neuropathy. *J Pain Symptom Manage.* 2010;40(6):883–891.
234. Nizard J, Lefaucheur JP, Helbert M, de Chauvigny E, Nguyen JP. Non-invasive stimulation therapies for the treatment of refractory pain. *Discov Med.* 2012;14(74):21–31.
235. Canavero S, Bonicalzi V, Dotta M, Vighetti S, Asteggiano G, Cocito D. Transcranial magnetic cortical stimulation relieves central pain. *Stereotact Funct Neurosurg.* 2002;78(3-4):192–196.
236. Di Rollo A, Pallanti S. Phantom limb pain: low frequency repetitive transcranial magnetic stimulation in unaffected hemisphere. *Case Report Med.* 2011;2011:130751.
237. Lefaucheur JP. Transcranial magnetic stimulation in the management of pain. *Suppl Clin Neurophysiol.* 2004;57:737–748.
238. Lefaucheur JP. The use of repetitive transcranial magnetic stimulation (rTMS) in chronic neuropathic pain. *Neurophysiol Clin.* 2006;36(3):117–124.
239. Lefaucheur JP. Use of repetitive transcranial magnetic stimulation in pain relief. *Expert Rev Neurother.* 2008;8(5):799–808.
240. Lefaucheur JP, Antal A, Ahdab R, et al. The use of repetitive transcranial magnetic stimulation (rTMS) and transcranial direct current stimulation (tDCS) to relieve pain. *Brain Stimul.* 2008;1(4):337–344.
241. Lefaucheur JP, Ayache SS, Sorel M, et al. Analgesic effects of repetitive transcranial magnetic stimulation of the motor cortex in neuropathic pain: Influence of theta burst stimulation priming. *Eur J Pain.* 2012;16(10):1403–1413.
242. Barr MS, Farzan F, Davis KD, Fitzgerald PB, et al. Measuring GABAergic inhibitory activity with TMS-EEG and its potential clinical application for chronic pain. *J Neuroimmune Pharmacol.* 2012;8(3):535–546.
243. Kocyigit F, Akalin E, Gezer NS, Orbay O, Kocyigit A, Ada E. Functional magnetic resonance imaging of the effects of low-frequency transcutaneous electrical nerve stimulation on central pain modulation: a double-blind, placebo-controlled trial. *Clin J Pain.* 2012;28(7):581–588.
244. Hurlow A, Bennett MI, Robb KA, Johnson MI, Simpson KH, Oxberry SG. Transcutaneous electric nerve stimulation (TENS) for cancer pain in adults. *Cochrane Database Syst Rev.* 2012;3:CD006276.
245. Potash M, Breitbart W. Affective disorders in advanced cancer. *Hematol Oncol Clin North Am.* 2002;16(3):671–700.
246. Wasteson E, Brenne E, Higginson IJ, et al. Depression assessment and classification in palliative cancer patients: a systematic literature review. *Palliat Med.* 2009;23(8):739–753.
247. O'Connor M, White K, Kristjanson LJ, Cousins K, Wilkes L. The prevalence of anxiety and depression in palliative care patients with cancer in Western Australia and New South Wales. *Med J Aust.* 2010;193(5 suppl):S44–S47.
248. Delgado-Guay M, Parsons HA, Li Z, Palmer JL, Bruera E. Symptom distress in advanced cancer patients with anxiety and depression in the palliative care setting. *Support Care Cancer.* 2009;17(5):573–579.
249. Pantilat SZ, O'Riordan DL, Dibble SL, Landefeld CS. Longitudinal assessment of symptom severity among hospitalized elders diagnosed with cancer, heart failure, and chronic obstructive pulmonary disease. *J Hosp Med.* 2012;7(7):567–572.
250. Mitchell AJ, Chan M, Bhatti H, et al. Prevalence of depression, anxiety, and adjustment disorder in oncological, haematological,

and palliative-care settings: a meta-analysis of 94 interview-based studies. *Lancet Oncol.* 2011;12(2):160–174.

251. Kolva E, Rosenfeld B, Pessin H, Breitbart W, Brescia R. Anxiety in terminally ill cancer patients. *J Pain Symptom Manage.* 2011;42(5):691–701.
252. Pasquini M, Biondi M, Costantini A, et al. Detection and treatment of depressive and anxiety disorders among cancer patients: feasibility and preliminary findings from a liaison service in an oncology division. *Depress Anxiety.* 2006;23(7):441–448.
253. Ford DE, Kamerow DB. Epidemiologic study of sleep disturbances and psychiatric disorders. An opportunity for prevention? *JAMA.* 1989;262(11):1479–1484.
254. Breslau N, Roth T, Rosenthal L, Andreski P. Sleep disturbance and psychiatric disorders: a longitudinal epidemiological study of young adults. *Biol Psychiatry.* 1996;39(6):411–418.
255. Paffenbarger RS, Jr., Lee IM, Leung R. Physical activity and personal characteristics associated with depression and suicide in American college men. *Acta Psychiatr Scand Suppl.* 1994;377:16–22.
256. Weissman MM, Greenwald S, Nino-Murcia G, Dement WC. The morbidity of insomnia uncomplicated by psychiatric disorders. *Gen Hosp Psychiatry.* 1997;19(4):245–250.
257. Johnson EO, Roth T, Breslau N. The association of insomnia with anxiety disorders and depression: exploration of the direction of risk. *J Psychiatr Res.* 2006;40(8):700–708.
258. Ohayon MM, Roth T. Place of chronic insomnia in the course of depressive and anxiety disorders. *J Psychiatr Res.* 2003;37(1):9–15.
259. Bin YS, Marshall NS, Glozier N. The burden of insomnia on individual function and healthcare consumption in Australia. *Aust N Z J Public Health.* 2012;36(5):462–468.
260. Barnes EA, Bruera E. Fatigue in patients with advanced cancer: a review. *Int J Gynecol Cancer.* 2002;12(5):424–428.
261. Theobald DE. Cancer pain, fatigue, distress, and insomnia in cancer patients. *Clin Cornerstone.* 2004;6(suppl 1D):S15–S21.
262. Sela RA, Watanabe S, Nekolaichuk CL. Sleep disturbances in palliative cancer patients attending a pain and symptom control clinic. *Palliat Support Care.* 2005;3(1):23–31.
263. Gibbins J, McCoubrie R, Kendrick AH, Senior-Smith G, Davies AN, Hanks GW. Sleep-wake disturbances in patients with advanced cancer and their family carers. *J Pain Symptom Manage.* 2009;38(6):860–870.
264. Delgado-Guay M, Yennurajalingam S, Parsons H, Palmer JL, Bruera E. Association between self-reported sleep disturbance and other symptoms in patients with advanced cancer. *J Pain Symptom Manage.* 2011;41(5):819–827.
265. Goforth HW, Lowery J, Cutson TM, McMillan ES, Kenedi C, Cohen MA. Impact of bereavement on progression of AIDS and HIV infection: a review. *Psychosomatics.* 2009;50(5):433–439.
266. Prasertsri N, Holden J, Keefe FJ, Wilkie DJ. Repressive coping style: relationships with depression, pain, and pain coping strategies in lung cancer outpatients. *Lung Cancer.* 2011;71(2):235–240.
267. Spina E, Santoro V, D'Arrigo C. Clinically relevant pharmacokinetic drug interactions with second-generation antidepressants: an update. *Clin Ther.* 2008;30(7):1206–1227.
268. Hayes BD, Klein-Schwartz W, Clark RF, Muller AA, Miloradovich JE. Comparison of toxicity of acute overdoses with citalopram and escitalopram. *J Emerg Med.* 2010;39(1):44–48.
269. Skljarevski V, Zhang S, Iyengar S, et al. Efficacy of duloxetine in patients with chronic pain conditions. *Curr Drug Ther.* 2011;6(4):296–303.
270. Kast RE. Mirtazapine may be useful in treating nausea and insomnia of cancer chemotherapy. *Support Care Cancer.* 2001;9(6):469–470.
271. Thompson DS. Mirtazapine for the treatment of depression and nausea in breast and gynecological oncology. *Psychosomatics.* 2000;41(4):356–359.
272. Theobald DE, Kirsh KL, Holtsclaw E, Donaghy K, Passik SD. An open-label, crossover trial of mirtazapine (15 and 30 mg) in cancer patients with pain and other distressing symptoms. *J Pain Symptom Manage.* 2002;23(5):442–447.
273. Cankurtaran ES, Ozalp E, Soygur H, Akbiyik DI, Turhan L, Alkis N. Mirtazapine improves sleep and lowers anxiety and depression in cancer patients: superiority over imipramine. *Support Care Cancer.* 2008;16(11):1291–1298.
274. Kim SW, Shin IS, Kim JM, et al. Effectiveness of mirtazapine for nausea and insomnia in cancer patients with depression. *Psychiatry Clin Neurosci.* 2008;62(1):75–83.
275. Ersoy MA, Noyan AM, Elbi H. An open-label long-term naturalistic study of mirtazapine treatment for depression in cancer patients. *Clin Drug Investig.* 2008;28(2):113–120.
276. Riechelmann RP, Burman D, Tannock IF, Rodin G, Zimmermann C. Phase II trial of mirtazapine for cancer-related cachexia and anorexia. *Am J Hosp Palliat Care.* 2010;27(2):106–110.
277. Davis MP, Kirkova J, Lagman R, Walsh D, Karafa M. Intolerance to mirtazapine in advanced cancer. *J Pain Symptom Manage.* 2011;42(3):e4–e7.
278. Mittur A. Trazodone: properties and utility in multiple disorders. *Expert Rev Clin Pharmacol.* 2011;4(2):181–196.
279. Davis MP. Does trazodone have a role in palliating symptoms? *Support Care Cancer.* 2007;15(2):221–224.
280. Tanimukai H, Murai T, Okazaki N, et al. An observational study of insomnia and nightmare treated with trazodone in patients with advanced cancer. *Am J Hosp Palliat Care.* 2012;30(4):359–362.
281. De Wit S, Cremers L, Hirsch D, Zulian C, Clumeck N, Kormoss N. Efficacy and safety of trazodone versus clorazepate in the treatment of HIV-positive subjects with adjustment disorders: a pilot study. *J Int Med Res.* 1999;27(5):223–232.
282. Razavi D, Kormoss N, Collard A, Farvacques C, Delvaux N. Comparative study of the efficacy and safety of trazodone versus clorazepate in the treatment of adjustment disorders in cancer patients: a pilot study. *J Int Med Res.* 1999;27(6):264–272.
283. Ventafridda V, Bonezzi C, Caraceni A, et al. Antidepressants for cancer pain and other painful syndromes with deafferentation component: comparison of amitriptyline and trazodone. *Ital J Neurol Sci.* 1987;8(6):579–587.
284. Cipriani A, Furukawa TA, Salanti G, et al. Comparative efficacy and acceptability of 12 new-generation antidepressants: a multiple-treatments meta-analysis. *Lancet.* 2009;373(9665):746–758.
285. Sood A, Barton DL, Loprinzi CL. Use of methylphenidate in patients with cancer. *Am J Hosp Palliat Care.* 2006;23(1):35–40.
286. Bruera E, Driver L, Barnes EA, et al. Patient-controlled methylphenidate for the management of fatigue in patients with advanced cancer: a preliminary report. *J Clin Oncol.* 2003;21(23): 4439–4443.
287. Breitbart W, Rosenfeld B, Kaim M, Funesti-Esch J. A randomized, double-blind, placebo-controlled trial of psychostimulants for the treatment of fatigue in ambulatory patients with human immunodeficiency virus disease. *Arch Intern Med.* 2001;161(3):411–420.
288. Schwartz AL, Thompson JA, Masood N. Interferon-induced fatigue in patients with melanoma: a pilot study of exercise and methylphenidate. *Oncol Nurs Forum.* 2002;29(7):E85–E90.
289. Kerr CW, Drake J, Milch RA, et al. Effects of methylphenidate on fatigue and depression: a randomized, double-blind, placebo-controlled trial. *J Pain Symptom Manage.* 2012; 43(1):68–77.
290. Yennurajalingam S, Palmer JL, Chacko R, Bruera E. Factors associated with response to methylphenidate in advanced cancer patients. *Oncologist.* 2011;16(2):246–253.
291. Bruera E, Valero V, Driver L, et al. Patient-controlled methylphenidate for cancer fatigue: a double-blind, randomized, placebo-controlled trial. *J Clin Oncol.* 2006;24(13):2073–2078.
292. Kennedy SH, Andersen HF, Lam RW. Efficacy of escitalopram in the treatment of major depressive disorder compared with conventional selective serotonin reuptake inhibitors and venlafaxine XR: a meta-analysis. *J Psychiatry Neurosci.* 2006;31(2):122–131.
293. Breimer DD. Pharmacokinetics and metabolism of various benzodiazepines used as hypnotics. *Br J Clin Pharmacol.* 1979;8(1):7S–13S.

294. Maher AR, Theodore G. Summary of the comparative effectiveness review on off-label use of atypical antipsychotics. *J Manag Care Pharm.* 2012;18(5 suppl B):S1–S20.
295. Casey DE. Atypical antipsychotics: enhancing healthy outcomes. Arch Psychiatr Nurs. 2002 Jun;16(3 Suppl 1):S12–19.
296. Kohler S, Unger T, Hoffmann S, Steinacher B, Fydrich T, Bschor T. Comparing augmentation with non-antidepressants over sticking to antidepressants after treatment failure in depression: a naturalistic study. *Pharmacopsychiatry.* 2012; 46(2):69–76
297. Gartlehner G, Hansen RA, Thieda P, et al.Comparative Effectiveness of Second-Generation Antidepressants in the Pharmacologic Treatment of Adult Depression. Portland (OR): Oregon Health & Science University; 2008.
298. Huh J, Goebert D, Takeshita J, Lu BY, Kang M. Treatment of generalized anxiety disorder: a comprehensive review of the literature for psychopharmacologic alternatives to newer antidepressants and benzodiazepines. *Prim Care Companion CNS Disord.* 2011;13(2):pii.
299. Maher AR, Maglione M, Bagley S, et al. Efficacy and comparative effectiveness of atypical antipsychotic medications for off-label uses in adults: a systematic review and meta-analysis. *JAMA.* 2011 28;306(12):1359–1369.
300. Zammit GK, Corser B, Doghramji K, et al. Sleep and residual sedation after administration of zaleplon, zolpidem, and placebo during experimental middle-of-the-night awakening. *J Clin Sleep Med.* 2006 15;2(4):417–423.
301. Dimsdale JE, Ball ED, Carrier E, et al. Effect of eszopiclone on sleep, fatigue, and pain in patients with mucositis associated with hematologic malignancies. *Support Care Cancer.* 2011;19(12):2015–2020.
302. Roth T, Price JM, Amato DA, Rubens RP, Roach JM, Schnitzer TJ. The effect of eszopiclone in patients with insomnia and coexisting rheumatoid arthritis: a pilot study. *Prim Care Companion J Clin Psychiatry.* 2009;11(6):292–301.
303. Walsh JK, Krystal AD, Amato DA, et al. Nightly treatment of primary insomnia with eszopiclone for six months: effect on sleep, quality of life, and work limitations. *Sleep.* 2007;30(8): 959–968.
304. Krystal AD. Antidepressant and antipsychotic drugs. *Sleep Med Clin.* 2010;5(4):571–589.
305. Haria M, Fitton A, McTavish D. Trazodone. A review of its pharmacology, therapeutic use in depression and therapeutic potential in other disorders. *Drugs Aging.* 1994;4(4):331–355.
306. Krystal AD, Lankford A, Durrence HH, et al. Efficacy and safety of doxepin 3 and 6 mg in a 35-day sleep laboratory trial in adults with chronic primary insomnia. *Sleep.* 2011;34(10): 1433–1442.
307. Stiefel F, Stagno D. Management of insomnia in patients with chronic pain conditions. *CNS Drugs.* 2004;18(5):285–296.
308. Krystal AD, Goforth HW, Roth T. Effects of antipsychotic medications on sleep in schizophrenia. *Int Clin Psychopharmacol.* 2008;23(3):150–160.
309. Laird BJ, Boyd AC, Colvin LA, Fallon MT. Are cancer pain and depression interdependent? A systematic review. *Psychooncology.* 2009;18(5):459–464.
310. Kroenke K, Zhong X, Theobald D, Wu J, Tu W, Carpenter JS. Somatic symptoms in patients with cancer experiencing pain or depression: prevalence, disability, and health care use. *Arch Intern Med.* 2010;170(18):1686–1694.
311. Kroenke K, Theobald D, Wu J, Loza JK, Carpenter JS, Tu W. The association of depression and pain with health-related quality of life, disability, and health care use in cancer patients. *J Pain Symptom Manage.* 2010;40(3):327–341.
312. Chen ML, Chang HK. Physical symptom profiles of depressed and nondepressed patients with cancer. *Palliat Med.* 2004;18(8):712–718.
313. Wang HL, Kroenke K, Wu J, Tu W, Theobald D, Rawl SM. Predictors of cancer-related pain improvement over time. *Psychosom Med.* 2012;74(6):642–647.
314. Badr H, Milbury K. Associations between depression, pain behaviors, and partner responses to pain in metastatic breast cancer. *Pain.* 2011;152(11):2596–2604.
315. Rawdin B, Evans C, Rabow MW. The relationships among hope, pain, psychological distress, and spiritual well-being in oncology outpatients. *J Palliat Med.* 2012;16(2):167–172.
316. Mystakidou K, Tsilika E, Parpa E, et al. Exploring the relationships between depression, hopelessness, cognitive status, pain, and spirituality in patients with advanced cancer. *Arch Psychiatr Nurs.* 2007;21(3):150–161.
317. O'Mahony S, Goulet J, Kornblith A, et al. Desire for hastened death, cancer pain and depression: report of a longitudinal observational study. *J Pain Symptom Manage.* 2005;29(5):446–457.

SECTION VII

OTHER DISORDERS

24.

HEADACHE

Hossein Ansari and Samer Narouze

CASE PRESENTATION

A 25-year-old woman presents with a history of right-sided headache for the past 3 years. She had been diagnosed with migraine. After a motor vehicle collision in which she was rear-ended 6 months ago, the headache worsened and became more frequent. This headache starts in the back of the head/upper neck area and radiates behind the right eye. It occurs on more than half of the days in the month and is associated with nausea and photophobia. It is not relieved by ibuprofen, indomethacin, or other nonsteroidal anti-inflammatory drugs (NSAIDs). The patient is currently on sumatriptan, ergotamine, and hydrocodone. Her use of hydrocodone/APAP 5/325 has escalated from an average of 60 tablets per month to 240 tablets per month over the past 6 months. She is referred to the Interdisciplinary Pain Medicine clinic.

Past medical history is significant for anxiety and a heart murmur.

Social history is significant for drinking alcohol socially; she denies illicit drug use. She works as a part-time secretary. She is involved in litigation related to the motor vehicle collision.

Review of systems is significant for snoring at night and daytime sleepiness.

On examination, the patient weighs 92 kg and is 156 cm tall. Her neurologic exam is unremarkable. She has increased muscle tone over the trapezius and a slightly decreased range of motion of the cervical spine in lateral rotation.

Imaging studies obtained last month, including C-spine magnetic resonance imaging (MRI) and X-ray series, as well MRI/MRA/MRV of the brain, are within normal limits.

QUESTIONS

1. What is the differential diagnosis in this case?
   a. What further history may be helpful in making the diagnosis?
   b. What are red flag symptoms?
2. What is the definition of cervicogenic headache (CeH)?
3. How is CeH differentiated from migraine?
4. What is the epidemiology of CeH?
5. What is the pathophysiology of CeH?
6. What stepwise approach would be followed to manage this patient?
   a. Behavioral
   b. Pharmacological
   c. Interventional
   d. Rehabilitation

WHAT IS THE DIFFERENTIAL DIAGNOSIS IN THIS CASE?

The first step in this case is to clarify the patient's underlying headache syndrome: this patient carries the diagnosis of migraine. If we examine the International Headache Society classification (ICHD-II) for migraine (Box 24.1) along with the case history, we are *unable* to classify the patient's current headache as migraine.

The patient may have had migraine in the past, per the history, but we cannot make the diagnosis without obtaining further history. The following information needs to be gathered:

- Duration of each headache attack
- Quality of pain: pulsating (throbbing) versus nonthrobbing
- Maximum intensity of pain: does the pain affects patient's daily activities?
- Whether pain is aggravated by routine physical activities

Obtaining a family history is also very important because migraine is a complex genetic disorder, and the presence of a family history of migraine will be helpful.

Asking about the possibility of migraine aura also is important. If the patient describes the symptoms fulfilling

Box 24.1 ICHD-II DIAGNOSTIC CRITERIA FOR MIGRAINE WITHOUT AURA

A. At least 5 attacks fulfilling criteria B–D:
B. Headache (HA) attacks lasting 4–72 h (untreated or unsuccessfully treated)
C. HA has at least two of the following characteristics:
  1. Unilateral location
  2. Pulsating quality (throbbing)
  3. Moderate or severe pain intensity
  4. Worsening with exertion
D. During headache at least 1 of the following:
  1. Nausea and/or vomiting
  2. Photophobia and phonophobia

the criteria for any type of aura (visual, sensory, language, or motor), it is not only very helpful to make the diagnosis, but also will be important during patient counseling.

Asking about the positional component of the headache is very important in this patient. For example, it is helpful to know whether her headache is worse upon waking in the morning or if it improves or worsens while lying flat. Considering the patient's body size (body mass index [BMI] >35), increased intracranial hypertension (pseudotumor cerebri) is one of the differentials.

In addition, the following questions should be asked:

- What are triggering or alleviating factors? Does neck and head movement make it worse? Do any particular head positions improve the pain?
- Does her headache respond to sumatriptan or ergotamine? If so, why did she begin using opiates?
- Has she tried any preventative medication? If so, which medication? What dose? How long was the medication taken?
- What is the history of heart murmur? Is it a chronic problem? Has she had a workup for it?
- Is there any history of blurry or double vision, specifically with worsening of her headache?
- Has she had any workup for her sleep problem? Is this a new or chronic issue?
- How long has she been obese? Did her headache worsen after weight gain?
- How long has she been using hydrocodone/APAP at an average 60 tablets per month?

After obtaining all this information, we will be able to characterize our patient's underlying headache syndrome. The most important red flag symptom in the history is the "side-lock appearance" of this patient's headache, without shifting the side.

Despite the fact that unilaterality is one of the criteria for migraine (Box 24.1), usually the side of headache shifts in patients with migraine. Also, in migraine patients whose headache always starts on one side, usually the pain evolves to the other side at least during some of their attacks. It seems that, in this patient, the headache is locked to the right side without moving to the left at all.

Migraines are still the most common side-locked headaches seen in the clinic due to the high prevalence of migraine. However, in patients with side-locked headache without side shift, other differential diagnoses need to be considered.

First and foremost, we must consider the secondary etiology of headache, such as tumor, cyst, vascular anomalies (including aneurysm or venous thrombosis), and the like Considering that this patient had normal brain MRI/MRA/MRV, these possibilities are already ruled out.

Despite the fact that a few reports of side-locked tension-type headache (TTH) are available in literature,[1,2] TTH is commonly a bilateral headache, which typically responds to simple analgesics. The fact that this patient's headaches do not respond to regular analgesics coupled with the fact that she needs opiates to relieve her pain makes this diagnosis very unlikely.

The headache category of trigeminal autonomic cephalalgia (TAC) is almost always side-locked, and so it is included in the differential. This includes three subtypes:

- Short-lasting unilateral neuralgiform headache attacks with conjunctival injection and tearing (SUNCT) and short-lasting unilateral neuralgiform headache attacks with cranial autonomic symptoms (SUNA)
- Cluster headache (CH)
- Paroxysmal hemicrania (PH)

As made clear by its name, the key feature of this headache category is the presence of autonomic symptoms. In this patient, the lack of any autonomic features rules out this diagnosis.

Hemicrania continua (HC) is always the differential for side-locked headache, as is clear by its name (hemicrania). However, HC is one of the indomethacin-responsive headaches, and the fact that this patient's headache did not respond to indomethacin rules out this possibility as well.

The CeH headache syndrome is usually unilateral and spreads from the back of the head to the frontal and temporal regions. It is triggered by certain movements or sustained provocative head positions.[3]

Considering the available data with this patient, CeH is the most likely diagnosis for her underlying headache syndrome. However, with the number of headache days she experiences and the amount of opioid analgesics she uses, chronic daily headache (CDH) in the setting of medication overuse headache (MOH) is her main diagnosis at this point.

Chronic Daily Headache (CDH)

CDH is a general categorical term defined as the presence of headache on more than 15 days per month for more than 3 months. CDH could be primary or secondary (Table 24.1)

Table 24.1 **PRIMARY VERSUS SECONDARY CHRONIC DAILY HEADACHE (CDH)**

PRIMARY CDH	SECONDARY CDH
Chronic tension type headache (CTTH)	Medication overuse headache (MOH)
Chronic migraine (CM)	Trauma (post traumatic headache)
Chronic cluster headache	Sleep disorder (e.g., sleep apnea)
New daily persistent headache (NDPH)	Cerebrospinal fluid pressure abnormality (low or high)
Hemicrania continua	Structural abnormalities:
Primary stabbing headache	*Cervical spine (cervicogenic headache)*
	Temporomandibular joint disorder
	Sinusitis and other rhinonasal abnormalities

Box 24.2 **MEDICATION-OVERUSE HEADACHE CRITERIA FROM ICHD-II, REVISED**

A. Headache ≥15 d/mo
B. Regular overuse for >3 months of ≥1 acute/symptomatic treatment drugs:
   1. Ergotamine, triptans, opioids, or combination analgesic medications on ≥10 d/mo on a regular basis for >3 months
   2. Simple analgesics or any combination of ergotamine, triptans, or analgesics opioids on ≥15 d/mo on a regular basis for >3 months without overuse of any single class alone
C. Headache developed or markedly worsened during medication overuse

MOH, which used to be called "rebound headache," is the most common subtype of secondary CDH.

Medication-Overuse Headache (MOH)

MOH is a secondary CDH described by the International Classification of Headache Disorders, Second Edition (ICHD-II. Box 24.2) as "an interaction between a therapeutic (analgesic) agent used excessively and susceptible patient overuse." "Susceptible patient" means that the patient needs analgesic medication for either another headache type or another pain issue.

With the number of headache days per month (more than half of the days per month for last 6 months), our patient clearly fulfills the criteria for CDH in which MOH is the major component of her CDH. Even prior to her motor vehicle collusion, the amount of her analgesic use, specifically opiate use, was much higher than recommended.

However, most patients with MOH have other types of headaches as well. In reviewing Table 24.1, there are four other possibilities that could be suggested for her CDH.

1. *Chronic migraine*: this patient carries the diagnosis of migraine. Despite the fact that we do not have enough information to confirm this diagnosis, patients with episodic migraine who do not begin preventative treatment at the appropriate time have an increased likelihood of transforming from episodic to chronic migraine. Also, comorbid condition(s) can facilitate this transformation. In this patient, there are a few significant comorbid conditions. These include:
   Obesity (BMI >35)[4]
   Sleep issue with snoring and daytime sleepiness
   History of anxiety disorder
2. *Sleep disorder* (e.g., sleep apnea): in this patient, considering her body habitus, the possiblity of sleep apnea based on given history is high. Sleep apnea not only could be a reason for secondary CDH by itself (Table 24.2), but it could also be a triggering factor for other headache disorders, specifically migraine, as discussed earlier. This possiblity needs to be further investigated by performing a sleep study.
3. *Trauma* (post-traumatic headache): Patients with migraine and other headache syndromes can experiencing worsening headaches after truma. However, we cannot call it post-traumatic headache in our patient because she clearly exeperienced some underlying headache syndrome prior to trauma.
4. *CeH*: in this chapter, we will discuss this type of headache because it seems to be the most likely diagnosis in our case.

In our case, the underlying headache syndrome is probably CeH. Due to misdiagnosis, our patient has not been treated appropriately. Because her headache continued, she used excessive amounts of analgesics, including opiates. This contributed to the development of MOH and trapped her in the cycle of CDH. Then, after her car accident and due to her other pain issues, she increased the use of opiates and made the MOH cycle worse. Even prior to her motor vehicle collision, her amount of opiate use was significantly higher than the recommended amount.

WHAT IS THE DEFINITION OF CEH?

Head pain that is referred from bony structures or soft tissues of the neck defines CeH.[5] Despite the fact that the hypothesis of CeH was suggested more than 30 years ago by Sjaastad et al.[5] and later diagnostic criteria were introduced (Table 24.2),[6] the controversies and uncertainties associated with this condition continue. The clinical overlap between CeH and other headache syndromes, specifically migraine, probably is the most likely reason for this controversy. In CeH, digital pressure over a triggering area at the upper nuchal region produces the spontaneous pain pattern.[3] Because cervical trigger(s) are also very common in migraine, patients with migraine could further confuse the CeH picture.

The International Headache Society (IHS) created another set of criteria for the diagnosis of CeH (Box 24.3).

Table 24.2 CERVICOGENIC HEADACHE INTERNATIONAL STUDY GROUP CRITERIA

Major criteria[a]	I. Symptoms and signs of neck involvement Ia. Precipitation of head pain, similar to the usually occurring one: Ia(1) by neck movement and/or sustained awkward head positioning, and/or: Ia(2) by external pressure over the upper cervical or occipital region on the symptomatic side. Ib. Restriction of range of motion (ROM) in the neck. Ic. Ipsilateral neck, shoulder, or arm pain of a rather vague, nonradicular nature, or occasionally arm pain of a radicular nature II. Confirmatory evidence by diagnostic anesthetic blockades III. Unilaterality of the pain, without side shift
Head pain characteristics	IV. Moderate-severe, nonthrobbing pain, usually starting in the neck. Episodes of varying duration or fluctuating, continuous pain
Other characteristics of some importance	V. Only marginal effect or lack of effect of indomethacin. Only marginal effect or lack of effect of ergotamine and sumatriptan. Not infrequent occurrence of head or indirect neck trauma by history, usually of more than only medium severity
Other features of less importance	VI. Various attack-related phenomena, only occasionally present and/or moderately expressed when present: (a) nausea, (b) phono- and photophobia, (c) dizziness, (d) ipsilateral "blurred vision," (e) difficulties swallowing, (f) ipsilateral edema, mostly in the particular area

[a]It is obligatory that one or more of phenomena Ia–Ic are present

HOW IS CEH DIFFERENTIATED FROM MIGRAINE?

A detailed history and examination are needed to differentiate CeH from migraine. Helpful features include:

- Pain is usually throbbing (pulsating) in migraine versus CeH, where the pain is nonthrobbing.
- CeH is usually side-locked *without side shift*. In migraine, despite the fact that unilaterality is one of diagnostic criteria (Box 24.1), side-lock appearance is uncommon.

Box 24.3 INTERNATIONAL CLASSIFICATION OF HEADACHE DISORDERS-II CRITERIA FOR CEH

A. Pain, referred from a source in the neck and perceived in one or more regions of the head and/or face, fulfilling criteria C and D.
B. Clinical, laboratory, and/or imaging evidence of a disorder or lesion within the cervical spine or soft tissues of the neck known to be, or generally accepted as, a valid cause of headache.
C. Evidence that the pain can be attributed to the neck disorder or lesion based on at least one of the following:
   1. Demonstration of the clinical signs that implicate a source of pain in the neck
   2. Abolition of headache following diagnostic blockade of a cervical structure or its nerve supply using placebo or other adequate controls
D. Pain resolves within 3 months after successful treatment of causative disorder or lesion.

- Presence of associated symptoms is mostly suggestive of migraine. Despite the fact that photophobia or phonophobia could be seen in CeH or any other type of headache, the presence of both photophobia and phonophobia is almost always suggestive of migraine.
- In migraine patients, in addition to cervical trigger points, other trigger point(s) include temporal, frontal, and supraorbital, and these can usually be determined during physical examination.

Always remember that nausea, vomiting, photophobia, and even phonophobia are possible in CeH. Therefore, the detailed history and examination need to differentiate CeH from migraine or other primary headache disorders because CeH can resemble them.[7–9]

WHAT IS THE EPIDEMIOLOGY OF CEH?

Due to diagnostic uncertainties, the epidemiology of CeH is not very clear. The prevalence of CeH varies considerably depending on the applied diagnostic criteria. Based on available data, the prevalence of cervicogenic headache in the general population is estimated at between 0.4% and 4%.[10–13] However, the prevalence will be different based on criteria used. For example, in one study that used Sjaastad's revised criteria (Table 24.2), the frequency of CeH was 8.0% among 298 patients with chronic headache.[14]

The prevalence of CeH in a population with chronic headache increased to 15–20%. CeH affected women more often than men.[13]

Co-occurrence of migraine and/or tension-type headache further complicates the diagnostics of CeH.[15,16]

WHAT IS THE PATHOPHYSIOLOGY OF CEH?

The anatomic locus for cervicogenic headache is the trigeminocervical nucleus in the upper cervical spinal cord. Sensory nerve fibers in the descending tract of the trigeminal nerve (trigeminal nucleus caudalis) are believed to interact with sensory fibers from the upper cervical roots. Only structures innervated by C1–C3 have been shown to be capable of causing headache.[17] This functional intersection of upper cervical and trigeminal sensory pathways is thought to allow the bidirectional transmission of pain signals between the neck and the trigeminal sensory receptive fields of the face and head.

The trigeminocervical nucleus is the essential structure for headache. At the lower end of this nucleus, trigeminal afferents overlap with those of the upper three cervical segments (C1–C3).This overlap seems to be the main mechanism for CeH. This anatomical connection between cervical and trigeminal innervation systems would explain the frontal or retro-orbital pain seen in the patient with CeH (like the patient in this chapter's case presentation).This frontal or retro-orbital distribution of headache is one reason that CeH is commonly mistaken as migraine or tension-type headache.

CeH usually happens without any demonstrable abnormality in cervical or brain imaging.[18,19] Most cervical lesions induce sparse episodes of neck and mostly radicular pain without or with very few complain of headache.[20]

Cervical radiculopathy is related to headache in 9.7% of patients.[21]Also, pain related to facet joints often occurs in the neck, shoulder, and mid-back, without headache.[22] Of the many potential painful structures in the neck area, facet joints (zygapophysial joints) appear to be the most important pain generators. Referred pain from facet joints does not include the trigeminal nerve.[23,24]

Only the pain stemming from the articulations between the first three cervical vertebrae can lead to CeH: atlanto-occipital, atlanto-axial (C1–C2), and C2–C3 facet joints.

In this case of CDH, in addition to MOH and possible sleep apnea, the underlying headache syndrome is most likely CeH, based on available history. The key features that are highly suggestive of CeH in her history are:

Side-lock appearance of her headache

Origination of pain from back of the head/upper neck

Increased muscle tone over the trapezius with some decreased range of motion of the cervical spine

Lack of response to indomethacin

Migraine is still a possibility, but, with the available history, we cannot make the diagnosis of migraine in this patient. Based on ICHD-II (Table 24.1), we do not have information about the duration of each attack (section B). Also from Table 24.1 section C, we only have information about unilateral location. Because we need at least two of the four criteria in section C, this patient clearly does not fulfill the diagnostic criteria of migraine. In addition, it seems that she did not respond to sumatriptan and ergotamine and was started on opioids. This is also against the diagnosis of migraine.

In summarizing this case's diagnosis based on available history we can tell that she is suffering from multifactorial CDH:

- Her underlying headache syndrome is most likely cervicogenic headache (CeH).
- Because she was not diagnosed and treated appropriately, her headache worsened; then, with excessive opiate use, she developed MOH, which made her headache even worse.
- Her car accident may have some impact on her CDH, although it was probably indirect by increasing the use of opiates and worsening the MOH cycle.
- Her possible sleep problem, which is most likely obstructive sleep apnea, plays an important role in her CDH, either directly (see Table 24.2) or indirectly by triggering her underlying headache syndrome.

WHAT STEPWISE APPROACH WOULD BE FOLLOWED TO MANAGE THIS PATIENT?

In this case, we are dealing with at least two main issues: CeH and MOH. Therefore, this requires parallel management of the two conditions.

BEHAVIORAL

Because MOH is the main driver of her headache at this point, without its management it will be impossible to control her underlying headache. Therefore, we need to focus on this first. MOH treatment involves three major steps: weaning, education, and establishing a preventative approach.[25]

Weaning Off Overused Medication

This step needs extensive discussion with the patient. She needs to understand the importance of this step. The patient and her family need to be educated regarding this major step.

Weaning can be done either slowly over 4–6 weeks or abruptly, with a bridge to blunt withdrawal symptoms. Also, based on the class of overused medication, some sort of detoxification program may be needed.

Barbiturate and opioid overuse are the worst because of the higher chances of withdrawal symptoms that can sometimes be life-threatening (especially with barbiturates).

In summary, high-dose narcotics, barbiturates, and benzodiazepines require special weaning skills and may require the implementation of an interdisciplinary program, whether day hospital or inpatient, based on the dose and duration of overuse. The interdisciplinary program should be formally structured and involve multiple medical subspecialties, such as neurology, pain management, primary care, psychology, skilled nursing, infusions, and physical therapy.

Other behavioral treatments include regular lifestyle habits, including light aerobic exercise on a scheduled basis, headache trigger avoidance, and active patient participation. Some types of mind-body exercises, such as yoga and meditation, can be particularly helpful when routinely practiced within an interdisciplinary pain rehabilitation program.

Education

It is important to take the time to educate the patient. When appropriate, patients need reassurance that they are not addicts, and it is important to differentiate abuse from overuse and dependence. Explain that treatment takes time and that return visits are necessary. Encourage the patient to bring family and friends into the treatment program.

> This patient has overused opioids for long duration with a relatively high dose. Therefore, she will benefit from an interdisciplinary program until she stops using narcotics. This will be the first step to manage her headache. Discuss with her that this is not an addiction program and provide enough information regarding the program in which she is enrolled.
>
> In the meantime, the patient is scheduled for a polysomnogram (PSG) to, first, confirm the possible diagnosis of sleep apnea and, second, to assess its severity. Based on the result of the PSG, she will need appropriate treatment, which will most likely be a CPAP machine.

Establishing Preventative Approach

A preventative approach could be medical or behavioral. Here, we discuss a behavioral approach; we discuss pharmacological treatment later. Regarding behavioral treatment, the first step usually will be psychiatric/psychological counseling to make sure no secondary gain exists. During this step, the possibility of other mood and anxiety disorders, which can play an important role in the intractability of headache, will be evaluated. Psychologists can counsel patients for anticipatory anxiety; provide biofeedback, relaxation therapy, and cognitive-behavioral therapy; and also help shift the locus of control to the patient.

One important reason for behavioral management in MOH is risk of relapse. Multiple studies show that after treatment of medication overuse and withdrawal of the offending medication, relapse occurs within months or years in a relatively high proportion of patients (30–40% at 1 year; 40–70% after 4–5 years).[26–31]

This suggests that MOH might be prompted and sustained by some psychological states and behavioral disorders, including fear of headache, anticipatory anxiety of attacks, and psychological drug dependence.[32]

> In our patient, due to her past medical history of anxiety disorder and her current involvement in litigation relative to motor vehicle collision, psychological counseling is very important. The patient should establish a psychiatry or psychology source for herself on regular basis, and she needs to continue regular follow-up with them.

PHARMACOLOGICAL TREATMENT

Appropriate abortive and preventative treatment needs to start simultaneously with a behavioral approach and during the weaning-off period. In terms of preventative treatment for CeH there very few studies have been completed. When using acute (abortive) agents, limitations need to be given clearly to the patient. Depending on the type of underlying headache, different medications could be used. NSAIDs are a good choice in CeH and are also a first-line agent in patients with migraine. Limitations for this class of medication could be up to 15–20 days per month. Most patients who use over-the-counter NSAIDs use a subtherapeutic dose, so it is always better to give a prescription to ensure that patients are using correct dosages.

We usually use three different classes of medication as preventative treatment in CeH:

- Muscle relaxants: specifically tizanidine
- Tricyclic antidepressants (TCAs)
- Calcium channel (voltage-gated) modulators: gabapentin and pregabalin

The choice of medication is based on the clinical scenario and examination. For example, in the patient with localized pain and tenderness in the neck and occipital area and presence of significant spasm in the examination, muscle relaxants may be the better choice.

On the other hand, in patients whose pain radiates from the back and neck to the front of the head, patients who have migrainous features (photophobia, nausea, etc.), and those with underlying mood and anxiety disorders, TCAs might be the better choice.

Gabapentin and pregabalin may be a better option for the patient who has some obvious anatomical abnormality in the imaging of cervical spine, or if they have concomitant shoulder/joint pain.

> In this case, due to the limited history, our working diagnosis is CeH. The use of naproxen sodium 550 mg as needed, with limitation to a maximum of 15–20 days per month is an appropriate acute treatment. Other NSAIDs also could be used at the correct dosage.
>
> Regarding preventative therapy, considering that her pain radiates from the back and neck to the front of her head, the migrainous features (nausea, photophobia), and past medical history of anxiety, low-dose amitriptyline (10 mg at bedtime) is an appropriate option. The dose is titrated by 10 mg per week. Usually, 50 mg/d is a good target point. The other reason to choose a TCA in this patient is questionable migraine. As

discussed earlier, considering her limited history, we cannot rule out the diagnosis of migraine until we obtain a more detailed history. TCAs are also used for migraine prevention.

INTERVENTIONAL

Nerve blocks have been used for both diagnostic and therapeutic purposes in CeH. As outlined in ICHD-II criteria (Box 24.3; section C-2), the blockade of a cervical structure or its nerve supply is used as one of the diagnostic criteria. Also, in the Cervicogenic Headache International Study Group Criteria classification, anesthetic block is confirmatory (Table 24.2).

Occipital Nerve Blocks (ONBs)

ONBs are effective in treating in a variety of headache disorders, including CeH, migraine, and cluster headaches as well as occipital neuralgia ONBs can be used for acute headache relief and to break an intractable headache cycle when medications have failed or are contraindicated due to comorbid medical conditions. ONBs also are used as a transitional therapy to assist weaning of medications in MOH, as in our patient. Recently, two consensus statements concerning ONBs from the Interventional Procedures Special Interest Section of the American Headache Society were published.[33,34]

Patients who experience relief with ONBs, even if short-lived, should be considered good candidates for radiofrequency (RF) ablation of the occipital nerves or occipital nerve stimulation.

Occipital Neurostimulation

Occipital neurostimulation (ONS) offers the potential for a minimally invasive, low risk, and reversible approach to managing intractable headache disorders (contrary to more invasive and more permanent neuroablative techniques). ONS has been used successfully in the treatment of chronic migraines,[35] as well as in CeH.[36]

Recently, two multicenter, prospective, randomized, blinded controlled studies were published supporting the safety and efficacy of ONS for treatment of intractable chronic migraine.[37,38]

C2–C3 Zygapophysial Joint and Third Occipital Headache

The C2–C3 zygapophyseal joint is innervated by the third occipital nerve, which is the superficial medial branch of the dorsal ramus of C3. Pain stemming from this joint (called *third occipital headache*) is seen in 27% of patients presenting with CeH after whiplash injury.[39] Tenderness over the C2–C3 joint is the only suggestive physical examination finding, and a diagnostic third occipital nerve block is mandatory to confirm the diagnosis.

One report showed that these blocks can lead to significant pain relief in more than 90% of the patients [40] If the diagnostic third occipital nerve blockade is temporarily successful in providing complete pain relief, more invasive procedures like RF neurotomy of the third occipital nerve in appropriate patients may be used. With improved RF techniques, complete relief was obtained in 88% of patients with third occipital headache.[41]

C2–C3 zygapophyseal joint intra-articular steroid injection was effective in one study. [42] On the other hand, Barnsley et al.[43] reported a lack of efficacy of intra-articular steroids for chronic pain stemming from the cervical zygapophyseal joints.

Atlanto-axial (C1–C2) Joint

The lateral atlanto-axial joint, which is innervated by the C2 ventral ramus, may account for 16% of patients with CeH.[44] Clinical presentations suggestive of pain originating from the lateral atlanto-axial joint include occipital or suboccipital pain, focal tenderness over the suboccipital area or over the transverse process of C1, restricted painful rotation of C1 on C2, and pain provocation by passive rotation of C1. The only means of establishing a likely diagnosis is a diagnostic block with intra-articular injection of local anesthetic.[44]

There is no conservative treatment for lateral atlanto-axial joint pain. However, intra-articular steroids are effective in short-term relief of pain originating from the lateral atlanto-axial joint.[45] Long-lasting pain relief may require arthrodesis of the lateral atlanto-axial joint.[46,47]

Cervical Discogenic Pain

C2–C3 provocative discography, but not at the lower levels, can reproduce CeH.[48] RF lesioning was shown to be effective in obtaining some pain relief for a few months in one study.[49] However, cervical disc interventions are not commonly performed because of the potential for serious complications.

In our case, trigger point injections (trapezius and cervical paraspinal muscles)[33] and greater ONB could be very helpful, and this should be considered the first step because these injections can be very helpful and are generally very safe.[50,51]

If our patient responds to the ONB, we will perform a repeated series of blocks. Based on the clinical response, we will proceed with the next step. Most of the time, if a patient emerges from the MOH cycle, a, combination of repeated blocks, appropriate abortive and preventative agents, and physical therapy is sufficient.

If she does not respond to ONB, we will consider diagnostic C1–C2, C2–C3 facet injections or third occipital nerve block, considering the location of her pain and the clinical presentation. RF neurotomy is always an option in this case, based on the response to the diagnostic block and the duration of her pain-free episodes.

REHABILITATION

Physical therapy is the preferred initial treatment because it is noninvasive and may provide long-term improvement for CeH. Physical treatment is better tolerated when initiated with gentle muscle stretching and manual cervical traction. Therapy can be slowly advanced as tolerated to include strengthening and aerobic conditioning.

Some techniques, specifically biofeedback, are very helpful in patients with CeH. The mobilization of the upper cervical joint using different techniques seems to be relatively safe and helpful. Using anesthetic blockade for temporary pain relief may enhance patient tolerance of physical therapy.

Chiropractic manipulation of neck should be used with extreme caution due to possible serious complications, specifically vertebral artery dissection.[52]

In this patient, regular physical therapy 3 days per week for 6 weeks is a good start. After 6 weeks, based on her clinical response, the frequency could be altered. Considering her increased tone in trapezius muscle plus history of anxiety, muscle relaxation techniques and biofeedback should to be a major part of her physical therapy sessions.

In addition to physical therapy, we will recommend participating in a regular exercise program to help reduce her weight. We will consider a nutritional consult as well. Weight loss is a very important step in this patient's management.

SURGERY FOR CEH

There is limited available data on the indications and efficacy of surgical interventions in CeH. In general, surgery is suggested for C2 spinal nerve compression by vascular/ligamentous structures,[53] osteoarthritis of the lateral atlanto-axial joint,[46,47] and upper cervical intervertebral disc pathology.[48,49]

In our case, since her C-spine X-ray and MRI are within normal limits, there is no indication to consider surgery at this point.

With a history of a rear-ended motor vehicle accident in our patient and some decreased range of motion in the examination, the question of whiplash injury is raised. It is not uncommon for patients with preexisting headache syndrome to experience worsening of headache after trauma. However, in this case, with her involvement in litigation relative to motor vehicle collision, compensation in the context of whiplash must be considered.[54] Schrader et al.[55] suggested that chronic symptoms are not usually caused by car accidents. Expectation of disability and attribution of preexisting symptoms to the trauma may be more important determinants for the evolution of late whiplash syndrome.

REFERENCES

1. Choi YC, Kim WJ, Kim CH, Lee MS. A clinical study of chronic headaches: Clinical characteristics and depressive trends in migraine & tension-type headaches. *Yonsei Med J.* 1995;36:508–514.
2. Wober-Bingol C, Wober C, Karwautz A, et al.Tension-type headache in different age groups at two headache centers. *Pain.* 1996;67:53–58.
3. Vincent MB. Headache and neck. *Curr Pain Headache Rep.* 2011;15(4):324–331.
4. Bigal ME, Tsang A, Loder E, Serrano D, Reed ML, Lipton RB. Body mass index and episodic headaches: a population-based study. *Arch Intern Med.* 2007;167(18): 1964–1970.
5. Sjaastad O, Saunte C, Hovdahl H, Breivik H, Grønbaek E. Cervicogenic headache. An hypothesis. *Cephalalgia.* 1983;3(4):249.
6. Sjaastad O, Fredriksen TA, Pfaffenrath V. Cervicogenic headache: diagnostic criteria. *Headache.* 1990;31:725–726.
7. Vincent MB, Luna RA. Cervicogenic headache: a comparison with migraine and tension-type headache. *Cephalalgia.* 1999;19(suppl 25):11–16.
8. Sjaastad O, Bovim G. Cervicogenic headache. The differentiation from common migraine. An overview. *Funct Neurol.* 1991;6(2):93–100.
9. Pfaffenrath V, Dandekar R, Pöllmann W. Cervicogenic headache—the clinical picture, radiological findings and hypotheses on its pathophysiology. *Headache.* 1987;27(9):495.
10. Sjaastad O. Cervicogenic headache: comparison with migraine without aura; Vågåstudy. *Cephalalgia.* 2008;28(suppl 1):18–20.
11. Nilsson N. The prevalence of cervicogenic headache in a random population sample of 20-59 year olds. *Spine* (Phila Pa 1976). 1995;20(17):1884.
12. Sjaastad O, Fredriksen TA. Cervicogenic headache: criteria, classification and epidemiology. *Clin Exp Rheumatol.* 2000;18(2 suppl 19):S3.
13. Haldeman S, Dagenais S. Cervicogenic headaches: a critical review. *Spine J.* 2001;1(1):31.
14. Aaseth K, Grande RB, Kvaerner KJ, Gulbrandsen P, Lundqvist C, Russell MB. Prevalence of secondary chronic headaches in a population-based sample of 30-44-year-old persons. The Akershus study of chronic headache. *Cephalalgia.* 2008;28(7): 705–701.
15. Sjaastad O, Fredriksen T, Pareja JA, Stolt-Nielsen A, Vincent M. Coexistence of cervicogenic headache and migraine without aura. *Funct Neurol.* 1999;14:209–218.
16. Vincent MB, Luna RA. Cervicogenic headache: a comparison with migraine and tension-type headache. *Cephalalgia.* 1999;19(suppl 25):11–16.
17. Bogduk N. The anatomical basis for cervicogenic headache. *J Manipulative Physiol Ther.* 1992;15(1):67.
18. Fredriksen TA, Fougner R, Tangerud A, Sjaastad O. Cervicogenic Headache: radiological investigations concerning head/neck. *Cephalalgia.* 1989;9:1–8.
19. Frese A, Evers S. Biological markers of cervicogenic headache. *Cephalalgia.* 2008;28 (suppl 1):21–23.
20. Harrop JS, Hanna A, Silva MT, Sharan A. Neurological manifestations of cervical spondylosis: an overview of signs, symptoms, and pathophysiology. *Neurosurgery.* 2007;60(1 suppl 1) S14–20.
21. Abbed KM, Coumans JV. Cervical radiculopathy: pathophysiology, presentation, and clinical evaluation [review]. *Neurosurgery.* 2007;60(1 suppl 1):S28–S34.
22. Kirpalani D, Mitra R. Cervical facet joint dysfunction: a review. *Arch Phys Med Rehabil.* 2008;89(4):770–774.
23. Dwyer A, Aprill C, Bogduk N. Cervical zygapophyseal joint pain patterns. I: a study in normal volunteers. *Spine* (Phila Pa 1976). 1990;15(6):453–457.
24. Fukui S, Ohseto K, Shiotani M, Ohno K, Karasawa H, Naganuma Y, Yuda Y. Referred pain distribution of the cervical zygapophyseal joints and cervical dorsal rami. *Pain.* 1996;68(1):79–83.
25. Tepper, S. Medication-overuse headache. *Continuum.* 2012;18(4):807–822.
26. Schnider P, Aull S, Baumgartner C, et al. Long-term outcome of patients with headache and drug abuse after inpatient withdrawal: five-year follow-up. *Cephalalgia.* 1996;16:481–485.
27. Fritsche G, Eberl A, Katsarava Z, Limmroth V, Diener HC. Drug-induced headache: long-term follow-up of withdrawal therapy and persistence of drug misuse. *Eur Neurol.* 2001;45: 229–235.

28. Pini LA, Cicero AF, Sandrini M. Long-term follow-up of patients treated for chronic headache with analgesic overuse. *Cephalalgia*. 2001;21:878–883.
29. Katsarava Z, Limmroth V, Finke M, Diener HC, Fritsche G. Rates and predictors for relapse in medication overuse headache: a 1-year prospective study. *Neurology*. 2003;60:1682–1683.
30. Bigal ME, Rapoport AM, Sheftell FD, Tepper SJ, Lipton RB. Transformed migraine and medication overuse in a tertiary headache centre. Clinical characteristics and treatment outcomes. *Cephalalgia*. 2004;24:483–490.
31. Katsarava Z, Muessig M, Dzagnidze A, Fritsche G, Diener HC, Limmroth V. Medication overuse headache: rates and predictors for relapse in a 4-year prospective study. *Cephalalgia*. 2005;25:12–15.
32. Saper JR, Hamel RL, Lake AE. Medication overuse headache (MOH) is a biobehavioral disorder. *Cephalalgia*. 2005;25:545–546.
33. Ashkenazi A, Blumenfeld A, Napchan U, et al. Interventional Procedures Special Interest Section of the American. Peripheral nerve blocks and trigger point injections in headache management: a systemic review and suggestions for future research. *Headache*. 2010; 50:943–952.
34. Blumenfeld A, Ashkenazi A, Napchan U, et al. Recommendations for the performance of peripheral nerve blocks for headaches—a consensus statement from the American Headache Society Interventional Procedures Section. *Headache*. 2013;53:437–446.
35. Serra G, Marchioretto F. Occipital nerve stimulation for chronic migraine: a randomized trial. *Pain Physician*. 2012;15(3): 245–253.
36. Rodrigo-Royo MD, Azcona JM, Quero J, Lorente MC, Acín P, Azcona J. Peripheral neurostimulation in the management of cervicogenic headache: four case reports. *Neuromodulation*. 2005;8:241–248.
37. Saper JR, Dodick DW, Silberstein SD, McCarville S, Sun M, Goadsby PJ, ONSTIM Investigators. Occipital nerve stimulation for the treatment of intractable chronic migraine headache: ONSTIM feasibility study. *Cephalalgia*. 2011;31(3):271–285.
38. Silberstein SD, Dodick DW, Saper J, et al. Safety and efficacy of peripheral nerve stimulation of the occipital nerves for the management of chronic migraine: results from a randomized, multicenter, double-blinded, controlled study. *Cephalalgia*. 2012;32(16):1165–1179.
39. Lord S, Barnsley L, Wallis B, Bogduk N. Third occipital headache: a prevalence study. *J Neurol Neurosurg Psychiatr*. 1994;57:1187–1190.
40. Zhou L, Hud-Shakoor Z, Hennessey C, Ashkenazi A. Upper cervical facet joint and spinal rami blocks for the treatment of cervicogenic headache. *Headache*. 2010;50(4):657–663.
41. Govind J, King W, Baily B. Bogduk N. Radiofrequency neurotomy for the treatment of third occipital headache. *J Neurol Neurosurg Psychiatr*. 2003;74:88–93.
42. Slipman CW, Lipetz JS, Plastara CT, et al. Therapeutic zygapophyseal joint injections for headache emanating from the C2-3 joint. *Am J Phys Med Rehabil*. 2001; 80:182–188.
43. Barnsley L, Lord SM, Wallis BJ, et al. Lack of effect of intraarticular corticosteroids for chronic pain in the cervical zygapophyseal joints. *N Engl J Med*. 1994; 330:1047–1050.
44. Aprill C, Axinn MJ, Bogduk N. Occipital headaches stemming from the lateral atlanto-axial (C1-2) joint. *Cephalalgia*. 2002;22(1):15–22.
45. Narouze SN, Casanova J, Mekhail N. The longitudinal effectiveness of lateral atlanto-axial intra-articular steroid injection in the management of cervicogenic headache. *Pain Med*. 2007;8:184–188.
46. Schaeren S, Jeanneret B. Atlantoaxial osteoarthritis: case series and review of the literature. *Eur Spine J*. 2005;14(5):501.
47. Ghanayem AJ, Leventhal M, Bohlman HH. Osteoarthrosis of the atlantoaxial joints- long term follow up after treatment with arthrodesis. *J Bone Joint Surg* (Am). 1996;78:1300–1307.
48. Grubb SA, Kelly CK. Cervical discography: clinical implications from 12 years of experience. *Spine*. 2000;25:1382–1389.
49. Blume HG. Cervicogenic headaches: radiofrequency neurotomy and the cervical disc and fusion. *Clin Exp Rheumatol*. 2000;18:S53–S58.
50. Naja ZM, El-Rajab M, Al-Tannir MA, Ziade FM, Tawfik OM. Occipital nerve blockade for cervicogenic headache: a double-blind randomized controlled clinical trial. *Pain Pract*. 2006;6(2):89–95.
51. Tobin J, Flitman S. Headache. Occipital nerve blocks: when and what to inject? *Headache*. 2009;49(10):1521–1533.
52. Rothwell DM, Bondy SJ, Williams JI. Chiropractic manipulation and stroke: a population-based case-control study. *Stroke*. 2001;32(5):1054–1060.
53. Pikus HJ, Phillips JM. Characteristics of patients successfully treated for cervicogenic headache by surgical decompression of the second cervical root. *Headache*. 1995;35(10):621.
54. Awerbuch MS.Whiplash in Australia: illness or injury? *Med J Aust*. 1992;157(3):193–196.
55. Schrader H, Obelieniene D, Bovim G, et al. Natural evolution of late whiplash syndrome outside the medicolegal context. *Lancet*. 1996;347(9010):1207–1211.

25.

COMPLEX REGIONAL PAIN SYNDROME (CRPS)

Salim M. Hayek, Binit J. Shah, Mehul J. Desai, Howard S. Smith, and Thomas C. Chelimsky

CASE PRESENTATION

A 61-year-old woman falls and sustains a left wrist Colle's fracture. She is treated with short-acting opioid analgesics and immobilization at a local emergency room. Over the following weeks, she complains of increasing pain, burning in nature, and a tight feeling inside the cast. She notes swelling, discoloration, and sweating in the left hand with decreased ability to move all digits. Removing the cast 6 weeks later does not alleviate her symptoms; radiologic studies show good alignment and adequate healing. She is noted to have decreased range of motion (ROM), not only of the left wrist, but also of the fingers. She is treated with hydrocodone/APAP 5/500 mg PO q6h PRN, naproxen 500 mg PO BID, and cyclobenzaprine 10 mg PO TID and referred for more occupational therapy. Pain persists, and, after another 6 weeks, the patient is referred to the Interdisciplinary Pain Medicine Clinic.

Past medical history is significant for migraine, asthma, and hypertension.

Past surgical history: left total knee arthroplasty.

Current medications include albuterol inhaler and lisinopril.

On examination: the left hand is swollen, discolored, mottled, and noticeably warmer than the right hand (Figure 25.1). Fingernails are noticeably longer on the left hand than the right. A fine tremor is noted only in the left hand. The patient is reluctant to move the hand or wrist. A marked decrease in the ROM is noted, and finger tapping is severely impaired. No allodynia is noted, but deep tissue hyperalgesia is observed in a nondermatomal pattern up to the mid-arm level.

A diagnosis of complex regional pain syndrome (CRPS) type 1 is established.

QUESTIONS

1. What is the definition and history of CRPS?
2. What is the pathophysiology of CRPS?
3. What is the incidence of CRPS?
4. What is the natural history of CRPS?
5. What are the clinical manifestations of CRPS, how is it diagnosed, and what are its subtypes?
6. How is CRPS managed?
   a. Rehabilitation
   b. Pharmacological management
   c. Interventional procedures
   d. Psychiatric interventions
7. In the event of surgery, how is the CRPS patient managed perioperatively?

WHAT IS THE DEFINITION AND HISTORY OF CRPS?

The entity now known as CRPS was first described in the medical literature in the late 1700s by the British surgeon Percivall Potts who was the first to note "atrophy and burning pain in an injured extremity."[1] This same condition was noted by Denmark who, in 1813, suggested that amputation may be a treatment for this condition.[2] Despite observations that predated him by decades, there was no notion that this was a distinct clinical syndrome. It was during the American Civil War that Army neurologist S. Weir Mitchell introduced the term "erythromelalgia" in 1864, before settling on the name "causalgia" in 1867 (from the Greek *kausos* for heat and *algos* for pain) to describe the ongoing color changes, swelling, and burning type of pain experienced by soldiers following major peripheral nerve injury.[3] Even then, Mitchell noted the strong association between emotional state and pain: "every strong moral emotion made him worse—anger or disappointment expressing themselves cruelly in the aching limb."[4] In 1900, Sudeck described cases of extremity pain, redness, and osteoporotic changes as "Sudeck's atrophy."[5] Based on the clinical findings on a series of 57 patients, Evans intuited the role of

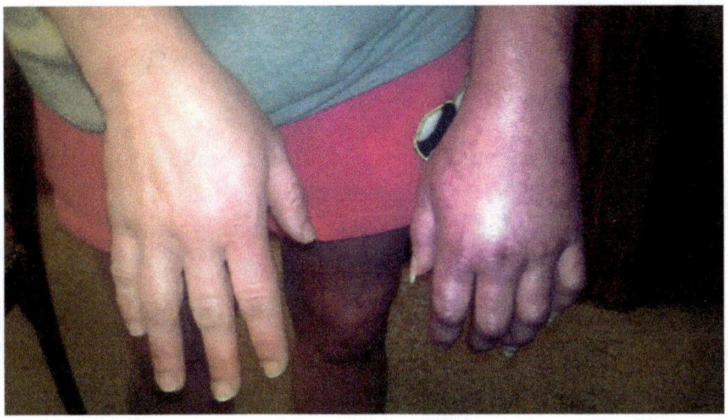

Figure 25.1 Appearance of the patient's left hand upon presentation to the Interdisciplinary Pain Medicine Clinic.

sympathetic nervous system dysfunction and coined the term "reflex sympathetic dystrophy" (RSD) in 1947.[6] The French surgeon Rene Leriche took this evolving concept of sympathetic dysfunction to the next logical step and showed that sympathectomy resulted in dramatic pain relief.[7] Although knowledge and interest in causalgia and RSD was expanding, research efforts were hampered by the lack of a widely accepted definition and homogeneous patient samples. The term *complex regional pain syndrome* (CRPS) was adopted by the International Association for the Study of Pain (IASP) in 1994 to replace older terms of RSD and causalgia.[8]

WHAT IS THE PATHOPHYSIOLOGY OF CRPS?

The etiopathogenesis of CRPS remains unclear. Two main mechanisms have been proposed: inflammatory (in particular, neurogenic inflammation) and neuropathic (with dysfunction of the somatic and autonomic nervous systems). Various modifying factors have been proposed to contribute to the pathogenesis of CRPS: genetic susceptibility, environmental factors resulting in facilitated neuroinflammation, alterations in the sympathetic nervous system responsiveness with up-regulation of α-adrenergic receptors, and central nervous system reorganization. Additionally, hypoxia and psychological factors have been implicated as potential contributors to CRPS pathogenesis. Recent implications of the immune system and of the cholinergic system raise intriguing prospects of an autoimmune etiology of CRPS.

In 1900, Paul Sudeck, a German surgeon, was the first to suggest an inflammatory etiology for the condition.[5] However, systemic markers of inflammation such as white blood count, C-reactive protein, antigen titers, and sedimentation rate are, for the most part, within normal limits in CRPS patients, suggesting that inflammation in CRPS is not a systemic event.[9] Instead, local neurogenic inflammation, a consequence of injury to peripheral tissue, appears to be exaggerated in CRPS. In response to trauma, hydrogen ions, adenosine triphosphate (ATP), serotonin, acetylcholine, and other mediators are released from damaged endothelial cells and platelets. These activate peripheral nociceptors that, in turn, through a local axon reflex arc, release local inflammatory mediators including substance P and calcitonin gene-related peptide (CGRP). These latter substances cause histamine release from mast cells and increase vascular permeability, thus triggering an inflammatory cascade and the formation and release of prostaglandins, cytokines, growth factors, tumor necrosis factor (TNF)-α, complement factors C3a and C5a, platelet-activating factor, neutrophil chemotactic factor, fibrinopeptides, and leukotrienes leading to increased vascular permeability and migration of local leukocytes into the interstitial space.[10] Although most patients heal after peripheral injury, neurogenic inflammation is more intense in CRPS patients, persists longer, and affects a wider area. Local elevation in inflammatory mediators has been demonstrated in studies of interstitial fluids from artificial blisters obtained by applying suction cups to CRPS-affected extremities.[11,12] CGRP levels were found to be systemically elevated in some CRPS patients,[9] but cerebrospinal fluid levels of inflammatory mediators were no different between CRPS patients with dystonia and controls.[13] However, pain and hyperalgesia were independent of increased neuropeptide concentration in chronic CRPS.[14–16] Interestingly, the vasoconstrictive neuropeptide endothelin-1 was found to be significantly increased in blister fluid in patients with early chronic CRPS when compared to the contralateral extremity, whereas nitric oxide levels were decreased.[17]

A growing body of literature suggests a role for the immune system in the pathophysiology of CRPS. A number of reports have shown an association of human leukocyte antigen (HLA) alleles with CRPS.[18–22] Although not diagnostic of an autoimmune process, a number of autoimmune conditions have HLA associations. Significantly, autoantibodies to a surface epitope in autonomic neurons, likely a cholinergic receptor, have been identified in a significant proportion of CRPS patients,[23] suggesting that CRPS could be an autoimmune disorder. Another preliminary study also identified autoantibodies in CRPS patients.[24] Furthermore, a double-blind, placebo-controlled randomized trial, albeit with small numbers of patients, demonstrated efficacy of intravenous immunoglobulin (IVIG) over saline in long-standing CRPS patients.[25] A randomized controlled trial (RCT) comparing 40 mg prednisolone to 20 mg piroxicam in CRPS patients following stroke revealed significant improvement in 83% of patients receiving steroids at 1 month compared to 17% in the piroxicam group. Additionally, the magnitude of improvement in pain scores was 6.47 for the prednisolone group compared to 0.47 for the piroxicam group.[26] Further support for an inflammatory role in the pathogenesis of CRPS comes from open-label reports involving the use of anti-TNF-α antibodies[27,28] and thalidomide,[29,30] an anti-TNF-α agent, in the treatment of CRPS patients. In a large epidemiological study from the Netherlands, the use of angiotensin-converting enzyme (ACE) inhibitors was associated with increased risk of CRPS. The authors hypothesized that ACE inhibitors alter the neuroinflammatory response in these patients by inhibiting the degradation of bradykinin and substance P and up-regulating the bradykinin (B_2) receptor.[31] Additionally, CRPS was found to be strongly associated with migraine and with asthma, both conditions sharing common neurogenic inflammation and increased mast cell activity with CRPS.[32] Hence, clearly, a significant role is played by the immune and inflammatory systems in the initiation and maintenance of CRPS.

On the other hand, neuropathic pain features are present in a large percentage of CRPS patients. Supportive evidence for neuropathic processes in CRPS patients comes from punch biopsies that showed a 29% reduction in small fibers in CRPS-affected limbs compared to nonaffected limbs,[33] as well as histological and immunohistochemistry markers of neuropathic pain in amputated limbs of two CRPS patients.[34] Necrosis and dysfunction of small-diameter nerve fibers may occur consequent to TNF-α and other cytokine release locally, which also affects sympathetic cutaneous vasoconstrictors.[33,34] Thus, an association may exist between the inflammatory and neuropathic factors involved in CRPS. Recent data suggest that an underactive peripheral effect of the cholinergic system may play a role in the pathogenesis of CRPS, partly by leading to overproduction of TNF-α. Peripheral acetylcholine release is mediated through immune cells (B cells, T cells, dendritic cells, neutrophils), keratinocytes, and vascular endothelial cells.[35–37] The recent finding of autoantibodies against a surface-binding inducible cholinergic autoantigen in 30–40% of CRPS patients warrants further study into an autoimmune etiology of CRPS(Kohr et al., 2009).[23]

The patient appears to display features of neuropathic pain and inflammation by history and physical examination. Additionally, her past medical history is significant for migraine and asthma, both conditions associating with CRPS. Furthermore, she is on an ACE inhibitor for hypertension, a factor associated also with CRPS development.

WHAT IS THE INCIDENCE OF CRPS?

To date, there have been only two population-based epidemiological studies of CRPS. In 2003, Sandroni et al. found that CRPS was rare, with an incidence of 5.46 cases per 100,000 and a high rate of spontaneous resolution.[38] A larger, more recent population-based study from the Netherlands using IASP diagnostic criteria found an incidence of 16.8 cases per 100,000, suggesting that CRPS was much less rare.[39] With an estimated U.S. population of 300 million, this suggests more than 50,000 new cases of CRPS annually. Although differences in incidence were noted, both studies found that CRPS is more common in females, had the highest incidence in the 50–70 age range, that fractures and sprains were the most common precipitating events, and that CRPS more commonly affected the upper extremities.[40] CRPS develops in 18% of patients after a wrist fracture and in up to 31% after ankle fractures.[41–43] The upper limb is more often involved, although the reasons are unclear. Schmalbruch showed that upper limb nerves contain a larger number of sympathetic fibers and a higher fiber density, and this morphologic difference may partly explain the difference.[44] Although fracture and sprain have consistently been found to be inciting events, in approximately 10% of patients there is no identifiable history of injury.[39,45]

The most common sign and symptom was swelling (in >90%) and color changes (in >70%), whereas sensory abnormalities were the least common clinical finding (~19%). In the vast majority of cases, CRPS remains confined to one limb, with spreading occurring in only 4–10% of cases.[38,46] Although once thought of as rare, movement disorders (including loss of voluntary control, bradykinesia, dystonia, myoclonus, and tremor) occur in approximately 25% of patients with CRPS, with prevalence increasing as disease duration lengthens.[22,45,47,48] Dystonia is the most common of these, with some evidence indicating female gender as a risk factor.[48,49]

Although there is certainly no "typical" CRPS patient, this case demonstrates many of the more commonly seen factors. Her age, race, and gender are in line with those who are most commonly affected. Females are affected 2–5 times more commonly than males,[45,49] and the overwhelming majority are Caucasian.[50,51] Our patient is a postmenopausal female, who may be at increased risk of developing CRPS after injury.[39,52] In addition, she has a movement disorder (tremor), which occurs more often in female patients.

WHAT IS THE NATURAL HISTORY OF CRPS?

The clinical presentation and outcomes of CRPS are varied and may be difficult to accurately predict. Galer and colleagues published the results of 31 CRPS patient self-report questionnaires. At a mean of 3.3 years from symptom onset, a majority reported no overall improvement or worsening of symptoms over time.[53] Schwartzman and coworkers in a retrospective review of 656 CRPS patients demonstrated no spontaneous remission of symptoms in any of the patients and suggested that CRPS is a progressive disease. At 1 year, the majority of the signs and symptoms were well developed and demonstrated only moderate increases with disease duration.[54] De Mos et al. reported that at 5.8 years after initiating injury, CRPS patients continued to demonstrate higher symptom and sign prevalence than reference patients with the same precipitating injury.[55] Furthermore, these rates did not seem to decrease significantly with longer duration since disease onset; 64% of patients still fulfilled IASP criteria at an average of 5.8 years after initial injury. These authors also reported the impact of the disease on the ability to work; 31% were permanently incapable of work, and 28% required work accommodations.[55] This contrasted with an Olmstead County, Minnesota-based work by Sandroni et al. which reported job restrictions in only 11% of cases.[38]

CRPS was hypothesized to have three sequential stages: an early inflammatory stage, followed by a dystrophic stage and a late atrophic stage.[56] However, no evidence for sequential temporal staging for CRPS patients could be ascertained in cluster analyses of 113 patients with CRPS.[57] Instead, Veldman and colleagues, in a prospective study of 829 CRPS patients, suggested that CRPS may be divided according to clinical presentation into warm and cold subtypes.[45] Skin temperature is increased with reddish discoloration in warm CRPS; blue discoloration with cool, shiny, and thin skin is observed in cold CRPS. The vast majority of patients at presentation had warm CRPS, and only 13% of patients presented with cold CRPS, suggesting an important inflammatory role.[45] Cold CRPS type 1 patients exhibited poorer clinical pain outcomes and persistent signs of central sensitization, correlating with disease progression, 8 years after diagnosis.[58] De Mos also reported worse outcome in patients with upper extremity involvement, precipitating injuries other than fracture, and cold CRPS.[55]

Even though CRPS involves typically one extremity at onset, spread has been described in CRPS patients and may involve ipsilateral, contralateral, or diagonal spread.[59,60] A recent tertiary-center study from the Netherlands examined 185 CRPS patients (160 females). More than one limb was affected by CRPS in 48% of patients, although CRPS started in one limb in 88% of patients. Spread of CRPS symptoms often occurs spontaneously, and contralateral spread is twice as likely as ipsilateral spread; diagonal spread is rare and usually the result of a new trauma. Patients with CRPS in multiple limbs were on average 7 years younger and more often had movement disorders. Patterns of spread implicate spinal cord and/or supraspinal mechanisms rather than systemic mechanisms.[60]

Given her recent history of injury, our patient is clearly in the early stages of CRPS. Her presentation of a "warm" extremity is a good prognostic sign, and this should be discussed with her. Although the focus of treatment is necessarily her left hand, high suspicion for spread should be entertained, and the patient educated to report any possible symptoms in her right hand so that early and aggressive treatment can be initiated.

WHAT ARE THE CLINICAL MANIFESTATIONS OF CRPS, HOW IS IT DIAGNOSED, AND WHAT ARE ITS SUBTYPES?

Clinical manifestations of CRPS involve a triad of sensory, autonomic, and motor signs and symptoms.

Sensory signs and symptoms characterized by intense pain and hyperesthesia are the hallmark of CRPS.[53,61] The pain, characterized as aching, burning, pricking, or shooting, is localized deep in the somatic tissue.[62] Evoked abnormal sensations of hyperalgesia, predominantly to mechanical stimuli or upon joint movement, and allodynia are frequently present.[61,62] Sensory deficits are common.[63,64] Hemisensory impairment with decreased temperature and pinprick sensation ipsilateral to the affected limb has been observed.[63]

Swelling, color and temperature changes, and sweating abnormalities consistent with autonomic changes have been reported.[61,65] These are often exacerbated by physical loading, painful stimuli, and temperature changes. Temperature asymmetry of up to 1°C between affected and unaffected limbs is often observed. Sweating abnormalities are observed in 59% of patients.[66]

Motor dysfunction in CRPS includes weakness, decreased ROM, tremor, dystonia, and myoclonus. Grip strength is often affected.[67] Early in disease, joint effusion affects ROM; later contracture and fibrosis are the culprits.[62] Twenty-four to sixty percent of patients exhibit tremor.[61,66] Dystrophic changes include changes in nail and hair growth, fibrosis of the skin, hyperkeratosis, and thin glossy skin.[65] Fifty-six to sixty-one percent of patients have myofascial components.[68,69] This is more common in the upper extremity, with a direct relationship to duration of symptoms.[68]

The diagnosis of CRPS is made purely on clinical grounds. A plethora of tests have been proposed to diagnose CRPS, however, none has clinically meaningful sensitivity or specificity. In 1994, the IASP taxonomy committee adopted *complex regional pain syndrome* (CRPS) as the newer nomenclature replacing older terms (RSD and causalgia) and established the diagnostic criteria for CRPS. Two types of CRPS were described with identical diagnostic criteria, with the exception of type 2 having the added criterion of evidence of identifiable nerve injury (Box 25.1). Hence, CRPS type 1 is

Box 25.1 ORIGINAL IASP DIAGNOSTIC CRITERIA FOR CRPS

CRPS Type 1(Reflex Sympathetic Dystrophy)

1. The presence of an initiating noxious event, or a cause of immobilization
2. Continuing pain, allodynia, or hyperalgesia with which the pain is disproportionate to any inciting event
3. Evidence at some time of edema, changes in skin blood flow, or abnormal sudomotor activity in the region of the pain
4. This diagnosis is excluded by the existence of conditions that would otherwise account for the degree of pain and dysfunction.
   - Criteria 2–4 must be satisfied

CRPS Type 2 (Causalgia)

1. The presence of continuing pain, allodynia, or hyperalgesia after a nerve injury, not necessarily limited to the distribution of the injured nerve
2. Evidence at some time of edema, changes in skin blood flow, or abnormal sudomotor activity in the region of the pain
3. This diagnosis is excluded by the existence of conditions that would otherwise account for the degree of pain and dysfunction
   - All three criteria must be satisfied

Adapted from Merskey H. *Classification of Chronic Pain: Description of Chronic Pain Syndromes and Definition of Pain Terms.* Seattle: IASP Press; 1994; Stanton-Hicks M., Janig W, Hassenbusch S, Haddox JD, Boas R, Wilson P. Reflex sympathetic dystrophy: changing concepts and taxonomy. *Pain.* 1995;63:127–133.

the newer nomenclature replacing RSD, and CRPS type 2 replaces causalgia.[8,70] These criteria were soon criticized, however, for being ambiguous (especially the expression "at some time") and overinclusive, thus possibly leading to overdiagnosis of CRPS.[61,71,72] Indeed, although diagnostic sensitivity using these criteria was very high (98%), specificity was quite low (36%), and a CRPS diagnosis could be made correctly in as few as 40% of patients using these criteria.[61,71]

Principal component factor analysis suggested that separating sudomotor and vasomotor manifestations from sensory symptoms, along with inclusion of motor manifestations, would potentially improve diagnostic utility of the criteria.[61,71] In addition to clinical symptoms, signs of sensory, vasomotor, sudomotor, and motor disturbance as documented by physical examination were thought to be of further diagnostic value.[61,73] Requiring three of four symptoms and two of four signs resulted in the best compromise, with respectable sensitivity (0.85) and specificity (0.69) for diagnosing CRPS clinically.[74] These have become known since as the *Budapest clinical criteria*, in reference to the meeting location at which consensus over these criteria was reached. Patients not meeting these criteria but thought to have CRPS as the most likely diagnosis were suggested to fall into a CRPS-NOS subtype. More recently, Harden and colleagues validated the Budapest criteria with data from a multinational study of 113 CRPS type 1 patients and 47 non-CRPS neuropathic pain patients. Applying the original IASP criteria (Box 25.1)[70] to this population resulted again in outstanding sensitivity (1.00) but poor specificity (0.41). However, applying the Budapest criteria (Box 25.2)[74] retained exceptional sensitivity (0.99) while greatly improving the specificity (0.68).[75] To increase specificity further for research purposes, requiring four of four symptoms and two of four signs resulted in the best permutation for improved specificity while retaining acceptable sensitivity (sensitivity values of 0.70[74] and 0.78[75]; specificity values of 0.94[74] and 0.79.[75] In 2012, the IASP adopted the Budapest criteria as the new diagnostic criteria for CRPS (Box 25.2).

Box 25.2 **NEW IASP CLINICAL DIAGNOSTIC CRITERIA (BUDAPEST) FOR CRPS**

i. Continuing pain, which is disproportionate to any inciting event
ii. Must report at least one symptom in three of the four following categories:
   1. Sensory: reports of hyperesthesia and/or allodynia
   2. Vasomotor: reports of temperature asymmetry and/or skin color changes and/or skin color asymmetry
   3. Sudomotor/edema: reports of edema and/or sweating changes and/or sweating asymmetry
   4. Motor/trophic: reports of decreased ROM and/or motor dysfunction (weakness, tremor, dystonia) and/or trophic changes (hair, nail, skin)
iii. Must display at least one sign at time of evaluation in two or more of the following categories:
   1. Sensory: evidence of hyperalgesia (to pinprick) and/or allodynia (to light touch and/or deep somatic pressure and/or joint movement)
   2. Vasomotor: evidence of temperature asymmetry and/or skin color changes and/or asymmetry
   3. Sudomotor/edema: evidence of edema and/or sweating changes and/or sweating asymmetry
   4. Motor/trophic: evidence of decreased ROM and/or motor dysfunction (weakness, tremor, dystonia) and/or trophic changes (hair, nail, skin)
iv. There is no other diagnosis that better explains the signs and symptoms

Adapted from Harden RN, Bruehl S, Stanton-Hicks M, Wilson PR. Proposed new diagnostic criteria for complex regional pain syndrome. *Pain Med.* 2007;8:326–331.

HOW IS CRPS MANAGED?

Utilizing the original IASP diagnostic criteria, our patient shows an initiating noxious event (left wrist fracture) followed by immobilization (casting), continuing pain, changes in skin blood flow (mottling of the hand, edema [swollen hand]), and no other explanation for her symptoms. Considering the new diagnostic (Budapest) criteria, the patient reports swelling, color asymmetry, and decreased ROM, and, on examination, swelling, changes in skin color, and tremor (motor dysfunction) is evident. She therefore qualifies for a diagnosis of CRPS under the original and the new IASP criteria.

REHABILITATION

At its core, management of CRPS centers on the concept of functional restoration. Increased use and subsequent normalization of use of the affected extremity is the goal of most therapies. To this end, rehabilitation is at the core of CRPS management. The principle of functional restoration is based on an algorithmic progression from very basic active movements toward weight-bearing, depending on the affected extremity. This progresses to movements that involve more active load bearing along with gradual desensitization to sensory stimuli while managing edema to optimize ROM.[76,77] It is imperative for the provider to demonstrate flexibility throughout this process; accessing adequate analgesia and providing encouragement and education may ensure greater success with physical therapy methods. Furthermore, selectively utilizing other therapies (i.e., pain management interventions and/or psychological interventions) may provide opportunities for progress (Figure 25.2). Occupational, physical, vocational, and recreational therapists may play a role in implementing a course of functional restoration.

OCCUPATIONAL THERAPY

Ideally, the occupational therapist takes a leading role in the functional restoration process.[78] It is essential to evaluate baseline function at the onset of any therapeutic

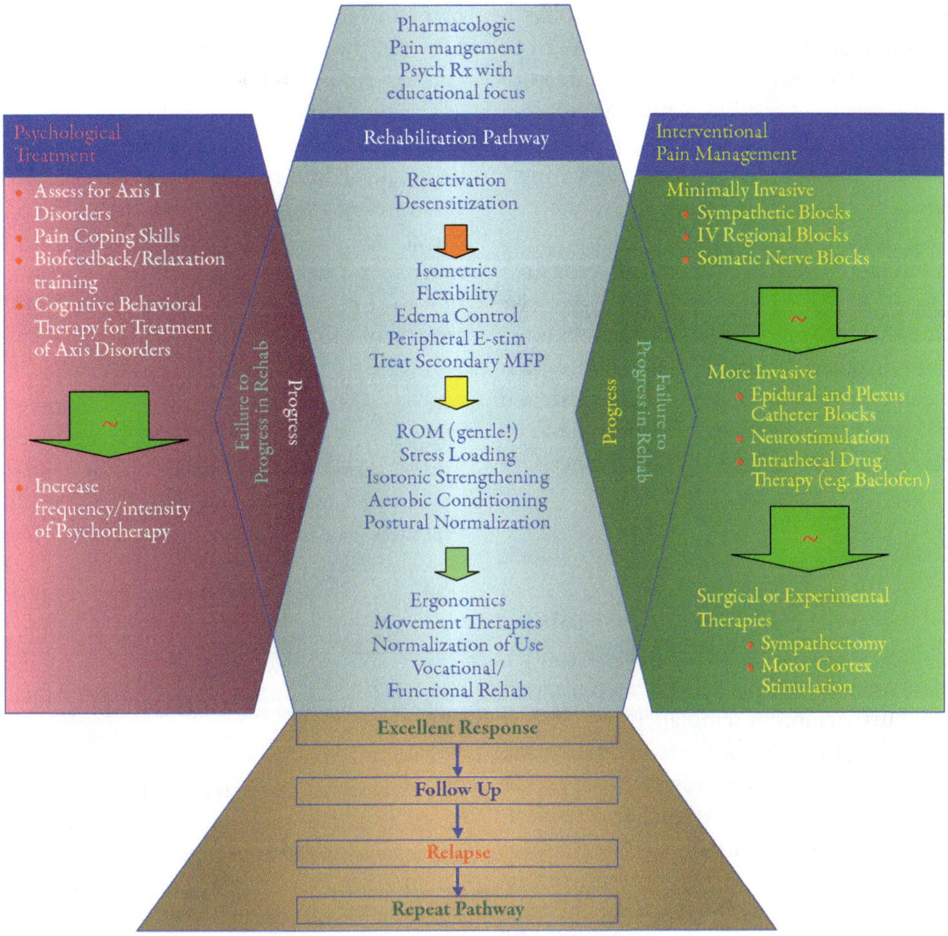

Figure 25.2 Complex regional pain syndrome (CRPS) management centers on a structured rehabilitation pathway. Failure to progress in the rehabilitation path because of pain invokes the use of interventional procedures, while failure to progress due to psychiatric issues should prompt psychological interventions. Adapted from Stanton-Hicks MD, Burton AW, Bruehl SP, et al. An updated interdisciplinary clinical pathway for CRPS: report of an expert panel. *Pain Pract.* 2002;2:1–16.

intervention. This assessment should include active ROM, edema, coordination/dexterity, skin/vasomotor changes, pain/sensation, and use of the extremity during activities of daily living[79] (ADLs). Treatment centers on minimizing edema while normalizing sensation. Encouraging normal positioning and decreasing muscle guarding may combine to increase functional use and promote independence for the patient. Some cases of CRPS may necessitate the use of functional splinting to promote circulation and nutrition and to facilitate more normal tissue length/positioning during the rehabilitation process.[80] The initial approach to therapeutic management includes minimizing edema, initiating gentle active movement, and beginning desensitization.[76] Next, a stress loading program is initiated to improve active movement and compression of the affected joints.[81] Initially, this may result in transient worsening within days; however, a decrease in pain and swelling should become evident. Stress loading consists of two principles: scrubbing and carrying. Scrubbing consists of moving the affected extremity in a back-and-forth motion while bearing weight through the extremity.[81] The amount of weight placed through the affected extremity and the duration of the activity are gradually increased. Carrying is the second component in stress loading. Increased weight-bearing can be accomplished with verbal/physical cueing or by having the patient carry a weighted object on the affected side. Loading can also be facilitated by engaging the patient in activities that promote weight shifting/balance (i.e., ball toss) or by placing the nonaffected foot onto a small footstool during static standing tasks. Once the patient is actively engaged in an edema management and stress loading program, treatment can progress toward increasing functional use of the extremity. As the pain and edema decrease, the patient will be better able to tolerate and participate in active ROM, coordination/dexterity, and strengthening tasks.[76]

PHYSICAL THERAPY

The goal of physical therapy is gentle exercise to improve ROM and flexibility to the patient's tolerance. Often, overly aggressive strengthening and stabilization programs may result in significant setbacks adversely impacting patient progress and trust in the therapeutic plan. Therefore, the therapist's role in this setting is one of balance; avoiding inactivity while also guarding against overuse. The goal of the exercise program is a gradual increase in strength and flexibility while emphasizing weight-bearing. Active or active-assisted exercises can be accomplished with a variety of devices that assist in introducing weight-bearing in a stepwise fashion. Other approaches include mat exercises and aquatic therapy. These options provide similar goals to land-based therapies while providing a break from land-based exercises in a setting where most of the exercises can be replicated while combating boredom and over-repetition. Myofascial pain is present in the affected limb in the majority of patients with advanced CRPS. Aggressive treatment of myofascial pain may require hands-on techniques including massage and myofascial release.[69,82] Modalities that are often utilized include electrostimulation, ultrasound, and contrast baths. These techniques have a relative dearth of evidence for use but are anecdotally effective.[83,84] Lymph massage may be helpful in some cases to decrease the edema.

RECREATIONAL THERAPY

Recreational therapy may provide a bridge to CRPS patients to initiate increased mobility by means of enjoyable activities. Often, the use of adaptive modified equipment is required to re-engage the patient. Furthermore, a semblance of control is returned to the patient, thus allowing for the freedom to make decisions. Recreational therapy may also provide the opportunity to reinforce goals set during occupational and physical therapy in real-world or pleasurable situations. Creativity is the hallmark of recreational therapy, providing subtle direction with regards to treatment goals while providing a distraction for patients. All in all, recreational therapy in a CRPS treatment session may be crucial to combat kinesophobia and encourage increased movement. Most importantly, recreational therapy can assist patients in making a smooth transition back into a balanced leisure lifestyle.[79]

VOCATIONAL REHABILITATION

The goal of vocational therapy is to intervene early to coordinate future efforts with members of the treatment team. Working to assess and simulate work activities while understanding the patient's prior job description and requirements is integral to guiding the patient back to work. Return to work is the apex of functional restoration, requiring careful coordination of vocation retraining and possible work hardening while operating within the work capacity of the patient. Furthermore, assisting the patient in negotiating a myriad of obstacles, including employer resistance due to periods of long unemployment or reluctance to employ workers with chronic pain, medicolegal issues, workplace adaption, and adequate educational background. Vocational counseling is also important in helping the patient understand the benefits of work.[79]

EVOLVING THERAPIES

One of the more promising therapies currently under investigation for use in CRPS is mirror therapy. This technique previously demonstrated promising efficacy in the setting of phantom limb pain, and, due to the similarities shared between these clinical states, mirror therapy has been recently adapted for use in CRPS.[85–87]

In summation, an interdisciplinary therapeutic approach with careful coordination between appropriate therapists may be ideal for implementing an algorithmic approach to functional restoration for patients with CRPS, particularly given the complexities of this disease state.[77] In general, therapists must seek a balance between too little activity and overexertion to continue to guide the patient's transition through the treatment spectrum.

> At this juncture, our patient has been essentially immobilized for 12 weeks, 6 weeks of which were spent in a cast. An appropriate initial therapeutic plan would include desensitization with contrast baths, manual tactile means, and the utilization of varying textures (i.e., fabrics). Furthermore, with regards to the patient's hand swelling, mild retrograde massage should be considered. Additionally, gentle active-assisted ROM of the hand and fingers should be part of the initial therapy prescription.

PHARMACOLOGIC MANAGEMENT OF CRPS

Pharmacologic approaches to the treatment of CRPS are vitally important and tend to be utilized in an overwhelming majority of patients with CRPS. In 2004, Burton et al. published a survey largely of practicing anesthesiology pain specialists who, on average, treat 14.9 (SD = 16.8) CRPS patients per month.[88] These providers utilized pharmacotherapy as an initial treatment 85% of the time.[88]

There are few RCTs of pharmacologic agents performed in CRPS patients. Most published CRPS pharmacologic studies are small in scale, noncontrolled, or have only been reported in poster form at meetings. Despite these obstacles, there is a myriad of pharmacologic agents that have been used to treat CRPS.[89] Two reviews on evidence-based guidelines have been published recently.[90,91]

ANTIEPILEPTIC DRUGS (AEDS)

One of the first literature reports to describe the efficacy of gabapentin was a case series of CRPS patients.[92] In a randomized, blinded trial in 58 patients with CRPS, gabapentin had a mild effect on pain.[93] In the largest placebo-controlled trial of gabapentin that included CRPS patients (85 of the 305 participants studied), gabapentin was shown to cause a significant reduction in pain compared to placebo.[94] Of note, although there was a 1.5-point improvement in pain with the gabapentin group, there was only a 0.5-point difference (0–10 point pain scale) between the placebo and gabapentin groups. This is less a reflection of lack of efficacy with gabapentin (or many other antineuropathic pain medicines) and more a testament to the power of placebo. In a placebo crossover study of gabapentin, van de Vusse et al. noted a mild benefit with gabapentin as well as a reduction in mechanical sensory deficits.[93]

Carbamazepine is an older AED indicated for trigeminal neuralgia that has been studied in CRPS in an RCT (seven of the 38 neuropathic pain patients studied had CRPS). Administration of 600 mg/d of carbamazepine over 8 days resulted in significant pain reductions compared with placebo.[95]

Sodium Channel Blockers

Intravenous lidocaine has strong sodium channel-blocking properties and has demonstrated efficacy in several uncontrolled studies of neuropathic pain and CRPS.[96,97] Pain severity and patient age may potentially identify those most likely to respond to IV lidocaine, with each decade of advancing age increasing the odds of being a lidocaine responder by 36%.[96] It is also conceivable that a "heavy" pain quality may identify patients with enhanced lidocaine response.[96] For example, Wallace et al. found that IV lidocaine reduced spontaneous pain and specific characteristics of evoked pain.[98]

IV lidocaine was administered in an escalating dose schedule to 49 severely affected CRPS patients in a monitored setting continuously over 5 days. Evaluation of pain parameters and other signs and symptoms of CRPS were obtained during the infusion and at 1, 3, and 6 months following therapy.[99] The majority of patients demonstrated a significant decrease in pain parameters and other symptoms and signs of CRPS. The pain reduction lasted an average of 3 months. Lidocaine may be particularly effective for thermal and mechanical allodynia. Intravenous lidocaine administration titrated to 5 mg/L demonstrated a significant decrease in mechanical and thermal allodynia for 3 months, lessened associated inflammatory components of CRPS, and only minimal side effects and no severe complications.[99]

Bisphosphonates

Bisphosphonates (e.g., pamidronate, clodronate, alendronate) inhibit bone resorption and have demonstrated efficacy in the treatment of CRPS in small, open,[100,101] and placebo-controlled studies.[102–104] In two placebo-controlled trials of bisphosphonates for the treatment of CRPS, either alendronate[102] (7.5 mg/d IV for 3 days) or clodronate[105] (300 mg/d IV for 10 days), it has been demonstrated that bisphosphonates may lead to improvement in pain, active movement, and motor function compared with placebo.

Robinson and colleagues conducted a double-blind, randomized, placebo-controlled trial in efforts to assess the efficacy of IV pamidronate 60 mg for CRPS type 1.[104] They compared single-dose administration of IV pamidronate 60 mg or normal saline, and patients were assessed at 1 and 3 months. Overall improvements in pain score, patient's global assessment of disease severity score, and physical function (SF-36) score were noted in the pamidronate group at 3 months, and improvements in role physical (SF-36) score were noted at 1 and 3 months.

Manicourt and colleagues conducted an 8-week randomized, double-blind, placebo-controlled study of alendronate therapy (per os 40 mg/d orally daily) for post-traumatic CRPS type 1, a condition associated with regional osteoclastic overactivity.[103] In contrast to placebo-treated patients ($n = 20$), all of the alendronate-treated patients ($n = 19$) exhibited a marked and sustained improvement in levels of spontaneous pain, pressure tolerance, and joint mobility at weeks 4 and 8. The improvement was maintained at week 12.[103]

In 2009, Brunner and colleagues published a systematic review of all RCTs to assess the benefit of bisphosphonates in the treatment of CRPS type 1 patients with bone loss.[106] Four trials of moderate-quality fulfilled their inclusion criteria. In total, 118 patients (intervention group $n = 59$, control group $n = 59$) with CRPS type 1 were treated. The participants were treated either with oral ($n = 1$)[103] or IV administration ($n = 3$)[102,104,105] of a bisphosphonate compound. With respect to function and quality of life there was a trend in favor of bisphosphonates, but differences in outcome assessment impeded pooling of results. Two trials provided sufficient data to pool pain outcomes. Bisphosphonates reduced pain intensity by 22.4 and 21.6 mm on a visual analog scale (VAS) after 4 and 12 weeks of follow-up.[106]

Tran et al. conducted a narrative review.[107] The search criteria yielded 41 RCTs with a mean of 31.7 participants per study. Only bisphosphonates appear to offer clear benefits for patients with CRPS. Improvement has been reported with dimethyl sulfoxide, steroids, epidural clonidine, intrathecal baclofen, spinal cord stimulation, and motor imagery programs, but further trials are required. The available evidence does not support the use of calcitonin, vasodilators, or sympatholytic and neuromodulative IV regional blockade (Bier Block).[107] In this review, no study was excluded based on factors such as sample size justification, statistical power, blinding, definition of intervention allocation, or clinical outcomes. Thus, evidence derived from "weaker" trials may be overemphasized.[107]

Anecdotal reports continue to periodically appear that seem to support the beneficial effects of bisphosphonate therapy for CRPS.[108–110]

Opioids

The only available randomized placebo-controlled trial of opioids specifically in CRPS found that sustained-release morphine did not reduce pain significantly relative to placebo over an 8-day trial, although this finding may have been affected by design limitations on the upward dose titration allowed.[95]

Corticosteroids

Small RCTs indicate that a pulse of oral corticosteroids may significantly improve symptomatology in acute CRPS.[111,112] After early reports of success with systemic steroids,[113] Christensen et al. studied 23 patients and reported that 30 mg/d of oral prednisone was significantly better than placebo.[112]

All studies evaluating the use of corticosteroids for the treatment of CRPS reported significantly positive results on overall clinical improvement. This included three case series, of which one showed improvement of clinical scores after one or two cycles of corticosteroids,[114] and two case series that showed good to excellent clinical results in, respectively, 59%[115] and 62%[116] of CRPS type 1 patients. Intramuscular corticosteroids were reported to provide an increase in proximal interphalangeal joint movement in 68% of the patients at a 1-year follow-up.[117] Two RCTs of moderate quality comparing corticosteroids to placebo[111,112] and a high-quality RCT comparing corticosteroids to piroxicam[26] reported significant differences in favor of corticosteroid treatment.

Zyluk and Puchalski admitted patients with early CRPS (<4 months), and they received treatment with 10% mannitol 250 mL/d BID and 8 mg dexamethasone per day for 1 week.[118] Measurements assessed included pain, range of finger movements, grip strength, and their own clinical severity scoring system for CRPS type 1 (CRPS score). The results were assessed at 1 week and, finally, at a mean of 9 (range 8–12) months. At 1-week assessment, all variables decreased significantly: pain from a mean VAS of 6.7 to 2.3, loss of finger flexion (6–0.3 cm), and the CRPS score (7.6–2.2 points). Total grip strength did not improve. At the final assessment of 70 patients, the VAS score was a mean of 1.8, loss of finger flexion a mean of 0.1 cm, the CRPS score was a mean of 1.6 and grip strength a mean of 34% of the strength of the unaffected hand. All these variables showed statistically significant improvement.[118]

Unlike the analgesic effects of intrathecal corticosteroids in postherpetic neuralgia,[119] Munts and colleagues found negative results in a double-blind, randomized, placebo-controlled parallel-group trial with single-dose intrathecal administration of 60 mg methylprednisolone in CRPS.[120]

Free Radical Scavengers

Free radical scavengers reduce the burden of inflammation and may improve CRPS symptoms. A prospective crossover study with 20 patients receiving dimethylsulphoxide (DMSO) locally five times a day during 1 week versus a placebo during 1 week, found a positive effect of DMSO on the function of the affected limb.[121] A randomized double-blind trial conducted with 32 CRPS type 1 patients receiving a fatty cream with or without 50% DMSO showed that five-times daily use of DMSO provided significantly better results on CRPS type 1 symptoms than placebo after 2 months of treatment.[122] A randomized double-blind study in 146 CRPS type 1 patients found comparable results for DMSO cream and N-acetylcysteine.[123] In general, DMSO generates lower (direct and indirect) costs than N-acetylcysteine. Subgroup analysis indicates that N-acetylcysteine is more cost effective in patients with a cold form of CRPS type 1 than DMSO. The opposite holds for warm forms of CRPS type 1.[124]

N-METHYL-D-ASPARTATE ANTAGONISTS: KETAMINE

Ketamine is a potent N-methyl-D-aspartic acid (NMDA) antagonist that has been used intravenously for the treatment of CRPS and a variety of neuropathic pain conditions.[89] Perhaps the most significant mechanism by which ketamine contributes to analgesia is via blocking the NMDA receptor by binding to its phencyclidine site. Ketamine has other actions, some of which may also contribute to its analgesic effects. These include interactions with other calcium and sodium channels, dopamine receptors, cholinergic transmission, and effects on noradrenergic and serotoninergic reuptake (intact descending inhibitory pathways are necessary for analgesia), together with opioid-like and anti-inflammatory effects.[125,126]

Correll et al. used relatively low IV doses (10–30 mg/h) of ketamine in CRPS patients for several days to 2 weeks in an inpatient setting. In their retrospective study, they noted significant long-term benefit from an open-label infusion protocol.[127]

Kiefer et al. evaluated 20 patients suffering from refractory CRPS who received ketamine in anesthetic dosage over 5 days in an open trial.[128] Anesthesia was induced by bolus injection of ketamine (1–1.5 mg/kg) and midazolam (2.5–7.5 mg), and treatment was maintained by infusions of ketamine over 5 days, starting at 3 mg/kg/h followed by gradual titration up to a final dose of 7 mg/kg/h with supplemental midazolam as appropriate; most patients were intubated and mechanically ventilated. Outcome criteria were pain relief, effect on the movement disorder, quality of life, and ability to work at baseline and at up to 6 months following treatment. Significant pain relief was observed at 1, 3, and 6 months following treatment (93.5 +/− 11.1%, 89.4 +/− 17.0%, 79.3 +/− 25.3%; $p < 0.001$). Complete remission from CRPS was observed at 1 month in all patients, at 3 months in 17, and at 6 months in 16 patients. If relapse occurred, significant pain relief was still attained at 3 and 6 months (59.0 +/− 14.7%, $p < 0.004$; 50.2 +/− 10.6%, $p < 0.002$). Quality of life, the associated movement disorder, and the ability to work significantly improved in the majority of patients at 3 and 6 months.[128]

Sigtermans and colleagues studied 60 CRPS type 1 patients with severe pain in a double-blind, randomized, placebo-controlled parallel-group trial.[129] Patients were given a 4.2-day IV infusion of low-dose ketamine ($n = 30$) or placebo ($n = 30$) using an individualized stepwise tailoring of dosage based on effect (pain relief) and side effects (nausea/vomiting/psychomimetic effects). The drug infusion rate was started at 1.2 mcg $kg^{-1}min^{-1}$ (or .5 mg/h for a 70 kg patient) and titrated at regular intervals (max. thrice daily) to a maximum of 7.2 mcg $kg^{-1}min^{-1}$ (or 30 mg/h for a 70 kg patient). The primary outcome of the study was the pain score (numerical rating score: 0–10) during the 12-week study period. The median (range) disease duration of the patients was 7.4 (0.1–31.9) years. At the end of infusion, the ketamine dose was 22.2+/− 2.0 mg/h/70 kg. Pain scores over the 12-week study period in patients receiving ketamine were significantly lower than those in patients receiving placebo ($p < 0.001$). The lowest pain score was at the end of week 1: ketamine 2.68+/− 0.51, placebo 5.45+/− 0.48.[129]

Schwartzman and colleagues conducted a randomized, double-blind, placebo-controlled trial designed to evaluate the effectiveness of IV ketamine in the treatment of CRPS.[130] All subjects were infused intravenously with normal saline with or without ketamine for 4 h (25 mL/h) daily for 10 days and followed for 3 months. The maximum ketamine infusion rate was 0.35 mg/kg/h, not to exceed 25 mg/h over a 4 h period. Subjects in both the ketamine and placebo groups were administered clonidine and versed. This study showed that IV ketamine administered in an outpatient setting resulted in statistically significant ($p < 0.05$) reductions in many pain parameters.[130]

> Several options were discussed with the patient. First, it is recommended to discontinue the use of hydrocodone, naproxen, and cyclobenzaprine as none of these medications has strong support for first-line treatment. As various medication options were reviewed, the patient voiced her desire to avoid multiple medications (given her unsatisfying experience with hydrocodone/naproxen/cyclobenzaprine) and gave further history of recent asthma exacerbation. Therefore, the decision was made to start a course of oral corticosteroids. Additional considerations include an antiepileptic agent (such as gabapentin, pregabalin, or topiramate) and PRN tramadol. A trial of DMSO cream and bisphosphonates may be undertaken. If pain is refractory, ketamine infusions may be considered.

INTERVENTIONAL APPROACHES

Sympathetic Blockade

Sympathetic blockade has become a nearly first-line treatment in CRPS since Leriche demonstrated the efficacy of sympathectomy 60 years ago.[7] Despite how commonly the procedure is performed, there has been a paucity of high-quality evidence to support it in the medical literature. In a 2005 Cochrane Database review, Cepeda found there was a "scarcity of published evidence to support the use of local anesthetic sympathetic blockade as the 'gold treatment' for CRPS" and that "no conclusion concerning the effectiveness of the procedure could be drawn."[131] A closer evaluation, however, shows that this was based on only two small randomized, double-blind, crossover studies that evaluated 23 patients in total. A more recent 2010 Cochrane Database review visited this issue again; however, it mistakenly evaluated sympathectomy for *any* neuropathic pain and CRPS together. The authors found only one double-blind, randomized, controlled trial and concluded that "sympathectomy for neuropathic pain and CRPS is based on very little high quality evidence."[132] This appears to be in stark contrast with clinical experience and nonblinded studies, which show tremendous benefit.[133] One must keep in mind that, when high-quality evidence is lacking, this does not equate to lack of efficacy: transforaminal epidural steroid injections have been used for decades to relieve lumbar radicular pain based on pathophysiological theory and excellent clinical response. It was only in 2010 that the first randomized trial took place.[134] Similarly, we should allow our collective clinical experience to guide our use of this safe, pain-relieving modality in patients with CRPS rather than forgo it due to "lack of evidence" while at the same time pursuing high-quality efficacy research. This thought process can be inferred in the most recently published (at the time of this writing) evidence-based review on interventional procedures in CRPS that recommends "sympathetic block [as] the interventional treatment of first choice."[135] A recent double-blind, placebo-controlled, crossover design study was undertaken in 23 children with CRPS. CRPS patients aged 10–18 years received IV lidocaine and lumbar sympathetic saline or lumbar sympathetic lidocaine and IV saline. A significant reduction in mean pain intensity of allodynia to brush and to pinprick temporal summation with lidocaine treatment via the lumbar sympathetic blockade was noted compared to the IV route. The latter did not produce significant changes in spontaneous and evoked pain intensity measurements compared to pretreatment values, unlike the lumbar sympathetic blockade with lidocaine.[136]

Spinal Cord Stimulation

There is strong evidence for long-term effectiveness of spinal cord stimulation (SCS) in CRPS patients. The best study comes from the Netherlands, whereby Kemler and colleagues studied refractory CRPS patients who had failed multiple treatment modalities including surgical sympathectomy (a procedure no longer advocated). They prospectively randomized 54 refractory CRPS patients to SCS and physical therapy (SCS + PT group) or to physical therapy alone (PT group) in a 2:1 ratio. Of the 36 randomized to SCS + PT, 24 (two-thirds) had a successful SCS trial, and 22 proceeded to permanent implant. However, all patients who underwent a SCS trial (even those who failed it and did not proceed to an implant) were included in the comparative analysis as part of the SCS + PT versus the 18 patients in the PT-alone group because that was an intent-to-treat analysis. At 6 months after initiation of treatment, both pain scores and the much-improved score (subscale 6) of the Global Perceived Effect (GPE, a 7-scale outcome measure ranging from worst ever to best ever) were significantly improved.[137] A follow-up study, looking at results 2 years after initiation of therapy, reported persistent significant improvements in pain scores and the much-improved score of the GPE.[138] It is noteworthy that although there was statistically significant improvement in pain and GPE, no significant functional improvement was noted.[137,138] Another analysis of the study participants was undertaken up to 5 years after initiation of therapy. At that time, 10 patients were excluded from the study, and the analysis thus compared 31 patients in the SCS + PT group with 13 controls in the PT-alone group. No statistically significant difference in pain scores was noted between both groups at 3, 4, or 5 years after initiation of therapy, thus leading the authors to conclude that the pain-alleviating effect of SCS in CRPS decreases with time and there is no longer a statistically significant difference compared to PT after 3 years.[139] However, this analysis was criticized for its intent-to-treat nature because nine of the patients in the SCS + PT group had failed the stimulation trial and never received an SCS implant but were included in the intent-to-treat analysis. Hence, an as-treated analysis was undertaken comparing the 22 patients in the SCS + PT group who had received an implant to the 13 patients in the PT-alone group. VAS pain scores decreased by an average of 2.5 points in the SCS + PT group versus 1.0 point in the PT-alone group ($p = 0.06$). Improvements in GPE scores were statistically significant in favor of the SCS + PT group ($p = 0.02$). In addition, the authors commented that "18 (90%) of 20 patients with an implant indicated that they had positively responded to the treatment, and 19 patients (95%) reported that they would undergo the treatment again for the same result."[140]

A number of other studies reported significantly positive analgesic effects of SCS on CRPS patients. In a prospective trial, Harke and colleagues assessed the long-term effects of SCS on pain and improvement of functional status in CRPS patients who had sympathetically maintained pain. They studied 29 patients with a mean CRPS duration of 5.4 years; 16 with cervical and 13 with thoracic lead placements. The outcomes examined were VAS scores for deep pain and allodynia, changes in Pain Disability Index (PDI) to quantify impairments in activities of daily living, and changes in analgesic medication consumption during SCS therapy. Patients were followed for an average of 35.6 ± 21 months after implant. They reported that all patients had a complete resolution of allodynia at 12 months and a significant improvement in deep pain. Furthermore, nearly three-quarters of the patients showed a significant decrease in the PDI with more than 50% improvement in scores.[141] Other prospective studies[142] including successful SCS in patients with upper-extremity CRPS[143,144] have been reported. Stimulation of both upper and lower extremities with cervically placed SCS electrodes has also been reported in patients with CRPS involving upper and lower extremities.[145]

SCS has been found to be cost-effective. Even though the cost of SCS therapy was $4,000 higher than non-SCS therapy during the first year, in the lifetime analysis, SCS was more effective than conventional therapy and less expensive (by about $60,000 per patient).[137] Similar findings were reported in a systematic review of SCS studies on CRPS patients.[146] A more recent study from the United Kingdom found incremental cost-effectiveness of SCS compared with conventional medical management (CMM) at about £3,562 per quality-adjusted life year (QALY).[147]

Other Neuromodulation Interventions

Limited effectiveness for peripheral nerve stimulation (PNS) and motor cortex stimulation (MCS) has been reported in CRPS based on uncontrolled, relatively small series of patients. Indeed, there is only one study that specifically examined long-term efficacy of each of these two modalities in CRPS. In a prospective study by Hassenbusch and colleagues, 32 CRPS patients were trialed with PNS systems, and 30 of those had a successful trial with significant pain relief. The study reported a 63% success rate at 3 years after implant in patients with advanced disease who had failed all other modalities except a trial of SCS. Of the 30 patients implanted with permanent PNS systems, eight (27%) required a revision of the electrode; placement of additional electrodes was carried out in six patients. There were 11 pain relief failures, mostly early on at 1.3 ± 0.1 years. According to this study, the best application of PNS appears to be for a small group of patients with localized pain along the distribution of a single major nerve.[148] However, when CRPS spreads and the perceived pain area increases,[59] further surgical revisions might be necessary. Although there might be a place for PNS in the treatment algorithm of CRPS, particularly CRPS type 2, well-designed randomized trials are necessary to assess its long-term effectiveness. Velasco and colleagues reported a case series of five CRPS patients, four of whom benefited from MCS implant. VAS and McGill pain questionnaire scores diminished significantly throughout the follow-up and worsened when MCS was turned off for 30 days (in a double-blinded fashion because patients do not experience paresthesias with MCS). In addition, there was resolution of allodynia and sympathetic signs lasting for more than 1 year.[149]

There are case series of successful management of intractable dystonia and pain in CRPS patients with intrathecal drug delivery systems using, respectively, baclofen[150] and ziconotide.[151] However, a high complication rate is reported in this patient group, and intrathecal pump implant should be considered carefully and only in refractory cases in this patient population.[152]

> Our patient was recommended to undergo a left stellate ganglion block. It was discussed with her that if she had a positive, prolonged response (weeks to months), stellate ganglion block could be continued as needed in conjunction with occupational therapy, provided longer lasting pain relief occurs with successive blocks. Should pain relief be short lasting with sympathetic blocks, consideration may be given to oral $\alpha 1$ blockers such as phenoxybenzamine or terazosin.[153,154] Neuromodulation interventions may be too early in the course of disease in this patient because there are no data indicating that early neurostimulation may reverse the course of the condition. However, should the pain be refractory to pharmacological management and sympathetic blockade, neurostimulation may be considered.

PSYCHOLOGICAL INTERVENTION

Before addressing psychiatric and behavioral modalities that can be implemented in patients with CRPS, one must have an understanding of the differences between CRPS and non-CRPS chronic pain patients. In a thorough literature review covering from the 1800s to the time of publication in 1992, Lynch concluded there was "no worthwhile evidence to substantiate the claim that psychological factors or certain personality traits predispose one to develop RSD."[155] Similar findings were reported in a large epidemiological study by de Mos and colleagues.[32] When patients with CRPS are directly compared to those with non-CRPS limb pain, it has been found that there are no statistically different findings on the Minnesota Multiphasic Personality Inventory (MMPI)[156,157] or the Symptom Checklist-90 (SCL-90).[158] Although one study did find increased reports of distress and pain severity among CRPS patients compared to low back pain patients, there was no difference between

CRPS and non-CRPS limb pain patients.[159] Ciccone compared patients with CRPS to those with low back pain and chronic neuropathy and found "patients with RSD did not display a unique or unusual pattern of psychological dysfunction."[50] Therefore, the evidence does not support the commonly held belief that CRPS patients have higher level of psychological dysfunction than other chronic pain patients. This fact becomes relevant when designing and implementing psychological treatment, allowing the practitioner to draw from the wealth of psychological treatments that may not be CRPS specific.

Only one randomized trial has specifically evaluated psychological intervention in CRPS patients. In it, Fialka et al. compared physical therapy to physical therapy plus once weekly autogenic training.[160]Although both groups improved across all domains measured (pain, ROM, edema), there were no significant differences. Based on clinical expertise and literature review, Bruehl has proposed a flowchart outlining psychological treatment (Figure 25.3).[161] Education should be provided early on for all patients and their families regarding pathophysiology of disease, active self-management, and the need to keep the limb active/mobile.

> At her initial visit, the patient completed a Beck Depression Inventory and Beck Anxiety Inventory, scoring 37 and 30, respectively. This was suggestive of levels of depression/anxiety of clinical concern, and that fact was discussed with her. She gave a further history of mild depression treated in the remote past and notes that since struggling with worsening pain and functional limitations, her mood has worsened. The patient denied suicidal ideation and was referred to a pain psychiatrist for further evaluation and co-management.

IN THE EVENT OF SURGERY, HOW IS THE CRPS PATIENT MANAGED PERIOPERATIVELY?

Surgery is a common cause for CRPS development, with varied percentages between 3% and 24% reported depending on the surgery, clinical setting, and reporting clinicians.[77,162] However, surgery on a CRPS-afflicted limb is generally avoided because of likelihood of CRPS exacerbation.[163] Nonetheless, 6–10% of CRPS patients may require surgery on the affected extremity. There are no definite guidelines regarding the optimal perioperative management of these patients to avoid CRPS exacerbation. In general, regional anesthesia is thought to be superior to general anesthesia in reducing the likelihood of CRPS exacerbation.[164,165]Additional treatments are geared at optimizing the condition of the CRPS-afflicted limb prior to surgery. Physical therapy, analgesics, sympatholysis, and vasodilators have been used to optimize the clinical status and temperature of the affected limb.[163,166]

There is strong evidence for vitamin C in preventing CRPS after wrist fractures. A randomized, double-blind, placebo-controlled trial was undertaken in 123 adults with 127 wrist fractures who were treated with 500 mg of vitamin C or placebo and were followed for 1 year. Patients were managed nonsurgically with casting and immobilization and assessed for signs and symptoms of CRPS. The incidence of CRPS in the vitamin C group was 7% versus 22% in the placebo group.[52] Another study evaluated the effectiveness of vitamin C in 195 patients who underwent intrafocal pinning for distal radius fractures. The first 100 patients received no vitamin C, and the last 95 patients received 1 g/d vitamin C for 45 days starting on the day of fracture. The incidence of CRPS was 2.1% in the vitamin C group versus 10% in the

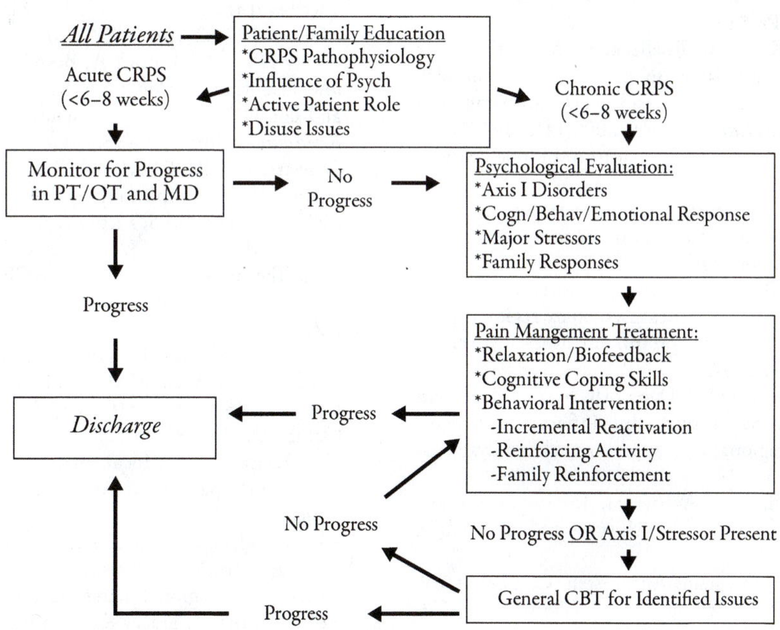

Figure 25.3 Complex regional pain syndrome (CRPS) rehabilitation with a focus on psychological interventions. Adapted from Bruehl S, Harden RN, Galer BS, Saltz S, Backonja M, Stanton-Hicks M. Complex regional pain syndrome: are there distinct subtypes and sequential stages of the syndrome? *Pain*. 2002;95:119–124.

group that did not receive vitamin C.[167] Similar results were demonstrated in a recent placebo-controlled trial.[168] Another prospective trial demonstrated no CRPS cases in patients receiving 500 mg vitamin C daily for 50 days, starting 2 days before surgery for basal thumb prosthesis.[169] Vitamin C, 1 g/d, appeared to prevent CRPS after foot and ankle surgery in a recent large study by Besse and colleagues of 420 operations in 392 patients.[170] The incidence of CRPS was 1.6% in the vitamin C group versus 9.6% in the group that did not receive vitamin C.[170]

Perioperative tunneled epidural catheter placement with continuous epidural infusion of local anesthetics and opioids has been advocated and offers the potential for outpatient maintenance of the infusion in refractory cases and for prevention of symptom exacerbation in the event of surgery on the affected CRPS limb.[77,171] However, the risk-benefit ratio of using this approach should be weighed carefully, given potential for epidural space infection in the CRPS patient population.[172]

REFERENCES

1. Casten DF, Betcher AM. Reflex sympathetic dystrophy. *Surg Gynecol Obstet.* 1995;100:97–101.
2. Speigel IJ, Milowsky JL. Causalgia. *JAMA.* 1945;127:9–15.
3. Turf RM, Bacardi BE. Causalgia: clarifications in terminology and a case presentation. *J Foot Surg.* 1986;25:284–295.
4. Mitchell SW. *Injuries of Nerves and Their Consequences.* New York: Dover Publications; 1872.
5. Sudeck P. Ueber die akute enzundiche Knochenatrophie. *Arch Klin Chir.* 1900;62:147–156.
6. Evans JA. Reflex sympathetic dystrophy; report on 57 cases. *Ann Intern Med.* 1947;26:417–426.
7. Leriche R. Treatment of pain by sympathectomy. *Rev Neurol* (Paris). 1950;83:41–42.
8. Merskey H, Bogduk N, eds. *Classification of Chronic Pain: Description of Chronic Pain Syndromes and Definition of Pain Terms.* Seattle, WA: IASP Press; 1994.
9. Schinkel C, Scherens A, Koller M, Roellecke G, Muhr G, Maier C. Systemic inflammatory mediators in post-traumatic complex regional pain syndrome (CRPS I)—longitudinal investigations and differences to control groups. *Eur J Med Res.* 2009;14:130–135.
10. Julius D, Basbaum AI. Molecular mechanisms of nociception. *Nature.* 2001;413:203–210.
11. Huygen FJ, De Bruijn AG, De Bruin MT, Groeneweg JG, Klein J, Zijlstra FJ. Evidence for local inflammation in complex regional pain syndrome type 1. *Mediators Inflamm.* 2002;11:47–51.
12. Munnikes RJ, Muis C, Boersma M, Heijmans-Antonissen C, Zijlstra FJ, Huygen FJ. Intermediate stage complex regional pain syndrome type 1 is unrelated to proinflammatory cytokines. *Mediators Inflamm.* 2005:366–372.
13. Munts AG, Zijlstra FJ, Nibbering PH, Daha MR, Marinus J, Dahan A, van Hilten JJ. Analysis of cerebrospinal fluid inflammatory mediators in chronic complex regional pain syndrome related dystonia. *Clin J Pain.* 2008;24:30–34.
14. Birklein F, Schmelz M, Schifter S, Weber M. The important role of neuropeptides in complex regional pain syndrome. *Neurology.* 2001;57:2179–2184.
15. Wesseldijk F, Huygen FJ, Heijmans-Antonissen C, Niehof SP, Zijlstra FP. Six years follow-up of the levels of TNF-alpha and IL-6 in patients with complex regional pain syndrome type 1. *Mediators Inflamm.* 2008a:469439.
16. Wesseldijk F, Huygen FJ, Heijmans-Antonissen C, Niehof SP, Zijlstra FJ. Tumor necrosis factor-alpha and interleukin-6 are not correlated with the characteristics of Complex Regional Pain Syndrome type 1 in 66 patients. *Eur J Pain.* 2008b;12:716–721.
17. Groeneweg JG, Huygen FJ, Heijmans-Antonissen C, Niehof S, Zijlstra FJ. Increased endothelin-1 and diminished nitric oxide levels in blister fluids of patients with intermediate cold type complex regional pain syndrome type 1. *BMC Musculoskelet Disord.* 2006;7:91.
18. de Rooij AM, Florencia Gosso M, Haasnoot GW, et al. HLA-B62 and HLA-DQ8 are associated with Complex Regional Pain Syndrome with fixed dystonia. *Pain.* 2009;145:82–85.
19. Kemler MA, van de Vusse AC, van den Berg-Loonen EM, Barendse GA, van Kleef M, Weber WE. HLA-DQ1 associated with reflex sympathetic dystrophy. *Neurology.* 1999;53:1350–1351.
20. Mailis-Gagnon A, Nicholson K, Blumberger D, Zurowski M. Characteristics and period prevalence of self-induced disorder in patients referred to a pain clinic with the diagnosis of complex regional pain syndrome. *Clin J Pain.* 2008;24:176–185.
21. van de Beek WJ, Roep BO, van der Slik AR, Giphart MJ, van Hilten BJ. Susceptibility loci for complex regional pain syndrome. *Pain.* 2003;103:93–97.
22. van Hilten JJ, van de Beek WJ, Roep BO. Multifocal or generalized tonic dystonia of complex regional pain syndrome: a distinct clinical entity associated with HLA-DR13. *Ann Neurol.* 2000b;48:113–116.
23. Kohr D, Tschernatsch M, Schmitz K, et al. Autoantibodies in complex regional pain syndrome bind to a differentiation-dependent neuronal surface autoantigen. *Pain.* 2009;143:246–251.
24. Goebel A, Vogel H, Caneris O, et al. Immune responses to Campylobacter and serum autoantibodies in patients with complex regional pain syndrome. *J Neuroimmunol.* 2005;162:184–189.
25. Goebel A, Baranowski A, Maurer K, Ghiai A, McCabe C, Ambler G. Intravenous immunoglobulin treatment of the complex regional pain syndrome: a randomized trial. *Ann Intern Med.* 2010;152:152–158.
26. Kalita J, Vajpayee A, Misra UK. Comparison of prednisolone with piroxicam in complex regional pain syndrome following stroke: a randomized controlled trial. *QJM.* 2006;99:89–95.
27. Bernateck M, Rolke R, Birklein F, Treede RD, Fink M, Karst M. Successful intravenous regional block with low-dose tumor necrosis factor-alpha antibody infliximab for treatment of complex regional pain syndrome 1. *Anesth Analg.* 2007;105:1148–1151.
28. Huygen FJ, Niehof S, Zijlstra FJ, van Hagen PM, van Daele PL. Successful treatment of CRPS 1 with anti-TNF. *J Pain Symptom Manage.* 2004;27:101–103.
29. Ching DW, McClintock A, Beswick F. Successful treatment with low-dose thalidomide in a patient with both Behcet's disease and complex regional pain syndrome type I: case report. *J Clin Rheumatol.* 2003;9:96–98.
30. Schwartzman RJ, Chevlen E, Bengtson K. Thalidomide has activity in treating complex regional pain syndrome. *Arch Intern Med.* 2003;163:1487–1488; author reply 1488.
31. de Mos M, Huygen FJ, Stricker BH, Dieleman JP, Sturkenboom MC. The association between ACE inhibitors and the complex regional pain syndrome: suggestions for a neuro-inflammatory pathogenesis of CRPS. *Pain.* 2009a;142:218–224.
32. de Mos M, Huygen FJ, Dieleman JP, Koopman JS, Stricker BH, Sturkenboom MC. Medical history and the onset of complex regional pain syndrome (CRPS). *Pain.* 2008;139:458–466.
33. Oaklander AL, Rissmiller JG, Gelman LB, Zheng L, Chang Y, Gott R. Evidence of focal small-fiber axonal degeneration in complex regional pain syndrome-I (reflex sympathetic dystrophy). *Pain.* 2006;120:235–243.
34. Albrecht PJ, Hines S, Eisenberg E, et al. Pathologic alterations of cutaneous innervation and vasculature in affected limbs from patients with complex regional pain syndrome. *Pain.* 2006;120:244–266.
35. Rosas-Ballina M, Tracey KJ. Cholinergic control of inflammation. *J Intern Med.* 2009a;265:663–679.
36. Rosas-Ballina M, Tracey KJ. The neurology of the immune system: neural reflexes regulate immunity. *Neuron.* 2009b;64:28–32.

37. Tracey KJ. Reflex control of immunity. *Nat Rev Immunol.* 2009;9:418–428.
38. Sandroni P, Benrud-Larson LM, McClelland RL, Low PA. Complex regional pain syndrome type I: incidence and prevalence in Olmsted county, a population-based study. *Pain.* 2003;103:199–207.
39. de Mos M, de Bruijn AG, Huygen FJ, Dieleman JP, Stricker BH, Sturkenboom MC. The incidence of complex regional pain syndrome: a population-based study. *Pain.* 2007;129:12–20.
40. Bruehl S, Chung OY. How common is complex regional pain syndrome-Type I? *Pain.* 2007;129:1–2.
41. Atkins RM, Duckworth T, Kanis JA. Algodystrophy following Colles' fracture. *J Hand Surg Br.* 1989;14:161–164.
42. Bickerstaff DR, Kanis JA. Algodystrophy: an under-recognized complication of minor trauma. *Br J Rheumatol.* 1994;33:240–248.
43. Sarangi PP, Ward AJ, Smith EJ, Staddon GE, Atkins RM. Algodystrophy and osteoporosis after tibial fractures. *J Bone Joint Surg Br.* 1993;75:450–452.
44. Schmalbruch H. Fiber composition of the rat sciatic nerve. *Anat Rec.* 1986;215:71–81.
45. Veldman PH, Reynen HM, Arntz IE, Goris RJ. Signs and symptoms of reflex sympathetic dystrophy: prospective study of 829 patients. *Lancet.* 1993;342:1012–1016.
46. Veldman PH, Goris RJ. Multiple reflex sympathetic dystrophy. Which patients are at risk for developing a recurrence of reflex sympathetic dystrophy in the same or another limb. *Pain.* 1996;64:463–466.
47. van Hilten JJ. Movement disorders in complex regional pain syndrome. *Pain Med.* 2010;11:1274–1277.
48. van Rijn MA, Marinus J, Putter H, van Hilten JJ. Onset and progression of dystonia in complex regional pain syndrome. *Pain.* 2007;130:287–293.
49. Schwartzman RJ, Kerrigan J. The movement disorder of reflex sympathetic dystrophy. *Neurology.* 1990;40:57–61.
50. Ciccone DS, Bandilla EB, Wu W. Psychological dysfunction in patients with reflex sympathetic dystrophy. *Pain.* 1997;71:323–333.
51. Mailis A, Wade J. Profile of Caucasian women with possible genetic predisposition to reflex sympathetic dystrophy: a pilot study. *Clin J Pain.* 1994;10:210–217.
52. Zollinger PE, Tuinebreijer WE, Kreis RW, Breederveld RS. Effect of vitamin C on frequency of reflex sympathetic dystrophy in wrist fractures: a randomised trial. *Lancet.* 1999;354:2025–2028.
53. Galer BS, Henderson J, Perander J, Jensen MP. Course of symptoms and quality of life measurement in Complex Regional Pain Syndrome: a pilot survey. *J Pain Symptom Manage.* 2000;20: 286–292.
54. Schwartzman RJ, Erwin KL, Alexander GM. The natural history of complex regional pain syndrome. *Clin J Pain.* 2009b;25:273–280.
55. de Mos M, Huygen FJ, van der Hoeven-Borgman M, Dieleman JP, Stricker BH, Sturkenboom MC. Outcome of the complex regional pain syndrome. *Clin J Pain.* 2009b;25:590–597.
56. Escobar PL. Reflex sympathetic dystrophy. *Orthop Rev.* 1986;15:646–651.
57. Bruehl S, Harden RN, Galer BS, Saltz S, Backonja M, Stanton-Hicks M. Complex regional pain syndrome: are there distinct subtypes and sequential stages of the syndrome? *Pain.* 2002; 95:119–124.
58. Vaneker M, Wilder-Smith OH, Schrombges P, de Man-Hermsen I, Oerlemans HM. Patients initially diagnosed as "warm" or "cold" CRPS 1 show differences in central sensory processing some eight years after diagnosis: a quantitative sensory testing study. *Pain.* 2005;115:204–211.
59. Maleki J, LeBel AA, Bennett GJ, Schwartzman RJ. Patterns of spread in complex regional pain syndrome, type I (reflex sympathetic dystrophy). *Pain.* 2000;88:259–266.
60. van Rijn MA, Marinus J, Putter H, Bosselaar SR, Moseley GL, van Hilten JJ. Spreading of complex regional pain syndrome: not a random process. *J Neural Transm.* 2011;118:1301–1309.
61. Harden RN, Bruehl S, Galer BS, et al. Complex regional pain syndrome: are the IASP diagnostic criteria valid and sufficiently comprehensive? *Pain.* 1999;83:211–219.
62. Birklein F, Handwerker HO. Complex regional pain syndrome: how to resolve the complexity? *Pain.* 2001;94:1–6.
63. Rommel O, Gehling M, Dertwinkel R, Witscher K, Zenz M, Malin JP, Janig W. Hemisensory impairment in patients with complex regional pain syndrome. *Pain.* 1999;80:95–101.
64. Thimineur M, Sood P, Kravitz E, Gudin J, Kitaj M. Central nervous system abnormalities in complex regional pain syndrome (CRPS): clinical and quantitative evidence of medullary dysfunction. *Clin J Pain.* 1998;14:256–267.
65. Wasner G, Backonja MM, Baron R. Traumatic neuralgias: complex regional pain syndromes (reflex sympathetic dystrophy and causalgia): clinical characteristics, pathophysiological mechanisms and therapy. *Neurol Clin.* 1998;16:851–868.
66. Birklein F, Sittl R, Spitzer A, Claus D, Neundorfer B, Handwerker HO. Sudomotor function in sympathetic reflex dystrophy. *Pain.* 1997;69:49–54.
67. Zyluk A. The sequelae of reflex sympathetic dystrophy. *J Hand Surg Br.* 2001;26:151–154.
68. Allen G, Galer BS, Schwartz L. Epidemiology of complex regional pain syndrome: a retrospective chart review of 134 patients. *Pain.* 1999;80:539–544.
69. Rashiq S, Galer BS. Proximal myofascial dysfunction in complex regional pain syndrome: a retrospective prevalence study. *Clin J Pain.* 1999;15:151–153.
70. Stanton-Hicks M, Janig W, Hassenbusch S, Haddox JD, Boas R, Wilson P. Reflex sympathetic dystrophy: changing concepts and taxonomy. *Pain.* 1995;63:127–133.
71. Bruehl S, Harden RN, Galer BS, et al. External validation of IASP diagnostic criteria for Complex Regional Pain Syndrome and proposed research diagnostic criteria. *Pain.* 1999;81:147–154.
72. van de Beek WJ, Schwartzman RJ, van Nes SI, Delhaas EM, van Hilten JJ. Diagnostic criteria used in studies of reflex sympathetic dystrophy. *Neurology.* 2002;58:522–526.
73. Galer BS, Bruehl S, Harden RN. IASP diagnostic criteria for complex regional pain syndrome: a preliminary empirical validation study. International Association for the Study of Pain. *Clin J Pain.* 1998;14:48–54.
74. Harden RN, Bruehl S, Stanton-Hicks M, Wilson PR. Proposed new diagnostic criteria for complex regional pain syndrome. *Pain Med.* 2007;8:326–331.
75. Harden RN, Bruehl S, Perez RS, et al. Validation of proposed diagnostic criteria (the "Budapest Criteria") for Complex Regional Pain Syndrome. *Pain.* 2010;150:268–274.
76. Stanton-Hicks M, Baron R, Boas R, et al. Complex Regional Pain Syndromes: guidelines for therapy. *Clin J Pain.* 1998;14:155–166.
77. Stanton-Hicks MD, Burton AW, Bruehl SP, et al. An updated interdisciplinary clinical pathway for CRPS: report of an expert panel. *Pain Pract.* 2002;2:1–16.
78. Severens JL, Oerlemans HM, Weegels AJ, van 't Hof MA, Oostendorp RA, Goris RJ. Cost-effectiveness analysis of adjuvant physical or occupational therapy for patients with reflex sympathetic dystrophy. *Arch Phys Med Rehabil.* 1999;80:1038–1043.
79. Harden RN, Swan M, King A, Costa B, Barthel J. Treatment of complex regional pain syndrome: functional restoration. *Clin J Pain.* 2006;22:420–424.
80. Phillips ME, Katz JA, Harden RN. The use of nerve blocks in conjunction with occupational therapy for complex regional pain syndrome type I. *Am J Occup Ther.* 2000;54:544–549.
81. Watson HK, Carlson L. Treatment of reflex sympathetic dystrophy of the hand with an active "stress loading" program. *J Hand Surg Am.* 1987;12:779–785.
82. Crombez G, Vlaeyen JW, Heuts PH, Lysens R. Pain-related fear is more disabling than pain itself: evidence on the role of pain-related fear in chronic back pain disability. *Pain.* 1999;80:329–339.
83. Kumar K, Toth C, Nath RK. Deep brain stimulation for intractable pain: a 15-year experience. *Neurosurgery.* 1997;40:736–746; discussion 746–737.
84. Portwood MM, Lieberman JS, Taylor RG. Ultrasound treatment of reflex sympathetic dystrophy. *Arch Phys Med Rehabil.* 1987;68:116–118.

85. McCabe CS, Haigh RC, Ring EF, Halligan PW, Wall PD, Blake DR. A controlled pilot study of the utility of mirror visual feedback in the treatment of complex regional pain syndrome (type 1). *Rheumatology* (Oxford). 2003;42:97–101.
86. Ramachandran VS, Rogers-Ramachandran D. Synaesthesia in phantom limbs induced with mirrors. *Proc Biol Sci.* 1996;263:377–386.
87. Sato K, Fukumori S, Matsusaki T, Maruo T, et al. Nonimmersive virtual reality mirror visual feedback therapy and its application for the treatment of complex regional pain syndrome: an open-label pilot study. *Pain Med.* 2010;11:622–629.
88. Burton AW, Hassenbusch SJ 3rd, Warneke C, Racz G, Stanton-Hicks M. Complex regional pain syndrome (CRPS): survey of current practices. *Pain Pract.* 2004;4:74–83.
89. Mackey S, Feinberg S. Pharmacologic therapies for complex regional pain syndrome. *Curr Pain Headache Rep.* 2007;11:38–43.
90. Perez RS et al. Evidence based guidelines for complex regional pain syndrome type 1. *BMC Neurol.* 2010;10:20.
91. Harden RN et al. Complex regional pain syndrome: practical diagnostic and treatment guidelines, 4th edition. *Pain Med.* 2013; 14(2):180–229.
92. Mellick GA, Mellick LB. Reflex sympathetic dystrophy treated with gabapentin. *Arch Phys Med Rehabil.* 1997;78:98–105.
93. van de Vusse AC, Stomp-van den Berg SG, Kessels AH, Weber WE. Randomised controlled trial of gabapentin in Complex Regional Pain Syndrome type 1 [ISRCTN84121379]. *BMC Neurol.* 2004;4:13.
94. Serpell MG. Gabapentin in neuropathic pain syndromes: a randomised, double-blind, placebo-controlled trial. *Pain.* 2002;99:557–566.
95. Harke H, Gretenkort P, Ladleif HU, Rahman S, Harke O. The response of neuropathic pain and pain in complex regional pain syndrome I to carbamazepine and sustained-release morphine in patients pretreated with spinal cord stimulation: a double-blinded randomized study. *Anesth Analg.* 2001;92:488–495.
96. Carroll I, Gaeta R, Mackey S. Multivariate analysis of chronic pain patients undergoing lidocaine infusions: increasing pain severity and advancing age predict likelihood of clinically meaningful analgesia. *Clin J Pain.* 2007;23:702–706.
97. Galer BS, Miller KV, Rowbotham MC. Response to intravenous lidocaine infusion differs based on clinical diagnosis and site of nervous system injury. *Neurology.* 1993;43:1233–1235.
98. Wallace MS, Ridgeway BM, Leung AY, Gerayli A, Yaksh TL. Concentration-effect relationship of intravenous lidocaine on the allodynia of complex regional pain syndrome types I and II. *Anesthesiology.* 2000;92:75–83.
99. Schwartzman RJ, Patel M, Grothusen JR, Alexander GM. Efficacy of 5-day continuous lidocaine infusion for the treatment of refractory complex regional pain syndrome. *Pain Med.* 2009c; 10:401–412.
100. Kubalek I, Fain O, Paries J, Kettaneh A, Thomas M. Treatment of reflex sympathetic dystrophy with pamidronate: 29 cases. *Rheumatology* (Oxford). 2001;40:1394–1397.
101. Pappagallo M, Breuer B, Schneider A, Sperber K. Treatment of chronic mechanical spinal pain with intravenous pamidronate: a review of medical records. *J Pain Symptom Manage.* 2003;26:678–683.
102. Adami S, Fossaluzza V, Gatti D, Fracassi E, Braga V. Bisphosphonate therapy of reflex sympathetic dystrophy syndrome. *Ann Rheum Dis.* 1997;56:201–204.
103. Manicourt DH, Brasseur JP, Boutsen Y, Depreseux G, Devogelaer JP. Role of alendronate in therapy for posttraumatic complex regional pain syndrome type I of the lower extremity. *Arthritis Rheum.* 2004;50:3690–3697.
104. Robinson JN, Sandom J, Chapman PT. Efficacy of pamidronate in complex regional pain syndrome type I. *Pain Med.* 2004;5:276–280.
105. Varenna M, Zucchi F, Ghiringhelli D, Binelli L, Bevilacqua M, Bettica P, Sinigaglia L. Intravenous clodronate in the treatment of reflex sympathetic dystrophy syndrome. A randomized, double blind, placebo controlled study. *J Rheumatol.* 2000;27:1477–1483.
106. Brunner F, Schmid A, Kissling R, Held U, Bachmann LM. Biphosphonates for the therapy of complex regional pain syndrome I—systematic review. *Eur J Pain.* 2009;13:17–21.
107. Tran de QH, Duong S, Bertini P, Finlayson RJ. Treatment of complex regional pain syndrome: a review of the evidence. *Can J Anaesth.* 2010;57:149–166.
108. Cassisi G, Sartori L. Efficacy of intramuscular clodronate in Complex Regional Pain Syndrome type I: description of a case located in the astragalus in a patient with psoriatic arthritis. *Acta Biomed.* 2009;80:268–277.
109. Gremeaux V, Herisson C, Pelissier J. Complex regional pain syndrome of the knee: early and beneficial action of diphosphonates on pain and function. *Ann Readapt Med Phys.* 2007;50:240–243.
110. Simm PJ, Briody J, McQuade M, Munns CF. The successful use of pamidronate in an 11-year-old girl with complex regional pain syndrome: response to treatment demonstrated by serial peripheral quantitative computerised tomographic scans. *Bone.* 2010;46:885–888.
111. Braus DF, Krauss JK, Strobel J. The shoulder-hand syndrome after stroke: a prospective clinical trial. *Ann Neurol.* 1994;36:728–733.
112. Christensen K, Jensen EM, Noer I. The reflex dystrophy syndrome response to treatment with systemic corticosteroids. *Acta Chir Scand.* 1982;148:653–655.
113. Kozin F, McCarty DJ, Sims J, Genant H. The reflex sympathetic dystrophy syndrome. I. Clinical and histologic studies: evidence for bilaterality, response to corticosteroids and articular involvement. *Am J Med.* 1976;60:321–331.
114. Bianchi C, Rossi S, Turi S, Brambilla A, Felisari G, Mascheri D. Long-term functional outcome measures in corticosteroid-treated complex regional pain syndrome. *Eura Medicophys.* 2006;42:103–111.
115. Glick EN. Reflex dystrophy (algoneurodystrophy): results of treatment by corticosteroids. *Rheumatol Rehabil.* 1973;12:84–88.
116. Glick EN, Helal B. Post-traumatic neurodystrophy. Treatment by corticosteroids. *Hand.* 1976;8:45–47.
117. Grundberg AB. Reflex sympathetic dystrophy: treatment with long-acting intramuscular corticosteroids. *J Hand Surg Am.* 1996;21:667–670.
118. Zyluk A, Puchalski P. Treatment of early complex regional pain syndrome type 1 by a combination of mannitol and dexamethasone. *J Hand Surg Eur Vol.* 2008;33:130–136.
119. Kotani N, Kushikata T, Hashimoto H, et al. Intrathecal methylprednisolone for intractable postherpetic neuralgia. *N Engl J Med.* 2000;343:1514–1519.
120. Munts AG, van der Plas AA, Ferrari MD, Teepe-Twiss IM, Marinus J, van Hilten JJ. Efficacy and safety of a single intrathecal methylprednisolone bolus in chronic complex regional pain syndrome. *Eur J Pain.* 2010;14:523–528.
121. Goris RJ, Dongen LM, Winters HA. Are toxic oxygen radicals involved in the pathogenesis of reflex sympathetic dystrophy? *Free Radic Res Commun.* 1987;3:13–18.
122. Zuurmond WW, Langendijk PN, Bezemer PD, Brink HE, de Lange JJ, van Loenen. Treatment of acute reflex sympathetic dystrophy with DMSO 50% in a fatty cream. *Acta Anaesthesiol Scand.* 1996;40:364–367.
123. Perez RS, Zuurmond WW, Bezemer PD, et al. The treatment of complex regional pain syndrome type I with free radical scavengers: a randomized controlled study. *Pain.* 2003;102:297–307.
124. van Dieten HE, Perez RS, van Tulder MW, et al. Cost effectiveness and cost utility of acetylcysteine versus dimethyl sulfoxide for reflex sympathetic dystrophy. *Pharmacoeconomics.* 2003;21:139–148.
125. Kawasaki C, Kawasaki T, Ogata M, Nandate K, Shigematsu A. Ketamine isomers suppress superantigen-induced proinflammatory cytokine production in human whole blood. *Can J Anaesth.* 2001;48:819–823.
126. Meller ST. Ketamine: relief from chronic pain through actions at the NMDA receptor? *Pain.* 1996;68:435–436.

127. Correll GE, Maleki J, Gracely EJ, Muir JJ, Harbut RE. Subanesthetic ketamine infusion therapy: a retrospective analysis of a novel therapeutic approach to complex regional pain syndrome. *Pain Med.* 2004;5:263–275.
128. Kiefer RT, Rohr P, Ploppa A, et al. Efficacy of ketamine in anesthetic dosage for the treatment of refractory complex regional pain syndrome: an open-label phase II study. *Pain Med.* 2008;9:1173–1201.
129. Sigtermans MJ, van Hilten JJ, Bauer MC, Arbous MS, Marinus J, Sarton EY, Dahan A. Ketamine produces effective and long-term pain relief in patients with Complex Regional Pain Syndrome Type 1. *Pain.* 2009;145:304–311.
130. Schwartzman RJ, Alexander GM, Grothusen JR, Paylor T, Reichenberger E, Perreault M. Outpatient intravenous ketamine for the treatment of complex regional pain syndrome: a double-blind placebo controlled study. *Pain.* 2009a;147:107–115.
131. Cepeda MS, Carr DB, Lau J. Local anesthetic sympathetic blockade for complex regional pain syndrome. *Cochrane Database Syst Rev.* 2005:CD004598.
132. Straube S, Derry S, Moore RA, McQuay HJ. Cervico-thoracic or lumbar sympathectomy for neuropathic pain and complex regional pain syndrome. *Cochrane Database Syst Rev.* 2010:CD002918.
133. Yucel I, Demiraran Y, Ozturan K, Degirmenci E. Complex regional pain syndrome type I: efficacy of stellate ganglion blockade. *J Orthop Traumatol.* 2009;10:179–183.
134. Ghahreman A, Ferch R, Bogduk N. The efficacy of transforaminal injection of steroids for the treatment of lumbar radicular pain. *Pain Med.* 2010;11:1149–1168.
135. van Eijs F, Stanton-Hicks M, Van Zundert J, et al. Evidence-based interventional pain medicine according to clinical diagnoses. 16. Complex regional pain syndrome. *Pain Pract.* 2011;11:70–87.
136. Meier PM, Zurakowski D, Berde CB, Sethna NF. Lumbar sympathetic blockade in children with complex regional pain syndromes: a double blind placebo-controlled crossover trial. *Anesthesiology.* 2009;111:372–380.
137. Kemler MA, Barendse GA, van Kleef M, et al. Spinal cord stimulation in patients with chronic reflex sympathetic dystrophy. *N Engl J Med.* 2000;343:618–624.
138. Kemler MA, De Vet HC, Barendse GA, Van Den Wildenberg FA, Van Kleef M. The effect of spinal cord stimulation in patients with chronic reflex sympathetic dystrophy: two years' follow-up of the randomized controlled trial. *Ann Neurol.* 2004;55:13–18.
139. Kemler MA, de Vet HC, Barendse GA, van den Wildenberg FA, van Kleef M. Spinal cord stimulation for chronic reflex sympathetic dystrophy—five-year follow-up. *N Engl J Med.* 2006;354:2394–2396.
140. Kemler MA, de Vet HC, Barendse GA, van den Wildenberg FA, van Kleef M. Effect of spinal cord stimulation for chronic complex regional pain syndrome Type I: five-year final follow-up of patients in a randomized controlled trial. *J Neurosurg.* 2008; 108:292–298.
141. Harke H, Gretenkort P, Ladleif HU, Rahman S. Spinal cord stimulation in sympathetically maintained complex regional pain syndrome type I with severe disability. A prospective clinical study. *Eur J Pain.* 2005;9:363–373.
142. Oakley JC, Weiner RL. Spinal cord stimulation for complex regional pain syndrome: a prospective study of 19 patients at two centers. *Neuromodulation.* 1999;2:47–50.
143. Calvillo O, Racz G, Didie J, Smith K. Neuroaugmentation in the treatment of complex regional pain syndrome of the upper extremity. *Acta Orthop Belg.* 1998;64:57–63.
144. Forouzanfar T, Kemler MA, Weber WE, Kessels AG, van Kleef M. Spinal cord stimulation in complex regional pain syndrome: cervical and lumbar devices are comparably effective. *Br J Anaesth.* 2004;'92:348–353.
145. Hayek SM, Veizi IE, Stanton-Hicks M. Four-limb neurostimulation with neuroelectrodes placed in the lower cervical epidural space. *Anesthesiology.* 2009;110:681–684.
146. Taylor RS, Van Buyten JP, Buchser E. Spinal cord stimulation for complex regional pain syndrome: a systematic review of the clinical and cost-effectiveness literature and assessment of prognostic factors. *Eur J Pain.* 2006;10:91–101.
147. Kemler MA, Raphael JH, Bentley A, Taylor RS. The cost-effectiveness of spinal cord stimulation for complex regional pain syndrome. *Value Health.* 2010;13:735–742.
148. Hassenbusch SJ, Stanton-Hicks M, Schoppa D, Walsh JG, Covington EC. Long-term results of peripheral nerve stimulation for reflex sympathetic dystrophy. *J Neurosurg.* 1996;84:415–423.
149. Velasco F, Carrillo-Ruiz JD, Castro G, et al. Motor cortex electrical stimulation applied to patients with complex regional pain syndrome. *Pain.* 2009;147:91–98.
150. van Hilten BJ, van de Beek WJ, Hoff JI, Voormolen JH, Delhaas EM. Intrathecal baclofen for the treatment of dystonia in patients with reflex sympathetic dystrophy. *N Engl J Med.* 2000[a];343:625–630.
151. Kapural L, Lokey K, Leong MS, et al. Intrathecal ziconotide for complex regional pain syndrome: seven case reports. *Pain Pract.* 2009;9:296–303.
152. van Rijn MA, Munts AG, Marinus J, et al. Intrathecal baclofen for dystonia of complex regional pain syndrome. *Pain.* 2009; 143:41–47.
153. Inchiosa MA Jr, Kizelshteyn G. Treatment of complex regional pain syndrome type I with oral phenoxybenzamine: rationale and case reports. *Pain Pract.* 2008;8:125–132.
154. Muizelaar JP, Kleyer M, Hertogs IA, DeLange DC. Complex regional pain syndrome (reflex sympathetic dystrophy and causalgia): management with the calcium channel blocker nifedipine and/or the alpha-sympathetic blocker phenoxybenzamine in 59 patients. *Clin Neurol Neurosurg.* 1997;99:26–30.
155. Lynch ME. Psychological aspects of reflex sympathetic dystrophy: a review of the adult and paediatric literature. *Pain.* 1992;49:337–347.
156. Haddox DJ, Abram SE, Hopwood MH. Comparison of Psychometric Data in RSD and Radiculopathy. *Regional Anesthesia and Pain Medicine.* 1988;13:27.
157. Zucchini M, Alberti G, Moretti MP. Algodystrophy and related psychological features. *Funct Neurol.* 1989;4:153–156.
158. DeGood DE, Cundiff GW, Adams LE, Shutty MS Jr. A psychosocial and behavioral comparison of reflex sympathetic dystrophy, low back pain and headache patients. *Pain.* 1993; 54:317–322.
159. Bruehl S, Husfeldt B, Lubenow TR, Nath H, Ivankovich AD. Psychological differences between reflex sympathetic dystrophy and non-RSD chronic pain patients. *Pain.* 1996;67:107–114.
160. Fialka V, Korpan M, Saradeth T, et al. Autogenic training for reflex sympathetic dystrophy: a pilot study. *Complementary Therapies in Medicine.* 1996;4:103–105.
161. Bruehl S, Chung OY. Psychological and behavioral aspects of complex regional pain syndrome management. *Clin J Pain.* 2006;22:430–437.
162. de Mos M, Sturkenboom MC, Huygen FJ. Current understandings on complex regional pain syndrome. *Pain Pract.* 2009c;9:86–99.
163. Katz MM, Hungerford DS. Reflex sympathetic dystrophy affecting the knee. *J Bone Joint Surg Br.* 1987;69:797–803.
164. Rocco AG. Sympathetically maintained pain may be rekindled by surgery under general anesthesia. *Anesthesiology.* 1993;79:865.
165. Viel EJ, Pelissier J, Eledjam JJ. Sympathetically maintained pain after surgery may be prevented by regional anesthesia. *Anesthesiology.* 1994;81:265–266.
166. Veldman PH, Goris RJ. Surgery on extremities with reflex sympathetic dystrophy. *Unfallchirurg.* 1995;98:45–48.
167. Cazeneuve JF, Leborgne JM, Kermad K, Hassan Y. Vitamin C and prevention of reflex sympathetic dystrophy following surgical management of distal radius fractures. *Acta Orthop Belg.* 2002;68:481–484.
168. Zollinger PE, Kreis RW, van der Meulen HG, van der Elst M, Breederveld RS, Tuinebreijer WE. No higher risk of CRPS after

external fixation of distal radial fractures—subgroup analysis under randomised vitamin C prophylaxis. *Open Orthop J.* 2010a;4:71–75.

169. Zollinger PE, Unal H, Ellis ML, Tuinebreijer WE. Clinical results of 40 consecutive basal thumb prostheses and no CRPS Type I after vitamin C prophylaxis. *Open Orthop J.* 2010b;4:62–66.
170. Besse JL, Gadeyne S, Galand-Desme S, Lerat JL, Moyen B. Effect of vitamin C on prevention of complex regional pain syndrome type I in foot and ankle surgery. *Foot Ankle Surg.* 2009;15:179–182.
171. Moufawad S, Malak O, Mekhail NA. Epidural infusion of opiates and local anesthetics for Complex Regional Pain Syndrome. *Pain Pract.* 2002;2:81–86.
172. Hayek SM, Paige B, Girgis C, et al. Tunneled epidural catheter infections in noncancer pain: increased risk in patients with neuropathic pain/complex regional pain syndrome. *Clin J Pain.* 2006;22:82–89.

26.

FIBROMYALGIA

Howard S. Smith, Kim D. Jones, Daniel J. Clauw, and Binit J. Shah

CASE PRESENTATION

L. H. is a 48-year-old woman who works as a social worker and is seeking medical attention for widespread moderate to severe pain for 5 years. She particularly notes significant chronic pain/tenderness in her neck, low back, right jaw, chest, right upper arm, left buttock, and left lower leg. She is still working but had to cut back to part-time work, and she just cancelled her vacation to Jamaica because of her pain. She states that she is also having some moderate problems with fatigue, low mood, and difficulty with insomnia and non-refreshing sleep. Recent stressors include a divorce 4 months ago and a teenage daughter engaging in disruptive behaviors at school. Her past medical history reveals that she also has been diagnosed with headaches/neck muscle spasms, irritable bowel syndrome, and interstitial cystitis.

Her primary care provider (PCP) started her on oxycodone CR 10 mg PO BID and naproxen 500 mg PO BID for pain relief and clonazepam 3 mg PO QHS to help her sleep, but she is on no other medications. Although these were 75% effective for the first 2 months, her symptoms have returned to baseline in the past 3 months. She asked her PCP to increase her dose of oxycodone CR, but, rather than do this, her PCP referred her to the Interdisciplinary Pain Medicine Clinic.

On examination: widespread tenderness/deep tissue hyperalgesia bilaterally over the posterior aspect of the cervical spine, lower thoracic and lumbar spine, all her painful areas, and all four extremities without true allodynia. Neurovascular examination is intact. Range of motion is mildly restricted. There is no synovitis.

A diagnosis of fibromyalgia (FM) was made.

QUESTIONS

1. What is the epidemiology of FM?
2. What is the prognosis for patients with FM?
3. What is the pathophysiology of FM?
4. What are the diagnostic criteria of FM?
5. How is FM managed using pharmacologic approaches?
6. How is FM managed using nonpharmacologic approaches?

WHAT IS THE EPIDEMIOLOGY OF FM?

FM is a debilitating chronic pain condition affecting approximately 15 million persons in the United States and is one of the more severe disorders on the continuum of persistent pain.[1-4] FM results in profound suffering, including widespread musculoskeletal pain and stiffness, fatigue, and disturbed sleep, and may include cognitive alterations/abnormalities (dyscognition), affective distress, and very poor quality of life (Figure 26.1).[5]

FM appears to have been identified in approximately 2–4% of the general population,[6,7] FM is predominantly diagnosed in patients between the ages of 20 and 60 years (mean age, 49) with approximately 80% of cases being female.[6,7] Women are more sensitive to painful stimuli than men and therefore have a greater response than men to the diagnostic tender point (TP) examination that is included in the American College of Rheumatology (ACR) 1990 criteria (tenderness on digital palpation at predestinated sites). As a result, men with chronic widespread pain (CWP) rarely meet ACR 1990 criteria for FM despite having a similar underlying pathologic process.[8] There is a high aggregation of FM in families of patients with FM. The odds ratio measuring the odds of FM in a relative of a proband with FM versus the odds of FM in a relative of a proband with rheumatoid arthritis was 8.5. The strong familial aggregation reported in FM, although not excluding a possible contribution by environmental factors, appears to point to a genetic basis as an important contributor to its etiology.[9] The mode of inheritance is unknown, but it is most probably polygenic.

Epidemiological studies of the historical component of the ACR criteria for FM, CWP, have been extremely instructive. CWP is typically operationalized as pain above and below the waist, involving the left and right sides of the body, and also involving the axial skeleton. Population-based studies of CWP suggest that 5–15% of the population has this symptom at any given point in time.[10-13] Chronic regional pain is found in 20–25% of the population. Both chronic widespread and regional pain occur about 1.5 times as commonly in women than in men.

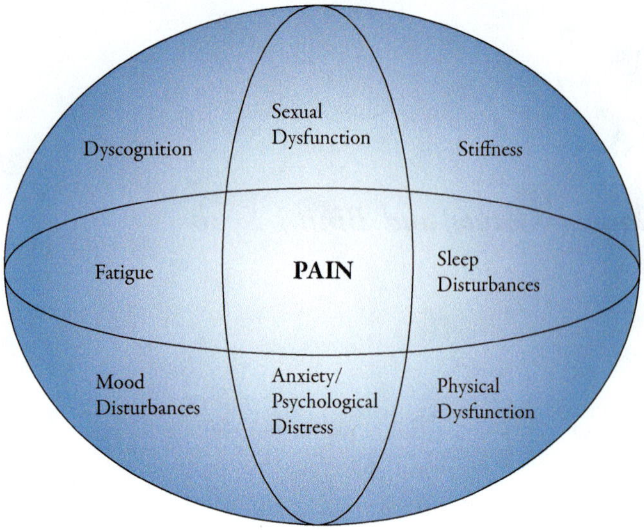

Figure 26.1 Fibromyalgia domains.

Among FM patients, 20–50% work few or no days despite being in their peak wage earning years.[14,15] Disability payments are received by 26–55% of FM patients, compared with a national average of 2% for disability payments from other causes.[14,16] Furthermore, healthcare costs are three times higher among FM patients compared to matched controls.[17]

Diminished aerobic fitness in FM has been documented for almost three decades, and recent studies report that the average 40-year-old with FM has fitness findings expected for a healthy 70- to 80-year-old; FM has now been associated with increased mortality.[1,3,18–21]

WHAT IS THE PROGNOSIS FOR PATIENTS WITH FM?

The prognosis of FM depends largely on where the individual falls on a continuum. On one end of the continuum are individuals in the population with CWP or individuals with FM who are seen in primary care, with the prognosis in these individuals being quite good.[22,23] On the other hand, individuals with FM seen in tertiary-care settings do quite poorly.[24] In this latter study, there was little change in symptoms over time, and no significant change in health satisfaction, symptoms, or functional disability.

With regard to function in FM, studies have reported varying disability rates from 9% to 44%.[24,25] Disability has been most strongly associated with functional and work status, pain, mood disturbances, coping ability, depression, pending litigation, and educational background.

WHAT IS THE PATHOPHYSIOLOGY OF FM?

Once FM is established, by far the most consistently detected objective abnormalities involve augmented pain and sensory processing systems. Because FM is defined in part by tenderness, considerable work has been performed exploring the potential reason for this phenomenon. Although the precise pathophysiology of FM remains uncertain, there are two different specific pathogenic mechanisms that may lead to a low pain threshold in FM and that have been identified using experimental pain testing: (1) increased wind-up or temporal summation and (2) a reduction of descending analgesic activity.

INCREASED WIND-UP IN FM

Early experimental pain testing studies also suggested that some individuals with FM might have evidence of wind-up, indicative of central sensitization.[26,27] More recent studies suggest that this does not occur as commonly in FM as diffuse hyperalgesia or decreased diffuse noxious inhibitory control (DNIC), but nonetheless this may help to further characterize patients.[28] In animal models, this finding is associated with increased glutamatergic and excitatory amino acid and substance P hyperactivity.[29,30]

Although experimental pain testing cannot yet identify individuals with increased glutamatergic or substance P activity contributing to FM pathogenesis, there is ample evidence that increased high levels of these neurotransmitters are playing some role in FM. Four independent studies have shown that patients with FM have approximately threefold higher concentrations of substance P in cerebrospinal fluid (CSF) when compared with normal controls.[31–34]

Glutamate (Glu) is a major excitatory neurotransmitter within the central nervous system, and CSF levels of Glu are twice as high in FM patients than in controls.[35] Not only are the CSF levels elevated, but several recent studies using proton spectroscopy demonstrated that the Glu levels in FM patients are also elevated in key pain processing areas of the brain, such as the insula, and change in response to changes in both clinical and experimental pain when patients are successfully treated.[36–39] A relatively new imaging study by Harris and colleagues suggests that the drug pregabalin is acting in part in FM by decreasing glutamatergic activity in the insula and thus decreasing functional connectivity between the default mode network (DMN) and insula.[40] In this study, individuals with the highest levels of Glu in the insula pretreatment were those most likely to respond to pregabalin. There is also evidence that subsets of patients respond to drugs known to be N-methyl-D-aspartic acid (NMDA)-receptor antagonists, inferring that glutamatergic activity is increased[41,42]; unfortunately these drugs, such as ketamine or dextromethorphan, are generally not well tolerated and thus not often practical for clinical use.

Foerster and colleagues evaluated 21 patients with FM and 27 healthy controls who underwent conventional magnetic resonance imaging (MRI) and dynamic susceptibility-weighted contrast-enhanced perfusion MRI (DSC).[43] Significant correlations were found between thalamic relative cerebral blood flow (rCBF) values and pain belief values, suggesting that there are baseline alterations of brain perfusion in patients with FM. rCBF values of the thalami exhibited lower correlations with respect to other brain regions thought to be involved in pain processing compared with those in healthy controls.[43] It is more likely that these changes in blood flow are "from" the processes that lead to FM rather than the "cause" of the condition.

Functional MRI (fMRI) and other imaging techniques may also be utilized to look at the extent that brain regions are "connected" to each other (i.e., simultaneously activated or deactivated).[44] This technique can either be applied to fMRI data acquired when individuals are "resting" (resting state analysis) or while performing a task. The advantage of resting state analysis is that it does not require giving the participant a stimulus, and thus it allows a window into potentially measuring brain changes associated with chronic, ongoing spontaneous pain. Another advantage is that there are many known neural networks that subserve different functions in the human brain, so the extent to which these networks are either intact or somehow disrupted by chronic pain can be examined. Napadow et al. used this technique to demonstrate that individuals with FM show increased connectivity between the DMN (a network active when the brain is "resting" and not performing any specific task) and the insula—a known "pro-nociceptive region of the brain.[45] Furthermore, in these studies, the degree of increased connectivity was related to the intensity of ongoing, spontaneous pain.[46] A different group has shown that during a painful stimulus connectivity is *decreased* between key antinociceptive regions (e.g., the brainstem—the origin of descending analgesic pathways) and a region they had previously identified to be a potential source of dysfunctional pain inhibition in FM.[47,48] Thus, these measures of connectivity hold considerable promise as potential biomarkers for pain intensity or mechanism, especially if they can be accurately and reliably measured using techniques, such as electroencephalogram (EEG), that are more practical for use at the point of care.

Studies of resting-state intrinsic brain connectivity in FM have demonstrated increased insular connectivity to the DMN, a network whose activity is increased during non-task states.[46] Moreover, increased insular connectivity to the DMN was associated with increased spontaneous pain levels. Napadow and colleagues evaluated 17 FM patients who underwent resting-state functional MRI at baseline and following 4 weeks of a nonpharmacologic intervention to diminish pain.[46] Clinical pain as assessed using the sensory scale of the SF-MPQ was reduced following therapy ($p = 0.02$). Intrinsic DMN connectivity to the insula was reduced, and this reduction correlated with reductions in pain (corrected $p < 0.05$) suggesting that intrinsic brain connectivity can be used as a candidate objective marker that reflects changes in spontaneous chronic pain within individual FM patients.[46]

Positron emission tomography (PET) has been used in several studies in FM. In a very early such study, Yunus and colleagues simply used PET as a crude marker of neuronal activity and failed to show any differences in regional cerebral blood flow between FM patients and controls.[49] However, Wood and colleagues used PET to show that attenuated dopaminergic activity may be playing a role in pain transmission in FM, and Harris and colleagues showed evidence of decreased μ opioid receptor availability (possibly due to increased release of endogenous μ opioids) in FM.[50,51]

Fayed and colleagues utilized protein magnetic resonance spectroscopy (H-MRS) to evaluate the brain metabolite patterns in patients with FM and somatization disorder (STD) compared with healthy controls.[52] A significant increase was found in the Glu + glutamine (Glx) levels in the posterior cingulate cortex (PCC): 10.73 (standard deviation [SD]: 0.49) for FM and 9.67 (SD: 1.10) for STD 9.54 (SD: 1.46) compared with controls ($p = 0.043$). In the FM + STD group, a correlation between Glx and pain catastrophizing in PCC ($r = 0.397$; $p = 0.033$) and between quality of life and the myo-inositol-to-creatine ratio in the left hippocampus ($r = -0.500$; $p = 0.025$) was found.[52] In addition to the aforementioned used of H-MRS to show elevated Glu levels, Harris and colleagues also used this technique to show that the levels of γ-aminobutyric acid (GABA), an inhibitory neurotransmitter, are decreased in the insula in individuals with FM.[53]

Foerster and colleagues evaluated 16 FM patients and 17 age- and sex-matched healthy controls who underwent pressure-pain testing and a 3T proton MRS session in which the right anterior insula, right posterior insula, anterior cingulate, and occipital cortex were examined in subjects at rest.[53] GABA levels in the right anterior insula were significantly lower in FM patients compared with healthy controls (mean ± SD 1.17 ± 0.24 arbitrary institutional units versus 1.42 ± 0.32 arbitrary institutional units; $p = 0.016$). Within the right posterior insula, higher levels of GABA were positively correlated with pressure-pain thresholds in the FM patients (Spearman's rho = 0.63; $p = 0.02$), and they concluded that diminished inhibitory neurotransmission resulting from lower concentrations of GABA within the right anterior insula may play a role in the pathophysiology of FM and other central pain syndromes.[53]

WHAT ARE THE DIAGNOSTIC CRITERIA OF FM?

The 1990 ACR criteria for FM, originally proposed exclusively for research purposes, require that an individual has both a history of CWP and the finding of 11 or more of 18 possible TPs on examination. TPs represent nine paired, predefined regions of the body, often located over musculotendinous insertions.[54] If an individual reports pain when a region is palpated with 4 kg of pressure, this is considered a positive TP. Between 25% and 50% of individuals who have CWP will also have 11 or more TPs and thus meet criteria for FM.[12,55]In 2010 and 2011, alternative criteria for FM were established that did not require performing a TP count.[54,56] These new criteria are aligned with a more contemporary view of the "pain centralization phenotype," which acknowledges that the most discriminating features of FM and other centralized pain states are multifocal pain (i.e., involving many areas of the body rather than just a few) combined with other comorbid symptoms such as fatigue, memory difficulties, and sleep and mood disturbances.[57,58]

Recently proposed diagnostic criteria that assess widespread pain along with the severity of symptoms of fatigue, sleep disturbance, cognitive dysfunction, and the extent of somatic symptoms may improve diagnosis and treatment of FM.[54] Wolfe and colleagues have proposed simple clinical criteria for FM that do not require the use of TPs,[54] thus expanding the definition of FM to include symptoms other than pain and providing a measure to assess FM symptom-related severity.[54] Wolfe et al. performed a two-stage, 55-site multicenter study of 1,002 patients with FM and pain controls to develop simple clinical criteria for FM.[54] Patients underwent a detailed interview and examination, including TP examination and assessment of the extent of widespread pain using a 0–19 Widespread Pain Index (WPI) and also completed a detailed questionnaire.[54] These 19 locations include: jaw–L, chest, jaw–R, abdomen, forearm–L, forearm–R, upper leg–L, upper leg–R, lower leg–L, lower leg–R, upper arm–L, upper arm–R, upper back, hip–L, hip–R, shoulder–L, shoulder–R, neck, and low back. The WPI was the best predictor of FM. Analyses excluding WPI identified unrefreshed sleep, fatigue, cognitive difficulties, and the extent of somatic symptom reporting as the key FM predictors. Wolfe and colleagues combined the four categorical symptom variables into a 0 and 12 Symptom Severity (SS) scale. The SS scale correlated with the TP count ($r = 0.688$) and the WPI (0.733). Wolfe et al. proposed that FM may be diagnosed when WPI is greater than 6, WPI is 3–6 and SS is greater than 4, or SS is 9 or greater (Table 26.1).[54]

The patient appears to satisfy the preliminary 2010 ACR criteria for FM. She definitely clearly notes seven areas of pain that she has had over the last week; so that her WPI is 7 and her SS scale score is 7.

- Cognitive = 0 (No problem)
- Fatigue = 2 (Moderate level of fatigue)
- Waking unrefreshed = 3 (Severe level)
- Somatic symptoms = 2 = moderate number of symptoms [fatigue/tiredness, headache, insomnia, constipation, irritable bowel, chest pain, painful urination (interstitial cystitis)].

In 2011, Wolfe et al. proposed a modified version of the ACR preliminary diagnostic criteria for fibromylagia (2010) that made it possible to use the crtieria in epidemiologic and clinical studies without the need for an examiner (this version was not intended to be used for self-diagnosis.[56] These new criteria (often referred to as the "2011 criteria" or "survey criteria" eliminate the physician's estimate of the extent of somatic symptoms and substitute the sum of three specific self-reported symptoms. Therefore, a new item scored 0–3 that represents the sum of three items—the presence or absence of headaches, pain, or cramps in lower abdomen or depression symptoms during the previous 6 months—was substituted for the extent of somatic symptoms item of the SS scale score.[56] They also created a 0–31 FM Symptom (FS) scale by adding the WPI to the modified SS scale. An FS score of 13 or greater best separated criteria-positive and criteria-negative patients, classifying 93.0% correctly, with a sensitivity of 96.6% and a specificity of 91.8% in the study population.[56] Others have expressed concern that these criteria may allow highly symptomatic persons with regional pain states to be classified as having FM.[59]

By the modified ACR 2010 criteria, in our patient's new scoring the WPI is the same as ACR 2010 criteria (7), and modified SS scale score is:

- Cognitive = 0
- Fatigue = 2
- Waking unrefreshed = 3
- Heasdache during the previous 6 months = Present = 1
- Pain or cramps in lower abdomen (from intestitial cystitis) during the previous 6 months = Present = 1
- Depression during the previous 6 months = Present = 1
- Modified SS scale score = 8
- FS score = WPI + SS = 7 + 8 = 15 (which is >13 – c/w FM)

HOW IS FM MANAGED USING PHARMACOLOGIC APPROACHES?

TRICYCLIC ANTIDEPRESSANTS

The most frequently studied pharmacologic therapy for FM is low doses of tricyclic compounds (TCAs). Most TCAs increase the concentrations of serotonin and/or norepinephrine (noradrenaline) by directly blocking their respective reuptake. The effectiveness of TCAs, particularly amitriptyline and cyclobenzaprine (structurally extremely similar to amitriptyline), in treating the symptoms of pain, poor sleep, and fatigue associated with FM is supported by several randomized controlled trials (RCTs).[60] Dose escalation, changes in QT intervals—particularly in the elderly—and tolerability of side effects remain a challenge in this drug class. Tolerability can be improved by beginning at very low doses (e.g., 10 mg of amitriptyline or 5 mg of cyclobenzaprine), giving the dose a few hours before bedtime, and very slowly escalating the dose. Very low-dose cyclobenzaprine has recently been shown to be quite effective in a subset of individuals with FM with a specific sleep architecture, seemingly with less side effects than seen in some of the earlier studies of higher doses.[61]

SELECTIVE SEROTONIN REUPTAKE INHIBITORS (SSRIS)

Because of a better side-effect profile, newer antidepressants, the SSRIs, are frequently used in FM. The SSRIs fluoxetine, citalopram, and paroxetine have each been evaluated in randomized, placebo-controlled trials.[62–66] In general, the results of studies of SSRIs in FM have paralleled the experience in other pain conditions. The newer "highly selective" serotonin reuptake inhibitors (e.g., citalopram) seem to be less efficacious than the older SSRIs, which have

Table 26.1 1990 VERSUS 2010 ACR DIAGNOSTIC CRITERIA FOR FIBROMYALGIA (FM)

1990 ACR CRITERIA[144]	PRELIMINARY 2010 ACR CRITERIA[54]	MODIFIED PRELIMINARY 2010 ACR CRITERIA[56]
Widespread pain (bilateral pain above and below waist; axial skeletal pain involving cervical thoracic, lumbar spine, and anterior chest) present for 3 months or greater, with no known disorder to explain the pain. Pain in 11 of 18 tender points upon digital palpation with 4 kg of pressure: • occiput at the suboccipital muscle insertions • low cervical at the anterior aspects of the inter-transverse spaces at C5–C7 • trapezius at the midpoint of the upper border • the supraspinatus at the origins near the medial border • at the second rib, upper lateral to the second costochondral junction • lateral epicondyle, 2 cm distal to the epicondyles • gluteal, in the upper, outer quadrants of the buttocks in the anterior fold of the muscle • the greater trochanter, posterior to the trochanteric prominence • knee, at the medial fat pad, proximal to the joint line	A patient satisfies diagnostic criteria for FM if the following 3 conditions are met: 1) Either (A) or (B) below is met: (A) Widespread pain index (WPI) ≥7 and a Symptom Severity (SS) scale score of ≥5. (B) A WPI of 3–6 and an SS scale ≥9. 2) Symptoms have been present at a similar level for at least 6 months; and, 3) The patient does not have a disorder that would otherwise explain the pain. WPI: *Note the number of areas in which the patient has had pain over the last week.* 0–19 possible points (areas of pain in past week); areas include left/right for each: shoulder girdle, upper/lower arm, hip/buttock/trochanter, upper/lower leg, jaw, chest, abdomen, upper/lower back, neck Symptom Severity (SS) Scale: Score between 0 and 12 possible points SS scale score = sum of the 3 symptoms + extent of somatic symptoms SS Scale includes: Fatigue, waking unrefreshed, cognitive symptoms for each symptom patient rates severity of problem as: 0 = none, 1 = slight, mild, or intermittent, 2 = moderate, considerable, 3 = severe, life disturbing Somatic symptoms (such as muscle pain, irritable bowel, fatigue/tiredness, thinking/remembering problems, muscle weakness, headache, pain/cramps in abdomen, numbness/tingling, dizziness, insomnia, depression, constipation, nausea/vomiting/diarrhea, blurred vision, dry mouth, loss of appetite) rated as: 0 = no symptoms, 1 = few symptoms, 2 = moderate number of symptoms, 3 = great deal of symptoms	A patient satisfies diagnostic criteria for FM if the following 3 conditions are met: 4) Either (A) or (B) below is met: (A) Widespread pain index (WPI) ≥7 and a Symptom Severity (SS) scale score of ≥5. (B) A WPI of 3–6 and an SS scale ≥9. 5) Symptoms have been present at a similar level for at least 6 months; and, 6) The patient does not have a disorder that would otherwise explain the pain. WPI: *Note the number of areas in which the patient has had pain over the last week.* 0–19 possible points (areas of pain in past week); areas include left/right for each: shoulder girdle, upper/lower arm, hip/buttock/trochanter, upper/lower leg, jaw, chest, abdomen, upper/lower back, neck Modified Symptom Severity (SS) Scale: Score between 0 and 12 possible points SS scale score = sum of the 3 symptoms + sum of 3 items: the presence or absence of headaches, pain or cramps in lower abdomen, or depression symptoms during the previous 6 months SS Scale includes: Fatigue, waking unrefreshed, cognitive symptoms for each symptom patient rates severity of problem as: 0 = none, 1 = slight, mild, or intermittent, 2 = moderate, considerable, 3 = severe, life disturbing Possible 0–3: • Headaches during previous 6 months Present = 1; Absent = 0 • Pain or cramps in lower abdomen during previous 6 months Present = 1; Absent = 0 • Depression symptoms during previous 6 months Present = 1; Absent = 0

Adapted with permission from Firestone KA, Holton KF, Mist SD, Wright CL, Jones KD. Optimizing fibromyalgia management. *Nurse Pract.* 2012;37:12–21.

some noradrenergic activity at higher doses.[67] Although there is some statistical significant in studies, they do not reach the level of likely clinical benefit, a fact that has been shown in clinical practice. SSRIs have consistently shown to be of little benefit for painful conditions, in distinction to TCAs and selective serotonin norepinephrine reuptake inhibitors (SNRIs).

Because TCAs and high doses of certain SSRIs such as fluoxetine and sertraline that have the most balanced reuptake inhibition are the most effective analgesics, many have concluded that dual receptor inhibitors such as serotonin-NE and NE-serotonin reuptake inhibitors (SNRIs and NSRIs) may be of more benefit than pure serotonergic drugs.[67] These drugs are pharmacologically similar to some TCAs in their ability to inhibit the reuptake of both serotonin and NE, but they differ from TCAs in being generally devoid of significant activity at other receptor systems. This selectivity results in diminished side effects and enhanced tolerability. The first available SNRI, venlafaxine, has data to support its use in the management of neuropathic pain, and retrospective trial data demonstrate that this compound is also effective in the prophylaxis of migraine and tension headaches.[68] Two studies in FM have had conflicting results, with the one using a higher dose showing efficacy.[69]

Two newer SNRIs, duloxetine and milnacipran, have undergone recent multicenter trials and were shown to be effective in a number of outcome variables; both are now approved in the United States for the treatment of FM.[70,71] These drugs seem roughly comparable in their overall efficacy profiles, with studies generally noting modest improvement (although not reaching statistical significance in all studies) in domains such as pain, overall improvement, physical functioning, level of fatigue, and degree of reported physical impairment. For both compounds, these effects seem to be independent of the drugs' effect on mood, thus suggesting that the analgesic and other positive effects of this class of drugs in FM is not simply due to their antidepressant effects. Both these drugs are better tolerated if taken with food. Patients should be warned about likely initial nausea and counseled that this typically resolves in a week or so; if not, then they should discontinue the drug. The maximum approved dose of duloxetine is 60 mg/d but it was studied in trials at doses up to 120 mg and shown to be safe (similarly, the initial dose of milnacipran is 50 mg BID), but some patients will benefit from increasing the dose as high as 100 mg BID. Hypertension and tachycardia are more likely to be a problem with milnacipran, since it appears to be more noradrenergic; for these same reasons, it might be slightly more likely to help with symptoms such as fatigue or dyscognition.

Es-reboxetine (not available in the U.S. market), a selective norepinephrine reuptake inhibitor, was also tested and shown to be efficacious in FM.[72] This adds to emerging evidence suggesting that norepinephrine reuptake activity may be much more important than serotonergic reuptake for analgesic effects.

OTHER CENTRAL NERVOUS SYSTEM-ACTING DRUGS

Some antiepileptic drugs have been shown to be effective in the treatment of various chronic pain conditions, including postherpetic neuralgia and painful diabetic neuropathy.[73] Pregabalin and gabapentin have the same mechanism of action and bind to the $\alpha 2\delta$ subunit of calcium channels, and both are approved for the treatment of neuropathic pain, as well as for several other indications. Several studies show the efficacy of pregabalin against pain, sleep disturbances, and fatigue as compared to placebo in FM, leading to pregabalin being the first drug approved in the United States for use in this condition.[74,75] Gabapentin has been shown to have a very similar efficacy and side-effect profile in FM.[60] The tolerability of these drugs can be dramatically enhanced by beginning at a low dose and giving either two-thirds of the dose, or the entire dose, at bedtime. The maximally approved dose of pregabalin is 450 mg, but in trials it was studied at doses as high as 600 mg and shown to be safe and efficacious. The dose of gabapentin needed for analgesic is often 1,800–2,400 mg/day. Another antiepileptic compound, clonazepam, has demonstrated efficacy in treating temporal mandibular disorder and associated jaw pain and is useful in the treatment of restless leg syndrome[73]; it may be of value in FM.

Sedative-hypnotic compounds are widely used by FM patients. A handful of studies have been published on the use of certain nonbenzodiazepine hypnotics in FM, such as zopiclone and zolpidem.[76,77] These reports suggest that these agents can improve the sleep and, perhaps, fatigue of FM patients, although they had no significant effects on pain.

On the other hand, γ-hydroxybutyrate (also known as sodium oxybate), a precursor of GABA with powerful sedative properties, has been shown to be very efficacious in large multicenter phase III trials in FM. Patients reported improve fatigue, pain, physical function, and sleep architecture.[78–81]

Note, however, that this agent is a scheduled substance due to its abuse potential and was not approved by the U.S. Food and Drug Administration (FDA) for FM due to diversion concerns. Nonetheless, these studies, along with the H-MRS showing low GABA levels, suggest that other less toxic GABA agonists may have an important role in treating FM (especially, perhaps, for a subpopulation of patients with severe sleep disturbances/insomnia refractory to all other pharmacotherapy) (Figure 26.2).

Cannabinoids are another class of drugs in which there is renewed interest in chronic pain states. There have been two RCTs of synthetic cannabinoids in FM (both with nabilone), and both studies concluded that the drug was efficacious (in one study for both pain and sleep, in the other study at lower dose for only sleep).[82,83] This is not surprising because there is increased recognition that this class of drugs may have utility in pain of neural origin.[84]

Pramipexole is a dopamine agonist indicated for Parkinson disease that has shown utility in the treatment of periodic leg movement disorder.[85] One study suggested that this compound may improve both pain and sleep in FM patients, but these results have not been replicated with this or other dopamine agonists.[86] Because of this, this class of drug may be best reserved for individuals with other indications, such as comorbid restless legs syndrome.

Tizanidine is a centrally acting $\alpha 2$ adrenergic agonist approved by the FDA for the treatment of muscle spasticity associated with multiple sclerosis and stroke. Literature suggests that this agent is a useful adjunct in treating several chronic pain conditions, including chronic daily headaches and low back pain. A recent trial reported significant improvements in several parameters in FM, including sleep, pain, and measures of quality of life.[87] Of particular interest was the demonstration that treatment with tizanidine resulted in a reduction in substance P levels within the CSF of patients with FM.

OPIOID ANALGESICS

There have been no adequate, randomized, controlled clinical trials of opiates in FM, and most in the field (including the authors) have not found this class of compounds to be effective in anecdotal experience.[88–93] Opioids are not a recommended treatment based on any available practice guidelines. The use of opioids by patients with FM is associated with poorer health, worsened psychosocial status, and higher rates of substance abuse.[94] A recent 2-year, prospective study of FM patients (N = 131) compared outcomes in those treated with opioids versus not in a multidisciplinary pain clinic.[95] Patient taking opioids were more likely to be disabled, unemployed, and scored higher on all measures of symptom severity. The authors were unable to ascertain added benefit from opioids.

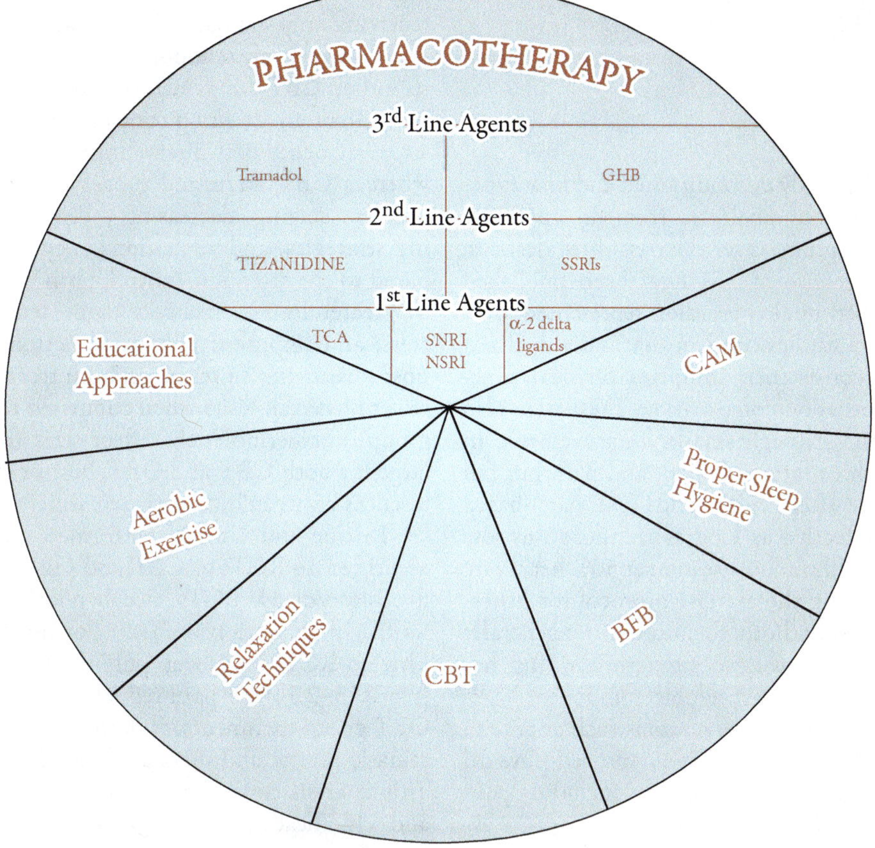

Figure 26.2 Potential therapies for fibromyalgia.

Abbreviations: BFB, biofeedback; CAM, complementary or alternative medicine; CBT, cognitive behavioral therapies; GHB, gamma hydroxybutyrate; NSRI, norepinephrine and serotonin reuptake inhibitor; SNRI, serotonin and norepinephrine reuptake inhibitor; TCA, tricyclic antidepressant

A 2013 review[96] on the use of opioids in FM concluded that "chronic opioid use is inappropriate in the treatment of FM." Despite the absence of evidence for effect, approximately 30% of patients with FM in the United States are on opioids.[97] This may, in part, be due to the fact that FM patients identify opioids as the most effective class of medications, specifically hydrocodone and oxycodone.[98]

Although it remains uncertain why the analgesia from opioids is generally poor for patients with FM, potential explanations may include the following: (1) enkephalin levels in the CSF are elevated; (2) μ opioid receptor (MOR) binding in neuroimaging study is decreased in the nucleus accumbens, amygdala, and dorsal anterior cingulated cortex,[51] suggesting that high levels of endogenous opioids may down-regulate MOR, which may lower the efficacy of opioids[99]; and, (3) although opioids generally activate serotonergic neurons to accelerate 5-hydroxytryptamine turnover ratio leading to facilitation of the serotonergic descending inhibitory pathways, animal model study suggests that in FM patients there is a loss of opioid-induced descending serotonergic activation.[99] In fact, it is conceivable that opioids may be counterproductive to the optimal efficency of the descending inhbitory pain pathways (with resultant reduced conditioned pain modulation), and it appears that opioid antagonists (e.g., naltrexone) may have a specific and clinically beneficial impact on FM pain.[100]

NONOPIOID ANALGESICS

Tramadol is a compound that has some opioid activity (weak μ agonist activity) combined with serotonin/norepinephrine reuptake inhibition. Tramadol is unscheduled or a schedule IV compound depending on the state. This compound was FDA approved for moderate to moderately severe pain based in part on two studies in FM but is not specifically approved for use in FM. Tramadol does appear to be somewhat efficacious in the management of FM as both an isolated compound[101] and as a fixed-dose combination with acetaminophen.[102] To date, there have only been a few small (i.e., underpowered) studies of nonsteroidal anti-inflammatory drugs (NSAIDs) in FM, and these have not been shown to be effective.

Several options were discussed with the patient. First, it was recommended to discontinue the OxyContin, naproxen, and clonazepam by gradual tapering, and the patient was started on cyclobenzaprine 5 mg PO QHS. The cyclobenzaprine was titrated up until the patient began to feel somewhat improved. Because the patient was still having moderate pain and trouble sleeping, pregabalin was initiated at 75 mg PO QHS and then titrated up gradually. The patient did reasonably well but was still complaining about persistent pain, headaches, and cervical paraspinal muscle spasms, at which point low-dose tizanidine was added.

HOW IS FM MANAGED USING NONPHARMACOLOGIC APPROACHES?

EXERCISE

Persons with FM are physically deconditioned and may experience some exercise-induced analgesia from an appropriately tailored exercise program. Over the past three decades, 125 clinical trials of exercise in FM have been published with increasingly higher quality studies represented over time. Most high-quality studies confirm that individualized low-intensity exercise consistently improves physical function more so than any other outcome marker. These trials also demonstrate significant although smaller improvements in key FM symptoms such as fatigue, mood, and pain but fail to significantly improve sleep. Both land- and water-based exercise studies were effective as long as the dose was low (generally twice weekly, 60 minutes/session at 50% heart rate maximum). Individualizing the exercise protocol for fitness level, regional pain states, and other comorbidities generally increases adherence.[103–105] Low-dose strength training has been found efficacious without an aerobic component.[106–112] Recently mind-body movement interventions such as tai chi, qigong, and yoga with mindfulness have improved physical function and a wider array of FM symptoms including pain and sleep.[103,104,113,114]

EDUCATIONAL APPROACHES

Most experts agree that an educational or psychoeducational treatment component is useful if not necessary when treating FM as part of a multimodal approach.[115] Burckhardt and colleagues assigned FM patients to an education-only condition, an education plus physical training condition, or a delayed treatment waitlist control.[116] Both active treatment groups improved on subjective ratings and reports of physical activity compared to controls. Rooks et al. [117] completed an RCT with 207 confirmed FM patients who were assigned to one of four groups: (1) an aerobic and flexibility exercise group; (2) a strength training, aerobic, and flexibility exercise group; (3) the FM Self-Help Course (FSHC) (Education group); or (4) a combination of the previous three groups. The primary outcome was change in physical function from baseline to completion of the intervention, and the combination group showed the greatest improvement.

COGNITIVE-BEHAVIORAL THERAPY (CBT)

Techniques such as pacing, graded activation, relaxation, pleasant activity scheduling, and sleep hygiene activities are commonly offered in CBT programs. Williams and colleagues[118] randomly assigned 145 patients with FM to either 4 weeks of group CBT (6 sessions) or standard medical care. Twenty-five percent of patients with FM receiving CBT met criteria for being a "treatment responder" (i.e., sustained improvement in functional status), compared to 12% of those receiving only standard medical care.

Thieme et al. randomly assigned 125 patients with FM to either CBT (n = 42), operant behavior therapy (OBT; n = 43), or an attention control group (n = 40).[119] OBT consisted of behavioral interventions to reduce pain behaviors, whereas CBT addressed modifying maladaptive thoughts, problem solving, decreasing psychological stress, pain coping strategies, and relaxation. They found that when compared to the attention control, both CBT and OBT resulted in greater improvement in pain, decreased emotional distress, and improved physical functioning for up to 1 year post-treatment.[119] Patients in both treatment groups also had fewer physician visits when compared to those in the control group. Furthermore, the effect sizes for improvement were large for both CBT and OBT, but for the most part the differences between both active treatments were not significant.

Thieme and Gracely performed a literature search that identified 14 RCTs of CBT and OBT, five relaxation RCTs, five biofeedback RCTs, five hypnotherapy RCTs, and two writing intervention RCTs.[120] For psychoanalytic therapy in FM, no RCTs have been published. The highest effect sizes (r = 0.53–2.14) for pain reduction are found after CBT and OBT group treatments.[120] Bernardy[121] published the first systematic review and meta-analysis of 14 CBT RCTs in FM. This analysis consistently revealed positive effects on mood and self-efficacy to control pain.

RELAXATION TECHNIQUES

In an RCT of 55 women with FM, it was found that those in the guided imagery arm (n = 17) had less pain compared to the control group.[122] In another study comparing a 6-week guided imagery intervention to treatment as usual, patients with FM receiving guided imagery demonstrated improved functional status and reported a greater sense of self-efficacy for managing pain although actual pain reports did not change.[123] In a study of 77 FM patients enrolled in a meditation-based stress reduction program, the authors reported that the scores of all patients completing the program improved, and 51% of completers had moderate to marked improvement.[124]

BIOFEEDBACK

Hassett and colleagues have attempted to use heart rate variability (HRV) biofeedback in the treatment of FM and found preliminary data suggesting some type of benefit.[125,126] Several studies also exist that similarly suggest some type of benefit using electromyogram (EMG) biofeedback [127–130] and EEG biofeedback[131] for patients with FM.

PATIENT SELF-MANAGEMENT IN FM

Unfortunately, not all patients have the resources for or the access to services from behavioral medicine specialists, physical therapists, and the like. Jones and colleagues reported a number of nonpharmacologic therapeutic measures that patients with FM can do in conjunction with pharmacotherapy in efforts to improve their quality of life.[132] They promoted self-management activities that included maximizing the relationship with the practitioner, pain management, self-administered cognitive-behavioral strategies, exercise, dietary approaches, and sleep management.[132]

The patient was counseled that a diagnosis of FM accounted for some of her pain and symptoms. She was educated about FM: the latest thoughts on FM pathophysiology, FM natural history and prognosis, and potential therapeutic options. She seemed somewhat relieved that she had a condition that explained some of her symptoms and was not fatal. Furthermore, once she understood more about FM, she felt more in control of her fate and better positioned to cope with adversity, as well as play a role in her own treatment. She gradually began an exercise program; initially in the water and later on land. She started seeing a behavioral medicine specialist who leveraged her knowledge of cognitive-behavioral techniques from her background as a social worker to improve mood, sleep, and self-efficacy to manage pain. Additionally, she joined a local FM support group and found that most others in the group with FM also had similar bowel and bladder issues, thus reducing her sense of fear and isolation.

At 6-month follow-up, she had sustained improvements in her function and decreased pain. Although she initially attributed her low mood to situational factors, there had been improvement in these domains, yet feelings of sadness became more pervasive. All financial matters regarding her divorce were settled, and her daughter had begun working with a school counselor, with significant improvement in behaviors and grades. On further discussion, the patient reports some continued difficulty with sleep initiation and occasionally sleep maintenance. She also notes some difficulty with sustained concentration/focus. This is not a new symptom, but she had previously felt it was due to the distracting quality of her constant pain. With her pain improved, she was at a loss as to why this would continue. She endorsed low appetite but did not notice any weight loss. Despite improvements in her physical activity levels, she endorsed mental fatigue and also anhedonia—she could now participate more regularly in activities (walking in the park) but didn't seem to enjoy them anymore.

Depression is one of the most common comorbid complaints among patients with FM. In fact, at one time, FM itself was seen as a variant manifestation of depression. Patients with FM are two to seven times more likely to have or develop an episode of major depressive disorder (MDD).[133] The lifetime prevalence of MDD is 62–86%.[134] Along with depression, they have increased rates of most Axis I and Axis II disorders. One prospective study found that approximately 48% had an Axis I disorder, with mood disorders in 22% and anxiety disorders in 32%. It also found a very high rate of personality disorders at 31%.[135] Interestingly, there have been no increased rates of bipolar disorder among patients with FM.

For any patient who presents with depressed mood, the differential should always include depressive disorders (major depressive disorder, adjustment disorder with depressed mood), bipolar depression, substance-induced depressive states, post-traumatic stress disorder, and psychotic disorders with mood components.

Through her description, the patient clearly meets criteria for a major depressive episode. She denies any symptoms that would be consistent with a manic or hypomanic episode (increased distractibility, grandiosity, flight of ideas, decreased need for sleep) and has no evidence of psychotic symptoms (paranoia, hallucinations, disorganized thinking). She is screened for and denies any history of physical or sexual abuse and has no military experience.

Once it has been established that the patient is presenting with true depression, a discussion should be had regarding treatment options. Overall, 60–70% of patients with depression who are treated with an antidepressant will improve.[136] Those with comorbid medical conditions, unfortunately, have lower response rates.[137] The practice guidelines from the American Psychiatric Association, Canadian Psychiatric Association, and the National Institutes of Health and Clinical Excellence all recommend either SSRI or SNRI medications as first-line treatment. Although there is no greater efficacy from SSRIs, they are better tolerated than SNRI medications. A comparative efficacy study found that escitalopram and sertraline have the best combination of tolerability and efficacy.[138] Discontinuation rates are similar among SSRIs (15–25%) but significantly higher for duloxetine (67%) and venlafaxine (40%).[139] Despite this, the initial agent in a patient with FM should be an SNRI because currently two SNRIs have been FDA approved for the treatment of FM: duloxetine and milnacipran. Milnacipran (Savella) should be considered as an SNRI and as an antidepressant because it also holds this indication in Europe. If the patient is unable to tolerate an SNRI, then another SNRI should be chosen for a trial. Although in the same "class," these agents are distinct enough that lack of response to one is not predictive of lack of response to another. If two SNRI medications have not been helpful, consideration should be given for the SSRIs fluoxetine, paroxetine, or escitalopram. The first two have moderate evidence for efficacy in FM,[140] whereas the last has been shown to have some promise in pain states (Table 26.2).[141,142]

Patients may have concern with beginning an antidepressant due to the fear of suicidality or suicidal thinking. The FDA instituted a "black-box" warning on all antidepressant medications in May 2007 warning of the increase in suicidality. This notes that the rate of suicidal thinking of behavior was 2% in those taking placebo and 4% in those taking medication. A 2012 reanalysis of all longitudinal suicidal event data from all published and unpublished placebo-controlled RCTs of fluoxetine and venlafaxine found *there is no increased suicide risk with treatment*.[143] In those 25 years of age and older, there were significant decreases in suicide risk measures. In those younger than 25, there was no increased risk but also no significant benefit regarding suicidality. Therefore, we can comfort patients with the knowledge that all the literature suggests the medication will help them and will not lead to suicidality.

Table 26.2 **DEPRESSION TREATMENT ALGORITHM IN FIBROMYALGIA**

First-line:	Dosing:	Maximum dose:
Duloxetine	30 mg/d PO with food × 1 week, then 60 mg/d thereafter	120 mg/d (as single or BID dosing
Venlafaxine XR	37.5 mg PO QAM with food × 1 week, then 75 mg PO QAM thereafter	225 mg/day
Milnacipran	12.5 mg QHS, titrate up to 50 mg BID	100 mg BID
Second-line:	5 mg/d PO	20 mg/d
Escitalopram	10 mg PO QAM × 1 week, then 20 mg PO QAM	80 mg/d (also available in a once-weekly oral formulation)
Fluoxetine		
Paroxetine	10 mg PO QHS × 1 week, then 20 mg PO QHS	60 mg QHS (there is a CR formulation available, but this has not been shown to be of any greater benefit)

After discussing risks, benefits, and alternatives, the patient was started on duloxetine 30 mg in the evening with food. She was educated regarding the most common side effects (nausea, dizziness, sweating) and that most of these would attenuate in 3–5 days. After 1 week, she was increased to 60 mg/d. At 1-month follow-up, the patient reported tolerating the medication well but was frustrated that she noticed no difference in her mood or pain. She was reminded that although some may notice improvement in 3–4 weeks, it may take up to 12 weeks to notice full benefits for both. The option at this point was to continue with 60 mg/d for another 4–8 weeks versus increasing to 90 mg/d. As she was tolerating it well, she opted to increased to 90 mg and follow-up in 4 weeks time. When next seen, she reported improvement in both mood and overall pain. She noted she was less irritable, less prone to crying, and more social. She was continued on medication without change and scheduled for follow-up in 2 months.

REFERENCES

1. Jain AK, Carruthers BM, van de Sande MI, et al. Fibromyalgia Syndrome: Canadian clinical working case definition, diagnostic and treatment protocols—a consensus document. *J Musculoskeletal Pain*. 2003;11:3–107.
2. Macfarlane GJ, McBeth J, Silman AJ. Widespread body pain and mortality: Prospective population based study. *BMJ*. 2001;323:662–665.
3. Macfarlane GJ, McBeth J, Silman AJ. Widespread pain and fibromyalgia: Should reports of increased mortality influence management? *Current Rheumatology Reports*. 2005;7:339–341.
4. White KP, Harth M. Classification, epidemiology, and natural history of fibromyalgia. *Curr Pain Headache Rep*. 2001;5:320–329.
5. Burckhardt CS, Bjelle A. Perceived control: a comparison of women with fibromyalgia, rheumatoid arthritis, and systemic lupus erythematosus using a Swedish version of the rheumatology attitudes index. *Scand J Rheumatol*. 1996;25:300–306.
6. Wolfe F, Ross K, Anderson J, Russell IJ, Hebert L. The prevalence and characteristics of fibromyalgia in the general population. *Arthritis Rheum*. 1995a;38:19–28.
7. Miedema HS, van der Linden SM, Rasker JJ, Valkenburg HA. National database of patients visiting rheumatologists in The Netherlands: the standard diagnosis register of rheumatic diseases. A report and preliminary analysis. *Br J Rheumatol*. 1998;37:555–561.
8. Clauw DJ. Fibromyalgia: update on mechanisms and management. *J Clin Rheumatol*. 2007;13:102–109.
9. Buskila D, Sarzi-Puttini P. Biology and therapy of fibromyalgia. Genetic aspects of fibromyalgia syndrome. *Arthritis Res Ther*. 2006;8:218.
10. Wolfe F, Ross K, Anderson J, Russell IJ. Aspects of fibromyalgia in the general population: sex, pain threshold, and fibromyalgia symptoms. *J Rheumatol*. 1995b;22:151–156.
11. Croft P, Rigby AS, Boswell R, Schollum J, Silman A. The prevalence of chronic widespread pain in the general population. *J Rheumatol*. 1993;20:710–713.
12. Coster L, Kendall S, Gerdle B, Henriksson C, Henriksson KG, Bengtsson A. Chronic widespread musculoskeletal pain—a comparison of those who meet criteria for fibromyalgia and those who do not. *Eur J Pain*. 2008;12:600–610.
13. McBeth J, Jones K. Epidemiology of chronic musculoskeletal pain. *Best Pract Res Clin Rheumatol*. 2007;21:403–425.
14. Ledingham J, Doherty S, Doherty M. Primary fibromyalgia syndrome-an outcome study. *Br J Rheumatol*. 1993;32:139–142.
15. Wolfe F, Anderson J, Harkness D, et al. Work and disability status of persons with fibromyalgia. *J Rheumatol*. 1997a;24:1171–1178.
16. Martinez JE, Ferraz MB, Sato EL, Atra E. Fibromyalgia versus rheumatoid arthritis: a longitudinal comparison of the quality of life. *J Rheumatol*. 1995;22:270–274.
17. Berger A, Dukes E, Martin S, Edelsberg J, Oster G. Characteristics and healthcare costs of patients with fibromyalgia syndrome. *Int J Clin Pract*. 2007;61:1498–1508.
18. Jones J, Rutledge DN, Jones KD, Matallana L, Rooks DS. Self-assessed physical function levels of women with fibromyalgia: a national survey. *Womens Health Issues*. 2008a;18:406–412.
19. Jones KD, King LA, Mist SD, Bennett RM, Horak FB. Postural control deficits in people with fibromyalgia: A pilot study. *Arthritis Res Ther*. 2011;13:R127.
20. Carbonell-Baeza A, Aparicio VA, Sjostrom M, Ruiz JR, Delgado-Fernandez M. Pain and functional capacity in female fibromyalgia patients. *Pain Med*. 2011a;12:1667–1675.
21. Panton LB, Kingsley JD, Toole T, et al. A comparison of physical functional performance and strength in women with fibromyalgia, age- and weight- matched controls, and older women who are healthy. *Phys Ther*. 2006;86:1479–1488.
22. Littlejohn G. The fibromyalgia syndrome. Outcome is good with minimal intervention [letter]. *BMJ*. 1995;310:1406.
23. Macfarlane GJ, Thomas E, Papageorgiou AC, Schollum J, Croft PR, Silman AJ. The natural history of chronic pain in the community: A better prognosis than in the clinic? *J Rheumatol*. 1996;23:1617–1620.
24. Wolfe F, Anderson J, Harkness D, et al. A prospective, longitudinal, multicenter study of service utilization and costs in fibromyalgia. *Arthritis Rheum*. 1997b;40:1560–1570.
25. Dinerman H, Goldenberg DL, Felson DT. A prospective evaluation of 118 patients with the fibromyalgia syndrome: prevalence of Raynaud's phenomenon, sicca symptoms, ANA, low complement,

and Ig deposition at the dermal-epidermal junction. *J Rheumatol.* 1986;13:368–373.
26. Staud R, Vierck CJ, Cannon RL, Mauderli AP, Price DD. Abnormal sensitization and temporal summation of second pain (wind-up) in patients with fibromyalgia syndrome. *Pain.* 2001;91:165–175.
27. Price DD, Staud R, Robinson ME, Mauderli AP, Cannon R, Vierck CJ. Enhanced temporal summation of second pain and its central modulation in fibromyalgia patients. *Pain.* 2002;99:49–59.
28. Potvin S, Paul-Savoie E, Morin M, Bourgault P, Marchand S. Temporal summation of pain is not amplified in a large proportion of fibromyalgia patients. Pain Res Treat. 2012: article 938595. doi:10.1155/2012/938595.
29. Woolf CJ, Thompson SW. The induction and maintenance of central sensitization is dependent on N-methyl-D-aspartic acid receptor activation: implications for the treatment of post-injury pain hypersensitivity states. *Pain.* 1991;44:293–299.
30. Xu XJ, Dalsgaard CJ, Wiesenfeld-Hallin Z. Spinal substance P and N-methyl-D-aspartate receptors are coactivated in the induction of central sensitization of the nociceptive flexor reflex. *Neuroscience.* 1992;51:641–648.
31. Liu Z, Welin M, Bragee B, Nyberg F. A high-recovery extraction procedure for quantitative analysis of substance P and opioid peptides in human cerebrospinal fluid. *Peptides.* 2000;21: 853–860.
32. Russell IJ, Orr MD, Littman B, Elevated cerebrospinal fluid levels of substance P in patients with the fibromyalgia syndrome. *Arthritis Rheum.* 1994;37:1593–1601.
33. Bradley LA, Alarcón GS. Is Chiari malformation associated with increased levels of substance P and clinical symptoms in persons with fibromyalgia? *Arthritis Rheum.* 1999;42:2731–2732.
34. Vaerøy H, Helle R, Førre O, Kåss E, Terenius L. Elevated CSF levels of substance P and high incidence of Raynaud phenomenon in patients with fibromyalgia: new features for diagnosis. *Pain.* 1988;32:21–26.
35. Sarchielli P, Di Filippo M, Nardi K, Calabresi P. Sensitization, glutamate, and the link between migraine and fibromyalgia. *Curr Pain Headache Rep.* 2007;11:343–351.
36. Harris RE, Sundgren PC, Pang Y, et al. Dynamic levels of glutamate within the insula are associated with improvements in multiple pain domains in fibromyalgia. *Arthritis Rheum.* 2008;58:903–907.
37. Harris RE, Sundgren PC, Craig AD, et al. Elevated insular glutamate in fibromyalgia is associated with experimental pain. *Arthritis Rheum.* 2009;60:3146–3152.
38. Fayed N, Garcia-Campayo J, Magallón R, et al. Localized 1H-NMR spectroscopy in patients with fibromyalgia: a controlled study of changes in cerebral glutamate/glutamine, inositol, choline, and N-acetylaspartate. *Arthritis ResTher.* 2010;12:R134.
39. Valdes M, Collado A, Bargallo N, et al. Increased glutamate/glutamine compounds in the brains of patients with fibromyalgia: a magnetic resonance spectroscopy study. *Arthritis Rheum.* 2010;62:1829–1836.
40. Harris RE. Elevated excitatory neurotransmitter levels in the fibromyalgia brain. *Arthritis Res Ther.* 2010;12:141.
41. Cohen SP, Verdolin MH, Chang AS, Kurihara C, Morlando BJ, Mao J. The intravenous ketamine test predicts subsequent response to an oral dextromethorphan treatment regimen in fibromyalgia patients. *J Pain.* 2006;7:391–398.
42. Noppers I, Niesters M, Swartjes M, et al. Absence of long-term analgesic effect from a short-term S-ketamine infusion on fibromyalgia pain: a randomized, prospective, double blind, active placebo-controlled trial. *Eur J Pain.* 2011;15:942–949.
43. Foerster BR, Petrou M, Harris RE, et al. Cerebral blood flow alterations in pain-processing regions of patients with fibromyalgia using perfusion MR imaging. *AJNR Am J Neuroradiol.* 2011;32:1873–1878.
44. Ploner M, Lee MC, Wiech K, Bingel U, Tracey I. Prestimulus functional connectivity determines pain perception in humans. *Proc Natl Acad Sci U S A.* 2010;107:355–360.
45. Napadow V, Lacount L, Park K, As-Sanie S, Clauw DJ, Harris RE. Intrinsic brain connectivity in fibromyalgia is associated with chronic pain intensity. *Arthritis Rheum.* 2010;62:2545–2555.
46. Napadow V, Kim J, Clauw DJ, Harris RE. Decreased intrinsic brain connectivity is associated with reduced clinical pain in fibromyalgia. *Arthritis Rheum.* 2012;64:2398–2403.
47. Jensen KB, Loitoile R, Kosek E, et al. Patients with fibromyalgia display less functional connectivity in the brain's pain inhibitory network. *Mol Pain.* 2012;8:32.
48. Jensen KB, Kosek E, Petzke F, et al. Evidence of dysfunctional pain inhibition in Fibromyalgia reflected in rACC during provoked pain. *Pain.* 2009;144:95–100.
49. Yunus MB, Young CS, Saeed AS, Aldag JC. Positron emission tomography (PET) imaging of the brain in fibromyalgia syndrome (FMS). *Arthritis Rheum.* 1997;40:S188.
50. Wood PB, Schweinhardt P, Jaeger E, et al. Fibromyalgia patients show an abnormal dopamine response to pain. *EurJNeurosci.* 2007;25:3576–3582.
51. Harris RE, Clauw DJ, Scott DJ, McLean SA, Gracely RH, Zubieta JK. Decreased central mu-opioid receptor availability in fibromyalgia. *J Neurosci.* 2007;27:10000–10006.
52. Fayed N, Andres E, Rojas G, et al. Brain dysfunction in fibromyalgia and somatization disorder using proton magnetic resonance spectroscopy: a controlled study. *Acta Psychiatr Scand.* 2012;126:115–125.
53. Foerster BR, Petrou M, Edden RA, et al. Reduced insular gamma-aminobutyric acid in fibromyalgia. *Arthritis Rheum.* 2012;64:579–583.##
54. Wolfe F, Clauw DJ, Fitzcharles MA, et al. The American College of Rheumatology preliminary diagnostic criteria for fibromyalgia and measurement of symptom severity. *Arthritis Care Res.* 2010;62:600–610.
55. Jacobsen S, Bredkjaer SR. The prevalence of fibromyalgia and widespread chronic musculoskeletal pain in the general population [letter; comment]. *Scand J Rheumatol.* 1992;21:261–263.
56. Wolfe F, Clauw DJ, Fitzcharles MA, et al. Fibromyalgia criteria and severity scales for clinical and epidemiological studies: a modification of the acr preliminary diagnostic criteria for fibromyalgia. *J Rheumatol.* 2011;38:1113–1122.
57. Williams DA, Clauw DJ. Understanding fibromyalgia: lessons from the broader pain research community. *J Pain.* 2009;10:777–791.
58. Phillips K, Clauw DJ. Central pain mechanisms in chronic pain states—maybe it is all in their head. *Best Pract Res Clin Rheumatol.* 2011;25:141–154.
59. Staud R, Price DD, Robinson ME. The provisional diagnostic criteria for fibromyalgia: one step forward, two steps back: comment on the article by Wolfe, et al. *Arthritis Care Res.* 2010;62:1675–1676; author reply 1676–1678.
60. Arnold LM, Goldenberg DL, Stanford SB, et al. Gabapentin in the treatment of fibromyalgia: a randomized, double-blind, placebo-controlled, multicenter trial. *Arthritis Rheum.* 2007;56:1336–1344.
61. Moldofsky H, Harris HW, Archambault WT, Kwong T, Lederman S. Effects of bedtime very low dose cyclobenzaprine on symptoms and sleep physiology in patients with fibromyalgia syndrome: a double-blind randomized placebo-controlled study. *J Rheumatol.* 2011;38:2653–2663.
62. Arnold LM, Hess EV, Hudson JI, Welge JA, Berno SE, Keck PE Jr. A randomized, placebo-controlled, double-blind, flexible-dose study of fluoxetine in the treatment of women with fibromyalgia. *Am J Med.* 2002;112:191–197.
63. Capaci K, Hepguler S. Comparison of the effects of amitriptyline and paroxetine in the treatment of fibromyalgia syndrome. *Pain Clin.* 2002;14:223–228.
64. Goldenberg D, Mayskiy M, Mossey C, Ruthazer R, Schmid C. A randomized, double-blind crossover trial of fluoxetine and amitriptyline in the treatment of fibromyalgia. *Arthritis Rheum.* 1996;39:1852–1859.

65. Nørregaard J, Volkmann H, Danneskiold-Samsoe B. A randomized controlled trial of citalopram in the treatment of fibromyalgia. *Pain.* 1995;61:445–449.
66. Anderberg UM, Marteinsdottir I, Von Knorring L. Citalopram in patients with fibromyalgia—a randomized, double-blind, placebo-controlled study. *Eur J Pain.* 2000;4:27–35.
67. Fishbain D. Evidence-based data on pain relief with antidepressants. *AnnMed.* 2000;32:305–316.
68. Adelman LC, Adelman JU, Von Seggern R, Mannix LK. Venlafaxine extended release (XR) for the prophylaxis of migraine and tension-type headache: A retrospective study in a clinical setting. *Headache.* 2000;40:572–580.
69. Grothe DR, Scheckner B, Albano D. Treatment of pain syndromes with venlafaxine. *Pharmacotherapy.* 2004;24:621–629.
70. Arnold LM, Lu Y, Crofford LJ, et al. A double-blind, multicenter trial comparing duloxetine with placebo in the treatment of fibromyalgia patients with or without major depressive disorder. *Arthritis Rheum.* 2004;50:2974–2984.
71. Clauw DJ, Mease P, Palmer RH, Gendreau RM, Wang Y. Milnacipran for the treatment of fibromyalgia in adults: a 15-week, multicenter, randomized, double-blind, placebo-controlled, multiple-dose clinical trial. *Clin Ther.* 2008;30:1988–2004.
72. Arnold LM, Hirsch I, Sanders P, Ellis A, Hughes B. Safety and efficacy of esreboxetine in patients with fibromyalgia: a fourteen-week, randomized, double-blind, placebo-controlled, multicenter clinical trial. *Arthritis Rheum.* 2012;64:2387–2397.
73. Wiffen P, Collins S, McQuay J, Carroll D, Jadad A, Moore A. Anticonvulsant drugs for acute and chronic pain. *Cochrane Database Syst Rev.* 2000;CD:001133.
74. Crofford LJ, Rowbotham MC, Mease PJ, et al. Pregabalin for the treatment of fibromyalgia syndrome: results of a randomized, double-blind, placebo-controlled trial. *Arthritis Rheum.* 2005;52:1264–1273.
75. Russell IJ, Crofford LJ, Leon T, et al. The effects of pregabalin on sleep disturbance symptoms among individuals with fibromyalgia syndrome. *Sleep Med.* 2009a;10:604–610.
76. Grönblad M, Nykänen J, Konttinen Y, Järvinen E, Helve T. Effect of zopiclone on sleep quality, morning stiffness, widespread tenderness and pain and general discomfort in primary fibromyalgia patients. A double-blind randomized trial. *Clin Rheumatol.* 1993;12:186–191.
77. Moldofsky H, Lue FA, Mously C, Roth-Schechter B, Reynolds WJ. The effect of zolpidem in patients with fibromyalgia: a dose ranging, double blind, placebo controlled, modified crossover study. *J Rheumatol.* 1996;23:529–533.
78. Scharf MB, Baumann M, Berkowitz DV. The effects of sodium oxybate on clinical symptoms and sleep patterns in patients with fibromyalgia. *JRheumatol.* 2003;30:1070–1074.
79. Russell IJ, Perkins AT, Michalek JE, Oxybate SXB-26 Fibromyalgia Syndrome Study Group. Sodium oxybate relieves pain and improves function in fibromyalgia syndrome: a randomized, double-blind, placebo-controlled, multicenter clinical trial. *Arthris Rhem.* 2009b;60:299–209.
80. Russell IJ, Holman AJ, Swick TJ, et al. Sodium oxybate reduces pain, fatigue, and sleep disturbance and improves functionality in fibromyalgia: Results from a 14-week, randomized, double-blind, placebo-controlled study. *Pain.* 2011;152:1007–1017.
81. Spaeth M, Bennter RM, Benson BA, Wang YG, Lai C, Choy EH. Extended report. Sodium oxybate therapy provides multidimensional improvement in fibromyalgia: results of an international phase 3 trial. *Ann Rheum Dis.* 2012;71:935–942.
82. Skrabek RQ, Galimova L, Ethans K, Perry D. Nabilone for the treatment of pain in fibromyalgia. *J Pain.* 2008;9:164–173.
83. Ware MA, Fitzcharles MA, Joseph L, Shir Y. The effects of nabilone on sleep in fibromyalgia: results of a randomized controlled trial. *Anesth Analg.* 2010;110:604–610.
84. Lynch ME, Campbell F. Cannabinoids for treatment of chronic non-cancer pain: a systematic review of randomized trials. *Br J Clin Pharmacol.* 2011;72:735–744.
85. Bennett JP Jr, Piercey MF. Pramipexole—a new dopamine agonist for the treatment of Parkinson's disease. *J Neurol Sci.* 1999;163:25–31.
86. Holman AJ, Myers RR. A randomized, double-blind, placebo-controlled trial of pramipexole, a dopamine agonist, in patients with fibromyalgia receiving concomitant medications. *Arthritis Rheum.* 2005;52:2495–2505.
87. Russell IJ, Michalek JE, Xiao Y, Hayes W, Vertiz R, Lawrence RA. Therapy with a central alpha 2-adrenergic agonist (tizanidine) decreases cerebrospinal fluid substance P, and may reduce serum hyaluronic acid as it improves the clinical symptoms of the fibromyalgia syndrome. *Arthritis Rheum.* 2002;46:S614.
88. Clauw DJ. Pharmacotherapy for patients with fibromyalgia. *J Clin Psychiatry.* 2008;69:25–29.
89. Lautenschlager J. Present state of medication therapy in fibromyalgia syndrome. *Scand J Rheumatol Suppl.* 2000;113:32–36.
90. Rao SG, Bennett RM. Pharmacological therapies in fibromyalgia. *Best Pract Res Clin Rheumatol.* 2003;17:611–627.
91. Rao SG, Clauw DJ. The management of fibromyalgia. *Drugs Today.* 2004;40:539–554.
92. Sorensen J, Bengtsson A, Backman E, Henriksson KG, Bengtsson M. Pain analysis in patients with fibromyalgia. Effects of intravenous morphine, lidocaine, and ketamine. *Scand J Rheumatol.* 1995;24:360–365.
93. Ngian GS, Guymer EK, Littlejohn GO. The use of opioids in fibromylagia. *Int J Rheum Dis.* 2011;14:6–11.
94. Fitzcharles MA, Ste-Marie PA, Gamsa A, et al. Opioid use, misuse, and abuse in patients labeled as fibromyalgia. *Am J Med.* 2011;124(10):955–960.
95. Fitzcharles MA, Faregh N, Ste-Marie PA, et al. Opioid use in fibromyalgia is associated with negative health related measures in a prospective cohort study. *Pain Rest Treat.* 2013; article 898493.
96. Painter JT, Crofford LJ. Chronic opioid use in fibromyalgia syndrome: a clinical review. *J Clin Rheumatol.* 2013;19(2):72–77.
97. Goldenberg DL, Ryan K, Chandran A, et al. What is the true cost of fibromyalgia to our society: results from a cross-sectional survey in the United States. *Arthritis Rheum.* 2009;60(suppl 10):104.
98. Bennett RM, Jones J, Turk DC, et al. An internet survey of 2,596 people with fibromyalgia. *BMC Musculoskel Dis.* 2007;8(27). doi: 10.1186/1471-2474-8-27.
99. Nishiyori M, Nagai J, Nakazawa T, Udea H. Absence of morphine analgesia amd its underlying descending serotonergic activation in an experimental mouse model of fibromyalgia. *Neurosci Lett.* 2010;472:184–187.
100. Younger J, Noor N, McCue R, Mackey S. Low-dose naltrexone for the treatment of fibromyalgia: findings of a small, randomized, double-blind, placebo-controlled, counterbalanced, crossover trial assessing daily pain levels. *Arthritis Rheum.* 2013; 65:529–538.
101. Russell IJ Kamin M, Bennet RM, Schnitzer TJ, Green JA, Katz QA. Efficacy of tramadol in treatment of pain in fibromyalgia. *J Clin Rheumatol.* 2000;6:250–257.
102. Bennett RM, Kamin M, Kamin R, Rosenthal N. Tramadol and acetaminophen combination tablets in the treatment of fibromyalgia pain: a double-blind, randomized, placebo-controlled study. *Am J Med.* 2003;114:537–345.
103. Häuser W, Klose P, Langhorst J, et al. Efficacy of different types of aerobic exercise in fibromyalgia syndrome: a systematic review and meta-analysis of randomised controlled trials. *Arthritis Res Ther.* 2010;12:R79.
104. Busch AJ, Webber SC, Brachaniec M, et al. Exercise therapy for fibromyalgia. *Curr Pain & Headache Rep.* 2011;15:358–367.
105. Jones KD, Liptan GL. Exercise interventions in fibromyalgia: Clinical applications from the evidence. *Rheum Dis Clin N Am.* 2009;35:373–391.
106. Kingsley JD, Panton LB, Toole T, Sirithienthad P, Mathis R, McMillan V. The effects of a 12-week strength-training program on strength and functionality in women with fibromyalgia. *Arch Phys Med Rehabil.* 2005;86:1713–1721.

107. Jones KD, Burckhardt CS, Clark SR, Bennett RM, Potempa KM. A randomized controlled trial of muscle strengthening versus flexibility training in fibromyalgia. *J Rheumatol.* 2002;29:1041–1048.
108. Figueroa A, Kingsley JD, McMillan V, Panton LB. Resistance exercise training improves heart rate variability in women with fibromyalgia. *Clin Physiol Funct Imaging.* 2008;28:49–54.
109. Valkeinen H, Alen M, Hakkinen A, Hannonen P, Kukkonen-Harjula K, Häkkinen K. Effects of concurrent strength and endurance training on physical fitness and symptoms in postmenopausal women with fibromyalgia: a randomized controlled trial. *Arch Phys Med Rehabil.* 2008;89:1660–1666.
110. Bircan C, Karasel SA, Akgun B, El O, Alper S. Effects of muscle strengthening versus aerobic exercise program in fibromyalgia. *Rheumatol Int.* 2008;28:527–532.
111. Hakkinen K, Pakarinen A, Hannonen P, et al. Effects of strength training on muscle strength, cross-sectional area, maximal electromyographic activity, and serum hormones in premenopausal women with fibromyalgia. *J Rheumatol.* 2002;29:1287–1295.
112. Valkeinen H, Hakkinen K, Pakarinen A, et al. Muscle hypertrophy, strength development, and serum hormones during strength training in elderly women with fibromyalgia. *Scand J Rheumatol.* 2005;34:309–314.
113. Langhorst J, Klose P, Dobos GJ, Bernardy K, Hauser W. Efficacy and safety of meditative-movement therapies in fibromyalgia syndrome: a systematic review and meta-analysis of randomized controlled trials. *Rheumatol Int.* 2013;33:193–207.
114. Mist DS, Firestone K, Jones KD. Complementary and alternative exercise for fibromyalgia: a meta-analysis. *J Pain Res.* 2013, in press.
115. Carville SF, Arendt-Nielsen S, Bliddal H, et al. EULAR evidence-based recommendations for the management of fibromyalgia syndrome. *Ann Rheum Dis.* 2008;67:536–541.
116. Burckhardt CS, Mannerkorpi K, Hedenberg L, Bielle A. A randomized, controlled clinical trial of education and physical training for women with fibromyalgia. *J Rheumatol.* 1994;21: 714–720.
117. Rooks DS, Gautam S, Romeling M, et al. Group exercise, education, and combination self-management in women with fibromyalgia: a randomized trial. *Arch Intern Med.* 2007;167: 2192–2200.
118. Williams DA, Cary MA, Groner KH, et al. Improving physical functional status in patients with fibromyalgia: a brief cognitive behavioral intervention. *J Rheumatol.* 2002;29:1280–1286.
119. Thieme K, Flor H, Tuck D. Psychological pain treatment in fibromyalgia syndrome: efficacy of operant behavioural and cognitive behavioural treatments. *Arthritis Res Ther.* 2006;8:121–132.
120. Thieme K, Gracely RH. Are psychological treatments effective for fibromyalgia pain? *Curr Rheumatol Rep.* 2009;11:443–450.
121. Bernardy K, Füber N, Köllner V, Häuser W. Efficacy of cognitive-behavioral therapies in fibromyalgia syndrome—a systematic review and metaanalysis of randomized controlled trials. *J Rheumatol.* 2010;37:1991–2005.
122. Fors EA, Sexton J, Götestam KG. The effect of guided imagery and amitriptyline on daily fibromyalgia pain: a prospective, randomized, controlled trial. *J Psychiatr Res.* 2002;36:179–187.
123. Menzies V, Taylor AG, Bourguignon C. Effects of guided imagery on outcomes of pain, functional status, and self-efficacy in persons diagnosed with fibromyalgia. *J Altern Complement Med.* 2006;12:23–30.
124. Kaplan KH, Goldenberg DL, Galvin-Nadeau M. The impact of a meditation-based stress reduction program on fibromyalgia. *Gen Hosp Psychiatry.* 1993;15:284–289.
125. Hassett AL, Radvanski DC, Vaschillo EG, et al. A pilot study of the efficacy of heart rate variability (HRV) biofeedback in patients with fibromyalgia. *Appl Psychophys Biof.* 2007;32:1–10.
126. Hassett AL, Radvanski DC, Sigal LH, Buyske S, Schlesinger N, Lehrer PM. Preliminary results from a randomized controlled trial of heart rate variability biofeedback in fibromyalgia. *Ann Rheum Dis.* 2008;67:S638.
127. Buckelew SP, Conway R, Parker J, et al. Biofeedback/relaxation training and exercise interventions for fibromyalgia: a prospective trial. *Arthritis Care Res.* 1998;11:196–209.
128. Babu AS, Mathew E, Danda D, Prakash H. Management of patients with fibromyalgia using biofeedback: a randomized control trial. *Indian J Med Sci.* 2007;61:455–461.
129. Mur E, Drexler A, Gruber J, Hartig F, Günther V. Electromyography biofeedback therapy in fibromyalgia. *Wein Med Wochenschr.* 1999;149:561–563.
130. Sarnoch H, Adler F, Scholz OB. Relevance of muscular sensitivity, muscular activity, and cognitive variables for pain reduction associated with EMG biofeedback in fibromyalgia. *Percept Mot Skills.* 1997;84:1043–1050.
131. Kayiran S, Dursun E, Ermutlu N, Dursun N, Karamürsel S. Neurofeedback in fibromyalgia syndrome. *Agri.* 2007;19:47–53.
132. Jones KD, Kindler LL, Liptan GL. Self-management in fibromyalgia. *JCRM M.* 2012b;3(1):59–68.
133. Henningsen P, Zimmermann T, Sattel H. Medically unexplained physical symptoms, anxiety, and depression: a meta-analytic review. *Psychosom Med.* 2003;65(4):528–533.
134. Arnold LM. Management of fibromyalgia and comorbid psychiatric disorders. *J Clin Psychiatry.* 2008;69[suppl 2]:14–19.
135. Uguz F, Cicek E, Salli A, et al. Axis I and Axis II psychiatric disorders in patients with fibromyalgia. *Gen Hosp Psychiatry.* 2010(32):105–107.
136. Trivedi MH, Rush AJ, Wisniewksi SR, et al. STAR*D study team: evaluation of outcomes with citalopram for depression using measurement-based care in STAR*D: implications for clinical practice. *Am J Psychiatry.* 2006;163:28–40.
137. Iosifescu D, Bankeir B, Fava M. Impact of medical comorbid disease on antidepressant treatment of major depressive disorder. *Curr Psychiatry Rep.* 2004;6:193–201.
138. Ciprianai A, Furukawa TA, Salanti G, et al. Comparative efficacy and acceptability of 12 new-generation antidepressants : a multiple treatments meta-analysis. *Lancet.* 2009;373:746–758.
139. Gartlehner G, Hansen RA, Morgan LC, et al. Comparative benefits and harms of second-generation antidepressants for treating major depressive disorder. *Ann Intern Med.* 2011;155:772–785.
140. Goldenberg DL, Burckhardt C, Crofford L. Management of fibromyalgia syndrome. *JAMA.* 2004;292:2388–2395.
141. Tsui JI, Herman DS, Kettavong M, et al. Escitalopram is associated with reductions in pain severity and pain interference in opioid dependent patients with depressive symptoms. *Pain.* 2011;152:2640–2644.
142. Mazza M, Mazza O, Pazzaglia C, et al. Escitalopram 20mg versus duloxetine 60mg for the treatment of chronic low back pain. *Expert Opin Pharmacother.* 2010;11(7):1049–1052.
143. Gibbons RD, Brown CH, Hur K, et al. Suicidal thoughts and behavior with antidepressant treatment. *Arch Gen Psychiatry.* 2012;69(6):580–587.
144. Wolfe F, Smythe HA, Yunus MB, et al. The American College of Rheumatology 1990 criteria for the classification of fibromyalgia. Report of the Multicenter Criteria Committee. *Arthritis Rheum.* 1990;33:160–172.

INDEX

A

Abatacept, for rheumatological disease pain, 107
Acetaminophen
 for postlaminectomy syndrome, 218, 219t
 for sacroiliac joint pain, 170–171
Acid-sensing ion channels, in myofascial pain syndrome, 74
Active trigger point, 70
Acupuncture
 for chemotherapy-induced neuropathy, 363
 for low back pain, chronic, 221
 for postherpetic neuralgia, 30
 for smoking cessation, 140
 for somatoform spectrum, 120
Acupuncture trigger point needling, for myofascial pain syndrome, 83
Acute pain
 Aδ fibers in, 341–342
 C fibers in, 341–342
 pathophysiology of, 341–342
 periaqueductal gray in, 342
Acyclovir, for postherpetic neuralgia, 23, 24t, 25
 prevention of, 23, 24t, 26
Adalimumab, for rheumatological disease pain, 100–102
Aδ fibers, 341–342
 in acute pain, 341–342
 in neuropathic pain, 359
 in small fiber neuropathy, 3, 9
Adenosine monophosphate, for postherpetic neuralgia, 25, 27
Adherence, 331
Adhesiolysis, epidural, for postlaminectomy syndrome, 222, 225, 225t
Adjacent segment disease, in postlaminectomy syndrome, 227–228
Afferent signals, 3
Alcohol use (abuse)
 management of, 345–346
 screening for, 346, 346t
 small fiber neuropathy with, 8
Alendronate
 for complex regional pain syndrome, 397
 for vertebral compression fracture prevention, 273
Allodynia, 341
 assessment of, with pelvic pain, 299
 definition of, 21
 in postherpetic neuralgia, 21
Amitriptyline. *See also* Tricyclic antidepressants (TCAs)
 for fibromyalgia, 410
 for post-herniorrhaphy pain, 344
Amyloidosis, small fiber neuropathy with, 10
Anesthesia dolorosa, facial, 41
Angina, chronic refractory, 303–315
 case presentation for, 303
  cost in, 308
  definition of CRA in, 304
  differential diagnosis in, 313
  landmarks in, 306
  management of, 315
  psychological factors in, 310–311
  risk factors in, 309
 conventional therapies and, 306–307
 cost and burden of, 308
 definition of, 304
 evaluation of patients with, 309–311, 410t
 follow-up parameters for, 311
 management of, 313–315
  angiogenesis, cell and gene therapy in, 315
  enhanced external counterpulsation in, 315
  heart transplantation in, 315
  left stellate ganglion block in, 314
  patient-centered *vs.* disease-centered, 313
  pharmacotherapeutics in, 314
  rehabilitation in, 313
  spinal cord stimulation in, 314
  thoracic epidural anesthesia in, 314–315
  transcutaneous electrical nerve stimuliation in, 314
  transmyocardial perfusion and vessel formation in, 315
 natural history and life expectancy with, 308–309
 pathophysiology of, 304–306
  brain imaging on, 306
  central pathway and mechanisms in, 305–306
  myocardial ischemia as trigger in, 305
  pain generator in, 305, 305f
  referred pain and spinal interneuron network in, 305
 prevalence and incidence of, 307
 psychological aspects of, 311–313
  aggravating factors in, 310–311
  differential diagnosis in, 313
  ER diagnosis and panic attack in, 312–313, 312t
  panic disorder in, 311
  psychiatric diagnoses in, 312
 revascularization ineligibility with, 306, 307b, 310
 stable *vs.* chronic refractory angina pain in, 306
 stable *vs.* refractory angina and, 307–308
Angina, stable *vs.* refractory, 307–308
Angiogenesis, chronic refractory angina and, 315
Angiokeratoma corporis, 9
Ankylosing spondylitis, 89–107. *See also* Rheumatological disease pain
Annular fissure, 133
Anticonvulsants. *See* Antiepileptic drugs (AEDs); *specific drugs*
Antidepressants. *See also specific drugs*
 for lumbar facet pain, 153
 for postlaminectomy syndrome, 218, 219t
 tricyclic (*See* Tricyclic antidepressants (TCAs))
Antiepileptic drugs (AEDs). *See also* Carbamazepine; Gabapentin; Pregabalin
 for cervical radicular pain, 260
 CNS depression from, with alcohol use, 345
 for complex regional pain syndrome, 396–397
 for fibromyalgia, 412
 for lumbar disc displacement, 200, 206
 for pancreatitis pain, chronic, 290, 295
 for postlaminectomy syndrome, 218, 220t
 for thoracic back pain, 274t
Anti-TNF inhibitors, for rheumatological disease pain, 100–102
Anxiety, with cancer pain
 diagnosis of, 363–364
 management of, 365–369, 366t
 on pain severity, 370
Arterial insufficiency, in neurogenic intermittent claudication, 187
Arthritis. *See specific types*
Arthrodesis, for discogenic back pain, 140–141
L-Ascorbic acid, for postherpetic neuralgia, 25, 27
Aspirin/diethyl ether, for postherpetic neuralgia, 24t, 25
 for prevention, 26
 for therapy, 27
Atlanto-axial headache, 387
Atypical antipsychotics
 for anxiety with cancer pain, 369
 for insomnia, 370
Atypical facial pain. *See* Persistent idiopathic facial pain
Autonomic nervous system
 on end organs, 4
 in myofascial pain syndrome, 79
Autonomic neuropathy
 chemotherapy-induced, 362
 small fiber, 3–4
Axial back pain *vs.* radicular leg pain, postlaminectomy, 214–217, 214f–216f. *See also under* Postlaminectomy syndrome
Axial manual traction test, for cervical radicular pain, 259

B

Back pain. *See also specific types*
 axial, postlaminectomy syndrome, 214–217, 214f–216f
 from disc herniation, causes of, 196–197
 discogenic, 127–141 (*See also* Discogenic back pain)
 low back (*See* Low back pain)
 pain generators in, 128–129
 red flags in, 147b
 from spondylolisthesis, 214, 214f
 thoracic, 264–280
Bakody maneuver, for facet-mediated neck pain, 249
Baldry's technique, for myofascial pain syndrome, 83
Baroreflex, 4
Beatty test, 240
Benzodiazepine-like agents, for insomnia, 369
Benzodiazepines
 for anxiety with cancer pain, 369
 for insomnia, 369
Berger procedure, for pancreatitis pain, 294
Berne procedure, for pancreatitis pain, 294
Biaculoplasty, for discogenic back pain, 135
Biofeedback, for fibromyalgia, 414
Biologic therapies, investigational, for rheumatological disease pain, 107
Biopsychosocial model, 331
Bipolar disorder
 clinical manifestations of, 242–243
 diagnosis of, 243
 piriformis syndrome and, 242–243
Bipolar radiofrequency, for sacroiliac joint pain, 175
Bisphosphonates
 for complex regional pain syndrome, 397
 for vertebral compression fracture prevention, 273
Blood pressure
 in dysautonomia, 7
 photoplethysmographic recordings of, 7
Bone scintigraphy
 for lumbar facet pain, 149
 for rheumatological disease pain, 93
Bony vibration test., 133
Botulinum toxin
 for myofascial pain syndrome, 83
 for piriformis syndrome, 242, 242f
 for postherpetic neuralgia, injected, 29
Brachial plexopathy, 358
Brachial plexus
 anatomy of, 356, 356f
 Pancoast tumors in, 356–357
Breast cancer surgery, 323–324
Breast-conserving surgery, 324
Breast innervation, 323, 323f
Breathing, deep, on heart rate, 7

Budapest clinical criteria, 394, 394b
Bupivacaine, for postsurgical thoracic pain, 330–331
Buprenorphine, for severe neuropathic cancer pain, 360–361
Bupropion
  for depression and anxiety with cancer pain, 366, 366t
  for smoking cessation, 139
Burning feet syndrome, familial, 9

C

C1–C2 headache, 387
C2–C3 headache
  cervical discogenic pain in, 387
  zygapophysial joint, 387
Calcitonin
  for lumbar spinal stenosis, 190, 191t
  for vertebral compression fractures, thoracic, 275
Calcitonin gene-related peptide (CGRP)
  in complex regional pain syndrome, 391
  in discogenic pain, 128
  in muscle overuse syndromes, 70, 71, 73, 74–75, 77
  in persistent postoperative pain, 342
Calcium, for vertebral compression fracture prevention, 273
Cancer pain, palliative, 355–371
  anxiety in
    diagnosis of, 363–364
    management of, 368–369
    on pain severity, 370
  for brachial plexopathy, 358
  case presentation for, 355
  chemotherapy-induced neuropathy in, 362–363
  demoralization in, 370–371
  depression in
    diagnosis of, 363–364
    management of, 365–368, 366t
    on pain severity, 370
  insomnia in, 365–368, 366t
    management of, 368–369
    on mood and pain perception, 365
  neuropathic, 358–362
    etiology and assessment of, 360
    management of, 360–362
    pathophysiology of, 358–360, 359f
  for Pancoast tumors, 356–357, 356f
  sleep disturbances in, 369–370
  for superior sulcus cancers, 357–358
Cannabinoids
  for chemotherapy-induced neuropathy, 363
  for fibromyalgia, 412
  for neuropathic pain, 24t, 329t
Capsaicin
  for chemotherapy-induced neuropathy, 363
  for persistent postsurgical pain, 343t, 344
  for post-herniorrhaphy pain, 343t
  for postherpetic neuralgia, 24t, 27, 31
  for postsurgical thoracic pain, 329, 329t
  for small fiber neuropathy, 12t
  for whiplash and cervical facet pain, 253
Capsaicin receptor (TRPV$_1$ receptor), 27, 329, 342
Carbamazepine
  on Aδ fibers, 48
  for cervical radicular pain, 260
  on C fibers, 48
  for complex regional pain syndrome, 397
Carpal tunnel anatomy, 60–61, 61f
Carpal tunnel syndrome, 60–65
  anatomy of, 60–61, 61f
  case presentation for, 60, 63–64, 65
  clinical findings in, 61–62
  definition and cause of, 61
  diagnostic studies of, 62–63, 63t
  differential diagnosis of, 62
  historical features of, 62
  management of, 63–65
    behavioral/psychiatric, 63–65
    interventional procedures in, 63
    pharmacological, 63
    rehabilitation and splinting in, 63
    surgical, 63
Cartesian model of pain, 304
Caudal epidural spinal injections (CESI)
  for lumbar disc displacement, 201–202, 204
  for postlaminectomy syndrome, 222, 224t
Causalgia, 390–402. *See also* Complex regional pain syndrome (CRPS)
Celecoxib. *See also* Cyclo-oxygenase 2 (COX-2) inhibitors
  for rheumatological disease pain, 100, 101t
Celiac disease, small fiber neuropathy in, 10
Celiac plexus blocks, for pancreatitis pain, 291, 292f
Cell therapy, for chronic refractory angina, 315
Centralization phenomenon, 133
Central sensitization, 324, 342
Cervical discogenic pain, headache from, 387
Cervical facet-mediated neck pain, 247–255. *See also* Whiplash associated disorder with cervical facet pain
  diagnosis of, 247–251, 249f
  incidence of, 251–252
  management of, 252–255
    interventional procedures in, 254–255, 255f
    pharmacological, 253–254
    rehabilitation in, 251–253
    surgery in, 255
Cervical facet palpation, 249
Cervical foraminal stenosis, facet-mediated neck pain from, 250
Cervical radicular pain, 258–262
  case presentation for, 258, 259, 260
  clinical examination for
    assessments in, 258–259, 259t
    imaging and electrophysiological tests in, 259
  epidural infiltration scheduling in, 258
  management of
    epidural interlaminar corticosteroids in, 260–261, 261f
    epidural transforaminal corticosteroids in, 261–262, 261f
    follow-up and registering outcome in, 262
    general, 259–260, 260t
  multidisciplinary evaluation for, 259
Cervicogenic headache (CeH), 382
  definition and criteria for, 383, 384b, 384t
  epidemiology of, 384–385
  management of
    behavioral, 385–386
    interventional, 387
    pharmacological, 386–387
    surgical, 388
  vs. migraine, 384
  pathophysiology of, 385
  prevention of, 386
C fibers, 341–342
  in acute pain, 341–342
  carbamazepine on, 48
  epidermal somatic, 3
  in facial pain, neuropathic, 39, 44
  in neuropathic pain, 359
  in small fiber neuropathy, 3–4, 9
  small, unmyelinated, functions of, 3
Chemotherapy-induced neuropathy, 362–363
Chest innervation, 324, 324f
Chickenpox, 16
Chinese medicine. *See* Traditional Chinese medicine
Chronic pain
  definition of, 321
  mechanisms of
    inflammatory pain in, 343
    neuropathic pain in, 342–343
  nervous system in, altered, 148
  neuronal sensitization in, 213–214
  neuropathic, 214
  pathophysiology of, 213–214, 300–301, 342–343
  persistent
    periaqueductal gray in, 300
    postoperative, 342–343
  post-herniorrhaphy, 342–343 (*See also* Post-herniorrhaphy pain)
  in postlaminectomy syndrome, 213–214
  in post-traumatic stress disorder, 154–155
  suffering response in, 106
Chronic pancreatitis pain, 289–295. *See also* Pancreatitis pain, chronic
Chronic pelvic pain, 297–302. *See also* Pelvic pain, chronic
Chronic refractory angina, 303–315. *See also* Angina, chronic refractory
Cimetidine, for postherpetic neuralgia, 25
Cinderella hypothesis, 73
Citalopram. *See also* Selective serotonin reuptake inhibitors (SSRIs)
  for carpal tunnel syndrome, 64
  for depression and anxiety with cancer pain, 366, 366t
  for fibromyalgia, 410–411
Claudication, vascular *vs.* neurogenic, 189, 189t
Clodronate, for complex regional pain syndrome, 397
Clomipramine, for carpal tunnel syndrome, 64
Clonidine
  for postherpetic neuralgia, 27
  for smoking cessation, 140
Cluster headache, 382–383
Cognitive behavioral therapy (CBT)
  for carpal tunnel syndrome, 64
  for cervical radicular pain, 258
  for chronic pain, 48–49, 48t
  for complex regional pain syndrome, 395f
  for fibromyalgia, 414, 415
  for headache prevention, 386
  for lumbar facet pain, 155
  for pancreatitis pain, chronic, 291
  for pelvic pain, chronic, 301
  for persistent postsurgical pain, 328
  for post-herniorrhaphy pain, 345
  for postlaminectomy syndrome, 221
  for tendinopathies, 120
  for thoracic back pain, 274, 275
  for thoracic pain, postsurgical, 331
  for trigeminal neuralgia, 48–50, 48t, 49t
Collagen type 1, 111
Combined somatic and sympathetic block, for postherpetic neuralgia, 28–29
Complex regional pain syndrome (CRPS), 390–402
  case presentation for, 390, 391f
    epidemiology and pathophysiology in, 392
    management in, 394, 396, 399, 400, 401
    natural history in, 393
    pathophysiology in, 392
  clinical manifestations of, 393
  definition and history of, 390–391
  diagnosis of, 393–394, 393b, 394b
  incidence of, 392
  management of, 394–402
    evolving therapies in, 396
    interventional, 399–400
    occupational therapy in, 394–395
    pharmacologic, 396–399
    physical therapy in, 395–396
    postoperative, 401–402
    psychological, 400–401
    recreational therapy in, 396
    rehabilitation in, 394, 395f, 401, 401f
    vocational rehabilitation in, 396
  natural history of, 392–393
  pathophysiology of, 391–392
Compliance, 331
Compression test, 167, 169f
Contingency management, for smoking cessation, 140
Control, locus of, 301
Cooled bipolar RFE, for discogenic back pain, 135
Corticosteroids
  for carpal tunnel syndrome, 63
  for complex regional pain syndrome, 397–398
  for postlaminectomy syndrome, 225, 226t
  for rheumatological disease, 100
Crohn disease, enteropathic arthritis in, 95t, 96–97
Cryoablation, for post-herniorrhaphy pain, 347
Cryoanalgesia, for postherpetic neuralgia, 30
Cupping, wet, for postherpetic neuralgia, 30
Cyclobenzaprine
  for fibromyalgia, 410
  for rheumatological disease pain, 100
Cyclo-oxygenase 2 (COX-2) inhibitors
  for lumbar spinal stenosis, 191
  for rheumatological disease pain, 100, 101t
  for thoracic back pain, 275
  for vertebral compression fractures, thoracic, 275

D

Deconditioning management, with lumbar facet pain, 152
Deep brain stimulation, for carpal tunnel syndrome, 64–65
Deep, dry needling, for myofascial pain syndrome, 80–81, 80t, 82–83
Delayed onset muscle soreness, muscle overload in, 73
Demand ischemia, 306
Demoralization, on cancer pain management, 370–371
Denervation, radiofrequency. *See* Radiofrequency denervation

Depression
with cancer pain
diagnosis of, 363–364
management of, 365–368, 366t
on pain severity, 370
with fibromyalgia, 415–416, 416t
with sacroiliac joint pain, 174
Dermatome, 16
Desipramine. *See also* Tricyclic antidepressants (TCAs)
for post-herniorrhaphy pain, 344
Dexamethasone, for complex regional pain syndrome, 397–398
Dextranomer, for postherpetic neuralgia, 25
Diabetes mellitus, small fiber neuropathy in, 7–8
Diffuse idiopathic skeletal hyperostosis (DISH), *vs.* rheumatological disease pain, 97, 98f
Dimethylsulphoxide (DMSO), for complex regional pain syndrome, 398
Disc decompression, percutaneous, 136
Disc displacement management, thoracic
options for, 274, 274b
pharmacologic, 275
physical rehabilitation in, 274–275
psychological, 275
Disc herniation
back pain from, causes of, 196–197
incidence of, 197
postlaminectomy, diagnosis of, 216
Disc herniation management, 199–208
classification in, 199
injection techniques in, 201–205, 201f, 202f
advantages and disadvantages of, 203–204
alternative imaging in, 203
complications of, 205
epidural techniques in, 201–202, 201f, 202f
outcomes of, 204–205
repetition of, necessity for, 205
risks and complications of, 202–203
steroids in, particulate *vs.* nonparticulate, 203
vascular anatomy in, 203
interventional limits of literature on, 200–201
other minimally invasive techniques in, 205–206
pharmacological, 200
physical therapy assessment in, 199–200
rehabilitation in, 199
surgery in, 206–208
complications of, 207–208
indications for, 207
postoperative care and rehabilitation in, 207
selection for, 216
surgical *vs.* conservative therapy outcomes in, 206–207
techniques in, 207
Discogenic back pain, 127–134
case presentation for, 127
clinical manifestations in, 134
diagnosis in, 131
epidemiology of, 132
management in, 138, 140, 141
natural history in, 132
pain generators in, 128
clinical manifestations of, 132–134
centralization phenomenon and bony vibration test in, 133
electromyographic testing in, 133
gold standard in, 134
history and physical examination in, 133
on MRI, 133–134
definition of, 129
diagnosis of
confirmation of, 128–131
CT in, post-discography, 129–130, 130f
discography in, analgesic, 131, 131f
discography in, provocative, 129–131, 129f
initial steps in, 128–129
likely, 127–128
historical perspective on, 129
incidence and prevalence of, 131–132
natural history of, 132
pain generators in, potential, 127–128
prognosis in, long-term, 141
Discogenic back pain management
interventional, 134–141
biaculoplasty, 135
biologic, 136–137
cooled bipolar RFE or intradiscal biacuplasty, 135
disc restorative solution, 136, 137f
filler substances, 137
intradiscal electrothermal annuloplasty or intradiscal thermal annuloplasty, 134–135
intradiscal electrothermal therapy, 134–135, 134f
intradiscal ozone, 136
intradiscal radiofrequency treatment or intradiscal radiofrequency thermocoagulation, 135
minimally invasive nuclear decompression, 135–136
nuclear bulking techniques, 137
percutaneous disc decompression, 136
psychiatric, 138–140, 139t
surgical, 140–141
Discography
analgesic, 131, 131f
provocative, 129–131, 129f
Disc, painful, postlaminectomy, 215–216
Disc restorative solution, for discogenic back pain, 136, 137f
Disease-modifying antirheumatic agents, for rheumatological disease pain, 100
Distraction test, 168f
Dorsal root ganglia (DRG)
in postherpetic neuralgia, 16, 22, 22f, 23f
stimulation of, for postlaminectomy syndrome, 230
sympathetic dysfunction at, 4
DREZ ablation, for postherpetic neuralgia, 29
Dry needling, deep, for myofascial pain syndrome, 80–81, 80t, 82–83
Duloxetine
for cancer pain, neuropathic, 361
for depression and anxiety with cancer pain, 366, 366t
for fibromyalgia, 411–412
for lumbar facet pain, 153
for post-herniorrhaphy pain, 344
for postsurgical thoracic pain, 329, 329t
DuVal procedure, for pancreatitis pain, 294
Dysautonomia
familial, 9 (*See also specific types*)
generalized, in small fiber neuropathy, 4

E

Efferent autonomic signals, 3
Elastin, 111
Electrodiagnostic testing (EDX). *See also specific disorders*
for carpal tunnel syndrome, 62–63, 63t
for disc displacement, 198–199
for discogenic back pain, 133
for small fiber neuropathy, 4–5
Electromyography. *See* Electrodiagnostic testing (EDX)
Endothelial progenitor cells, for chronic refractory angina, 315
Endplate noise, in trigger points, 77
Enhanced external counterpulsation, for chronic refractory angina, 315
Enteropathic arthritis, *vs.* rheumatological disease pain, 95t, 96–97
Enthesis, 89–90
Epidural adhesiolysis, for postlaminectomy syndrome, 222, 225, 225t
Epidural anesthesia, thoracic, for chronic refractory angina, 314–315
Epidural fibrosis, in postlaminectomy syndrome, 228
Epidural steroid injections (ESI). *See also specific disorders*
interlaminar
for cervical radicular pain, 260–261, 261f
safety of, 260–261
for thoracic radicular pain, 276, 276f
transforaminal, 261–262, 261f
Erythromelalgia, small fiber neuropathy in, 9
Escitalopram. *See also* Selective serotonin reuptake inhibitors (SSRIs)
for carpal tunnel syndrome, 64
for depression and anxiety with cancer pain, 366, 366t
Es-reboxetine, for fibromyalgia, 412
Estrogen replacement therapy, for vertebral compression fracture prevention, 273
Eszopiclone, for insomnia, 369
Etanercept
for post-herniorrhaphy pain prevention, 344
for rheumatological disease pain, 100–102
Exercise
for fibromyalgia, 414
for lumbar spinal stenosis, 190
for postlaminectomy syndrome, 221
for rheumatological disease pain, 104
for vertebral compression fracture prevention, weight-bearing, 272F
FABER (flexion abduction external rotation) test, 167, 169f
Fabry's disease, small fiber neuropathy in, 9
Facet arthropathy. *See also* Lumbar facet pain
diagnosis of, 147–148
Facet injection, for cervical facet pain, 254
Facet interventions, for postlaminectomy syndrome, 225, 226t, 227t
Facet joint, lumbar, anatomy of, 153f
Facet (joint) pain
etiology of, 149
lumbar (*See* Lumbar facet pain)
postlaminectomy, 216
Facet palpation, cervical, 249
Facial pain conditions, 38–57, 39
anatomical structures in, 44–46
in head pain, 44–45, 45f
sphenopalatine ganglion in, 45–46, 46f
trigeminal ganglion and trigeminal nerves in, 44–45, 45f
atypical facial pain in (*See* Persistent idiopathic facial pain)
clinical correlates of, 44
comorbidities of, 47, 47f
diagnostic studies for, 43–44, 44f
differential diagnosis of, 38–39
glossopharyngeal neuralgia, 42
history in, 42–43
management of, 47–56 (*See also under* Trigeminal neuralgia)
rehabilitation in, 56–57
neuropathic facial pain in, 39–41, 40b,40t, 41f
pathophysiology of, 46–47, 46f
persistent idiopathic facial pain in, 41–42, 41b,42t
symptoms and pain distribution in, 40–41, 40t, 41f
tic convulsif in, 41
trigeminal autonomic cephalgias in, 42
trigeminal neuralgia in, 39–41, 40b,40t, 41f (*See also* Trigeminal neuralgia)
Failed back surgery syndrome. *See* Postlaminectomy syndrome
FAIR test, for piriformis syndrome, 239, 240
Famciclovir, for postherpetic neuralgia, 23, 24t
Familial burning feet syndrome, 9
Familial dysautonomia, 9. *See also specific types*
Fatigue, cancer-related, 368
Fentanyl
for postsurgical thoracic pain, intrathecal, 330–331
for severe neuropathic cancer pain, 360–361
Fibromyalgia, 407–416
case presentation for, 407, 410
definition of, 407, 408f
depression in, 415–416, 416t
diagnostic criteria for, 409–410, 411t
epidemiology of, 407–408
management of, 410–416
nonpharmacologic, 414–416
pharmacologic, 410–413, 413f
pathophysiology of, 408–409
prognosis in, 408
Filler substances, for discogenic back pain, 137
5-HT (serotonin), in myofascial pain syndrome, 71, 73, 74
Fluoxetine. *See also* Selective serotonin reuptake inhibitors (SSRIs)
for carpal tunnel syndrome, 64
for depression and anxiety with cancer pain, 366, 366t
for fibromyalgia, 410–411
Fluvoxamine. *See also* Selective serotonin reuptake inhibitors (SSRIs)
for depression and anxiety with cancer pain, 366, 366t
Foraminal stenosis, postlaminectomy, radicular leg pain from, 215, 216f
Fortin finger test, 165, 173b
Fostering hope, for chronic pain, 106
Free radical scavengers, for complex regional pain syndrome, 398
Freiberg's sign, 240
Frey procedure, for pancreatitis pain, 294

G

Gabapentin. *See also* Antiepileptic drugs (AEDs)
for cancer pain, neuropathic, 361

Gabapentin (*Cont.*)
for cervical radicular pain, 260
for complex regional pain syndrome, 396
for fibromyalgia, 412
for headache, 386
for lumbar disc displacement, 200
for lumbar facet pain, 153
for lumbar spinal stenosis, 190, 191t
for post-herniorrhaphy pain, 343
for postherpetic neuralgia, 24t, 25, 26
for postsurgical thoracic pain, 328–329, 329t
Gaenslen's test, 167, 169f
γ-hydroxybutryrate, for fibromyalgia, 412
Gapping test, 168f
Gene therapy, for chronic refractory angina, 315
Gillet test, 167, 171f
Glia, in sensory neurotransmission, 360
Glossopharyngeal neuralgia, 42
Glutamate, in fibromyalgia, 408
Glycerol rhizolysis, for trigeminal neuralgia, 54
Golimumab, for rheumatological disease pain, 100–102
Granulomatous angiitis, 19
Guanosine analogues, for postherpetic neuralgia, 23

H

Headache, 381–388
C1–C2 (atlanto-axial), 387
C2–C3 zygapophysial joint, 387
case presentation of, 381
differential diagnosis in, 382, 383
management in, 386–388
pathophysiology in, 385
cervicogenic, 382
definition and diagnosis of, 383, 384b,384t
epidemiology of, 384–385
management of, surgical, 388
vs. migraine, 384
pathophysiology of, 385
prevention of, 386
chronic daily, primary *vs.* secondary, 382–383, 383t
cluster, 42, 43t, 382–383
differential diagnosis of, 381–382, 382t
hemicrania continua in, 382
management of, 385–388
behavioral, 385–386
interventional, 387
pharmacological, 386–387
rehabilitation in, 387–388
surgical, 388
medication-overuse, 383, 383t
tension-type, 382
third occipital, 387
trigeminal autonomic cephalalgia, 382
Head pain, anatomy of, 44–45, 45f
Head-up tilt table test, 7
Heart rate
deep breathing on, 7
in dysautonomia, 7
Valsalva maneuver on, 7
Heart rate response to deep breathing (HR_{DB}), 10–11
Heart transplantation, for chronic refractory angina, 315
Hemicrania continua, 42, 382
Hemicrania, paroxysmal, 42, 43t
Hereditary sensory autonomic neuropathies, small fiber neuropathy in, 9
Hernia surgery
pain after, 337–347 (*See also* Post-herniorrhaphy pain)
risk factors for, preoperative, 338–339
surgical risk factors in, 339–340
Herniated disc, *vs.* rheumatological disease pain, 95t, 97
Herpes zoster infection
herpes zoster ophthalmicus, 18–19, 18f
postherpetic neuralgia after, 16–32 (*See also* Postherpetic neuralgia)
Histamine, for insomnia, 370
HIV, small fiber neuropathy in, 10–11
HIZ, 133–134
Hope, fostering, for chronic pain, 106
Hospital Anxiety and Depression Scale (HADS), 363–364
Hutchinson's sign, 18
Hydromorphone
for postsurgical thoracic pain, intrathecal, 330–331
for severe neuropathic cancer pain, 360–361
Hyperactivity, nerve cell, 3
Hyperalgesia, 341
definition of, 21
in postherpetic neuralgia, 21
primary, 342
secondary, 342
Hyperlipidemia, small fiber neuropathy in, 8
Hypermobility, in myofascial pain syndrome, 76
Hypnosis, for smoking cessation, 140
Hypoactivity, nerve cell, 3
Hypothyroidism, small fiber neuropathy in, 8

I

Iceberg Theory, 111, 111f
Illness anxiety disorder, 118
Imipramine. *See also* Tricyclic antidepressants (TCAs)
for post-herniorrhaphy pain, 344
Inflammation (pain of)
in ankylosing spondylitis, 89, 90, 92, 93
in chronic regional pain syndrome, 391–393, 397, 398
in discogenic pain, 128, 133, 136, 137
in enteropathic arthritis, 96
in enthesitis, 89, 99
in facial neuropathic pain, 39
in fibromyalgia, 413
in lower back pain, 161t
in lumbar disc displacement, 197, 200
in lumbar facet pain, 149
in lumbar spinal stenosis, 189
mechanisms of, 343
in myocardial ischemia and angina pain, 305
in myofascial pain syndrome, 74
in osteoarthritis, 99
in pancreatitis pain, chronic, 289
in pelvic pain, chronic, 300
in post-herniorrhaphy pain, 337, 339, 340, 343
in postherpetic neuralgia, 19, 22, 31
postsurgical, 343
process of, 89
in reactive arthritis, 95
in rheumatologic disease, 89, 90, 92, 93, 98, 99
in sacroiliac joint pain, 164
in small fiber neuropathy, 10, 12t
in spondyloarthritis, 99–100
in tendinopathies, 111f, 113
in whiplash-associated disorder, 252
Infliximab, for rheumatological disease pain, 100–102
Infraneural epidural injections, for lumbar disc displacement, 201
Inguinal neural anatomy, 337–338, 339f, 339t
Insomnia
with cancer pain, 369–370
management of
with cancer pain, 365–368, 366t, 369–370
with chronic pelvic pain, 300
with lumbar facet pain, 152
on mood and pain perception, 365
primary, 369
Integrated hypothesis of the trigger point, Simons's, 70
Intercostobrachial neuralgia, post-mastectomy, 324–325, 326
Interferon, for postherpetic neuralgia, 25, 28
Interlaminar epidural spinal injections (ILESI)
for cervical radicular pain, 260–261, 261f
for lumbar disc displacement, 201–202, 202f, 203–205
for lumbar spinal stenosis, 185f
for postlaminectomy syndrome, 222, 223t
Internal mammary artery syndrome, 325, 326
Intradiscal biacuplasty (IDB), for discogenic back pain, 135
Intradiscal electrothermal annuloplasty (IDEA), for discogenic back pain, 134–135
Intradiscal electrothermal therapy (IDET)
for discogenic back pain, 134–135, 134f
for postlaminectomy syndrome, 225, 227
Intradiscal ozone, 136
Intradiscal radiofrequency thermocoagulation (IRFT), for discogenic back pain, 135
Intradiscal thermal annuloplasty (IDTA), for discogenic back pain, 134–135
Intra epidermal nerve fiber density, 5–6
Intrathecal drug delivery
for complex regional pain syndrome, 400
for postlaminectomy syndrome, 230–232, 231f, 232f
for postsurgical thoracic pain, 330–331
Ischemia
in chronic refractory angina (*See* Angina, chronic refractory)
demand, 306

K

Ketamine, IV
for chronic pain, 290
for complex regional pain syndrome, 398–399
for pancreatitis pain, chronic, 290
for postherpetic neuralgia, 27
for postsurgical thoracic pain, 329t, 330
for small fiber neuropathy, 12t
Ketamine, topical
for cancer pain, palliative, 363
for postherpetic neuralgia, 28
for small fiber neuropathy, 12t
Kyphoplasty, for thoracic vertebral compression fractures, 278–279, 278f

L

Lacosamide, for cancer pain, neuropathic, 361
Laminectomy, lumbar. *See also* Postlaminectomy syndrome
facet pain after, 149–150
Laparoscopic pain mapping, for pelvic pain, 300
Lasègue's sign, 240
Laser, low-level, for myofascial pain syndrome, 81
Latent trigger point, 70
Leflunomide, for rheumatological disease pain, 100
Leg length discrepancy, 166
Levodopa, for postherpetic neuralgia, 25
Lidocaine
for myofascial pain syndrome, 81–82
for postsurgical thoracic pain, 329–330, 329t
topical
for post-herniorrhaphy pain, 343–344
for postherpetic neuralgia, 24t,25, 27
for sacroiliac joint pain, 171
Lidocaine, IV
for complex regional pain syndrome, 397
for postherpetic neuralgia, as therapy, 26–27
for postsurgical thoracic pain, 329t, 330
Locus of control, 301
Low back pain, 128. *See also specific disorders*
differential diagnosis of, 146–147, 161, 161b
from disc herniation, 197 (*See also* Lumbar disc displacement)
discogenic (*See* Discogenic back pain)
Lumbar disc displacement (LDD), 196–208
back pain and radicular pain from disc herniation in, 196–197
case presentation for, 196
classification of, 199
clinical manifestations and diagnosis of, 197–199
definitions in, 197
general points on, 197
imaging in, 198–199
incidence of disc herniation in, 197
management of disc herniation in, 199–208 (*See also* Disc herniation management)
Lumbar facet joint
anatomy of, 150, 153f
pain referral from, 150f
Lumbar facet pain, 146–156
after lumbar surgery, prevalence of, 149–150
case presentation for, 146, 147, 148, 151, 154, 155
clinical manifestations and diagnosis of, 150–151, 153f
diagnostic modalities for, further, 148–149
differential diagnosis of, 146–148, 147b
etiology and prevalence of, 149
management of, 151–155
for deconditioning and weakness, 152
interventional procedures in, 153–154, 153f
mental health screening in, 149
for obesity, 151–152
pharmacological, 152–153
psychiatric, 154–155
for sleep impairment, 152
surgical, 155
prognosis in, long-term, 155–156

Lumbar laminectomy. *See also* Postlaminectomy syndrome
facet pain after, 149–150
Lumbar spinal stenosis (LSS), 183–193
case presentation for, 183, 184f, 185f
clinical manifestations and key indications of, 188–189, 189f
definition of, 185
differential diagnosis of, 189, 189t, 190t
epidemiology of, changing, 185–186
management of, 190–193
evolution of, expected, 193
nonsurgical, 190–191
surgical, 191–193, 192t, 195f
natural history of, 187–188, 188t
pain mechanism of, 186
microcirculatory derangement in, 187
neurovascular dysfunction in, 186–187
pathophysiology of, 187
progression of, 189–190
Lumbar spine surgery, persistent pain incidence after, 227
Lyme disease, small fiber neuropathy in, 11

M

Magnesium, for postherpetic neuralgia, 27, 29
Massage, for myofascial pain syndrome, 81
Mastectomy
modified radical, 324
radical, 323–324
Medial branch block (MBB)
for cervical facet pain diagnosis, 251
for lumbar facet pain diagnosis, 148, 151
for thoracic back pain, 271
for thoracic spondylosis, 277
Medial branch radiofrequency ablation, for lumbar facet pain, 153–154, 153f
Median nerve anatomy, 60–61
Medication-overuse headache (MOH), 383, 383t
management of
behavioral, 385–386
interventional, 387
pharmacological, 386–387
Membrane stabilizers. *See* Antiepileptic drugs (AEDs); *specific drugs*
Methadone. *See also* Opioid analgesics
for chemotherapy-induced peripheral neuropathy, 363
for postherpetic neuralgia, 23, 24t, 26
for postsurgical thoracic pain, 329t
for severe neuropathic cancer pain, 360–361
Methotrexate, for rheumatological disease pain, 100
Methylphenidate
for cancer-related fatigue, 368
for depression and anxiety with cancer pain, 367–368
Methylprednisolone. *See also* Corticosteroids; Steroids, injected
for carpal tunnel syndrome, 63
Mexiletine, for postherpetic neuralgia, 26–27
Microcirculatory derangement, in neurogenic intermittent claudication, 187
Microvascular arterial insufficiency, in neurogenic intermittent claudication, 187
Microvascular decompression, for trigeminal neuralgia, 50–52, 51f, 52b
Migraine headache. *See also* Headache
vs. cervicogenic headache, 384
diagnosis of, 381–382, 382t
without aura, diagnosis of, 381–382, 382t
Milnacipran, for fibromyalgia, 411–412
Minimally invasive nuclear decompression, 135–136
Mirtazapine
for depression and anxiety with cancer pain, 366–367, 366t
for insomnia, 370
Mitochondrial disorders, small fiber neuropathy in, 9
Monoclonal gammopathy, small fiber neuropathy in, 10
Mood. *See also* Anxiety; Depression
insomnia on, 365
Morphine. *See also* Opioid analgesics
for chemotherapy-induced peripheral neuropathy, 363
for complex regional pain syndrome, 397
for postherpetic neuralgia, 23, 24t, 26
for postsurgical thoracic pain, 329t
intrathecal, 330–331
for severe neuropathic cancer pain, 360–361
Motor cortex stimulation (MCS)
for complex regional pain syndrome, 400
for trigeminal neuralgia, 56
Moxibustion, for postherpetic neuralgia, 30
Muscle overuse syndromes, 72–75
acid-sensing ion channels in, 74
calcitonin gene-related peptide in, 70, 71, 74–75
inflammatory pain models in, 74
myofascial pain syndrome in, 70–72
pain initiation in, 73–74
pathophysiology of, 72–73
postural stresses in, 73
serotonergic mechanisms of, 74
spinal modulation in, 75
trigger points in, latent and active, 75
Muscle relaxants
for rheumatological disease pain, 100
for thoracic back pain, 275
MVO_2 balance, 305, 305f
Myelopathy, in postherpetic neuralgia, 19
Myocardial ischemia, as nociceptive trigger, 305
Myocardial oxygen consumption (MVO_2), 305, 305f
Myofascial pain syndrome, 69–84
case presentation for, 69
clinical manifestations of, 76–77
electrophysiology in, 77
range of motion in, 77
recruitment in, 77
sensory changes in, 77
trigger point identification in, 76
weakness in, 76–77, 79
definition and history of, 69–70
diagnosis of, 77–80
criteria for, 79, 79t
general points in, 77–78
history in, 78
physical examination in, 78–79
trigger point characteristics in, other, 79–80
trigger point reliability in, 80–81
epidemiology of, 75–76
gender differences in, 75–76
hypermobility in, 76
management of, 80–84
acupuncture trigger point needling in, 83
botulinum toxin in, 83
invasive, 82–83
noninvasive, nonmanual techniques in, 81–82
principles for, 80
provocative factors in, 84
restoration of normal function in, 84
structural and mechanical factors in, 84
trigger point injections and deep, dry needling in, 80–81, 80t, 82–83
trigger pont inactivation in, manual, 81
pathophysiology of, 70–75
central pathways in, 72
muscle overuse in, 70–72
muscle overuse syndromes in, 72–75 (*See also* Muscle overuse syndromes)
muscle pathology in, 72
taut band in, 70, 76
trigger points in, 70
post thoracic surgery, 326
Myofascial trigger point, 69–70. *See also* Myofascial pain syndrome

N

Neck Disability Index (NDI), 253
Neck pain, facet-mediated, 247–255. *See also* Whiplash associated disorder with cervical facet pain
diagnosis of, 247–251, 249f
incidence of, 251–252
management of, 252–255
interventional procedures in, 254–255, 255f
pharmacological, 253–254
rehabilitation in, 251–253
surgery in, 255
Needle electromyography, for carpal tunnel syndrome, 62
Needling, for myofascial pain syndrome
acupuncture, 83
deep, dry, 80–81, 80t, 82–83
Negative neuropathic symptoms, 3
Nerve blocks. *See also specific types*
for headache, 387
for post-herniorrhaphy pain, 347
sympathetic (*See* Sympathetic (ganglion) block)
Neuralgia. *See specific types*
Neurogenic intermittent claudication (NIC)
cardinal features of, 189, 190t
definition of, 185
differential diagnosis of, 189, 189t, 190t
management of, 190–193
evolution of, expected, 193
nonsurgical, 191
pain mechanism of, 186
microcirculatory derangement in, 187
neurovascular dysfunction in, 186–187
pathophysiology of, 187
vs. vascular claudication, 189, 189t
Neuroma pain, post-mastectomy, 326
Neuromodulation. *See also* Spinal cord stimulation (SCS); *specific types*
for sacroiliac joint pain, 176
Neuromuscular junction, in trigger points, 70–71
Neuronal sensitization, in chronic pain, 213–214
Neuropathic pain, 39
in cancer, 358–362
etiology and assessment of, 360
management of, 360–362
pathophysiology of, 358–360, 359f
chronic, 214
definition of, 321
mechanisms of, 342–343
Neuropathic pain syndrome, postsurgical, 321. *See also* Thoracic pain, postsurgical
Neuropathy. *See also specific types*
chemotherapy-induced, 362–363
small fiber, 3–13
Neurostimulation. *See also specific types*
for trigeminal neuralgia, 56
N-methyl-D-aspartate (NMDA) antagonists
for complex regional pain syndrome, 398–399
for postherpetic neuralgia, 23–25, 24t, 27
for postsurgical thoracic pain, 329t, 330
Nociception, 341
inhibitory pathways for, 359–360
neuroanatomy of, 359, 359f
Nociceptive pain, 39
Nonadherence, 331–334
definition of, 331
epidemiology of, 332
pain and, 333–334
reasons for, 332–333
Noncompliance, 331–334
definition of, 331
epidemiology of, 332
reasons for, 332–333
strategies for, 333
Nonsteroidal antiinflammatory drugs (NSAIDs). *See also specific disorders*
for lumbar disc displacement, 200
for lumbar facet pain, 152
for lumbar spinal stenosis, 190–191
for postherpetic neuralgia, 24t, 25, 28
for postlaminectomy syndrome, 218, 219t
for rheumatological disease pain, 100, 101t
for sacroiliac joint pain, 170–171
for thoracic back pain, 275
for vertebral compression fractures, thoracic, 275
Nortriptyline. *See also* Tricyclic antidepressants (TCAs)
for post-herniorrhaphy pain, 344
for smoking cessation, 140
Notalgia paresthetica, 326
Nuclear bulking techniques, for discogenic back pain, 137
Nuclear decompression, minimally invasive, 135–136
Nucleoplasty, 135–136
Nucleoside analogs. *See also specific agents*
for postherpetic neuralgia, 23, 24t
Nucleoside analogues, for postherpetic neuralgia, 23
Nutrition, for chronic pain, 106

O

Obesity management, for lumbar facet pain, 151–152
Obsessive-compulsive disorder (OCD)
carpal tunnel syndrome with, 64
diagnosis of, 64
Occipital nerve blocks, for headaches, 387
Occipital neurostimulation, for headaches, 387
Opioid analgesics. *See also* specific types
for cancer pain, neuropathic, 360–361
for chemotherapy-induced peripheral neuropathy, 363

Opioid analgesics (*Cont.*)
for complex regional pain syndrome, 397
for fibromyalgia, 412–413
for lumbar facet pain, 152–153
for post-herniorrhaphy pain, 344
for postherpetic neuralgia, 23, 24t, 26
for postlaminectomy syndrome, 218, 219t
for postsurgical thoracic pain, 329t, 330
intrathecal, 330–331
Orthostasis management, 13
Orthostatic hypotension, 4
Oxcarbazepine, for cervical radicular pain, 260
Oxycodone, for severe neuropathic cancer pain, 360–361
Ozone, intradiscal, 136

P

Pace sign, 240
Pain assessment, 360
Pain behaviors, 11
Painful disc. *See also* Disc entries
postlaminectomy, 215–216
Pain generators. *See specific disorders*
Pain mapping, laparoscopic, for pelvic pain, 300
Pain perception, insomnia on, 365
Palliative cancer pain, 355–371. *See also* Cancer pain, palliative
Pamidronate, for complex regional pain syndrome, 397
Pancoast tumor
management of, 357–358
presentation of, 356–357, 356f
Pancreaticojejunostomy, lateral, for pancreatitis pain, 294
Pancreatitis pain, chronic, 289–295
case presentation for, 289
clinical presentation in, 289–290
diagnosis of, 290
etiology of, 289
management of pain in, 290–294
conservative, 290–291
nerve blocks in, 291, 292f
psychological, 291
radiofrequency denervation in, 292–293, 293f
spinal cord stimulation in, 293–294
splanchinectomy in, 293
surgical, 294
pain generators in, 289
Panic attack
in chronic refractory angina, 312, 312t
differential diagnosis of, 312t, 313
Panic disorder, in chronic refractory angina, 311
Paracetamol, for cervical radicular pain, 259
Parasympathetic nervous system, on end organs, 4
Parathyroid hormone, for vertebral compression fracture prevention, 273
Paroxetine. *See also* Selective serotonin reuptake inhibitors (SSRIs)
for carpal tunnel syndrome, 64
for depression and anxiety with cancer pain, 366, 366t
for fibromyalgia, 410–411
for neuropathic pain, 329t
for persistent postsurgical pain, 343t, 344
Paroxysmal hemicrania, 42, 43t
Patient self-management
for complex regional pain syndrome, 401
for fibromyalgia, 414–415
for small fiber neuropathy, 11
Patrick's test, 167, 169f
Pedicular screw placement, postlaminectomy pain from, 216, 216f
Pelvic pain, chronic, 297–302
assessment of, 298–300
bedside sensory testing in, 298–299
family history in, 298
further, with visceral dysfunction suspected, 300
imaging in, 299–300
laboratory tests in, 299
case presentation for, 297–298, 300, 301
differential diagnosis of, 297–298
management of
affect and cognitive changes in, 301
for psychological aspects, 301–302
pathophysiology of, 300–301
Perception symmetry assessment, with pelvic pain, 298
Percutaneous balloon compression, for trigeminal neuralgia, 55
Percutaneous disc decompression, for discogenic back pain, 136
Percutaneous myocardial laser revascularization, for chronic refractory angina, 315
Percutaneous vertebroplasty, for thoracic vertebral compression fractures, 278
Performance enhancement, for chronic pain, 107
Periaqueductal gray (PAG)
in acute pain, 342
anterior cingulate cortex on, 301
in chemotherapy-induced neuropathy, 362
in chronic persistent pain, 300
Peripheral endplate function, in myofascial pain syndrome, 71
Peripheral nerve neurostimulation, for trigeminal neuralgia, 56
Peripheral nerve stimulation, for complex regional pain syndrome, 400
Peripheral neuropathic pain disorders, 39. *See also specific types*
Peripheral polyneuropathy
pathophysiology of, 3
small fiber neuropathy in, 3 (*See also* Small fiber neuropathy)
Persistent idiopathic facial pain, 38–39. *See also* Facial pain conditions
vs. trigeminal neuralgia, 42t
Persistent postoperative pain, 341–343
acute pain in, 341–342
chronic pain in, 342–343
general mechanisms of, 341
pathophysiology of, 342
persistent pain in, 342
Phalen's maneuver, in carpal tunnel syndrome, 61
Phantom breast pain, post-mastectomy, 324, 326
Photoplethysmographic blood pressure recordings, 7
Phrenic nerve, 324, 324t
Pinprick hyperalgesia assessment, with pelvic pain, 299
Piriformis injection, for piriformis syndrome, 242, 242f
Piriformis syndrome, 238–244
case presentation for, 238–239, 240, 243, 244
clinical manifestations of, 241
diagnosis of, 239–240
management of, 241–243
coordinated approach in, 241
interventional procedures in, 242, 242f
pharmacological, 242
psychiatric, 242–243
rehabilitation and physical therapy in, 241–242, 241b
surgical, 243
natural history of, 240–241
pain generators in, 238–239
prevalence of, 240
prognosis in, long-term, 244
Platelet rich plasma, for discogenic back pain, 136–137
Porphyria, small fiber neuropathy in, 9
Positive neuropathic symptoms, 3
Post-herniorrhaphy pain, 337–347
case presentation for, 337, 341, 343–347
diagnostic studies for, 340–341
differential diagnosis of, 337, 338t
exam findings in, pertinent, 340
history in, 337–338
inguinal neural anatomy in, 337–338, 339f, 339t
management of, 343–347
alcohol use, 345–346, 346t
behavioral, 345
interventional, 347
pharmacologic, 343–344, 343t
rehabilitation in, 347
surgical, 346–347
pathophysiology of, 341–343
acute pain in, 341–342
chronic pain in, 342–343
general points on, 341
persistent pain in, 342
risk factors for, 337, 338t, 339f
preoperative, 338–339
surgical, 339–340
Postherpetic neuralg23
natural history and phases of, 20
pain etiology in, 22, 22f, 23f
features of, 31
of rash, 21
prevention of, guidelines for, 24t, 31
risk factors and predisposing factors in, 21
for chronic pain, 22
Postherpetic neuralgia, 16–23
case presentation for, 16, 20, 22
clinical manifestations of, 17–20
cutaneous, 19
dermatomal distribution in, 17, 18f
disseminated, 20
neurologic, 19
ocular, 19
ophthalmic, 18–19, 18f
prodrome in, 17, 17f
progression in, 17, 17f
etiologic agent of, 16–17, 17f
incidence and prevalence of, 20, 20f, 21f
vaccination on, 21, 21f
Postherpetic neuralgia management, 23–31
complementary and alternative treatment in, 30
guidelines for, 23, 24t
interventional/surgical
for pain control and rash healing, 28
for prevention, 28
for therapy, 28–30
medications in
for pain control and rash healing, 23–25, 24t
for prevention, 25–26
for therapy, 26–28
psychosocial and rehabilitation, 30–31
Postlaminectomy syndrome, 213–233
appropriateness of index operation in, 217
axial back pain *vs.* radicular leg pain in, 214–217, 214f–216f
disc herniation in, 216
facet pain in, 216
foraminal stenosis in, 215
painful disc in, 215–216
pedicular screw placement in, 216, 216f
psychological factors in, 216–217
spinal instability in, 216
case presentation for, 213, 214f
management in, 217, 218, 221–222, 227, 228, 229f, 232–233
cause of pain in, 213
epidural fibrosis in, 228
spinal stenosis in, 228
spine instability and adjacent segment disease in, 227–228
management of, 217–233
chiropractic and spine manipulation therapy in, 221
DRG stimulation in, 230
epidural adhesiolysis in, 222, 225, 225t
epidural injections in, 222, 223t–224t
exercise in, 221
facet interventions in, 225, 226t, 227t
intrathecal drug delivery system in, 230–232, 231f, 232f
massage in, 221
for persistent pain, 227–228
pharmacotherapy, 217–218, 219t–220t
prognosis in, long-term, 233
rehabilitation in, pain, 232
rehabilitation in, techniques, 221
sacroiliac joint interventions in, 225
spinal cord stimulation in, 229–230, 231f
high-frequency, 230
thermal annular procedures in, 225, 227, 227f
transcutaneous electrical nerve stimuliation in, 221
workers compensation claims on outcome in, 233
pathophysiology of chronic pain in, 213–214
persistent pain incidence in, 227
reoperation for, 228
surgery for, revision, 228
Post-mastectomy pain syndrome, 322
clinical characteristics of, 325t, 326
etiology and pathophysiology of, 324–325, 325t
risk factors for, 322–323, 323t
Post-sternotomy pain syndrome, 322
clinical characteristics of, 326, 326t
etiology and pathophysiology of, 325, 326t
risk factors for, 322f, 323
Postsurgical neuropathic pain syndrome. *See also* Thoracic pain, postsurgical
definition of, 321
etiology and pathophysiology of, 324–325, 325t, 326t
prevalence of, 322
Postsurgical thoracic pain. *See* Thoracic pain, postsurgical
Post-thoracotomy pain syndrome, 322
clinical characteristics of, 325t, 326
etiology and pathophysiology of, 325, 325t
risk factors for, 323

Post-traumatic stress disorder (PTSD)
characteristics of, 154
chronic pain in, 154–155
treatment of, 155
Postural orthostatic tachycardia syndrome (POTS)
management checklist for, 13
quantitative sudomotor axon reflex test fir, 5
Postural stresses, in myofascial pain syndrome, 73
Pramipexole, for fibromyalgia, 412
Pregabalin. *See also* Antiepileptic drugs (AEDs)
for cancer pain, neuropathic, 361
for cervical radicular pain, 260
for fibromyalgia, 412
for headache, 386
for lumbar disc displacement, 200
for post-herniorrhaphy pain, 343
for postherpetic neuralgia, 26
for postsurgical thoracic pain, 328–329, 329t
Prolotherapy (proliferative therapy), for sacroiliac joint pain, 174
Prostaglandin E1 (PGE1), for postherpetic neuralgia, 27
Prostaglandin E2 (PGE2), in neuropathic pain, 360
Pseudo-sciatica, 90
Psoriatic arthritis, *vs.* rheumatological disease pain, 95, 95t
Psychological assessment, for chronic pain, 106
Psychological factors, 331–334. *See also specific disorders*
diagnostic criteria for, 331, 332t
nonadherence in, 331
noncompliance in, 331
Pterygopalatine ganglion radiofrequency ablation, for trigeminal neuralgia, 55–56, 56t
Puestow procedure, Partington-Rochelle modification, for pancreatitis pain, 294
Punch biopsy, in intra epidermal nerve fiber density, 5–6

Q

Quantitative sensory testing (QST)
for cancer pain
chemotherapy-induced neuropathy, 362
palliative, 360
for cervical radicular pain, 259
for persistent idiopathic facial pain, 42, 42t
for post-herniorrhaphy pain, 341
for postsurgical neuropathic pain, 328f
for small fiber neuropathy, 6
for trigeminal neuralgia, 44
Quantitative sudomotor axon reflex test (QSART), 6
for small fiber neuropathy, 5
for sudomotor autonomic function, 6

R

Radiation therapy, for postherpetic neuralgia, 30
Radicular pain
cervical, 258–262 (*See also* Cervical radicular pain)
definition of, 197
from disc herniation, 196–197
leg
vs. axial back pain, postlaminectomy, 214–217, 214f–216f
postlaminectomy, 215, 216f
vs. radiculopathy, 258
vs. whiplash with cervical facet pain, 248
Radiculopathy
definition and diagnosis of, 197
vs. radicular pain, 258
thoracic, 266, 266f
Radiofrequency treatment
for cervical facet pain, 254–255, 255f
for pancreatitis pain, 292–293, 293f
for post-herniorrhaphy pain, 347
for postlaminectomy syndrome, 225, 227t
for sacroiliac joint pain, 175, 175b,176, 177t
bipolar, 175
complications of, 176
conventional, 175
cooled, 176
for thoracic radicular pain, 275–276
for thoracic spondylosis, 277, 277f
for trigeminal neuralgia, 52–54, 54f
for vertebral compression fractures, thoracic, 277–278
Ramsay-Hunt syndrome, 18–19, 18f
Range of motion (ROM)
in myofascial pain syndrome, 77
trigger points on, 77, 79
Reactive arthritis, *vs.* rheumatological disease pain, 95–96, 95t
Recruitment, muscle, in myofascial pain syndrome, 77
Referred pain
in chronic refractory angina, 305
in lumbar facet pain, 150
in myofascial pain syndrome, 69, 72 (*See also* Myofascial pain syndrome)
elicitation of, 79
taut band in, 79
from sacroiliac joint, 165, 165f, 166f
Reflex sympathetic dystrophy, 390–402. *See also* Complex regional pain syndrome (CRPS)
Refractory angina, chronic, 303–315. *See also* Angina, chronic refractory
Reiter syndrome, 96
Relaxation techniques, for fibromyalgia, 414
Resisted abduction, 167, 170f
Retroneural epidural injections, for lumbar disc displacement, 201
Rheumatological disease pain, 89–100
case presentation for, 89, 91, 94, 97, 100
classification of, 99t
clinical manifestations of, 89–91
characteristics in, 90
physical examination in, 90–91
definition of, 89
diagnosis of, 91–92, 91t
diagnostic modalities in, 92–94
bone scintigraphy in, 93
computed tomography in, 93–94
laboratory, 92
magnetic resonance imaging in, 94
radiographs in, 92–93, 93f, 93t
ultrasound in, 94
differential diagnosis of, 94–97, 95t
diffuse idiopathic skeletal hyperostosis in, 97, 98f
enteropathic arthritis in, 95t, 96–97
herniated disc in, 95t, 97
psoriatic arthritis in, 95, 95t
reactive arthritis in, 95–96, 95t
epidemiology of, 91
pain characteristics in, 97–100, 99t
Rheumatological disease pain management, 100–107
goals of, 100
investigational biologic therapies in, 107
pharmacological, 100–102, 101t
physical therapy in, 102–105
education in, 105
examination in, 102–104
follow-up and goals in, 105
interventions in, 104
manual therapy in, 104–105
therapeutic exercises in, 104
psychological, 105–107
Rhizotomy
for facial pain and trigeminal neuralgia, 51, 51f
for thoracic back pain, 277
for thoracic spondylosis, 277, 277f
Rituximab, for rheumatological disease pain, 107

S

Sacroiliac joint
anatomy of, 161–162, 163f
innervation of, 162
surface landmarks of, 168f
Sacroiliac joint interventions, for postlaminectomy syndrome, 225
Sacroiliac joint pain, 160–170
anatomy of, 161–162, 163f
biomechanics of, 162–163
case presentation for, 160, 170
diagnosis of, 165–170
compression test in, 167, 169f
distraction (gapping) test in, 168f
evidence-based findings in, 167t
Fortin finger test in, 165, 173b
Gaenslen's test in, 167, 169f
Gillet (stork) test in, 167, 171f
historical perspectives on, 165, 165b
history of illness and clinical manifestations in, 165, 165f, 166b, 166f
IASP criteria in, 165, 165b
imaging in, 170, 173b
injections in, 168–170, 172t
inspection in, 165–166
muscle testing in, 167
neurovascular testing in, 167
palpation in, 166
Patrick's (FABER) test in, 167, 169f
provocative and mobility/alignment maneuvers in, 167, 168f–171f, 168t
range of motion in, 167
referred pain in, 165, 165f, 166f
resisted abduction in, 167, 170f
standing flexion (Vorlauf) test in, 167, 171f
thigh thrust test in, 167, 169f
Yeoman's test in, 167, 170f
differential diagnosis of, 161, 161b
disability from, 161
natural history and long-term prognosis of, 164
pathophysiology and etiology of, 164, 164b
postlaminectomy, 216
prevalence and incidence of, 161, 162t
Sacroiliac joint pain management, 170–178
acute-phase, 172–173
conservative, 172
interdisciplinary treatment paradigm in, 177b–178b
interventional
radiofrequency ablation, complications, 176
radiofrequency ablation, cooled, 176
radiofrequency, bipolar, 175
radiofrequency, conventional, 175
radiofrequency denervation, 175, 175b,176, 177t
steroid injections, 175
maintenance-phase, 173
manual medicine in, 174
neuromodulation in, 176
pharmacological, 170–172
prolotherapy in, 174
psychosocial, 174–175
recovery-phase, 173
surgical, 176
Sacroiliac joint transforaminal epidural spinal injections, for lumbar disc displacement, 201, 201f, 204–205
Salicylates, for rheumatological disease pain, 100, 101t
Sciatica, 197
Scrambler therapy, for postherpetic neuralgia, 29
Screw placement, pedicular, in postlaminectomy syndrome, 216, 216f
Sedative-hypnotics, for fibromyalgia, 412
Selective serotonin norepinephrine reuptake inhibitors (SNRIs)
for depression and anxiety with cancer pain, 366–367, 366t, 368
for fibromyalgia, 411–412
for lumbar facet pain, 153
Selective serotonin reuptake inhibitors (SSRIs). *See also specific agents*
for carpal tunnel syndrome, 64
for depression and anxiety with cancer pain, 366–367, 366t, 368
for fibromyalgia, 410–411, 415
Self-management, patient
for complex regional pain syndrome, 401
for fibromyalgia, 414–415
for small fiber neuropathy, 11
Self-regulation training, for chronic pain, 106
Sensitization
central, 324, 342
neuronal, in chronic pain, 213–214
Serotonin (5-HT), in myofascial pain syndrome, 71, 73, 74
Serotonin norepinephrine reuptake inhibitors (SNRIs)
for cancer pain, neuropathic, 361
for post-herniorrhaphy pain, 344
for postsurgical thoracic pain, 329, 329t
Sertraline. *See also* Selective serotonin reuptake inhibitors (SSRIs)
for carpal tunnel syndrome, 64
for depression and anxiety with cancer pain, 366, 366t
Shingles. *See* Herpes zoster infection; Postherpetic neuralgia
Short-lasting unilateral neuralgiform headache attacks with conjunctival injection and tearing (SUNCT), 42, 43t, 382
Short-lasting unilateral neuralgiform headache attacks with cranial autonomic features (SUNA), 42, 43t, 382
Shoulder abduction test, for cervical radicular pain, 259
Signals
afferent, 3
efferent autonomic, 3
Simons's integrated hypothesis of the trigger point, 70
Sjögren syndrome, small fiber neuropathy in, 9–10

Sleep disturbances. *See* Insomnia
Sleep, for chronic pain, 106
Small fiber neuropathy, 3–13
case presentation for, 3, 4, 7, 8
definition of, 3
differential diagnosis and testing for, 7–11
alcohol and toxins in, 8
amyloidosis in, 10
celiac disease in, 10
diabetes mellitus in, 7–8
erythromelalgia in, 9
Fabry's disease in, 9
hereditary sensory autonomic neuropathies in, 9
HIV in, 10–11
hyperlipidemia in, 8
infectious and immunologic causes in, 9–10
Lyme disease in, 11
metabolic, toxic, and genetic causes in, 7–9
monoclonal gammopathy in, 10
other causes in, 10–11
porphyria in, 9
Sjögren syndrome in, 9–10
thyroid abnormalities in, 8
vitamin B_{12} deficiency in, 8–9
idiopathic, 7, 11
management of, 11–13
for orthostasis, 13
for pain, 11–13, 12t
pathophysiology of, 3–4
patient evaluation in, 4–7
confirming measurable dysautonomia in, 6–7
electrodiagnostic test in, 4–5
etiology in, searching for, 7
intra epidermal nerve fiber density in, 5–6
photoplethysmographic blood pressure recordings in, 7
quantitative sensory testing in, 6
quantitative sudomotor axon reflex test in, 5
thermoregulatory sweat test in, 6
Smoking cessation, for discogenic back pain, 138–140, 139t
Sodium channel blockers. *See also* Lidocaine, IV
for complex regional pain syndrome, 397
Sodium fluoride, for vertebral compression fracture prevention, 273–274
Sodium oxybate, for fibromyalgia, 412
Somatic and sympathetic block, combined, for postherpetic neuralgia, 28
Somatic symptom disorder, 117–118
management of, 119–121
Somatization, 115–116
Sphenopalatine ganglion
neuroanatomy of, 45–46, 46f
radiofrequency ablation of, for trigeminal neuralgia, 55–56, 56t
Spinal cord neuroanatomy, 359, 359f
Spinal cord stimulation (SCS)
for chronic refractory angina, 314
for complex regional pain syndrome, 399–400
for pancreatitis pain, 293–294
for post-herniorrhaphy pain, 347
for postlaminectomy syndrome, 229–230, 231f
high-frequency, 230
for postsurgical thoracic pain, 330, 330f
for small fiber neuropathy, 12–13
for thoracic radicular pain, 276
Spinal interneuron network, in chronic refractory angina, 305
Spinal pain management, mental health screening in, 149
Spinal stenosis
definition of, 186
in postlaminectomy syndrome, 228
Spine instability
postlaminectomy, 216, 216f
in postlaminectomy syndrome, 227–228
Splanchinectomy, for pancreatitis pain, 293
Splanchnic nerve blocks, for pancreatitis pain, 291, 292f
Spondylolisthesis
back pain with, 214, 214f
discogenic pain with, 133
facet pain with, 216
lumbar facet pain with, 147
lumbar spinal stenosis with, 186, 192
postlaminectomy syndrome with, 214f, 216, 227, 229f, 233
from spinal instability, 216
Spondylosis management, thoracic
interventional, 276–277, 277f
options for, 274, 274b
pharmacologic, 275
physical rehabilitation in, 274–275
psychological, 275
surgery in, 279–280
Spontaneous electrical activity, in trigger points, 77
Spurling's maneuver
for cervical radicular pain, 259
for facet-mediated neck pain diagnosis, 249
Standing flexion test, 167, 171f
Stellate ganglion block
for chronic refractory angina, 314
for postsurgical thoracic pain, 331
Stereotactic radiosurgery, for trigeminal neuralgia, 54–55
Steroids, injected. *See also specific disorders; specific types*
for lumbar facet pain, 153–154
for postherpetic neuralgia, 29
for sacroiliac joint pain, 175
for thoracic spondylosis, 276–277
Stork test, 167, 171f
Straight leg raise, 240
STS (implanted field stimulation), for postherpetic neuralgia, 29
Sudek's atrophy. *See* Complex regional pain syndrome (CRPS)
Sudomotor fibers, in small fiber neuropathy, 3–4
Suffering response, in chronic pain, 106
Sulfasalazine, for rheumatological disease pain, 100
Superior sulcus cancers
management of, 357–358
presentation of, 356–357, 356f
Sweat pattern, 6
Sympathetic (ganglion) block
for complex regional pain syndrome, 395f, 399
for erythromelalgia, 9
for postherpetic neuralgia, 23, 28, 30
prevention of, steroid, 28
for postsurgical thoracic pain, 331
Sympathetic nervous system, on end organs, 4

T

Tapentadol, for neuropathic cancer pain, 360–361
Tarlov cysts, 205
Taut band
in myofascial pain syndrome, 76
generation of, 70
referred pain in, 79
palpation of, 78
Tendinopathies, 110–121
case presentation for, 110
clinical manifestations in, 112–113
comorbidities in, 118
management in, 113, 114
psychological state on symptoms in, 115, 119, 121
clinical manifestations of, distal biceps, 112–113, 112f, 113f
differential diagnosis of, 110
epidemiology of, 110–111
management of, 113–115
autologous blood or platelet-rich plasma tissue graft in, 114–115
eccentric loading in, 113
general points on, 113
glycerin trinitrite in, 113–114
tendon needle tenotomy/fenestration in, 114–115
pathophysiology of, 111, 111f
prognosis in, 115
psychological state on physical symptoms in, 115–119
clinician frustration on, 116–117
comorbidities in, 118–119
DSM classifications of, 117
illness anxiety disorder in, 118
management of, 119–121
outcomes on somatic symptoms in, 117
overview of, 115
somatic symptom disorder in, 117–118
somatization in, 115–116
Tendon anatomy, 111
Tension-type headache, 382. *See also* Headache
Thermal annular procedures, for postlaminectomy syndrome, 225, 227, 227f
Thermoregulatory sweat test (TST), 6
Thermorhizotomy of Gasserian ganglion, for trigeminal neuralgia, 52–54, 54f
Thigh thrust test, 167, 169f
Thioclochicoside, for myofascial pain syndrome, 82
Third occipital headache, 387
Thoracic back pain, 264–273
anatomy in, 265–266, 265f, 266f
clinical presentation of, 264, 267, 270, 271
definition of, 264
diagnosis in, confirming, 267–271, 271b
additional tests in, 269
diagnostic blocks in, 270–271
history in, 267–268, 268f, 269b, 269f
imaging in, 269–270, 270f, 271b
physical examination in, 268
differential diagnosis of, 266–267, 267b
pain generators and diagnosis in, 264–265
vertebral compression fracture in
clinical consequences of, 272
incidence of, 271–272
natural history of, 272
prevention of, 272–273, 273b
risk factors for, 273, 273b
Thoracic back pain management, 274–280
interventional
for radicular pain, 275–276, 275f
for spondylosis, 276–277, 277f
for vertebral compression fractures, 277–279, 278f
options for, 274, 274b
pharmacologic, 275
physical rehabilitation in, 274–275
psychological, 275
surgery in, 279–280, 280b
Thoracic disc displacement management
options for, 274, 274b
pharmacologic, 275
physical rehabilitation in, 274–275
psychological, 275
Thoracic epidural anesthesia, for chronic refractory angina, 314–315
Thoracic medial branch block (TMBB), 271
for thoracic spondylosis, 277
Thoracic pain, postsurgical, 321–334
breast cancer surgery type in, 323–324
breast innervation and, 323, 323f
case presentation for, 321
behavioral and psychological factors in, 331–334
clinical characteristics in, 326
definition in, 322
diagnosis in, 327
etiology and pathophysiology in, 326
prevention in, 327
risk factors in, 323
chest innervation and, 324, 324f
clinical characteristics of
in post-mastectomy pain syndrome, 325t, 326
in post-sternotomy pain syndrome, 326, 326t
in post-thoractomy pain syndrome, 325t, 326
definitions of
post-mastectomy pain syndrome in, 322
post-sternotomy pain syndrome in, 322
postsurgical neuropathic pain syndrome in, 321
post-thoracotomy pain syndrome in, 322
diagnosis of, 327
etiology and pathophysiology of, 324–325, 325t, 326t
in post-mastectomy pain syndrome, 324–325, 325t
in post-sternotomy pain syndrome, 325, 326t
in post-thoracotomy pain syndrome, 325, 325t
management of
behavioral and psychological, 331–334
interventional, 330–331, 330f
nonpharmacologic, 328
options for, 327–328
pharmacologic, 328–330, 329t
prevalence of, 322
prevention of, 327
risk factors for, 322–323, 322f
in post-mastectomy pain syndrome, 322–323, 323t
in post-sternotomy pain syndrome, 322f, 323
in post-thoracotomy pain syndrome, 323
thoracic surgery types and, 324
Thoracic surgery, 324
Thoracic vertebrae anatomy, 265, 265f
Threshold management, for chronic pain, 106–107

Thyroid abnormalities, small fiber neuropathy in, 8
Tic convulsif, 41
Tic douloureux, 41
Tinel's sign, in carpal tunnel syndrome, 61–62
Tizanidine, for fibromyalgia, 412
Tocilizumab, for rheumatological disease pain, 107
Tolosa-Hunt, 39
Total disc arthroplasty, for discogenic back pain, 141
Toxins, small fiber neuropathy from, 8
Traditional Chinese medicine, for postherpetic neuralgia, 30
Tramadol
  for cancer pain, neuropathic, 360–361
  for fibromyalgia, 413
  for post-herniorrhaphy pain, 344
  for postherpetic neuralgia, 24t, 26
Transcutaneous electrical nerve stimulation (TENS)
  for cancer care, palliative, 363
  for chronic refractory angina, 314
  for facial pain, 56
  for low back pain, chronic, 221
  for myofascial pain syndrome, 81
  for postherpetic neuralgia, 28, 29, 31
  for postlaminectomy syndrome, 221
  for small fiber neuropathy, 12
  for thoracic back pain, 274
Transforaminal epidural spinal injections (TESI)
  for cervical radicular pain, 261–262, 261f
  for lumbar disc displacement, 201, 201f, 204
  for postlaminectomy syndrome, 222, 223t
Transient receptor potential (TRP) channels, 342
Transient receptor potential vanilloid 1 receptor. *See* $TRPV_1$ receptor
Transmyocardial myocardial laser revascularization, for chronic refractory angina, 315
Trazodone
  for depression and anxiety with cancer pain, 367
  for insomnia, 369–370
Tricyclic antidepressants (TCAs)
  for cancer pain, neuropathic, 361
  for carpal tunnel syndrome, 64
  for cervical radicular pain, 259–260
  for fibromyalgia, 410
  for insomnia, 370
  for lumbar facet pain, 153
  for post-herniorrhaphy pain, 344
  for postherpetic neuralgia, 26
    prevention of, 24t, 25–26
  for postsurgical thoracic pain, 329, 329t
  for small fiber neuropathy, 11–12, 12t
Trigeminal autonomic cephalgia, 42, 382
Trigeminal ganglion anatomy, 44–45, 45f
Trigeminal nerve
  anatomy of, 44–45, 45f
  ophthalmic division of, 18, 18f
  in varicella-zoster virus infection, 17f, 18, 18f
Trigeminal neuralgia, 38–47
  anatomical structures in, 44–46
    in head pain, 44–45, 45f
    sphenopalatine ganglion in, 45–46, 46f
    trigeminal ganglion and trigeminal nerves in, 44–45, 45f
  case presentation for, 38, 49, 50
  clinical correlates of, 44
  comorbidities of, 47, 47f
  diagnostic studies for, 43–44, 44f
  differential diagnosis of, 38–39
  epidemiology of, 39
  etiology, classification, and diagnostic criteria for, 39–40, 40f, 40t
  history in, 42–43
  vs. neuropathic facial pain, 41
  pathophysiology of, 46–47, 46f
  vs. persistent idiopathic facial pain, 42t
  symptoms and pain distribution in, 40–41, 40t, 41f
Trigeminal neuralgia management, 47–56
  ablative
    choice, 52
    glycerol rhizolysis, 54
    neurostimulation, 56
    percutaneous balloon compression, 55
    radiofrequency ablation, 52–54, 54f
    sphenopalatine ganglion radiofrequency, 55–56, 56t
    stereotactic radiosurgery, 54–55
  algorithm for, 50–51, 50f
  cognitive and behavioral approaches in, 48–50, 48t, 49t
  medications in, 47–48
  microvascular decompression in, 50–52, 51f, 52b
  rehabilitation in, 56–57
Trigger point compression, for myofascial pain syndrome, 81
Trigger point injections, in myofascial pain syndrome, 80–81, 80t, 82
Trigger points. *See also* Myofascial pain syndrome
  active, 70
  biochemistry of, 71–72
  electrophysiology of, 77
  identification of, 76
  latent, 70
  management of
    deep dry needling in, 80–81, 80t, 82–83
    injections in, 80–81, 80t, 82
    invasive treatment in, 82–83
    manual inactivation in, 81
  in muscle overuse syndromes, latent and active, 70, 75
  muscle recruitment in, 77
  muscle weakness in, 76–77, 79
  neuromuscular junction in, 70–71
  on range of motion, 77, 79
  reliability of examination for, 80–81
  sensory changes in, 77
  taut band in, 70, 76
  twitch response in, local, 76
TRPV1, 342
  in persistent pain, 342
$TRPV_1$ receptor, 342
  capsaicin on, 27, 329, 342
  in myocardial ischemia, 305
Tumor necrosis factor α, for rheumatological disease pain, 100–102
12th rib syndrome, 267
Twitch response, local, in trigger points, 76

U
Ulcerative colitis, enteropathic arthritis in, 95t, 96–97
Ultrasound, for myofascial pain syndrome, 81
Ultraviolet B (UVB) therapy, for postherpetic neuralgia, 28, 30

V
Vaccination, varicella-zoster virus, on postherpetic neuralgia, 21, 21f
Vagus nerve, 324, 324t
Valacyclovir, for postherpetic neuralgia, 23, 24t
  prevention of, 23, 24t, 26
Valsalva maneuver, heart rate response to, 7
Varenicline, for smoking cessation, 139–140
Varicella zoster vasculopathy, 19
Varicella-zoster virus, in postherpetic neuralgia, 16–17, 17f
Varicella-zoster virus vaccine, on postherpetic neuralgia, 21, 21f
Vascular endothelial growth factor, for chronic refractory angina, 315
Vasculopathy, varicella zoster, 19
Venlafaxine
  for cancer pain, neuropathic, 361
  for depression and anxiety with cancer pain, 366, 366t
  for post-herniorrhaphy pain, 344
  for postsurgical thoracic pain, 329, 329t
Vertebral augmentation procedures, for thoracic vertebral compression fractures, 278–279, 278f
Vertebral compression fracture (VCF), thoracic. *See also* Thoracic back pain
  clinical consequences of, 272
  incidence of, 271–272
  management of, 277–279
    interventional, 277–279, 278f
    options for, 274, 274b
    pharmacologic, 275
    physical rehabilitation in, 274–275
    psychological, 275
    surgery in, 280, 280b
  natural history of, 272
  prevention of, 272–273, 273b
  risk factors for, 273, 273b
Vertebroplasty, percutaneous, for thoracic vertebral compression fractures, 278
Vitamin B_{12} deficiency, small fiber neuropathy in, 8–9
Vitamin C, for postherpetic neuralgia, 25, 27
Vitamin D, for vertebral compression fracture prevention, 273
Vorlauf test, 167, 171f

W
Weakness, muscle
  with lumbar facet pain, management of, 152
  in myofascial pain syndrome, 76–77, 79
Wet cupping, for postherpetic neuralgia, 30
Whiplash associated disorder (WAD)
  incidence of, 251–252
  management of, 252–255
    interventional procedures in, 254–255, 255f
    pharmacological, 253–254
    rehabilitation in, 251–253
    surgery in, 255
  natural history of, 252
Whiplash associated disorder with cervical facet pain, 247–255
  case presentation for, 247
  diagnosis of, 247–251, 249f
    anatomy and biomechanics in, 247–248
    cervical axial pain in, 249
    cervical extension or ipsilateral rotation in, 248
    contralateral cervical rotation in, 248
    facet palpation in, 249
    imaging in, 250
    localization of painful joint in, 248–249, 249f
    maneuvers in, 249–250
    medial branch block in, 251
    vs. radicular pain, 248
    sensation and innervation in, 250–251
  incidence of, 251–252
  management of, 252–255, 255f
  natural history of, 252
  pain generators in, 247
Whipple procedure, for pancreatitis pain, 294
Wind-up, in fibromyalgia, 408–409

X
X-STOP, 193

Y
Yeoman's test, 167geId="170">170f

Z
Zaleplon, for insomnia, 369
Ziconotide, for postsurgical thoracic pain, 331
Z-joint, 150
Zolpidem
  for fibromyalgia, 412
  for insomnia, 369
Zopiclone, for fibromyalgia, 412
Zygapophyseal joint (C2-C3), 150
  referred pain from, 238
Zygapophyseal joint (C2–C3) headache, 387